E.E. Vokes · H.M. Golomb

Oncologic Therapies

# Springer

*Berlin*
*Heidelberg*
*New York*
*Barcelona*
*Hong Kong*
*London*
*Milan*
*Paris*
*Singapore*
*Tokyo*

E.E. Vokes   H.M. Golomb (Eds.)

# Oncologic Therapies

With 39 Figures and 176 Tables

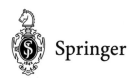 Springer

Prof. Everett E. Vokes, M.D.
University of Chicago
Medical Center
5841 S. Maryland Ave., MC 2115
Chicago, IL 60637-1470
USA

Prof. Harvey M. Golomb, M.D.
University of Chicago
Medical Center
5841 S. Maryland Ave., MC 2115
Chicago, IL 60637-1470
USA

ISBN   3-540-64052-5   Springer-Verlag Berlin Heidelberg New York
ISBN   3-387-64052-5   Springer-Verlag New York Berlin Heidelberg


Library of Congress Cataloging-in-Publication Data

**Oncologic therapies** [edited by] E. E. Vokes ; H. M. Golomb. -
      p.   cm.
   Includes bibliographical references and index.
   ISBN 3-540-64052-5 (softcover)
   1. Cancer--Treatment--Handbooks, manuals, etc.  I. Vokes, E. E.
(Everett E.), 1954– .  II. Golomb, Harvey M. (Harvey Morris),
1943–
   [DNLM: 1. Neoplasms--therapy.    QZ 266 0583 1999]
   RC270.8.053    1999
   616.99'406--dc21
   DNLM/DLC
   For library of Congress                                   98-37566
                                                             CIP

© Springer-Verlag Berlin Heidelberg 1999
Printed in Italy

The use of general descriptive names, registered names, trademarks, etc. in this publication does not imply, even in the absence of a specific statement, that such names are exempt from the relevant protective laws and regulations and therefore free for general use.

The publisher cannot assume any legal responsibility for given data, especially as far as directions for the use and the handling of chemicals are concerned. This information can be obtained from the instructions on safe laboratory practice and from the manufactures of chemical and laboratory equipment.

Typesetting: cicero Lasersatz, Dinkelscherben
SPIN: 10051930       9/3134 - 5 4 3 2 1 0  –  Printed on acid-free paper

# Preface

Our goal in this book is to provide a brief introduction to the principles and practice of oncology and to oncologic therapies. The book provides a description of the major treatment modalities, i.e., surgery, radiation therapy, and systemic therapies (including classic chemotherapy and biological therapies). It also provides a brief overview of supportive care and quality of life assessments. This is followed by a discussion of site-specific cancers covering the hematologic malignancies and solid tumors. Each chapter is designed to provide a brief discussion of background information including epidemiology, risk factors, and staging principles, followed by a description of standard therapies according to stage and current investigational approaches. While the major features of each disease are discussed, the emphasis of this book is clearly on the state-of-the-art therapy. As such, this book should be useful to general internists with an interest in oncology as well as to house staff and junior oncologists of all major oncologic modalities seeking a brief and focused patient management resource. References providing more in-depth discussion for each field are also provided. We recommend that any information pertaining to specific chemotherapy regimens and dosing be confirmed on the basis of a primary source, since we cannot exclude the possibility of an occasional typographical error.

The contributing authors represent nationally and internationally renowned programs in their respective fields. Many were chosen from our own faculty at the University of Chicago or collaborating institutions. We wish to thank all authors and co-authors for the high quality of their contributions and their timeliness. We also wish to thank Monika Schrimpf and Gisela Schmitt at Springer-Verlag for their help and support in generating this book. We would appreciate any feedback and suggestions to improve on this book for the second edition.

Chicago, September 1998          *Everett E. Vokes, Harvey M. Golomb*

# Contents

## Hepatobiliary Cancer

## Genitourinary Malignancies

## Gynecologic Cancers

## Brain Tumors

## Miscellaneous

## Ethical Issues

# Author List

Ain
Boyle
Brockstein
Butler
Cappuzzo
Crawford
Cummings
Daugherty
DeMario
Dragovich
Ewesuedo
Ferguson
Finiewicz
Flaherty
Fleming
Gajewski
Giles
Golomb
Grossman
Guitart
Helft
Herndon
Hesketh
Hoffman
Johnston
Kantarjian
Kindler
Kuzel
Lamont
Larson
Le Chevalier
Le Pechoux
Liebowitz
List

Macdonald
Mandel
Mani
Markman
Mauer
McCaffrey
Morganstern
Motzer
Mundt
Nicholas
Oh
Olopade
Papadimitrakopoulou
Peabody
Posner
Ratain
Rosen
Rudin
Ryan
Salloum
Schilsky
Shammo
Simon
Soltani
Stadler
Stupp
Szatrowski
Ultmann
Vargish
Vogelzang
Vokes
Waggoner
Williams
Zimmerman

# Contributors

K.B. Ain (e-mail: kbain1@pop.uky.edu,
Tel.: +1-606-323-5821, Fax: +1-606-323-5707)
Thyroid Nodule and Oncology Clinical Service, Division of
Endocrinology and Molecular Medicine, Department of Internal
Medicine, University of Kentucky Medical Center, and Thyroid Clinic,
Veterans Affairs Medical Center, Lexington, KY 40502. USA

F.M. Boyle
Royal North Shore Hospital, Pacific Hwy, St Leonards, Sydney 2065,
Australia

B.E. Brockstein
University of Chicago Medical Center, MC 2115, 5841 S. Maryland Ave.,
Chicago, IL 60637-1470, USA

P. Butler
Cancer Research Center, University of Chicago, MC 1140, 5841 S.
Maryland Ave., Chicago IL 60637, USA

F. Cappuzzo
Institut Gustave Roussy, 39 Rue Camille Desmoulins, 94805 Villejuif,
France

J. Crawford (e-mail: Crawf006@mc.duke.edu,
Tel.: +1-919-684-5621, Fax: +1-919-681-5864)
Medical Oncology/Hematology, Duke University Medical Center,
25177 Morris Bldg., Durham, NC 27710, USA

B.J. Cummings (e-mail: Bernard_Cummings@pmh.toronto.on.ca,
Tel.: +1-416-946-2129, Fax: +1-416-946-2038)
Princess Margaret Hospital, University of Toronto, Department of
Radiation Oncology, 610 University Avenue, Toronto, M5G 2M9, Canada

C.K. Daugherty (e-mail: ckdaughe@mcis.bsd.uchicago.edu,
Tel.: +1-773-702-4139, Fax: +1-773-702-0963)
Section of Hematology/Oncology, and the MacLean Center for Clinical
Medical Ethics, University of Chicago Medical Center, MC 2115,
5841 S. Maryland Ave., Chicago, IL 60637-1470, USA

M. DeMario (e-mail: mdemari@mcis.bsd.uchicago.edu,
Tel.: +1-773-702-4400, Fax: +1-773-702-0963)
Section of Hematology/Oncology, and Committee on Virology,
University of Chicago Medical Center, MC 2115, 5841 S. Maryland Ave.,
Chicago, IL 60637-1470, USA

T. Dragovich
University of Chicago Medical Center, MC 2115, 5841 S. Maryland Ave.,
Chicago, IL 60637-1470, USA

R.B. Ewesuedo
Fellow, Section of Pediatric Hematology-Oncology, Department of
Pediatrics, and Committee on Clinical Pharmacology, University of
Chicago Medical Center, MC 2115, 5841 S. Maryland Ave., Chicago,
IL 60637-1470, USA

M.K. Ferguson (e-mail: mferguso@surgery.bsd.uchicago.edu,
Tel.: +1-773-702-3551, Fax: +1-773-702-2642)
Department of Surgery, University of Chicago Medical Center, MC 2115,
5841 S. Maryland Ave., Chicago, IL 60637-1470, USA

K.J. Finiewicz (e-mail: kjfiniew@mcis.bsd.uchicago.edu,
Tel.: +1-773-702-4140)
University of Chicago Medical Center, 5841 S. Maryland Ave., Chicago,
IL 60637-1470, USA

J. Flaherty (e-mail: jflahert@medicine.bsd.uchicago.edu,
Tel.: +1-773-702-2712, Fax: +1-773-702-8998)
University of Chicago Hospital, Department of Medicine,
Section of Infectious Diseases, 5841 S. Maryland Ave. MC 5065, Chicago,
IL 60637, USA

G. Fleming
University of Chicago Medical Center, MC 2115, 5841 S. Maryland Ave.,
Chicago, IL 60637-1470, USA

T.F. Gajewski
Department of Pathology and Department of Medicine, Section of
Hematology/Oncology, University of Chicago Medical Center, MC 2115,
5841 S. Maryland Ave., Chicago, IL 60637-1470, USA

F.J. Giles
M.D. Anderson Cancer Center, 1515 Holcombe Boulevard, Box 61,
Houston, TX 77030-4095, USA

H.M. Golomb (Tel.: +1-773-702-6115, Fax: +1-773-702-3002)
University of Chicago Medical Center, 5841 S. Maryland Ave., Chicago,
IL 60637-1470, USA

S.A. Grossman (e-mail: grossman@welchlink.welch.jhu.edu,
Tel.: +1-410-955-8837, Fax: +1-410-955-0125)
Johns Hopkins Oncology Center, 600 N. Wolfe St., Baltimore, MD 21287,
USA

J. Guitart
Department of Dermatology, Lurie Comprehensive Cancer Center of
Northwestern University, 303 E. Chicago Avenue, Olson 8250,
Chicago, IL 60611, USA

P.R. Helft (Fax: +1-773-702-0963)
University of Chicago Hospitals, Department of Medicine, Section of
Hematology/Oncology, 5841 S. Maryland Ave. MC 2115, Chicago,
IL 60637, USA

J.E. Herndon II
Division of Biometry, Department of Community and Family Medicine,
Duke University Medical Center, Box 3958, and CALGB Statistical
Center, Trent Drive, Durham, NC 27708, USA

P.J. Hesketh
Tufts University School of Medicine, and Section of Medical Oncology,
St. Elizabeth's Medical Center, 736 Cambridge St., Boston MA 02135,
USA

P.C. Hoffman
Section of Oncology, Department of Medicine, University of Chicago,
5841 S. Maryland Ave., MC 2115, Chicago, IL 60637, USA

E.M. Johnston
Medical Oncology/Hematology, Duke University Medical Center,
25177 Morris Bldg., Durham, NC 27710, USA

T. Kuzel
Department of Medicine, Lurie Comprehensive Cancer Center of
Northwestern University, 303 E. Chicago Avenue, Olson 8250,
Chicago, IL 60611, USA

E.B. Lamont (Tel.: +1-773-702-4400, Fax: +1-773-702-0963)
Section of Hematology, Department of Medicine, University of Chicago,
5841 S. Maryland Ave., MC 2115, Chicago, IL 60637, USA

R.A. Larson (e-mail: ralarson@mcis.bsd.uchicago.edu,
Tel.: +1-773-702-6783, Fax: +1-773-702-0963)
University of Chicago Medical Center, Section of
Hematology/Oncology, and the Cancer Research Center, University of
Chicago, Chicago IL 60637-1470, USA

T. Le Chevalier (e-mail: tleche@igr.fr,
Tel.: +33-1-4211-4322, Fax: +33-1-4211-5219)
Institut Gustave Roussy, 39 Rue Camille Desmoulins, 94805 Villejuif,
France

C. Le Pechoux
Institut Gustave Roussy, 39 Rue Camille Desmoulins, 94805 Villejuif,
France

D.N. Liebowitz
Section of Hematology/Oncology, and Committee on Virology,
University of Chicago Medical Center, MC 2115, 5841 S. Maryland Ave.,
Chicago, IL 60637-1470, USA

M.A. List (e-mail: malist@mcis.bsd.uchicago.edu, Tel.: +1-773-702-6180,
Fax: +1-773-702-9311)
Cancer Research Center, University of Chicago, MC 1140, 5841 S.
Maryland Ave., Chicago IL 60637, USA

J.S. Macdonald (e-mail: jmacdona@svccc.salick.com,
Tel.: +1-212-367-1861, Fax: +1-212-462-2919)
Gastrointestinal Oncology Service, St. Vincents Comprehensive Cancer
Center, 111 Eighth Avenue, Suite 1513, New York, NY 10011, USA

H.D. Mandel
Section of Dermatology, University of Chicago Medical Center, MC 2115,
5841 S. Maryland Ave., Chicago, IL 60637-1470, USA

S. Mani
Department of Medicine, Section of Hematology/Oncology, University
of Chicago Medical Center, 5841 S. Maryland Ave., MC 2115, Chicago,
IL 60637, USA

M. Markman (e-mail: markmam@cesmtp.ccf.org,
Tel.: +1-216-445-6888, Fax: +1-216-444-9464)
Department of Hematology/Medical Oncology, Cleveland Clinic
Foundation, 9500 Euclid Ave., Cleveland, OH 44195, USA

A.M. Mauer (e-mail: ammauer@mcis.bsd.uchicago.edu,
Tel.: +1-773-702-4138, Fax: +1-773-702-0963)
University of Chicago Medical Center, MC 2115, 5841 S. Maryland Ave.,
Chicago, IL 60637-1470, USA

J.A. McCaffrey (e-mail: mccaffrj@MSKCC.org,
Tel.: +1-212-639-6414, Fax: +1-212-794-5813)
Memorial Sloan-Kettering Cancer Center, 1275 York Ave., New York,
NY 10021, USA


D.E. Morganstern
Tufts University School of Medicine, and Section of Medical Oncology,
St. Elizabeth's Medical Center, 736 Cambridge St., Boston MA 02135,
USA


R.J. Motzer
Memorial Sloan-Kettering Cancer Center, 1275 York Ave., New York,
NY 10021, USA


A.J. Mundt (e-mail: hyperlink mailto:mundt@rover.uchicago.edu,
Tel.: +1-773-702-4751, Fax: +1-773-702-0610)
Department of Radiation and Cellular Oncology, University of Chicago
Hospitals, 5758 S. Maryland Ave. 9006, Chicago IL 60637, USA


K. Nicholas (e-mail: knichola@neurology.bsd.uchicago.edu [with
hyperlink], Tel.: +1-773-834-1726, Fax: +1-773-702-9076)
University of Chicago Medical Center, MC 2030, 5841 S. Maryland Ave.,
Chicago, IL 60637-1470, USA


Y. Oh
University of Chicago Medical Center, MC 0926, 5841 S. Maryland Ave.,
Chicago, IL 60637-1470, USA


O. Olopade
University of Chicago Medical Center, MC 2115, 5841 S. Maryland Ave.,
Chicago, IL 60637-1470, USA


V. Papadimitrakopoulou (Fax: +1-713-796-8655)
M.D. Anderson Cancer Center, 1515 Holcombe Boulevard, Houston,
TX 77030, USA


T.D. Peabody
University of Chicago Medical Center, MC 2115, 5841 S. Maryland Ave.,
Chicago, IL 60637-1470, USA

M.C. Posner
Department of Surgery, University of Chicago Medical Center, MC 2115,
5841 S. Maryland Ave., Chicago, IL 60637-1470, USA

M.J. Ratain (e-mail: mjratain@mcis.bsd.uchicago.edu,
Tel.: +1-773-703-4400, Fax: +1-773-702-0963)
Section of Hematology/Oncology, Department of Medicine, Committee
on Clinical Pharmacology, and Cancer Research Center, University of
Chicago, 5841 S. Maryland Ave., MC 2115, Chicago, IL 60637, USA

S.T. Rosen (Tel.: +1-312-908-5250, Fax: +1-312-908-1372)
Department of Medicine, Lurie Comprehensive Cancer Center of
Northwestern University, 303 E. Chicago Avenue, Olson 8250, Chicago,
IL 60611, USA

C.M. Rudin (Tel.: +1-773-702-4142, Fax: +1-773-702-1576)
University of Chicago Hospitals, Department of Medicine, Section of
Hematology/Oncology, 5841 S. Maryland Ave. MC 2115, Chicago,
IL 60637, USA

C.W. Ryan
Section of Hematology/Oncology, Department of Medicine, University
of Chicago Medical Center, 5841 S. Maryland Ave., MC 2115 Chicago,
IL 60637, USA

R.M. Salloum
Section of General Surgery, University of Chicago Medical Center,
MC 2115, 5841 S. Maryland Ave., Chicago, IL 60637-1470, USA

R.L. Schilsky (Tel.: +1-773-702-6180, Fax: +1-773-702-9311)
Cancer Research Center, University of Chicago, 5841 S. Maryland Ave.,
Chicago, IL 60637-1470, USA

J.M. Shammo (Tel.: +1-773-702-6115, Fax: +1-773-702-3002)
University of Chicago Medical Center, 5841 S. Maryland Ave., Chicago,
IL 60637-1470, USA

K. Soltani (e-mail: k. Soltani@medicine.bsd.uchicago.edu,
Tel.: +1-773-702-6559, Fax: +1-773-702-8398)
Section of Dermatology, University of Chicago Medical Center, MC 2115,
5841 S. Maryland Ave., Chicago, IL 60637-1470, USA

W. Stadler (e-mail: wmstadle@mcis.bsd.uchicago.edu,
Tel.: +1-773-702-4150, Fax: +1-773-702-3163)
University of Chicago, 5841 S. Maryland, MC2115, Chicago, IL 60637, USA

R. Stupp (e-mail: Roger.Stupp@chuv.hospvd.ch,
Tel.: +41-21-314-0156, Fax: +41-21-314-0167)
University Hospital CHUV, Multidisciplinary Oncology Center,
46 Rue du Bugnon, Lausanne CH-1011, Switzerland

T.P. Szatrowski (Tel.: +1-212-746-2855)
Cornell University Medical College, New York Hospital, Division of
Hematology/Oncology, 1300 York Ave, C-606, NY, NY 10021, USA

J.E. Ultmann
University of Chicago Medical Center, 5841 S. Maryland Ave., Chicago,
IL 60637-1470, USA

T. Vargish
Department of Surgery, University of Chicago Medical Center, MC 2115,
5841 S. Maryland Ave., Chicago, IL 60637-1470, USA

N.J. Vogelzang
Section of Hematology/Oncology, Department of Medicine, University
of Chicago Medical Center, 5841 S. Maryland Ave., MC 2115 Chicago,
IL 60637, USA

E.E. Vokes (e-mail: eevokes@mcis.bsd.uchicago.edu,
Tel.: +1-773-702-9306, Fax: +1-773-702-2465)
University of Chicago Medical Center, MC 2115, 5841 S. Maryland Ave.,
Chicago, IL 60637-1470, USA

S.E. Waggoner (e-mail: swaggon@babies.bsd.uchicago.edu,
Tel.: +1-773-702-6722, Fax: +1-773-702-5411)
Department of Obstetrics and Gynecology, University of Chicago
Medical Center, MC 2115, 5841 S. Maryland Ave., Chicago, IL 60637-1470,
USA

S.F. Williams (e mail: sfwilla@mcis.bsd.uchicago.edu,
Tel.: +1-773-702-6956, Fax: +1-773-702-3002)
University of Chicago Medical Center, 5841 S. Maryland Ave., MC 2115,
Chicago, IL 60637-1470, USA


T. M. Zimmerman (e-mail: tmzimmer@mics.bsd.uchicago.edu,
Tel.: +1-773-702-4159, Fax: +1-773-702-3163)
Section of Hematology/Oncology, University of Chicago Medical
Center, MC 2115, 5841 S. Maryland Ave., Chicago, IL 60637-1470, USA

# Therapeutic Modalities

# Principles of Surgical Oncology

R.M. Salloum, M.C. Posner

Surgery remains the most effective treatment for patients with solid tumors and the only chance to cure the majority of patients with cancer. Reports of surgical treatment of various tumors was described as early as 1600 BC. In the modern era, the first report of an operation for an abdominal (ovarian) tumor dates to 1809 [1] when Dr. MacDowell removed a 22-lb ovarian tumor from Mrs. Jane Todd Crawford. The operation was performed on a kitchen table and the patient survived 30 years after her operation. Performing more sophisticated operations had to be delayed until the introduction of anesthesia (1846) and antisepsis (1867). Between 1860 and 1890, Theodore Billroth performed the first gastrectomy, esophagectomy, and laryngectomy for malignant disease.

Surgical oncology has evolved from being the only treatment modality for cancer patients to being one component, albeit an essential one, in the multi-modality approach to the management of patients with solid tumors. The role of the surgical oncologist now encompasses all areas of cancer care including, prevention, diagnosis, staging, treatment and palliation.

## Prevention

The role of the surgeon in general, and the surgical oncologist in particular, is not limited to the diagnosis and treatment of cancer but, instead, extends to intervening earlier in the natural history of malignant transformation. The surgical oncologist should be aware of all conditions that carry an increased incidence or risk for developing a malignancy. A subset of these conditions may require surgical intervention to prevent the development of invasive cancer. Examples of these situations are abundant in the surgical literature, the best example being the case of the familial

adenomatous polyposis coli (FAP) syndrome [2, 3]. This autosomal dominant disorder is characterized by the presence of innumerable adenomatous polyps of varying sizes (2 mm–2 cm in diameter) that carpet the
entire colon and rectum. Members of these kindred have a mutation of the
APC gene on chromosome 5 and are at increased risk of developing a
variety of malignancies, particularly colon cancer. These patients should
undergo prophylactic proctocolectomy to prevent the progression of their
disease to a malignant state. Ulcerative colitis (UC) is another disease that
carries an increased risk of malignancy [4]. UC is of unknown etiology
and is characterized by diffuse inflammation of the mucosal lining of the
colon and rectum. It has been well established that patients with this
disease are at increased risk of developing colon cancer and that the risk
increases markedly approximately 10 years after diagnosis. It is estimated
that the risk of developing cancer of the colon in UC patients is about 1%
per year starting at 10 years after diagnosis [4]. Patients with UC require
surveillance colonoscopies and prophylactic proctocolectomy as soon as
dysplasia is detected in any mucosal biopsy to prevent progression to invasive carcinoma. With the introduction of advanced techniques of ileo-anal
anastomosis, these patients are cured of their disease and their quality of
life is not compromised by the morbidity of a permanent stoma.

Another example where prophylactic surgery may be indicated is in
those patients with multiple endocrine neoplasia (MEN) IIA and IIB
syndromes. Patients with these syndromes are affected by medullary
thyroid carcinoma (MTC), pheochromocytoma, parathyroid hyperplasia
(MEN IIA) and mucosal neuromas (MEN IIB). The prognosis of these
patients essentially follows the course of the thyroid lesion. Hence, the
aggressiveness of the disease differs among kindreds. MEN IIA patients
usually follow a more indolent course than MEN IIB. The advent of genetic screening and the identification of germline mutations in the RET
proto-oncogene in patients with MEN IIA and MEN IIB has made
screening kindred members at risk relatively simple, requiring only the
collection of one peripheral blood sample for preparation of genomic
DNA. MTC develops in virtually all patients with MEN II and is the only
component of the syndrome that is invariably malignant. Based on these
facts, it is now recommended that patients with these disease specific
mutations undergo total thyroidectomy when they are as young as five
years of age [5].

Barrett's esophagus is defined as a change of the lining of the esophageal mucosa from normal squamous to columnar epithelium. Barrett's

esophagus is fairly common, occurring in 5%–10% of patients with gastro-esophageal reflux disease. Once Barrett's esophagus has been identified, patients require continuous endoscopic surveillance at regular intervals to screen for dysplasia. Approximately 50% of patients with high-grade dysplasia in Barrett's esophagus will have adenocarcinoma on pathologic examination of esophagectomy specimens and a large percentage of the remaining patients will go on to develop neoplasia [6]. Although controversial, the presence of high grade dysplasia in the setting of Barrett's esophagus is considered an indication for esophageal resection. Photodynamic ablation [7, 8] is currently being investigated as an alternate method to esophagectomy for treating Barrett's esophagus. Red light (630 nm) is delivered endoscopically to the diseased area of the esophagus with the addition of a photosensitizer (e.g. 5-ALA-induced protoporphyrin IX). This produces, initially, extensive mucosal damage to the treated areas followed by healing and regeneration of the normal squamous lining of the esophagus. Preliminary data suggest that photodynamic therapy may be effective in eliminating Barrett's esophagus or, at least, significantly reducing it [8].

The discovery of BRCA 1/2 genes has fueled a controversy regarding prophylactic mastectomy. It is estimated that patients carrying germline mutations of BRCA 1/2 have an 87% risk of developing breast cancer by age 70. The risk of developing ovarian cancer was estimated at approximately 44% by age 70 [9, 10]. Identified patients and family members with these mutations require close surveillance (mammography and pelvic US), in addition to genetic counseling. The role of surgical prophylaxis is as yet undefined but may be an appropriate option in select, properly informed patients.

## Diagnosis and Staging

Accurate diagnosis is essential to direct management of the cancer patient and the critical step of obtaining tissue for histopathologic examination frequently falls into the realm of the surgeon. With the incorporation of more sophisticated techniques of tissue analysis (e.g. immunohistochemistry, flow cytometry, hormone receptor analysis, mutational analysis, etc.), this process has become increasingly more important. The spectrum of procedures used to obtain tissue extends from simple needle aspiration to core needle and excisional biopsy. A fine needle aspirate may be sufficient to diagnose (or rule out) a malignant process by cytologic analysis in the breast, thyroid gland, parotid gland or cervical lymph node. Needle aspiration of a cystic breast mass that yields clear fluid and leads to the resolution of the mass allows the surgeon to reassure the patient that no malignant process exists. Conversely, if a solid mass is encountered, cytologic diagnosis is near 100% accurate and treatment can be instituted. With the increased use of routine screening mammography, early cancers are being detected with increased frequency. Suspicious microcalcifications noted on a mammogram require excision, usually by a needle localized breast resection to secure a pathologic diagnosis. An alternative method to biopsy suspicious microcalcifications is the stereotactic core needle biopsy. This procedure, usually performed in the radiology suite, has the advantage of lower cost and morbidity, with the major disadvantage being sampling error. The accuracy of core needle biopsy is similar to fine needle aspiration with sensitivity ranging from 79% to 94% and no reported false positives [11, 12]. Excisional biopsy consists of resecting all gross visible tumor. The procedure is recommended for enlarged lymph nodes and small tumor masses. In contrast to excisional biopsy, incisional biopsy consists of removing a small wedge of tissue from the tumor. This is the preferred method for diagnosing tumor masses such as extremity sarcomas where extensive dissection for biopsy purposes may compromise subsequent curative resection. Core needle biopsies have been shown to provide equivalent data (grade, tumor type) and have supplanted incisional biopsy in most instances [13].

With the advent of laparoscopy in the 1980s, cancer staging has been revolutionized in a number of solid tumor types [14]. The use of minimally invasive surgical techniques to provide staging information is associated with less morbidity (and possibly mortality) than open laparotomy and may decrease cost. The applications of laparoscopy for staging are multiple. One example is the use of laparoscopy in the management of patients with peripancreatic carcinoma. Prior to the routine use of laparoscopy, the majority of patients would undergo obligate celiotomy and only a very small proportion would be deemed resectable for cure. The use of laparoscopy as an initial staging tool has allowed many patients to avoid unnecessary laparotomy with its attendant morbidity. If, at the time of laparoscopy, any liver metastases, omental or peritoneal implants are found, resection is contraindicated. Locally advanced tumors that encase the portal vein, mesenteric vessels or the celiac axis can be identified with the use of laparoscopic ultrasound. Finally, palliative bypass procedures can be performed via minimally invasive approaches and spare the patient laparotomy.

Laparoscopy has been used in a similar fashion for the management of patients with gastric carcinoma. In the United States, gastric carcinoma continues to carry a poor prognosis with an overall 5-year survival of less than 20% [15]. Patients who undergo initial laparoscopy and are found to have peritoneal tumor implants, liver metastases, or malignant ascites that are not visualized on preoperative imaging studies can be spared laparotomy. Gastrectomy in these patients, if not performed for palliative intent (bleeding, obstruction and/or perforation) is meddlesome and has no impact on survival [14, 15].

The advent of video assisted thoracoscopic surgery (VATS) has proved to be useful in diagnosis and treatment of lung masses. VATS provides diagnostic information for both malignant and benign pulmonary processes with very high sensitivity and specificity [16]. VATS is a viable option in the management of metastatic disease to the lungs [17]. Finally, patients with primary lung tumors that present a prohibitive risk for routine thoracotomy may be candidates for thoracoscopic resection [18].

## Treatment and Cure

Surgery has been and remains the mainstay of treatment for most solid tumors. In the early and middle part of the 20th century, the principles of surgical oncology dictated performing more radical operations in an attempt to cure the patient and prevent recurrences both locally and systemically. The radical mastectomy, popularized by William Stewart Halsted, was based on the presumption that cancer progression was sequential from the breast to the lymph nodes to systemic sites. Decision making in the management of cancer patients has evolved markedly with the introduction of the clinical trial process as a means of applying the scientific method to define treatment based on tumor biology. As our understanding of the biology and natural history of breast cancer has evolved through the application of properly designed and conducted clinical trials, it is clear that the extent of local regional therapy is not the major determinant of outcome. Segmental mastectomy (lumpectomy), axillary lymph node dissection and postoperative radiation therapy have been demonstrated in prospective randomized trials to yield similar results to the modified radical mastectomy in terms of long-term survival [19, 20]. These more conservative operations decrease morbidity and result in less pain, smaller scars and a lower incidence of lymphedema. They are also less disfiguring and, therefore, more cosmetically acceptable, improving the patient's quality of life while not compromising longevity [16–21].

Similar concepts have been applied to the management of soft tissue sarcoma of the extremity. Amputation, considered routine two decades ago, has now been judiciously supplanted by limb sparing surgery in combination with adjuvant radiotherapy with equivalent survival rates [22, 23].

Likewise, the management of rectal cancer patients has also undergone considerable change. Abdominal-perineal resection (APR) with permanent colostomy was the "gold standard" treatment recommended for the vast majority of patients. Sphincter preservation is now the norm with a variety of techniques available (low anterior resection, transanal excision, etc.) to maintain intestinal continuity. With the advent of endorectal ultrasonography, patients with T1 (tumor invading the submucosa) and T2 (tumor invading the muscularis propria) lesions, can be carefully selected for local transanal excision, thus, avoiding laparotomy. Preliminary data suggests that two-year survival rates in this group of patients is comparable to those who undergo radical resection (APR) [24]. It should be noted, however, that few data exists regarding local recurrence rates and the benefit of salvage surgery in these patients. Adjuvant chemotherapy and radiation therapy have been proven effective in the treatment of rectal adenocarcinoma, with improved local control and overall survival confirmed in a number of phase III trials [25, 26]. Controversy still exists whether adjuvant modalities should be used preoperatively or postoperatively.

The introduction of sentinel lymph node biopsy has profoundly influenced the management of malignant melanoma [27]. Therapeutic lymph node dissection is efficacious and indicated in any melanoma patient with clinically palpable nodes. The issue of elective lymph node dissection (ELND) has been more problematic. Although several retrospective studies have suggested a benefit for ELND in patients with intermediate thickness melanoma (Breslow 1.0–4.0 mm) this has not been verified in any of the prospective randomized trials [28, 29]. The sentinel lymph node is the first node that drains a particular area or limb. Following intradermal injection of technetium 99$^m$ labeled sulfur colloid, the lymph node drainage of the area is defined using lymphoscintigraphy. In the operating room, the primary site is injected intradermally with iso-sulfan blue and then with the guidance of a hand held gamma probe and direct visualization of a blue-stained node, the sentinel node is identified and harvested. A histologically negative sentinel lymph node would indicate that there are no metastases to any other lymph node in the draining basin in greater than 95% of cases. Based on these data, the patients with negative sentinel nodes do not require lymph node dissection. Similarly, the biopsy of a sentinel node that reveals metastatic melanoma can be appropriately treated with a complete lymph node dissection and, more importantly, the patient is a candidate for adjuvant alpha-interferon [30] which has demonstrated efficacy in patients with Stage III disease.

Unresectable regional recurrence of malignant melanoma as well as intransit disease of the extremities can be effectively treated with isolated limb perfusion. This involves surgical isolation of the arterial and venous supply to the affected limb and placing the extremity on circulatory bypass. After this is accomplished, a continuous arterial infusion of cytotoxic agents combined with hyperthermia (40–41°) bathes the involved limb. The procedure is meant to deliver high concentrations of the drugs to the tumor while avoiding systemic toxicity [31]. The most commonly used agent is melphalan. Trials are currently being conducted to define the role of tumor necrosis factor (TNF) which, in phase II studies, enhances the clinical response rate. Response rates of up to 80% have been reported with melphalan alone [32]. Isolated limb perfusion may help avoid amputation in patients with advanced regional disease.

Counter intuitively, surgery is an effective method for treating select metastatic tumors. Resection of metastases can result in a long-term disease free state in certain instances (resection of pulmonary metastases from soft tissue and osteogenic sarcomas) in addition to providing effective palliation (debulking of metastatic carcinoid tumors to the liver). The most compelling data involves resection of hepatic colorectal metastases. Patients with three or fewer liver metastases and no evidence of extrahepatic disease have a 25%–30% 5-year survival following hepatic resection with tumor free margins. No form of systemic treatment can duplicate the flat tail on the survival curve indicating cure [33] that has been repeatedly demonstrated in large series of liver resection for colorectal metastases.

## Palliation

A significant percentage of patients with solid tumors are either not candidates for curative resection at the time of presentation or not "cured" by surgery. However, in many instances, surgery is an effective, if not the only, means of providing meaningful palliation of symptoms. An array of surgical techniques are available to improve the quality of life of cancer patients including resection (e.g. colectomy for an obstructing sigmoid lesion), bypass (e.g. gastroenteric and biliary enteric bypass for gastric outlet and common bile obstruction, respectively, secondary to locally advanced peripancreatic cancer) and stent placement (e.g. esophageal stent to relieve dysphagia associated with esophageal cancer). Frequently, the procedure designed to affect cure is, in reality, more likely to palliate (e.g. pancreaticoduodenectomy for pancreatic cancer). Suffice it to say that surgical intervention should be considered as one of the therapeutic modalities that can relieve the cancer patient's suffering.

## Summary

Surgery is a critical component of the multimodality treatment approach to most solid tumors. As more effective systemic and regional approaches, other than surgery, are developed, it is entirely possible that resection will no longer be the primary therapeutic modality for these malignancies but instead may be relegated to adjuvant status (e.g. squamous cell carcinoma of the anus). However, to date, surgery's seminal role in effecting cure for solid tumors has not been supplanted although it will continue to be appropriately refined.

## References

1. Hill GJ (1979) Historic milestones in cancer surgery. Semin Oncol 6:409
2. Haggitt RC, Reid BJ (1986) Hereditary gastrointestinal polyposis syndromes. Am J Surg Pathol 10:871
3. Caspari R, Friedl W, Mandl M et al. (1994) Familial adenomatous polyposis mutation at codon 1309 and early onset of colon cancer. Lancet 343:629
4. Devroede GJ, Taylor WF, Sawer WG (1971) Cancer risk and life expectancy in children with ulcerative colitis. N Engl J Med 285:17
5. Wells, SA, Chi DD, Toshimak et al. (1994) Predictive DNA testing and prophylactic thyroidectomy in patients at risk for MEN IIA. Ann Surg 220:237

6. Harvey JC, Kagan AR, Hause D, Sachs T, Frankl H (1990) Adenocarcinoma arising in Barrett's esophagus. J Surg Oncol 45:162

7. Overhold BF, Panjehpour M (1997) Photodynamic therapy for Barrett's esophagus. Gastrointestin Endosc Clinic North Am 7/2:207–220

8. Gossner L, Stolte M, Sroka R et al. (1998) Photodynamic ablation of high grade dysplasia and early cancer in Barrett's esophagus by means of 5 aminolevulinic acid. Gastroenterology 114/3:448–455

9. Ford D, Easton DF, Bishop DT (1994) Risks of cancer in BRCA 1 – mutation carriers: breast cancer linkage consortium. Lancet 19, 343 (8899): 692–695

10. Couch FJ, Deshano ML, Blackwood M et al. (1997) BRCA 1 mutations in women attending clinics that evaluate the risk of breast cancer. N Engl J Med 15/336 (20): 1409–1415

11. Gross M, Evans W, Peters G et al. (1995) Stereotactic breast biopsy as an alternative to open biopsy. Ann Surg Oncol 2:195

12. Minkowitz S, Moskowitz R, Khalif R et al. (1986) Tru cut needle biopsy of the breast and analysis of its specificity and sensitivity. Cancer 57:230

13. Heslin MJ, Lewis JJ, Woodruff JM, Brennan MF (1997) Core needle biopsy for diagnosis of extremity soft tissue sarcoma. Ann Surg Oncol 4/5:425–431

14. Lowy AM, Mansfield PF, Leach SD, Ajani J (1996) Laparoscopic staging for gastric cancer. Surgery 119/6:611–614

15. Meyers WC, Damiano RJ, Postlethwait RW, Rotolo FS (1987) Adenocarcinoma of the stomach. Ann Surg 205:1

16. Allen MS, Deschamps C, Lee RE, Trastek VF, Daly RC, Pairolero PC (1993) Video-assisted thoracoscopic stapled wedge excision for indeterminate pulmonary nodules. J Thorac Cardiovasc Surg 106/6:1048–1052

17. Dowling RD, Keenan RJ, Ferson PF, Landreneau RJ (1993) Video-assisted thoracoscopic resection of pulmonary metastases. Ann Thorac Surg 56/3:772–775

18. Landreneau RJ, Hazelrigg SR, Ferson PF et al. (1992) Thoracoscopic resection of 85 pulmonary lesions. Ann Thorac Surg 54/3:415–419

19. Fisher B, Bauer M, Margolese R et al. (1985) Five-year results of a randomized clinical trial comparing total mastectomy and segmental mastectomy with or without radiation in the treatment of breast cancer. N Engl J Med 14/312 (11): 665–673

20. Lichter AS, Lippman ME, Danforth DN Jr et al. (1992) Mastectomy versus breast-conserving therapy in the treatment of stage I and II carcinoma of the breast: a randomized trial at the National Cancer Institute. J Clin Oncol 10/6:986–983

21. Fisher B, Redmond C, Poissan R (1989) Eight year results of a randomized clinical trial comparing total mastectomy and lumpectomy with or without irradiation in the treatment of breast cancer. N Engl J Med 320:822

22. Rosenberg SA, Kent H, Costa J et al. (1978) Prospective randomized evaluation of the role of limb-sparing surgery, radiation therapy, and adjuvant chemoimmunotherapy in the treatment of adult soft-tissue sarcomas. Surgery 84/1:62–69

23. Rosenberg SA, Glatstein EJ (1981) Perspectives on the role of surgery and radiation therapy in the treatment of soft tissue sarcomas of the extremities. Semin Oncol 8/2:190–200

24. Faivre J, Chaume J, Pigot F, Trojani M, Bonichon F (1996) Transanal electroresection of small rectal cancer: a sole treatment? Dis Colon Rectum 39/3:270–278

25. Grage TB, Hill GJ, Cornell GN, Frelick RW, Moss SE (1978) Adjuvant chemotherapy in large-bowel cancer: demonstration of effectiveness of single agent chemotherapy in a prospectively controlled, randomized trial. Recent Results Cancer Res 68:222–230

26. Kemeny N, Saltz L, Cohen A (1997) Adjuvant therapy of colorectal cancer. Surg et al.Oncol Clin North Am 6/4:699–722

27. Morton DL, Wen D, Wong JH et al. (1992) Technical details of intraoperative mapping for early stage melanoma. Arch Surg 127:392
28. Sim FH, Taylor WF, Pritchard DJ et al. (1986) Lymphadenopathy in the management of stage I melanoma: a prospective randomized study. Mayo Clinic Proceedings 61:697
29. Veronesi V, Adamus J, Bandiera DC et al. (1977) Inefficacy of immediate lymph node dissection in stage I melanoma of the limb. N Engl J Med 297:627
30. Kirkwood J, Strawderman M et al. (1996) The Eastern Cooperative Oncology Group Trial 1684. J Clin Oncol 14/1:7–17
31. Lienard D, Eggermont AM, Kroon BB, Schraffordt Koops H, Lejeune FJ (1998) Isolated limb perfusion in primary and recurrent melanoma: indications and results. Semin Surg Oncol 14/3:202–209
32. Fraker DL, Alexander HR, Andrich M, Rosenberg SA: Treatment of patients with melanoma of the extremity using hyperthermic isolated limb perfusion with melphalan, tumor necrosis factor, and interferon gamma: results of a tumor necrosis factor dose-escalation study
33. Blake C, Rosen LJ, Steele GD et al. (1998) Surgical margin in hepatic resection for colorectal metastases. Ann Surg 227/4:566–571

# Principles of Radiation Oncology

A.J. Mundt

## Introduction

Radiation Oncology is a field devoted to the treatment of benign and malignant disease with ionizing radiation. The field was born not long after the discovery of X-rays by Wilhelm Roentgen in 1895 [1]. Radiation therapy (RT) was soon being used in a wide variety of malignant diseases [2, 3]. However, treatment was often associated with significant cutaneous toxicity and had limited applicability until the introduction of high energy (megavoltage) machines in the 1950s. Over the last twenty years, tremendous advances in imaging technology and treatment delivery have been seen allowing increased accuracy in dose delivery and sparing of normal tissues. RT currently occupies an important position in the management of benign and maligant diseases throughout the entire body in both children and adults, and offers an effective means of palliation when cure is not possible.

## Radiation Physics

### Types of Radiation

Two major types of radiation are used therapeutically: electromagnetic and particulate. Electromagnetic radiation (X-rays) is the most common type and is conceptually thought of as small packets of energy (photons). Examples of particulate radiation include electrons, neutrons, protons and heavy charged particles.

Radiation beams vary widely in terms of energy and depth of penetration. X-ray energies are expressed in kiloelectron volts and million electron volts. Superficial (10–125 KeV) and orthovoltage (125–400 KeV)

X-rays are relatively low energy beams and deposit most of their energy at the skin surface and within subcutaneous tissues. Megavoltage (4–24 MV) X-rays are high energy beams which deposit little energy in the superficial tissues, a phenomenon known as skin sparing. Megavoltage irradiation thus avoids the significant cutaneous toxicity seen with low energy treatment. Unlike X-rays, electrons are negatively charged particles that do not penetrate deeply and are thus ideal in the treatment of superficial tumors. Protons are positively charged, heavy particles that deposit their energy at a specific depth over a very limited range.

## Radiation Dose

Radiation dose is defined as the amount of energy deposited in a given mass of tissue. Traditionally, dose has been measured in rads or radiation absorbed dose. One rad is defined as the absorption of 0.01 J/kg. Dose is currently specified in grays. One Gy is defined as 1 J/kg and is equivalent to 100 rads. Practically, it is useful to report dose in centiGrays (1 cGy=1 rad). In special situtations, dose is defined in millicuries or milligram-hours.

### Treatment Delivery

RT is primarily delivered as either teletherapy or brachytherapy. Teletherapy is "treatment at a distance" and is synonymous with external beam RT. Brachytherapy ("close therapy") involves the placement of radioactive sources near or within a tumor. Unlike teletherapy, brachytherapy delivers high doses of radiation to a limited volume with a rapid falloff in surrounding tissues. Other means of treatment delivery include radiolabelled monoclonal antibodies and radioisotopes injected intraperitoneally or intravenously.

## Radiation Biology

Cellular Response to Radiation

The primary target of radiation is deoxyribonucleic acid (DNA) [4]. Damage to the nuclear membrane, however, may also be important. Radiation-induced DNA damage includes single and double strand breaks as well as formation of cross-links. The mechanism of DNA damage differs between the various radiation types. Electromagnetic radiation is indirectly ionizing. DNA damage results from the interaction of DNA with short-lived, free hydroxyl radicals produced primarily by the ionization of cellular H2o [5]. Protons and heavy particles are directly ionizing. DNA damage results from direct interaction of these particles with cellular DNA [6].

Radiation damage is primarily manifested by the loss of cellular reproductive integrity. Irradiated cells are thus said to undergo a reproductive death. Radiation may also kill cells via induction of apoptosis [7]. A cell that has sustained lethal damage may undergo one or two final cell divisions. Cell that are not lethally damaged may be repaired. While the exact molecular mechanism of DNA repair is not well understood, two types have been identified: sublethal (SLDR) [8] and potentially lethal (PLDR) [9] damage repair. Differences in DNA repair capacity have been postulated to explain differences in the sensitivity of many "radioresistant" tumors [10].

Modifiers of Radiation Response

The extent of DNA damage following radiation exposure is dependent on several factors. The most important is cellular oxygen [11]. Hypoxic cells are considerably less sensitive than aerated cells. The difference in radiosensitivity between hypoxic and aerated cells is known as the oxygen enhancement ratio (OER). Oxygen is believed to prolong the lifetime of the short-lived free radicals produced by the interaction of X-rays and cellular $H_2O$. Indirectly ionizing radiation is consequently less effective in tumors with significant areas of hypoxia and necrosis. In addition, hemoglobin levels have been correlated with tumor control rates in a variety of tumors [12, 13]. DNA damage is also dependent on the phase of the cell cycle. Radiosensitivity varies both between and within the various phases. The most sensitive phases are M and $G_2$; the least sensitive are G1 and S [14]. DNA damage following exposure to directly ionizing radiation is less dependent upon cellular oxygen levels and cell cycle phases [15].

Numerous chemicals have been shown to modify the effects of ionizing radiation. An important class of compounds are the hypoxic cell sensitizers which include metronidazole, misonidazole and etanidazole [16]. These agents mimic oxygen and have been shown in vitro to increase cell kill of hypoxic cells [17]. Clinical experience with these agents, however, has been mixed. Only two prospective trials have demonstrated a benefit to their use in conjunction with RT [18, 19]. Toxicity is common, particularly peripheral neuropathy. Promising results with less toxicity have been noted with the newest hypoxic sensitizer nimorazole [20].

A second promising class of radiation sensitizers are the thymidine analogues iododeoxyuridine (IUdR) and bromodeoxyuridine (BUdR) [21]. Both are incorporated into DNA in the place of thymdine and render DNA more susceptible to radiation damage. While non-randomized trials have been promising [22, 23], no prospective trial has demonstrated a benefit to their use. Of note, both are associated with significant acute toxicity.

Multiple chemotherapeutic agents sensitize cells to radiation including 5-fluorouracil, actinomycin-D, cisplatin, gemcitabine, fludarabine, paclitaxel, doxorubicin, hydroxyurea, mitomycin-C, topotecan and vinorelbine. The mechanism of radiosensitization varies between the different agents. Cisplatin inhibits both SLDR and PLDR [24]. Inhibition of repair may also explain the radiosensitizing properties of topotecan [25]. Doxorubicin increases cellular oxygen levels by inhibiting mitochondrial and tumor cell respiration [26]. Hydroxyurea is preferentially toxic to cells in S phase and inhibits entry of cells into S from $G_1$ [27]. Mitomycin-C is preferentially toxic to hypoxic cells [28]. Paclitaxel synchronizes cells in $G_2/M$ phase [29].

Other drugs act as radioprotectors protecting tissues from radiation damage while not affecting tumor radiosensitivity. The best known radioprotector is amifostine, a derivative of cysteamine which acts as a free radical scavenger. Following administration, amifostine quickly penetrates into normal tissue but only slowly into tumors resulting in a preferential protection of normal tissues. Promising results have been reported in head and neck cancer patients undergoing RT [30]. Amifostine has also been used to reduce chemotherapy related sequelae [31].

Fractionation

Early in this century, it became apparent that RT was equally efficacious but better tolerated when administered in divided doses [32], a concept known as fractionation. Fractionation spares normal tissues by allowing time for repair and repopulation of normal cells. In addition, fractionation increases tumor cell kill due to reoxygenation and reassortment of cells into sensitive phases of the cell cycle [33]. Conventional fractionation schemes involve a daily fraction of 1.8–2 Gy five days a week. Total treatment times depend upon the total dose prescribed ranging from 3 to 7 weeks. Hyperfractionation is the use of small doses given once or more daily. The total dose administered is higher and the total treatment time is unchanged. Accelerated fractionation is the use of conventional daily fractions given several times a day to similar or slightly reduced total doses over a shorter overall time. Hypofractionation is the use of large daily fractions given less than five days a week.

## Treatment Planning and Techniques

Simulation

Treatment planning begins with selection of treatment fields, patient positioning and fabrication of treatment aids including immobilization, a process known as simulation. While most patients are treated in the supine position, specific positions are indicated in a variety of tumors in order to minimize exposure of neighboring critical structures. Breast and lung cancer patients, for example, are treated with arms overhead to allow for the use of angled (oblique) beams which do not transverse the arms. Specialized positions include the "frog leg" position (vulvar cancer) and the "chin tuck" position (pituitary tumors). Patients are immobilized in the treatment position with the aid of thermoplastics, foam cradles, bite blocks, arm boards etc. Immobilization minimizes day-to-day variability in setup due to patient movement. Field borders are set at simulation under fluoroscopic guidance based on patient anatomy and knowledge of tumor spread.

Treatment Planning

The goal of treatment planning is to deliver a homogeneous dose to the target volume while minimizing dosage to the normal surrounding organs. Multiple variables (beam number, beam angles, radiation type) are evaluated to achieve this goal. In addition, treatment aids including shielding blocks and tissue compensators are considered. This process requires close cooperation with a radiation physicist and dosimetrist. In most tumors, multiple beams are used in order to minimize the dosage

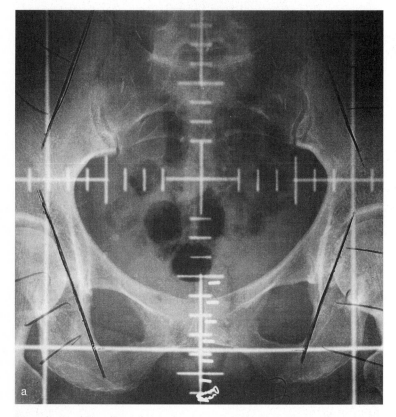

**Fig. 1a,b.** Simulation films of an early stage cervical carcinoma patient treated with whole pelvic radiotherapy. Darkened areas represent blocking.

to overlying critical structures. Prostate cancer, for example, is typically treated with four fields (opposed anterior-posterior and lateral fields). To further reduce exposure of surrounding organs (bladder and rectum), many centers now use six field techniques (opposed laterals and four oblique fields) [34]. Beam energy also depends upon the tumor site.

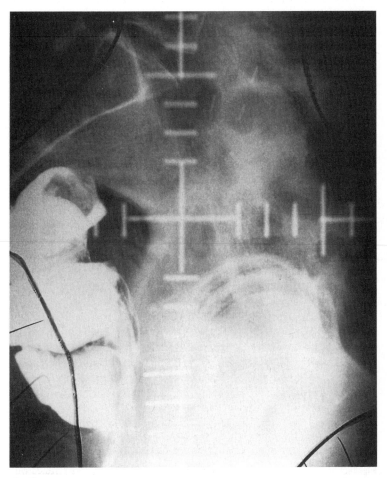

**Fig. 1b**

In general, low energy beams are used for superficial tumors, e.g. skin cancer. Most chest, abdomen and pelvic (deep seated) tumors require high energy (megavoltage) beams. In many cases, multiple beam energies and radiation types (photons and electrons) are used in the same patient. Treatment fields are shaped with the aid of lead alloys (Cerrobend) to minimize dose to critical organs. Figure 1 illustrates an example of a four field treatment of the pelvis in a patient with cervical cancer.

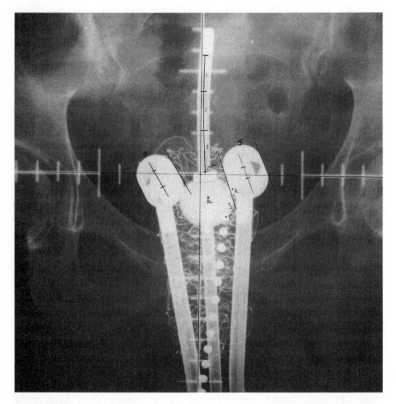

**Fig. 2.** Fletcher-Suit afterloading applicator in place in a patient with early stage cervical carcinoma.

Brachytherapy

Brachytherapy is typically performed in the operating room under general anesthesia. However, considerable pre-planning and imaging are required to ensure accurate delineation of the target volume. Radioactive sources are either placed within an existing body cavity, e.g. the vagina or uterus, in close proximity to a tumor (intracavitary therapy) or directly within a tumor (interstitial therapy). Intracavitary therapy is accomplished with the aid of specialized applicators, the best known example is the Fletcher-Suit applicator used in carcinoma of the cervix. Interstitial therapy involves the use of hollow needles placed within the tumor which are subsequently replaced by plastic catheters. Sources are placed either temporarily or permanently. A variety of isotopes are used including cesium ($^{137}$Cs), gold ($^{198}$Au), and iodine ($^{125}$I). Examples of temporary and permanent brachytherapy treatments are illustrated in Figures 2–4.

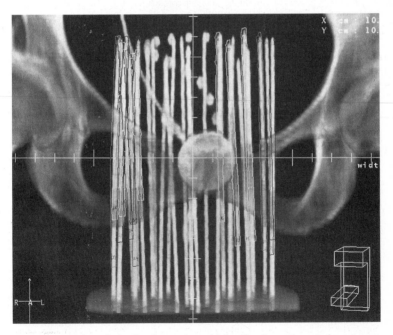

**Fig. 3.** Interstitial needle implant in a patient with locally advanced cervical carcinoma.

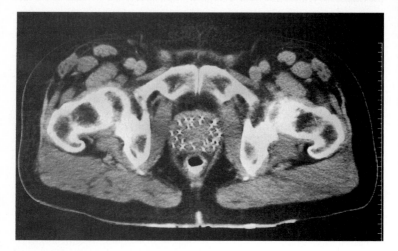

**Fig. 4.** Axial computed-tomography scan of a patient with early stage prostate carcinoma treated with a permanent implant.

New Technologies

Multiple technologic advances have been introduced in treatment planning and delivery over the last decade. Traditional simulation is being
replaced with computed-tomography (CT) simulation. CT-simulation
allows contouring of the tumor, suspected areas of microscopic disease
spread and critical normal structures on axial CT slices of a patient
immobilized in the treatment position. A 3-dimension (3D) treatment
plan is then generated on a treatment planning computer. Unlike traditional techniques, 3D treatment planning results in conformation of the
high dose region to the target volume in three dimensions. However,
considerable accuracy in patient positioning, immobilization and understanding of internal organ movement are required. 3D conformal RT
(3DCRT) is further enhanced with the aid of intensity modulation
(IMRT) and inverse treatment planning [35]. These approaches are particularly useful in the treatment of irregularly shaped target volumes. One
promising use of 3DCRT and IMRT is the exclusion of the contralateral
parotid gland in head and neck patients thereby reducing the risk of

xerostomia [36]. Conventional cerrobend blocking is also being replaced with multi-leaf collimation (MLC) in which small "leaves" whose position and movement is under computer control. Accuracy of patient positioning is improved with the aid of on-line electronic portal imaging [37].

Technologic advances have also been realized in brachytherapy. Brachytherapy is traditionally delivered over several days at a low dose rate (LDR), e.g. 50–70 cGy/h. High dose rate (HDR) techniques have been introduced using high activity iridium sources with dose rates exceeding 200 cGy/min. Unlike LDR, HDR is an outpatient procedure requiring only minimal anesthesia. It is particularly appealing in older patients with multiple medical problems. Promising results have been reported in many sites including head and neck [38], cervix [39], endometrium [40] and prostate [41]. Controversy exists regarding the increased potential of HDR for late complications [42, 43]. Further followup and randomized trials are needed to resolves this issue.

Special Techniques

A number of special techniques are available at large cancer centers. Stereotactic radiosurgery (SRS) is the use of large, single fractions of radiation focused on small intracranial volumes with high precision. Immobilization is assured with the aid of surgical pins placed in the skull [44]. Promising results have been reported in inoperable arteriovenous malformations [45], primary brain tumors [46] and isolated cerebral metastases [47]. Several centers are exploring stereotactic radiotherapy (SRT) using a relocatable frame (without pins placed in the skull) and fractionated irradiation [48]. Contact therapy is the use of low energy photons to treat superficial, localized rectal tumors without surgery [49]. Radimmunotherapy utilizes antibodies with specificity against tumor associated antigens to deliver radioactive nuclei to tumors. Promising results have been reported in non-Hodgkin's lymphoma [50] and hepatoma [51]. Intraperitoneal radiocolloids have been used in high risk early stage ovarian [52] and endometrial cancer with positive peritoneal cytology [53]. Hyperthermia is the use of heat (>42.5°C) to kill cancer cells and enhance the effects of both RT and select cytotoxic agents. This approach shows promise in a number of sites including locally recurrent breast [54] and cervical carcinoma [55].

## Role of Radiation Therapy

Definitive Therapy

RT alone as definitive therapy is used in a variety of tumors. Examples include early stage head and neck cancer [56], Hodgkin's disease [57] and cervical cancer [58]. Treatment may consist of external beam alone (Hodgkin's disease) or involve a combination of external beam and brachytherapy (head and neck cancer, cervix cancer). Definitive RT is also used in tumors in which surgery is the mainstay of therapy when a patient is unable to undergo or refuses surgery. Notable examples include early stage lung cancer [59] and endometrial cancer [60].

## Adjuvant Therapy

RT is commonly administered in conjunction with surgery and/or chemotherapy. When combined with surgery, RT is given prior to (preoperative), following (postoperative) or during (intraoperative) surgery. While common in the past, preoperative RT is used less often today and primarily large borderline resectable tumors, e.g. rectal cancer [61] and soft tissue sarcomas [62]. In contrast, postoperative RT is used in many sites including tumors of the central cervous system [63], head and neck [64], breast [65], lung [66], genitourinary [67] and gastrointestinal tract [68]. In resectable disease, postoperative RT is preferable because treatment is tailored to the pathology findings and higher doses can be administered. Moreover, there is reduced potential for interference in normal wound healing. Indications for postoperative RT include close/positive surgical margins, residual disease, and lymph node involvement. Potential disadvantages of postoperative RT include delaying therapy until wound healing is complete and reduced vascularity of tissues following surgery. Intraoperative RT (IORT) is the delivery of a single, large radiation fraction during surgery with either electrons or low energy X-rays [69]. This is accomplished with either a dedicated treatment machine in the operating room or by transporting the patient to the radiotherapy department during surgery. An important benefit is that normal tissues, e.g. small bowel, can be displaced out of the treatment field. A disadvantage, however, is that the total treatment is delivered in a single fraction obviating the benefits of fractionation. Promising results have been reported in retroperitoneal soft tissue sarcomas [70]. An alternative is the use of brachytherapy with catheters placed at surgery. It is imperative, however, to delay loading for several days to allow for adequate wound healing [71].

When RT and chemotherapy are combined, chemotherapy is administered either prior to (neoadjuvant), during (concomitant), or following (maintenance) RT. Chemoradiotherapy approaches aim to improve local control and to eradicate micro-metastatic disease. Neoadjuvant chemotherapy has been used in a number of disease sites including early stage Non-Hodgkin's lymphoma [72] and small cell lung cancer [73]. A potential benefit is that bulky disease sites can be cytoreduced allowing irradiation of smaller volumes. However, increasing evidence suggests that concomitant chemoradiotherapy is perferable in a variety of disease sites. Concomitant chemoradiotherapy is now commonplace in locally advanced cancer of the lung [74], head and neck [75], esophagus [76], bladder [77] and cervix [78]. Maintenance chemotherapy is used in Wilm's tumor and rhabdomyosarcoma.

In select sites, all three modalities are combined. A variety of schedules have been used. Examples include neoadjuvant chemotherapy, surgery and postoperative RT (locally advanced breast cancer) [79] and surgery followed by concomitant chemoradiotherapy (pancreas and rectum) [80, 81].

Palliative RT

RT is an important means of providing rapid and effective palliation due to local and/or metastatic disease. Osseous metastases secondary to breast, prostate and other tumors are treated with localized fields and short course regimens, e.g. 30 Gy in 10 fractions. Pain relief is achieved in over 70% of patients [82]. The optimal fractionation schedule, however, remains unclear. Rapid large fractions, e.g. 20 Gy over 5 days, are equivalent to more protracted regimens using smaller daily doses [83]. Such approaches are indicated in patients with symptomatic long bone sites not in close proximity to critical organs. More rapid schedules may be possible. The Radiation Therapy Oncology Group (RTOG) is currently comparing 8 Gy in 1 fraction to 30 Gy in 10 fractions in a randomized trial. Large field (hemibody) irradiation has been used in patients with widespread bone metastases [84]. Promising results have also been reported with intravenous 89Sr [85].

Whole brain RT is indicated in patients with cerebral metastases. Treatment is typically delivered over 10 days to total dose of 30 Gy. As with ossesous metastases, controversy exists over the optimal treatment regimen in these patients. Borgelt et al. reviewed various regimens ranging from 20 Gy in 5 fractions to 40 Gy in 20 fractions on two randomized trials. No differences were seen in terms of frequency or duration of response. Overall, 50% of patients had significant improvement in neurologic symptoms. However, the less protracted regimens resulted in more rapid overall response rates [86]. Protracted regimens are indicated, however, in patients with controlled primaries and solitary metastases.

Other indications for palliative RT include spinal cord compression [87], liver metastases [88], orbital metastases [89], and carcinomatous meningitis [90]. Palliative RT is also used in symptomatic locally advanced lung [91] and ovarian cancer [92]. Brachytherapy can be used in palliative treatment as well, e.g. bronchial [93], biliary [94] and esophageal [95] obstruction.

## Benign Disease

RT is used in a wide variety of benign tumors and conditions, e.g. keloids [96], hemangiomas [97], desmoids [98] and pterygium [99]. Other indications include renal [100] and cardiac [101] transplant rejection, macular degeneration [102] and heterotopic bone prophylaxis following arthroplasty [103]. Promising results have recently been reported in the prevention of re-stenosis in patients undergoing coronary angioplasty [104].

## Radiation Sequelae

### Acute Sequelae

Acute radiation sequelae, e.g. skin desquamation, mucositis and diarrhea, occur during or immediately following treatment. Such sequelae are believed to be due to the interruption of repopulation of rapidly proliferating tissues [105]. The type of reaction is dependent upon the site irradiated. The one exception is fatigue which occurs in almost all patients. Most acute sequelae are self-limited and respond to pharmacologic management, e.g. diphenoxy hydrochloride with atropine sulfate (diarrhea) and viscous lidocaine (esophagitis). It is imperative to control symptoms and avoid prolonged treatment breaks since treatment protraction has been correlated with worse tumor control in several disease sites [106, 107]. Prophylactic medication may also be helpful. Promising results have been reported using sulcralfate in patients undergoing thoracic irradiation to decrease the severity of esophagitis [108].

The severity of acute sequelae is dependent on a variety of factors. Two major factors are fraction size and treatment volume. Whenever large treatment volumes are used, it is thus imperative to reduce the daily fraction size to minimize acute sequelae. A commonly held belief is that older patients are at higher risk for acute sequelae. However, recent reports have disputed this belief [109, 110].

## Chronic Sequelae

Chronic reactions, e.g. fibrosis, fistulae and necrosis, occur months to years following treatment and are due, in part, to damage to slowly proliferating tissues. Other factors including vascular damage may also play a part in their development [111]. Chronic reactions, like acute reactions, are dependent upon the irradiated site. Chronic reactions, however, are often permanent. Sequelae vary widely in severity ranging from mild fibrosis to small bowel obstruction, fistulae and second malignancies. Overall, the risk of a second malignancy following RT is low. The notable exception is osteosarcoma arising in irradiated bones in children treated for retinoblastoma, particularly the hereditary type [112].

Select chronic radiation sequelae are responsive to medical management, e.g. pneumonitis is managed with bronchodialators and, if necessary, a course of corticosteroids. Recent evidence supports the role of angiotensin II receptor antagonist in the treatment and prevention of radiation nephritis [113]. Prophylactic medications may also decrease the risk of select late sequelae. Promising results have been reported with pilocarpine in head and neck cancer to decrease the incidence of xerostomia [114]. Recently, zinc sulfate has been found to reduce the risk of significant taste alterations in head and neck cancer patients [115]. The most important means of reducing the risk of chronic sequelae, however, is prevention. Strict attention to optimal technique is imperative. Soft tissue sarcoma patients, for example, should never receive treatment to the entire circumference of the extremity in order to reduce the risk of chronic edema. The risk of late sequelae is also reduced by avoiding the use of large daily fractions since fraction size is a major determinant of late effects [116]. As noted earlier, new approaches including 3DCRT, IMRT and inverse treatment planning should further aid in the reduction of the risk of late sequelae.

Future

Since its first use a century ago, the role of RT in the treatment of cancer has undergone tremendous changes. Its role will continue to change in the coming century. Definitive wide-field irradiation approaches will be replaced with small volume treatment delivered in conjunction with chemotherapy. In general, combined modality approaches will become more common, particularly organ preservation techniques [117]. RT will be increasingly integrated into high dose chemotherapy and stem cell programs providing imporved control of bulky and refractory disease sites [118, 119].

The next century will see increased understanding and application of radiobiologic concepts to clinical radiation oncology. Potential strategies include induction of apoptosis, modification of cellular resistance, modulation of cell cycle regulation and predictive assays for tumor control [120, 121]. An exciting area of research is radiogenetic therapy. Selected genes are linked to radioincuable promoters and integrated into tumor DNA. Expression of these genes can then be regulated by ionizing radiation and may improve the therapeutic ratio of RT [122]. These and other approaches will continue to solidify the importance of RT in the treatment of the cancer patient.

**References**

1. Roentgen WC: "On a new kind of rays (preliminary communication)." Translation of a paper read before the Physikalische-medicinischen Gesellschaft of Wurzburg on December 28, 1895. Br J Radiol 4:32, 1931
2. Coutard H: Roentgentherapy of epitheliomas of the tonsillar region, hypopharynx and larynx from 1920 to 1926. Am J Roentgenol 28:313–332, 1932

3. Paterson RP: The radical X-ray treatment of carcinomata. Br J Radiol 9:671–679, 1936

4. Dizdaroglu M: Measurement of radation-induced damage in DNA at the molecular level. Int J Radiat Biol 61:175, 1992

5. Ward JF: DNA damage produced by ionizing radiation in mammalian cells: identities, mechanisms of formation and reparability. Prog Nucleic Acids Mol Biol 35:95, 1988

6. Phillips MH, Griffin TW: Physics of high-linear energy transfer (LET) particles and protons. In Principles and practice of radiation oncology. Edited by Perez, CA and Brady LW. Lippincott-Raven Publishers, Philadelphia, PA, 1997

7. Hellman S, Weichselbaum RR: Radiation oncology and the new biology. Cancer J Sci Am 1:174–179, 1995

8. Elkind MM: Fractionated dose radiotherapy and its relathionship to survival curve shapes. Cancer Treat Rev 3:2, 1976

9. Phillips RA, Tolmach LJ: Repair of potentially lethal damage in x-irradiated HeLa cells. Radiat Res 29:413, 1966

10. Weichselbaum RR, Little JB, Nove J: Response of human osteosarcoma in vitro to irradiation. Evidence for unusual cellular repair activity. Int J Radiat Oncol Biol Phys 31:295, 1977

11. Littbrand B, Revesz L: The effect of oxygen on cellular survival and recovery after radiation. Br J Radiol 42:914, 1969

12. Bush RS, Jenkin RDT, Allt WEC, Beale FA, Beam H, Dembo AJ, Pringle JF: Definitive evidence for hypoxic cells influencing cure in cancer therapy. Br J Cancer 37 (suppl 3):302, 1978

13. Overgaard J, SandHansen H, Jorgenseon K, Hjelm-Hansen M: Primary radiotherapyt of larynx and pharynx carcinoma – an analysis of some factors influencing local control and survival. Int J Radiat Oncol Biol Phys 12:515, 1986

14. Terasima T, Tolmach LJ: Variations in several responses of HeLa cells to x-irradiation during the division cycle. Biophys J 3:11, 1963

15. Raju MR, Amols HI, Bain E et al. A heavy particle comparative study. III. OER and RBE. Br J Radiol 51:712–719, 1978

16. Chapman JD: Hypoxic sensitizers: implications for radiation therapy. N Engl J Med 301:1429–1432, 1979

17. Coleman CN, Bump EA, Kramer RA: Chemical modifiers of cancer therapy. J Clin Oncol 6:709, 1988

18. Lee DJ, Cosmatos D, Marcial V, Fu KK, Rotman M, Cooper JS, Ortiz HG, Beitler JJ, Abrams RA, Curran WJ: Results of an RTOG phase III trial (RTOG 85–27) comparing radiotherapy plus etandazole with radiotherapy alone for locally advanced head and neck carcinoma. Int J Radiat Oncol Biol Phys 32:567–576, 1995

19. Overgaard J, Hansen HS, Andersen AP, Hjelm-Hansen M, Jorgensen K, Sandberg E, Berthelsen A, Hammer R, Pedersen M: Misonidazole combined with split-course radiotherapy in the treatment of invasive carcinoma of the larynx and pharynx: report from the DAHANCA 2 study. Int J Radiat Oncol Biol Phys 16:1065–1068, 1989

20. Overgaard J, Hansen HS, Overgaard M, Bastholt L, Berthelsen A, Specht L, Lindelov B, Jorgensen K: A randomized double-blind phase III study of nimorazole as a hypoxic radiosensitizer of primary radiotherapy in supraglottic larynx and pharynx carcinoma. Results of the Danish Head and Neck Cancer Study (DAHANCA) Protocol 5–85,. Radiother Oncol 42:135–146, 1998

21. Kinsella TJ, Dobson PP, Mitchell JB et al. The use of halogenated thymidine analogs as clinical radiation sensitizers: rationale, current status and future prospects: non-hypoxic cell sensitizers. Int J Radiat Oncol Biol Phys 10:1399–1406, 1984

22. Phuphanich S, Levin EM, Levin VA: Phase I study of intravenous bromodeoxyuridine used concomitantly with radiation therapy in patients with primary malignant brain tumors. Int J Radiat Oncol Biol Phys 10:1769–1772, 1984

23. Chang AE, Kinsella TJ, Rowland TJ et al. A phase I study of intraarterial iododeoxyuridine in patients with colorectal liver metastases. J Clin Oncol 7:662–669, 1989

24. Dritschillo A, Pizo A, Kellman A et al. The effect of cisplatinum on the repair of radiation damage in plateau phase Chinese hamster (V-79) cells. Int J Radiat Oncol Biol Phys 5:1345–1349, 1979

25. Ng CE, Bussey AM, Raaphorst GP: Inhibition of potentially lethal damage and sublethal damage repair by camptothecin and etoposide in human melanoma cell lines. Int J Radiat Biol 66:49–57, 1994

26. Durand R: Adriamycin: a possible indirect radiosensitizer of hypoxic cells. Radiology 119:217–222, 1979

27. Sinclair WK: The combined effect of hydroxyurea and X-rays on Chinese hamster cells in vitro. Cancer Res 28:198–206, 1968

28. Gran C, Overgaard J: Radiosensitizing and cytotoxic properties of mitomycin-C in a C3H mouse mammary carcinoma in vivo. Int J Radiat Oncol Biol Phys 20:265–269, 1991

29. Geard C, Jones JM, Schiff PB et al. Taxol and radiation. Monogr Natl Cancer Inst 15:89–94, 1993

30. new amifostine h/n asco

31. Nagy B, Dale PJ, Grdina D: Protection against cis-diamminedichloroplatinum cytotoxicity and mutagenicity in V79 cells by 2 [(aminopropyl)amino]ethanethil. Cancer Res 46:1132, 1986

32. Regaud C, Ferroux R: Discordance des effects de rayons X, d'une part dans le testicule, par le fractionment de la dose. C R Soc Biol 97:431–434, 1927

33. Suit H, Witte R: Radiation dose fractionation and tumor control probability. Radiat Res 29:267, 1966

34. Neal AJ, Oldham M, Dearnaley DP: Comparison of treatment technique for conformal radiotherapy of the prostate using dose-volume histograms and normal tissue complication probabilities. Radiother Oncol 37:29–34, 1995

35. Mohan R, Leibel SA: Intensity modulation of the radiation beam. In Cancer: Principles and practice of oncology. Devita VT, Hellman S, Rosenberg SA (eds) Lippincott-Raven, Philadelphia, 1997

36. Hazuka M, Martel M, Marsh L et al. Preservation of parotid function after external beam irradiation in head and neck cancer patients: a feasibility study using 3-D treatment planning. Int J Radiat Oncol Biol Phys 27:731–737, 1993

37. Michalski JM, Wong JW, Gerber RL et al. The use of in-line image verification to estimate the variation in radiation therapy dose delivery. Int J Radiat Oncol Biol Phys 27:707–716, 1993

38. Inoue T, Teshima T, Muraya S, Shimizutani K, Fuchihata H, Furukawa S: Phase III trial of high and low dose rate interstitial radiotherapy for early oral tongue cancer. Int J Radiat Oncol Biol Phys 36:1201–1204, 1996

39. Stitt JA, Fowler JF, Thomadsen BR, Buchler DA, Paliwal BP, Kinsella TJ: High dose rate intracavitary brachytherapy for carcinoma of the cervix: the Madison System: I. Clinical and radiobiological considerations. Int J Radiat Oncol Biol Phys 24:335–348, 1992

40. Knocke TH, Kucera H, Weidlinger B, Holler W, Potter R: Primary treatment of endometrial carcinoma with high-dose-rate brachytherapy: results of 12 years of experience with 280 patients. Int J Radiat Oncol Biol Phys 37:359–365, 1997

41. Martinez A, Gonzalez J, Stromberg J et all: Conformal prostate brachytherapy: Initial experience of a phase I/II dose-escalating trial. Int J Radiat Oncol Biol Phys 35:1019–1027, 1995

42. Eifel PJ: High-dose-rate brachytherapy for carcinoma of the cervix: high tech or high risk? Int J Radiat Oncol Biol Phys 24:383–386, 1992

43. Orton CG, Seyedsadr M, Somnay A: Comparison of high and low dose rate remote afterloading for cervix cancer and the importance of fractionation. Int J Radiat Oncol Biol Phys 21:1425–1434, 1992

44. Wasserman TH, Rich KM, Drymala RE, Simpson JR: Steroetactic irradiation. In Principles and practice of radiation oncology. Edited by Perez, CA and Brady LW. Lippincott-Raven Publishers, Philadelphia, PA, 1997

45. Colombo F, Benedetti A, Fozza F, Marchetti C, Chierego G: Linear accelerator radiosurgery of cerebral arteriovenous malformations. Neurosurg 24:833–840, 1989

46. Engenhart R, Kimmig B, Hover KH, Wowra B, Sturm V, van Kaick G, Wannenmacher M: Stereotactic single high dose radiation therapy of benign intracranial meningiomas. Int J Radiat Oncol Biol Phys 19:1021–1026, 1990

47. Adler JR, Cox RS, Kaplan I, Martin DP: Stereotactic radiosurgery treatment of brain metastases. J Neurosurg 76:444–449, 1992

48. Corn BW, Curran WJ, Shrieve DC, Loeffler JS: Stereotactiv radiosurgery and radiotherapy: new developments and new directions. Sem Oncol 24:707–714, 1998

49. Gerard JP, Ayzac L, Coquard R, Romestaing P, Ardiet JM, Rocher FP, Barbet N, Cenni JL, Souquet JC: Endocavitary irradiation for early rectal carcinomas T1 (T2). A series of 101 patients treated with the Pappillon technique. Int J Radiat Oncol Biol Phys 34:775–783, 1996

50. Press OW, Eary JF, Badger CC et al. Treatment of refractory non-Hodgkin's lymphoma with radiolabelled MB-1 (anti-CD37) antibody. J Clin Oncol 7:1027–1038, 1989

51. Order S: Presidential Address: systemic radiotherapy. The new frontier. Int J Radiat Oncol Biol Phys 18:981–992, 1990

52. Young RC, Walton LA, Ellenberg SS: Adjuvant therapy in stage I and stage II epithelial ovarian cancer: results of two prospective randomized trials. N Engl J Med 322:1021–1027, 1990

53. Soper JT, Creasman WT, Clarke-Pearson DL et al. Intraperitoneal chromic phosphate 32P suspension therapy of malignant peritoneal cytology in endometrial carcinoma. Am J Obstet Gynecol 153:191, 1985

54. Perez CA, Gillespie B, Pajak T, Hornback NB, Emami B, Rubin P: Quality assurance problems in clinical hyperthermia and impact on therapeutic outcome: a report of the Radiation Therapy Oncology Group. Int J Radiat Oncol Biol Phys 16:551, 1989

55. Sharma S, Patel FD, Sandhu APS, Gupta BD, Yadav NS: A prospective randomized study of local hyperthermia as a supplement and radiosensitizer in the treatment of carcinoma of the cervix with radiotherapy. Endocuriether Hyperther Oncol 5:151, 1989

56. Lee WR, Mendenhall WM, Parsons JT et al. Carcinoma of the tonsillar region: a multivariate analysis of 243 patients treated with radical radiotherapy. Head Neck 15:283–288, 1993

57. Farah R, Ultmann J, Griem M et al. Extended mantle radiation therapy for pathologic stage I and II Hodgkin's disease. J Clin Oncol 6:1047–1052, 1988

58. Perez CA, Camel HM, Walz BJ et al. Radiation therapy alone in the treatment of carcinoma of the uterine cervix: a 20-year experience. Gynecol Oncol 23:127–140, 1986

59. Dosoretz D, Katin M, Blitzer P et al. Radiation therapy in the management of medically inoperable carcinoma of the lung: results and implications for treatment strategies. Int J Radiat Oncol Biol Phys 4:3–9, 1992

60. Grigsby PW, Kuske RR, Perez CA et al. Medically inoperable stage I adenocarcinoma of the endometrium treated with radiotherapy alone. Int J Radiat Oncol Biol Phys 13:483, 1987

61. Pahlman L, Glimelius B, Ginman C et al. Preoperative irradiation of primarily non-resectable adenocarcinoma of the rectum and rectosigmoid. Acta Radiol Oncol 24:35, 1985

62. Barkley H, Martin R, Romsdahl M, Lindberg R, Zagars G: Treatment of soft tissue sarcomas by preoperative irradiation and conservative surgical resection. Int J Radiat Oncol Biol Phys 14:693–699, 1988

63. Mirimanoff RO, Dosoretz DE, Linggood RM et al. Meningioma: analysis of recurrence and progression following neurosurgical resection. J Neurosurg 62:18–24, 1985

64. Peters LJ, Goepfert H, Ang KK, Byers RM, Maor MH, Guillamondegui O, Morrison WH, Weber RS, Garden AS, Frankenthaler RA et al. Evaluation of the dose for postoperative radiation therapy of head and neck cancer: first report of a prospective randomized trial. Int J Radiat Oncol Biol Phys 26:3–11, 1993

65. Heimann R, Powers C, Halpern HJ, Michel AG, Ewing CA, Wyman B, Recant W, Weichselbaum RR: Breast preservation in stage I and II carcinoma of the breast>The University of Chicago experience. Cancer 78:1722–1730, 1996

66. Lad T, Lung Cancer Study Group: The benefit of adjuvant treatment for resected locally advanced non-small cell lung cancer. J Clin Oncol 6:9–17, 1988

67. Anscher MS, Prosnitz LR: Postoperative radiotherapy for patients with carcinoma of the prostate undergoing radical prostatectomy with positive margins, seminal vesicle involvement and/or penetration through the capsule. J Urol 138:1407–1412, 1987

68. Hoskins RB, Gunderson LL, Dosoretz DE et al. Adjuvant postoperative radiotherapy in carcinoma of the rectum and rectosigmoid. Cancer 55:61, 1985

69. Gunderson LL, Willett CG, Harrison LB, Petersen IA, Haddock MG: Intraoperative irradiation: current and future status. Sem Oncol 24:715–731, 1998

70. Kinsella TJ, Sindelar WF, Lack E, et al. Preliminary results of a randomized study of adjuvant radiation therapy in resectable adult retroperitoneal soft tissue sarcomas. J Clin Oncol 6:18–25, 1988

71. Shiu M, Turnball A, Nori D, Hajdu S, Hilaris B: Control of locally advanced extremity soft tissue sarcomas by function saving resection and brachytherapy. Cancer 53:1385–1392, 1984

72. Glick J, Kim K, Earle J et al. An ECOG randomized phase III trial of CHOP vs CHOP + radiotherapy for intermediate grade early stage non-Hodgkin's lymphoma. Proc Am Soc Clin Oncol 14:391, 1995

73. Perry M, Eaton W, Propert K: Chemotherapy with or without radiation therapy in limited stage small-cell carcinoma of the lung. N Engl J Med 316:912–918, 1987

74. Schaake-Koning C, Van den Bogaert W, Dalesio O et al. Effects of concomitant cisplatin and radiotherapy in inoperable non-small cell cancer. N Engl J Med 326:524–530, 1992

75. Haraf DJ, Stenson K, List M, Witt ME, Weichselbaum RR, Vokes EE: Continuous infusion paclitaxel, 5-fluorouracil, and hydroxyurea with concomitant radiotherapy in patients with advanced or recurrent head and neck cancer. Semin Oncol 24 (suppl):S2-S68, 1997

76. Herskovic A, Martz K, Al-Sarraf M et al. Combined chemotherapy and radiotherapy compared with radiotherapy alone in patients with cancer of the esophagus. N Engl J Med 326:1593–1598, 1992

77. Shipley WU, Prout JR, Eisenstein AB et al. Treatment of invasive bladder cancer by cisplatin and irradiation in patients unsuited for surgery: a high success rate in clinical stage T2 tumors in a National Bladder Cancer Group trial: JAMA 258:931, 1987

78. Stehman FR, Bundy EN, Thomas G et al. Hydroxyurea versus misonidazole with radiation in cervical carcinoma: long-term follwup of a gynecologic oncology group trial. J Clin Oncol 11:1523–1528, 1993

79. Bonadonna G, Veronesi U, Bronhilla T et al. Primary chemotherapy to avoid mastectomy in tumors with diameters three centimeters or more. J Natl Cancer Instit 82:1539–1545, 1990

80. Kalser MH, Ellenberg SS, for Gastrointestinal Tumor Study Group: pancreatic cancer: adjuvant combined radiation and chemotherapy following curative resection. Arch Surg 120:899, 1985

81. Krook JE, Moertel CG, Gunderson LL et al. Effective surgical adjuvant therapy for high-risk rectal carcinoma. N Engl J Med 324:709, 1991

82. Price P, Hoskin PJ, Easton D: Low dose single fraction radiotherapy in the treatment of metastatic bone pain: a pilot study. Radiother Oncol 12:297–301, 1988

83. Tong C, Gilliack L, Hendrickson FR: The palliation of symptomatic osseous metastases: final results of the study by the Radiation Therapy Oncology Group. Cancer 50:893–896, 1982

84. Salazar OM, Rubin P, Hendrickson FR, Poulter C, Zagaras G, Feldman MI, Asbell S, Doss L: Single-dose half-body irradiation for the palliation of multiple bone metastases from solid tumors: a preliminary report. Int J Radiat Oncol Biol Phys 7:773–781, 1981

85. Scher HI, Chung LWK: Bone metastases: improving the therapeutic index. Semin Oncol 21:630–635, 1994

86. Borgelt BB, Gelber R, Brady LW, Griffin T, Hendrickson FR: The palliation of hepatic metastases: results of the Radiation Therapy Oncology Group pilot study. Int J Radiat Oncol Biol Phys 7:587–591, 1981

87. Findlay GFG: Adverse effects of the management of malignant spinal cord compression. J Neurol Neurosurg Psych 47:761–765, 1984

88. Liebel SA, Pajak TF, Massullo V, Order SE, Komaki RU, Chang CH, Wasserman TH, Phillips TL, Lipshutz J, Durbin LM: A comparison of misonidazole sensitized radiation therapy to radiation therapy alone for the palliation of hepatic metastases: results of the Radiation Therapy Oncology Group prospective trial. Int J Radiat Oncol Biol Phys 13:1057–1062, 1987

89. Dobrowsky W: Treatment of choroid metastases. Br J Radiol 61:140–144, 1988

90. Zachariah B, Zachariah SB, Vorghese R, Balducci L: Carcinomatous meningitis: clinical manifestations and mangement. Int J Clin Pharmacol Therp 33:7–12, 1995

91. Rees GJ, Tevrell CE, Barley VC, Newman HF: Palliative radiotherapy for lung cancer: two versus five fractions. Clin Oncol 9:90–95, 1997

92. Adelson MD, Wharton JT, Delclos L, Copeland L, Gershenson D: Palliative radiotherapy for ovarian cancer. Int J Radiat Oncol Biol Phys 13:531–535, 1993

93. Cotter GW, Larscy C, Ellingwood KE, Herbert D: Inoperable endobronchial obstructing lung cancer treated with combined endobronchial and external beam irradiation: a dosimetric analysis. Int J Radiat Oncol Biol Phys 27:531–535, 1993

94. Montemaggi P, Costamagna G, Dobelbower RR, Cellini N, Morganti AG, Mutignanui M, Perri V, Brizi G, Marano P: Intraluminal brachytherapy in the treatment of pancreas and bile carcinomas. Int J Radiat Oncol Biol Phys 32:437–441, 1995

95. Taal BG, Aleman BM, Koning CC, Boot H: High dose rate brachytherapy before external beam radiotherapy in inoperable oesophageal cancer. Br J Cancer 74:1452–1457, 1996

96. Kovalic J, Perez C: Radiation therapy following keloidectomy: a 20-year experience. Int J Radiat Oncol Biol Phys 17:77–80, 1989
97. Schild S, Buskirk S, Frick L, Cupps R: Radiotherapy for large symptomatic hemangiomas. Int J Radiat Oncol Biol Phys 21:729–735, 1991
98. Sherman N, Romsdahl M, Evans H, Zagars G, Oswald M: Desmoid tumors: a 20-year radiotherapy experience. Int J Radiat Oncol Biol Phys 19:37–49, 1990
99. Van den Brenck HAA: Results of prophylactic postoperative irradiation in 1300 cases of pterygium. Am J Roentgenol 103:723–727, 1968
100. Sutherland DER, Ferguson RM, Rynasiewicz JJ et al. Total lymphoid irradiation versus cyclosporin for retransplantation in recipients at high risk to reject renal allografts. Transplant Proc 15:460, 1983
101. Frist WH, Winterland AW, Gerhardt EB et al. Total lymphoid irradiation in heart transplantation: adjuvant treatment for recurrent rejection. Ann Thorac Surg 48:863, 1989
102. Berson AM, Finger PT, Sherr DL, Emery R, Alfieri AA, Bosworth JL: Radiotherapy for age-related macular degeneration: technique and preliminary subjective response. Int J Radiat Oncol Biol Phys 36:861–866, 1996
103. Ritter MA, Vaughn RB: Ectopic ossification after total hip arthroplasty: predisposing factors, frequency and effect on results. J Bone J Surg 59 A:345–348, 1977
104. Tierstein PS, Massullo V, Jani S, Popma JJ, Mintz GS, Russo RJ, Schatz RA, Guaneri EM, Steuterman S, Morris NB, Leon MB: Cather-based radiotherapy to inhibit restenosis after coronary stenting. N Engl J Med 336:1697–1703, 1997
105. Stevens KR: The Stomach and intestines. In Radiation Oncology, Rationale, Techniques. Edited by WT Moss and JD Cox. St Louis, CV Mosby, 1989, pp 362–408
106. Perez CA, Grigsby PW, Castro-Vita H et al. Carcinoma of the uterine cervix. I. Impact of prolongation of overall treatment time and timing of brachytherapy on outcome of radiation therapy. Int J Radiat Oncol Biol Phys 32:1275–1299, 1995
107. Skladowski K, Law MG, Maciejewski B et al. Planned and unplanned gaps in radiotherapy: the importance of gap position and gap duration. Radiother Onol 30:109–120, 1994
108. Meredith R, Salter M, Kim R, Spencer S, Wepelmann B, Rodu B, Smith J, Lee J: Sulcralfate for radiation mucositis: results of a double-blind randomized trial. Int J Radiat Oncol Biol Phys 37:275–279, 1997
109. Pignon T, Horiot JC, Bolla M, van Poppel H et al. Age is not a limiting factor for radical radiotherapy in pelvic malignancies. Radiother Oncol 42:107–120, 1997
110. Pignon T, Gregor A, Schaake-Koning C, Roussel A, Van Glabbeke M, Scalliet P: Age has no impact on acute and late toxicity of curative thoracic radiotherapy. Radiother Oncol 46:239–248, 1998
111. Weichselbaum RR, Hallahan DE, Chen GTY: Biological and physical basis to radiation oncology. In Holland J, Frei E, Bast R, Kufe D, Morton D, Weichselbaum RR (eds). Cancer Medicine. Lea & Febriger, Malvern, 1993
112. Smith LM, Donaldson SS, Egbert PR et al. Aggressive management of second primary tumors in survivors of hereditary retinoblastoma. Int J Radiat Oncol Biol Phys 17:499–505, 1989
113. Moulder JE, Fish BL, Cohen EP: Angiotensin II receptor antignosts in the treatment and prevention of radiation nephropathy. Int J Radiat Oncol Biol Phys 73:415–421, 1998
114. LeVeque FG, Montgomery M, Potter D, Zimmer MB, Rieke JW, Steiger BW, Gallahger SC, Muscoplat CC: A multicenter, randomized, double-blind, placebo-controlled, dose-titration study of oral pilocarpine for treatment of radiation-induced xerostomia in head and neck cancer patients. J Clin Oncol 11:1124–1131, 1993

115. Ripamonti C, Zecca E, Brunelli C, Fulfaro F, Villa S, Balzarini A, Bombardieri E, De Conno F: A randomized, controlled clinical trial to evaluate the effects of zinc sulfate on cancer patients with taste alterations caused by head and neck irradiation. Cancer 82:1938–1945, 1998

116. Withers HR, McBride WH: Biologic basis of radition therapy. In Principles and pracice of radiation oncology. Perez CA, Brady LW (eds). Lippincott-Raven Publsihers, Philadelphia, 1997

117. The Department of Veteran Affairs Laryngeal Cancer Study Group: Induction chemotherapy plus radiation compared with surgery plus radiation in patints with advanced laryngeal cancer. N Engl J Med 324:1685–1690, 1991

118. Mundt AJ, Sibley G, Williams S, Rubin S, Halpern H, Heimann R, Weichselbaum RR. Patterns of failure and outcome of complete responders following high-dose chemotherapy and autologous bone marrow transplantation for metastastic breast cancer. Int J Radiat Oncol Biol Phys 30:151–160, 1994

119. Mundt AJ, Sibley G, Williams SF, Hallahan DE: Patterns of failure and outcome following high-dose chemotherapy and bone marrow transplantation with involved field radiotherapy for relapsed/refractory Hodgkin's disease. Int J Radiat Oncol Biol Phys 33:261–270, 1995

120. Coleman CN: Beneficial liaisons: radiobiology meets cellular and molecular biology. Radiother Oncol 28:1–15, 1993

121. Iliakis G: Cell cylce regulation in irradiated and nonirradiated cells. Sem Oncol 24:602–615, 1998

122. Advani SJ, Chmura SJ, Weichselbaum RR: Radiogenetic therapy: on the interaction of viral therapy and ionizing radiation for improving local control of tumors. Sem Oncol 24:626–632, 1998

# Cancer Chemotherapy

M.J. Ratain, R.B. Ewesuedo

## General Principles of Cancer Chemotherapy

The use of anticancer drugs as part of the treatment strategy for cancer has greatly improved the overall prognosis of cancer. Though the principles of cancer chemotherapy stem from, with rare exceptions, empirical observations made in early clinical trials involving children, the overall approach to cancer chemotherapy will continue to evolve as more clinical protocols adapt to emerging knowledge about carcinogenesis.

There are several drugs and compounds that are in use or in different stages of clinical trials, however, only a few of these usually get approved for treatment of common oncologic malignancies. A concise overview of drugs that are approved or in advanced stages of development will be presented, and whence indicated, relevant or significant clinical trial information will also be provided.

Antineoplastic agents will be classified based on mechanism(s) of tumor cell kill or by their origin into the following; antimetabolites, alkylating agents, anthracyclines and related intercalators, hormonal agents, microtubule targeting agents or plant alkaloids, DNA topoisomerase inhibitors or as miscellaneous agents. A summary of the common antineoplastic drugs and mechanism(s) of action are listed with each subgroup of drugs.

As a cancer specialist, it is imperative that the approach to using any antineoplastic agent be based on sound scientific principles that should be considered in the application of any drug or treatment modality for cancer therapy.

## Chemotherapy Principles

Over the years, continued research in the basic as well as applied sciences have led to a greater understanding of the differences between cancer cells and normal cells. Such differences provide insight into the basis for activation of growth pathways and inactivation of growth control pathways/mechanism of genetic alteration of oncogenes and cancer suppressor genes, thus providing much understanding into the cause and pathogenesis of many forms of cancer. However, only a few treatments have been based on this new frontier of cancer biology. To date, most anticancer drugs are nonselective in their mechanism of action, and are directed at essential components or metabolic pathways that are crucial to both the malignant and normal cells.

As more knowledge accrues about the biology of tumors and the pharmacology of anticancer agents, the use of chemotherapy will hopefully become more efficacious. In clinical practice, chemotherapy for cancer often requires a combination of drugs. The selection of standard chemotherapy combination regimens to treat individual patients is based solely on tumor histology and extent of disease [1]. Therefore, understanding the clinical pharmacology of anticancer drugs is imperative for achieving optimal benefits from use of these agents. Clinical trials are usually performed to fully understand the clinical pharmacology of an anticancer agent. The initial or dose-finding study (phase I trial) determines drug toxicity relative to dose, and subsequent studies define the spectrum of activity of the drug. These studies employ empirical methodology; adopting a trial and error method to determine significant antitumor activity in a variety of tumor types in the latter process. Nevertheless, experiences from the clinics have been and will continue to be an invaluable source of advancement in the principles of anticancer drug development.

## Treatment Strategies

Three principles underlie the general approach to designing specific regimens for the treatment of cancer. These principles are: (a) drugs are more effective when used in combination, (b) drugs are more effective at higher doses and (c) drugs should be used in conjunction with local therapies such as surgery and radiation.

*Combination Chemotherapy*

The usefulness of this strategy in cancer chemotherapy is based on early observations made in the treatment of acute lymphoblastic leukemia [2]. Anticancer drugs in general are more effective when used in combination. To achieve maximum therapeutic benefit, selected drug combinations should incorporate the most active single agents known to have produced complete remissions in early clinical studies in the tumor type being treated. It is desirable to avoid an overlap of major toxicities, mechanism of action and resistance mechanism(s). Also, it is desirable to administer most drugs at their maximum tolerated doses with minimum time intervals between such doses. The major advantages of combining chemotherapeutic drugs are that it may promote additive or possible synergism through biochemical interactions and, also decrease the emergence of resistance in early tumor cells which would have been otherwise responsive to initial chemotherapy with a single agent. An example of the use of biochemical interactions in selecting drug combinations is demonstrated by the administration of leucovorin to increase the binding of an active intracellular metabolite of 5-fluorouracil to its target, thymidylate synthase, thus increasing its cytotoxic effects [3].

*Dose Intensity/Density*

Dose intensity refers to the amount of drug administered per unit time, typically reported as milligrams per square meter per week, regardless of the schedule used [4]. Application of this principle in the usage of anticancer drugs is very important in the success of any chemotherapy regimen. There is overwhelming evidence to suggest that drug resistant tumor cells may be selected from a larger tumor population by the use of sub-optimal doses of an anticancer drug. Unfortunately, the resistance that is acquired herein is not always specific to the particular anticancer agent. A steep-dose response curve is demonstrated between the dose of anticancer agent and degree of tumor cell kill, even with small increases in dose [5], leading to the paradigm of maximizing dose intensity/density in treatment protocols in humans. Nevertheless, the use of dose intensification in humans should always take into account existing conditions in a patient, such as organ dysfunction or prior toxicities, performance status and other medical problems that would otherwise warrant some degree of modification of the standard dose.

Hryniuk et al. and other investigators have shown in several analyses the relationship of survival to dose intensity in advanced adult cancers such as breast cancer and pediatric cancers [6–9]. An offspring of this realization, is the application of loco-regional chemotherapy for the treatment of ovarian cancer, using intraperitoneal cisplatin [10], intraarterial therapy for the treatment of hepatic primary or secondary tumors and intrathecal administration of methotrexate and/or asparaginase for prophylaxis or treatment of central nervous system leukemia. The achievement of maximum dose intensity is often a key goal in the design of treatment regimens for cancer.

It is worth noting however, that while the main goal of dose intensification is to achieve supratherapeutic concentrations of cytotoxic drug(s), such concentrations may or may not be reached. In solid tumors, the use of dose intensification chemotherapy either alone or with cytokine support has not been shown to significantly improve outcome and should not be considered standard therapy [11, 12].

Nevertheless, the potential benefits for the use of increased dose intensity/density of anticancer drugs continues to evolve as research continues in the areas of design of treatment regimens, use of colony-stimulating factors (filgrastim, sargramostim), use of hematopoietic stem cell transplantation for rescue therapy after the use of myeloablative doses, and improvement in the management of infections and supportive care of patients.

## Adjuvant Chemotherapy

Since micrometastases often develop prior to diagnosis, chemotherapy is often administered before or after local therapy with radiation or surgery. Animal and clinical experience have shown that regimens producing the most dramatic responses in metastatic or recurrent disease have the greatest likelihood of being curative in the adjuvant setting [13].

There are ample theoretical considerations and experimental evidence supporting the use of adjuvant chemotherapy [14–16]. However, while this form of therapy shows definite benefit in a subset of patients with breast cancer and colo-rectal cancers [17–20], this does not appear to be true for a variety of other malignancies [21]. In order to improve the efficacy of adjuvant chemotherapy, it is increasingly being investigated, as neoadjuvant therapy, prior to primary surgery (neoadjuvant chemotherapy), especially in cancer of the breast, esophagus and head and neck [22–24]. In pediatrics, neoadjuvant therapy has demonstrated efficacy in the treatment of a variety of solid tumors [25].

## Pharmacologic Principles

A vast number of anticancer drugs/agents continue to be available to the practicing cancer specialist. Clearly, the task of maximizing the potential benefits of any of these drugs requires a thorough understanding of the clinical pharmacology of the drug along with the pathogenesis and natural history of the disease. These principles will include general mechanism(s) of drug action, pharmacokinetics, pharmacodynamics and drug resistance.

### *General Mechanism of Action*

The mechanism of action of anticancer drugs is largely through the alteration of signal pathways in cancer cells. In most cases the signals are also affected in normal dividing cells. Many of the antimetabolites (e.g. 5-fluorouracil, methotrexate, 6-thioguanine) and alkylating agents (cisplatin, melphalan) require chemical or enzymatic activation intracellularly before cytotoxicity can be achieved. Thus the presence of the required activating enzymes in any tumor type is a prerequisite for effectiveness of such a drug.

It is fundamental that for any drug to be useful it has to be present and be maintained at adequate concentrations at its site of action. Thus physical characteristics, such as plasma protein binding, route of administration, first-pass metabolism, and diffusion characteristics will influence delivery of anticancer drugs to their site of action. To produce cytotoxicity, most anticancer drugs require uptake into the cell. A notable exception is L-asparaginase, a bacterial enzyme that inhibits cell growth by depletion of circulating L-asparagine [26].

Both normal and cancer cells undergo division through the same phases. A genetic predisposition or environmental factor results in the dysregulation of the normal cell division, resulting in a proliferative advantage for the malignant population in cancer. This is fundamentally true of most cancers, for example, a mutation or deletion in the $p^{53}$ tumor suppressor gene results in the disruption of $G_1$ to S phase in the cell cycle. Cells expressing normal $p^{53}$ are arrested in $G_1$ phase in response to DNA damage secondary to cytotoxic drugs, allowing for repair of the DNA damage [27, 28]

There are a number of mechanisms by which anticancer drugs result in cytotoxicity. Advances in the molecular sciences continue to increase the spectrum of mechanisms of action of new anticancer agents. Broadly, cancer chemotherapeutic agents act on cancer cells largely by interacting with DNA or its precursors, inhibiting the synthesis or function of new nucleic materials, DNA and RNA, or irreparable damage to vital nucleic acids by intercalation (anthracyclines), alkylation (cyclophosphamide, chloroethyl-nitrosoureas) or enzymatic inhibition mechanisms. Other mechanisms of cytotoxicity include targeting the proliferative process by disrupting membranes, microtubules (vinca alkaloids) and hormone receptors (antiestrogens). Also, there is increasing interest in the use of biochemical modulators to potentiate the action of some anticancer drugs, e.g. the use of $O^6$-benzylguanine to prevent cellular repair of DNA damage caused by chloroethylnitrosoureas (CENUs). It is logical that anticancer drug combination regimen, take advantage of the knowledge of biochemical and cytokinetic profiles of cancer cells to inhibit intracellular signal processes that will result in cytotoxicity.

*Pharmacokinetics*

Optimization of cancer chemotherapy requires minimizing the toxicity associated with any anticancer drug while increasing the efficacy of such a drug either when used alone or in combination with other drugs or modalities of treatment. Understanding how an administered anticancer drug is absorbed, distributed, metabolized or excreted from the body is critical in achieving optimal therapy with the drug. Since most anticancer drugs are administered intravenously, the problem with absorption is minimally encountered, particularly in the inpatient setting. However, the oncologist is likely to be increasingly confronted with cancer patients on oral therapies, who are at risk for variable absorption of oral anticancer drugs. There may be abnormalities in drug absorption due to vomiting, prior surgery, chemotherapy or radiotherapy.

Dosing of anticancer drugs is usually empirical, based on mg/m$^2$ or mg/kg. This basis of dosing does not take into consideration any biological or physiological inter-patient variability parameters. Consequently, the exposure of a tumor mass to a drug over a time period (AUC) may vary significantly between patients. Thus, any anticipated antineoplastic effects are subject to fluxes in attainable concentrations, secondary to variability in drug handling between and amongst individual patients. This factor is further compounded by the narrow therapeutic index of most of these drugs and the lack of good surrogate markers of toxicity or response. The realization that significant inter-individual variability in the metabolism of anticancer drugs leads to differences in systemic exposure to cancer chemotherapy has led to attempts to individualize the treatment regimens in patients based on clinical and biological characteristics [29, 30], and the monitoring of methotrexate concentrations with leucovorin rescue after the use of high dose methotrexate. Along this line, there are several studies attempting to individualize therapy with drugs such as etoposide, 5-fluorouracil, topotecan and irinotecan.

Understanding the different pharmacokinetic parameters should aid the oncologist in determining an optimal dose and schedule for any drug to be used. For the majority of anticancer drugs, the oncologist should be particularly mindful of three pharmacokinetic parameters as they relate to a particular drug. These parameters include half-life ($t_{1/2}$) of a drug, clearance (CL) and the area under the concentration-time curve (AUC).

Half-life refers to the time it takes for the plasma concentration or the amount of drug in the body to be decreased by 50%. In most clinical trials the concentration in the plasma is used to calculate this parameter. Thus, a stated half-life in the plasma or central compartment is not always reflective of the drug concentration in other compartments (e.g. pleural effusion or ascitic fluid) in the body of a given patient. The half-life of an anticancer drug may be affected by major organ dysfunction such as the kidneys or liver depending on the main route of elimination or metabolism.

The other parameters to consider are clearance (CL) and area under the concentration-time curve (AUC). For clinical or therapeutic purposes, these are the main pharmacokinetic parameters to be aware of, since they are reflective of the degree of total drug exposure. Clearance is the apparent plasma volume cleared of the drug per unit time. It is a function of both distribution and total body elimination (hepatic, renal, pulmonary, etc). For practical purposes clearance is calculated according to the following formulae:

$$\text{clearance (ml/min)} = \text{dose(mg)}/\text{AUC (mg ml}^{-1} \text{min}^{-1}),$$

or:

$$\text{CL}=\text{infusion rate}/\text{Css}.$$

The AUC represents the integration of both plasma concentration and time. It is also an important parameter for pharmacodynamic correlates or drug toxicity [31]. From the above formulae, AUC is directly related to the administered dose of a drug.

Factors which are known to contribute to significant inter or intra-individual variability in anticancer drug disposition include physiological conditions such as obesity and "biological age" (greater than 60 years of age and less than 15 years) [32–34].

Renal dysfunction may result in drug accumulation and increased toxicity of drugs for which this is the major route of elimination. Dosing when using any such drug(s) should take into consideration the glomerular filtration rate or degree of renal impairment in the patient.

Hepatic function is also important in anticancer drug treatment. The use of laboratory tests to monitor liver functions is not generally regarded as sensitive tools for predicting plasma drug concentrations. However, the use of drugs, which are mainly metabolized in the liver or excreted by the biliary system such as the vinca alkaloids, may easily result in increased toxicity [35].

Hypoproteinaemia, especially when using drugs, which show a high affinity for proteins (such as cisplatin), is also a factor to consider. The cytotoxicty of a drug is more closely related to the free-drug level than to the total drug concentration [35]. The oncologist should be aware that the presence of a "third space" such as ascites, edema, pericardial effusion or pleural effusion could affect the pharmacokinetics of a drug [35].

There is increasing interest in the role of pharmacogenetics in drug disposition. Pharmacogenetic variation in biotransformation enzyme systems that are known to metabolize chemotherapeutic compounds can be an important determinant in the toxicity or efficacy of a drug, such as mercaptopurine (thiopurine methyltransferase), fluorouracil (dihydropyrimidine dehydrogenase), and irinotecan (UGT1A1) [36–38].

*Drug Interactions*

Anticancer drugs are usually given in combinations. Conceivably, there is a great potential for drug-drug interactions between the anticancer drugs and other prescribed drugs for the patient. Some of these interactions are well described but others are probably yet to be discovered. It is imperative that oncologists should be very familiar with such interactions and exploit it where it can be beneficial to the patient, for instance, the combination of fluorouracil and leucovorin or the use of cyclosporine to modulate the biliary excretion of SN-38, the active metabolite of irinotecan [39]. More importantly, knowledge of such interactions does help in predicting severe toxicities or antagonism that can diminish a drug's antitumor effect.

*Drug Resistance*

One of the major problems in anticancer chemotherapy is the development of drug resistance. Resistance in this instance arises from one of two possible origins. There is a kinetic component, which results from tumor cells that are non-dividing or dormant, and secondly, a genetic based resistance brought about by a spontaneous generation of drug-resistant clones as a consequence of a mutation, gene deletion, gene amplification, translocation, or chromosomal rearrangement [40].

Unlike the type of drug resistance encountered with antimicrobials, this is often a phenomenon of pleotrophic drug resistance, or simultaneous resistance to unrelated drugs (multidrug resistance, MDR). Goldie and Coldman alluded to the possibility of a genetic basis for the development of this type of drug resistance [40]. Possible mechanisms responsible for MDR [41] include reduced intracellular drug accumulation (P-glycoprotein [Pgp; *mdr I* gene]) and the MDR-associated protein (*mrp*) gene], drug detoxification (glutathione-S-transferase gene), altered targets (topoisomerase II), and alteration in drug-induced apoptosis (bcl-2 pathway).

In an attempt to define the role MDR mechanisms play in cancer response to chemotherapy, several studies have and continue to be undertaken to characterize the proteins that confer MDR to tumor cells. The *mdr-1* and MRP genes are identified as members of a superfamily of ATP-binding membrane-associated transport protein [ATP-binding cassette (ABC) transporters] genes widely distributed in all kingdoms of life. Due to the non-specificity of the MDR mechanism, it is speculated that P-gp interacts directly with a broad range of hydrophobic compounds in the lipid bilayer and transports them directly into the exterior of the cell using ATP and the intrinsic ATPase for energy [41].

There are studies correlating the presence of P-gp in tumor cells with outcome to chemotherapy [42, 43]. While the presence of the P-gp is of prognostic significance, thresholds for clinically significant levels of expression of this protein would be needed for adequate chemotherapy strategies in situations where the protein is detected.

There are a number of compounds, which have been found to reverse P-gp-mediated MDR phenotype in vitro. However application of some of these compounds in combination with conventional chemotherapy have demonstrated limited success. In clinical trials of verapamil, there was evidence of reversal of drug resistance in patients with multiple myeloma and non-Hodgkin's lymphoma [44, 45]. However, the dose-limiting cardiac toxicity of verapamil prevented the achievement of drug concentrations in the range required to reverse doxorubicin resistance [46]. Results such as this and other studies have led to the suggestions that the inclusion of a P-gp modulator affects the pharmacokinetics of the anticancer drug and the reversing agent, probably as a result of inhibition of P-gp in the liver and other tissues. This type of possible drug-drug interaction could potentially affect the disposition of any of the drugs.

## Alkylating Agents and Platinum Compounds (Covalent DNA-Binding Drugs)

The drugs in this class share the ability to exert cytotoxic effects mainly by forming covalent bonds between a reactive alkyl group and cellular macromolecules such as DNA. This leads to damage of the DNA template and inhibition of DNA replication and transcription [47]. There is generally no cell cycle phase specificity in their action [48]. Alkylation is either *bifunctional* (two alkyl groups involved) or *monofunctional* (single alkyl group involved). It is believed that the cytotoxicity of bifunctional alkylators correlates with interstrand cross-linkage of DNA [49]. Because these agents often have a steep dose-response curve with no plateau in cytotoxic effect, high doses of alkylators can be used in chemotherapy regimen in conjunction with stem cell transfusion rescue.

Though these agents differ in their patterns of antitumor activity, the major toxicity associated with the commonly used alkylating agents is a dose-related acute myelosuppression. However, the severity of this effect varies with the individual agents. Thus, while busulfan, thiotepa, melphalan, carmustine and cyclophosphamide are commonly used as myeloablative agents in many stem cell transplant induction regimens, the other alkylators are not. Given that the alkylating agents also have cytotoxic effects on other rapidly dividing cells, damage to the gastrointestinal tract, hair follicles and bladder epithelia are sites of manifested signs of toxicity. There is an estimated risk of 1% to 1.5% per year, from 2 to 9 years after long-term treatment with alkylating agents, of developing secondary leukemia [50]. Other toxicities that are unique to the individual agents will be pointed out in the review of such drugs in the text.

Mechanisms that have been implicated for the development of resistance to the alkylating agents include, increased activity of DNA repair enzymes [51], alterations in drug delivery, transport and/or metabolism by the cell [52, 53], increased production of gluthatione (GSH; competes with targeted DNA for alkylation) [54, 55] and increased enzymatic catabolism of activated forms of alkylating agents to inactive metabolites [56]. While these mechanisms might explain resistance to alkylating agents, it has been suggested that the acquired resistance to this group of compounds is multifactorial [57].

There are six major types of alkylating agents (covalent DNA-binding drugs) in clinical use, including nitrogen mustards, nitrosoureas, alkyl sulfonates, triazenes, ethyleneimines and platinum compounds (see Table 1).

## Nitrogen Mustards

The nitrogen mustards are widely used in cancer treatment. The antineoplastics that are included in this group include cyclophosphamide and it analogue ifosfamide, chlorambucil, melphalan and mechlorethamine. These compounds are known to cause treatment related malignancies.

### *Cyclophosphamide*

Cyclophosphamide differs from most other alkylating agents in that it is an inactive prodrug. It is a phosphorylated mustard compound with two (*bifunctional*) alkyl groups. It expresses its antitumor activity only after biotransformation by hepatic microsomal oxidation (by CYP2B6) to 4-

hydroxycyclophosphamide [58]. This metabolite is in spontaneous equilibrium with the open ring aldehyde aldophosphamide, which gets converted to acrolein and phosphoramide mustard, the respective principal toxic and active products.

Cyclophosphamide is one of the most widely used antineoplastic agents [59]. The clinical spectrum of activity for cyclophosphamide is very broad. Cyclophosphamide is mostly used in combination with other drugs or modalities of therapy for the treatment of leukemias, carcinomas of the lung, breast, ovary, cervix and Ewing's sarcoma, lymphomas, retinoblastoma, neuroblastoma, multiple myeloma and mycosis fungoides [60]. Improving the efficacy of cyclophosphamide is the goal of several clinical studies. High doses of the drug are commonly used in preparative regimens for hematopoeitic stem cell transplantation.

Standard doses for cyclophosphamide depend on the treatment and cancer type. In general, a single intravenous dose of 400–1800 mg/m² per treatment course (1–5 days) every 2–4 weeks is used. The maximum single dose without BMT is 7 g/m² single agent therapy. On the contrary, regimens associated with BMT use 5–7 g/m² per day given over 2–4 days. Oral doses are 50–100 mg/m² per day.

Cyclophosphamide is well absorbed orally in the usual dose range. Plasma concentrations of the drug increase with increasing parenteral doses, however with higher doses such as in BMT; many patients will exhibit Michaelis-Menten kinetics [61]. A large fraction of the drug is eliminated by hepatic metabolism. The metabolites are mainly eliminated through the kidneys. The half-life of cyclophosphamide varies with age; it is 2.4–6 h in children, and averages 7 h in adults [62].

The dose-limiting toxicity is usually neutropenia with less severe thrombocytopenia, unless high doses are used. Other toxicities include altered mental status due to syndrome of inappropriate antidiuretic hormone secretion (SIADH), chemical hemorrhagic cystitis due to irritant effect of acroelin on the bladder epithelium (mesna in combination with adequate bladder irrigation reduces this risk), mucosal ulceration, nausea and vomiting, increased skin pigmentation, transverse ridging of the nails, interstitial pulmonary fibrosis, gonadal failure and rarely cardiotoxicity. Cyclophosphamide is also known to have a propensity to lead to treatment related acute myeloid leukemia [50].

**Table 1.** Alkylating agents and platinum compounds

| Drugs | Mode of action | Potential uses | Side effects |
|---|---|---|---|
| *Nitrogen mustards* | | | |
| Cyclophospha-mide | Cross-linking DNA | Leukemia, lymphoma, sarcomas, Ca breast, ovary, cervix and lung, multiple myeloma, retinoblastoma, mycosis fungoides | Hemorrhagic cystitis, myelosuppression, nausea, vomiting, alopecia infertility, pulmonary fibrosis, treatment-related leukemia |
| Ifosfamide | Cross-linking DNA | Germ cell testicular Ca, sarcomas, pediatric solid tumors resistant to cyclophosphamide, lymphoma | Neurotoxicity, alopecia, hemorrhagic cystitis, Fanconi's anemia, cardiotoxicity |
| Melphalan | Cross-linking DNA | Multiple myeloma, ovarian Ca, sarcomas, AL-amyloidosis, lymphoma, breast Ca, neuroblastoma | Myelosuppression, mucositis enterocolitis, SIADH, veno-occlussive disease, pulmonary toxicity, leukemia |
| Chlorambucil | Cross-linking DNA | Chronic lymphocytic leukemia, Waldenstrom's macroglobulinemia, lymphoma, Ca of breast, testis, ovary and choricarcinoma, nephrosis | Azospermia, myelosuppression, amenorrhea, pulmonary fibrosis, neurotoxicity, dermatitis, nausea, vomiting |
| Mechlorethamine | Cross-linking DNA | Lymphoma, cutaneous histiocytosis | Myelosuppression, nausea, vomiting, diarrhea, diaphoresis, lacrimination, infertility |
| *Nitrosoureas* | | | |
| Carmustine (BCNU) | Cross-linking DNA | Brain tumors lymphoma, melanoma, GI tumors | Myelosuppression, hepatotoxicity, pulmonary toxicity, nausea, vomiting, renal failure, neurotoxicity |
| Lomustine (CCNU) | Similar to CCNU | Melanoma, brain tumors, colon Ca, lymphoma | Delayed myelosuppression delayed renal and pulmonary toxicity |
| Fotemustine | Cross-linking DNA | Brain tumors, lung Ca, melanoma | Myelosuppression |

| Streptozocin | Inhibition of DNA synthesis by methylation of DNA | Carcinoid tumors, pancreatic islet cell Ca | Hepatotoxicity, proximal renal tubular-damage |
| **Ethyleneimine** | | | |
| Thiotepa | Cross-linking DNA | Ca breast, ovary, brain tumors lymphoma, Ewing's sarcoma (?), leptomeningeal metastases | Dermatitis, myelosuppression hyperpigmentation, stomatitis alopecia, nausea, vomiting |
| Hexamethylamine | Cross-linking DNA | Ovarian carcinoma | Neurotoxicity, mood disorder |
| **Alkane sulfonates** | | | |
| Busulfan | Cross-linking DNA | Chronic myelogenous leukemia | Myelosuppression with prolonged thrombocytopenia, impotence, sterility, nausea, vomiting |
| Treosulfan | Cross-linking DNA | Ovarian carcinoma | Myelosuppression |
| **Tetrazine** | | | |
| Temozolomide | Cross-linking DNA | Brain tumors, melanoma | Myelosuppression |
| Dacarbazine | Multifactorial, but includes DNA alkylation | Melanoma, lymphoma, brain tumors, sarcomas | Photosensitivity, flu-like illness myelosuppression, vomiting |
| Procarbazine | Cross-linking DNA | Lymphoma, glioma, melanoma | Infertility, peripheral neuropathy, myelosuppression |
| Mitomycin C | Alkylation of DNA | Anal squamous cell carcinoma, Ca of breast, prostate and lung | Myelosuppression, mucositis, hemolytic uremic syndrome pulmonary toxicity, renal fail nausea, vomiting |
| **Platinum compounds** | | | |
| Cisplatin | Inhibits DNA precursors by crosslinking | Most adult solid tumors and osteosarcoma, brain, tumors neuroblastoma in pediatrics | Vomiting, nephrotoxicity, Mg and potassium wasting ototoxicity |
| Carboplatin | Similar to cisplatin | Similar to cisplatin | Thrombocytopenia, ototoxicity nephrotoxicity, vomiting |

*Ifosfamide*

Ifosfamide is an analogue of cyclophosphamide. It is also a *bifunctional* alkylating agent, which undergoes hydroxylation mainly by hepatic microsomal oxidation (by CYP3A) to form an active metabolite. One of its metabolites, chloroacetaldehyde is neurotoxic. Ifosfamide has a similar clinical spectrum of activity as cyclophosphamide. It is widely used in the treatment of germ cell neoplasia and pediatric and adult sarcomas. Ifosfamide has demonstrated significant antitumor activity as salvage treatment against pediatric solid tumors resistant to cyclophosphamide [63]. It also has activity, in combination with other drugs, in the treatment of refractory lymphomas, carcinoma of the ovary, lung and head and neck [62].

Because of side effects frequently associated with orally administered ifosfamide, the drug is usually given with mesna by the intravenous route. Usual doses are 700–2000 mg/m$^2$ day for 5 days or 2400 mg/m$^2$ day for 3 days or 5000 mg/m$^2$ as a single dose. In children, however, ifosfamide is usually administered in fractionated doses or as a continuous 5-day infusion in doses of 1200–1800 mg/m$^2$ per day. Treatment cycles are usually every 3–4 weeks.

Elimination of the drug is mainly hepatic. The elimination half-life of ifosfamide ranges from 5.5–7.7 h with a mean of 7 h [64]. Significant adverse effects associated with ifosfamide include bladder toxicity, alopecia, nausea and vomiting, Fanconi's syndrome and central nervous system toxicity, which ranges from irritability to coma. Methylene blue has been shown to be an effective agent for reversal of, and prophylaxis against the central nervous system toxicity [65]. Cardiotoxicity can result from high doses.

*Melphalan*

Melphalan is an analogue of the amino acid phenylalanine. It is rapidly taken up by cells through an active carrier mediated process, that is independent of the mechanism used by other alkylating agents [66]. This uptake mechanism is affected by the intracellular concentration of calcium. After uptake, melphalan is converted intracellularly to 4-(glutathionyl) phenylalanine [67]. Melphalan used as a single agent or in combination with other drugs demonstrates significant activity in ovarian cancer, multiple myeloma, soft tissue sarcomas and amyloidosis [68, 69]. High doses are often used as consolidation therapy with autologous bone marrow support in the treatment of ovarian cancer, Hodgkin's disease, breast cancer, neuroblastoma, Ewing's sarcoma and myeloma [68].

The required doses vary with age, route of administration, disease type and treatment protocol. In children, the usual dose is 4–20 mg/m$^2$ per day for 1–21 days by mouth. Adults with multiple myeloma may receive 0.15 mg/kg per day for 7 days every 4–6 weeks. For intravenous use much higher doses are recommended such as 10–35 mg/m$^2$ per dose every 21–28 days for pediatric patients with soft tissue sarcoma and 16 mg/m$^2$ infused over 15–20 min every 2 weeksx4 doses for treating multiple myeloma. Doses up to 200 mg/m$^2$ are administered in bone marrow transplant protocols for multiple myeloma [70].

Oral bioavailability is unpredictable. There is significant interindividual variability in the clearance of the drug; children and patients on hyperhydration demonstrate increased clearance [71, 72]. Elimination half-life ranges from 17–75 min at doses of 140–180 mg/m$^2$ [68]. In addition, for single doses of 120–140 mg/m$^2$, elimination half-life is estimated to be 1.3 (0.2 h [73]). This drug is excreted in urine and in feces as well probably due to active biliary excretion. Up to 15% of a given dose is excreted unchanged in the urine [74]. Dosing adjustment is required in patients with renal impairment.

The main toxicity associated with melphalan is myelosuppression (neutropenia and thrombocytopenia) with a prolonged time to recovery, usually 28–35 days. The AUC of high dose melphalan correlates very well with the severity of myelosuppression.

Others include mucositis and enterocolitis especially in high doses, syndrome of inappropriate antidiuretic hormone, hepatic venoocclusive disease, interstitial pneumonitis, pulmonary fibrosis and secondary leukemias.

*Chlorambucil*

Chlorambucil is a phenylbutyrate derivative of nitrogen mustard. Cells rapidly take up the drug by simple diffusion mechanism [75], after which it is converted intracellularly to an active alkylating metabolite (phenylacetic acid mustard). Its cytotoxicity is related to its cross-linking DNA properties.

Chlorambucil is used for the treatment of chronic lymphocytic leukemia and Waldenstrom's macroglobulinemia. It is also used in combination with steroids in the treatment of minimal change nephrotic syndrome. Though it has demonstrable activity against Hodgkin's and non-Hodgkin's lymphomas, choriocarcinoma, testicular carcinoma, breast carcinoma and ovarian neoplasms, its main application is in the treatment of lymphoproliferative disorders.

Route of administration is oral. Absorption is rapid, with peak concentrations occurring within 1 h [76]. Age of the patient is important in dosing. For adults 0.1–0.2 mg/kg for a minimum of 3 weeks is the initial starting dose; adjustments are made based on blood count. Children generally require 0.1–0.2 mg/kg per day or in the case of CLL, 0.4 mg/kg biweekly with increases of 0.1 mg/kg every 2 weeks, or monthly regimens of 0.4 mg/kg with increases of 0.2 mg/kg every 4 weeks until clinical response or myelosuppression occur.

The drug is well absorbed when taken orally. The active metabolite has a half-life of 2.5 h, and it is primarily excreted in the urine. It is about 99% bound to plasma protein and tissue. Associated adverse effects are, myelosuppression, azospermia that could be prolonged on rare occasions [77], amenorrhea, pulmonary fibrosis, hepatotoxicity, reversible neurologic toxicities, seizures, dermatitis and gastrointestinal discomfort.

## Mechlorethamine

Mechlorethamine is a bifunctional alkylator. It is the most reactive of the nitrogen mustards, and has a strong predisposition to react with the $N^7$ position of guanosine [47]. Uptake by cells is by an active mechanism involving choline transporter. Intracellular biotransformation is rapid, resulting in a very short half-life of the drug.

Therapeutic indications for mechlorethamine primarily involve use of the drug in combination chemotherapy regimen with vincristine (oncovin), procarbazine and prednisone (MOPP) as standard therapy for Hodgkin's disease and malignant lymphomas. Topical mechlorethamine is also effective in treating the cutaneous lesions of histiocytosis [78].

Administration of the drug is by rapid intravenous infusions over 3 min. Dosing is normally 6 mg/m$^2$ on days 1 and 8 of a 28-day cycle.

Dose limiting toxicity for mechlorethamine is myelosuppression. Cumulative doses could result in prolonged pancytopenia. Other noted adverse effects include nausea and vomiting which usually occur within minutes of administration, diarrhea, diaphoresis, and lacrimation. Thrombophlebitis and/or thrombosis are a potential complication of therapy. High doses have also been associated with neurotoxicity. Like other nitrogen mustards, it may produce secondary malignancies and menstrual irregularities and oligospermia.

## Nitrosoureas

The nitrosourea drugs include carmustine (BCNU), lomustine (CCNU), semustine (methyl-CCNU), fotemustine (FM) and the naturally occurring antibiotic streptozocin.

BCNU, CCNU, methyl CCNU and fotemustine are chloroethylnitrosoureas (CENUs). Streptozocin is a naturally occurring methyl nitrosourea.

The central antitumor activity of the CENUs is thought to be due to the formation of $O^6$-chloroethylguanine adducts, with subsequent formation of covalent interstrand cross-links and secondly by protein carbamoylation [79]. The ability of the CENUs to cross-link nuclear macromolecules is thought to be responsible for the increased cytotoxic potential when compared with the methyl nitrosoureas [80, 81].

These compounds are lipid soluble and share the common ability to cross the blood-brain barrier and penetrate deeply into neoplastic tissues. They have established clinical activity for a variety of human malignancies, including acute lymphocytic leukemia, lymphomas, melanoma, multiple myeloma, gliomas, and gastrointestinal neoplasms [81].

A major mechanism of resistance to chemotherapy by the CENUs has been shown to be through $O^6$-methylguanine-DNA methyltransferase (MGMT) and gluthatione (GST). Subsequently, there have been a number of studies using other compounds for biochemical modulation [82, 83].

## Carmustine

Cytotoxicity of BCNU is not cell cycle phase specific. This drug is widely used as a component of multimodality treatment of glioblastoma multiforme and metastatic tumors of the brain. It is used in combination with other drugs for the treatment of lymphomas, melanoma and gastrointestinal tumors. There are ongoing studies attempting to increase the efficacy of BCNU, by using modulators of MGMT, to ameliorate de novo tumor resistance, in patients with relapsed high-grade gliomas and other solid tumors [77].

Carmustine is usually administered intravenously. The dose for adults is $150-200$ mg/m$^2$ every 6 weeks or $75-100$ mg/m$^2$ per day for 2 days every 6 weeks. For children the usual doses range from $200-250$ mg/m$^2$ every 4–6 weeks. BCNU rapidly crosses the blood-brain barrier producing peak CSF levels simultaneously with peak plasma levels [84]. It undergoes a rapid biotransformation by both enzymatic and spontaneous chemical processes to active chemotherapeutic moieties. The plasma elimination pattern is biphasic with a short terminal half-life of about 20 min and a secondary half-life of 4.26 h [85, 86].

Myelosuppression, hepatic toxicity and pulmonary toxicity [87] limit systemic efficacy of carmustine. The associated myelosuppression is characteristically delayed. Other reported adverse effects are immediate gastrointestinal toxicity, renal failure and encephalopathy with high dose [84], and treatment related leukemias.

To decrease the systemic toxicity of BCNU when it is used for the treatment of brain tumors, several attempts are being made to administer the drug intracranially [88]

## Lomustine

Lomustine is an analogue of carmustine. The primary advantage over BCNU is that it is administered orally and it has a rapid and complete absorption [89]. The spectrum of antitumor activity is same with BCNU. Lomustine is used in combination with other agents/treatment modalities for the treatment of malignant brain tumors, lymphomas, colon cancer and melanoma.

The usual dose is $100-130$ mg/m$^2$ orally every 6–8 weeks. Lomustine crosses the blood-brain barrier. It is rapidly metabolized in the liver by hydroxylation to two active metabolites (trans- and cis-4$^?$-hydroxy CCNU); elimination half-life with low or high doses range from 1.3–4 h [90]. This might account for the large interindividual variability in exposure to the CCNU metabolites observed by Kastrissios et al. [90].

Lomustine causes delayed myelossuppresion, late renal and pulmonary adverse effects in therapeutic doses.

## Fotemustine

Fotemustine is a member of the CENU class of alkylating agents. Compared to the other nitrosoureas, it has a higher permeability through cell membranes and the blood-brain barrier [91]. Used singly or in combination therapy regimens, it has proven antitumor activity against advanced or disseminated malignant melanoma, primary brain tumors and non-small cell lung cancer [92–95]. Cytotoxicity of fotemustine is thought to be through the formation of two DNA-reactive intermediates [96].

The conventional dose is 100 mg/m² intravenously every week for 3 weeks, followed by maintenance doses of 100 mg/m² every 3 weeks. High doses of 300–500 mg/m² per dayx2 days have been used with autologous bone marrow rescue [91]. Hepatic arterial administration has also been used at doses of 100 mg/m² as a 4-h infusion every weekx4 doses and then, after a 5 week rest period, every 3 weeks until toxicity is observed [92]. This drug has a wide range of interindividual variability with a biphasic disposition pattern and short plasma half-life, ranging from 13.2–63.8 min [91, 97]. The dose limiting toxicity of fotemustine is usually a delayed and reversible myelosuppresion [91, 95].

## Streptozocin

Streptozocin is a naturally occurring methylnitrosourea produced by fermentation of Streptomyces achromogenes [81]. It is less toxic to the bone marrow than the CENUs. The main use of the drug is in the treatment of malignant pancreatic islet cell carcinoma and carcinoid tumors. Though streptozocin has been shown to modulate $O^6$-alkylguanine transferase activity [98], it did not modulate resistance to BCNU in pretreated patients with metastatic colon or rectal cancer [99]. Of note is the fact that while streptozocin can transfer methyl groups to DNA (for cytotoxicity) it does not form cross-links [81].

Administered intravenously, it is rapidly metabolized with an elimination half-life ranging from 15–85 min, and close to 80% of the dose is excreted as metabolites in the urine [100, 101]. The usual dose as a single agent is 1–1.5 g/m$^2$ per week for 6 weeks followed by a 4 week recovery period or in combined regimen, 0.5–1 g/m$^2$ per day for 5 days to be followed by an observation period of 4 weeks. Dose adjustment is required for patients with renal impairment.

The major toxicities of streptozocin are hepatic toxicity and proximal tubular damage that is usually reversible. Severe nausea and vomiting is a frequent side effect. Other less severe side effects are anemia, neutropenia and thrombocytopenia.

## Other alkylators

### Thiotepa

Thiotepa is an *ethyleneimine* with delayed hematologic toxicity in comparison to most alkylating agents. There is a resurgence of interest in this drug given the role it plays in bone marrow transplantation. Thiotepa has antitumor activity in superficial bladder cancer [102] and has also been used as a component of high dose chemotherapy regimens for patients with advanced ovarian cancer, breast cancer, aggressive oligodendroglioma, Ewing's sarcoma and non-Hodgkin's lymphoma [62, 103–107]. Though intrathecal thiotepa is recommended for the treatment of pediatric leptomeningeal metastases, there are data suggesting limited efficacy [108].

Conventional doses are up to 80 mg/m$^2$. High doses are usually 300 mg/m$^2$ per day for 3 days in children and 500–700 mg/m$^2$ for adults. Thiotepa can be administered intravenously or loco-regionally into the appropriate cavity or space. It is rapidly metabolized to TEPA, with a mean elimination half-life of 125 min [109]. In higher doses as used in bone marrow transplant it has been suggested that there is less conversion of the drug to TEPA [110]. Apparently, when administered intravesically, the drug is not only absorbed through the bladder lining but it can also recirculate into the bladder. The mean elimination half-life is 81–110 min [102], with less than 2% of a given dose excreted in the urine [109].

Toxicities associated with thiotepa are delayed myelosuppresion, alopecia, and severe dermatitis with subsequent hyperpigmentation, stomatitis, mucositis, nausea and vomiting.

## Hexamethylamine (Altretamine)

Altretamine is an alkylating agent used both as a single agent and in combined regimen for the treatment of primary or refractory ovarian cancer [111]. It is administered orally at a dose of 260 mg/m² per day for 14 days every 4 weeks. Elimination is mainly by hepatic metabolism, but this is very variable between patients. Elimination half-life ranges from 5 to 13 h [112]. The main clinical toxicity is neurologic disturbances. Rarely, peripheral neuropathy, mood disorders, gait abnormalities are reported.

### Alkane Sulfonates

#### Busulfan

Busulfan is the most commonly used *alkane sulfonate* in clinical practice. It is a bifunctional alkylator. The drug is commonly used in the treatment of chronic granulocytic leukemia. High doses are used in combination with high doses of cyclophosphamide, for myeloablative preparative regimens, for the treatment of chronic myelogenous leukemia. This has the advantage in children of avoiding the growth inhibitory effects of radiation [113].

Busulfan is available in oral formulation, and as an investigational parenteral formulation. The usual dose is 0.06–0.12 mg/kg per day for remission induction in children and 4–8 mg/day in adults, with maintenance doses of 1–4 mg/day. For myeloablative therapy, the dose is 16 mg/kg (range of 600–650 mg/m²] or 1 mg/kg per dose every 6 hx16 doses. Busulfan is well absorbed orally; however, there is wide interindividual variability in drug disposition in children and adults [114, 115]. The half-life in children ranges from 1.3 to 8.5 h [114]. Age is a significant factor in the disposition of busulfan. Children under 6 years have a higher clearance and volume of distribution, while above age 6 the disposition is similar to adults [115]. The wide inter-patient variability in drug handling has led to attempts at individualizing high dose therapy, with the goal of establishing uniform drug exposure among patients; thus minimizing toxicity and improving antitumor activity [116].

Toxic effects associated with busulfan are mainly myelosuppression with prolonged thrombocytopenia, sterility, impotence and gastrointestinal distress. The major toxicity associated with higher dose regimens as used in BMT, is a reversible hepatic venoocclusive disease that correlates with busulfan disposition [114, 117]. However, it has been suggested that the propensity to develop this phenomenon might be related to the use of high-doses of other alkylating agents used in such conditioning regimens and/or drug interaction [114].

Other Covalent DNA-Binding Drugs

*Temozolomide*

Temozolomide is an imidazotetrazine derivative, which spontaneously decomposes, in aqueous solution to the active metabolite of dacarbazine [118]. The antitumor activity of the drug is due to the methylation of DNA at $N^7$-guanine, $O^6$-guanine and $N^3$-adenine [119]. Temozolomide has shown significant antitumor activity against high-grade gliomas [120] and malignant melanoma [121] in clinical studies. The antitumor effect of this drug is tempered by three DNA-repair activities including, repair of methyl adducts by MGMT [122], base excision repair and poly (ADP-ribose) polymerase [123] and DNA-mismatch repair [119]. To potentiate the activity of the drug, there are a number of studies using modulation of DNA repair process to circumvent the ability of tumor cells to repair induced DNA methylation [122, 123].

For ongoing clinical trials the drug is administered orally on a 4 week cycle, first 150 mg/m$^2$ per day is given over 5 days if no myelosuppresion after 3 weeks, the dose is increased to 200 mg/m$^2$ per day. There is rapid absorption with complete bioavailability (range of 67% to 136%, mean of 109%], and elimination is monocompartmental with a half-life of 1.81hours [124]. Hepatic clearance of the drug is minimal. Future studies will further define adequate dosing pattern or schedule for the drug, since its activity is schedule dependent. Dose limiting toxicity from clinical trials is myelosuppresion.

*Dacarbazine*

Dacarbazine is a prodrug that is demethylated by CYP3A4 to a monomethyl species. This metabolite spontaneously decomposes to an active methylating compound. Though the exact mechanism of action is thought to be multifactorial, tumor cell kill is not cell cycle specific. This drug is therapeutically effective for the treatment of metastatic melanoma [125], Hodgkin's lymphoma, malignant brain tumors [79] and it is also used in combination chemotherapy (with doxorubicin and ifosfamide) for the treatment of adult sarcoma.

Because of the rather slow and erratic oral absorption, it is always administered intravenously. The usual dose for intravenous administration is disease specific. For malignant melanoma 200–250 mg/m² per day for 5 days every 3 week cycle is used. While 150 mg/m² per day for 5 days every 4 weeks is considered standard therapy for Hodgkin's disease. The dose for children is different. In this population, 200–470 mg/m² per day for 5 days every 3 weeks is used for most solid tumors, and 375 mg/m² on days 1 and 15, repeated every 28 days is recommended for Hodgkin's disease. Doses of 1.2 g/m² and 2.0 g/m² have been used for locoregional therapy for melanoma [126]. Plasma disposition is biexponential, with a terminal elimination half-life of 5 h [85] and renal excretion accounts for up to 50% of the administered dose [127].

Myelosuppression, vomiting and photosensitivity reactions and flu like syndrome are the major side effects associated with the use of this drug.

### Procarbazine

Procarbazine is a *methylhydrazine derivative* (pro-drug) that undergoes metabolic activation to generate reactive metabolites, which methylate DNA at the $O^6$ and $N^7$ positions of guanine [128]. The main use of this drug is in combination chemotherapy (MOPP) for the treatment of Hodgkin's disease. It however has demonstrated antitumor activity against melanoma, small cell carcinoma of the lung, non-Hodgkin's lymphoma and in pre-treated gliomas when used in combination therapy [62, 129].

Administration is orally. Recommended dose is 100–200 mg/m² per day (in MOPP) for 14 days every 4 weeks, for the treatment of Hodgkin's disease. There is a rapid oral absorption, with a very short half-life of about 7 min [85].

There is a high incidence of hypersensitivity reactions associated with this drug, when used in combination with anticonvulsants. This is thought to be due to a reactive intermediate generated by CYP3A isoform induction [130]. Procarbazine is also a weak *MAO inhibitor*, thus foods containing high amounts of tyramine should be avoided, as well as caution should be exercised when used with other drugs to avoid untoward reactions. Azospermia, infertility, myelosuppression, peripheral neuropathy and parasthesia are also known toxicities of the drug.


Platinum Compounds

Platinum containing drugs enter cells slowly by passive diffusion and partly through facilitated diffusion [131]. Once intracellular, these compounds undergo a series of intermediate reactions to form platinum complexes. The platinum complexes then react with DNA to form intra~ and inter~strand cross-links, majority of which are at the $N^7$-guanine position. The DNA platinum adducts lead to inhibition of DNA replication and transcription resulting ultimately in cell death.

Cisplatin and carboplatin are currently the two drugs in this class of compounds that are widely used in cancer chemotherapy. There are many analogues that are in clinical trials including oxaliplatin, enloplatin, lobaplatin, ormaplatin, zeniplatin, JM-216, 254-S, CI-973, DWA2114R and liposome-entrapped analogues. The platinum compounds remain the key agents in the systemic treatment of germ cell cancers.

Resistance mechanisms that have been postulated for clinical resistance are decreased drug uptake/transport [132], increase in capacity for DNA tolerance or repair [133] and increased cytoplasmic detoxification through an induction of glutathione [134].


*Cisplatin*

This was the first platinum compound to be introduced into clinical practice. However due to the significant toxicities associated with the drug, there have been attempts to develop analogues that will increase the therapeutic index of the drug.

Cisplatin is used in combination chemotherapy for the treatment of a wide range of cancer types including anal carcinoma, testicular cancer, ovarian carcinoma, cervical carcinoma, endometrial carcinoma, bladder carcinoma, head and neck cancers, breast carcinoma, osteosarcoma, melanoma, mesothelioma, myeloma, small cell carcinoma and non-small cell lung cancer, neuroblastoma, glioblastoma, esophageal, gastric cancer and lymphoma [62, 79].

The drug is administered intravenously at doses of 30–100 mg/m$^2$ once every 2–3 weeks, or 60 mg/m$^2$x2 days every 3–4 weeks (for recurrent brain tumors) in children. In adults, doses range from 50–120 mg/m$^2$ every 3–4 weeks, with the exception of testicular cancer cases where 10–20 mg/m$^2$ per day for 5 days every 3 weeks is recommended. Intraperitoneal use requires 90–270 mg/m$^2$. The plasma disposition profile of the drug is biphasic with a terminal elimination half-life of greater than 24 h [135]. Renal excretion accounts for up to 90% of an administered dose.

Nephrotoxicity with wasting of magnesium and potassium, ototoxicity and emesis are the major toxicities associated with cisplatin. In order to circumvent nephrotoxicity, hyperhydration and diuresis must be employed. Other rare toxicities reported are hypersensitivity reactions and peripheral neuropathy with repeated dosing.

## Carboplatin

Carboplatin is an analogue of cisplatin. Its potential for nephrotoxicity and emetogenesis are lower than those of cisplatin. Though its mechanism of action and antitumor spectrum are similar to those of cisplatin, it is less potent in producing interstrand DNA cross-links compared to cisplatin.

The drug is well tolerated clinically. The clinical applications of the drug parallel those of cisplatin. Antitumor activity has been confirmed in advanced ovarian carcinoma, cervical carcinoma, testicular cancer, bladder cancer, small cell lung carcinoma, mesothelioma, malignant pediatric brain tumors, osteosarcoma, sarcoma, neuroblastoma and head and neck cancers.

A unique feature of the drug in clinics is the ability to reasonably predict systemic drug exposure produced by any dose of the drug in a given patient, on the basis of the patient's renal function [29]. Thus the following calculation (Calvert formula) is used for dosing in *adults*: dose (mg)=target AUCx(GFR+25); however, for the *pediatric* population a modified formula by Newell et al. [136] can be used: dose (mg)=target AUCx(GFR+(0.36xBW [kg]).

The usual target AUC is in the range of 5–7 mg min/ml for both adults and children. Notwithstanding, the recommended dose for children with solid tumors is 600 mg/m$^2$ every 4 weeks. The Calvert formula is particularly relevant in patients with compromised renal function. In using the Calvert formula, the best estimation of a patients' GFR is obtained by using 51 chromium-EDTA ($^{51}$Cr-EDTA) clearance [30]; however, in clinical practice estimation of renal function (GFR) is commonly based on creatinine clearance using the Cockcroft-Gault method. To minimize interpatient variability in the disposition of carboplatin due to errors in predicting a patients' GFR, Chatelut et al. [30] have proposed a formula for predicting carboplatin clearance (CL), thus:

$$CL\ (ml/min) = 0.134 \times weight + [218 \times weight\ (1-0.00457 \times age) \times (1-0.314 \times sex)]/serum\ creatinine\ (\mu M)$$

(with weight in kg, age in years, and sex=0 if male and sex=1 if female). This formula takes into account an individual's morphological and biological characteristics, and in obese patients the mean value between the ideal and actual weights is better suited for the formula [137]. Nevertheless, this formula does not apply to pediatric patients or patients on hemodialysis.

For intraperitoneal administration 200–650 mg/m$^2$ has been used. The pharmacokinetics of carboplatin has been studied extensively using different dosing schedules and locoregional administration techniques. The drug exhibits linear pharmacokinetics with a mean terminal half-life ranging from 2–6 h [138, 139].

Dose limiting toxicity for carboplatin is a delayed thrombocytopenia. Rare toxicities with high doses are rash, alopecia and hepatotoxicity.

*Mitomycin C*

Mitomycin C is a naturally occurring antibiotic with antitumor activity. Anticancer activities in humans were first confirmed in Japan [140]. The primary mechanism responsible for cytotoxicity appears to be alkylation of DNA at the N$^6$ position of adenine and at the O$^6$ and N$^7$ positions of guanine, producing cross-linkages and adduct formation [141]. This drug is used in combination chemotherapy for the treatment of anal squamous cell carcinoma, breast, lung and prostate cancer. It is occasionally used with curative intent in the treatment of superficial bladder carcinoma.

Mitomycin C is usually administered intravenously. Recommended dose is 20 mg/m$^2$ every 6 weeks as single agent therapy and 10 mg/m$^2$ every 6 weeks for combination therapy. After administration, the drug is rapidly activated by quinone reduction to a quinone methide [140], and the terminal half-life ranges from 25 to 90 min [142].

The major clinical toxicity is prolonged myelosuppression and dose dependent hemolytic uremic syndrome [143]. Other observed toxicities are mucositis, prolonged nausea, vomiting and anorexia, skin induration, neurological abnormalities, interstitial pneumonia, pulmonary fibrosis, renal failure and potentiation of anthracycline cardiotoxicity [79].

## Antimetabolites

Antimetabolites are generally structural analogs of naturally occurring intracellular metabolic intermediates essential for the normal function of a cell (*pyrimidines or purines*). Such similarities allow for these drugs or their metabolites to serve as substrates for key intracellular enzymes. The substrate substitution ultimately results in the inhibition of key enzymes necessary for synthesis of folic acid, pyrimidine or purine for DNA or RNA formation in neoplastic cells. Since DNA synthesis occurs in the S phase of cell division, most antimetabolites are termed S-phase specific in their action. In many cases, they are best administered by prolonged infusion. The antimetabolites that are of established use and significance in oncology include, folic acid analogues e.g. methotrexate (amethopterin), pyrimidine analogs (5-fluorouracil), cytarabine, purine analogs and gemcitabine, a nucleoside analog. While some of these drugs have broad applications in oncology, others are used mainly for the treatment of hematological malignancies (see Table 2).

### Pyrimidine Analogues

#### 5-Fluorouracil

5-Fluorouracil (5-FU) is a pyrimidine analogue with the capacity to inhibit the biosynthesis of pyrimidine nucleotides. Following rapid transport into the cell, a significant amount of the drug is converted by ribosylation and phosphorylation reactions to three metabolites, two of

**Table 2.** Antimetabolites

| Drug | Mode of action | Potential uses | Side effects |
|---|---|---|---|
| *Pyrimidine analogues* | | | |
| 5-Fluorouracil | Inhibits DNA and RNA synthesis by: incorporation of active metabolites, 5-FUTP into RNA and inhibition of thymidylate synthase | Head/neck, colorectal, breast, pancreatic GI cancers liver, | Myelosuppression, mucositis, diarrhea, hand-foot syndrome |
| Gemcitabine | Inhibits DNA synthesis by: termination of DNA chain, elongation through competitive inhibition by GEM-TP and GEM-DP | Locally advanced and metastaticpancreatic cancer, head- and neckcancer, lymphoma | Myelosuppression, $\uparrow$ liver enzymes, flu-like syndrome, nausea/vomiting |
| Cytosine arabinoside | Inhibits DNA synthesis by direct inhibition of DNA polymerase | Leukemia, lymphoma | Myelosuppression, seizures, conjunctivitis, nausea/emesis, megaloblastic anemia |
| *Purine analogues* | | | |
| 6-Mercaptopurine, 6-thioguanine | Inhibits DNA synthesis by blockade of purine synthesis, through incorporation of 6-TGN into DNA and RNA templates | Leukemia | Myelosuppression, hepatotoxicity nausea/emesis |
| Fludarabine | Inhibits purine synthesis by inhibiting DNA polymerase and ribonucleotide reductase enzymes | Chronic leukemia | Myelosuppression, chills, myalgia, gastrointestinal prolonged immunosuppression, pulmonary toxicity, autoimmune hemolytic anemia |
| Pentostatin | Inhibits purine synthesis by inhibiting adenosine deaminase | Hairy cell leukemia | Renal failure, lethargy, myelosuppression, dermatitis, hepatotoxicity |

| Drug | Mode of action | Potential uses | Side effects |
|---|---|---|---|
| *Other antimetabolites* | | | |
| Cladribine | Inhibition of DNA synthesis by formation of DNA breaks, NAD and ATP depletion | Hairy cell leukemia AML, CLL, lymphoma, Waldenstrom's macroglobinemia | Myelosuppression, dermatitis immunosuppression, fever |
| Hydroxyurea | Inhibits DNA synthesis and repair | CML, acute leukemia with hyperleukocytosis, sickle hemoglobinopathy, essential thrombocytosis, polycythemia vera | Myelosuppression, anemia |
| *Chelate analogues* | | | |
| Methotrexate | Inhibition of purine and thymidylate synthesis by inhibiting DHFR enzyme | Sarcomas, Ca of breast, head/neck, colon, ovarian bladder and lung, leukemia, lymphoma | Stomatitis, nausea, emesis myelosuppression |
| Trimetrexate | Similar to methotrexate | Brainstem gliomas, neuroblastoma, renal cell Ca | Mucositis hepatotoxicity |

which, fluorouridine triphosphate (5-FUTP) and fluorodeoxyuridine monophsophate (5-dFUMP), are known to be active. Cytotoxicity of the drug occurs subsequent to the incorporation of 5-FUTP directly into RNA, and/or the inhibition of thymidylate synthase activity by 5-dFUMP, which is enhanced by reduced folates. The latter reaction depletes the cell of thymidine triphosphate (TTP), a necessary precursor of DNA synthesis [144, 145]. A third mechanism of action for this drug has been proposed, the inhibition of pre-rRNA processing (an essential step for protein synthesis) by 5-FU [146]. Nevertheless, since the relative contribution of each of the mentioned mechanisms is not clear, it is conceivable that specific mechanisms will be tumor specific based on intratumoral metabolic pattern of 5-fluorouracil.

5-FU is used in combination with other compounds in the treatment strategies of a variety of carcinomas including, colorectal cancer with or without metastases, breast cancer, hepatic tumors, head and neck cancers, carcinoma of the ovary, cervix, urinary bladder, vulva and pancreatic cancer [147].

Several mechanisms have been purported for observed resistance to 5-FU by tumor cells. These include loss or decreased activity of the key enzyme required for its activation, increased clearance, overproduction of thymidylate synthase (acquired resistance) through gene amplification, over-expression or mutation [148]. Other mechanisms involve the use of "salvage pathways" of purine or pyrimidine synthesis [149] which circumvent pathways of de novo synthesis and, as a function of DNA damage response due to the loss of p53 function in tumor cells [148, 150]. In attempts to circumvent resistance to 5-FU by tumor cells, a number of modulators have been used to increase the cytotoxicity of the drug including folinic acid and eniluracil [151].

The pharmacokinetics of 5-FU in humans has been studied extensively. Because of the poor and erratic oral bioavailability, which ranges from 0% to 74% (mean of 28%) [152], the drug is normally administered intravenously. However, subcutaneous administration has also been used, which has a bioavailability of about 93% [153]. It has a short plasma half-life ranging from 13 to 20 min after intravenous bolus administration [154]. Kissel et al. [155] reported differences in the intratumoral retention ("trapping") of the drug in patients with liver metastases from colorectal adenocarcinoma. 5-FU has a first-pass clearance of up to 50% [156]. It is mainly metabolized in the liver, approximately 5% of a given dose are excreted unchanged in urine up to 6 h, and a large amount is excreted as $CO_2$ from the lung.

The recommended dosing for 5-fluorouracil varies with different schedules depending on the type of cancer, however, some of the representative schedules are shown in Table 3.

Toxicity includes myelosuppression, severe mucositis and diarrhea especially with leucovorin combination. The gastrointestinal toxicity is more severe with continuous infusion regimens. Other toxicities include alopecia, nail changes, dermatitis, acute cerebellar syndrome, cardiac toxicity, hyperpigmentation over the vein used for infusion and hand-foot syndrome especially with continuous infusion schedules. Pseudomembranous colitis has been reported with 5-FU monotherapy [157].

**Table 3.** Dosing schedules of 5-fluorouracil in combination chemotherapy regimens (from [342])

| Dose | Usual 5-FU dose schedule |
| --- | --- |
| Initial | 400–500 mg/m$^2$ X 4–5 days (single iv or continuous infusion; maximum dose = 800 mg/day) |
| Maintenance regimens | 200–250 mg/m$^2$ QOD X 4 days, every 4 weeks or 500–600 mg/m$^2$ weekly (single iv or continuous infusion) |

*Administered with regimen containing*[a]

| | |
| --- | --- |
| Leucovorin | 370 mg/m$^2$/day X 5 days, or 500–1000 mg/m$^2$ every 2 weeks, or 600 mg/m$^2$ weekly X 6 weeks |

(administer leucovorin 1 h before 5-FU dose)

| | |
| --- | --- |
| Methotrexate | 600 mg/m$^2$ days 1 and 8 (repeated every 3–4 weeks) 5-FU usually given before methotrexate |
| Cisplatin | 1000 mg/m$^2$ continuous infusion X 4 days (weeks 1, 5, 8, 11) with radiation therapy |
| Levamisole | 450 mg/m$^2$/day X 5 days 450 mg/m$^2$/week [weeks 4–52] |
| Interferon-α and interleukin-2 | 750 mg/m$^2$ day 1 [weeks 5–8] schedule repeated every 2 months |
| Mitomycin C | 750–1000 mg/m$^2$ days X 4 days (days 1–4, 29–32) with radiation therapy |

* Dosing of 5-FU could vary with the addition of two or more chemotherapy agents or other treatment modalities.
[a] Dosing schedules with these drugs differ from the general schedules.

*Oral Fluoropyrimidines*

Oral fluoropyrimidines are prodrug formulations of 5-fluorouracil, which are designed to achieve selective high concentrations of 5-FU or an active metabolite, in a tumor after enzymatic conversion. The commonly used oral fluoropyrimidines include doxifluridine, tegafur and the combination of tegafur and uracil (UFT). These drugs are being studied extensively in the clinics as alternatives to prolonged intravenous infusions of 5-fluorouracil in the treatment of malignant tumors of the digestive tract, pancreas, head and neck and breast. In such cases, they have been found to be especially useful in patients with incurable diseases [158, 159].

*Tegafur* is absorbed from the small intestine and converted to 5-FU. It has demonstrated significant antitumor activity against neoplasms sensitive to 5-FU [158]. A new formulation of this drug, S-1, has been shown to have a greater therapeutic index than tegafur in preclinical studies [160].

*UFT* is a 4:1 concentration combination of uracil and tegafur. Uracil in this combination prevents the catabolism of 5-FU, by competitively inhibiting uracil dehydrogenase enzyme, predominantly in the tumor cells [158, 160]. UFT has shown significant antitumor activity in neoplasms sensitive to 5-FU. There are clinical studies designed to modulate UFT with leucovorin [161, 162]. Toxicities associated with UFT include nausea, vomiting and myelosuppression. There are reports of possible myocardial ischemia associated with the use of this drug [163].

*Doxifluridine* is an oral fluoropyrimidine that is converted to 5-FU in tumor cells, where it is selectively cytotoxic [159]. It has been combined with leucovorin for the palliative treatment of advanced gastric and pancreatic cancer, with 15% and 4% objective responses lasting up to 4 months, observed in patients previously treated with 5-FU. Its major dose limiting toxicity is diarrhea [159].

*S-1* is a new oral formulation of tegafur, which in addition to tegafur is also composed of 5-chloro-2, 4-dihydroxypyridine (CDHP) and potassium oxonate (Oxo) in a molar ratio of 1:0.4:1; in this combination, CDHP and Oxo act as modulators of 5-FU [160]. CDHP is a potent inhibitor of 5-FU degradation (by inhibiting dihydropyrimidine dehydrogenase) and Oxo is an inhibitor of 5-FU phosphorylation [159]. Preclinical studies by Takechi et al. [160] suggest that Oxo locally protects the gastrointestinal tract from 5-FU induced toxicity without decreasing the antitumor effect of the drug. Dose limiting toxicities include leukopenia, diarrhea and stomatitis.

*Capecitabine* is also an orally administered prodrug of 5-FU. This drug was developed to avert the gastrointestinal toxicity associated with 5-FU. It is preferentially activated into 5-FU at the tumor site [164]. Capecitabine was recently recommended for FDA approval for the treatment of breast cancer. Clinical trials are ongoing to further define other clinical activities. Toxicity observed after a course of 14 days was mild edema [164].

The pharmacokinetics of 5-FU have been suggested to be a factor limiting the efficacy of the drug [165]. This is because 5-FU is rapidly and extensively catabolized by dihydropyrimidine dehydrogenase (DPD) [166]. Eniluracil (776C85 and 776 C), an oral mechanism based inactivator of DPD, has been used to significantly increase the oral bioavailability of 5-FU, as well as tegafur, a prodrug [167–169]. In clinical studies, neutropenia was the principal toxicity of the combination therapy [167, 168].

## Gemcitabine

Gemcitabine is a deoxycytidine (nucleoside) analogue. Following intracellular uptake, it is phosphorylated to two active metabolites gemcitabine-triphosphate (GEM-TP) and gemcitabine diphosphate (GEM-DP). Cytotoxicity is mainly due to GEM-TP competitive inhibition of deoxycytidine triphosphate, resulting in termination of DNA chain elongation, DNA fragmentation and cell death [170, 171].

Gemcitabine is approved in the United States for the treatment of locally advanced and metastatic pancreatic cancer. However, it has shown significant antitumor activities when used either as monotherapy or in combination with other drugs in the treatment of non-small cell lung, head and neck, ovarian and breast carcinoma [172–177]. Preliminary data also suggest antitumor activity of the drug in cancer of the urothelium, and Hodgkin's and non-Hodgkin's lymphoma [178, 179].

The commonly used dose for gemcitabine is an initial dose of 1000 mg/m² per week given as a 30 min infusionx3 every 4 weeks. Individual patients may tolerate dose escalations of 25–50 per cent before observing any dose limiting toxicity. Though a repeated 4-week cycle is usual for treatment of non-small cell lung carcinoma, an initial 8-week cycle followed by a 4-week cycle is suggested in patients with pancreatic cancer. Optimizing the efficacy of this drug is the subject of various ongoing clinical studies.

Studies involving patients with different types of malignancies show a linear pharmacokinetic profile of the drug for doses up to 1000 mg/m$^2$ [180, 181]. Incorporation of the drug into DNA is both time and dose dependent, and increasing the dose beyond 350 mg/m$^2$ over a 30 min infusion time, does not show a significant effect on the intracellular AUC for gemcitabine-triphosphate (GEM-TP), thus suggesting intracellular saturation with the nucleotide at this point [181]. The plasma half-life of this drug is about 0.3 h, and clearance is mainly by renal route, which accounts for up to 96% of an administered dose [174]. The clearance of gemcitabine decreases with age and is about 30% lower in women [174].

Toxicities associated with gemcitabine reported from clinical trials include myelosuppression, transient elevation of liver enzymes, nausea and vomiting, flu like symptoms and fatigue. A case of delayed anemia and thrombocytopenia was recently reported [182].

## Cytarabine (Cytosine Arabinoside)

This drug is an analogue of 2'-deoxycytidine. It is one of the most effective induction agents in the treatment of acute leukemia. It is also used for prophylaxis and treatment of CNS leukemia. Cytarabine has shown activity in patients with chronic lymphocytic leukemia, non-Hodgkin's lymphoma and myelodysplastic syndrome. To be cytotoxic, the drug is sequentially phosphorylated intracellularly to Ara-CTP by the action of deoxycytidine kinase and other appropriate nucleotide kinases. Ara-CTP is incorporated into DNA, resulting in a direct inhibition of DNA synthesis [183]. A correlation exists between clinical response and the pharmacokinetics of ara-CTP in leukemia cells during therapy [184]. Also, it is known that retention of ara-CTP in circulating lymphoblasts is associated with both a sustained inhibition of DNA synthesis and clinical response [185]. Thus, it is necessary to administer the drug as a prolonged infusion when high doses are not used.

Two standard schedules are routinely used for adults and children: intravenous administration of 200 mg/m$^2$ per day for 5 days at 2-week intervals, or 100–200 mg/m$^2$ every 12 h for 5–10 days or every day until remission. For prophylaxis or treatment of CNS leukemia, intrathecal administration of 5–75 mg/m$^2$ every 4 days is used pending normalization of CNS findings. High-dose therapy requires 1–3 g/m² every 12 hx6–12 doses for acute non-lymphoblastic leukemia or refractory leukemias or refractory non-Hodgkin's lymphoma. The drug is metabolized mainly in the liver to ara-CTP and it has a terminal elimination half-life of 0.5–2.5 h. Close to 85% of the dose is excreted in the urine as metabolites.

Dose limiting toxicity is myelosuppression. Other toxicities include seizures with intrathecal administration, dermatitis, conjunctivitis with high doses, megaloblastic anemia, hepatic dysfunction, fever and pneumonitis.

Purine Analogs

*6-Mercaptopurine*

6-Mercaptopurine (6-MP) is a prodrug, which is used widely in the treatment of acute lymphoblastic leukemia. The drug is initially converted intracellularly through three separate metabolic pathways (involving thiopurine methyltransferase (TPMT), xanthine oxidase (XO), and hypoxanthine-guanine phosphoribosyltransferase (HPRT)) to different thionucleotide metabolites. Further metabolism of the mercaptopurine nucleotide through the TPMT pathway results in the formation of thioguanine nucleotides (6-TGN) [186]. The anticancer activity of 6-mercaptopurine is mainly through the incorporation of formed 6-TGN into DNA and RNA templates, resulting in cell death [187, 188].

Individual differences in the levels of these key enzymes (genetic or otherwise), resulting in differences in intracellular accumulation of 6-MP metabolites do account for significant differences in anti-leukemic effect and toxicity [186, 189, 190]. Nevertheless, only the red blood cell thioguanine levels have been found to be a significant predictor of toxicity [191].

6-MP is administered orally at a dose of 75 mg/m² in children and 2.5–5 mg/kg per day or 1.5–2.5 mg/kg per day for induction and maintenance therapy respectively in adults. 6-Mercaptopurine is metabolized in the liver and intestinal wall. There is significant interindividual variability in oral bioavailability ranging from 15% to 50% and this is largely due to the significant amount of first pass effect and genetic polymorphism in the catabolic enzymatic pathway [192]. The use of 6-MP intravenously as a way to avert the problem with oral bioavailability is being investigated in the pediatric population [193].

Dose limiting toxicities include myelosuppression, gastrointestinal distress, hepatotoxicity that is due to the accumulation of the drug and its metabolites in the liver [194].

## Thioguanine

6-Thioguanine (6-TG) is a purine (guanine) analog and cytotoxic antimetabolite. It is used mainly in the treatment of leukemia and has been suggested to have antitumor activity in patients with breast cancer [195]. This drug is also used as an immunosuppressive agent in patients with nephrosis and collagen vascular diseases.

6-TG exerts its cytotoxic effects first by being converted intracellularly to 6-thioguanine monophosphate (6TGMP) by the enzyme hypoxanthine-guanine phosphoribosyl transferase (HGPRT). Through a series of other reactions including incorporation of 6TGMP into DNA and RNA templates, DNA replication is inhibited, resulting ultimately in cell death [196].

Conventional doses for children and adults are 75–200 mg/m$^2$ per day for 5–7 days or until remission of leukemia. In infants the normal dose is 3.3 mg/kg per day for 4 days. Oral absorption is incomplete, with bioavailability of about 30%. It is extensively metabolized in the liver and plasma half-life is from 0.5 to 6 h [197].

Dose limiting toxicity is myelosuppression and gastrointestinal distress. The observed toxicities in different organs systems is dependent of the HPRT status of the tissue [196].

## Other Purine Analogues

*Fludarabine* is a purine analogue of adenine arabinoside. It is the most active drug in the treatment of chronic lymphocytic leukemia. It has also shown activity in the treatment of malignant lymphomas [198, 199]. Though the precise mechanism by which fludarabine exerts it cytotoxic effect is not clear, it is thought to be through an active phosphorylated metabolite 2-fluoro-Ara-ATP, by inhibiting DNA polymerase and ribonucleotide reductase enzymes [200]. It has been suggested that deoxycytidine kinase (dC) released from lyzed leukemic cells, when present in clinically relevant amounts, contributes to drug resistance [201].

A dose of 20–30 mg/m$^2$ per day x 5 days is usually administered intravenously. O'Rourke et al. [202] administered fludarabine orally and obtained a bioavailability of 58%. The terminal elimination half-life is about 22 h and approximately 40% is excreted through the renal route.

Clinical toxicities include myelosuppression, gastrointestinal distress, chills and myalgia, pulmonary toxicity, autoimmune hemolytic anemia and prolonged immunosuppression that could be life threatening.

*Covidarabine (pentostatin, deoxycoformycin)* is used for the treatment of hairy cell leukemia. Its precise mechanism of action is not well defined. Notwithstanding, it is a known potent inhibitor of adenosine deaminase, and by so doing cells accumulate deoxyadenosine triphosphate, which ultimately inhibits ribonucleotide reductase [147]. It has been suggested that the cytotoxicity of this drug is probably due to an imbalance in intracellular purine nucleotide pools [77]. Covidarabine is used as intravenous injections of 4 mg/m$^2$. Plasma disposition is biphasic with a terminal elimination half-life of about 6 h. Elimination is mainly by renal route.

Dose-limiting toxicity includes myelosuppression, renal failure in high doses, fatigue, lethargy, dermatitis, immunosuppression and abnormal hepatotoxicity.

*Cladribine (2-CDA)* is a synthetic deaminase-resistant purine analog. It is indicated as first line treatment for hairy cell leukemia. It also has activity in acute myelogenous leukemia, chronic lymphocytic leukemia, lymphomas and Waldenstrom's macroglobulinemia [147]. It is readily transported intracellularly, where it is phosphorylated by deoxycytidine kinase. Subsequently, it is incorporated into DNA leading to inhibition of DNA synthesis, DNA breaks, incorporation into DNA, and NAD and ATP depletion [203].

The dose is 3–10 mg/m$^2$ per day for 5 days for children. In adults, the commonly cited dose is 0.09 mg/kg per day for 7 days, or 0.1 mg/kg per day for 5–7 days, administered as a 24-h continuous infusion [147, 204]. However, until recently an optimal dose schedule was not known. Larson et al. [205] have defined a maximally tolerated dose, by daily 1 h infusion for 5 days, of 21.5 mg/m$^2$ in patients with advanced hematological malignancies. Administered orally or subcutaneously, cladribine's bioavailability is 37%–51% or 100% respectively [206]. The plasma disposition profile of cladribine is biphasic. The terminal elimination half-life is between 6 and 20 h [207, 208]. The drug is eliminated mainly by the kidneys. Toxicities associated with this drug include myelosuppression which is dose limiting, nausea, dermatitis, headache, fever and immunosuppression.


Ribonucleotide Reductase Inhibitor

*Hydroxyurea*

Hydroxyurea is used in oncology mainly for the treatment of chronic myelogenous leukemia and acute leukemia with hyperleucocytosis. However, it is also being investigated as a biochemical modulator to increase the efficacy of 5-fluorouracil based regimens [209], as an adjunct to radiation [210, 211], and for modulation of drug resistance mediated by gene amplification. Hydroxyurea exerts it cytotoxic effect by two mechanisms, mainly as an *inhibitor of ribonucleotide reductase*, which results in an arrest of DNA synthesis, and prevention of damaged DNA repair [212]. The cytotoxic effect of the drug is S-phase specific.

Hydroxyurea is also used in the treatment of non-malignant conditions such as sickle cell anemia (recently approved for pediatrics), polycythemia vera, and essential thrombocytosis.

The dose is 20–50 mg/kg for initial treatment of hyperleukocytosis, decreased to 20–30 mg/kg per day for maintenance therapy, or 20–30 mg/kg for treatment of solid tumors. Another dosing scheme is to administer 80 mg/kg once every 3 days. Despite the near complete oral bioavailability of hydroxyurea, the attainable peak concentration, and time to reach peak concentration varies by two- to fourfold between patients; to avert possible interindividual variability in drug absorption, the drug has been administered using different intravenous dosing schedules ranging from 72 to 120 h [213]. Tracewell et al. [214] reported nonlinear kinetics for intravenous doses over 2 g/m$^2$ per day, however this was not observed by Newman et al. using intravenous doses between 1 and 3.2 mg/m$^2$ per day [213]. Nevertheless, the elimination half-life ranges from 3.3 to 5.5 h. About 50% of a given dose is excreted in the urine. Thus dose adjustment is recommended in patients with significant renal impairment.

Myelosuppression is the dose limiting toxicity, and it increases with increasing duration of intravenous administration [213]. An idiopathic megaloblastic anemia is known to occur. Extensive dermatological reactions, which are preventable with premedication with steroids and antihistamine, have been associated with prolonged infusion [213]. However, increased corticosteroid secretion through cytokines has also been observed with hydroxyurea in animal models, and this effect is thought to afford protection to the toxic effects of the drug [215].

Antifolates

*Methotrexate*

Methotrexate is a folic acid analogue that is used extensively in the treatment of a variety of solid tumors. It is a specific inhibitor of the enzyme dihydrofolate reductase (DHFR), which plays a critical role in intracellular folate metabolism [216]. This reaction leads to an increase in the intracellular dihydrofolate pool, and subsequent inhibition of purine and thymidylate synthesis in both malignant and normal cells.

Methotrexate is used as monotherapy or in combination with other antineoplastics in the treatment of leukemia and a variety of solid tumors such as breast cancer, head and neck cancer, small cell lung cancer, bladder cancer, ovarian carcinoma, rhabdomyosarcoma, colon cancer and osteosarcoma [147, 217].

For oncologic therapy, methotrexate is usually administered in high doses intravenously along with leucovorin to minimize toxicity. Three schedules of dosing are available for the use of this drug. The conventional dose of 30–50 mg/m$^2$ is used weekly, intermediate dosing is 50–150 mg/m$^2$ i.v push every 2–3 weeks or 240 mg/m$^2$ infusions followed with leucovorin rescue every 4–7 days or 500–1000 mg/m$^2$ infusions every 2–3 weeks. High dose regimens use 1–18 g/m$^2$ followed with leucovorin rescue every 1–3 weeks. Oral regimens are variable, but may include using 15–20 mg/m$^2$ twice weekly or 15 mg/day for 5 days every 2–3 weeks.

The pharmacokinetics of methotrexate vary significantly depending on the route of administration and the dose. Oral absorption is rapid but unpredictable with bioavailability ranging from 50% to 90% indicating about a fivefold interindividual variability. Absorption after intramuscular and subcutaneous administration is also rapid and complete [218]. Methotrexate is widely distributed in the body. It is approximately 50%

protein bound and elimination from the body is both age and dose dependent [147]. Distribution of MTX is in three phases. The terminal half-life is 3–10 h for low doses, 8–15 h for doses more than 30 mg/m², and up to 55 h in patients with pleural effusion [147, 77, 218].

There are recognized mechanisms for intrinsic and acquired resistance to MTX in human tumors. These mechanisms generally involve increased levels of DHFR due to gene amplification [219], mutant DHFR with reduced affinity for MTX, or decreased uptake or polyglutamylation of the drug [220].

Toxicities arising from the use of MTX include myelosuppression, which tends to be severe in the presence of folate deficiency or impaired renal function. Leucovorin given within 42 h of MTX will decrease the degree of myelotoxicity. Alternatively, carboxypeptidase $G_2$ has been used for rescue after high doses [221]. Other common toxicities are mucositis, elevated hepatic enzymes and renal failure especially with high doses. Renal toxicity is due to the precipitation of the drug and its metabolites in the renal tubules in the presence of an acidic urine and inadequate hydration (urine pH <7, urine output <100 ml/h). Rare toxicities reported with the use of MTX include acute or subacute neurologic disorders, headache, fever, meningismus and encephalopathy with intrathecal administration.

### Other Folate Analogs

To increase the therapeutic potentials of folate analogues, a number of drugs have been developed and are in various stages of clinical trials. Preliminary results indicate comparable or better antitumor activities (see review by Hum and Kamen [222]).

*Edatrexate* is a new folate analog is structurally similar to methotrexate, it inhibits dihydrofolate reductase (DHFR). It has shown promising antitumor activity in combination therapy regimens (especially cyclophosphamide) in a variety of adult solid tumors. The dose limiting toxicity is mucositis, and mild myelosuppression.

*Trimetrexate* is a lipophilic antifolate. Its mechanism of action is similar to MTX, in that it binds tightly to DHFR and inhibits the enzyme. It is approved in the United States for the treatment of Pneumocystis carinii pneumonia. It has shown activity in pediatric patients with refractory solid tumors including brainstem glioma, neuroblastoma and renal cell carcinoma. Its oral bioavailability ranges from 19% to 67% (mean 44%) [223]; thus it has the potential for development as an outpatient therapy. Dose-limiting toxicity is mucositis and mild hepatotoxicity.

*Raltitrexed* is a folate analog. It exerts its cytotoxic action by a direct, specific and non-competitive inhibition of thymidylate synthase [222, 224]. It does not require metabolic conversion for activity. Transport into cells is through the same active transport mechanisms used by folate and methotrexate. Unlike methotrexate, it does not inhibit dihydrofolate reductase enzyme.

In clinical trials it has shown promising antitumor activity in a range of tumor types including breast, pancreatic, non-small cell lung and refractory ovarian cancer [224], this is especially significant in patients with advanced breast and colorectal cancers [225].

Recommended dose in adults is single intravenous injections of 3 mg/m$^2$ every 3 weeks. Dose limiting toxicity is neutropenia. Other adverse effects include nausea, vomiting, diarrhea, transient elevation of liver enzymes and malaise.

## Anthracyclines and Related Intercalators

The anthracyclines are widely regarded as essential anticancer agents in different combination chemotherapy regimens. Their continued success as first-and second-line treatment of metastatic disease has led to their use for adjuvant or neoadjuvant chemotherapy [226]. Despite the significant impact these compounds have made in cancer chemotherapy and their years of usage, the major mechanism(s) contributing to their cytotoxicity in tumor cells remains unclear. What is known is that these compounds can intercalate with DNA thereby preventing DNA and RNA synthesis. Several mechanisms/targets have been suggested to explain observed cytotoxicity including inhibition of DNA topoisomerases [227, 228], generation of toxic free radicals [229], inhibition of helicases, alteration of membrane structure and function and endonucleolytic cleavage [230].

The major toxicity with the use of these compounds is an insidious dose-related cardiotoxicity, the precise mechanism of which is unclear. However, several hypotheses have been put forward foremost of which is that, free radical formation by anthracyclines [231] enhance the susceptibility of cardiac tissue to lipid peroxidation [232] leading to a progressive dose-related irreversible vacuolization and myocyte necrosis in response to the anthracyclines. Recently, a novel mechanism for cardiotoxicity was demonstrated by Bottone et al. [233], indicating that anthracyclines increase the maximal tension in cardiac muscle fibers by direct interaction with the actin-myosin cross-bridges; thus contributing to destruction of the contractile machinery of cardiac muscle.

At present, doxorubicin, daunorubicin, epirubicin, and idarubicin are the anthracyclines commonly used in the clinics (Table 4). These drugs are usually administered intravenously. A rapid distribution phase and a slow elimination phase characterize their plasma disposition profiles. Metabolism is mainly hepatic, with excretion mostly through the bile, implying that care should be taken in their use in patients with hepatic dysfunction [234].

Clinical resistance to the anthracyclines is thought to be through four possible mechanisms including overexpression of MDR1 gene (p-glycoprotein), MDR-associated protein, lung resistance-associated protein (LRP) and tumor variability in the content or activity of topoisomerase II enzyme [226]. The correlation of these attributes to either intracellular drug concentration of anthracyclines or the degree of cytotoxicity is yet to be conclusive.

Toxicities common to the anthracyclines are myelosuppression, mucositis and cardiomyopathy, which is characterized by a gradual loss in contractile force. Mediastinal irradiation or administration of high doses of cyclophosphamide or multiple anthracyclines increases the risk of cardiomyopathy. The total lifetime cumulative dose for doxorubicin is thought to be $450–550$ mg/m$^2$ [235]. Doxorubicin is more cardiotoxic than idarubicin or epirubicin, but daunorubicin might be equi- or less cardiotoxic [236].

## Doxorubicin (Adriamycin)

This is the most widely used anthracycline. It is an analogue of daunorubicin. This drug has a broad spectrum of anticancer activity against leukemias, lymphomas, and solid tumors [236]. It has been used in combination with other agents as adjuvant chemotherapy in the treatment of osteosarcoma, soft tissue sarcoma and breast carcinoma [236, 237].

Dosing schedule will depend on individual protocol. In general, doses used for children are $35–75$ mg/m$^2$ once every 3 weeks or $20–30$ mg/m$^2$ per week or $60–90$ mg/m$^2$ continuous infusion over 96 h. For adults a

**Table 4.** Anthracyclines and related intercalators

| Drugs | Mode of action | Potential uses | Side effects |
|---|---|---|---|
| *Anthracyclines* Doxorubicin | Inhibition of DNA/RNA synthesis, by intercalating DANN | Breast Ca, sarcomas | Cardiotoxicity, mucositis, myelosuppression, nausea, vomiting, alopecia |
| Daunorubicin | Inhibition of DNA synthesis | Acute leukemia, sarcomas, melanoma | Cardiotoxicity, mucositis, nausea, vomiting |
| Epirubicin | Similar to doxorubicin | Breast cancer, bladder Ca | Myelosuppression, cardiotoxicity, nausea, vomiting, mucositis |
| Idarubicin | Same as daunorubicin | acute leukemia | Cardiotoxicity, myelosuppression, nausea, vomiting, mucositis, alopecia |
| *Mitoxantrone* | Inhibition of DNA synthesis by topo II inhibition and intercalating DNA | Acute leukemia, lymphoma | Cardiotoxicity, mucositis, myelosuppression, alopecia |

one-time dose of 60–75 mg/m² every 3 weeks or 20–30 mg/m² per day for 2–3 days every 4 weeks or 20 mg/m² weekly is commonly prescribed. The usual recommended maximum cumulative lifetime dose is 550 mg/m² or 450 mg/m² in patients with prior radiation therapy to the mediastinal areas. Nevertheless, there are ongoing studies attempting to optimize dosing schedules of doxorubicin in different combination chemotherapy regimen [237], or administering doxorubicin in conjunction with car-dioprotective agent dexrazoxane [238].

The plasma disposition profile is multiexponential with terminal eli-mination half-life of 30 h. Renal excretion of the drug is less than 10% of an administered dose [234], but this is usually enough to color the urine red. Acute manifestations of toxicity are myelosuppression, mucositis, alopecia, nausea, vomiting with the major chronic toxicity being car-diomyopathy and acute leukemia.

## Daunorubicin

Daunorubicin is the initial anthracycline that prompted the search for analogues that will have greater antitumor potentials in this class of drugs. The main application of this drug is in combination therapy for the induction regimens of acute nonlymphocytic and acute lymphocytic leukemias. The dose is usually 25–45 mg/m² per day for 3 days in child-ren or 30–60 mg/m² per day for 3–5 days in adults. After an intravenous dose, the drug is rapidly biotransformed to its major metabolite daun-orubicinol. Plasma disposition is biexponential, with terminal half-life of 15–20 h and about 30 h for the parent drug and its main metabolite res-pectively [239, 240].

The dose limiting toxicities are myelosuppression, mucositis, stoma-titis, nausea, and vomiting and cumulative dose-related cardiomyopathy.

## Idarubicin

Idarubicin is an analogue of daunorubicin. It induces a time and con-centration dependent increase in DNA breaks in tumor cells [241, 242]. Use of this drug is mainly in *combination with cytarabine* for the treat-ment of leukemia. It is also used for palliative therapy in patients with breast carcinoma and lymphoma.

Dosing is either intravenous or by oral route; 8–12 mg/m$^2$ per day for 3 days is used for intravenous administration, and 45–60 mg/m$^2$ once every 2–4 weeks is used for oral administration. The pharmacokinetics of idarubicin is similar to that of daunorubicin with terminal half-lives of 15–20 h and 40–60 h for the parent drug and its major metabolite respectively, regardless of the route of administration [243]. Bioavailability of idarubicin ranges between 20% and 30%, however, given the fact that the major metabolite is also active the total bioavailability of the active species is estimated at about 40%–50% [243]. Toxicities associated with this drug are similar to those of the other anthracyclines, however the propensity to cause cardiomyopathy is much less.

*Epirubicin*

Epirubicin is an analogue of doxorubicin. It has a spectrum of antitumor activity similar to doxorubicin. It is among the most active single agents used in the treatment of early and advanced breast cancer [244]. It has also been shown to be an effective prophylactic treatment against superficial bladder cancer [245].

The optimal dosing schedule is still the subject of ongoing clinical trials. Antitumor activity of epirubicin is directly related to the dose of the drug [244]. Compared to doxorubicin much higher doses of epirubicin are required to achieve the same antitumor effects [246]. To enhance its therapeutic effect, several studies have used single infusions every 3 weeks, with MTD at 150–180 mg/m$^2$ [246]. Galvez et al. [247] have reported significant antitumor activity when the drug is used at a dose of 120 mg/m$^2$ intravenously every 21/28 daysx6 cycles, for the treatment of metastatic breast cancer.

Epirubicin is rapidly metabolized to epirubicinol, epirubicinol-glucuronide and aglycones. The major dose limiting adverse effects are myelosuppression and cumulative dose-related cardiomyopathy, however, these effects are less severe when compared to equimolar doses of doxorubicin [244]. Other toxicities include, mucositis, nausea, vomiting and alopecia.

## Mitoxantrone

Mitoxantrone is an anthracenedione with limited cardiotoxicity compared with the anthracyclines. Its exerts its antitumor action by inhibition of topoisomerase II enzyme and by interacting with DNA. It has been used in high doses in combination therapy in the treatment of refractory solid tumors [248]. Mitoxantrone is used mainly in the treatment of acute leukemia, non-Hodgkin's lymphoma and prostate cancer. For palliative therapy, it has been used in patients with a variety of solid tumor types including carcinoma of the breast, liver, head and neck and osteogenic and soft tissue sarcomas.

A dose of 18–20 mg/m$^2$ every 3–4 weeks is used for children and 12 to 14 mg/m$^2$ every 3–4 weeks for adults. Maximum allowable dose is usually 150 mg/m$^2$. The toxicity profile is similar to doxorubicin.

## Dactinomycin (Actinomycin D)

This was the first antibiotic antitumor agent to be used in cancer chemotherapy. It is a very potent antineoplastic agent. Cytotoxicity of this drug is thought to be through two mechanisms. First, it intercalates between adjacent guanine-cytosine base pairs resulting in blockade of DNA transcription by RNA polymerase [249], and the second mechanism involves a possible inhibition of topoisomerase II enzyme through a free radical intermediate [250].

Dactinomycin is an important component of chemotherapy regimen or modalities in the curative treatment of pediatric solid tumors including Ewing's sarcoma, rhabdomyosarcoma and Wilm's tumor [251, 252]. It has shown significant antitumor activity against osteogenic sarcoma, soft tissue sarcomas, Kaposi's sarcoma, choriocarcinoma and germ cell tumors of the ovary and testis. This drug is of limited value in adult oncology.

Usually 10–15 μg/kg per day for 5 days is administered intravenously. This schedule might be repeated every 3–6 weeks if there is no evidence of toxicity, or 0.75–2 mg/m$^2$ once, at intervals of 1–4 weeks. This drug is minimally metabolized in the body. Plasma half-life is about 36 h and it is excreted predominantly through the bile (up to 50%) and urine (up to 10%).

Dose-limiting toxicities are severe myelosuppression, gastrointestinal distress, oral ulcerations, proctitis, alopecia and dermatitis.

## Antimitotic (Anti-Microtubular Drugs)

This class of drugs includes the naturally occurring *vinca* alkaloids including vincristine and vinblastine and their semi-synthetic analogues including vinorelbine, and the *taxanes*, paclitaxel and docetaxel (Table 5). Most of the antimitotics are plant alkaloids.

The microtubules are an essential part of the cytoskeleton of the eukaryotic cells. They are involved in chromosome movement, intracellular transport, and the regulation of cell shape and motility [253, 254]. Microtubules are normally assembled from a pool of heterodimeric ($\alpha/\beta$) globular protein called tubulin. Two processes are involved in the normal mitotic events in the cell; namely polymerization and depolymerization of the mitotic spindle microtubules.

The vinca alkaloids bring about their cytotoxic activities by binding specifically to $\beta$-tubulin subunits, thus blocking the ability of the protein to polymerize into microtubules. On the contrary, the taxanes specifically bind to the ($\beta$-tubulin subunit of microtubules and prevent depolymerization of this key cytoskeletal protein, thus chromosomes are prevented from moving to the metaphase plate, and their correct segregation during anaphase is undermined [255], this leads to an arrest of mitosis. Therefore, both groups of drugs are cell-cycle specific anticancer agents.

Taxanes

*Paclitaxel*

Paclitaxel was the first of the taxanes to be used for cancer treatment. It promotes (inducer) rather than inhibits microtubular formation. This drug is cytotoxic during mitosis (M-phase). As a result drugs that prevent the normal progression of a cell through DNA synthesis and into mitosis, will antagonize the cytotoxic effect of this drug. In addition cytotoxic activity is related to length of exposure.

Paclitaxel has demonstrated significant antitumor activity against a variety of tumor types including breast, non-small cell and small cell lung, head and neck, ovarian [256], bladder [257, 258], cervical [259] and gastric carcinomas [260], as well as lymphoma [261]. There are several ongoing clinical trials attempting to delineate schedules for its optimal

**Table 5.** Antimitotic antineoplastic agents (Antimicrotubular Drugs)

| Drugs | Mode of action | Potential uses | Side effects |
|---|---|---|---|
| *TAXANES* | | | |
| Taxol | Inhibits DNA synthesis by stabilizing microtubule assembly | Ca breast, ovary, cervix, prostate NSCLC, gastric carcinoma, lymphoma | Mucositis, neurotoxicity abdominal pain, alopecia cardiotoxicity, nausea, vomiting, pancreatitis, diarrhea |
| Taxotere | Similar to taxol | Sarcomas, head and neck Ca, ovarian, breast and pancreatic cancer | Pleural effusion, alopecia myalgia, edema, myelosuppression |
| *VINCA ALKALOIDS* | | | |
| Vincristine | Inhibit DNA synthesis by blockade of tubulin assembly | Leukemia, lymphoma, brain tumors, Ca of Breast, lung, liver and multiple myeloma | Peripheral neuropathy, SIADH constipation, alopecia, hepatotoxicity |
| Vinblastine | Similar to vincristine | Prostate carcinoma | Myelosuppression, SIADH, mucositis, nausea, vomiting, alopecia, |

use either as a single agent or in combination with other antineoplastics or treatment modalities.

The basis for clinical drug resistance is not known, however, there are preliminary data suggesting that this phenomenon might be related to the level of HER-2/neu expression in the tumor [262] and/or P-glycoproteins [263].

Paclitaxel is given intravenously. Dosing depends on the cancer type. Usual doses range from 100 to 200 $mg/m^2$ infusions over periods of 3–24 h depending on the protocol. Higher doses might be needed in patients on anticonvulsants [264]. Also, in patients with ovarian cancer, paclitaxel dosages of 100 $mg/m^2$ could be administered safely into the peritoneal cavity [265]. *Pre-medication with antihistamines, steroids and $H_1$ and $H_2$ blockers are recommended to minimize hypersensitivity reactions known to occur with administration of paclitaxel.* Suffice it to say that given the plethora of ongoing clinical trials, modification of dosing schedules will evolve as more anticancer agents or treatment modalities are used in combination with the drug.

Results from various clinical trials suggest substantial interpatient variability in the disposition of the drug, with complex nonlinear pharmacokinetics [266, 267]. Observed terminal elimination half-life ranges from 1.3 to 49.7 h, depending on the dose and dose schedule [256, 264–267]. Hepatic metabolism is by *CYP2C8 and CYP3A*, subsequent biliary excretion probable accounts for the bulk of systemic clearance of an administered dose. Renal clearance is minimal (<10%) [256, 267]. Dose adjustments are required in patients with hepatic impairment [268].

For clinical use, paclitaxel is formulated in 50% dehydrated alcohol and 50% polyethoxylated castor oil (Cremophor EL). This diluent has a tendency to leach the plasticizer diethylhexylphthalate (DEHP) from plastic solution bags and PVC tubings, as such the drug be administered only in glass or polyolefin containers and polyethylene lined, nitroglycerin tubing.

Dose limiting toxicity is leucopenia, mucositis, peripheral neuropathy characterized by numbness and parasthesia, and severe abdominal pain when administered intraperitoneally [265]. Other toxicities include nausea, vomiting, hyperbilirubinemia, headache, cardiac arrhythmia and alopecia. Pulmonary toxicity has also been reported with the use of the drug [269]. In the pediatric population neuropathy was found to be the dose limiting toxicity [270]; other toxicities unique to this age group include hemorrhagic cystitis, diarrhea and pancreatitis.

*Docetaxel*

Doxetaxel is a semisynthetic analogue of paclitaxel. Its mechanism of tumor cell kill and spectrum of clinical activity is similar to that of paclitaxel [271], in that, it acts as a spindle poison by promoting and stabilizing microtubule assembly [272]. However, its cytotoxicity is S-phase specific, as such, it is ineffective during mitosis [273]. Docetaxel has demonstrated significant antitumor activity in patients with anthracycline pretreated metastatic breast cancer, ovarian carcinoma, cancer of the head and neck, and lungs [266].

The usual dose for docetaxel ranges from 60 to 100 mg/m² given as a 1-hour infusion every 3 weeks. It is advisable to administer dexamethasone (8 mg BID) for 5 days, beginning 1 day before treatment to reduce the side effects. Higher doses are being studied in ongoing clinical trials involving pediatric patients [274]. Unlike paclitaxel the disposition of docetaxel is not schedule dependent. It has a linear multi-exponential pharmacokinetic profile, with a terminal half-life of between 11.3 and 13.6 h [275]. The drug undergoes extensive metabolism in the liver mainly by CYP3A isoenzymes. Excretion occurs almost exclusively in the feces via the biliary route [276].

The major dose-limiting toxicity includes a dose dependent myelosuppression with platelet sparing, cutaneous toxicity, edema, pleural effusions, alopecia and severe myalgias especially in pediatric patients.

Dose adjustments are required for patients with febrile neutropenia, hepatic dysfunction or in the presence of severe peripheral neuropathy or cutaneous reactions.

Vinca Alkaloids

The vinca alkaloids are widely used for cancer chemotherapy. Cytotoxicity by these agents is cell-cycle dependent, and unlike the taxanes, they arrest cells at metaphase by blocking the assembly of tubulins [277]. Commonly used vinca alkaloids include vincristine, vinblastine and vinorelbine. There is incomplete cross-resistance between the vinca alkaloids. However, drug resistance to the vinca alkaloids is thought to result from mutations in tubulin subunits that prevent effective binding of the drug to the target site [278], gene amplification [279], and through membrane transporters mediating multidrug resistance [280]. A large volume of distribution and long terminal half-life generally characterize the plasma disposition of vinca alkaloids, and there is significant inter-individual variability in drug handling [281].

## Vincristine

This drug has a potent and selective effect on tumor tissue. It is used widely as an important component of combination chemotherapy regimens for treating childhood and adult leukemias, pediatric solid tumors, Hodgkin's and non-Hodgkin's lymphomas, hepatoblastoma, brain tumors, breast carcinoma, multiple myeloma and small cell lung carcinomas [77].

Vincristine is administered intravenously as a rapid injection at a dose of 1–2 mg/m$^2$ weekly (maximum dose of 2 mg). It is extensively bound to tissue. Vincristine is extensively metabolized by the liver and eliminated via the hepatobiliary system. Renal excretion accounts for less than 15% of a given dose [282]. The plasma disposition is triphasic in both children and adults, with terminal elimination half-life of 23–85 h [281–283].

Major toxicity from vincristine usage is peripheral neuropathy, and constipation associated with abdominal pain. These toxicities are usually reversible when the drug is stopped. Other toxicities include alopecia, SIADH, and rarely ischemic cardiac toxicity.

## Vinblastine

While the pharmacology of this drug parallels those of vincristine, it is used mainly for the treatment of testicular carcinomas and lymphomas. Preliminary data suggest antitumor activity, in combination chemotherapy regimens, for the treatment of hormone refractory prostate carcinoma [284, 285].

The usual dose is 4–20 mg/m$^2$ every 7 days or as a 5 day continuous infusion at 1.4–1.8 mg/m$^2$ per day. The pharmacokinetic profile of vinblastine is same as that of vincristine. Hepatic metabolism is mainly by CYP3A isoenzymes [281]. Toxicities associated with vinblastine are myelosuppression, gastrointestinal distress, syndrome of inappropriate antidiuretic hormone (SIADH), mucositis, alopecia and rarely ischemic cardiotoxicity.

## *Vinorelbine*

Vinorelbine is a semisynthetic analogue of the vinca alkaloids. It is used for the treatment of non-small cell lung cancer and breast cancer. In ongoing clinical trials, it also has demonstrated antitumor activity in combined chemotherapy regimens against ovarian carcinoma, Hodgkin's disease, Kaposi's sarcoma and head and neck cancer [286–289].

The usual dose is 30 mg/m$^2$ intravenously weekly or every 2–3 weeks. The pharmacokinetic profile is the same as the other vinca alkaloids. The major toxicity is myelosuppression. Unlike the other vinca alkaloids neurotoxicity is less frequent.

## Topoisomerase Inhibitors

Topoisomerases are DNA enzymes involved in controlling the topology of supercoiled DNA double helix during cellular functions, namely transcription and replication of cellular genetic materials. There are two classes of topoisomerases, topoisomerase I and II [290] (see Table 6). Drugs, which prevent the functions of these enzymes, are generally referred to as inhibitors, however, a drug might bind to one of these enzymes and prolong the existence of formed DNA cleavages. In such situations, the term topoisomerase poison is increasingly being used, since it is thought to be more descriptive of the molecular action of the drug.

Sabotaging the function of one or both of these enzymes plays an important role in cancer chemotherapy. Camptothecin and its water-soluble derivatives are used to specifically inhibit topoisomerase I [291], whereas the epipodophyllotoxins achieve cytotoxicity by inhibiting topoisomerase II. The topoisomerase I inhibitors approved for clinical use are irinotecan (CPT-11) and topotecan, and the epipodophyllotoxins (topoisomerase II inhibitors) commonly used in the clinics are etoposide and teniposide.

### Topoisomerase I Inhibitors

The topoisomerase I inhibitors prevent the cleavage of a strand of DNA, a process required for the replicative mechanism of the cell, this subsequently results in irreversible DNA replication defect with cell cycle

**Table 6.** Topoisomerase inhibitors

| Drugs | Mechanism of action | Potential uses | Side effects |
|---|---|---|---|
| *Topoisomerase (topo) I inhibitors* | | | |
| Irinotecan (CPT-11) | Inhibition of DNA synthesis by inhibiting topo I enzyme | 5-FU refractory colorectal carcinoma | Diarrhea, myelosuppression |
| Topotecan | Similar to irinotecan | Cisplatin refractory ovarian carcinoma | Granulocytopenia, dermatitis, nausea, vomiting, conjunctivitis |
| *Topoisomerase (topo) II inhibitors* | | | |
| Etoposide (VP-16) | Inhibition of DNA synthesis by inhibiting topo II enzyme | Leukemia, lymphoma, Kaposi's sarcoma, cancer of lung, testis | Myelosuppression, nausea, alopecia, hepatotoxicity, diarrhea, treatment-related leukemia, hypotension |
| Teniposide | Similar to etoposide | Refractory leukemia | Hypotension, nausea, vomiting, alopecia |

arrest and cell death [292]. These drugs are presumed to have significant activity against tumors that express high levels of the topoisomerase I enzyme, however, a critical factor that influences this premise is the length of exposure of the tumor to the drug [292]. Thus the efficacy of these agents is likely going to be schedule dependent.

*Irinotecan (CPT-11)*

This is a semisynthetic analogue of camptothecin. It has significant antitumor activity against 5-FU refractory metastatic colorectal cancer [293]. In clinical trials it has also demonstrated antitumor activity in patients with a variety of solid tumors [293–295]. Irinotecan is approved in the United States for the treatment of refractory metastatic colorectal cancer.

Assigning a dosing schedule to CPT-11 is the subject of several clinical studies, since the dose limiting toxicity is schedule dependent. While the generally accepted dose in the United States is intravenous infusions of 125 mg/m$^2$ weeklyx4 doses, with a two-week rest period between chemotherapy cycles, in Europe 30 min infusion of 350 mg/m$^2$ once every three weeks is used [296]. CPT-11 is metabolized mainly in the liver and to a lesser extent by carboxylesterase in tumor cells, to an active metabolite, 7-ethyl-10-hydroxycamptothecin (SN-38) [297, 298]. The pharmacokinetic profile of CPT-11 is multiexponential with a terminal half-life of 12 h. SN-38 undergoes enterohepatic circulation, and about 17% of CPT-11 dose and only 0.23% of SN-38 are excreted in the urine [299].

The dose limiting toxicity of CPT-11 is myelosuppression, and a dual (early- and late-) phase diarrhea that is directly related to the "biliary index" of its metabolite, SN-38 [300]. SN-38 is normally conjugated by uridine diphosphate glucuronosyl transferase (UGT 1A1) to form the glucuronide, SN-38G [38], and the ratio of SN-38G to SN-38 varies widely among patients [300]. This observation has been noted to have potential clinical implications including that of: the modulation of the biliary excretion of SN-38 with drugs such as cyclosporine A or phenobarbital to increase the therapeutic index of the drug [39, 301], and that interpatient variability in the glucuronidation of the SN-38 may determine the risk of dose-limiting toxicity. Thus patients with a deficiency of UGT 1A1 (as in Gilbert syndrome) or compromised liver function, are hypothesized to be at increased risk of toxicity. For such group of patients, concomitant administration of an inducer of SN-38 conjugation may prove beneficial.

*Topotecan*

Topotecan is a water-soluble semisynthetic analogue of camptothecin. It is approved in the United States for the treatment of cisplatin-refractory ovarian carcinoma. Topotecan has also demonstrated antitumor activity in patients with leukemia, and a variety of solid tumors including adult and pediatric patients with brain tumor [293].

There are ongoing studies trying to identify the optimal dosing schedule for topotecan. It is administered intravenously and orally. The oral bioavailability is 30% $\pm/-7.7\%$ [302]. There is significant interindividual variability in drug handling. The plasma disposition pattern is biexponential, with a terminal half-life of 2–3 h. Elimination appears to be primarily by the renal route [303].

Dose limiting toxicity for topotecan is granulocytopenia. Other adverse effects associated with the use of topotecan include nausea, vomiting, diarrhea, dermatitis, conjunctivitis, peripheral neuropathy, headache and psychiatric symptoms.

Epipodophyllotoxins (as Topoisomerase II Poisons)

Etoposide and teniposide are semisynthetic glycosides of the mandrake plant extract podophyllotoxin. They have demonstrated significant antitumor activity by formation of cleavable complexes with the topoisomerase II enzyme, the target of a number of other antineoplastic agents. Topoisomerase II enzyme mediates the passage of double DNA strands during replication. By forming a ternary complex with the enzyme and DNA, these drugs inhibit the religation of the cleaved DNA strands. The persistence of the topoisomerase II DNA cleavable complexes results in cell cycle arrest and cell death. These drugs demonstrate significant antitumor activity in a variety of cancers including leukemias, Hodgkin's and non-Hodgkin lymphoma, and small cell carcinomas of the lung and testicular tumors.

Over the years considerable evidence have clearly implicated epipodophyllotoxins as a cause of secondary or therapy related myeloid leukemias (t-AML), with a short latent period [304, 305]. The predominant FAB subtypes observed are M4 and M5, and balanced chromosome aberrations involving bands 11q23 and 21q22 are frequently found.

## Etoposide (VP-16–213)

Etoposide is commonly used in oncology. It has been suggested to have synergistic activity with cisplatin [306]. Etoposide has significant activity as a single agent therapy or in combination therapy regimens in the first-line treatment of lung (small cell and non-small cell) cancer, testicular cancer, lymphoma, leukemia, and Kaposi's sarcoma. It continues to be studied in the clinics for the treatment of other malignancies [306].

Given the spectrum and degree of its activity, dosing of etoposide normally depends on the cancer type and existing protocol. In general weekly or twice weekly doses are less effective than treatment regimens given over 3–5 days [306]. There are a number of ongoing clinical trials focusing on prolonged dosing schedules. A pharmacokinetic/pharmacodynamic relationship does exist with infusional dosing [307]. Nevertheless, there are three primary determinants of etoposide disposition and possibly pharmacological effect including elimination (renal), metabolism (hepatic), and protein binding. Thus factors that influence any of these factors would potentially affect the pharmacological response [308].

Oral bioavailability of the drug is very variable. Etoposide is eliminated by both hepatic metabolism and renal excretion, with approximately 40%–60% of an administered dose recovered intact in urine. The plasma disposition of the drug is biphasic with a terminal half-life of 6–8 h in patients with normal renal function [309]. In patients with hepatic and renal dysfunction, creatinine clearance and serum albumin are the best predictors of systemic clearance of the drug [309], thus, dosing adjustment is needed in patients with severe renal insufficiency. Resistance to etoposide is thought to result from decreased intracellular accumulation of etoposide due to efflux from the cell by multidrug resistance (MDR), and/or changes in the amount or activity of topoisomerase II (at-MDR).

The dose limiting toxicity of etoposide is myelosuppression with mild thrombocytopenia. Other toxicities encountered with the use of etoposide include mucositis at very high doses, nausea, vomiting, diarrhea, and transient hypotension with infusion therapy, alopecia and hepatotoxicity.

## Teniposide

Though the mechanism of action of teniposide is the same as etoposide, the use of this drug in the clinic is mainly in combination with cytosine arabinoside for the salvage treatment of refractory leukemia. Notwithstanding, it has significant antitumor activity in patients with Hodgkin's and non-Hodgkin's lymphomas, neuroblastoma, glioma, bladder carcinomas and familial erythrophagocytic lymphohistiocytosis [310, 311].

The dose schedule for teniposide is still evolving, however doses of 50 mg/m$^2$ per day for 5 days or 150–200 mg/m$^2$ per day twice weekly for 4 weeks, is used for leukemia treatment. Teniposide is eliminated primarily by hepatic metabolism; thus its clearance will likely be influenced by the concurrent use of anti-convulsants.

Dose limiting toxicity includes myelosuppression, nausea, vomiting, and hypotension following rapid infusion, alopecia and rarely pulmonary toxicity.

## Miscellaneous Antineoplastics

A sizeable number of compounds are used in cancer chemotherapy to potentiate or modulate the antitumor activity of combined chemotherapy regimens or treatment modalities, yet others are useful in chemoprevention strategies. As more knowledge becomes available about the molecular biology of tumor cells, there is the likelihood that more agents will be used in clinical trials to better the outcome of cancer treatment. While some of these compounds have demonstrated significant antitumor activity as single agents, others antagonize mechanisms that tumor cells need for metastasis or continued growth. This broad category of compounds includes *differentiation agents, angiogenesis inhibitors, interferons and related cytokines, hormones, antisense oligonucleotides and modified genes.*

### Differentiation Agents

The agents that are frequently implied by this class of drugs are mainly derivatives of vitamin A (retinoids). These agents play a critical role in the development and maintenance of normal epithelial tissues. They also play a vital role in cancer chemotherapy by their antiproliferative and cytodifferenting effects on tumor cells towards a normal phenotype. Retinoids have the ability to inhibit malignant transformation and restore normal morphology to metaplastic tissues, for this reason, they have been used as chemopreventive agents [312]. The adverse effects associated with the retinoids are usually headache, pseudotumor cerebri, leucocytosis, hepatotoxicity, respiratory distress, and derangement in lipid metabolism and cardiovascular toxicity.

## Tretinoin (All-trans Retinoic Acid)

Though the main use of this drug is in the treatment of acute promyelocytic leukemia, they have been several studies looking at the antitumor activity of this drug in solid tumors. The results have showed minor activity in gliomas, Kaposi's sarcoma and cervical cancer [313, 314]. The drug is usually given orally using doses of 45–60 mg/m$^2$, however, because of the lack of antitumor activity and observable toxicity in this dose range, there are studies using much higher doses. Bioavailability is incomplete and there is significant interindividual variation in drug handling, the drug is rapidly metabolized and leads to autoinduction of its metabolism through the cytochrome P450 system. The mean elimination half-life is about 36 h [315]. The most common side effect of this agent if headache which occurs a couple of hours after drug ingestion.

## 13-cis Retinoic Acid

This is the most widely studied of the retinoids. Most of the significant antitumor activity of this agent is in combination therapy especially with interferon alpha. There are ongoing clinical studies looking into the chemopreventive and definitive treatment role of this agent [316, 317]. The most common side effects of 13 cis-retinoic acid are mucositis and dry skin.

## Fenretinide

Fenretinide differs from other agents retinols because it does not bind to any retinoid receptor. It has been shown to inhibit carcinogen-induced malignant transformation of mammary cells [318]. In preclinical studies, fenretinide has been shown to be an effective chemopreventive agent against carcinoma of the bladder, oral cavity, prostate and breast [319, 320]. The characteristic side effect of this drug is night blindness, and dosing schedules are normally interrupted for up to 4 days each month to prevent this effect.

### Interferon-Alpha

Interferon alpha originally intended for treatment of viral diseases has been shown to have significant biological activity in a variety of cancers including cancer of the head and neck, bladder cancer, ovarian cancer, cervical carcinoma, colorectal carcinoma, renal cell carcinoma, malignant melanoma, and Kaposi's sarcoma [321]. It is used as first line treatment in hairy cell leukemia, chronic myelogenous leukemia and condylomata acuminata. Though the mechanism of action of the antitumor activity of interferon alpha is unknown, it is inferred to involve a carry-over from the inhibition of protein synthesis, from immunological enhancement, as well as an alteration in the expression of several oncogenes [321]. Interferon can be administered by intravenous, intramuscular or subcutaneous route. Drug absorption from a site of injection is the rate-limiting factor for the elimination of the drug. However, the bioavailability of the drug is approximately 100% irrespective of the route of administration [322]. The drug is metabolized in the kidneys; the plasma half-life ranges from 2.3 to 5.1 h but its biological effects usually lasts up to 7 days.

The use of interferon is associated with a flu-like syndrome, skin rash, nausea, vomiting, dry mouth and mild myelosuppression. Other side effects are peripheral neuropathy, hepatotoxicity and blurred vision.

### Hormones

The discovery that certain tumor types characteristically express significant amounts of hormone receptors has led the use of receptor blockade as a tool to modulate the growth of such tumors. Conversely, the observation that an increase in the physiological levels of some hormones result in a down regulation of receptor expressivity has also led to the use of hormone analogues for the treatment of certain tumor types.

Though these manipulations have met with limited success, overall they have come to be common place in chemoprevention strategies as well as part of curative or palliative treatment regimens of a variety of advanced cancers, especially cancer of the breast and prostate.

*Antiestrogens*

Tamoxifen and Related Analogs

Tamoxifen is a *nonsteriodal antiestrogen*. It is prescribed commonly as first-line therapy for hormonal treatment of disseminated, receptor~positive breast cancer in addition to being used as a chemopreventive in women at high risk of developing breast cancer. Clinical studies using tamoxifen in combination regimens, suggest modest activity of the drug, in the treatment of prostate cancer and platinum~refractory ovarian cancer [323]. The antitumor activity of this drug is attributed mainly to its active metabolite 4-hydroxytamoxifen [323].

Tamoxifen and its metabolite act as competitive inhibitors of estradiol binding to the estrogen receptor. Through binding a conformational change exist in the receptor, thus preventing any binding to estrogen-responsive elements on DNA. The subsequent result is the inhibition of two processes: blockade of the estrogen mediated stimulation of breast carcinoma tumor growth and growth factor-mediated proliferation of the tumor [324]. While this explains an antagonistic effect of the drug, tamoxifen is also known to have agonist effects of the estrogen receptor, and it is this paradox that is thought to be partly responsible for the endometrial proneoplastic effects of the drug [323].

Tamoxifen is usually taken in 10–20 mg doses twice daily. It is readily absorbed and metabolized by *CYP3A isoenzyme*. Thus, the potential exists for significant drug-drug interactions with substrates of this CYP450 isoenzyme. Steady-state levels of the drug are achieved at 4–6 weeks [325].

Common adverse effects associated with tamoxifen include hot flushes, nausea and vomiting, menstrual irregularities, dermatitis, thromboembolic events. Tamoxifen is increasing being implicated as a cause of secondary endometrial carcinoma in patients who have been taking the drug on a chronic basis, and it is also known to cause hepatocellular carcinoma in rats [325, 326].

Notwithstanding, there are known benefits to using tamoxifen including decrease in total serum cholesterol, low circulating-LDL which potentially decrease the risk of myocardial infarction and decrease in the rate of development of osteoporosis.

Based on the known pharmacology of this drug, there are a number of antiestrogen compounds that are being developed. Preliminary data show that while these compounds have a high affinity for the estrogen receptor and less estrogenic properties on the uterus, their antitumor activities are inferior to tamoxifen [327]. While some of these agents are developed for the treatment of breast cancer (*clorotamoxifen, 3-hydroxytamoxifen*) a specific estrogen receptor modulator (SERM) *raloxifene* is being developed for the treatment of osteoporosis.

## Adrenocorticosteroids

The adrenocorticosteroids are used extensively in cancer chemotherapy in three major situations, in the treatment of pediatric acute leukemias and malignant lymphomas, in conjunction with radiation therapy to control symptoms of brain edema in brain tumors, and for the secondary hematological or respiratory complications of lymphomas and chronic leukemia. The cytotoxicity of glucocorticoids is thought to be via inhibition of mitosis in lymphocytes, and induction of apoptosis mediated through transcription interference [328, 329].

The drugs included in this class of compounds are hydrocortisone, dexamethasone, prednisone, prednisolone, methylprednisone and cortisone acetate. Of these agents, dexamethasone is used commonly in conjunction with radiation therapy to reduce the effect of secondary edema in critical areas like the central nervous system. The discontinuation of glucocorticoid therapy requires a gradual tapering of the dose.

## Antiandrogens

The use of this modality of treatment is considered one of the safest forms of cancer chemotherapy. It is mainly for the palliative treatment of metastatic prostate cancer. These agents produce their effect by competitive inhibition of nuclear binding of androgens to the cytosolic DHT receptors. The drugs that are currently approved for use are flutamide and bicalutamide.

*Flutamide* is normally used in combination with GNRH analogues or finasteride, in doses of 250 mg three times daily. It is well absorbed orally. The major side effect is abdominal discomfort and anemia.

*Bicalutamide* is a nonsteroidal antiandrogen, which appears to have fewer side effects than flutamide [330]. It is administered once a day because of its long half-life [331].

## Aromatase Inhibitors

Aromatase inhibitors are unique in their mechanism of action. They act in the early cascade of adrenal steroidogenesis by inhibiting the conversion of cholesterol to pregnenolone, affecting the initial step in synthesis of cortisol, aldosterone and androgens. These drugs are used in the palliative treatment of advanced prostate and estrogen receptor-positive breast carcinomas.

*Aminoglutethimide* is the prototype aromatase inhibitor. The major indication is as second or third line treatment of estrogen-receptor positive advanced breast carcinoma. It has also been used in the treatment of adrenocortical carcinoma. Aminoglutethimide is usually administered orally at a dose of 250 mg four times daily. The associated side effects are blurring of vision, lethargy, drowsiness and gait disturbances.

*Anastrozole* is a new third generation aromatase inhibitor. Clinical studies suggest significant antitumor activity in patients with advanced breast cancer [332], the disease stage for which it is approved. Its mechanism of action parallels that of aminoglutethimide. It is not associated with weight gain or thromboembolic events.

*Letrozole* is also a third generation aromatase inhibitor approved for use in advanced breast cancer in postmenopausal women. Usual dose is 2.5 mg once daily. Side effects are mild hot flashes, nausea and diarrhea.

## *Other Hormonal Agents*

There are other hormonal agents used in cancer chemotherapy that are of interest to the oncologist. These include:

*Estrogens*, which in physiological doses have beneficial effects in patients with metastatic prostate and breast cancer. The side effects associated with its use are gastrointestinal distress, tender gynecomastia, fluid retention, menstrual irregularities and hyperpigmentation of skin folds. Included in this group of drugs are: *diethylstilbestrol, estradiol, conjugated estrogen and esterified estrogens.*

*Progestins* are used in the treatment of cancer of the endometrium, ovary, prostate and breast, as well as hot flashes in survivors of breast cancer [333–337], prostate cancer and ovarian cancer. Side effects are feminization and weight gain. The commonly used progestins include *megestrol acetate, hydroxyprogesterone coproate and medroxyprogesterone acetate.*

*LHRH analogues (GNRH)* are used for medical castration. They are used mainly in patients with advanced prostate cancer. Side effects are hot flushes, decrease libido and impotence. LHRH analogues are *leuprolide acetate and goserelin acetate.*

## Enzymes

### L-Asparaginase

L-asparaginase is used in the induction chemotherapy regimen for acute lymphoblastic leukemia. Its cytolytic effect is through the depletion of L-asparagine in tumor cells, which leads to rapid inhibition of protein synthesis, and cell death. Because sensitive tumor cells lack asparagine synthetase, they cannot regenerate L-asparagine after depletion, however, the resistant tumor cells which normally have asparagine synthetase do regenerate L-asparagine. The antileukemic effect of the drug is schedule dependent, thus when administered with a drug such as methotrexate, synergistic cytotoxicity results only when methotrexate precedes L-asparaginase.

Administration is usually by intramuscular injection using a dose of 6000 IU/m$^2$ every other day for 3–4 weeks. However it can also be given intravenously. The elimination half-life varies from 8 to 30 h for iv dosing to up to a week for PEG L-asparaginase. Bioavailability after intramuscular administration is between 10 and 50% [338].

Adverse effects associated with use are associated with hypersensitivity reactions to the drug. Other side effects are secondary to inhibition of protein synthesis in normal tissues such hyperglycemia due to insulin deficiency, hepatotoxicity, and thrombotic events affecting the central nervous system and other hemorrhagic complications due to reduction in hemostatic and clotting factors [339] (including fibrinogen, factors IX, XI, AT III, protein C and S). The drug can also result in direct neurotoxicity.

## Bleomycin

Bleomycins are a group of related *antibiotic antitumor* agents. The commonly used drug in this family is a combination of the two copper-chelating peptides, bleomycin $A_2$ and $B_2$. The cytotoxic action of bleomycin results from single strand scission of DNA [340]. Given the unique mechanism of action and the lack of overlapping toxicity with other chemotherapy agents, bleomycin is commonly used in combination chemotherapy. Though this drug has cell-cycle specific cytocidal effects, it is not clear if this action is phase specific [340].

Bleomycin has significant antitumor activity against germ cell tumors of the testis and ovary, Hodgkin's disease and non-Hodgkin's lymphoma. The most common use of this drug is in combination therapy for the treatment of lymphomas. This drug is also a radiosensitizer.

Bleomycin is one of a few anticancer agents that can be administered using a variety of routes including intravenous, intramuscular, subcutaneous or locoregional (bladder, pleural, peritoneal or pericardial), and yet achieve antitumor effects. The recommended dose is 10–20/U/m² once or twice a week as single agent therapy. Dose modifications are required in combination therapy regimens. Maximum cumulative lifetime dose should not exceed 400/U and total doses exceeding 250/U should be administered with caution to minimize pulmonary toxicity. Bleomycin is rapidly metabolized by hydrolase. Depending on a patient's renal function status, the terminal half-life ranges from 9 h in a patient with normal renal function to 30 h in patients with renal failure [341].

The most serious toxicity encountered with bleomycin use is pulmonary toxicity, which could progress to pulmonary fibrosis. Other toxicities include fever chills, urticaria anaphylaxis/anaphylactoid reactions, flushing of the face, cutaneous toxicity, Raynaud's phenomenon and coronary artery disease, hyperthermia, and nausea and vomiting.

# References

1. Chabner BA (1990) Clinical strategies for cancer treatment: the role of drugs. In: Chabner BA, Collins JM (eds) Cancer Chemotherapy. Principles and Practice. Philadelphia: JB Lippincott, pp 1–15
2. Henderson EH, Samaha RJ (1969) Evidence that drugs in multiple combinations have materially advanced the treatment of human malignancies. Cancer Res 29:2272–2280
3. Erlichman C, Fine S, Wong A et al (1988) A randomized trial of fluorouracil and folinic acid in patients with metastatic colorectal carcinoma. J Clin Oncol 6:469–475
4. Hryniuk WM, Bush H (1984) The importance of dose intensity in chemotherapy of metastatic breast cancer. J Clin Oncol 2:1281–1288
5. Frei E III, Canellos G (1980) Dose: a critical factor in cancer chemotherapy. Am J Med 69:585–594
6. Hryniuk WA, Figueredo A, Goodyear M (1987) Applications of dose intensity to problems in chemotherapy of breast and colorectal cancer. Semin Oncol 14 (Suppl 4):3–11
7. Ayash L, Elias A, Ibrahim J et al (1997) High-dose multimodality therapy with autologous stem cell support for stage IIIB breast cancer: the DFC/BIH experience. Proc Am Soc Clin Oncol 16:90
8. Smith MA, Ungerleider RS, Horowitz ME et al (1991) Influence of doxorubicin dose intensity on response and outcome for patients with osteogenic sarcoma and Ewing's sarcoma. J Natl Cancer Inst 83:1460–1470
9. Cheung N-KV, Heller G (1991) Chemotherapy dose intensity correlates strongly with response, median survival, and median progression-free survival in metastatic neuroblastoma. J Clin Oncol 9:1050–1058
10. Howell SB (1988) Intraperitoneal chemotherapy for ovarian carcinoma. J Clin Oncol 6:1673–1675
11. Savarese DMF, Hsieh C, Stewart FM (1997) Clinical Impact of Chemotherapy Dose Escalation in Patients With Hematologic Malignancies and Solid Tumors. J Clin Oncol 15:2981–2995
12. Wrigley E, Weaver A, Jayson G et al (1996) A randomized trial investigating the dose intensity of primary chemotherapy in patients with ovarian carcinoma: a comparison of chemotherapy given every four weeks with the same chemotherapy given at three week intervals Ann Oncol 7:705–711
13. Wittes RE (1986) Adjuvant chemotherapy – clinical trials and laboratory models. Cancer treat Rep 70:87–103
14. Martin DS (1981) The scientific basis for adjuvant chemotherapy. Cancer Treat Rev. 8:169–189
15. Berg SL, Grisell DL, DeLaney TF et al (1991) Principles of treatment of pediatric solid tumors. Pediatr Clin North Am 38:249–267
16. Goldie JH, Coldman AJ (1986) Theoretical considerations regarding the early use of adjuvant chemotherapy. Recent Results Cancer Res;103:30–35
17. Early Breast Cancer Trialists' Collaborative Group (1988). Effects of adjuvant tamoxifen and of cytotoxic therapy on mortality in early breast cancer. N Engl J Med 319:1681–1692
18. Weiss GR, Coltman CA (1990) Conference summary overview. In: Salmon SE (ed). Adjuvant therapy of cancer VI. Philadelphia: WB Saunders. pp 623–629
19. Moertel CG, Fleming TR, Macdonald JS et al (1990) Levamisole and fluorouracil for adjuvant therapy of resected colon carcinoma. N Engl J Med 322:352–358
20. O'Connell MJ, Gunderson LL, Fleming TR (1988) Surgical adjuvant therapy of rectal cancer. Semin Oncol 15:138–145

21. Gilewski T, Bitran JD (1996) Adjuvant Chemotherapy. In: Perry MC (ed). The Chemotherapy Source Book. Williams & Wilkins, Baltimore, MD. pp 79–100

22. Ragaz J, Baird R, Rebbeck P et al (1997) Preoperative (neoadjuvant-PRE) versus postoperative (POST) adjuvant chemotherapy (CT) for stage I-II breast cancer (SI-II BC). Long term analysis of British Columbia randomized trial. Proc Am Soc Clin Oncol 16:142

23. Belani CP, Luketich J, Landreneau RJ et al (1997) Efficacy of paclitaxel, 5-fluorouracil and cisplatin (PFT) regimen for carcinoma of the esophagus. Proc Am Soc Clin Oncol 16:283

24. Wanebo HJ, Chougule P, Akerley W et al (1997) Preoperative paclitaxel, carboplatin and radiation in advanced head and neck cancer (stage III and IV) induces a high rate of complete pathologic response (CR) at the primary site and high rate of organ preservation. Proc Am Soc Clin Oncol 16:391

25. Balis FM, Holcenberg JS, Poplack DG (1997) General Principles of Chemotherapy In: Pizzo PA, Poplack DG (eds). Principles and Practice of Pediatric Oncology. Lippincott-Raven Publishers. Philadelphia. pp 215–272

26. Miller AA, Ratain MJ, Schilsky RL (1996) Principles of Pharmacology. In: Perry MC (ed). The Chemotherapy Source Book. Williams & Wilkins, Baltimore, MD. pp 27–41

27. Kohn KW, Jackman J, O'Connor PM (1994) Cell cycle control and cancer chemotherapy. J Cell Biochem 54:440–452

28. O'Connor PM, Kohn KW (1992) A fundamental role for cell cycle regulation in the chemosensitivity of cancer cells?. Semin Cancer Biol 3:409–416

29. Calvert AH, Newell DR, Grumbell LA et al (1989) Carboplatin dosage: prospective evaluation of a simple formula based on renal function. J Clin Oncol. 7:1748–56

30. Chatelut E, Canal P, Brunner V et al (1995) Prediction of carboplatin clearance from standard morphological and biological patient characteristics. J Natl Cancer Inst. 87:573–580

31. Ratain MJ, Schilsky RL, Conley BA et al (1990) Pharmacodynamics in cancer therapy. J Clin Oncol 8:1739–1753

32. Cockcroft DW, Gault MN (1976) Prediction of clearance from serum creatinine. Nephron 16:31–41

33. Borsi JD, Moe PJ (1987) Prognostic importance of systemic clearance of methotrexate in childhood. Cancer Chemother. Pharmacol. 19:261–264

34. Lind MJ, Margison JM, Cerny T et al (1989) Prolongation of ifosfamide elimination half-life in obese patients due to altered drug distribution. Cancer Chemother. Pharmacol. 25:139–42

35. Freyer G, Ligneua B, Tranchand B et al (1997) Pharmacokinetic studies in cancer chemotherapy: Usefulness in clinical practice. Cancer Treat Rev. 23:153–169

36. Krynetski EY, Tai HL, Yates CR et al (1996) Genetic polymorphism of thiopurine S-methyltransferase: clinical importance and molecular mechanisms. Pharmacogenetics 6:279–290

37. Wei X, μleod HL, McMurrough J et al (1996) Molecular basis of human dihydropyrimidine dehydrogenase deficiency and 5-fluorouracil toxicity. J Clin Invest 93:610–615

38. Lalitha I, King CD, Whitington PF et al (1998) Genetic Predisposition to the Metabolism of Irinotecan (CPT-11) Role of Uridine Diphosphate Glucuronosyltransferase Isoform 1A1 in the Glucuronidation of its Active Metabolite (SN-38) in Human Liver Microsomes. J Clin Invest 101:847–854

39. Gupta E, Safa AR, Wangxet al (1996) Pharmacokinetic modulation of irinotecan and metabolites by cyclosporin A. Cancer Res 56:1309–1314

40. Goldie JH, Coldman AJ (1984) The genetic origin of drug resistance in neoplasms: implications for systemic therapy. Cancer Res;44:3643–3653

41. Ling V (1997) Multidrug resistance: molecular mechanisms and clinical relevance. Cancer Chemother Pharmacol 40 (supp l):S3-S8

42. Chan HSL, Thorner P, Haddad G et al (1990) Immunohistochemical detection of P-glycoprotein: prognostic correlation in soft tissue sarcoma of childhood. J Clin Oncol 8:689-704

43. Chan HSL, Haddad G, Thorner PS et al (1991) P-glycoprotein as a predictor of the outcome of therapy for neuroblastoma. N Engl J Med 325:1608-1614

44. Durie BGM, Dalton WS (1988) Reversal of drug resistance in multiple myeloma with verapamil. Br J Hematol 68:203-206

45. Dalton WS, Grogan TM, Meltzer PS et al (1989) Drug resistance in multiple myeloma and non-Hodgkin's lymphoma: Detection of P-glycoprotein and potential circumvention by addition of verapamil to chemotherapy. J Clin Oncol 7:415-424

46. Ozols RF, Cunnion RE, Klecker RW et al (1987) Verapamil and Adriamycin in the treatment of drug-resistant ovarian cancer patients. J Clin Oncol;5:641-647

47. Hall AG, Tilby MJ (1992) Mechanisms of action of, and modes of resistance to, alkylating agents used in the treatment of hematological malignancies. Blood Rev 6:163-173

48. Bruce WR, Meeker BE, Valeriote FA (1966) Comparison of the sensitivity of normal hematopoietic and transplanted lymphoma colony-forming cells to chemotherapeutic agents administered in vivo. J Natl Cancer Inst. 37, 233-245

49. Garcia ST, McQuillan, A, Panasci l (1988) Correlation between the cytotoxicity of melphalan and DNA crosslinks as detected by the ethidium bromide fluorescence assay in the F1 variant of B16 melanoma cells. Biochem Pharmacol 37:3189-3192

50. Pedersen-Bjergaard J, Ersb? II J, S?rensen HM et al (1985) Risk of acute nonlymphocytic leukemia and preleukemia in patients treated with cyclophosphamide for non-Hodgkin's lymphoma. Comparison with results obtained in patients treated for Hodgkin's disease and ovarian carcinoma with other alkylating agents. Ann Intern Med 103:195-200

51. Calsou P, Salles B (1993) Role of DNA repair in the mechanisms of cell resistance to alkylating agents and cisplatin. Cancer Chemother Pharmacol 32:85-89

52. Hare CB, Elion GB, Colvin OM et al (1997) Characterization of the mechanisms of busulfan resistance in a human glioblastoma multiforme xenograft. Cancer Chemother Pharmacol 40:409-414

53. Friedman HS, Skapek SX, Colvin OM et al (1988) Melphalan transport, glutathione levels, and gluthatione-S-transferase activity in human medulloblastoma. Cancer Res 48:5397-5402

54. Colvin OM, Friedman HS, Gamcsik MP et al (1993) Role of gluthatione in cellular resistance to alkylating agents. Adv Enzyme Regul 33:19-26

55. Ahmad S, Okine L, Le B et al (1987) Elevation of gluthatione in phenylalanine mustard-resistant murine L1210 leukemia cells. J Biol Chem 262:15048-15053

56. Robson CN, Lewis AD, Wolf CR et al (1987) Reduced levels of drug-induced DNA cross-linking in nitrogen mustard-resistant Chinese hamster ovary cells expressing elevated gluthatione-S-transferase activity. Cancer Res 47:6022-6027

57. Goldberg GJ, Moore MJ (1997) Nitrogen mustards. In: Teicher B (ed) Cancer Therapeutics: Experimental and Clinical Agents Humana Press Inc., Totowa, NJ. pp 3-22

58. Chang TKH, Weber GF, Crespi CL et al (1993) Differential activation of cyclophosphamide and ifosphamide by cytochromes P-450 2B and 3 A in human liver microsomes. Cancer Res. 53:5629-5637

59. Colvin M (1981) Cyclophosphamide and analogues. In: Crooke ST, Prestayko AW (eds). Cancer and Chemotherapy, vol. III. New York: Academic. pp 25-36

60. Wright JE (1997) Phosphoramide and Oxazaphosphorine Mustards. In: Teicher B (ed) Cancer Therapeutics: Experimental and Clinical Agents Humana Press Inc. Totowa, NJ. pp 23–80

61. Chen TL, Passos-Coelho JL, Noe DA et al (1995) Non-linear pharmacokinetics of cyclophosphamide in patients with metastatic breast cancer receiving high-dose chemotherapy followed by autologous bone marrow transplantation. Cancer Res 55:810–817

62. Grochow LB (1996) Covalent DNA-Binding Drugs. In: Perry MC (ed). The Chemotherapy Source Book. Williams & Wilkins, Baltimore, MD. pp 293–316

63. Dechant KL, Brogden RN, Pilkington T et al (1991) Ifosfamide/Mesna. A review of its antineoplastic activity, pharmacokinetic properties and therapeutic efficacy in cancer. Drugs 42:428–467

64. Kaiser GP, Beijnen JH, Bult A et al (1994) Ifosfamide metabolism and pharmacokinetics (review). Anticancer Res 14:517–532

65. Kupfer A, Aeschlimann C, Wermuth B et al (1994) Prophylaxis and reversal of ifosfamide encephalopathy with methylene-blue. Lancet 343:763–764

66. Goldenberg GJ, Lee M, Lam HYP et al (1977) Evidence for carrier-mediated transport of melphalan by L5178Y lymphoblasts in vitro. Cancer Res 37:755–760

67. Dulik DL, Fenselau C (1987) Conversion of melphalan to 4- (glutathionyl)phenylalanine: a novel mechanism for conjugation by glutathione-S-transferases. Drug Metab Dispos 15:195–199

68. Samuels BL, Bitran JD (1995) High-dose intravenous melphalan: a review. J Clin Oncol 13:1786–99

69. Nagura E, Ichikawa A, Kamiya O et al (1997) A randomized study comparing VMCP and MMPP in the treatment of multiple myeloma. Cancer Chemother Pharmacol 39:279–285

70. Cunningham D, Paz-Ares L, Milan S et al (1994) High dose melphalan and autologous bone marrow transplantation as consolidation in previously untreated myeloma. J Clin Oncol 12:759–763

71. Gouyette A, Hartman O, Pico JL (1986) Pharmacokinetics of high dose melphalan in children and adults. Cancer Chemother Pharmacol. 16:184–189 72 Ardiet C, Tranchand B, Biron P et al (1986) Pharmacokinetics of high dose intravenous melphalan in children and adults with forced diuresis: report in 26 cases. Cancer Chemother Pharmacol 16:300–305

73. Bengala C, Tibaldi C, Pazzagli I et al (1997) High-dose (HD) thiotepa and melphalan (L-PAM) with hemopoietic progenitor support as consolidation treatment following paclitaxel (TXL)-containing chemotherapy in metastatic breast cancer (MBC): a phase II study with pharmacokinetic profile analysis. Proc Am Soc Clin Oncol 16:98

74. Alberts DS, Chang SY, Chen HSG et al (1979) Kinetics of intravenous melphalan. Clin. Pharmacol. Ther. 26:73–80

75. Begleiter A, Goldenberg GJ (1983) Uptake and decomposition of chlorambucil by L5178Y lymphoblasts in vitro. Biochem Pharm 32:535–539

76. Alberts DS, Chang SY, Chen HSG et al (1980) Comparative pharmacokinetics of chlorambucil and melphalan in man. Recent Results in Cancer Research 74:124–127

77. Marmour D, Grob-Menendez F, Duyck F et al (1992) Very late return of spermatogenesis after chlorambucil therapy: case reports. Fertility and Sterility. 58:845–46

78. Wong E, Holden CA, Broadbent V et al (1986) Histiocytosisxpresenting as intertrigo and responding to topical nitrogen mustard. Clin Exp Dermatol 11:183–187

79. Chabner BA, Allegra CJ, Curt GA et al (1996) Antineoplastic Agents In: Hardman GH, Gilman AG, Limbird LE (eds). Goodman and Gilman's The Pharmacological Basis of Therapeutics. The μgraw-Hill Co Inc. New York, NY.pp1233–1287

80. Bradley MO, Sharkey NA, Kohn KW (1980) Mutagenicity and cytotoxicity of various nitrosoureas in V-79 Chinese hamster cells. Cancer Res 40:2719–2725

81. Mitchell EP, Schein PS (1986) Contributions of Nitrosoureas to Cancer Treatment. Cancer Treat Rep. 70:31–41

82. Dolan ME, Roy SK, Fasanmade AA et al (1998) O⁶-Benzylguanine in Man: Metabolic, Pharmacokinetic and Pharmacodynamic Findings. J Clin Oncol (*in press*)

83. Egyhazi S, Edgren MR, Hansson J et al (1997) Role of O⁶-Methylguanine- DNA Methyltransferase, Glutathione Transferase M3–3 and Glutathione in Resistance to Carmustine in a Human Non-small Cell Lung Cancer Cell Line. Eur. J Cancer 33:447–452

84. Burger PC, Kamenar E, Schold SC et al (1981) Encephalopathy following high-dose BCNU therapy. Cancer 48:1318–1327

85. Lind MJ, Ardiet C (1993) Pharmacokinetics of alkylating agents. Cancer surveys 17:157–188

86. Levin VA, Hoffman W, Weinkam RJ (1978) Pharmacokinetics of BCNU in man: preliminary study of 20 patients. Cancer Treat Rep 62:1305–1312

87. Kornblith P, Walker M (1988) Chemotherapy for malignant gliomas. J Neurosurg 68:1–17

88. Sipos EP, Tyler B, Piantadosi S et al (1997) Optimizing interstitial delivery of BCNU from controlled release polymers for the treatment of brain tumors. Cancer Chemother Pharmacol 39:383–389

89. Sponzo RW, DeVita VT, Oliverio VT (1973) Physiologic disposition of 1-(2- chloroethyl)-3-cyclohexyl-1-nitrosourea (CCNU) and 1-(2-chloroethyl)-3-(4-methylcyclohexyl)-1-nitrosourea (MeCCNU) in man. Cancer 31:1154–1156

90. Kastrissios H, Chao NJ, Blaschke TF (1996) Pharmacokinetics of high-dose oral CCNU in bone marrow transplant patients Cancer Chemother Pharmacol 38:425–430

91. Iliadis A, Launay-Iliadis M-C, Lucas C et al (1996) Pharmacokinetics and Pharmacodynamics of Nitrosourea Fotemustine: A French Cancer Centre Multicentric Study. Eur J Cancer 32 A (3):455–460

92. Leyvraz S, Spataro V, Bauer J et al (1997) Treatment of Ocular Melanoma Metastatic to the Liver by Hepatic Arterial Chemotherapy. J Clin Oncol 15:2589–2595

93. Jacquillat C, Khayat D, Banzet P et al (1990) Final report of a french multicenter Phase II study of nitrosourea fotemustine in 153 evaluable patients with disseminated malignant melanoma including patients with cerebral metastases. Cancer 66:1873–1878

94. Frenay M, Giroux B, Khoury S et al (1991) Phase II study of fotemustine in recurrent supra-tentorial malignant gliomas. Eur J cancer 27:852–856

95. Cotto C, Berille J, Souquet PJ et al (1996) A Phase II Trial of Fotemustine and Cisplatin in Central Nervous System Metastases From Non-small Cell Lung Cancer. Eur J Cancer 32 A (1):69–71

96. Hayes MT, Bartley J, Parsons PG et al. (1997) Mechanism of Action of Fotemustine, a New Chloroethylnitrosourea Anticancer Agent: Evidence for the Formation of Two DNA-Reactive Intermediates Contributing to Cytotoxicity. Biochemistry, 36:10646–10654

97. Tranchard B, Lucas C, Biron P et al (1993) Phase I pharmacokinetics study of high-dose fotemustine and its metabolite 2-chloroethanol in patients with high-grade gliomas. Cancer Chemother Pharmacol 32:46–52

98. Marathi UK, Kroes RA, Dolan ME et al (1993) Prolonged depletion of $O^6$- Methylguanine-DNA Methyltransferase Activity following Exposure to $O^6$-Benzylguanine with or without Streptozocin Enhances 1,3-Bis (2-chloroethyl)-1-nitrosourea Sensitivity in Vitro. Cancer Res 53:4281–4286

99. Wilson JKV, Haag JR, Trey JE et al (1995) Modulation of $O^6$-Alkylguanine Alkyltransferase Directed DNA Repair in Metastatic Colon Cancers. J Clin Oncol 13:2301–2308

100. Schein P, Kahn R, Gorden P et al (1973) Streptozocin for malignant insulinomas and carcinoid tumor. Arch Intern Med 132:555–561

101. Adolphe AB, Glasofer ED, Troetel WM et al (1977) Preliminary pharmacokinetics of streptozocin, an antineoplastic antibiotic. J Clin Pharmacol 17:379–388

102. Masters JRW, McDermott BJ, Harland S et al (1996) ThioTEPA pharmacokinetics during intravesical chemotherapy: the influence of dose and volume of instillate on systemic uptake and dose rate to the tumor. Cancer Chemother Pharmacol 38:59–64

103. Bilgrami SA, Tutschka PJ, Tuck D et al (1997) Busulfan, thiotepa, and carboplatin followed by autologous stem cell rescue in metastatic carcinoma of the breast. Proc Am Soc Clin Oncol 16:99

104. Smith A, Rosenfeld S, Dropcho W et al (1997) High-dose thiotepa with hematopoietic reconstitution for recurrent aggressive oligodendroglioma. Proc Am Soc Clin Oncol 16:409

105. Hawkins D, Sanders J, Bensinger W et al (1997) Busulfan, melphalan, and thiotepa (MuBelTt) (total marrow irradiation (TM) with hematopoietic stem cells (HSC) for Ewing's sarcoma family tumors (ES). Proc Am Soc Clin Oncol 16:522

106. Cairncross G, Swinnen L, Stiff P et al (1997) High-dose thiotepa with hematopoietic reconstitution (deferring radiation) for newly diagnosed aggressive oligodendroglioma. Proc Am Soc Clin Oncol 16:388

107. Goto S, Takeshita A, Sactome T et al (1997) Total body irradiation (TBI), VP-16, and thiotepa as a preparative regimen for autologous peripheral stem cell transplantation (PBSCT) in adult poor prognosis non-Hodgkin's lymphoma (NHL): a preliminary report. Proc Am Soc Clin Oncol 16:122

108. Fischer PG, Kadan-Lottick, Korones DN (1997) Treatment of pediatric leptomeningeal metastases with intrathecal thiotepa: a retrospective clinical study. Proc Am Soc Clin Oncol 16:523

109. Cohen BE, Egorin MJ, Kohlhepp EA et al (1986) Human-plasma pharmacokinetics and urinary-excretion of thiotepa and its metabolites. Cancer Treat Rep 70:859–864

110. Ackland SP, Choi KE, Ratain MJ et al (1988) Human-plasma pharmacokinetics of thiotepa following administration of high-dose thiotepa and cyclophosphamide. J Clin Oncol 6:1192–1196

111. Manetta A, Tewari K, Podczaski ES (1997) Hexamethylamine as a Single Second-Line Agent in Ovarian Cancer: Follow-up Report and Review of the Literature. Gynecol Oncol 66:20–26

112. D'Incalci M, Bolis G, Mangoni C et al (1978) Variable oral absorption of hexamethylmelamine in man. Cancer Treat Rep. 62:2117–2119

113. Wingard JR, Plotnick LP, Freemer CS (1992) Growth in children after bone marrow transplantation; busulfan plus cyclophosphamide versus cyclophosphamide plus total body irradiation. Blood 79:1068–1073

114. Vassal G, Koscielny S, Challine D et al (1996) Busulfan disposition and hepatic veno-occlusive disease in children undergoing bone marrow transplantation. Cancer Chemother Pharmacol 37:247–253

115. Jones RJ, Grochow LB (1995) Pharmacology of Bone Marrow Transplantation Conditioning Regimens. Annals NY Acad Sci 770:237–241
116. Meresse V, Hartman O, Vassal G et al (1992) Risk factors for hepatic veno- occlusive disease after high-dose busulfan-containing regimens followed by autologous bone marrow transplantation: a study in 136 children. Bone Marrow Transplant 10:135–141
117. Grochow LB, Jones RJ, Brundrett RB et al (1989) Pharmacokinetics of busulfan: correlation with veno-occlusive disease in patients undergoing bone marrow transplantation. Cancer Chemother Pharmacol 25:55–61
118. Stevens MFG, Hickman JA, Langdon SP et al (1987) Antitumor activity and pharmacokinetics in mice of 8-carbomyl-3-methyl-imidazo [5, 1-d]-1, 2, 3, 5 terazin-4 (3H)-one (CCRG 81045;M&B 39831), a novel drug with potential as an alternative to dacarbazine. Cancer Res 47:5846–5852
119. Newlands ES, Stevens MFG, Wedge SR et al (1997) Temozolomide: a review of its discovery, chemical properties, pre-clinical development and clinical trials. Cancer Treat Rev 23:35–61
120. Newlands ES, O'Reilly SM, Glaser MG et al (1996) The Charing Cross Hospital Experience with Temozolomide in Patients with Gliomas. Eur J Cancer 32 A:2236–2241
121. Bleehen NM, Newlands ES, Lee SM et al (1995) Cancer Research Campaign Phase II trial of temozolomide in metastatic melanoma. J Clin Oncol 13:910–913
122. Baer JC, Freeman AA, Newlands ES et al (1993) Depletion of $O^6$- alkylguanine-DNA alkyltransferase correlates with potentiation of temozolomide and CCNU toxicity in human tumor cells. Br J Cancer 67:1299–1302
123. Tentori L, Orlando L, Lacal PM et al (1997) Inhibition of $O^6$- Alkylguanine DNA-Alkyltransferase or Poly (ADP-ribose) Polymerase Increases Susceptibility of Leukemic Cells to Apoptosis Induced by Temozolomide. Mol Pharmacol 52: 249–258
124. Newlands ES, Blackledge GRP, Slack JA et al (1992) Phase I trial of temozolomide (CCRG 81045: M&B 39831: NSC 362856). Br J Cancer 65:287–291
125. Punt CJA, van Herpen CML, Jansen RHL et al (1997) Chemoimmunotherapy with bleomycin, vincristine, lomustine, dacarbazine (BOLD) plus interferon (for metastatic melanoma: a multicentre phase II study. Br J Cancer 76:266–269
126. Didolkar MS, Jackson A, Lesko L et al (1996) Pharmacokinetics of Dacarbazine in the Regional Perfusion of Extremities With Melanoma. J Surg Oncol 63:148–158
127. Breithaupt H, Dammann A, Aigner K (1982) Pharmacokinetics of dacarbazine (dtic) and its metabolite 5-aminoimidazole-4-carboxamide (aic) following different dose schedules. Cancer Chemother Pharmacol 9:103–109
128. Souliatis VL, Kaila S, Boussiotis VA et al (1990) Accumulation of $O^6$- Methylguanine in human blood leukocyte DNA during exposure to procarbazine and its relationships with dose and repair. Cancer Res 50:2759–2764
129. Brandes A, Scelzi E, Ermani M et al (1997) Procarbazine plus high-dose tamoxifen in recurrent high-grade gliomas: a phase II trial. Proc Am Soc Clin Oncol 16:394
130. Lehman DF, Hurteau TE, Newman N et al (1997) Anticonvulsant usage is associated with an increased risk of procarbazine hypersensitivity reactions in patients with brain tumors. Clin Pharmacol Ther 62:225–229
131. Gately DP, Howell SB (1993) Cellular accumulation of the anticancer agent cisplatin: a review. Br J Cancer 67:1171–1176
132. Loy SY, Mistry P, Kelland LR et al (1992) Reduced drug accumulation as a major mechanism of acquired resistance to cisplatin in human ovarian carcinoma cell line: circumvention studies using novel platinum (II) and (IV) ammine/amine complexes. Br J Cancer 66:1109–1115

133. Scanlon KJ, Kashani-Sabet M, Tone T et al (1991) Cisplatin resistance in human cancers. Pharmacol Ther 52:385–406
134. Mistry P, Kelland LR, Abel G et al (1991) The relationships between glutathione, glutathione-S-transferase and cytotoxicity of platinum drugs and melphalan in eight human ovarian carcinoma cell lines. Br J Cancer 64:215–220
135. Himmelstein KJ, Patton TF, Belt RJ et al (1981) Clinical kinetics of intact cisplatin and some related species. Clin Pharmacol Ther 29:658–664
136. Newell DR, Pearson ADJ, Balmano K et al (1993). Carboplatin pharmacokinetics in children: the development of a pediatric dosing formula. The United Kingdom Children's Cancer Study Group. J Clin Oncol 11:2314–2323
137. Bénézet S, Guimbaud R, Chatelut E et al (1997) How to predict carboplatin clearance from standard morphological and biological characteristics in obese patients. Ann Oncol 8:607–609
138. Ando Yuichi, Minami H, Saka H et al (1997) Pharmacokinetic study of Carboplatin Given on a 5-Day Intravenous Schedule. Jpn J Cancer Res 88:517–521
139. van Warmerdam LJC, Huizing MT, Giaccone G et al (1997) Clinical Pharmacology of Carboplatin Administered in Combination With Paclitaxel. Sem Oncol 24 (Suppl 2):S2–97-S2–104
140. Cummings J, Spanswick VJ, Smyth JF (1995) Re-evaluation of the Molecular Pharmacology of Mitomycin C. Eur J Cancer; 31 A:1928–1933
141. Verweij J, den Hartigh J, Pinedo HM (1990) Antitumor antibiotics. In: Chabner BA Longo DL (eds). Cancer Chemotherapy: Principles and Practice, Lippincott, Philadelphia. pp 382–396
142. Dorr RT (1988) New findings in the pharmacokinetic, metabolic, and drug-resistance aspects of mitomycin C. Semin Oncol 15 suppl 4:32–41
143. Wu DC, Liu JM, Chen YM et al (1997) Mitomycin-C Induced Hemolytic Uremic Syndrome: a Case Report and Literature Review. Jpn J Clin Oncol 27:115–118
144. Sommer A, Santi DV (1974) Purification and amino acid analysis of an active site peptide from thymidylate synthetase containing covalently bound 5'-fluoro-2'-deoxyuridylate and methylene tetrachloride. Biochem Biophys Res Commun. 57:689–696
145. Mandel G (1969) The incorporation of 5-fluorouracil into RNA and its molecular consequences. In Hahn FE (ed). Progress in Molecular and Subcellular Biology, Springer: New York. pp. 82–135
146. Ghoshal K, Jacob ST (1997) An Alternative Molecular Mechanism of Action of 5-Fluorouracil, a Potent Anticancer Drug. Biochem Pharmacol 53:1569–1575
147. Gutheil J, Kearns C (1996) Antimetabolites. In: The Chemotherapy Source Book. Michael C Perry (ed). Williams & Wilkins, Baltimore, MD. Pp 317–343
148. Kinsella AR, Smith D, Pickard M (1997). Resistance to chemotherapeutic antimetabolites: a function of salvage pathway involvement and cellular response to DNA damage. Br J Cancer 75:935–945
149. Weber G (1993) Biochemical strategy of cancer cells and the design of chemotherapy: GHA Clowes Memorial Lecture. Cancer Res 43:3466–3492
150. Pickard M, Dive C, Kinsella AR (1996) Differences in resistance to 5-FU as a function of cell cycle delay and not apoptosis. Br J Cancer 72:1389–1396
151. Fischel JL, Formento P, Etienne MC et al (1997) Dual Modulation of 5-fluorouracil Cytotoxicity Using Folinic Acid with a Dihydropyrimidine Dehydrogenase Inhibitor. Biochem Pharmacol 53:1703–1709
152. Christophidis N, Vadja FJE, Lucas I et al (1978). Fluorouracil therapy in patients with carcinoma of the large bowel: a pharmacokinetic comparison of various rates and routes of administration. Clin Pharmacokinet 3:330–336
153. Eatock MM, Carlin W, Dunlop DJ et al (1996) Bioavailability of subcutaneous 5-fluorouracil: a case report. Cancer Chemother Pharmacol 38:110–112

154. Heggie GD, Sommadossi J-P, Cross DS et al (1987) Clinical pharmacokinetics of 5-fluorouracil and its metabolites in plasma, urine and bile. Cancer Res 47:2203–2206

155. Kissel J, Brix G, Belleman ME (1997) Pharmacokinetic Analysis of 5-[18F]Fluorouracil Tissue Concentrations Measured with Positron Emission Tomography in Patients with Liver Metastases from Colorectal Adenocarcinoma. Cancer Res 57:3415–3423

156. Ensminger WD, Rosowsky A, Raso V et al (1978). A clinical-pharmacological evaluation of hepatic arterial infusions of 5-fluoro-2'-deoxyuridine and 5-fluorouracil. Cancer Res 38:3784–3792

157. Trevisani F, Simoncini M, Alampi G et al (1997) Colitis Associated to Chemotherapy with 5-Fluorouracil. Hepatogastroenterology 44:710–712

158. Feliu J, González-Bari M, Alampi G et al (1997) Colitis Associated to Chemotherapy with 5-Fluorouracil. Hepatogastroenterology 44:710–712 ine and 5-fluorouracil. Cancer Res 38:3784–3792 Colorectal

159. Di Bartolomeo M, Bajetta E, Somma L et al (1996) Doxifluridine as Palliative Treatment in Advanced Gastric and Pancreatic Cancer Patients Oncology 53:54–57

160. Takechi T, Nakano K, Uchida J et al (1997) Antitumor activity and low intestinal toxicity of S-1, a new formulation of oral tegafur, in experimental tumor models in rats. Cancer Chemother Pharmacol 39:205–211

161. Abad A, Navarro M, Sastre J et al (1997) A preliminary report of a phase II trial. UFT plus oral folinic acid as therapy for metastatic colorectal cancer in older patients. Spanish Group for the Treatment of Gastrointestinal Tumors (TTd Group). Oncology (Huntingt) 11 (9 Suppl 10):53–57

162. González-Bar(9 Suppl 10):53–57 l (1997) A preliminary report of a phase II trial. UFT plus oral folinic acid as therapy for metastatic colorectal cancer in older patients. Spanish Group for the Trea

163. Camps C, Godes M, Soler JJ (1990) Possible cardiotoxicity induced by orally administered fluoropyrimidines. An Med Interna 7:525–527

164. Bajetta E, Carnaghi C, Somma L et al (1996) A pilot safety study of capecitabine, a new oral fluoropyrimidine, in patients with advanced neoplastic disease. Tumori 82:450–452

165. Keizer HJ, De Bruijin EA, Tjaden UR et al (1994 Inhibition of fluorouracil catabolism in cancer patients by the antiviral agent (E)-5-(2-bromovinyl)-2'-deoxyuridine. J Cancer Res Clin Oncol 120:545–549

166. Daher GC, Harris BE, Diaso RB (1990) Metabolism of pyrimidine analogues and their nucleosides. Pharmacol Ther 48:189–222

167. Baker SD, Khor SP, Adjei AA et al (1996) Pharmacokinetic, oral bioavailability, and safety study of fluorouracil in patients treated with 776C85, an inactivator of dihydropyrimidine dehydrogenase. J Clin Oncol 14:3085–3096

168. Khor SP, Amyx H, Davis ST et al (1997) Dihydropyrimidine dehydrogenase inactivation and 5-fluorouracil pharmacokinetics: allometric scaling of animal data, pharmacokinetics and toxicodynamics of 5-fluorouracil in humans. Cancer Chemother Pharmacol 39:233–238

169. Cao S, Baccanari DP, Joyner SS et al (1995) 5-Ethynluracil (776C85): Effects on the Antitumor Activity and Pharmacokinetics of Tegafur, a Prodrug of 5-Fluorouracil. Cancer Res 55:6227–6230

170. Huang P, Plunkett W (1995) Fludarabine and gemcitabine-induced apoptosis: incorporation of analogs into DNA is a critical event. Cancer Chemother Pharmacol 36:181–188

171. Ruiz van Haperen VWT, Veerman G, Vermorken JB et al. (1993) 2', 2'-Difluoro-deoxycytidine (gemcitabine) incorporation into RNA and DNA of tumor cell lines. Biochem Pharmacol 46:762–766

172. Manegold C, Drings P, von Pawel J et al. (1997) A Randomized Study of Gemcitabine Monotherapy Versus Etoposide/Cisplatin in the Treatment of Locally Advanced or Metastatic Non-Small Cell Lung Cancer. Semin Oncol 24 (suppl 8):S8–13-S8–17

173. Anderson H, Lund B, Bach F et al (1994) Single-agent activity of weekly gemcitabine in advanced non-small cell lung cancer: a phase II study. J Clin Oncol. 12:1821–1826

174. Noble S, Goa KL (1997) Gemcitabine. A review of its pharmacology and clinical potential in non-small cell lung cancer and pancreatic cancer. Drugs 54:447–472

175. Catimel G, Vermorken JB, Clavel M et al (1994) A phase II study of Gemcitabine (LY 188011) in patients with advanced squamous cell carcinoma of the head and neck. Ann Oncol 5:543–547

176. Lund B, Hansen OP, Theilade K et al (1994) Phase II study of gemcitabine (2', 2'-difluoro-deoxycytidine) in previously treated ovarian cancer patients. J Natl Cancer Inst 86:1530–1533

177. Carmichael J, Walling J (1997) Advanced breast cancer: Investigating role of gemcitabine. Eur J Cancer 33 (suppl 1):S27–30

178. Stadler WM, Kuzel T, Roth B et al (1997) Phase II study of single-agent gemcitabine in previously untreated patients with metastatic urothelial cancer. J Clin Oncol 11:3394–3398

179. Santoro A, Devizzi L, Bonfante V et al (1997) Phase II study with gemcitabine in pretreated patients with Hodgkin's (HD) and no-Hodgkin's lymphomas (NHL): results of a multicenter study. Proc Am Soc Clin Oncol 16:21

180. Abbruzzese JL, Grunewald R, Weeks EA et al (1991) A phase I clinical, plasma and cellular pharmacology study of gemcitabine. J Clin Oncol 9:491–8

181. Grunewald R, Abbruzzese JL, Tarassoff P et al (1991) Saturation of 2', 2'-difluorodeoxycytidine 5'-triphosphate accumulation by mononuclear cells during a phase I trial of gemcitabine. Cancer Chemother Pharmacol 27:258–62

182. Malayeri R, Krajnik G, Ohler L et al (1997) Delayed Anemia and Thrombocytopenia After Treatment With Gemcitabine. J Natl Cancer Inst. 89:1164

183. Cozzarelli NR (1977) The mechanism of action of inhibitors of DNA synthesis. Annu Rev Biochem 46:641–668

184. Estey E, Keating MJ, McCredie KB et al (1990) Cellular ara-CTP pharmacokinetics, response and karyotype in newly-diagnosed acute myelogenous leukemia. Leukemia 4:95–99

185. Plunkett W, Gandhi V (1994) Evolution of the Arabinosides and the Pharmacology of Fludarabine. Drugs 47 (suppl 6):30–38

186. Lennard L, Lilleyman JS (1996) Individualizing Therapy with 6-Mercaptopurine and 6-Thioguanine Related to the Thiopurine Methyltransferase Genetic Polymorphism. Ther Drug Monit 18:328–334

187. Bostrom B, Erdmann (1993) Cellular Pharmacology of 6-Mercaptopurine in Acute Lymphoblastic Leukemia. Pediatr Hematol Oncol 15:80–86

188. Nelson JA, Carpenter JW, Rose LM et al (1975) Mechanisms of action of 6- thioguanine, 6-mercaptopurine, and 8-azaguanine. Cancer Res 35:2872–2878

189. Koren G, Ferrazini G, Sulh H et al (1990) Systemic Exposure to Mercaptopurine as a Prognostic Factor in Acute Lymphocytic Leukemia in Children. N Engl J Med 323:17–21

190. Schmiegelow K, Bruunshuus I (1990) 6-Thioguanine nucleotide accumulation in red blood cells during maintenance chemotherapy for childhood acute lymphoblastic leukemia, and its relation to leukopenia. Cancer Chemother Pharmacol 26:288–292
191. Aarbakke J, Janka-Schaub G, Elion GB (1997) Thiopurine biology and pharmacology. Trends Pharmacol Sci 18:3–7
192. Lennard L (1992) The clinical Pharmacology of 6-mercaptopurine. Eur J Clin Pharmacol 43:329–339
193. Pinkel D (1993) Intravenous Mercaptopurine: Life Begins at 40. J Clin Oncol 11:1826–1831
194. Berkovitch M, Matsui D, Zipursky A et al (1996) Hepatotoxicity of 6-Mercaptopurine in Childhood Acute Lymphocytic Leukemia: Pharmacokinetic Characteristics. Med Pediatr Oncol 26:85–89
195. Ingle JN, Twito D, Suman VJ et al (1997) Evaluation of Intravenous 6-Thioguanine as First-Line Chemotherapy in Women with. Metastatic Breast Cancer. Am J Clin Oncol 20:69–72
196. Aubrecht J, Goad MEP, Schiestl RH (1997) Tissue Specific Toxicities of the Anticancer Drug 6-Thioguanine Is Dependent on the Hprt Status in Transgenic Mice. J Pharmacol Exp Ther. 282:1102–1108
197. Lu K, Benvenuto JA, Bodey GP et al (1982) Pharmacokinetics and metabolism of beta-2'-deoxythioguanosine and 6-thioguanine in man. Cancer Chemother Pharmacol 8:119–123
198. Adkins JC, Peters DH, Markham A (1997) Fludarabine. An update of its pharmacology and use in the treatment of hematological malignancies. Drugs 53:1005–1037
199. Decaudin D, Bosq J, Tertian G et al (1998) Phase II trial of fludarabine monophosphate in patients with mantle-cell lymphomas. J Clin Oncol 16:579–583
200. Brockman RW, Cheng YC, Schabel FM Jr et al (1980) Metabolism and chemotherapeutic activity of 9-beta-D-arabinofuranosyl-2-fluoroadenine against murine leukemia L1210 and evidence for its phosphorylation by deoxycytidine kinase. Cancer Res. 40:3610–3615
201. Cohen JD, Strock DJ, Braun TJ (1997) Deoxycytidine in human plasma: protection of leukemic cells during chemotherapy. Proc Am Soc Clin Oncol 16:4
202. O'Rourke TJ, Burris HA, Rodriguez GI et al (1997) Phase I pharmacokinetic and bioavailability study of five daily intravenous and oral doses of fludarabine phosphate in patients with advanced cancer. Proc Am Soc Clin Oncol 16:210
203. Griffig J, Koob R, Blakey RL (1989) Mechanisms of inhibition of DNA synthesis by 2-chlorodeoxyadenosine in human lymphoblastic cells. Cancer Res 49 (24 pt 1):6923–6928
204. Kong LR, Samuelson E, Rosen ST et al (1997) 2-Chlorodeoxyadenosine in cutaneous T-cell lymphoproliferative disorders. Leuk. Lymphoma 26:89–97
205. Larson RA, Mick R, Spielberger RT et al (1996) Dose-escalation trial of cladribine using five daily intravenous infusions in patients with advanced hematologic malignancies. J Clin Oncol 14:188–195
206. Liliemark J (1997) The clinical pharmacokinetics of cladribine. Clin Pharmacokinetic 32:120–137
207. Liliemark J, Juliusson G (1991) On the pharmacokinetics of 2-chloro-2'-deoxyadenosine in humans. Cancer Res 51:5570–5572
208. Kearns CM, Blakley RL, Santana VM et al (1994) Pharmacokinetics of cladribine (2-chlorodeoxyadenisine) in children with acute leukemia. Cancer Res 54:1235–1239

209. Di Costanzo F, El-Taani H, Parriani D et al (1996) Hydroxyurea May Increase the Activity of Fluorouracil plus Folinic Acid in Advanced Gastrointestinal Cancer: Phase II Study. Cancer Invest 14:234–238

210. Stehman FB, Bundy BN, Kucera PR et al (1997) Hydroxyurea, 5-Fluorouracil Infusion, and Cisplatin Adjunct to Radiation Therapy in Cervical Carcinoma: A Phase I-II Trial of the Gynecologic Oncology Group. Gynecol Oncol 66:262–267

211. Brockstein B, Haraf DJ, Stenson K et al (1998) Phase I Study of Concomitant Chemoradiotherapy With Paclitaxel, Fluorouracil, and Hydroxyurea With Granulocyte Colony-Stimulating Factor Support for Patients With Poor-Prognosis Cancer of the Head and Neck. J Clin Oncol 16:735–744

212. Yarbro JW (1992) Mechanism of action of hydroxyurea. Semin Oncol 19 (3 suppl 9):1–10

213. Newman EM, Carroll M, Akman SA et al (1997) Pharmacokinetics and toxicity of 120-hour continuous-infusion hydroxyurea in patients with advanced solid tumors. Cancer Chemother Pharmacol 39:254–258

214. Tracewell WG, Trump DL, Vaughan WP et al (1995) Population pharmacokinetics of hydroxyurea in cancer patients. Cancer Chemother Pharmacol 35:417–422

215. Navarra P, Grohmann U, Nocentini G et al (1997) Hydroxyurea Induces the Gene Expression and Synthesis of Proinflammatory Cytokines In Vivo. J Pharmacol Exp Ther 280:477–482

216. Allegra CJ (1990) Antifolates. In: Chabner BA and Collins JA (eds). Cancer Chemotherapy. Principles and Practice. Lippincott: Philadelphia. pp 110–153

217. Delpine N, Delepine G, Bacci G et al (1996) Influence of methotrexate dose intensity on outcome of patients with high grade osteogenic sarcoma. Analysis of the literature. Cancer 78:2127–2135

218. Egan LJ, Sandborn WJ (1996) Methotrexate for inflammatory Bowel Disease: Pharmacology and Preliminary Results. Mayo Clin Proc 71:69–80

219. Lonn U, Lonn S, Nilsson B et al (1996) Higher frequency of gene amplification in breast cancer patients who received adjuvant chemotherapy. Cancer 77:107–12

220. Huennekens FM (1994) The methotrexate story: a paradigm for development of cancer chemotherapeutic agents. Adv Enzyme Regul 34:397–419

221. DeAngelis LM, Tong WP, Lin S et al (1996) Carboxypeptidase $G_2$ Rescue After High-Dose Methotrexate. J Clin Oncol 14:2145–2149

222. Hum and Kamen (1996) Folate, antifolates, and folate analogs in Pediatric Oncology. Invest New Drugs 14:101–111

223. Rogers P, Allegra CJ, Murphy RF et al (1988) Bioavailability of oral trimetrexate in patients with acquired immunodeficiency syndrome. Antimicrob Agents Chemother 32:324–326

224. Judson IR (1997) Tomudex (raltitrexed) development: preclinical, phase I and II Studies. Anticancer Drugs 8 (suppl 2):S5-S9

225. Cunningham D, Zalcberg J, Smith I et al (1996) 'Tomudex' (ZD 1694): a novel thymidylate synthase inhibitor with clinical antitumor activity in a range of solid tumors. 'Tomudex' International Study Group. Ann Oncol 7:179–182

226. Gianni L (1997) Anthracycline Resistance: The Problem and Its Current Definition. Semin Oncol 24 (4 Suppl 10):S10–11-S10–17

227. Fogleson PD, Reckford C, Swink S (1992) Doxorubicin inhibits human DNA topoisomerase I. Cancer Chemother Pharmacol 30:123–125

228. Linn SC, Pinedo HM, Van Ark-Otte J et al (1997) Expression of Drug Resistance Proteins in Breast Cancer, in Relation to Chemotherapy. Int J Cancer 71:787–795

229. Bachur NR, Gordon SL, Gee MW (1977) Anthracycline antibiotic augmentation of microsomal electron transport and free radical formation. Mol Pharmacol 13:901–910

230. Sweatman TW, Israel M (1997) Anthracyclines. In: Teicher B (ed). Cancer Therapeutics: Experimental and Clinical Agents. Humana Press Inc. Totowa, NJ pp 113–136

231. Doroshow JH (1983) Effect of anthracycline antibiotics on oxygen radical formation in rat heart. Cancer Res 43:460–472

232. Myers CE, µguire WP, Liss RH et al (1977) Adriamycin: the role of lipid peroxidation in cardiac toxicity and tumor response. Science 197:165–167

233. Bottone AE, de Beer EL, Voest EE (1997) Anthracyclines Enhance Tension Development in Cardiac Muscle by Direct Interaction with the Contractile System. J Mol Cell Cardiol 29:1001–1008

234. Robert J, Gianni L (1993) Pharmacokinetics and Metabolism of Anthracyclines. Cancer Surveys 17:219–252

235. von Hoff DD, Rozencweig M, Leyard M et al (1977) Daunomycin-induced cardiotoxicity in children and adults. A review of 110 cases. Am J Med. 62:200–208

236. Riggs, Jr CE. (1996) Antitumor Antibiotics and Related Compounds. In: Perry MC (ed) The Chemotherapy Source Book.. Williams & Wilkins, Baltimore Maryland pp 345–385

237. Antoine E, Chollet Ph, Montardini S et al (1997) Sequential administration of docetaxel (D) followed by doxorubicin (A) in combination with cyclophosphamide (C) as first-line chemotherapy for metastatic breast cancer (MBC): preliminary results. Proc Am Soc Clin Oncol 16:159

238. Speyer J, Green MD, Kramer E et al (1988) Protective effect of the bispiperazinedione ICRF-187 against doxorubicin-induced cardiac toxicity in women with advanced breast cancer. N Engl J Med 319:745–752

239. Rahman A, Goodman A, Foo W et al (1984) Clinical pharmacology of daunorubicin in phase I patients with solid tumors: development of an analytical methodology for daunorubicin and its metabolites. Semin Oncol 11 (suppl 3):36–44

240. Riggs CE (1984) Clinical pharmacology of daunorubicin in patients with acute leukemia. Semin Oncol 11 (suppl 3):2–11

241. Capranico G, De lsabella P, Penco S et al (1989) Role of DNA breakage in cytotoxicity of doxorubicin, 9-deoxydoxorubicin, and 4-demethyl-6-deoxydoxorubicin in murine leukemia P388 cells. Cancer Res 49:2022–2027

242. Woods KE, Ellis AL, Randolph JK et al (1989) Enhanced sensitivity of the rat hepatoma cell to the daunorubicin analogue 4-demethoxydaunorubicin associated with the induction of DNA damage. Cancer Res 49:4846–4851

243. Camaggi CM, Strocchi E, Carisi P et al (1992) Idarubicin metabolism and pharmacokinetics after intravenous and oral administration in cancer patients: a crossover study. Cancer Chemother Pharmacol 30:307–316

244. Coukell AJ, Faulds D (1997) Epirubicin. An updated review of its Pharmacodynamic and pharmacokinetic properties and therapeutic efficacy in the management of breast cancer. Drugs 53:453–482

245. Sengör F, Beysel M, Erdogan K et al (1996) Intravesical epirubicin in the prophylaxis of superficial bladder cancer. Int Urol Nephrol 28:201–206

246. Budman DR, Lichtman SM (1996) Investigational Drugs. In: Perry MC (ed). The Chemotherapy Source Book. Williams & Wilkins, Baltimore, MD. pp 479–555

247. Galvez C, Bonicatto S, Cavarra G et al (1997) High-dose epirubicin in advanced Breast Cancer patients. Proc Am Soc Clin Oncol 16:169

248. Ballestrero A, Ferrando F, Garuti A et al (1997) High-dose mitoxantrone with peripheral blood progenitor cell rescue: toxicity, pharmacokinetics and implications of dosage and schedule. Br J Cancer 76:797–804

249. Sobell HM (1973) The stereochemistry of actinomycin binding to DNA and its implications in molecular biology. Prog Nucleic Acid Res Mol Biol 13:153–190

250. Waksman Conference on Actinomycins (1974) Their potential for cancer chemotherapy. Cancer Chemother Rep 58:1–123
251. Frei E (1974) The clinical use of actinomycin. Cancer Chemother Rep 58:49–54
252. Mehta MP, Bastin KT, Wiersma SR (1991) Treatment of Wilm's tumor. Current Recommendations. Drugs 42:766–780
253. Manfredi JJ, Horwitz SB (1984) Taxol: An antimitotic agent with a new mechanism of action. Pharm Ther 25:83–125
254. Hyams JS, Lloyd CW (1993) In: Harford JB (ed). Microtubules, Modern Cell biology Series, vol. 13. New York: Wiley Liss. p 460
255. Wadsworth P (1993) Mitosis: spindle assembly and chromosome motion. Current Opinion Cell Biol 5:123–128
256. Rowinsky EK, Wright M, Monsarrat B et al (1993) Taxol: Pharmacology, Metabolism and Clinical Implications. Cancer Surveys 17:283–304
257. Roth BJ, Finch DE, Birhle R et al (1997) A phase II trial of ifosfamide + paclitaxel (IT) in advanced transitional cell carcinoma of the urothelium. Proc Am Soc Clin Oncol 16:324
258. Schnack B, Grbovic M, Brodowicz T et al (1997) High effectivity of a combination of Taxol with carboplatin in the treatment of metastatic urothelial cancer. Proc Am Soc Clin Oncol 16:325
259. Rose PG, Blessing JA, Gershenson DM (1997) Paclitaxel and cisplatin as first-line therapy in recurrent or advanced squamous cell carcinoma of the cervix: a Gynecologic Oncology Group (GOG) study. Proc Am Soc Clin Oncol 16:363
260. Ajani JA, Fairweather J, Dumas P et al (1997) A phase II study of Taxol in patients with advanced untreated gastric carcinoma. Proc Am Soc Clin Oncol 16:263
261. Younes A, Preti A, Romaguera J et al (1997) Activity of Taxol and high-dose Cytoxan with granulocyte colony-stimulating factor (G-CSF) in 54 patients with relapsed/refractory non-Hodgkin's lymphoma (NHL). Proc Am Soc Clin Oncol 16:21
262. Colomer R, Montere S, Lluch A et al (1997) Circulating HER-2/neu predicts resistance to Taxol/Adriamycin in metastatic breast carcinoma: preliminary results of a multicentric prospective study. Proc Am Soc Clin Oncol 16:140
263. Rowinsky E, Smith L, Chaturvedi P et al (1997) Pharmacokinetic (PK) and toxicologic interactions between the multidrug resistance reversal agent VX-710 and paclitaxel (P) in cancer patients. Proc Am Soc Clin Oncol 16:218
264. Kuhn J, Rizzo J, Chang S et al (1997) Effects of anticonvulsants (Acs) on the pharmacokinetics (PK) and metabolic profile of paclitaxel. Proc Am Soc Clin Oncol 16:224
265. Markman M, Rowinsky E, Hakes T et al (1992) Phase I trial of taxol administered by the intraperitoneal route: a Gynecologic Oncology Group study. J Clin Oncol 10:1485–1491
266. Huizing MT, Misser VHS, Pieters RC et al (1995) Taxanes: A New Class of Antitumor Agents. Cancer Inv 13 (4):381–404
267. Gianni L, Kearns C, Gianni A et al (1995) Nonlinear pharmacokinetics and metabolism of paclitaxel and its pharmacokinetic/pharmacodynamic relationships in humans. J Clin Oncol. 13:180–190
268. Venook AP, Egorin MJ, Rosner GL et al (1998) A phase I and pharmacokinetic trial of paclitaxel in patients with hepatic dysfunction: CALGB 9264. J Clin Oncol, in press
269. Cagnoni PJ, Nieto Y, Shpall EJ et al (1997) Pulmonary toxicity secondary to paclitaxel (PAC)-containing high-dose chemotherapy (HDC). Proc Am Soc Clin Oncol 16:232

270. Hurwitz A, Relling M, Ragab A et al (1993) Phase I trial of taxol in children with refractory solid tumors: A Pediatric Oncology Group study. Proc Am Soc Clin Oncol 12:1410

271. Ringel I, Horwitz SB (1991) Studies with RP 56976 (Taxotere): A semisynthetic analogue of Taxol. J Natl Cancer Inst 83:288–291

272. Horwitz SB (1992) Mechanism of action of taxol. Trends Pharmacol Sci 13:134–136

273. Hennequin N, Giocanti N, Favaudon V (1995) S-phase specificity of cell killing by docetaxel (Taxotere) in synchronized HeLa cells. Br J Cancer 71:1194–1198

274. Seibel NL, Blaney SM, O'Brien M et al (1997) Pediatric phase I trial of docetaxel (D) with G-CSF: A Collaborative pediatric branch, NCI and Children's Cancer Group trial. Proc Am Soc Clin Oncol 16:220

275. Bruno R, Sanderink GJ (1993) Pharmacokinetics and Metabolism of Taxotere™ (Docetaxel). Cancer Surveys 17:305–313

276. De Valeriola D, Brassinne C, Cpillard C (1993) Study of excretion balance, metabolism and protein binding of $C^{14}$ radiolabelled Taxotere (RP 56976, NSC 628503) in cancer patients. Proc Am Assoc For Cancer Res 34:373

277. Gelmon K (1994) The taxoids: paclitaxel and docetaxel.: Lancet 344:1267–1272

278. Cabral FR, Barlow SB (1991) Resistance to the antimitotic agents as genetic probes of microtubule structure and function. Pharmacol Ther 52:159–171

279. Endicott JA, Ling V (1989) The biochemistry of P-glycoprotein-mediated multidrug resistance. Ann Rev Biochem. 58:137–171

280. Kuss BJ, Deeley RG, Cole SPC et al (1994) Deletion of gene for multidrug resistance in acute myeloid leukemia with inversion in chromosome 16: prognostic implications. Lancet 343:1531–1534

281. Rahmani R, Zhou X-J (1993) Pharmacokinetics and metabolism of Vinca Alkaloids. Cancer Surveys 17:269–281

282. Bender RA, Castle MC, Margileth DA et al (1977) The pharmacokinetics of [³H]-vincristine in man. Clin Pharmacol Ther 22:430–438

283. Rowinsky EK, Donehower RC (1991) The clinical pharmacology and use of antimicrotubule agents in cancer chemotherapeutics. Pharmacol Ther 52:35–84

284. Wehbe T, Akerley W, Stein B et al (1997) Strontium-89, estramustine and vinblastine (SEV) in hormone refractory prostate carcinoma (HRPC): concurrent chemoradiotherapy. Proc Am Soc Clin Oncol 16:312

285. Hudes G, Roth B, Loehrer P et al (1997) Phase II trial of vinblastine versus vinblastine plus estramustine phosphate for metastatic hormone refractory prostate cancer (HRPC). Proc Am Soc Clin Oncol 16:316

286. Bonfante V, Santoro A, Viviani S et al (1997) Ifosfamide (IFX) and vinorelbine (VNR), an active regimen potentially effective in detecting sensitive relapses in Hodgkin's disease (HD). Proc Am Soc Clin Oncol 16:9

287. Errante D, Spina M, Tavio M et al (1997) Evidence of activity of vinorelbine (VNR) in patients (pts) with previously treated epidemic Kaposi's sarcoma (KS). Proc Am Soc Clin Oncol 16:42

288. Oliveira J, Geoffrois L, Rolland F et al (1997) Activity of Navelbine on lesions within previously irradiated fields in patients with metastatic and/or local recurrent squamous cell carcinoma of the head and neck (SCHNC): an EORTC-ECSG study. Proc Am Soc Clin Oncol 16:406

289. Canfield VA, Saxman SB, Kolodzei MA et al (1997) Phase II trial of vinorelbine in advanced or recurrent squamous cell carcinoma (SCCa) of the head and neck. Proc Am Soc Clin Oncol 16:387

290. Chen AY, Liu LF (1994) DNA topoisomerases: essential enzymes and lethal targets. Annu Rev Pharmacol Toxicol 34:191–218

291. Beck WT, Kim R, Chein M (1994) Novel actions of inhibitors of DNA topoisomerase II in drug-resistant tumor cells. Cancer Chemother Pharmacol 34 (suppl):S14-S18
292. Yves P (1996) Eukaryotic DNA topoisomerase I: genome gatekeeper and its intruders, camptothecins. Semin Oncol 23 (suppl 3):3-10
293. Ewesuedo R, Ratain MJ (1997) Topoisomerase I Inhibitors. The Oncologist 2:359-364
294. Shimada Y, Rothenberg M, Hilsenbeck SG et al (1994) Activity of CPT-11 (irinotecan hydrochloride), a topoisomerase I inhibitor, against human tumor colony-forming units. Anticancer Drugs 5:202-206
295. Wagener DJ, Verdonk HE, Dirix et al (1995) Phase II trial of CPT-11 in patients with advanced pancreatic cancer, an EORTC early clinical trials group study. Ann Oncol 6:129-132
296. Saltz LB (1997) Clinical Use of Irinotecan: Current Status and Future Considerations. The Oncologist 2:402-409
297. Lavelle F, Bissery MC, Andre S et al (1996) Preclinical evaluation of CPT-11 and its active metabolite SN-38. Semin Oncol 23 (suppl 3):11-20
298. Takaoka K, Ohtsuka K, Jin M et al (1997) Conversion of CPT-11 to its active form, SN-38, by carboxylesterase of non-small cell lung cancer. Proc Am Soc Clin Oncol 16:252a
299. Chabot GG, Abigerges D, Catimel G et al (1995) Population pharmacokinetics and pharmacodynamics of irinotecan (CPT-11) and active metabolite SN-38 during phase I trials. Ann Oncol 6:141-151
300. Gupta E, Lestingi TM, Mick R et al (1994) Metabolic Fate of Irinotecan in Humans: Correlation of Glucuronidation with Diarrhea. Cancer Res 54:3723-3725
301. Gupta E, Wang X, Ramirez J et al (1997) Modulation of glucuronidation of SN-38, the active metabolite of irinotecan, by valproic acid and phenobarbital. Cancer Chemother Pharmacol 39:440-444
302. Schellens JH, Creemers AJ, Beijnen JH et al (1996) Bioavailability and pharmacokinetics of oral topotecan: a new topoisomerase I inhibitor. Br J Cancer 73:1268-1271
303. Herben VM, ten Bokkel Huinink WW, Beijnen JH (1996) Clinical Pharmacokinetics of topotecan. Clin Pharmacokinet 31:85-102
304. Pui CH, Behm FG, Raimondi SC et al (1989) Secondary acute myeloid leukemia in children treated for acute lymphoid leukemia. N. Engl J Med 321:136-142
305. Ratain, MJ, Kaminer LS, Bitran JD et al (1987) Acute nonlymphocytic leukemia following etoposide and cisplatin combination chemotherapy for advanced non-small-cell carcinoma of the lung. Blood 70:1412-1417
306. Joel S (1996) The clinical pharmacology of etoposide: an Update. Cancer Treat Rev 22:179-221
307. Ratain MJ, Mick R, Schilsky RL et al (1991) Pharmacologically based dosing of etoposide: a means of safely increasing dose intensity. J Clin Oncol 9:1480-1486
308. Stewart CF (1994) Use of etoposide in patients with organ dysfunction: Pharmacokinetic and pharmacodynamic considerations. Cancer Chemother Pharmacol 34 (suppl):S76-S83
309. Arbuck SG, Douglas HO, Crom WR et al (1986) Etoposide pharmacokinetics in patients with normal and abnormal organ functions. J Clin Oncol 4:1690-1695
310. Macbeth FR (1982) VM 26: phase I and II studies. Cancer Chemother Pharmacol 7:87-91
311. Henter JI, Elinder G, Finkel Y et al (1986) Successful induction with chemotherapy including teniposide in familial erythrophagocytic lymphohistiocytosis. Lancet 2:1402

312. Hong WK, Lippman SM, Itri LM et al (1990) Prevention of Secondary primary tumors with isotretinoin in squamous-cell carcinoma of the head and neck. N Engl J Med 323:795–801

313. Atiba J, Jamil S, Meyskens FJ et al (1994) Transretinoic acid (tRA) in the treatment of malignant gliomas (MG): a phase II study. Proc Am Soc Clin Oncol 13:178

314. Weiss GR, Liu PY, Alberts DS et al (1997) A randomized phase II trial of 13-*cis*-retinoic acid (CRA) or all-*trans*-retinoic acid (ATRA) plus interferon alpha 2a (IFN) for metastatic or recurrent squamous/adenosquamous carcinoma of the uterine cervix: a Southwest Oncology Group study. Proc Am Soc Clin Oncol 16:355

315. Sutton LM, Warmuth MA, Petros WP et al (1997) Pharmacokinetics and clinical impact of all-*trans* retinoic acid in metastatic breast cancer: a phase II trial. Cancer Chemother Pharmacol 40:335–341

316. Khuri FR, Winn RJ, Lee JJ et al (1997) Run in phase: an effective screening tool for a randomized chemoprevention trial. Proc Am Soc Clin Oncol 16:539

317. DiPola RS, Weiss R, Goodin S et al (1997) The clinical and biological effects of 13 cis-retinoic acid (CRA) and alpha interferon (IFN-A) in patients with prostate-specific antigen (PSA) progression after initial local therapy for prostate cancer. Proc Am Soc Clin Oncol 16:332

318. Chatterjee M, Banerjee MR (1982) Influence of hormones on N-(4- hydroxy-phenyl) retinamide inhibition of 7, 12-dimethyl-benz (a)-anthracene transformation of mammary cells in organ culture. Cancer Lett 16:239–245

319. Moon RC, Mehta RG (1989) Chemoprevention of experimental carcinogenesis. Prev Med 18:576–591

320. Pienta KJ, Nguyen NM, Lehr JE (1993) Treatment of prostate cancer in the rat with a synthetic retinoid fenretinide. Cancer Res 53:224–226

321. Dorr RT (1993) Interferon-(in malignant and Viral Diseases: A Review. Drugs 45 (2):177–211

322. Wills RJ, Dennis S, Spiegel HE et al (1984) Interferon kinetics and adverse reactions after intravenous, intramuscular, and subcutaneous injection. Clin Pharmacol Ther. 35:722–727

323. Gallo MA, Kaufman D (1997) Antagonistic and Agonistic Effects of Tamoxifen: Significance in Human Cancer. Semin Oncol 24 (1suppl 1):S1–71–S1–80

324. Wosikowski K, Kung W, Hasmonn M et al (1993) Inhibition of growth factor activated proliferation by anti-estrogens and effects on early gene expression by MCF-7 cells. Int J Cancer 53:290–297

325. Jordan VC (1982) Metabolites of tamoxifen in animals and man: identification, pharmacology, and significance. Breast Cancer Res Treat 2:123–138

326. Wogan GN (1997) Review of the Toxicology of Tamoxifen. Semin Oncol 24 (1 suppl 1):S1–87–S1–97

327. Gradishar WJ, Jordan VC (1997) Clinical Potential of New Antiestrogens. J Clin Oncol 15:840–852

328. Galili U (1983) Glucocorticoids induced cytolysis of human normal and malignant lymphocytes. J Steroid Biochem 19:483–490

329. Yang-Yen HF, Chambard JC, Sun Y-L et al (1990) Transcriptional interference between C-jun and the glucocorticoid receptor: mutual inhibition of DNA binding due to direct protein-protein interaction. Cell 62:1205–1221

330. Strum SB, McDermed JE, Scholz MC et al (1997) Anemia associated with androgen deprivation (AAAD) in prostate cancer (PC) patients (pts) receiving combination hormone blockade (CHB). Proc Am Soc Clin Oncol 16:345

331. Blackledge G (1993) Casodex-mechanisms of action and opportunities for usage. Cancer Suppl 72:3830–3833

332. Buzdar A, Jonat W, Howell A et al (1997) Significant improved survival with Arimidex (anastrozole) versus megestrol acetate in postmenopausal advanced breast cancer: updated results of two randomized trials. Proc Am Soc Clin Oncol 16:157

333. Greven KM, Corn BW (1997) Endometrial cancer. Curr Probl Cancer 21:65–127

334. Gadducci A, Fanucchi A, Cosio S et al (1997) Hormone Replacement therapy and gynecological cancer. Anticancer Res 17:3793–3798

335. Cersosimo RJ, Carr D (1996) Prostate cancer: current and evolving strategies. Am J Health Syst Pharm 53:381–396

336. Vogel CL (1996) Hormonal approaches to breast cancer treatment and prevention: an overview. Semin Oncol 23 (suppl 9):2–9

337. Lucerno MA, McCloskey WW (1997) Alternatives to estrogen for the treatment of hot flushes. Ann Pharmacother 31:915–917

338. Asselin BL, Whitin JC, Coppola DJ et al (1993) Comparative pharmacokinetic studies of three asparaginase preparations. J Clin Oncol 11:1780–1786

339. Lyss AP (1996) Hormones and Enzymes. In: Perry MC (ed). The Chemotherapy Source Book. Williams & Wilkins, Baltimore, MD. pp 459–478

340. Lazo JS, Sebti SM (1994) Bleomycin. Cancer Chemother Biol Response Modif 15:44–50

341. Dalgleish AG, Woods RL, Levi JA (1984) Bleomycin pulmonary toxicity: its relationship to renal dysfunction. Med Pediatr Oncol 12:313–317

342. Dorr VJ, Morris D, Lorber M (1996) Chemotherapy Programs. In: Perry MC (ed) The Chemotherapy Source Book. Williams & Wilkins, Baltimore, MD. pp 845–887

# A Brief Review of Cancer Chemoprevention

Y. Oh, V. Papadimitrakopoulou

## Rationale for Chemoprevention

Chemoprevention is the use of natural or synthetic chemical compounds to inhibit the development of invasive cancer. Carcinogenesis has been attributed to the clonal propagation of cumulative genetic damage over latent periods of a decade or more. Chemopreventive agents are meant to interrupt this clonal propagation of aberrant cells by blocking DNA damage, retarding or reversing malignant phenotype, or inducing apoptosis in the damaged cells of premalignant lesions [1]. In addition to a sound biomolecular rationale, acceptable chemopreventive agents must possess little or no toxicity, since they will be used by an essentially healthy cohort of people at high risk for cancer. Several categories of compounds such as retinoids, cyclooxygenase inhibitors, and sex hormone antagonists have proven helpful in the prevention of various epithelial cancers, especially for the primary prevention of cancers in high-risk individuals or the secondary prevention of metachronous cancers in prior cancer patients [1].

Two complementary concepts in cancer biology pose a strong rationale for the practice of chemoprevention. Multistep carcinogenesis is a concept that models the progression from normal epithelium to cancerous tissue as a result of cumulative genetic alterations that inactivate tumor suppressor genes (e.g., *p53, p16, MMAC*) or activate growth- and invasion-promoting oncogenes (e.g., *K-ras, c-Myc, Her2-neu*). Such a genetic progression model has been described for colonic carcinogenesis by Vogelstein, and similar models for progression of other cancers are being elucidated (Fig. 1). These genetic alterations or their epigentic manifestations (e.g., loss of heterozygosity, increased cell proliferation, increased epidermal growth factor receptor expression, or genomic instability) can serve as biomarkers of ongoing carcinogenesis allowing

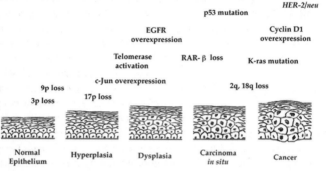

**Fig. 1.** A genetic progression model for lung carcinogenesis, indicating the accrual of various genetic abnormalities and the stages at which they are thought to arise.

the efficacy of chemopreventive therapy to be monitored. Since these genetic and phenotypic changes leading to cancer accumulate over more than a decade, a sizeable window of time exists during which cancer biomarkers can be identified in the epithelium of susceptible patients allowing early pharmacological intervention [2–5].

Another concept supporting the practice of chemoprevention is that of field cancerization, which recognizes chronic carcinogen exposure over epithelial surfaces as the etiology of multiple synchronous and metachronous neoplastic lesions of some cancers, such as those of the aerodigestive tract or colonic mucosa [6–8]. After sufficient genetic damage has been done, even cessation of carcinogen exposure does not appear to eliminate the increased susceptibility to cancer in these areas, as illustrated by study of former smokers [2]. People at increased risk of new or recurrent cancer on the basis of this field cancerization effect would then optimally benefit from chemopreventive therapy [1, 3, 4, 9].

One of the greatest obstacles to designing a randomized, placebo-controlled chemoprevention trial used to be the prohibitively long period of patient follow-up necessary for outcomes assessment. To shorten the time span needed for a prospective chemoprevention trial, surrogate end points are now being utilized. Instead of end points such as cancer detection, recurrence, or disease-related death, surrogate end points such as oral leukoplakia, colon polyp formation, intraepithelial neoplasia, epithelial cell proliferation, and levels of prostate specific antigen or carcinoembryonic antigen, can be measured in a shorter timeframe. These biomarkers of early cancer development or promotion might be alternative end points for examination of the efficacy of chemopreventives in patients.

## Selected Agents and Their Toxicity

Three categories of compounds have been used for chemoprevention in randomized patient trials: retinoids, cyclooxygenase inhibitors, and sex hormone antagonists. Of these agents, the retinoids have been the most extensively studied, especially in the chemoprevention of aerodigestive cancers, and they may be efficacious in the prevention of a broad range of cancers.

### Retinoids and Carotenoids

The vitamin A family of dietary agents includes provitamin A, or carotenoids (e.g., $\beta$-carotene), and preformed vitamin A, or retinoids (including retinol, retinal, retinoic acid, retinyl esters, and their derivatives). Retinoids are naturally found in animal products, whereas carotenoids are found in fruits and vegetables. The role of carotenoids in cancer chemoprevention is still controversial, but retinoids are proving beneficial in the prevention and treatment of a growing range of malignancies (Table 1).

Various retinoids in different experimental systems have been shown to induce $G_1$ arrest, apoptosis, or differentiation in transformed or malignant cells, but the molecular mechanisms by which retinoids inhibit the development of cancers is still poorly understood. Retinoids elicit a broad, complex network of biological activities that are just beginning to be elucidated. Retinoid-bound receptors are internalized into the cell nucleus where they bind DNA and can act as transcription factors. Retinoids have also been shown to downregulate the activity of AP-1, a transcription factor important in cell proliferation. Functional retinoid receptors are homodimers or heterodimers of RAR ($\alpha$, $\beta$ or $\gamma$) and/or RXR ($\alpha$, $\beta$ or $\gamma$) receptors. Different receptor dimerizations confer effector specificity to different cells.

**Table 1.** Retinoid chemoprevention trials

| Author | Population | Intervention | End point | Result |
|---|---|---|---|---|
| Hong et al. [474] | Oral leukoplakia | 13cRA | Regression vs. placebo | 67% vs. 10% |
| Stich et al. [169] | Oral leukoplakia | Vitamin A vs. placebo | Regression | 57% vs. 3% (CR) |
| Han et al. [230] | Oral leukoplakia | 4HPR vs. placebo | Regression | 87% vs. 17% (CR) |
| Lippman et al. [172] | Oral leukoplakia | 13cRA vs. B-carotene | Progression after13cRA induction | 8% vs. 55% |
| Chiesa et al. [174] | Oral leukoplakia | 4HPR vs. no treatment | Recurrence or new lesion | 6% vs. 30% |
| Zaridze et al. [170] | Oral leukoplakia | β-Carotene + retinol + vitamin E vs. placebo | Leukoplakia prevalence | OR 0.632 (0.39–0.98) |
| | Esophagitis | | Progression/stable vs. regression | OR 0.65 (0.29–0.48) |
| Hong et al. [176] [231] | Prior HNSCC | 13cRA vs. placebo | Second Primary tumor | 4% (32 mo), 14% (55 mo), 24% (82 mo), 31% (S5 mo) |
| Bolla et al. [232] | Prior HNSCC | Etretinate vs. placebo | Second primary tumor | 18% vs. 18% (41 mo) |
| McLarty et al. [233] | Male asbestos workers | Retinol q.o.d. + β-carotene vs. placebo | Sputum atypia | OR 1.24 (0.78–1.96) |
| Arnold et al. [234] | Bronchial metaplasia | Etretinate vs. placebo | Improvement | 32% vs. 30% |
| Lee et al. [235] | Bronchial metaplasia | 13cRA vs. placebo | Improvement | 54% vs. 59% |
| Omenn [54] | Smokers, asbestos workers | β-Carotene + retinol | Lung cancer vs. placebo | RR 1.28 (1.04–1.57) |
| Pastorino et al. [60] | Prior NSCLC | Retinyl palmitate vs. Longer time to primary tumor | Second primary tumor no treatment | Second primary tumor |
| De Palo et al. [136] | Prior breast cancer | 4HPR vs. no treatment | Ovarian cancer | 0 vs. 6 (52 mo) |
| Moriarty et al. [236] | Actinic keratoses | Etretinate vs. placebo | Regression | 84% vs. 5% |
| Watson [198] | Actinic keratoses | Etretinate vs. placebo | Regression | 93% vs. 13% |
| Klignan and Thorne [237] | Actinic keratoses | Topical ATRA (0.05%) vs. vehicle control | | Regression 42% vs. 13% |
| Klignan and Thorne [287] | Actinic keratoses | Topical ATRA (0.1%) vs. vehicle control | | Regression 55% vs. 41% |
| Tangrea et al. [238] | Prior basal cell carcinoma | 13cRA vs. placebo | Second basal cell cancer | 0.94 vs. 0.96 tumor/patient year |

**Table 1.** Continued

| Author | Population | Intervention | End point | Result |
|---|---|---|---|---|
| Moon et al. [239] Prior basal cell, squamous cell cancer | Prior actinic keratoses | Retinol vs. placebo 13cRA + retinol vs. placebo | Skin cancer negative Second skin cancer negative | |
| Bouwes Bavinck et al. [240] | Renal transplant | Acitretin vs. placebo | Skin cancer | 2 vs. 0 patients |
| Lamm et al. [191] | Prior bladder cancer, TCC | Megadose vitamins + retinol vs. RDA vitamins | Recurrence | 41% |
| Alffhan et al. [182] | Prior bladder cancer | Etretinate vs. placebo | Rate of recurrence prevention | 73% vs. 27% |
| Pederson et al. [181] | Prior bladder cancer | Etretinate vs. placebo | Nonrecurrence | 27% vs. 87% (8 mo) |
| Studer [183] | Prior bladder cancer | Etretinate vs. placebo | Recurrence at 3/12/24 mo. | 29%/35%/29% vs. 40%/55%/56% |
| Meyskens et al. [167] | CIN 2, 3 | Topical ATRA vs. placebo | Complete response | 43%, 125% vs. 27%, 131% (CIN 2, CIN 3) |
| Munoz et al. [241] | High-risk GE cancer (Huxian, China) | Retinol, riboflavin, and zinc vs. placebo | Precancerous esophageal lesions | 48.9% vs. 45.3% |
| Muto et al. [210] [242] | Resected or EtOH injected hepatocellular cancer | Polyprenoic acid vs. placebo | New or recurrent hepatoma | 27% vs. 49% (median 38 mo) |

13cRA, 13-*Cis* retinoic acid; CR, complete remission; 4HPR, fenretinide; OR, odds ratio; RR, relative risk; NSCLC, non-small-cell lung cancer; ATRA, all-*trans* retinoic acid; TCC, transitional cell carcinoma; RDA, recommended daily allowance; CIN, cervical intraepithelial.

One important effect of retinoids on premalignant and malignant cells of the head and neck is the upregulation of RAR-β. Of all the retinoid receptor types, RAR-β exhibits the most marked alterations in expression between normal, dysplastic, and malignant oral tissue, decreasing in expression with progressive cellular atypia and transformation [10]. RAR-β mRNA expression can be detected in 100% of normal control tissue, but in only 40% of oral premaligannt lesions. Transcription of RAR-β is tightly modulated by endogenous retinoid levels, and reduced expression of RAR-β in premalignant lesions has been found to be a result of defective intracellular vitamin A metabolism and diminished retinoic acid levels [11]. Pharmacologic doses of retinoic acid (RA) are able to correct the expression of RAR-β, which also corroborates the finding that the defect in RAR-β expression is not attributable to gene mutation or deletion [11].

Following 3 months of high-dose 13cRA therapy as part of a chemoprevention trial, RAR-β mRNA and protein expression in oropharyngeal tumor biopsies from patients increased from 40% to 90% [12]. Furthermore, upregulation of RAR-β was more likely to occur (82%) in lesions responding to treatment than in non-responding lesions (47%) [12], suggesting that RAR-β upregulation may be one means by which retinoids suppress malignant cell growth. Other studies support the notion that RAR-β expression may inhibit tumor cell proliferation [13].

Carotenoids may also have cancer preventative effect in some situations, although pharmacologic doses in large clinical trials have failed to show benefit. Carotenoids have demonstrated antioxidant activity, immune enhancement, inhibition of malignant transformation, and regression of premalignant lesions in various experimental models. The mechanism of action is even less understood than that of retinoids, although carotenoids may indirectly act through RAR and RXR receptors after being converted to retinoids. The ability of carotenoids to quench oxygen singlets and free radicals may help prevent mutagenesis, but their antioxidant effect is weak. There is evidence that b carotene administration enhances lymphocyte maturation and proliferation [14, 15] and also induces apoptosis of transformed cells [16, 17] in vitro.

Unlike β-carotene, retinoids in pharmacologic doses have shown benefit in preventing cancers of the head and neck and lung. The toxicity of retinoid compounds is similar to that of hypervitaminosis A and includes varying severity of cheilitis, facial erythema, dry/peeling skin, conjunctivitis, and hypertriglyceridemia [18, 19]. This toxicity is being ameliorated in some studies by the addition of a-tocopherol (800 IU/day) without any loss of retinoid activity [20]. Whereas overall toxicity is milder with fenretinide (also called 4-HPR), this retinoid has the additional adverse effect of "night blindness, or impaired visual adaptation to darkness, an effect which appears to be related to the lowering of serum retinol levels [21]. This reversible ocular toxicity of fenretinide occurs in about 25% of patients, is asymptomatic in 50% of affected patients [22], and can be minimized or averted by allowing drug holidays for 3 days a month [23].

## Tamoxifen

Long-term tamoxifen treatment has been associated with few side effects, most of which are mild, such as dizziness and hot flashes. Tamoxifen's partial estrogenic effects provide fortuitous clinical effects such as lowering the risk of osteoporosis, myocardial infarction, and cardiovascular disease in general [24, 25]. However, estrogenic effects also appear to be related to rare serious side effects such as thrombosis (increased serum fibrinogen and imbalance of coagulation factors) [26]. Crystalline retinal deposits, macular edema, corneal changes, and cataracts are also reported with increasing frequency after prolonged use [27]. Routine screening for ocular effects, however, is only recommended every two years unless symptoms develop [28]. Enhancement of radiotherapy-related lung fibrosis is another potential toxicity of tamoxifen and may be related to stimulation of TGF-b secretion [29]. A relative risk of 2.0 was noted in patients receiving simultaneous tamoxifen and radiotherapy versus radiotherapy alone.

   One controversial long-term adverse effect of tamoxifen therapy is the potential development of second primary malignancies. Although at least one case-controlled study has suggested no association between tamoxifen therapy and an increased risk of second primary cancers [30], other studies of tamoxifen therapy, including the National Surgical Adjuvant Breast and Bowel Project (NSABP) B-14 study, have reported a relative risk of 6 to7 for endometrial cancer [25, 31]. Reports of increased colorectal and stomach cancer incidence from the Stockholm Breast Cancer Study Group have not yet been corroborated by any prospective data [32].

COX Inhibitors

The rationale for chemoprevention of colonic neoplasia using cyclooxygenase (COX) inhibitors arose from epidemiologic data regarding aspirin usage [33, 34] and from animal experiments using the non-steroidal
anti-inflammatory drug (NSAID) sulindac [35, 36]. Although the large
prospective trials to date have employed nonspecific COX inhibitors
(sulindac or aspirin), experimental evidence suggests that the cyclooxygenase COX-2 is the target of NSAID chemoprevention therapy. Both
COX-1 and COX-2 are cyclooxygenases (also known as prostaglandin
endoperoxide synthases), however COX-1 appears to be constitutively
produced and distributed throughout normal human tissues, whereas
COX-2 appears to be inducible and expressed in inflamed tissues only
[37, 38]. Colon cancer and neoplasia are also associated with inflammation and increased prostaglandin production [39], and in animal models
colon cancer is accompanied by increased levels of COX-2 activity [36,
38].

The significance of COX-2 in the setting of cancer is uncertain, but it
appears to prevent apoptosis of proliferating inflammatory cells as well
as cancer cells [40]. In a mouse model of human familial adenomatous
polyposis, a specific inhibitor of COX-2 was able to reduce the number of
colonic polyps [38,] just as nonspecific inhibitors have been shown to do
[36]. If the use of specific COX-2 inhibitors can be applied to chemoprevention of human colon cancer, much of the toxicity of current NSAID
therapy could be avoided.

Finasteride

Finasteride is an inhibitor of 5-a reductase, the enzyme responsible for
the conversion of testosterone to dihydrotestosterone (DHT), the form of
the hormone which effects secondary sexual characteristics [41]. Five-
alpha reductase is present in the cells of target organs such as pubic skin,
scalp hair, and prostate [41]. Treatment with finasteride was shown not
only to reduce hormone-dependent growth of benign prostatic hyperplasia [42, 43] and of prostate cancer [44], but also potentially to affect
male-pattern baldness [41]. About 3% of patients treated with finasteride
for prostate cancer or benign prostatic hypertrophy (BPH) experienced
impotence, decreased libido, and decreased ejaculate volume at 3 years of

follow-up [45, 46]. Adverse effects observed in less than 1% of patients included dysuria, dizziness, headache, asthenia, abdominal pain, diarrhea, rash, and breast pain; no drug interactions are yet known [46]. Gynecomastia is the most common adverse effect of finasteride, occurring in up to 30% of patients but with a delayed onset of 14 days to 2.5 years (median: 180 days) [46]. Although gynecomastia resolved either completely or partially in 80% of patients after finasteride was discontinued, in at least two of these patients primary intraductal breast carcinoma subsequently developed (overall incidence ~0.28%) [46].

## Specific Cancers

Non-Small Cell Lung Cancer

Beta-carotene ($\beta$-carotene) was one of the first vitamin A-related compounds to be tested for efficacy in cancer chemoprevention. It was selected because epidemiologic and dietary studies showed elevated $\beta$-carotene serum levels and intake to be associated with a decreased incidence of lung cancer and because it has a favorable toxicity profile [47–50]. One placebo-controlled randomized trial in heavy smokers using $\beta$-carotene at 50 mg per day demonstrated a decrease in the frequency of micronuclei in sputum, suggestive of decreased DNA damage [51], but failed to show a decrease in urinary excretion of 8-oxo-7,8-dihydro-2'-deoxyguanosine, suggesting that $\beta$-carotene was not exerting an antioxidant effect [52].

However, two separate multicenter, randomized, double-blind, placebo-controlled trials actually found an increase in lung cancer incidence among patients who received pharmacologic $\beta$-carotene supplementation [48, 53, 54]. The $\beta$-carotene and retinol efficacy trial (CARET) reported a 28% increase in lung cancer incidence in $\beta$-carotene-supplemented subjects and a 17% higher mortality rate [54]. Similarly, the Alpha-Tocopherol, $\beta$-Carotene Cancer Prevention Study (ATBC Study) reported a 16% increase in lung cancer incidence in subjects who received $\beta$-carotene supplementation [53, 54].

Why $\beta$-carotene in large doses appears to increase lung cancer development is unknown. Inhibition of absorption of other nutrients by large doses of $\beta$-carotene has been proposed as a possible explanation for this finding [56]. Some studies suggest that $\beta$-carotene under high oxygen tension, especially at high concentrations, can lose its antioxidant effect and exert autocatalytic prooxidant activity that could further damage the lungs of smokers [56]. No animal models or mechanistic studies of β-carotene cancer prevention were done prior to the two large chemoprevention trials, emphasizing the importance of adequate preclinical data prior to human studies.

Unlike β-carotene, several different retinoids have been shown to be effective in preventing the development of lung cancers; however success has only been demonstrated for secondary prevention and not for primary prevention. Lung cancer primary prevention has not been demonstrated using retinoids; however success in secondary prevention has been shown. One randomized, placebo-controlled primary prevention trial of chronic smokers using 13-cis retinoic acid (isotretinoin) at a 1 mg/kg dose for 6 months [57] did not show change in the incidence of squamous metaplasia or dysplasia on random bronchoscopic biopsies. Smoking cessation was associated with decrease in incidence of squamous metaplasia. Another such study using etretinate at 25 mg/day did not show any change in the incidence of sputum atypia in chronic smokers after 6 months [58]. Despite these negative results, because isotretinoin was useful in secondary chemoprevention of oral squamous cell cancers, low-dose 13-cis retinoic acid is being evaluated in an Intergroup National Cancer Institute (NCI) phase III trial for secondary chemoprevention of non-small cell lung cancer after complete resection of stage I tumors [59]. Retinyl palmitate, on the other hand, has already shown efficacy in secondary prevention of lung cancer. In a randomized placebo-controlled study of 307 patients following resection of a stage I non-small cell lung cancer, retinyl palmitate was given at 30,000 IU/day for a year with a median follow-up period of 46 months. Advantages in the treatment arm versus the placebo arm included a 64% versus 51% 5-year survival, an 11.8% versus 18.6% second primary rate, and a statistically significant increase in the time to second primary development and the disease-free interval [60]. An ongoing European multicenter study, the Euroscan trial, is a phase III 2x2 factorial-design study. This trial is currently comparing the efficacy of retinyl palmitate with that of N-acetyl cysteine or both in combination in secondary tumor prevention after resection of primary head and neck or lung cancer [61].

Regional delivery of retinoids is a novel approach to early lung cancer intervention that is being developed as an answer to the frequent and debiliitating side effects associated with chronic oral retinoid administration. The advantage is a significantly greater therapeutic index than that of systemic retinoids, and inhalational forms of retinoids are currently under development [62].

COX-2 inhibitors may also be chemopreventive or therapeutic agents for non small cell lung cancer. Preliminary work has demonstrated that COX-2 in non small cell lung cancer cells catalyzes an intense production of prostagandin E2 (PGE2) which in turn induces the production of IL-10 by macrophages and lymphocytes and simultaneously suppresses the production of IL-12 by macrophages [63]. These findings lead to speculation that COX-2 inhibitor therapy might modify the cytokine microenvironment of lung cancer cells in ways that could increase their immunogenicity or reduce their neovascularity.

## Breast Cancer

The antiestrogen tamoxifen has been evaluated widely as an agent for the chemoprevention of secondary breast cancer. The drug was tested in large clinical trials as adjuvant therapy in early stage breast cancer, and recipients of tamoxifen demonstrated a lower incidence of development of contralateral breast cancer [25, 32, 64]. Long-term disease-free survival was also shown to be prolonged in pathologic node-negative patients receiving adjuvant tamoxifen following definitive treatment of primary breast cancer [64]. Postmenopausal patients with early-stage breast cancer with or without positive axillary lymph nodes have also been shown to experience statistically significant improvements in event-free and overall survival rates on adjuvant tamoxifen in single studies and meta-analyses [25, 65]. Adjuvant treatment for 5 years appears to be more advantageous than treatment for only two years [25]. Tamoxifen is more effective at preventing recurrence of estrogen- and progesterone-receptor-positive tumors but is still beneficial for patients with receptor-negative tumors [65].

Tamoxifen has also been validated as a primary chemopreventive agent for breast cancer (NIH news release, April 6, 1998). An NCI trial evaluating tamoxifen in healthy women at increased risk for breast cancer (on the basis of age >60, first-degree relatives diagnosed with breast cancer, late age at first pregnancy, history of frequent breast lumps and/or atypical hyperplasia, early menarche, history of lobular carcinoma in situ) has demonstrated a 45% reduction in breast cancer mortality in subjects on tamoxifen after 1 to 5 years of follow-up observation. Tamoxifen-treated patients versus placebo-treated patients had an increased risk of endometrial cancer, pulmonary embolism, and deep venous thrombosis (relative risks: 2.35, 2.83, 1.58, respectively), but patients under the age of 50 in the tamoxifen arm experienced no excess risk of adverse effects. This cohort of patients will continued to be followed by the National Surgical Adjuvant Breast and Bowel Project (NSABP) in North America. Similar primary chemoprevention trials are also under way in the United Kingdom and Italy [26].

Retinoids are also being evaluated for secondary prevention of breast cancer. Preclinical data suggest that all-trans retinoic acid (ATRA) can induce apoptosis or differentiation in cultured breast cancer cells [66] while only mediating growth arrest in normal mammary epithelial cells [67]; however, ATRA has not been shown to have activity in metastatic breast cancer [68] and has not been implemented in chemoprevention. Fenretinide (4HPR), on the other hand, has demonstrated preclinical activity in breast cancer and has been advanced to secondary chemoprevention trials [23, 69]. A particularly useful characteristic of fenretinide is that it accumulates in breast tissue [23]. Fenretinide like tamoxifen lowers serum levels of insulin like growth factor I (IGF-I), a hormone that is thought to protect cancer cells from apoptosis and stimulate their proliferation [68]. An Italian study begun in 1993 randomized 2,972 patients with stage I breast cancer after definitive treatment to receive either fenretinide or tamoxifen plus fenretinide for 5 years; serum IGF-I levels are used as one surrogate marker of chemopreventive efficacy [22]. Another phase III trial involving fenretinide plus tamoxifen in prevention of contralateral breast cancer is under way at the NCI.

Prostate Cancer

Multiple lines of evidence suggest that prostate cancer develops under androgen stimulation from precursor lesions called prostate intraepithelial neoplasia (PIN). Foci of PIN are associated with an average level of prostate specific antigen (PSA) intermediate between normal and prostate cancer, and they tend to occur in the periphery of the gland (as does prostate cancer) and often in close proximity to a focus of cancer [70]. The presence of PIN on a random biopsy or a transurethral prostatectomy (TURP) specimen is associated with a high risk for metachronous prostate cancer development [70, 71]. PIN lesions express androgen receptors [72] and have been shown to undergo apoptosis [73] and a decrease in number in the glands of patients receiving long-term androgen ablation treatment for prostate cancer [74, 75]. The PIN lesions that persist after months of androgen ablation still express androgen receptors [71], supporting the rationale for prolonged antiandrogen therapy to suppress PIN and prevent prostate cancer.

Androgen blockade with first generation nonsteroidal antiandrogens like flutamide is associated with too many adverse effects to be considered for chemoprevention [76–78]. Finasteride, however, the first available 5-a reductase inhibitor has efficacy, a relatively low-toxicity profile, and appears to be an acceptable choice for chemoprevention [45, 46, 79, 80]. Use of finasteride for 6 months or more results in a 50% reduction in serum PSA levels whether or not treatment is given for BPH or for prostate cancer [81], but doubling the PSA value of patients on finasteride allows direct comparison with the normal reference range without any apparent loss in the sensitivity of detecting a growing prostate cancer [81, 82].

The Prostate Cancer Prevention Trial (PCPT) was initiated in 1995 as a chemoprevention trial of finasteride with a primary end point of biopsy-proven presence or absence of prostate cancer [82]. The trial was intended to run for 9 years using the same maximally effective dose of finasteride used for BPH and prostate cancer, 5 mg/day. If preliminary results are favorable for prevention of prostate cancer, finasteride also might be considered for an intermittent dosing schedule [83]. The efficacy of intermittent hormone therapy for patients with metastaf the vitamin D receptor associated with a lower risk of osteoporosis [86] has now been found to be associated with a lower rate of aggressive prostate cancer [87]. Homozygosity for the t allele of the vitamin D receptor, which correlates with higher circulating levels of active vitamin D and higher bone density [86], also has been associated with one third the risk for prostate cancer requiring prostatectomy, compared with men who are either heterozygous or homozygous for the T allele [87]. Some the vitamin D receptor associated with a lower risk of osteoporosis [86] has now been found to be associated with a lower rate of aggressive prostate cancer [87]. Homozygosity for the t allele of the vitamin D receptor, which correlates with higher circulating levels of active vitamin D and higher bone density [86], also has been associated with one third the risk for prostate cancer requiring prostatectomy, compared with men who are either heterozygous or homozygous for the T allele [87]. Some in vitro studies have shown growth inhibition of prostate cancer cells by 1α, 25-dihydroxyvitamin D (calcitriol) [88], and others have shown a reduced secretion of type IV collagenases (MMP-2 and MMP-9) and inhibition of invasive cell growth [89]. Based on these results, calcitriol may become beneficial in the chemoprevention or treatment of prostate cancer, particularly tumors with the higher risk tT or TT receptor polymorphism.

Other agents also await further clinical testing for chemoprevention. Treatment with fenretinide, or 4HPR, in a ras+myc-induced murine prostate cancinogenesis model reduced tumor incidence by 49% and tumor mass by 52% [90]. A phase II trial of fenretinide in 22 patients, however, resulted in eight patients being biopsy-positive for neoplastic lesions after 1 year of therapy, and the study was closed [91].

Lycopene is a non-provitamin A carotenoid that has potent antioxidant activity. It can be found in vegetables, most prominently in tomatoes, and its consumption has been associated with a prostate cancer risk reduction of 22% [92, 93]. In a Health Professionals Follow-up Study report, it was shown that greater consumption of tomatoes and related food products resulted in a lower the risk for prostate cancer (RR=0.65), and lycopene was the only one of five carotenoids tested that was associated with a prostate cancer risk reduction [92]. Isomers and derivatives of lycopene are currently being developed for improved efficacy in chemoprevention of prostate cancer [93].

Linomide is a water-soluble, low-molecular-weight molecule found to immunomodulate the severity of multiple sclerosis and other autoimmune diseases [94, 95]. It has now been found to have antiangiogenic activity in tumors [94, 96–99]. Despite disappointing results in phase II trials for renal cancer [100, 101], linomide's activity in prostate cancer and in chemoprevention are not yet known. Preclinical models of linomide in prostate cancer are encouraging, and because the invasive phase of prostate cancer behavior is so dependent on angiogenesis, linomide may be effective in preventing this malignant progression [96, 98, 99].

Colorectal Cancer

Surveillance techniques are particularly useful in diagnosing and monitoring colorectal cancer because the lesions are readily visible and easily biopsied in the premalignant and early malignant stages. Many investigators have thus focused on colorectal adenomatous polyps as a biological end point of chemoprevention trials.

Case reports of adenomatous polyp regression in patients with familial adenomatous polyposis (FAP) who take the NSAID sulindac led to a randomized, placebo-controlled, double-blind crossover study of sulindac in 10 FAP patients [102]. All patients had undergone total colectomy with ileorectal anastomosis and were monitored for rectal polyp formation. A statistically significant decrease in rectal polyps was seen in the sulindac-treated group within 4 months of treatment. Crossover to placebo treatment resulted in a resurgence of rectal polyps again within 4 months. Statistically significant changes in polyp growth were again reported in a larger randomized, placebo-controlled, double-blinded trial of 22 FAP patients of whom 18 still had an intact colon [103]. After 9 months of sulindac therapy, the mean number of polyps decreased to 44% of baseline, and the mean diameter of polyps decreased to 35% of baseline.

Suppression of adenomatous polyp growth by sulindac in FAP patients has not been reproduced in sporadic polyps occurring in the general population [104]; however, a number of studies suggest that aspirin, another COX-inhibitor, reduces the growth of sporadic adenomatous polyps. A prospective analysis of 793 subjects with a history of at least one previous colonic polyp demonstrated a lower incidence of new adenomas at 1 year follow-up in patients who reported regular aspirin use [33]. A case control study from the Melbourne colorectal cancer group also published a lower prevalence of colorectal cancer in regular users of aspirin, with a relative risk of 77% [34].

An overall decreased incidence of colon cancer in regular aspirin users has also been demonstrated by most large prospective studies [105–108]. A cohort study by the American Cancer Society followed 662,424 adults for 6 years [107]. Those who reported taking 16 or more aspirins per month for at least 1 year were found to have about a 40% decrease in colon cancer related deaths. In the Male Health Professionals Study of the United States, men who were regular users of aspirin (two per week) at the beginning of the study at 4 years follow-up demonstrated a 38% decrease in the incidence of colon cancer and a 49% decrease in the incidence of metastatic colon cancer respectively [109]. Similarly, in the Nurse's Health Study, women taking two aspirin per week had a 44% decrease in the incidence of colon cancer that was statistically significant but only after 20 or more years of follow-up [108]. Maximal reduction in risk was observed in women who took four to six tablets per week or a higher dose.

Only two large prospective studies have failed to demonstrate a significant inverse correlation between aspirin intake and colorectal cancer incidence [110]. In the Physicians Health Study, 325 mg of aspirin every other day was used predominantly for myocardial protection, at a dose of 325 mg tablet every other day, a lower dose than what has been protective for colon cancer in other studies, and no reduction in colorectal cancer was seen at 5-year median follow-up. Also, the Leisure World cohort, from a California retirement community consisting of 22,781 residents, demonstrated an increased risk for colorectal cancer at 6.5-, 8- and 11-year follow-up [111, 112]. The mean age of this cohort was 73 years, which was significantly higher than that of the other cohort studies. Despite these two exceptions, most prospective studies suggest that colorectal cancer incidence can be curtailed by aspirin consumption. These last two studies further suggest that the benefit of aspirin is dose- and duration-dependent and possibly limited to a younger age group.

Calcium and vitamin D are controversial dietary factors implicated in the prevention of colorectal cancer. Indirect epidemiologic studies suggest a reduced risk of colorectal cancer associated with calcium and/or vitamin D consumption or vitamin D supplementation related to sun exposure [113, 114]. One prospective observational study of about 2,000 men in Chicago found an inverse correlation between calcium and vitamin D (dairy product) consumption and colorectal cancer risk after a 19-year follow-up [115]. More recently, the U.S. Health Professionals Study with 47,935 participants reported a relative risk of 58% for colon cancer in subjects with the highest dietary calcium or vitamin D intake; but after adjusting for confounding variables, this result was not statistically significant after 6 years of follow-up [116]. In a randomized, double-blinded, placebo-controlled study in which patients with a history of adenomatous colon polyps received 1,200 mg of calcium per day, colonic epithelial proliferation was evaluated after 6 months as a biomarker of cancer promotion [117]. Whereas total epithelial proliferation was the same in both calcium- and placebo-treated arms, calcium-treated patients normalized the distribution of proliferation to the lower epithelial crypt. To further evaluate the effect of calcium supplementation on the risk of colorectal cancer, the European Cancer Prevention Organization has begun accruing patients for a randomized trial giving 2 g of calcium with dietary fiber daily and measuring metachronous polyp development [118].

Other dietary factors may be equally useful in the chemoprevention of colorectal cancer. Population studies have long shown a lower risk of colon cancer associated with high fiber intake [119, 120]. Several large prospective studies have also corroborated this finding [121–123]. Dietary fiber may reduce exposure of the colonic mucosa to ingested carcinogens or endogenous carcinogens, such as secondary bile acids, by binding the carcinogens, diluting carcinogens in increased stool bulk, and therefore reducing the time of exposure of the mucosa to the carcinogens. Dietary fiber also may contain compounds active against malignant cells or release such compounds upon degradation by bacterial microbes. Garlic is a source of fiber noted to be particularly associated with a reduced risk of distal colon cancer [121], and the diallyl sulfides found in garlic have been shown to induce apoptosis in human colon cancer cells [124]. Folic acid supplementation may be beneficial in chemoprevention of ulcerative colitis according to a preliminary 3-month trial looking at upper colonic crypt proliferation as a biological marker of cancer promotion [125]. Other vitamins and antioxidants have been evaluated for chemoprevention of colorectal cancer, and vitamins A, C, and E in combined supplementation as well as Lactulose have shown benefits [126]. Preliminary results of an ongoing trial evaluating vitamins A, C, E, or N-acetylcysteine show up to a 40% decrease in polyp formation [126].

## Ovarian and Endometrial Cancer

Oral contraceptives (OC) are moderately effective in reducing the risk for ovarian cancer with an acceptable toxicity profile. In various studies, the incidence of ovarian cancer in women who have used OC for 5 to 8 years can be shown to be diminished by 50–70% [127–129]. This protection appears to increase with duration of treatment with OC [127, 129] and may persist for up to 15 years after their discontinuation [128]. Furthermore, women who are at higher risk for ovarian cancer because of nulliparity or family history have been shown to normalize their risk for ovarian cancer after 5 and 8 years respectively of OC use [129]. Oral contraceptive use thus may be a valid chemopreventive therapy for patients with a high lifetime risk, such as the BRCA-1 or BRCA-2 gene or other strong family history of ovarian cancer.

For the prevention of sporadic ovarian cancer or disease in patients with lesser risk factors, such as nulliparity, infertility, or antiestrogen use, the course of action is less certain. Ovarian cancer accounts for only 4% of cancers in women, and the lifetime risk of ovarian cancer in the general population is only 1.4% [130, 131]. With this low prevalence of disease, even the relatively nontoxic and inexpensive OC treatment is not safe enough or cost-effective for universal usage. Better screening methods are needed both to detect early disease [131, 132] and to determine populations at risk for disease in the general population. Some promising reports measuring the effectiveness of serial serum markers OVX-1, M-CSF, and the second generation CA-125 for this purpose have been published [133]. For now, women with the lesser risk factors (noted above) should be counseled about the option for OC chemoprevention for ovarian cancer and informed about the risks involved.

First-generation OCs consisted of only estrogens, which resulted in unopposed estrogen stimulation of endometrium and actually produced an increased risk of endometrial hyperplasia and cancer [127, 128]. Lowering the estrogen dose of OCs and adding low-dose progesterone not only reversed this effect but also reduced the incidence of endometrial cancer by as much as 50–90% [127, 128, 134]. Because endometrial growth is so exquisitely sensitive to hormonal modulation, OC treatment can also reverse very early hyperplasia [135]. In conjunction with endometrial sampling techniques, OC treatment may become a useful chemopreventive strategy for women with known risk factors for endometrial cancer, such as obesity or nulliparity [134]. Prevention trials of women in their reproductive years are being designed and need to undergo feasibility and cost-benefit studies [135].

Fenretinide also has shown promise in preventing ovarian cancer. Preliminary follow-up of 3,000 women enrolled in a placebo-controlled secondary chemoprevention trial with fenretinide for breast cancer has demonstrated that this drug has an incidental protective effect for ovarian cancer [23]. Pending further data, fenretinide may become an alternative to OC for women at high risk for ovarian cancer if they are on tamoxifen for a history of breast cancer or if they otherwise have a contraindication for estrogen or progesterone therapy [136].

Esophagus and Stomach

Antioxidant micronutrients may be useful in preventing gastroesophageal (GE) cancer, according to the results of large nutritional intervention studies completed in Linxian, an area of relative malnourishment in north-central China that has one of the world's highest rates of gastroesophageal (GE) cancer [47]. Four different micronutrient supplements were given to 30,000 inhabitants over a 5-year period, and the combination of antioxidants, β-carotene, α-tocopherol, and selenium was found to reduce the prevalence of esophageal cancer by 42%, the incidence of esophageal and gastric cancer deaths by 4% and 21%, respectively, and total cancer deaths by 13% [46, 137–139]. The combination of retinol and zinc also was associated with a 62% reduction in gastric cancer prevalence, but no significant change in cancer-related deaths [139].

   Although extrapolation of the Linxian experience to well-nourished countries may not be wholly accurate, the developed world also shows an association between GE cancer and deficiency of certain dietary factors, especially antioxidants such as ascorbic acid, β-carotene, folate [140–142], vitamin E and selenium [143]. Antioxidants may inhibit mutagenic damage of gastric mucosa by oxygen free radicals [144], prevent activation of carcinogens [145], modifiy Helicobacter pylori mediated injury [145], and preserve immunologic surveillance of developing malignancies [146]. All these theoretical effects may contribute to the efficacy of antioxidants in GE cancer protection.

   Onions [147] and garlic [148] also have been reported as having a cancer-preventive effect, but which phytochemicals are responsible for this effect is unknown. The diallyl sulfides found in garlic may have a similar effect in GE cancer as they do in colon cancer [124]. Garlic and onions have the potential for offering an inexpensive, large-scale chemoprevention for GE cancer in developing countries. Teachings from Chinese herbal apothecaries have led to the investigation of green tea [149, 150] or Chelidonium majis L. (Papaveraceae) herb extract [151] as a preventive agent for gastric cancer, and trials with these preparations are beginning.

   Now that H. pylori infection has been implicated in the etiology of stomach cancer, large population studies need to be done to evaluate the impact of eradicating infection on the incidence of gastric cancer [152]. Intermediate markers for follow-up in these studies can be premalignant lesions or polyps, which will require careful evaluation and standardization of histologic criteria to avoid misclassification [153]. Of note, allium vegetables such as garlic have antibiotic activity and have been shown to kill H. pylori organisms [148]. In addition, two trials ongoing in Latin America and the one planned in Europe, all deal with the effect of anti-oxidants, with or without H. pylori eradication, on the progression/regression rate of precancerous lesions of the stomach [154].

Cervical Cancer

Many epidemiologic and case-control studies have implicated poor nutrition in the pathogenesis of cervical cancer, variably reporting an increased risk with poor intake of vitamins A, C, E, folate, β-carotene, and selenium [155–159]. Some of these associations have been dismissed as a consequence of selection bias because of the typically lower socioeconomic status of cervical cancer patients. Folate deficiency had received some attention as a facilitator of carcinogenesis by aiding the incorporation of oncogenic human papillomavirus (HPV) genomes at a fragile chromosome site [160]. Thereafter, a phase III trial of folate supplementation (5 mg/day) in women with cervical intraepithelial neoplasia (CIN) lesions failed to show any role for folate in inducing regression of the neoplasia [161], however folate supplementation may have been given too late in this trial to be beneficial. Some studies evaluating β-carotene for cervical cancer prevention have shown no benefit [162]; a more recent study showed a reversible regression of some CIN lesions during β-carotene supplementation at 30 mg/day over 6 months [163].

Topical treatments also have been found to be protective for cervical cancer. The use of vaginal spermicide with or without a barrier contraceptive for 5 or more years has been associated with a 30% to 50% reduction in invasive cervical cancer [164, 165]. Because spermicides are able to block the transmission of many sexually transmitted pathogens by their detergent effect on bacterial cell membranes and viral envelopes, they also were thought to kill or inhibit the growth of HPV, which is implicated in the etiology of the vast majority of cervical cancers. However, the most common spermicidal active agent, nonoxynol-9, does not appear to inhibit the growth or transforming ability of related herpes DNA viruses [166], and the mechanism of spermicides on cervical cancer is unknown.

Topical ATRA 0.372% by collagen sponge delivery for 4 days then for 2 days every 3 months has been reported to increase the regression rate of moderate and severe CIN from 27% to 43% [167]. Despite experimental evidence for the inhibition of growth and induction of apoptosis in cervical cancer cells by retinoids [167, 168], little clinical chemoprevention data is available for systemic retinoid treatment.

Head and Neck Cancer

The concept of cancer chemoprevention first entered practice in head and neck cancer patients with the use of retinoids, and some of the first studies to suggest a role for retinoids were carried out in Uzbekistan of the former Soviet Union. Subjects at high risk for oropharyngeal cancer from chewing tobacco-containing betel quids were randomized to either placebo, β-carotene, or α-carotene plus retinol (100,000 IU). After 6 months of follow-up, the rate of oral leukoplakia regression was significantly better in the treatment groups than in the placebo groups with a greater response rate in the β-carotene/retinol arm (28.5% versus 14.8% versus 3%) [169]. The development of new leukoplakias during the 6-month period also was lowest in the β-carotene/retinol arm versus the β-carotene or placebo arm (7.8%, 14.8%, and 21.2% respectively). Another study in a Uzbekistan population demonstrated a significant decrease in the prevalence (odds ratio) of oral leukoplakia to 62% in subjects given a combination of retinol (100,000 IU), b-carotene, and vit E compared with those given only riboflavin or a combination of riboflavin, retinol, β-carotene, and vit E [170].

In the developed western world, retinoid chemoprevention of oropharyngeal malignancy was first demonstrated with 13-cis retinoic acid 13cRA (or isotretinoin) [171]. After a dose of 1 to 2 mg/kg/day for 3 months 13cRA was found to effect a major regression of oral leukoplakia in 67% of patients, whereas placebo was only associated with a 10% spontaneous regression rate. Drug toxicity was fully reversible with dose reduction or discontinuation of the study drug, yet 8% of patients were unable to tolerate them. In addition, >50% of patients manifested recurrence of their lesions within 3 months of treatment cessation [171]. To reduce toxicity and to address the need for maintenance therapy, 13cRA was given at a dose of 1.5 mg/kg/day for only 3 months then the 84% of patients with stable or regressing lesions were given maintenance therapy for nine months with 13cRA at 0.5 mg/kg/day or β-carotene at 30 mg/day [172]. On the low-dose 13cRA regimen 92% of patients continued to have stable or regressing lesions at the end of the treatment period in contrast to only 45% of the patients on b-carotene maintenance. Five invasive squamous cell carcinomas developed in the β-carotene group versus none in the 13cRA group [172]. After long-term follow-up at 5 years, however, the incidence of oral squamous cell carcinoma had equalized in both groups (22% in the 13cRA group and 27% in the β-carotene group), suggesting that long-term treatment is necessary for chemoprevention [173].

Fenretinide (4HPR) also has shown benefit for the secondary prevention of oral leukoplakias following surgical resection [174]. The Istituto Nazionale Tumori (INT) of Milan reported preliminary data of an ongoing trial randomizing post-resection patients to receive either fenretinide at 200 mg/day or nothing. After 1 year of treatment the fenretinide group demonstrated ~13% local recurrence rate compared with a ~29% recurrence rate in untreated patients. About 10% of fenretinide patients had to interrupt treatment because of toxicity. A preliminary updated report after patient accrual to 153 revealed a 6% new or recurrent oral leukoplakia incidence versus 30% for the untreated cohort [23].

Premalignant laryngeal lesions and advanced premalignant lesions of the oral cavity (moderate or severe dysplasia) portend a high rate of progression to invasive cancer and also to single-agent retinoid resistance. To provide a chemoprevention strategy for this higher risk group, a combination of a interferon and 13cRA with a tocopherol was evaluated [175]. Preliminary results of the study show efficacy of the treatment combination in preventing progression of the laryngeal lesions but not of the oral lesions. After 6 to 12 months of treatment, laryngeal sites showed an 83% complete histologic response rate, with a 67% major clinical response rate. In contrast, oral cavity sites showed no complete histologic responses, and three patients progressed to invasive cancer. The oral lesions showed significantly higher levels of chromosome polysomy, p53 protein and Ki67 labeling (a proliferation marker) compared to laryngeal lesions. In addition, loss of heterozygosity at 9p21 persisted in post-treatment specimens despite evidence of complete clinical and histologic response. These genetic alterations are biomarkers that can be followed over time even in the absence of measurable disease and may become a means to monitor the activity of carcinogenesis and the efficacy chemopreventive therapy [175].

When secondary head and neck malignancies are used as the primary end point of chemoprevention, 13cRA has again demonstrated benefit [176]. After curative resection and/or radiotherapy of head and neck squamous cell carcinomas, patients were randomized to receive placebo or 13cRA at 50–100 mg/m2/day for 1 year. Despite a lack of difference between the study arms in the rate of primary tumor recurrence or survival, second primary incidence was significantly lower at 4% in the 13cRA group versus 24% in the placebo group. At least three other centers have also begun trials to evaluate the usefulness of β-carotene in the chemoprevention of secondary head and neck malignancies [177–179].


Bladder Cancer

Retinoids have demonstrated activity in preventing recurrent superficial bladder cancer. When 13-cRA was first tried by the National Bladder Cancer Group as a chemopreventive agent in bladder cancer, retinoid toxicity was so severe and universal that the study was terminated early without recordable activity [180]. Etretinate also has been evaluated for prevention of recurrent superficial bladder cancer, and in two of three randomized, placebo-controlled trials it has shown a modest protective effect becoming significant after 1 year of follow-up [181–183]. Mucocutaneous toxicity of etretinate was prominent but tolerable in most patients. A phase IIa study of fenretinide in patients treated for superficial bladder cancer also appears to show activity when DNA flow cytometry changes were used as an intermediate end point; clinical end points for fenretinide treatment are still pending [184].

Many miscellaneous agents are also showing promise in preventing recurrent bladder cancer. Difluoromethylornithine (DFMO) is a chemopreventive agent shown to have efficacy in animal tumor models of early bladder cancer [185, 186] and other cancers. DFMO is currently being tested in a phase I trial for patients who have had cystoscopically resected superficial bladder cancer [186]. Bropirimine is an oral immunostimulant that promotes the endogenous production of $\alpha$ interferon [187]. In a phase II trial for patients with carcinoma in situ (CIS) of the bladder, 17/29 (59%) complete responses have been reported with a flu-like syndrome reminiscent of interferon toxicity [187].

Bropirimine therapy also has been effective in patients who had recurrences following standard treatment with intravesical Bacillus Calmette-Guerin (BCG), suggesting it to be a good salvage therapy for recurrent bladder CIS and potentially an effective firstline chemopreventive agent as well [187].

An oral preparation of lactobacillus casei (BLP) has been shown to prevent recurrence of superficial bladder cancer with minimal or no toxic effects, extending the 50% recurrence-free interval up to 1.8 times that of the control group [188, 189]. BLP is speculated to work by altering the intestinal flora, particularly because enteric bacteria can be involved in producing or processing carcinogens such as nitroso compounds associated with bladder carcinogenesis [190].

Another virtually nontoxic preventative therapy may be megadose vitamins. A double-blind clinical trial comparing a recommended daily allowance (RDA) of multivitamins versus an RDA of multivitamins supplemented with an antioxidant combination of retinol 40,000 IU, pyridoxine 100 mg, ascorbic acid 2000 mg, alpha-tocopherol 400 units, and zinc 90 mg resulted in a 91% bladder cancer recurrence rate in the unsupplemented group versus 41% in the antioxidant-supplemented group [191].

Preclinical studies also point to the potential of even more compounds for bladder cancer prevention, including oltipraz [192]; natural carotenoids such as astaxanthin and canthaxanthin [193]; and nonsteroidal anti-inflammatory drugs, such as indomethacin [194] or piroxicam [185] in conjunction with fenretinide and DFMO.

Skin Cancer

Retinoids have a record of activity on premalignant skin lesions and in the prevention of skin cancers [195, 196]. Lesions such as actinic keratoses, keratoacanthoma, and epidermodysplasia verruciformis have been treated with orally administered retinoids [196]. In patients with actinic keratosis randomized to receive etretinate, 37/44 (84%) showed a complete or partial regression, whereas only 2/42 (4.8%) patients receiving placebo had spontaneous regressions [197]. Patients with multiple actinic keratoses who have large areas at risk for squamous cell carcinoma were treated on an 8-month, double-blinded, crossover trial with etretinate (4 months placebo/4 months etretinate assigned randomly) [198]. Unlike the lesion progression seen during placebo therapy, significant mild lesion regression was seen during etretinate therapy. Furthermore, no significant new lesion development was noted during the 4-month follow-up period after etretinate treatment, suggesting that intermittent therapy may be sufficient for actinic keratoses [198].

Retinoids are especially efficacious in patients with Xeroderma pigmentosum, a rare autosomal recessive disease characterized by defective DNA repair, increased sun sensitivity, and a 1000-fold increased risk for skin cancers. A small cohort of these patients when treated with high-dose isotretinoin (13 cRA, or Accutane) for 2 years exhibited a nearly 80% reduction in the incidence of skin cancers [191]; however, upon cessation of the study drug, skin cancer frequency increased by 850% [195, 199].

Topical agents for skin cancer chemoprevention also are available. Sunscreens with high sun protection factors (spf) have long been recommended as protective for actinic skin damage and skin cancer [200]; however, recent epidemiologic and laboratory studies are beginning to question the true efficacy of blocking ultraviolet light (UV) exposure with sunscreens and clothing in preventing the initiation of skin cancer, especially melanoma [201, 202]. The amount of UV exposure necessary to initiate melanoma in predisposed individuals may be orders of magnitude lower than that required for sunburn or typical actinic damage, demanding other measures in addition to UV blockade to protect these individuals [202].

The retinoid etretinate has been applied topically for five patients at high risk for melanoma because of dysplastic nevi syndrome [203]. Areas of skin treated with etretinate for 6 months showed dysplastic changes in only 25% of nevi as opposed to 81% of nevi on untreated skin [204]. Larger studies with disease-defined end points will be needed to further assess the efficacy of topical etretinate as well as the general tolerability of the skin inflammation associated with its usage [204].

An apparently nontoxic topical therapy that shows promise in preventing skin cancer is based on green tea extract. Animal studies have shown that the polyphenolic fraction isolated from green tea contains compounds that when applied topically reduce the incidence of experimental skin cancer [205]. At least one active ingredient, (-)-epigallocatechin-3-gallate (EGCG), an antioxidant compound, has been purified and found to reduce the incidence of UV-induced skin cancer in animal models when applied topically [206]. The evaluation of topically used EGCG for chemoprevention of skin cancer is commencing phase II trials.

Hepatocellular Carcinoma

Oltipraz (oltipraz [4-methyl-5-(2-pyrazinyl)-1,2-dithiole-3-thione]) is a substituted dithiolethione that induces activity of the hepatic detoxification enzymes, glutathione S-transferase [207]. It appears to reduce the mutagenicity of carcinogens by augmenting their detoxification and clearance from the liver; in particular, olitpraz has been found to inhibit aflatoxin-mediated hepatocarcinogenesis in the rat [207]. Oltipraz treatment in mouse models of hepatic carcinogenesis results in reduced hepatic levels of aflatoxin-DNA adducts and elevated levels of aflatoxin metabolites excreted in urine and bile (the depurination product aflatoxin-N7-guanine and aflatoxin-glutathione conjugates in urine and bile, respectively) [207].

The daily and weekly administration of oltipraz to 234 adults from Qidong, Jiangsu Province, People's Republic of China was evaluated in a placebo-controlled phase II trial. Both aflatoxin exposure and hepatocellular carcinoma are wide-spread in this area [208]. Twenty percent of the subjects experienced toxic effects consisting of a reversible extremity syndrome during the 8-week treatment interval. Aflatoxin-albumin adducts were measured in patient samples as surrogate biomarker end points in the 8-week follow-up period and were found to correlate with treatment; however, these adduct levels did not correlate with risk for development of hepatocellular carcinoma [209]. Longer treatment periods, longer follow-up periods, or both may be needed to demonstrate an effect of oltipraz treatment, and alternative biomarkers may need to be evaluated.

Polyprenoic acid is a semi-synthetic acyclic retinoid that has been shown in preclinical studies to inhibit hepatocarcinogenesis and to induce differentiation or apoptosis in hepatoma cell lines. A randomized, placebo-controlled study in 89 patients whose tumors were surgically resected or percutaneously injected with ethanol demonstrated a significant reduction in recurrent or new hepatomas after a median follow-up of 38 months in the polyprenoic acid arm [210]. New or recurrent hepatomas were seen in 27% of polyprenoic acid-treated patients versus 49% of placebo-treated patients [210]. Larger studies utilizing polyprenoic acid for secondary prevention of hepatoma and primary prevention in individuals at high-risk are pending.

## New Agents

New chemical compounds are constantly being evaluated for their efficacy and feasibility as chemopreventive agents. Based on their known mechanisms of action and previous applications, most of these compounds could likely have activity in more than one tumor type. Some new agents are semi-synthetic variants or modifications of existing chemopreventive agents, such as carotenoids and retinoids; others constitute novel classes of chemical compounds discovered by investigation of biochemical pathways or purification of plant extracts. A description of some promising new agents follows; these agents also are outlined in Table 2.

Lycopene, as discussed earlier, is the major carotenoid found in tomatoes, and its consumption has been associated with prostate-cancer-risk reduction [92, 93]. Laboratory studies, however, also show it to be effective in suppressing the growth of endometrial, mammary, and lung cancer cells in vitro with much greater efficacy than $\beta$- or $\alpha$-carotene [211]. Furthermore, lycopene appears to inhibit IGF-I-stimulated growth as well, suggesting that it might act synergistically with other chemopreventive agents known to decrease IGF-1 levels, such as fenretinide [22, 69, 211].

Retinoids and their derivatives are continuing to prove useful for chemoprevention. The synthetic acyclic retinoid polyprenoic acid, as already described, appears to show promise in the prevention of hepatocellular carcinoma [210]. A novel retinoid 6-[3-(1-adamantyl)-4-hydroxyphenyl]-2-naphthalenecarboxylic acid (AHPN) which has been shown to inhibit breast and lung cancer and leukemia cell growth in vitro appears to be more potent than ATRA and 9cRA in inhibiting growth of ovarian cancer cells [212] and to kill leukemia cells resistant to retinoic acid [205]. AHPN appears to mediate tumor-cell apoptosis by increasing cyclin-dependent kinase inhibitor p21 (waf1/cip1) independently of any known retinoid receptor [212, 213].

The compound alpha-Difluoromethylornithine (DFMO) has been adopted for evaluation in chemoprevention based on its ability to block polyamine synthesis in mammalian cells. Polyamines (putrescine, spermidine, and spermine) play a critical role in cell growth and transformation. Ornithine decarboxylase (ODC), by catalyzing the synthesis of putrescine, regulates the biosynthesis of higher polyamines such as spermidine and spermine, which are apparently crucial to the regulation of

**Table 2.** Chemopreventive agents and mechanisms of action

| Class/subclass of agent | Mechanism of action | Examples | Potential cancer targets |
|---|---|---|---|
| **Vitamin A-related** | | | |
| Retinoids | Growth inhibition<br>Neoplastic cell differentiation<br>Malignant cell apoptosis<br>Upregulating retinoic acid receptor β | Isotretinoin | Head and neck, lung |
| | | Retinyl palmitate | Head and neck, cervix, lung |
| | | All *trans*-retinoic acid | Head and neck, skin |
| | | Fenretinide | Head and neck, lung, ovarian, breast, bladder |
| | | | Hepatocellular |
| | | Polyprenoic acid | Prostate, breast, lung |
| Carotenoids | Growth inhibition | Lycopene | |
| | | Astaxanthin and canthaxanthin | Bladder |
| **Prostaglandin metabolism** | | | |
| Nonsteroidal anti-inflammatory drugs | Apoptosis of proliferating inflammatory and malignant cells | Aspirin | Colorectal |
| Cyclooxygenase-2 inhibitors | Modulation of prostaglandin E$_2$ and cytokine microenvironment<br>Apoptosis of proliferating inflammatory and malignant cells | Sulindac<br>Colecoxib | Colorectal<br>Lung, colorectal |
| **Hormonal agents** | | | |
| Antiestrogens | Blockade of hormone-dependent growth | Tamoxifen | Breast |
| 5α-Reductase inhibitors | Preventing hormone-mediated growth | Finasteride | Prostate |
| Estrogen/ progesterone | | Oral contraceptive combinations | Ovarian, endometrial |

| Class/subclass of agent | Mechanism of action | Examples | Potential cancer targets |
| --- | --- | --- | --- |
| Antioxidants Micronutrients | Reducing oxygen free radical mediated mutagenesis | Vitamin C Vitamin E Selenium Folate | All carcinomas |
| Others | Reducing oxygen free radical mediated mutagenesis | N-Acetylcysteine Diallyl sulfides Curcumin | Gastric, colorectal |
| Miscellaneous Polyphenols | Antioxidant Anti-inflammatory Inhibition of phenolsulfotransferase Malignant cell growth inhibition Tyrosine kinase inhibition (genistein) | Epigallocatechin 3-gallate Genistein Curcumin | Lung, skin Lung, prostate, colorectal |
| Vitamin D | Malignant cell growth inhibition Reduced secretion type IV collagenases (metalloproteinase 2 and 9) Calcium-mediated normalization of crypt cell proliferation | | Prostate cancer |
| Oltipraz | Induction of glutathione S-transferase Increased clearance of glutathione-conjugated carcinogens | | Bladder cancer |
| Difluormethyl ornithine | Block polyamine synthesis necessary for regulation of cell transformation and growth | | Cervical, breast, bladder, skin, colorectal |
| H. pylori regimens | Eradication of an early cofactor in gastric carcinogenesis | | Gastic cancer |
| Hepatitis B vaccine | Eradication of the most common promoter of hepatic carcinogenesis | | Hepatocellular cancer |

cell growth and transformation. Because of its critical role in cell transformation, ODC is considered a proto-oncogene worth targeting in chemoprevention [204, 206].

DFMO is an irreversible inhibitor of ODC that is active in preventing carcinogen-induced epithelial cancers and their metastases, including those of the skin, colon, breast, and urinary bladder in animal models [214–218]. DFMO treatment also lowers polyamine levels in blood and tissue, readily providing a biomarker of its activity in vivo [214, 216, 217]. The monitoring of N1-acetylspermidine levels may be particularly useful, because this derivative polyamine is produced predominantly in malignant cells and not in normal cells [212]. Phase II trials of DFMO for the chemoprevention of cervical cancer in patients with cervical intraepithelial neoplasia grade 3 CIN and of colon cancer have been initiated, all of which show appropriate lowering of polyamine levels in blood and tissue samples [204, 216, 218, 219]. Toxicity of DFMO seems to be limited to a reversible elevation in the auditory threshold, particularly for low frequencies, which is dose- and duration-dependent [220]; in general, however, no significant toxic effects are reported at doses of 0.5 to 1 g/m2 which are still biochemically efficacious [214, 218, 221]. The long-term endpoints of these trials will determine the usefulness of DFMO as a chemopreventive agent and to validate the measurement of polyamine levels as a surrogate end point.

Unlike the logical step-wise development of DFMO as a potential chemopreventive agent, most other new agents are recruited empirically. A growing multitude of aromatic compounds purified from plant products are beginning to be analyzed for their biologic activity, and many of these novel phytochemicals appear to be anti-carcinogenic in preclinical studies. A few examples of the compounds currently being studied include the flavonoid polyphenolic compounds, quercetin, ellagic acid, curcumin, and genistein, all of which inhibit P-form phenolsulfotransferase, a detoxification enzyme of the human liver [222]. By preventing sulfoconjugation of certain harmful chemicals, these agents may be able to block the activation of some carcinogens [222], much as oltipraz is thought to prevent activation of aflatoxin in hepatic carcinogenesis by blocking glutathione S-transferase.

But the polyphenols seem to have other mechanisms of action as well. Curcumin, the yellow pigment in the rhizome of turmeric, an ingredient of curry spice, exhibits a variety of pharmacological effects, including antiinflammatory, antiinfectious, and antitumor activities [40, 223–225].

Curcumin has been shown to modulate apoptosis in tumor cells [40] and to inhibit colon cancer cell proliferation by arresting cells in the $G_2/M$ phase of the cell cycle [224]. The compound (-)-Epigallocatechin 3-gallate (EGCG), a polyphenolic constituent of green tea that also has been shown to inhibit growth of various cancer cell lines, such as lung, mammary, and stomach, also may work by arresting tumor cells in $G_2/M$ phase [226]. Genistein, a polyphenol found in soy, has been found to be a naturally occurring inhibitor of tyrosine kinases, enzymes which are essential for mediating cell growth factor signals [226]. Because the incidence of breast and prostate cancers is three- to fourfold lower in far eastern countries [130] where genistein consumption is estimated to be 7–80 times higher [227] than in the United States, genistein in the form of soy products is being considered for chemoprevention trials. Genistein in combination with curcumin also shows synergistic inhibition of mammary carcinoma cell growth stimulated by pesticides or 17-β estradiol [228], hinting at the possibility of mixing various active phytochemicals to optimize their anticancer action. Curcumin's antioxidant activity alone might be helpful in the prevention of hepatocellular carcinoma, because curcumin and other antioxidant food additives, including butylated hydroxyanisole (BHA), butylated hydroxytoluene (BHT) and ellagic acid, can all inhibit aflatoxin-mediated mutatgenesis in Salmonella mutagen screening assays [62].

## Future Prospects

Chemoprevention is still in its infancy. Even as more specific strategies for chemoprevention develop, physicians should continue to relay to patients the NCI's recommendations for the most basic chemopreventive regimen, a healthful diet that consists of abundant servings of fresh fruits and vegetables, dietary fiber, and decreased fat and meat. Meanwhile, the field of oncology is rediscovering and reinventing nature's pharmacopoeia by semi-synthetic chemistry. The number of natural products purified and modified each year is multiplying quickly as automated techniques are employed. High throughput screening of novel compounds using end points such as antioxidant activity, mutagenesis assays, tumor cell growth inhibition assays, and apoptosis assays also should hasten the search for efficacious agents. Progress in chemoprevention trials will also be achieved as new biological insight and clinical experience determine more accurate surrogate end points for each individual cancer type, expediting and improving the predictive value of human drug studies. New molecular diagnostic techniques also may lead to identification of drug targets and biomarkers that are specific for the chemoprevention and follow-up of individual patients. Technological progress and resources should behoove developed nations to devise inexpensive, possibly food-based agents to be widely disseminated for the chemoprevention of hepatocellular and gastric cancers that heavily afflict the rest of the world. The development of chemoprevention will be shaped by all of these advances, and the practice of chemoprevention is anticipated to decrease dramatically society's burden of cancer in the coming millennium.

## References

1. Hong WK & Sporn MB (1998) Recent Advances in the Chemoprevention of Cancer. Science 278:1073–1077
2. Mao L, et al. (1997) Clonal genetic alterations in the lungs of current and former smokers. J Natl Cancer Inst 89 (12):857–62
3. Lippman SM, et al. (1994) Cancer Chemoprevention. J Clin Oncol, 12:851.
4. Greenwald P. (1996) Chemoprevention of cancer. Sci Am 275 (3):96–9
5. Lippman SM, et al. (1990) Biomarkers as intermediate end points in chemoprevention trials. J Natl Cancer Inst 82 (7):555–60
6. Papadimitrakopoulou VA, et al. (1996) Molecular and cellular biomarkers for field cancerization and multistep process in head and neck tumorigenesis. Cancer Met Rev 15 (1):53–76
7. Sozzi G, et al. (1995) Genetic evidence for an independent origin of multiple preneoplastic and neoplastic lung lesions. Cancer Res 55 (1):135–40
8. Tomlinson I,et al. (1997) Molecular genetics of colon cancer. Cancer Metastasis Rev 16 (1–2):67–79
9. Hong WK, et al. (1995) Cancer chemoprevention. J Natl Cancer Inst. Monogr (17):49–53
10. Xu X-C, et al. (1994) Differential expression of nuclear retinoic acid receptors in normal, premalignant, and malignant head and neck tissues. Cancer res, 54:3580
11. Xu X-C, Zile MH, et al. (1995) Anti-retinoic acid (RA) Ab binding to human premalignant oral lesions,which occurs less frequently than binding to normal tissue,increases after 13cRA treatment in vivo & is related to RAR-b expresssion, Cancer Res, 55:5507
12. Lotan R, et al. (1995) Suppresssion of Retinoic acid receptor-b in premaliganant oral lesions & its upregulation by isotretinoin. N Engl J Med, 332:1405
13. Frangioni JV, et al. (1994) The DNA binding domain of retinoic acid receptor beta is required for ligand-dependent suppression of proliferation. Application of general purpose mammalian coexpression vectors. J Cell Science, 107 (Pt4): 827–38
14. Chew BP, et al. (1996) Effects of conjugated dienoic derivatives of linoleic acid and beta-carotene in modulating lymphocyte and macrophage function. Anticancer Res 17 (2 A):1099–106

15. Murata T, et al. (1994) Effect of long-term administration of beta-carotene on lymphocyte subsets in humans. Am J Clin Nutr. 60 (4):597–602
16. Toba T, et al. (1997) Growth suppression and induction of heat-shock protein-70 by 9-cis beta-carotene in cervical dysplasia-derived cells. Life Sciences. 61 (8):839–45
17. Muto Y, et al. (1995) Growth retardation in human cervical dysplasia-derived cell lines by beta-carotene through down-regulation of epidermal growth factor receptor. Amer J Clin Nutr62 (6 Suppl):1535S-1540 S
18. Levin AA (1995) Receptors as tools for understanding the toxicity of retinoids. Toxicol Lett 82–83:91–7
19. Silverman AK,et al. (1987) Hypervitaminosis A syndrome: a paradigm of retinoid side effects. J Amer Acad Dermatol 16 (5 Pt 1):1027–39
20. Dimery IW, et al. (1997) Phase I trial of alpha-tocopherol effects on 13-cis-retinoic acid toxicity. Ann Oncol 8 (1):85–9
21. Mariani L, et al. (1996) Chemoprevention of breast cancer with fenretinide (4-HPR): study of long-term visual and ophthalmologic tolerability. Tumori 82 (5): 444–9
22. Decensi A, et al. (1993) Breast cancer chemoprevention: studies with 4-HPR alone and in combination with tamoxifen using circulating growth factors as potential surrogate endpoints. J Cell Biochem – Suppl 17G:226–33
23. Costa A, et al. (1994) Prospects of chemoprevention of human cancers with the synthetic retinoid fenretinide. Cancer Res 54:2032 S
24. Cobelli S, et al. (1997) Long-term toxicity in adjuvant treatment with tamoxifen. J Chemother 9 (4):300–3
25. Swedish Breast Cancer Cooperative Group (1996) Randomized trial of two versus five years of adjuvant tamoxifen for postmenopausal early stage breast cancer. J Natl Cancer Inst 88 (21):1543–9
26. Vogel CL, et al. (1996) Hormonal approaches to breast cancer treatment and prevention: an overview. Semin Oncol 23 (4 Suppl 9):2–9
27. Nayfield SG, et al. (1996) Tamoxifen-associated eye disease. J Clin Oncol 14 (3): 1018–26
28. Therssen R, et al. (1995) Screening for tamoxifen ocular toxicity: a prospective study. Eur J Ophthalmol 5 (4):230–4
29. Bentzen SM, et al. (1996) Radiotherapy-related lung fibrosis enhanced by tamoxifen. J Nat Cancer Inst 88 (13):918–22
30. Cook LS, et al. (1995) Population-based study of tamoxifen therapy and subsequent ovarian, endometrial, and breast cancers. J Natl Cancer Inst 87 (18):1359–64
31. Fisher B, et al. (1994) Endometrial cancer in tamoxifen-treated breast cancer patients: findings from the National Surgical Adjuvant Breast and Bowel Project (NSABP) B-14.    J Natl Cancer Inst 86 (7):527–37
32. Rutqvist LE, et al. (1995) Adjuvant tamoxifen therapy for early stage breast cancer and second primary malignancies. Stockholm Breast Cancer Study Group. J Natl Cancer Inst 87 (9):645–51
33. Greenberg ER, (1993) Reduced risk of large bowel adenomas among aspirin users. J Natl Cancer Inst 85:912–16
34. Kune GA, et al. (1988) Case-control results from the Melbourne Colorectal Cancer study. Cancer Res 48:4399–4404
35. Moorghen M, et al. (1988) A protective effect of sulindac against chemically-induced primary colonic tumours in mice. J Pathol 156:341–347
36. Boolbol SK, et al. (1996) Cyclooxygenase-2 overexpression and tumor formation are blocked by sulindac in a murine model of familial adenomatous polyposis. Cancer Res 56 (11):2556–60

37. Seibert K, et al. (1994) Pharmacological and biochemical demonstration of the role of cyclooxygenase-2 in infalmmation and pain. Proc Natl Acad Sci USA 91:12013–7
38. Oshima M, et al. (1996) Suppression of intestinal polyposis in Apc delta716 knockout mice by inhibition of cyclooxygenase 2 (COX-2). Cell 87 (5):803–9
39. Rigas B, et al. (1993) Altered eicosinoid levels in human colon cancer. J Lab Med 122:518–523
40. Samaha HS, et al. (1997) Modulation of apoptosis by sulindac, curcumin, phenylethyl-3-methylcaffeate, and 6-phenylhexyl isothiocyanate: apoptotic index as a biomarker in colon cancer chemoprevention and promotion. Cancer Res 57 (7):1301–5
41. Gormley GJ (1995) Finasteride: a clinical review. Biomedical Pharmacology 49 (7–8) 319–24
42. Nickel JC, et al. (1997) Efficacy and safety of finasteride therapy for benign prostatic hyperplasia: results of a 2-year randomized controlled trial (the PROSPECT study). PROscar Safety Plus Efficacy Canadian Two year Study. Can Med Assoc J 155 (9): 1251–9
43. Polat O, et al. (1997) Pharmacotherapy of benign prostatic hyperplasia: inhibitor of 5 alpha-reductase. Int Urol Nephrol 29 (3):323–30
44. Brufsky A, et al. (1997) Finasteride and flutamide as potency-sparing androgen-ablative therapy for advanced adenocarcinoma of the prostate. Urology 49 (6):913–20
45. Steiner JF (1996) Clinical pharmacokinetics and pharmacodynamics of finasteride. Clin Pharmacokinet 30 (1):16–27
46. Green L, et al. (1996) Gynecomastia and breast cancer during finasteride therapy. N Engl J Med 335:823
47. Blot WJ, et al. (1993) Nutritioin intervention trials in Linxian, china: supplementation with specific vitamin/mineral combinations, cancer incidence, and disease-specific mortality in the general population. J Natl Cancer Inst, 85:1483
48. Albanes D, et al. (1995) Effects of alpha-tocopherol and beta-carotene supplements on cancer incidence in the Alpha-Tocopherol Beta-Carotene Cancer Prevention Study. Am J Clin Nutr 62 (6 Suppl): 1427S-1430 S
49. Ocke MC, et al. (1997) Repeated measurements of vegetables, fruits, beta-carotene, and vitamins C and E in relation to lung cancer. The Zutphen Study. Amer J Epidemiol 145 (4): 358–65
50. Goodman GE, et al. (1996) The association between participant characteristics and serum concentrations of beta-carotene, retinol, retinyl palmitate, and alpha-tocopherol among participants in the Carotene and Retinol Efficacy Trial (CARET) for prevention
51. Van Poppel G,et ål. (1992) β-carotene supplementation in smokers reduces the frequency of micronuclei in sputum. Br J Cancer 66:1164
52. Van Poppel G, (1995). No influence of B-carotene on oxidative DNA damage in male smokers. J Natl Cancer Inst. 86:310
53. The Alpha-Tocopherol, β-carotene, Cancer Prevention Study Group. (1994) The effect of vitamin E and β-carotene on the incidence of lung cancer and other cancers in male smokers. N Engl J Med, 330:1029
54. Omenn GS, et al. (1996) Effects of a combination of beta carotee and vitamin A on lung cancer and cardiovascular disease. N Engl J Med 334 (18): 1150–5
55. Olson JA (1996) Benefits and liabilities of vitmin A and carotenoids. J Nutr 126:12085
56. Burton GW & Ingold KU (1984) β-Carotene: an unusual type of lipid antioxidant. Science 224 (4649):569–73

57. Lee JS, et al. (1994) Randomized placebo-controlled trial of isotretinoin in chemo-prevention of bronchial squamous metaplasia. J Clin Oncol 12:937
58. Arnold AM, et al. (1992) The effect of the synthetic retinoid etretinate on sputum cytology: results from a randomized trial. Br J Cancer 65:737
59. Lippman SM (1993) Not yet standard: retinoids versus second primary tumors J Clin Oncol 11:1204
60. Pastorino U, et al. (1993) Adjuvant treatment of stage I lung cancer with high-dose vitamin A. J Clin Oncol 11:1216
61. De Vries N, et al. (1991) The Euroscan study. Br J Cancer, 64:985
62. Mulshine JL, et al. (1998) Regional delivery of retinoids: A new approach to early lung cancer intervention. In Clinical and Biological Bsis of Lung Cancer Prevention, ed. Martinet Y, Hirsdi FR, Martinet N, Viguaud JM, Mulshine JL; Birkhauser Verlag Basel/Switzerland
63. Huang M, et al. (1998) Non-small cell lung cancer cyclooxygenase-2-dependent regulation of cytokine balance in lymphocytes and macrophages: up-regulation of interleukin 10 and down-regulation of interleukin-12 production. Cancer Res 58:1208–1216
64. Stewart HJ (1992) The Scottish trial of adjuvant tamoxifen in node-negative breast cancer. Scottish Cancer Trials Breast Group. J Natl Cancer Inst (11):117–20
65. Muss HB, et al. (1994) The role of chemotherapy and adjuvant therapy in the management of breast cancer in older women. Cancer 74 (7 Suppl):2165–71
66. Toma S, et al. (1997) Effects of all-trans-retinoic acid and 13-cis-retinoic acid on breast-cancer cell lines: growth inhibition and apoptosis induction. Int J Cancer 70 (5):619–27
67. Seewaldt VL, et al. (1997) All-trans-retinoic acid mediates G1 arrest but not apoptosis of normal human mammary epithelial cells. Cell Growth Different 8 (6):631–41
68. Sutton LM, et al. (1997) Pharmacokinetics and clinical impact of all-trans retinoic acid in metastatic breast cancer: a phase II trial. Cancer Chemother Pharmacol 40 (4):335–41
69. Torrisi R, et al. (1993) The synthetic retinoid fenretinide lowers plasma insulin-like growth factor I levels in breast cancer patients. Cancer Res 53 (20):4769–71
70. Haggman MJ, et al. (1997) The relationship between prostatic intraepithelial neo-plasia and prostate cancer: critical issues. J Urol 158 (1):12–22
71. Pacelli A & Bostwick DG (1997) Clinical significance of high-grade prostatic intra-epithelial neoplasia in transurethral resection specimens. Urology 50 (3):355–9
72. van der Kwast TH & Tetu B (1996) Androgen receptors in untreated and treated prostatic intraepithelial neoplasia. Eur Urol 30 (2):265–8
73. Montironi R, et al. (1995) Apoptotic bodies in prostatic intraepithelial neoplasia and prostatic adenocarcinoma following total androgen ablation. Pathol Res Pract 191 (9):873–80
74. Wheeler TM (1996) Influence of irradiation and androgen ablation on prostatic intraepithelial neoplasia. Eur Urol 30 (2):261–4
75. Ferguson J, et al. (1994) Decrease of prostatic intraepithelial neoplasia following androgen deprivation therapy in patients with stage T3 carcinoma treated by radi-cal prostatectomy. Urology 44 (1):91–5
76. Wallace C, et al. (1993) Hepatotoxicity complicating flutamide treatment of hirsu-tism. Ann Intern Med 119:1150
77. Wysowski DK, et al. (1993) Fatal and nonfatal hepatotoxicity associated with fluta-mide. Ann Intern Med 118:860–4
78. Leroy D, et al. (1996) Flutamide photosensitivity. Photodermatol Photoimmunol Photomed 12 (5):216–8

79. Gormley GJ, et al. (1995) The potential application of finasteride for chemoprevention of prostate cancer. Ann N Y Acad Sci 768:163–9
80. Gormley GJ, et al. (1992) Chemoprevention strategies for prostate cancer: the role of 5 alpha-reductase inhibitors. J Cell Biochem- Suppl 16H:113–7
81. Guess HA, et al. (1996) The effect of finasteride on prostate specific antigen: review of available data. J Urol 155 (1):3–9
82. Oesterling JE, et al. (1997) Biologic variability of prostate-specific antigen and its usefulness as a marker for prostate cancer: effects of finasteride. The Finasteride PSA Study Group. Urology 50 (1):13–8
83. Feigl P, et al. (1995) Design of the Prostate Cancer Prevention Trial (PCPT). Controlled Clinical Trials 16 (3):150–63
84. Oliver RT, et al. (1995) Intermittent endocrine therapy and its potential for chemoprevention of prostate cancer. Cancer Surveys 23:191–207
85. Homma Y, et al. (1997) Inhibition of rat prostate carcinogenesis by a 5 alpha-reductase inhibitor, FK143. J Natl Cancer Inst 89 (11):803–7
86. Morrison et al. (1994) Prediction of bone density from vitamin D receptor alleles. Nature (Lond.) 367 (6460): 284–7
87. Taylor JA, et al. (1996) Association of prostate cancer with vitamin D receptor gene polymorphism. Cancer Res 56 (18):4108–10
88. Feldman D, et al. (1995) Vitamin D and prostate cancer. Adv Exp Med Biol 375:53–63
89. Schwartz GG, et al. (1997) 1 alpha,25-Dihydroxyvitamin D (calcitriol) inhibits the invasiveness of human prostate cancer cells. Cancer Epidemiol Biomarkers Prev 6 (9):727–32
90. Slawin K, et al. (1993) Dietary fenretinide, a synthetic retinoid, decreases the tumor incidence and the tumor mass of ras+myc-induced carcinomas in the mouse prostate reconstitution model system. Cancer Res 53 (19):4461–5
91. Pienta KJ, et al. (1997) Phase II chemoprevention trial of oral fenretinide in patients at risk for adenocarcinoma of the prostate. Am J Clin Oncol 20 (1):36–9
92. Giovannucci E, et al. (1995) Intake of carotenoids and retinol in relation to risk of prostate cancer. J Natl Cancer Inst 87 (23):1767–76
93. Clinton SK, et al. (1996) cis-trans lycopene isomers, carotenoids, and retinol in the human prostate. Cancer Epidemiol Biomarkers Prev 5 (10):823–33
94. Lehmann D, et al. (1997) Inhibition of the progression of multiple sclerosis by linomide is associated with upregulation of CD4+/CD45RA+ cells and downregulation of CD4+/CD45RO+ cells. Clin Immununol Immunopath 85 (2):202–9
95. Bergh JC, et al. (1997) The first clinical pilot study of roquinimex (Linomide) in cancer patients with special focus on immunological effects. Cancer Invest 15 (3):204–11
96. Hartley-Asp B, et al. (1997) Anti-angiogenic treatment with linomide as adjuvant to surgical castration in experimental prostate cancer. J Urol 158 (3 Pt 1):902–7
97. Borgstrom P, et al. (1995) Inhibition of angiogenesis and metastases of the Lewislung cell carcinoma by the quinoline-3-carboxamide, Linomide. Anticancer Res 15 (3):719–28
98. Vukanovic J & Isaacs JT (1995) Human prostatic cancer cells are sensitive to programmed (apoptotic) death induced by the antiangiogenic agent linomide. Cancer Res 55 (16):3517–20
99. Joseph IB, et al. (1996) Antiangiogenic treatment with linomide as chemoprevention for prostate, seminal vesicle, and breast carcinogenesis in rodents. Cancer Res 56 (15):3404–8

100. Pawinski A, et al. (1997) An EORTC phase II study of the efficacy and safety of linomide in the treatment of advanced renal cell carcinoma. Eur J Cancer 33 (3):496–9

101. de Wit R, et al. (1997) EORTC phase II study of daily oral linomide in metastatic renal cell carcinoma patients with good prognostic factors. Eur J Cancer 33 (3):493–5

102. Labayle D, et al. (1991) Sulindac causes regression of rectal polyps in familial adenomatous polyposis. Gastroenterol 101:635–9.

103. Giardiello FM, et al. (1993) Treatment of colonic and rectal adenomas with sulindac in familial adenomatous polyposis. N Engl J Med 328:1313–6.

104. Ladenheim J, et al. (1995) Effect of sulindac on sporadic colonic polyps. Gastroenteology 108:1083–7.

105. Schreinmachers DM, et al. (1994) Aspirin use and lung, colon and breast cancer incidence in a prospective study. Epidemiology 5:138–46

106. Thun MJ, et al. (1993) Aspirin use and risk of fatal cancer. Cancer Res 53:1322–7

107. Thun MJ, et al. (1991) Aspirin use and reduced risk of fatal colon cancer. N Engl J Med 325:1593–1596.

108. Giovannucci E, et al. (1995) Aspirin and the risk of colorectal cancer in women. N Engl J Med 333:609–14.

109. Giovannucci E, et al. (1994) Aspirin use and the risk ofr colorectal cancer and adenoma in male health professionals. Ann Intern Med 121:241–6

110. Gann PH, et al. (1993) Low-dose aspirin and incidence of colorectal tumors in a randomized trial. J Natl Cancer Inst 85:1220–4.

111. Paganini-Hill A, et al. (1991) Aspirin use and incidence of large-bowel cancer in a California retirement community. J Natl Cancer Inst 83:1182–1183

112. Paganini-Hill, et al. (1995) The Leisure World cohort revisited. Prev Med 24:113–5

113. Slattery ML, et al. (1988) Dietary calcium intake as a mitigating factor in colon cancer. Am J Epidemiol 128:504–14

114. Garland C & Garland FC (1979) Do sunlight and vitamin D reduce the likelihood of colon cancer? Int J Epidemiol 27:155

115. Garland C, et al. (1985) Dietary vitamin D and calcium and risk of colorectal cancer: A 19 year prospective study in men. Lancet 1:307–9

116. Kearney J, et al. (1996) Calcium, vitamin D, and dairy foods and the occurrence of colon cancer in men. Am J Epidem 143 (9):907–17

117. Bostick RM, et al. (1995) Calcium and colorectal epithelial cell proliferation in sporadic adenoma patients. A randomized, double-blinded, placebo- controlled clinical trial. J Natl Cancer Inst 87:1307–15

118. Faivre J, et al. (1997) Chemoprevention of metachronous adenomas of the large bowel: design and interim results of a randomized trial of calcium and fibre. ECP Colon Group. Eur J Cancer Prev 6 (2):132–8

119. Burkitt DP (1971) Epidemiology of cancer of the colon and rectum. Cancer 28:3–13

120. Reddy BS, et al. (1978) Metabolic epidemiology of large bowel cancer: Fecal bulk and constituents of high risk North American and low-risk Finnish populations. cancer 42:2832–8

121. Steinmetz KA, et al. (1994) Vegetables, fruit and colon cancer in the Iowa Women's Health Study. Am J epidemiol 139:1–15

122. Willett WC, et al. (1990) Relation of meat, fat, and fiber intake to the risk of colon cancer in a prospective study among young women. N Engl J Med 323:1664–72

123. Giovannucci E, et al. (1992) Relationship of diet to risk of colorectal adenoma in men. J Natl Cancer Inst 84:91–8

124. Sundaram SG, et al. (1996) Diallyl disulfide induces apoptosis of human colon tumor cells. Carcinogenesis 17:669–73
125. Biasco G, et al. (1997) Folic acid supplementation and cell kinetics of rectal mucosa in patients with ulcerative colitis. Cancer Epidemiol Biomarkers Prev 6 (6):469–71
126. Ponz de Leon M, et al. (1997) Chemoprevention of colorectal tumors: role of lactulose and of other agents. Scand J Gastroenterol Suppl 222:72–5
127. Hulka BS (1997) Epidemiologic analysis of breast and gynecologic cancers. Prog Clin Biol Res 396:17–29
128. Vessey MP & Painter R (1995) Endometrial and ovarian cancer and oral contraceptives-findings in a large cohort study. Br J Cancer 71 (6):1340–2
129. Gross TP & Schlesselman JJ (1994) The estimated effect of oral contraceptive use on the cumulative risk of epithelial ovarian cancer. Obstet Gynecol 83 (3):419–24
130. Landis SH, et al. (1998) Cancer Statistics, in CA: A Cancer Journal for Clinicians 48 (1): 6–9
131. Gershenson DM, et al. (1996) Ovarian intraepithelial neoplasia and ovarian cancer. Obstet Gynecol Clin North Am 23 (2):475–543
132. Anonymous, (1995) NIH consensus conference. Ovarian cancer. Screening, treatment, and follow-up. NIH Consensus Development Panel on Ovarian Cancer. JAMA 273 (6):491–7
133. Bast RC Jr, et al. (1995) Molecular approaches to prevention and detection of epithelial ovarian cancer. J Cell Biochem 23 (Suppl): 219–22
134. Sulak PJ (1997) Endometrial cancer and hormone replacement therapy. Appropriate use of progestins to oppose endogenous and exogenous estrogen. Endocrinol Metabo Clin North Am 26 (2):399–412
135. Burke TW, et al. (1996) Endometrial hyperplasia and endometrial cancer. Obstet Gynecol Clin North Amer 23 (2):411–56
136. De Palo G, et al. (1995) Can fenretinide protect women against ovarian cancer? J Natl Cancer Inst 87:46
137. Li J-Y, et al. (1993) Nutrition intervention trials in Linxian, China: multiple vitamin/mineral supplementation, cancer incidence, and disease-specific mortality among adults with esophageal dysplasia. J Natl Cancer Inst, 85:1492
138. Dawsey SM, et al. (1994) Effects of vitamin/mineral supplementation on prevalence of histological dysplasia & early cancer of the esophagus and stomach: results from the dysplasia trial, Linxian, China. Cancer Epidemiol Biomarkers Prev 3:167
139. Taylor PR, et al. (1994) Prevention of esophageal cancer: the nutrition intervention trials in Linxian, China. Linxian Nutrition Intervention Trials Study Group. Cancer Res 54 (7 Suppl):2029s-2031 s
140. Eichholzer M, et al. (1996) Prediction of male cancer mortality by plasma levels of interacting vitamins: 17-year follow-up of the prospective Basel study. Int J Cancer 66 (2):145–50
141. La Vecchia C, et al. (1994) Selected micronutrient intake and the risk of gastric cancer. Cancer Epidemiol Biomarkers Prev 3 (5):393–8
142. Gonzalez CA, et al. (1994) Nutritional factors and gastric cancer in Spain. Amer J Epidemiol 139 (5):466–73
143. Kono S & Hirohata T (1996) Nutrition and stomach cancer. Cancer Causes Control 7 (1):41–55
144. Drake IM, et al. (1996) Ascorbic acid may protect against human gastric cancer by scavenging mucosal oxygen radicals. Carcinogenesis 17 (3):559–6

145. Phull PS, et al. (1995) A radical view of the stomach: the role of oxygen-derived free radicals and anti-oxidants in gastroduodenal disease. Eur J Gastroenterol Hepatol 7 (3):265–74

146. Zhang YH, et al. (1995) Possible immunologic involvement of antioxidants in cancer prevention. Am J Clin Nutr 62 (6 Suppl):1477S-1482 S

147. Dorant E, et al. (1996) Consumption of onions and a reduced risk of stomach carcinoma. Gastroenterology 110 (1):12–20

148. Sivam GP, et al. (1997) Helicobacter pylori-in vitro susceptibility to garlic (Allium sativum) extract. Nutr Cancer 27 (2):118–21

149. Gao YT, et al. (1994) Reduced risk of esophageal cancer associated with green tea consumption. J Natl Cancer Inst 86 (11):855–8

150. Xu GP, et al. (1993) Effects of fruit juices, processed vegetable juice, orange peel and green tea on endogenous formation of N-nitrosoproline in subjects from a high-risk area for gastric cancer in Moping County, China. Eur J Cancer Prev 2 (4): 327–35

151. Kim DJ, et al. (1997) Potential preventive effects of Chelidonium majis L. (Papaveraceae) herb extract on glandular stomach tumor development in rats treated with N-methyl-N'-nitro-N nitrosoguanidine (MNNG) and hypertonic sodium chloride. Cancer Lett

152. Hirohata T & Kono S (1997) Diet/nutrition and stomach cancer in Japan. Int J Cancer 10 (suppl):34–6

153. Plummer M, et al. (1997) Histological diagnosis of precancerous lesions of the stomach: a reliability study. Int J Epidemiol 26 (4):716–20

154. Buiatti E & Munoz N (1996) Chemoprevention of stomach cancer. IARC Sci Pub (136):35–9

155. Potischman N & Brinton LA (1996) Nutrition and cervical neoplasia [published erratum appears in Cancer Causes Control. Cancer Causes & Control. 7 (1):113–26 7 (3):402]

156. Herrero R, et al. (1991) A case-control study of nutrient status and invasive cervical cancer. I. Dietary indicators. Am J Epidemiol 134 (11):1335–46

157. Ziegler RG, et al. (1991) Diet and the risk of in situ cervical cancer among white women in the United States. Cancer Causes Control 2 (1):17–29

158. Slattery ML, et al. (1990) Dietary vitamins A, C, and E and selenium as risk factors for cervical cancer. Epidemiology 1 (1):8–15

159. Brock KE, et al. (1988) Nutrients in diet and plasma and risk of in situ cervical cancer. J Natl Cancer Inst 80 (8):580–5

160. Butterworth CE Jr. (1992) Effect of folate on cervical cancer. Synergism among risk factors. Ann N Y Acad of Sci 669:293–9

161. Childers JM, et al. (1995) Chemoprevention of cervical cancer with folic acid: a phase III Southwest Oncology Group Intergroup study. Cancer Epidemiol Biomarkers Prev 4 (2):155–9

162. DeVet HCW, et al. (1991)The effect of β-carotene on the regression & progression of cervical dysplasia: A clinical experiment. J Clin Epidemiol 44:273

163. Manetta A, et al. (1996) beta-Carotene treatment of cervical intraepithelial neoplasia: a phase II study. Cancer Epidemiol Biomarkers Prev 5 (11):929–32

164. Grimes DA & Economy KE (1995) Primary prevention of gynecologic cancers. Amer J Obstet Gyn 172 (1 Pt 1):227–35

165. Hildesheim A, et al. (1990) Barrier and spermicidal contraceptive methods and risk of invasive cervical cancer. Epidemiology 1 (4):266–72

166. Hermonat PL, et al. (1992) The spermicide nonoxynol-9 does not inactivate papillomavirus. Sex Transm Dis 19 (4):203–5

167. Meyskens FL, et al. (1994) Enhancement of regression of cervical intraepithelial neoplasia II (moderate dysplasi) with topically applied all-trans-retinoc acid: a randomized trial. J Natl Cancer Inst, 86:539

168. Oridate N, et al. (1995) Inhibition of proliferation and induction of apoptosis in cervical carcinoma cells by retinoids: implications for chemoprevention. J Cell Biochem 23 (Suppl):80–6

169. Stich HF, et al. (1988) Remission of oral leukoplakias and micronuclei in tobacco/betel quid chewers treated with β-carotene and with β-carotene plus vitamin A. Int J Cancer 42:195

170. Zaridze D, et al. (1993) Chemoprevention of oral leukoplakia and chronic esophagitis in an area of high incidence of oral and esophageal cancer. 70 Ann Epidemiol 3:225

171. Hong WK, et al. (1986) 13-cis retinoic acid in the treatment of oral leukoplakia. N Engl J Med 315:1501

172. Lippman SM, et al. (1993) Comparison of low-dose isotretinoin with β-carotene to prevent oral carcinogenesis. N Engl J Med 328:15

173. Papadimitrakopoulou VA, et al. (1997) low-dose isotretinoin versus beta-carotene to prevent oral carcinogenesis – long-term follow-up. J Natl Cancer Inst 89 (3):257–258

174. Chiesa F, et al. (1993) 4HPR in chemprevention of oral leukoplakia. J Cell Biochem Suppl 17F:255

175. Papadimitrakopoulou V, et al. (1997) Efficacy of biochemoprevention in the devleopment of laryngeal and advanced oral premalignant lesions. Proceedings of the American Society of Clinical Oncology 16:383 A, abstract #1366

176. Hong WK, et al. (1990) Prevention of second primary tumors with 13cRA in squamous-cell carcinoma of the head and neck. N Engl J Med 323:795

177. Bairati I, et al. (1996) Prevention of second primary cancer with vitamin supplementation in patients treated for head and neck cancers. Bulletin du Cancer. Radiotherapie 83 (1):12–6

178. Toma S, et al. (1995) Effectiveness of beta-carotene in cancer chemoprevention. Eur J Cancer Prevent 4 (3):213–24

179. Mayne ST, et al. A population-based trial of chemoprevention of head and neck cancer. In: Newell GR, and Hong WK, eds. The biology and prevention of aerodigestive tract cancers. New York: Plenum, 1992:119

180. Prout GR Jr & Barton BA (1992) 13-cis-retinoic acid in chemoprevention of superficial bladder cancer. The National Bladder Cancer Group. J Cell Biochem 16I (suppl):148–52

181. Pedersen H, et al. (1984) Administration of a retinoid as prophylaxis of recurrent non-invasive bladder tumors. Scand J Urol Nephrol 18:121

182. Alfthan O, et al. (1983) Tigason (etretinate) in prevention of recurrence of superficial bladder tumors. Eur Urol 9:6

183. Studer UE, et al. (1984) Prevention of recurrent superficial bladder tumors by oral etretinate: preliminary results ofa randomized, double blind multicenter tiral in Switzerland. J Urol, 131:47

184. Decensi A, et al. (1994) Phase IIa study of fenretinide in superficial bladder cancer, using DNA flow cytometry as an intermediate end point. J Natl cancer Inst 86:138

185. Moon RC, et al. (1993) Chemoprevention of OH-BBN-induced bladder cancer in mice by piroxicam. Carcinogen 14 (7):1487–9

186. Loprinzi CL, et al. (1992) A prospective clinical trial of difluoromethylornithine (DFMO) in patients with resected superficial bladder cancer. 6 J Cell Biochem 16I (suppl):153–5

187. Sarosdy MF (1997) Oral bropirimine immunotherapy of rodent prostate cancer. Eur Urol 31 (Suppl) 1:5–9

188. Aso Y, et al. (1995) Preventive effect of a Lactobacillus casei preparation on the recurrence of superficial bladder cancer in a double-blind trial. The BLPStudy Group. Eur Urol 27 (2):104–9

189. Aso Y & Akazan H (1992) Prophylactic effect of a Lactobacillus casei preparation on the recurrence of superficial bladder cancer. BLP Study Group. Urol Internat 49 (3):125–9

190. Akaza H (1997) New strategy of bio-chemoprevention on recurrence of superficial bladder cancer based on a hypothesis of the mechanism of recurrence. Gan to Kagaku Ryoho [Japanese Journal of Cancer Chemotherapy]. 24 Suppl 1:253–6

191. Lamm DL, et al. (1994) Megadose vitamins in bladder cancer: a double-blind clinical trial. J Urol, 151:21

192. Moon RC, et al. (1994) Chemoprevention of OH-BBN-induced bladder cancer in mice by oltipraz, alone and in combination with 4-HPR and DFMO. Anticancer Res 14 (1 A):5–11

193. Tanaka T, et al. (1994) Chemoprevention of mouse urinary bladder carcinogenesis by the naturally occurring carotenoid astaxanthin. Carcinogenesis 15 (1):15–9

194. Shibata MA, et al. (1993) Chemoprevention by indomethacin of tumor promotion in a rat urinary bladder carcinogenesis model. Int J Cancer 55 (6):1011–7

195. Kraemer KH, et al. (1992) Chemoprevention of skin cancer in xeroderma pigmentosum. J Derm 19 (11):715–8

196. Lippman SM, et al. (1988) Nonsurgical treatments for skin cancer: retinoids and alpha-interferon. J Derm Surg Oncol 14 (8):862–9

197. Moriarty M, et al. (1982) Etretinate in treatment of actinic keratosis: a double blind crossover study. Lancet 1:364

198. Watson AB (1986) Preventative effect of etretinate therapy on multiple actinic keratoses. Cancer Detect Prev 9 (1–2):161–69

199. Kraemer KH, et al. (1988) Prevention of skin cancer in xeroderma pigmentosum with the use of oral isotretinoin. N Engl J Med 318:1633

200. Naylor MF & Farmer KC (1997) The case for sunscreens. A review of their use in preventing actinic damage and neoplasia. Arch Dermatol 133 (9):1146–54

201. Harvey I, et al. (1996) Non-melanoma skin cancer and solar keratoses II analytical results of the South Wales Skin Cancer Study. Brit J Cancer 74 (8):1308–12

202. Ley RD & Reeve VE (1997) Chemoprevention of ultraviolet radiation-induced skin cancer. Environ Health Perspect 105 Suppl 4:981–4

203. Meyskens FL Jr., et al. (1986) Role of topical tretinoin in melanoma and dysplastic nevi. J Am Acad Dermatol 15 (4 Pt 2):822–5

204. Halpern AC, et al. (1994) Effects of topical tretinoin on dysplastic nevi. J Clin Oncol 12 (5):1028–35

205. Katiyar SK, et al. (1997) Protection against induction of mouse skin papillomas with low and high risk of conversion to malignancy by green tea polyphenols. Carcinogenesis 18 (3):497–502

206. Gensler HL, et al. (1996) Prevention of photocarcinogenesis by topical administration of pure epigallocatechin gallate isolated from green tea. Nutr Cancer 26 (3):325–35

207. Kensler TW, et al. (1997) Chemoprevention by inducers of carcinogen detoxication enzymes. Environ Health Perspect 105 Suppl 4:965–70

208. Jacobson LP, et al. (1997) Oltipraz chemoprevention trial in Qidong, People's Republic of China: study design and clinical outcomes. Cancer Epidemiol Biomarkers Prev 6 (4):257–65

209. Kensler TW, et al. (1997) Predictive value of molecular dosimetry: individual versus group effects of oltipraz on aflatoxin-albumin adducts and risk of liver cancer. Cancer Epidemiol Biomarkers Prev 6 (8):603–10

210. Muto Y, et al. (1996) Prevention of second primary tumors by an acyclic retinoid, polyprenoic acid, in patients with hepatocellular carcinoma. Hepatoma Prevention Study Group. N Engl J Med 334 (24):1561–7

211. Levy J, et al. (1995) Lycopene is a more potent inhibitor of human cancer cell proliferation than either alpha-carotene or beta-carotene. Nutr Cancer 24 (3):257–66

212. Chao WR, et al. (1997) Effects of receptor class- and subtype-selective retinoids and an apoptosis-inducing retinoid on the adherent growth of the NIH:OVCAR-3 ovarian cancer cell line in culture. Cancer Lett 115 (1):1–7

213. Nishioka K, et al. (1995) Polyamines as biomarkers of cervical intraepithelial neoplasia. J Cell Biochem 23 (suppl):87–95

214. Hsu CA, et al. (1997) Retinoid induced apoptosis in leukemia cells through a retinoic acid nuclear receptor-independent pathway. Blood 89 (12):4470–9

215. Pegg AE, et al. (1995) Ornithine decarboxylase as a target for chemoprevention. J Cell Biochem 22 (suppl):132–8

216. Meyskens FL Jr, et al. (1994) Dose de-escalation chemoprevention trial of alpha-difluoromethylornithine in patients with colon polyps. J Natl Cancer Inst 86 (15):1122–30

217. Manetta A, et al. (1988) Effect of alpha-difluoromethylornithine (DFMO) on the growth of human ovarian carcinoma. Eur J Gynaecol Oncol 9 (3):222–7

218. Meyskens FL Jr & Gerner EW (1995) Development of difluoromethylornithine as a chemoprevention agent for the management of colon cancer. J Cell Biochem 22 (suppl):126–31

219. Boiko IV, et al. (1997) DNA image cytometric measurement as a surrogate end point biomarker in a phase I trial of alpha-difluoromethylornithine for cervical intraepithelial neoplasia. Cancer Epidemiol Biomarkers Prev 6 (10):849–55

220. Pasic TR, et al. (1997) alpha-difluoromethylornithine ototoxicity. Chemoprevention clinical trial results. Arch Otolaryn Head Neck Surg 123 (12):1281–6

221. Loprinzi CL, et al. (1997) Toxicity evaluation of difluoromethylornithine: doses for chemoprevention trials. Cancer Epidemiol Biomarkers Prev 5 (5):371–4

222. Eaton EA, et al. (1997) Flavonoids, potent inhibitors of the human P-form phenolsulfotransferase. Potential role in drug metabolism and chemoprevention. Drug Metabol Dispos 24 (2):232–7

223. Yamamoto H, et al. (1997) Inhibitory effect on curcumin on mammalian phospholipase D activity. FEBS Letters 417 (2):196–8

224. Hanif R, et al. (1997) Curcumin, a natural plant phenolic food additive, inhibits cell proliferation and induces cell cycle changes in colon adenocarcinoma cell lines by a prostaglandin-independent pathway. J Lab Clin Med 130 (6):576–84

225. Venkatesan N, et al. (1997) Curcumin protects bleomycin-induced lung injury in rats. Life Sciences. 61 (6):PL51–8

226. Okabe S, et al. (1997) Mechanisms of growth inhibition of human lung cancer cell line, PC-9, by tea polyphenols. Jap J Cancer Res 88 (7):639–43

227. Barnes S, et al. (1995) Rationale for the use of genistein-containing soy matrices in chemoprevention trials for breast and prostate cancer. J Cell Biochem- Suppl 22:181–7

228. Verma SP, et al. (1997) Curcumin and genistein, plant natural products, show synergistic inhibitory effects on the growth of human breast cancer MCF-7 cells Induced by estrogenic pesticides. Biochem Biophys Res Comm 233 (3):692–6

229. Soni KB, et al. (1997) Protective effect of food additives on aflatoxin-induced mutagenicity and hepatocarcinogenicity. Cancer Lett 115 (2):129–33

230. Han, et al (1990) Evaluation of N-4-(hydroxycarbophenyl) retinamide as a cancer prevention agent and as a cancer chemotherapeutic agent. In Vivo 4:153

231. Benner, et al. (1994) Prevention of second primary tumors with isotretinoin in patents with squamous cell carcinoma of the head and neck: long term follow-up. J Natl Cancer Inst 86:140

232. Bolla, et al. (1994) Prevention of second primary tumors with etretinate in squamous cell carcinoma of the oral cavity and oropharynx: results of a multicentric double-blind randomized study. Eur J Cancer 30 A:767

233. McLarty, et al. (1995) β-Carotene, vitamin A, and lung cancer chemoprevention: results of an intermediate end point study. Am J Clin Nutr 62 (Suppl): 1431 S

234. Arnold, et al. (1992) The effect of the synthetic retinoid etretinate on sputum cytology; from a randomized trial. Br J Cancer 65:737

235. Lee, et al. (1994) Randomized placebo-controlled trial of isotretinoin in chemoprevention of bronchial squamous metaplasia. J Clin Oncol 12:937

236. Moriarty, et al. (1982) Etretinate in treatment of actinic keratosis; a double blind crossover study. Lancet 1:364

237. Kigman & Theme (1991) Topical therapy of actinic keratosis with tretinoin. In: Marks R, ed. Retinoids in cutaneous malignancy Cambridge1 MA: Blackwell Scientific, 1991:66

238. Tangrea et al. (1992) Long term therapy with low-dose isotretinoin for prevention of basal cell carcinoma: a multicenter clinical trial. J Natl Cancer [nst 84:328

239. Moon, et al. (1993) The Arizona Skin Cancer Study Group. Chemoprevention and etiology of non-melanoma skin cancers. Program and abstracts, 1 7th Annual Meeting of the American Society of Preventive Oncology, March, 1993

240. Bouwes Bavinck, et al. (1995) Prevention of skin cancer and reduction of keratotic skin lesions during aceitretin therapy in renal transplant recipients: a double-blind placebo-controlled study. J Clin Oncol 13:1933

241. Munoz, et al. (1985) No effect of riboflavin, retinol and zinc on prevalence of precancerous lesions of esophagus: randomized double-blind intervention study in high-risk population of China. Lancet 2:111

242. Munoz, et al. (1987) Effect of ribofavin, retinol and zinc on micronuclel of buccal mucosa and oesophagus: A randomized double-blind intervention study in China. J Natl Cancer Inst 79:687

# High-Dose Chemotherapy

S.F. Williams

## High-Dose Chemotherapy Regimens

The rationale for the use of high-dose chemotherapy begins with experimental observations on dose-response effects. As their dose is linearly increased certain agents demonstrate logarithmic tumor cell killing [1]. Some chemotherapeutics demonstrate a steep dose-response curve where for small increments in dose one sees logarithmically increased cell killing. Alkylating agents such as cyclophosphamide, thiotepa, and nitrosoureas, are examples and are commonly used in high-dose regimens. It has also been demonstrated in the laboratory that combinations of alkylating agents can be synergistic in tumor cell killing and high doses can overcome drug resistance [2]. There are certain factors that can effect this dose-response and include; the type of chemotherapeutic agent, the drug schedule, the tumor type and volume being treated, and the emergence of drug resistance [3]. Thus, many treatment programs are designed to optimize these factors to fully exploit dose-response effects.

Since alkylating agents have been the primary agents utilized myelosuppression has been a major dose limiting toxicity. To overcome this investigators have employed hematopoietic stem cells and/or myeloid growth factors. These stem cells can come from marrow, blood or cord blood. They can be collected from the patient (autologous), from a matched donor (allogeneic) or identical twin (syngeneic). In the autologous setting these stem cells are strictly a rescue from the severe myelosuppressive effects of high-dose chemotherapy but in the allogeneic setting they are not only a hematologic rescue but may be useful immunologically to suppress minimal residual disease (so-called graft versus leukemia or tumor effect).

To summarize, agents chosen for high-dose chemotherapy have certain characteristics that underline their usefulness. These characteristics include the demonstration of a steep dose-response curve, myelosuppression as the major acute toxicity with reversible non-myeloid side effects, lack of cross resistance with previously administered agents and ideally minimal long term toxicity.

## Collection and Processing of Stem Cells

As mentioned there are three practical sources of hematopoietic stem cells; marrow, blood, and cord blood. Traditionally, marrow has been collected both in the allogeneic and autologous settings but currently blood has become the most accepted source. This has become possible for several reasons which involve the ability to "mobilize" stem cells, progenitors and precursors into the peripheral circulation to allow collection through large bore catheters by continous blood flow cell separators (apheresis). Cord blood in adults as a rescue remains investigational and will not be covered in detail here.

Mobilization became possible because of the observation that as patients recover from hematologic nadir from agents such as cyclophosphamide, hematopoietic progenitors as measured by colony assays increase dramatically in peripheral blood [4]. This has lead to the process of chemotherapy moblization. One can also increase the numbers of circulating progenitors in the blood stream by administering myeloid growth factors such as G- or GM-CSF and after a certain number of days collect these progenitors through apheresis [5]. A combination of chemotherapy and myeloid growth factors also yields a high number of progenitors.

It has been shown by numerous investigators that mobilized blood progenitors (or peripheral blood progenitors) leads to faster hematologic recovery after high-dose chemotherapy which also leads to less antibiotic usage, less transfusion support and shorter hospital stays [6]. It also appears that there is faster immune reconstitution after high-dose therapy [7]: (a) more rapid hematologic recovery, (b) reduced rate of infection, (c) reduced transfusion support, (d) reduced hospital stays, (e) faster immunologic reconstitution. However, compared to marrow collection more time is required for an adequate collection and many patients need large bore central venous catheters.

Thus, there are three ways to mobilize progenitor and stem cells from the marrow cavity to the blood stream. One involves chemotherapy alone where these cells are collected during rebound from hematologic nadir. This method is unpredictable in terms of scheduling collections as one has to wait for blood counts to recover; however, it does permit the patient to receive additional chemotherapy which if properly chosen can further treat the underlying malignancy. The second method utilizes myeloid growth factors which offer predictable timing of collections and is useful in collecting progenitor cells from normal donors in the allogeneic setting so these donors are not exposed to chemotherapy. The third method combines chemotherapy and myeloid growth factors allowing for collections with high percentages of progenitors and stem cells [8]:

- Collection during recovery from hematologic nadir after myelosuppressive chemotherapy
  - Unpredictable timing of apheresis
  - Toxicity of chemotherapy
  - Additional anti-neoplastic benefit
- Stimulation of progenitors into circulation with myeloid growth factors
  - Predictable timing of apheresis
  - Good yields of progenitor cells
  - No additional anti-neoplastic benefit
- Combination of recovery from myelosuppressive chemotherapy and stimulation with myeloid growth factors
  - Very high yields of progenitors
  - Unpredictable timing of apheresis
  - Toxicity of chemotherapy is less with use of growth factors
  - Additional anti-neoplastic benefit

Progenitors can be assayed in two ways: bioassays such as colony assays or flow cytometry. Bioassays can quantify clonogenic progenitors but can take weeks to be evaluable since colony formation is measured. A more rapid method involves quantification of the number of cells expressing the CD34 antigen. This antigen is present on stem cells and committed progenitors but as hematopoietic cells differentiate and lose their replicative capacity they lose expression of CD34. Through flow cytometry one can quantify the number of CD34 positive cells present in the product. It has been shown that at least $1-2 \times 10^6$ CD34 positive cells per kilogram patient body weight will lead to rapid, sustained hematologic recovery after high-dose chemotherapy [9].

## Phases of High-Dose Chemotherapy with Stem Cell Rescue

The phases of stem cell transplantation are as follows.

Preparation or Conditioning
– Make space
– Treatment
– Immunosuppresion (allo-setting)
– High-dose therapy: drugs
    – Cyclophosphamide
    – Busulfan
    – Thiotepa
    – VP-16
    – BCNU
    – Melphalan
– High-dose therapy: radiation
    – Total body radiotherapy
    – Total lymphoid radiotherapy
Stem Cell Transplant: Transplant/Rescue
– Allogeneic: graft versus leukemia
– Autologous: hematopoietic rescue
Posttransplant Care: Supportive Care
– Cytokines
– Blood products
– Antibiotics
– Nutrition
– Acute GvH prophylaxis treatment (allo-setting)
– Manage diarrhea
– Mucositis
– Consolidation
    – Radiotherapy
    – Immunotherapy

Once a soure of stem cells is secure, the first phase involves the administration of the high-dose therapy also called the preparative or conditioning regimen. The main goal is to treat the underlying malignant condition. However, in the allogeneic setting this conditioning also involves making space in the marrow cavity for new stem cells and immunosuppressing the host (patient) to prevent graft rejection.

After conditioning the progenitor cells are infused. In the autologous setting these cells are collected prior to high-dose therapy and cryopreserved in DMSO and stored in liquid nitrogen to maintain viability. The cryopreserved cells are then rapidly thawed at the bedside and reinfused into the patient. The major side effects of reinfusion relate to potential DMSO toxicity and include flushing, dyspnea and chest discomfort. In the allogeneic setting the cells are obtained fresh from the donor and reinfused as soon as available after conditioning.

The post-infusion period following administration of stem cells requires medical care of acute toxicities of the high-dose therapy and includes support of a pancytopenic period of approximately 10–14 days. In the allogeneic setting once engraftment of donor stem cells occurs graft versus host disease (GVHD) can intervene. Acute GVHD manifests itself in the skin, liver or GI tract with a characteristic rash, jaundice or voluminous diarrhea. Prophylactic immunosuppressive therapy with cyclosporine, steroids and/or methotrexate is begun before engraftment occurs to minimize this condition. The older the patient and the more disparate the HLA match between donor and patient the greater the likelihood of severe and sometimes fatal GVHD. After 100 days chronic GVHD can occur. The clinical manifestations of this disorder are more autoimmune in nature and include sclerodermatous skin changes, infections, and bronchiolitis obliterans with organizing pneumonia.

Additionaly as more patients undergo high-dose chemotherapy and survive longer there are other potential long term complications that may require specific medical intervention. These include effects the chemotherapy could have on endocrine function and fertility as well as the cardiopulmonary and hepatic systems. Therapy related myelodysplastic syndromes, leukemias and solid tumors have been reported [10, 11]. The use of long term steroids to treat some of the manifestations of GVHD can lead to aseptic necrosis of the femoral and/or humeral heads and cataracts. Thus, patients require long term follow-up with a specialist cognizant of these conditions.

## Results of High-Dose Chemotherapy

There are many indications for this therapeutic modality and include acute and chronic leukemias, lymphomas, myeloma and solid tumors such as breast cancer, ovarian cancer, testis cancer and neuroblastoma.

Each section will cover specific results of high-dose chemotherapy for each malignant disorder. The leading indication in North America for high-dose chemotherapy with stem cell rescue is breast cancer [12]. There are few randomized clinical trials of this therapy to support its routine use in many of these disorders. There are small trials in myeloma, lymphoma and breast cancer [13, 14, 15]. However, especially in breast cancer the results of larger randomized trials are pending further accrual. Further studies are necessary before high-dose chemotherapy can be considered non-investigational therapy in many settings including most solid tumors.

## Complications

Acute complications are related to the chemotherapeutic agents utilized but in general, nausea, vomiting, mucositis and diarrhea can occur. In patients who receive high-dose cyclophosphamide, hemorrhagic cystitis and cardiomyopathy are possible and require careful monitoring. Veno-occlusive disease of the liver can occur with any high-dose regimen. The clinical manifestations include jaundice, painful hepatomegaly and weight gain. Treatment is supportive in nature. Pulmonary complications can manifest as interstitial pneumonitis associated with cytomegalovirus infections in the allogeneic setting to diffuse alveolar hemorrhage treatable with steroids in the autologous setting.

Infectious complications can be problematic. Early in the course infections are related to the neutropenic state. Immune function nadirs 1–4 months post stem cell transplant. Immune reconstitution usually occurs about 6 months after an autologous reinfusion to 12 months after an uncomplicated allogeneic transplant. Cytomegalovirus infection can be very serious in allogeneic recipients and prophylaxis should be undertaken through appropriate transfusion support and antiviral thearpy. Herpes zoster can occur in up to 25% of patients after high-dose chemotherapy with stem cell rescue [16].

## Future Directions

As the results of large randomized clinical trials become available determination of appropriate patient groups who will benefit from this modality will be better defined. Additionally the introduction of newer chemotherapeutic agents such as the taxanes may improve upon clinical outcome. Further refinements in stem cell identification, processing and ex vivo culturing will further improve safety and increase the therapeutic index of this modality in clinical oncology.

**Acknowledgements.** I appreciate the secretarial skills of Karen Gordon in preparing this chapter.

### References

1. Frei E III, Teicher BA, Holden SA et al (1988) Preclinical studies and clinical correlation of the effect of alkylating dose. Cancer Res 48:6417–6423
2. Teicher BA, Cucci CA, Lee JB et al (1986) Alkylating agents in vitro studies of cross resistance patterns in human cell lines. Cancer Res 46:4379–4383
3. Henderson IC, Hayes DF, Gelman R (1988) Dose-response in the treatment of breast cancer: a critical review. J Clin Oncol 6:1501–1515
4. Richman CM, Weiner RS, Yankee RA (1976) Increase in circulating stem cells following chemotherapy in man. Blood 47, 1031–1039
5. Gianni Am, Siena S, Bregni M et al (1989) Granulocyte-macrophage colony-stimulating factor to harvest circulating stem cells for autotransplant. Lancet 2:58–585
6. Zimmerman TM, Mick R, Myers S et al (1995) Source of stem cells impacts upon hematopoietic recovery after high dose chemotherapy. Bone Marrow Trans 15:973–927
7. Talmadge JE, Reed E, Ino K, et al (1997) Rapid immunologic reconstitution following transplantation with mobilized peripheral blood stem cells as compared to bone marrow. Bone Marrow Trans 19:161–172
8. Bender JG, Williams SF, Myers S, et al (1992) Characterization of chemotherapy mobilized peripheral blod progenitor cells for use in autologous stem cell transplantation. Bone Marrow Transpl 10:281–285
9. Bender JG, To LB, Williams SF et al (1992) Defining a therapeutic dose of peripheral blood stem cells. J Hematother 1:329–341
10. Vose JM, Kennedy BC, Bierman PJ et al (1992) Long-term sequelae of autologous bone marrow or peripheral stem cell transplantation for lymphoid malignancies. Cancer 69:784–789
11. Curtis RE, Rowlings PA, Deeg HJ, et al (1997) Solid cancers after bone marrow transplantation. N Engl J Med 336, 897–904
12. Antman KH, Rowlings PA, Vaughan WP et al (1997) High-dose chemotherapy with autologous hematopoietic stem-cell support for breast cancer in North America. J Clin Oncol 15:1870–1879
13. Attal M, Harousseau J-L, Stoppa A-M, et al (1996) A prospective, randomized trial of autologous bone marrow transplantation and chemotherapy in multiple myeloma. N Engl J Med 335:91–97
14. Philip T, Guglielmi C, Hagenbeek A, et al (1995) Autologous bone marrow transplantation as compared with salvage chemotherapy in relapses of chemotherapy-sensitive non-Hodgkins lymphoma. N Engl J Med 333:1540–1545

15. Bezwoda WR, Seymour L, Dansey RD: High-dose chemotherapy with hematopoie-
    tic rescue as primary treatment for metastatic breast cancer: A randomized trial. J
    Clin Oncoll 13:2483–2489
16. Schuchter L, Wingard J, Piantadosi S, et al (1989) Herpes zoster infection after auto-
    logous bone marrow transplantation. Blood 74:1424–1427

# Cancer Immunotherapy

T.F. Gajewski

## Introduction

The remarkable specificity of the adaptive immune system has long attracted immunologists to seek application in the treatment of cancer. The era of immunosuppressive drugs and AIDS has revealed that an intact immune system is required for protection against many cancers, particularly those with a viral origin. Animal models have demonstrated the powerful capability of an appropriately activated cellular immune response to reject established tumors. Immunomodulatory cytokines, monoclonal antibodies, and antigen-specific vaccination approaches have entered the clinical arena in the treatment of melanoma, renal cell carcinoma, breast cancer, and lymphoma, among others. Immune-based therapy is thus emerging as a valid fourth therapeutic modality in cancer treatment.

## History

The hypothesis that the immune system might be capable of promoting regression of human cancers was proposed a century ago when William Coley treated sarcomas with bacterial extracts, generating response rates of approximately 15% [1]. Specific immunity against experimental tumors was first reported by Gross in 1943 [2]. In that model, implantation of methylcholanthrene-induced sarcomas into syngeneic mice followed by surgical resection led to immunologic protection of those mice against rechallenge with the same tumor but not against other related tumors. Similar results have since been obtained with tumors induced by other carcinogens, including 3, 4-benzopyrene, ultraviolet light, or viruses, and also with spontaneous murine tumors [3, 4]. T cell-deficient nude mice were found to be unable to mount such tumor protection, arguing that T lymphocytes were required for rejection. The absence of cross-protection of mice against other tumors similar to the initial implant suggested that the dominant immune response in these models was against antigens unique to each tumor.

The existence of shared tumor antigens that might have broader therapeutic implications was first suggested by the tumor-minus (tum⁻) experiments by Boon and colleagues in the 1970s. Treatment of several different established tumor cell lines that normally grew progressively in syngeneic mice with the mutagen *N*-methyl-*N*=-nitro-*N*-nitrosoguanidine rendered them susceptible to rapid immune-mediated rejection [5]. Apparently, a mutational event resulted in new antigens that stimulated a stronger immune response. Importantly, most mice rejecting these mutated tum⁻ cells also rejected a challenge with the non-mutated parental tumor, suggesting that at least one antigen was shared between the two tumor variants. It appeared that shared antigens existed in the parental tumors but were less capable of initiating an immune response on their own. Cytolytic T lymphocytes (CTL) could be identified from protected mice that either recognized uniquely the mutated tumor or recognized both the mutated variant and the parental line [6]. These observations suggested that CTL might comprise the effector population mediating the final tumor rejection event, and also provided a tool for identifying the antigens themselves.

The field of tumor immunology gained a respectable footing upon the successful molecular cloning of genes encoding tumor antigens recognized by CTL [7]. The first tumor antigen genes identified were those encoding unique antigens expressed by the immunogenic murine tum⁻ variants [8]. These neoantigens appeared to arise from point mutations in normal genes [9, 10]. The first gene encoding a shared antigen was identified from the mouse mastocytoma P815 and is designated P1 A [11, 12]. This gene is expressed in several mouse tumor lines tested but appears to be silent in normal tissues except for the testis and placenta [13]. In those tissues, P1 A is present in cells that lack expression of class I molecules encoded by the major histocompatibility complex (MHC), making them invisible to the host immune system [13]. Thus, this antigen can be considered to be truly tumor-specific, and provides one of the most useful preclinical models for studying anti-tumor immunity.

The molecular validation that shared, non-mutated tumor antigens could exist in murine tumors paved the way for the identification of similar antigens from human cancers. The first human tumor antigen gene cloned was isolated from a melanoma cell line and was designated MAGE-1 [14]. MAGE-1 was the first identified member of a family of at least 12 genes, most of which, like the mouse P1 A gene, are expressed only in tumor cells and in the testis [15]. The powerful technique of expression cloning utilizing specific CTL that recognize the desired antigen as a detection method has since been applied to many additional tumors, and has led to the identification of multiple human tumor antigens that could serve as targets for specific immunotherapy in patients. As such, these efforts at precise antigen characterization constitute a major accomplishment in modern tumor immunology.

In parallel with the identification of specific tumor antigens, the molecular understanding of T lymphocyte biology exploded in the 1980s. In particular, the identification of cytokines produced by T cells and other cell types of the immune system allowed for a dissection of the complex regulatory interactions that control the initiation, expansion, quiescence, and memory of specific immune responses. The molecular cloning of the cDNAs encoding these immunoregulatory molecules provided a means for large-scale production by the biotechnology industry, thus allowing their testing in human clinical trials. The pioneering efforts by Rosenberg and colleagues demonstrated that administration of the T cell growth factor interleukin-2 (IL-2) induced major clinical responses in patients with metastatic renal cell carcinoma and melanoma [16], providing the first real evidence that interventions aimed at potentiating the cellular immune response could constitute a viable treatment strategy for human malignancy. Similar clinical experience with leukocyte-derived interferon-α (IFN-α) has demonstrated responses in patients with a variety of malignancies, and has led to the first effective treatment in the post-surgical adjuvant setting for melanoma [17]. A multitude of additional recombinant cytokines has since been examined in human clinical trials, and logical combinations of factors are being explored to control specific events involved in generating specific immunity.

Most efforts in cancer immunotherapy are currently focused on initiating tumor antigen-specific T cell or antibody responses using vaccination strategies, and modulating the host immune response by the administration of cytokines.

## General Principles of Anti-tumor Immunity

Effector Mechanisms

There are several routes by which the immune system can destroy tumors. The most straightforward to conceptualize is that mediated by antibodies. Antibodies recognize antigens directly in solution. With respect to tumors, this property restricts the role of antibodies to the binding of surface proteins expressed on the tumor cell membrane. Once bound, antibodies can theoretically promote tumor destruction through complement activation, or by activating leukocytes via Fc receptors that are ligated by a domain in the heavy chain of the antibody molecule. The technology to produce monoclonal antibodies developed in the 1970s by Cesar Milstein and Georges Kohler has provided a means to generate the large quantities necessary for administration to human patients, and earned a Nobel Prize for those investigators in 1984. Passively administered monoclonal antibodies can be conjugated to chemical or radioactive toxins, providing a novel alternative effector mechanism for promoting tumor destruction that does not technically rely on normal immunologic functions. Other non-immunologic ways in which antibodies might influence tumor growth is by ligating a receptor that delivers a pro-apoptotic signal, or through blocking a growth factor receptor that leads to apoptotic death secondary to growth factor deprivation.

Antibody responses are normally generated to protect against bacterial and viral pathogens. In contrast, T cell responses are generated against tissue grafts, intracellular pathogens, and chronic infections. As such, a T cell-mediated immune response may be more useful for attempting to eliminate a long-standing tumor mass. Unlike antibodies, an antigen-specific T cell receptor (TCR) does not recognize whole antigen in solution, but rather sees a peptide fragment of an antigen bound to a groove in a specific MHC molecule. There are two major subclasses of T cells, those that express CD4 and those that express CD8. CD4+ T cells recognize antigenic peptides bound to class II MHC molecules, whereas CD8+ T cells recognize peptides presented by class I MHC molecules. This property of MHC-restriction of T cell recognition was a major breakthrough in immunology that earned a Nobel Prize for Rolph Zinkernagel and Peter Doherty in 1996. The crystal structure of each type of MHC molecule bound to peptides has been solved, and has provided invaluable information about the nature of TCR ligands.

Expression of class II MHC molecules is generally restricted to professional antigen-presenting cells, such as dendritic cells, B cells, and macrophages. In contrast, essentially all nucleated cells express class I MHC molecules. Therefore, most tumors are class I$^+$ but class II$^-$, implying that CD8$^+$ T cells represent the predominant effector cell for tumor-specific cellular immunity. CD8$^+$ T cells are generally cytolytic, and kill target cells via one of two mechanisms. The first is by releasing granules that contain a protein called perforin that forms a pore in the target cell membrane, along with other enzymes called granzymes that pass through that pore and initiate apoptosis in the affected cell [18, 19]. The second lytic mechanism is mediated by expression of Fas-ligand on the surface of the T cell which ligates Fas expressed on the target cell, initiating a programmed apoptotic pathway resulting in death [20]. Activated T cells also can express armed Fas, giving rise to the unusual situation that both the effector T cells and the tumor cells may be competing for Fas-mediated death.

Natural killer (NK) cells also possess cytolytic activity. The receptor expressed by NK cells that triggers their lytic machinery is poorly characterized. In contrast to T cells, NK cells do not appear to kill targets in an MHC-restricted fashion. Rather, many NK cells have been shown to be inhibited by particular class I MHC molecules, through ligation of a killer inhibitory receptor [21]. Thus, NK cells are thought to be activated when the target cell *lacks* MHC molecules. This property might be critical under situations in which CD8$^+$ CTL select for antigen-loss or MHC-loss tumor cell variants.

Lymphokine-activated killer (LAK) cells were developed as a nonspecific cytolytic cell population. They are derived by long-term culture of lymphocytes in IL-2, and appear to have the ability to kill a broad array of tumor cell types. The lineage and phenotype of LAK cells is not completely clear, and their potential role in a normal immune response also is uncertain. Nonetheless, they have been utilized therapeutically in attempts to treat established tumors in vivo.

Macrophages can participate in the effector phase of an anti-tumor immune response through the release of inflammatory cytokines, oxygen radicals, nitrates, and other mediators. One important cytokine that activates macrophage function is interferon-$\gamma$ (IFN-$\gamma$), which is produced by a subset of effector T cells and by NK cells. It is thought that macrophages also participate in the remodeling of blood vessels, both positively and negatively, and therefore might be involved in regulating tumor neovascularization. Neutrophils and eosinophils also have been proposed to participate in anti-tumor immune responses, but like macrophages, this relationship might be either antagonistic or augmentative for tumor growth.

Cytokines in some circumstances can be considered effector molecules for tumor regression. For example, tumor-necrosis factor-$\alpha$ (TNF-$\alpha$) can result in tumor microvessel destruction, thus indirectly causing tumor cell death. IFN-$\alpha$ and IFN-$\gamma$ can exert direct antiproliferative effects on tumor cells, and also upregulate the expression of MHC molecules on the surface of tumor cells.

## Induction of T Cell Responses

In order to understand the rationale behind some of the current immunotherapeutic interventions being performed in cancer treatment, it is necessary to appreciate some of the central events in T cell activation and differentiation. Naive, resting T cells do not possess effector function but must differentiate into effector cells following encounter with antigen in a secondary lymphoid organ. This initial activation event is performed by professional antigen-presenting cells (APC), the most potent of which is called a dendritic cell (DC). APCs pick up exogenous antigen, process it into peptide fragments, and re-present it on the cell surface bound to MHC molecules. DCs are resident in most normal tissues, and under inflammatory conditions become activated and carry endocytosed antigen to regional draining lymph nodes. There, circulating naive T cells percolate through, sampling the array of antigenic peptides present on the relocated DCs. Any T cells that bear a specific TCR that recognizes that peptide antigen/MHC complex are retained in the lymph node and become activated.

In addition to ligation of the TCR, the APC provides other signals that are critical for T cell activation and differentiation. These include adhesion molecules, such as ICAM-1 that engages LFA-1 on the T cell surface; and also costimulatory molecules, such as B7–1 and B7–2 that ligate the costimulatory receptor CD28 on the responding T cell [22–24]. Engagement of the TCR without providing B7-family costimulation not only fails to completely activate T cells, but paradoxically can induce an unresponsive state termed clonal anergy [25–27].

Cytokines produced by the APC also control T cell differentiation. IL-12 is a critical cytokine that promotes the acquisition of cytolytic machinery and the capability of a T cell to produce high quantities of the inflammatory cytokines IFN-γ and TNF-α[23, 28]. T cells with this particular functional phenotype are designated Th1 or Tc1 cells, if they are CD4+ or CD8+, respectively [29–31]. In contrast, T cells activated in the presence of IL-4 differentiate into a Th2/Tc2 phenotype, characterized by the ability to produce IL-4, IL-5, and IL-10, and possessing inferior cytolytic activity [31, 32]. Th2 cells appear to promote optimal B cell activation, particularly to produce antibodies of the IgE isotype. It is generally thought that optimal tumor rejection will be mediated by Th1/Tc1 cells [33, 34].

Once the initial activation sequence of naive T cells begins, the activated cells produce IL-2, which drives T cell proliferation and expansion via autocrine as well as paracrine pathways. The expanded, differentiated effector cells then leave the lymph node via the efferent lymphatics and re-enter the peripheral circulation. Effector T cells are capable of penetrating into inflamed tissues by crossing the vascular endothelium. This transmigration is dependent upon homing receptors and adhesion molecules on the T cells interacting with specific counterreceptors on the endothelial cells. Migration is guided by chemoattractant factors called chemokines, different types of which cooperate to attract various subtypes of leukocytes, including T cells, into sites of inflammation. Once in the inflamed tissue, the effector T cells might be triggered to die by apoptosis soon after they execute their effector function, which may limit the duration of their efficacy.

Interventions which augment or promote each of these requisite steps in T cell activation and effector function are being explored in preclinical and clinical studies. These include strategies that stimulate non-specific tissue inflammation, DC expansion and activation, antigen processing and presentation, B7 costimulation, appropriate T cell differentiation, T cell expansion, T cell trafficking into tumors, and effector T cell survival.

## Immunotherapeutic Approaches

A convenient way to segregate immunotherapy approaches is by whether they are passive or active, and specific or non-specific. *Passive* immunotherapy implies direct administration of effector molecules or cells to the patient, whereas *active* approaches attempt to elicit that effector phase from the host's own immune system. *Non-specific* immunotherapy aims to induce inflammation or otherwise amplify immune responses that are present in the host, whereas *specific* approaches rely on antigen recognition by antibodies or T cells. This general categorization is summarized in Table 1, and major examples will be discussed in the context of this framework. Most advances in the translation of information learned from preclinical studies into clinical application have been made in melanoma. However, it should be emphasized that, with a few important exceptions, immunologic approaches are largely experimental and still in the development stages.

Passive, Non-specific

*LAK Cells*

LAK cells were first generated in murine models by stimulating lymphocytes in vitro with high concentrations of IL-2. These cells were capable of killing a variety of murine tumor cells in vitro, and also mediated tumor rejection following adoptive therapy (along with IL-2) into mice in vivo [35, 36]. In light of success in preclinical models, Rosenberg and colleagues initiated clinical trials of human autologous LAK cells plus IL-2 in patients with advanced cancer. Overall, approximately 25% of patients with renal cell carcinoma or melanoma exhibited a clinical response, with 5%–10% experiencing a durable complete res-

**Table 1.** Categorization of immunotherapeutic approaches

| Approach | Examples |
| --- | --- |
| Passive, non-specific | LAK cells |
| | Ex vivo expanded, non-specific T cells |
| | Cytokines |
| Passive, specific | Monoclonal antibodies |
| | Antibody-toxin conjugates |
| | Ex vivo expanded, specific T cells |
| Active, non-specific | BCG, *C. parvum* |
| | Anti-CD3 mAb |
| | Cytokines |
| | In vivo gene transfer |
| Active, specific | Tumor cell-based vaccines |
| | CTL epitope-based vaccines |
| | Ganglioside and other antibody-inducing vaccines |

ponse. However, subsequent studies using IL-2 alone resulted in similar response rates [16]. Randomized clinical trials have since been performed in both renal cell carcinoma and in melanoma comparing IL-2 with or without LAK cells, demonstrating no significant improvement in survival for the patients receiving LAK cells [37]. Thus, the clinical results achieved with this regimen can be attributed to IL-2. Although the underlying premise that LAK cells were important mediators of tumor rejection was not validated, these studies nonetheless provided the important conclusion that administration of a cytokine that acts on T cells could result in meaningful clinical responses in cancer.

*Non-specific T Cells*

It has been suggested that cancer patients become generally immunosuppressed, particularly in the setting of advanced disease. This is evidenced clinically by a high incidence of anergy to skin testing for recall antigens. Several investigators have documented specific T cell signaling defects in patients with advanced cancers of several histologies [38]. It is thus reasoned that removing T cells from that immunosuppressive environment, activating them in vitro, and reinfusing them might bypass that immunosuppressive block. Pan-activation of T cells using anti-CD3 mAb (which ligates the invariant signal-transducing $\epsilon$ chain associated with the TCR) in vitro followed by reinfusion into mice has resulted in regression of large established tumors [39]. This approach has been examined in a phase I clinical trial in patients with advanced cancer, with interesting preliminary results [40].

As mentioned previously, optimal T cell activation requires not only ligation of the T cell receptor but also the engagement of costimulatory receptors such as CD28. June and colleagues have demonstrated that human T cells can be expanded logarithmically for an extended period of time using a combination of anti-CD3 and anti-CD28 mAb coupled to beads [41]. In preliminary studies, autologous T cells expanded with this regimen have been reinfused back into HIV patients in an attempt to restore T cell numbers, with promising results. Similar studies have recently been initiated in cancer patients to assess the anti-tumor efficacy of this adoptive therapy regimen. It is anticipated that T cells activated with anti-CD3 plus anti-CD28 mAb may have superior anti-tumor activity compared to T cells activated with anti-CD3 mAb alone.

## Cytokines

Cytokines are produced by T lymphocytes, macrophages, dendritic cells, and other cells, and mediate communication between the participants of an inflammatory response. The biologic effect of cytokines can be either stimulatory or inhibitory for particular immunologic functions. Multiple cytokines that might augment immune responses or inhibit tumor growth have been examined in pre-clinical and clinical studies. Examples of clinical trials utilizing cytokines having immunopotentiating or direct anti-proliferative properties are depicted in Table 2.

Several cytokines are thought to act, in part, as direct effector molecules that cooperate to suppress tumor growth or cooperate to induce cytotoxicity. The two principal examples are the interferons and TNF-$\alpha$. Both IFN-$\alpha$ and IFN-$\gamma$ can induce upregulation of MHC molecule expression on the surface of tumor cells, and also may augment expression of genes encoding other proteins involved in antigen processing, such as TAP and components of the proteosome [42]. Interferons also have anti-proliferative activity and may induce direct tumor cell death [43]. It is probably through this direct anti-tumoral activity that IFN-$\alpha$ has found application in the treatment of CML, hairy cell leukemia, lymphoma, Kaposi's sarcoma, and other malignancies [43]. The possibility that an immunologic mechanism participates even in these effects is suggested by the observation that IFN-$\alpha$ therapy of Kaposi's sarcoma in HIV patients is only effective in those individuals with CD4 T cell counts greater than 200/$\mu$l [44].

TNF-$\alpha$ has demonstrated anti-tumor activity as a single agent in murine preclinical studies. However, systemic administration to human

**Table 2.** Important immunologically active cytokines explored in human clinical trials

| Cytokine | Tumor type | Reference |
|---|---|---|
| IL-2 | Renal cell, melanoma | [16, 65] |
| IL-4 | Renal cell, melanoma | [134] |
| IL-6 | Various | [135] |
| IL-12 | Various | Studies ongoing |
| TNF-$\alpha$ | Various | [46, 50, 136] |
| IFN-$\alpha$ | Renal cell, melanoma | [17, 43, 137, 138] |
| IFN-$\gamma$ | Renal cell, melanoma | [136, 139, 140] |
| M-CSF | Various | [141, 142] |
| GM-CSF | Melanoma | [75, 76] |
| Flt3-L | Various | Studies ongoing |

cancer patients has revealed unacceptable toxicity at biologically active doses. To overcome this limitation, TNF-α also has been administered locally, by installation into the peritoneum or pleural space for malignant effusions, or at high concentrations in isolated limb perfusion for the treatment of melanoma or sarcoma confined to the extremity. TNF-α in combination with melphalan and IFN-γ administered by limb perfusion has resulted in response rates exceeding 90% [45, 46], allowing surgical limb sparing in the majority of patients with sarcoma and melanoma. However, recurrence at distal sites is still common, and overall survival may not be affected. In addition, the procedure is cumbersome and expensive, requiring coordinated efforts of surgeons, cardiac bypass equipment and support staff, nuclear medicine specialists to monitor for limb leak, and individuals experienced in cytokine administration. Isolated limb perfusion should thus be considered investigational. The mechanism by which TNF-α exerts its anti-tumor effect at high doses appears to be through blockade of neovascularization, in part by decreasing binding of the integrin αvβ3 [47], a critical cell surface molecule for angiogenesis [48].

## Passive, Specific

### Monoclonal Antibodies

Specific immunotherapy involves participation of either antibodies or T lymphocytes, both of which have the potential for recognizing particular antigens with tremendous precision. Passive, specific immunotherapy relies on the adoptive transfer of tumor antigen-specific antibodies or T cells into a recipient, with the goal of directly mediating tumor regression or protection.

Many antibodies have been examined in clinical trials in almost every malignancy, and a list of some of the most promising agents is depicted in Table 3. Two of these antibodies have shown rather dramatic effects in common solid tumors and warrant further discussion. The first is against the Her-2/*neu* gene product. Her-2/*neu* is a proto-oncogene expressed in approximately 25% of breast and ovarian cancers, as well as some other tumors [49], that encodes a 185 kd cell surface protein resembling the epidermal growth factor receptor. mAbs against the Her-2/*neu* protein have been examined in clinical trials in the setting of metastatic

**Table 3.** Important tumor-specific antibodies examined in human clinical trials

| Tumor type | Antibody specificity | Reference |
|---|---|---|
| Breast cancer | Her-2/neu | [50, 51] |
| Colon carcinoma | gp72 (RTA-conjugated) | [143] |
| Lymphoma | CD20 | [52, 53] |
| B-lymphoid malignancies | CD19 (blocked-ricin-conjugated) | [144] |
| Melanoma | Gangliosides GD2, GD3 | [145, 146] |

breast cancer, revealing some therapeutic efficacy as a single agent [50]. Recent studies of systemic chemotherapy with or without anti-Her-2/*neu* mAb have shown a striking advantage for the combination, with response rates of 36% for chemotherapy alone versus 62% for the chemotherapy plus anti-Her-2/*neu* mAb [51]. It should be noted that this mAb is not necessarily functioning via an immunologic mechanism, but may be blocking binding of a putative growth factor to this receptor or over-ligating the molecule, predisposing the tumor cells to apoptosis.

A second important antibody demonstrating clinical efficacy is directed against the CD20 marker expressed on B cell lymphomas. As a single agent, response rates of approximately 50% have been observed in patients with relapsed low-grade non-Hodgkin's lymphoma (NHL) [52]. Combination of anti-CD20 mAb plus CHOP chemotherapy has yielded responses near 100% in intermediate- and high-grade NHL [53], with demonstration of molecular CR in the majority of patients. Based on these and other similar results, the Rituximab anti-CD20 mAb has recently been approved by the FDA for the treatment of relapsed or refractory low-grade NHL. It is not clear if this agent is functioning through an immunologic mechanism or by ligating CD20 and inducing apoptosis in the tumor cells.

## Specific T Cells

In parallel with studies utilizing non-specifically activated T cells, other investigators have pursued the approach of expanding specific T cells that only recognize specific antigens present on the tumor cells of the recipient. The proof of concept for this approach was nicely demonstrated by Greenberg and colleagues with virus-specific T cells in the post-allogeneic bone marrow transplant setting. Such patients are often immunosuppressed for prolonged periods, and can develop life-threatening infections with cytomegalovirus (CMV). CMV-specific CTL were developed from the peripheral blood of bone marrow donors and infused into the recipient patients [54]. Persistent anti-viral immunity was detected in the blood of recipients, demonstrating that adoptive specific T cell therapy was safe and functional. Preclinical studies in cancer models have shown regression of established tumors using this approach, suggesting that clinical trials in patients with advanced cancer will be forthcoming.

As an alternative to deriving specific T cell clones from the peripheral blood of patients, Rosenberg and colleagues have expanded T cells isolated from melanoma tumors for adoptive therapy. These so-called tumor-infiltrating lymphocyte (TIL) populations contain a high proportion of T cells that recognize tumor antigens expressed by the melanoma cells, and can be expanded in vitro with IL-2. Treatment of melanoma patients with TILs plus IL-2 has generated clinical responses in patients who failed therapy with IL-2 alone, suggesting that the addition of tumor-specific T cells to IL-2 therapy may be beneficial [55]. Randomized clinical trials have yet to be performed.

## Active, Non-specific

### Bacillus Calmette-Guerin

BCG activates macrophages and DC to promote a Th1/Tc1-type immune response, and therefore might be considered a good adjuvant to consider for inducing anti-tumor effects. Initial attempts in melanoma utilizing BCG given systemically, either combined with chemotherapy in patients with metastatic disease or as post-surgical adjuvant treatment in high risk stage III patients, failed to show improved response rates or survival [56, 57]. Of interest is the observation that patients who converted to a positive PPD during therapy appeared to have a longer survival, arguing that immune modulation, when successful, did confer benefit. BCG also has been injected intralesionally into cutaneous melanoma tumors, yielding a 33% response rate [58]. This local effect of BCG has perhaps had the greatest effect in the intravesicular treatment of superficial bladder cancer, decreasing post-surgical recurrence rate from 70% to 30% [59]. Installation of BCG has thus become a standard therapy for this disease.

Although the success of conventional BCG has been limited, its use has been reconsidered as a component of antigen-specific vaccines. The technology to generate recombinant BCG organisms having genes encoding specific antigens incorporated into their genome has allowed the transformation of a non-specific immune stimulator into a specific vaccination vector [60]. Clinical application of this approach to cancer treatment has yet to be performed.

## Anti-CD3 mAbs

One way to augment T cell responses in vivo is to administer activating doses of anti-CD3 mAb, which binds to the invariable ε chain of the TCR-associated CD3 complex. Although high doses of this mAb deplete T cells and are immunosuppressive, low doses trigger cytokine release without compromising the T cell pool. Preclinical murine models demonstrated that this approach of activating T cells non-specifically could generate significant tumor regression responses [61]. However, pilot human clinical trials have failed to confirm such results with cancer patients [62], and anti-CD3 mAb plus IL-2 was not more effective than IL-2 alone in melanoma and renal cell carcinoma [63]. It is conceivable that the murine tumor models utilized in the preclinical experiments were particularly sensitive to TNF, which is produced in substantial quantities following treatment with low-dose anti-CD3 mAb in vivo. As an extension of this approach, hybrid antibodies have been constructed such that one binding site recognizes CD3ε and the other binds to a surface-expressed tumor-specific antigen. Such heteroconjugate antibodies should bring T cells into the vicinity of a tumor cell expressing the targeted antigen and activate them in situ. Preclinical murine studies with some these reagents have been promising [64].

## Cytokines

Based on the hypothesis that some patients have initiated generation of a low-level but ineffective anti-tumor immune response spontaneously, cytokines have been administered in an attempt to amplify or modify that response with the hope of promoting tumor regression. A multitude of cytokines has been administered systemically to cancer patients, the most important of which are listed in Table 2. Several of these have interesting properties and warrant further discussion. These are IL-2, IL-12, GM-CSF, and Flt3-ligand.

IL-2 is a growth factor for T lymphocytes and NK cells, and is thought to amplify pre-existing immune effector cells that in turn induce tumor cell killing. IL-2 was first explored as a bolus intravenous infusion in patients with advanced malignancies, and clinical responses were seen predominantly in patients with melanoma and renal cell carcinoma [16]. Overall, the response rate is approximately 15%–20% in those patients, with about 5% of patients achieving complete responses, most of them durable. IL-2 is the most effective single agent in metastatic renal cell carcinoma, and it is approved by the FDA for this indication. It is usually administered as 600,000 IU/kg every 8 h by IV infusion for 5 days for 14 total doses followed by 9 days of rest and a second identical course. More recently, this regimen was shown to produce responses in metastatic melanoma comparable to those seen in renal cell carcinoma [65], prompting recent FDA approval for this indication as well. Other less toxic dosing regimens for IL-2 have been examined and are discussed in the chapters regarding those specific malignancies. Occasional clinical responses to IL-2 have also been observed in patients with lymphoma and colon carcinoma.

IL-12 is a cytokine normally produced by dendritic cells and macrophages, and acts predominantly on T cells and NK cells. T cells undergoing antigen-specific activation are directed by IL-12 to differentiate into a Th1/Tc1 phenotype, producing high levels of IFN-$\gamma$ and TNF-$\alpha$ and having high cytolytic capability [66–68]. In murine pre-clinical models, IL-12 has shown potent anti-tumor activity in several tumor systems that is dependent on T cells and, in some models, on NK cells [69, 70]. IL-12 also has anti-angiogenic properties [71]. In tumor models that are relatively resistant to IL-12 alone, co-administration of IL-12 during tumor antigen immunization schemes results in complete tumor regression that is dependent on cytotoxic T cells [72–74]. Phase I and phase II clinical trials have been completed with IL-12 as a single agent, and studies are underway utilizing IL-12 to potentiate tumor antigen vaccines.

GM-CSF was originally developed for clinical application as a hematopoietic growth factor to protect against chemotherapy-induced myelosuppression. However, this cytokine also has an immunologic activity, as it stimulates the expansion and activation of dendritic cells, which might be expected to result in enhanced presentation of tumor antigens promoting tumor-specific T cell activation. Second generation clinical trials are underway using GM-CSF alone or in combination with other agents to capitalize on its immunopotentiating properties [75, 76]. Flt3-ligand is another hematopoietic growth factor that potently expands dendritic cells in vivo [77]. In preclinical models, administration of Flt3-ligand can induce significant tumor regression [78, 79]. Clinical trials in cancer patients are underway to assess the anti-tumor activity of Flt3-ligand in humans.

## In Vivo Gene Transfer

One method being developed in an attempt to promote tumor regression involves intralesional injection of an expression vector encoding an allogeneic class I MHC molecule. Conceptually, this should initiate activation of alloreactive T cells that should kill the successfully transduced tumor cells. It is thought that this tumor cell death might result in delivery of new antigens to the host immune system and initiate a second wave of T cell responses against tumor-specific antigens, which in turn might kill non-transduced tumor cells. Pilot clinical trials utilizing HLA-B7 have been completed in renal cell carcinoma, colon carcinoma, and melanoma, which have demonstrated that in vivo gene expression can be achieved [80, 81]. In addition, some clinical responses have been observed in the injected tumor of some patients, but regression of non-injected tumors has only rarely been observed. This technology also is being utilized to introduce cytokine genes into tumor lesions.

## Active, Specific

### Tumor Cell-Based Vaccines

The ultimate goal of active, specific immunotherapy is to vaccinate a patient such that a long-lived, tumor-specific immune response is induced that causes rejection of active disease as well as protective immunologic memory. The simplest source of tumor antigens to consider is from tumor cells themselves, and vaccination with lethally irradiated autologous or allogeneic tumor cell lines has been examined for a number of years in both preclinical and clinical studies. The advantage of this approach is that the immunization will include all the hypothetical antigens present in the patient's tumor. However, the disadvantages include potential expression of low levels of MHC molecules that might be insufficient to initiate T cell priming; possible secretion of inhibitory factors, such as TGF-β, that can prevent T cell activation; expression of molecules such as Fas-ligand, that can kill activated T cells expressing Fas; and lack of tumor expression of B7-family costimulator molecules, that may result in induction of specific T cell anergy rather than activation. Despite these limitations, immunization with irradiated tumor cells is indeed effective at inducing tumor-specific protection in some murine models, although clinical trials in melanoma utilizing irradiated autologous tumor cells have shown only an occasional response [82]. Combining adjuvants, such as BCG, with autologous melanoma cells has generated higher response rates of approximately 15% [82], suggesting that other factors from the host immune system are necessary in addition to antigen for initiation of T cell priming. Determining the status of the immune response in these patients and whether it correlates with disease outcome may help identify the critical factors required for a successful anti-tumor response, but this is difficult using whole tumor cell-based vaccination approaches due to lack of knowledge of the dominant tumor antigens present in the vaccine.

To overcome the difficulty of obtaining tumor cells from every patient to be treated, Morton and colleagues have utilized pooled allogeneic melanoma cell lines as a common source of tumor antigens. Response rates of 20% have been observed in patients with metastatic melanoma, with maximal benefit being seen in patients with small metastases [83]. This vaccine also is being used in patients following surgical resection of isolated metastases, as an adjuvant to prevent disease recurrence, with promising preliminary results.

In order to increase the immunogenicity of tumor cells, Berd and colleagues have pursued an approach of haptenization of autologous melanoma cells prior to their injection back into the patient. The rationale is that coupling of the tumor surface proteins with dinitrophenyl (DNP), which is strongly antigenic, will help elicit a stronger immune response against the tumor antigens as well. Several clinical responses have been seen in patients treated with DNP-modified autologous melanoma cells plus BCG [84, 85]. This vaccine approach has been examined in the post-surgical adjuvant setting, yielding a 5-year survival rate of over 50% [86]. Survival was greatest for patients who developed a DTH response to the vaccine, and in patients who showed an inflammatory response in metastatic lesions. Comparison of this adjuvant treatment to other therapies, such as IFN-$\alpha$, should be forthcoming.

Another methodology for augmenting immune responses against tumor cell-based vaccines is by transfection to express immunomodulatory molecules. By this approach, cytokines and costimulatory molecules normally produced by APC or helper T cells can be produced locally wherever the injected tumor cell transfectants migrate. A multitude of cDNAs encoding cytokines and other molecules has been transfected into murine tumor cells, with some remarkable effects in preclinical studies in vivo [87, 88]. Several of these deserve further comment: those engineered to express B7, GM-CSF, or IL-12. These molecules have been studied extensively in preclinical systems, the success of which suggests that clinical application to cancer patients will be undertaken in the near future.

As mentioned previously, B7 is a costimulatory molecule expressed by APC that engages CD28 on T cells. Ligation of CD28 augments cytokine production and proliferation, and prevents induction of T cell anergy [26, 89, 90]. Expression of B7-family molecules in several different mouse tumors that normally grow progressively resulted in potent regression in vivo, via a mechanism dependent upon CD8$^+$ T cells [91–93]. In addition, immunization with lethally irradiated B7-transfectants has protected mice against challenge with wildtype tumors [94], indicating that immunologic memory was induced.

As an alternative to expressing a molecule on the tumor cell that makes it function as a better APC, one might envision expressing a molecule that recruits and activates host APC to the vaccine site. During a screen of multiple different cytokine transfections in the Renca tumor model, Dranoff and colleagues observed that irradiated tumor cells expressing GM-CSF were particularly immunogenic [95]. Consistent with the known property of GM-CSF to activate DC, immunization appeared to depend upon host APC [96]. The safety of, and prior experience with, GM-CSF in cancer patients makes it an attractive candidate for clinical application.

The ability of IL-12 to promote the desired Th1/Tc1-type T cell response has promoted its examination in tumor transfectant vaccines as well. Immunization with irradiated IL-12-transfectants was shown not only to protect mice against subsequent tumor challenge but also eliminated large pre-established tumors [73, 97]. This anti-tumor effect was antigen-specific, as it depended upon shared antigens between the growing tumor in the mouse and the IL-12-transfectant used to vaccinate. The completion of phase I and phase II clinical trials using IL-12 makes it possible to consider the use of this factor as a vaccine adjuvant in patients.

## CTL Epitope Tumor Antigen Vaccines

The possibility that tumor cells, which are derived from self tissues, could express antigens recognizable by T cells from the same host was an elusive concept for many years. The cloning of genes encoding human tumor antigens has eliminated remaining doubt, and has opened the possibility of designing antigen-specific vaccines that do not rely on tumor cells as an immunogen. As mentioned previously, these antigens are recognized by CD8+ CTL in the form of short peptides bound to particular class I MHC molecules. For clinical application, tumor biopsy material can be obtained to assay for antigen expression by RT-PCR or immunohistochemistry. In addition, the patient can be HLA-typed to know which of the defined CTL epitopes from the antigen of interest should be utilized for immunization and to allow measurement of the relevant specific CTL activity from the blood of vaccinated patients. Thus, the availability of defined antigens has rendered tumor vaccine development much more precise, providing a means by which correlations between clinical outcome and antigen-specific immunologic parameters can be attempted [98].

Tumor antigens apparently can arise by a variety of mechanisms, as listed in Table 4. Unique antigens can be created by point mutations in normal genes or by differential splicing of mRNA species. Antigens that could potentially be shared in common with tumors from different individuals can result from re-expression of genes normally expressed during fetal development, overexpression of oncogenes, expression of fusion proteins resulting from common chromosomal translocations, overexpression of tissue-specific differentiation antigens, altered glycosylation of normal proteins, or expression of viral proteins resulting from viral infection. Antigens from each of these classes have been examined as potential targets for vaccination in pre-clinical models, and human counterparts to some of these antigens have entered clinical testing. Shared antigens hold more promise for wide applicability to patients.

**Table 4.** Examples of tumor antigens defined by T lymphocyte recognition

| Antigen type | Murine examples | Human examples |
|---|---|---|
| Probable embryonic genes expressed in tumor | P1 A [11] | MAGE, BAGE, GAGE [15, 147, 148]; CEA, PSA |
| Point mutations | P198 [9], P91 A [10] | β-Catenin [149] connexin [150], L9 [151] |
| Intronic sequences | | gp75 [152], MUM-1 [153] |
| Mutated oncogenes/ tumor suppressors | p53 [109, 154] | Ras [155], p53 [156] |
| Fusion proteins | | Bcr-abl [157] |
| Differentiation antigens | Trp-2 [158], Trp-2 [161] | Melan-A/MART-1 [159], tyrosinase [160], gp100 [103] |
| Differentially glycosylated normal proteins | | MUC-1 [162] |
| Viral proteins | | HPV 16 E6/E7 [99, 120], Adeno E1 A [163] |

Although methodologies for vaccination to generate antibody responses have been known for many years, the optimal approach for vaccination to induce specific CTL is not known. For this reason, multiple methodologies have been investigated in preclinical models, and several of these approaches have entered clinical study. The principal vaccination techniques being studied are depicted in Table 5; the rationale for their use warrants some discussion. As mentioned previously, the initial activation of specific T cells depends on presentation of antigen by host APCs. Therefore, each vaccination modality must target antigen to APCs, either directly or indirectly. A simple approach is to emulsify antigenic peptide or protein in an oil-based adjuvant, or mixed with particular cytokines,

**Table 5.** Immunization modalities to induce tumor antigen-specific CTL

| Modality | Reference |
|---|---|
| Tumor cells/transfectants | [87, 95] |
| Peptide/protein in adjuvant | [99–101] |
| Peptide plus cytokines | [76, 164–166] |
| Heat shock proteins | [105, 106] |
| Recombinant viruses | [107–110, 112] |
| Recombinant bacteria | [60, 113, 114] |
| Plasmid DNA | [115–117] |
| Peptide-loaded APCs | [119–123] |
| Transfected APCs | [125, 126] |

that promotes uptake by dendritic cells that transport the antigen to draining lymph nodes. Preclinical studies with incomplete or complete Freund's adjuvant have resulted in the generation of CTL in some experimental models [99–101]. Clinically, a European phase I vaccine study utilizing a peptide derived from the melanoma antigen MAGE-3 dissolved only in saline resulted in a surprising 25% response rate in patients with metastatic melanoma [102]. Another recent clinical trial using vaccination with a melanoma antigen peptide in incomplete Freund's adjuvant followed by IL-2 administration resulted in a response rate of approximately 40% [103]. These studies suggest that these relatively simple immunization approaches may be sufficient to potentiate a specific anti-tumor immune response in some patients.

Antigenic peptides or proteins mixed with particular immunomodulatory cytokines might be expected to augment responses to the vaccine. Preclinical studies of IL-12 mixed with model antigens has demonstrated improved T cell activation in vivo [104]. Tumor antigen peptides mixed in oil-based adjuvants along with IL-12 also is being explored. GM-CSF has been combined with the dominant Melan-A/MART-1 peptide in a pilot clinical trial in Europe, which has demonstrated successful immunization and tumor regression in some patients [76].

As an alternative to using defined antigens, Srivastava and colleagues have utilized heat shock proteins isolated from tumor cells, which appear to have a sampling of the array of cellular peptides bound to them. Immunization with tumor-isolated gp96 induces specific CTL responses and tumor protection in mice via a mechanism dependent upon host APCs [105, 106]. The potential advantage of this approach is that identity of the antigens is not necessary, making it usable in tumors from which specific antigens have not yet been defined.

Recombinant viruses have been developed for use in human gene replacement clinical trials. However, in most studies, gene expression has been of limited duration because of the immune response generated against the virus, limiting therapeutic efficacy. With respect to tumor immunity, it has been possible to take advantage of the natural immunogenicity of viruses by incorporating cDNAs encoding tumor antigens into the viral genome, so that the immune response developed against the virus includes a CTL response against the desired tumor antigen epitope. Successful preclinical studies have been performed using recombinant adenovirus [76], vaccinia virus [107, 108], canarypox virus [109], and fowlpox virus [110]. Concomitant expression of B7 by vaccinia virus or co-administration of IL-12 resulted in potentiation of the immune response observed [111]. One nagging limitation of this approach is the induction of neutralizing antibodies against the injected virus, such that subsequent booster immunizations fail to augment CTL activity [112]. Patients with pre-existing antibodies against the viral vector may fail to generate a CTL response even with the first vaccination. Nonetheless, clinical trials have been initiated in patients with melanoma utilizing most of these viral vectors.

Like recombinant viruses, bacteria can be engineered to express tumor antigens. Recombinant BCG has been engineered to encode model antigens, resulting in antigen-specific T cell responses in murine studies [60]. *Listeria monocytogenes* has been constructed to encode a tumor antigen, resulting in potent systemic immunity in mice [113]. Interestingly, recombinant *Listeria* also was effective when given orally [114], making it the first of these engineered vectors demonstrated to be effective via this route. Bacterial delivery systems take advantage of the natural adjuvant properties of the organisms, which promote non-specific activation of immune cells.

Rather surprisingly, naked plasmid DNA encoding tumor antigens induces protective CTL when injected into mice [115, 116]. Generation of this CTL response depends upon host APC, and appears to be a natural response against sequences present within bacterial DNA [117, 118]. Exogenous cytokines, such as IL-12, augment this immune response as in other vaccination systems. The ease by which DNA can be prepared in a form suitable for administration to patients makes this delivery system especially attractive for clinical application.

Finally, rather than utilizing immunization approaches that depend upon antigen uptake by host APCs in vivo, this step has been bypassed by loading antigen directly onto APCs in vitro. This approach avoids the potential deleterious consequences of antigen presentation by cells other than professional APC. Immunization of mice with purified DC pulsed with peptides derived from mutant p53 [119], HPV [120], or P91 [121], as well as with the model antigens β-galactosidase [122] and ovalbumin [123], has been shown to induce specific immunity and/or protection against tumor challenge in vivo. Co-administration with IL-12 appears to augment considerably the responses observed [74, 124]. Rather than pulsing with peptides, DC also have been transfected with either DNA encoding tumor antigens or RNA isolated from tumor specimens [125, 126]. Transfection of DC to express IL-12 also is being explored. Expansion of

DC from the peripheral blood of human patients has been achieved [127], providing the technology necessary for creating DC-based vaccines for human application. A recent study in Europe utilizing peptide-loaded DCs injected intralymphatically into patients with metastatic melanoma demonstrated over a 30% clinical response rate [128]. Thus, optimization of this approach may provide the most efficacious vaccine methodology to date.

*Ganglioside and Other Antibody-Inducing Vaccines*

As an alternative to vaccine approaches aiming to induce tumor-specific CTL, other investigators have focused on immunization to generate antibodies that recognize cell surface molecules expressed on tumor cells. The most developed of these approaches is designed to induce antibodies against gangliosides expressed on melanoma cells and other tumors. Melanoma patients who naturally generate antibodies against the GM2 ganglioside have a longer survival than patients who do not [129]. Clinical trials have been performed in stage III melanoma patients following lymph node resection by Livingston and colleagues using GM2 coupled to BCG, with an improvement in overall survival [129]. As an improvement on this approach, GM2 has been conjugated to keyhole limpet hemocyanin (KLH), an immunogenic carrier protein, and emulsified in the adjuvant QS21. This vaccine has successfully induced anti-GM2 antibodies in 100% of patients immunized, and is currently being tested in a randomized phase III study in resected stage III melanoma patients. Whether methodologies to induce tumor-specific antibody responses or those that induce CTL responses are superior has yet to be determined.

**Future Directions**

The molecular characterization of tumor antigens, a better understanding of immune regulation, and the creation of various antigen delivery systems all have generated renewed excitement about the possibility of effective immunologic strategies for the treatment of cancer. Although significant advances have been made, several obstacles remain. It is apparent that patients with advanced cancer are generally immunosuppressed, and unlocking or overcoming that immunosuppressed state will be necessary for optimal immunization of patients with advanced disease. As can be judged by the wealth of clinical trials being performed, the optimal methodology for vaccinating to induce specific CTL against tumor antigens is not yet known, and further clinical testing will be required to arrive at an ideal strategy. The advantage of defined epitope-based vaccines is that immune responses against the antigen can be assessed independently from clinical response, thus allowing determination of whether generation of T cell responses is sufficient on its own to induce tumor regression. However, the optimal readout of successful immunization is not clear. Most investigators are measuring CTL activity, but the cytokine phenotype of the activated T cells also may be important, as well as the duration of the T cell lifespan. The recent development of class I MHC tetramers bound to specific antigenic peptides should allow quantitation of tumor antigen-specific T cells in the peripheral blood by simple flow cytometric analysis [130].

Generation of activated CD8+ CTL is probably an important component to an optimal anti-tumor immune response, but that alone may not be sufficient. It is possible that induction of CD4+ T cells also will be critical, to provide the requisite help for maintenance of long-term survival of the CTL. Currently, there are few class II MHC-binding tumor antigen epitopes defined, and more work is required in this area. Once generated, effector T cells must penetrate into the tumor site. This activity might not be optimal under normal circumstances, as a slowly growing tumor mass may appear innocuous to the host, lacking the non-specific inflammatory response characteristic of infections. Provision of chemokines that attract inflammatory cells into the tumor mass may be useful in this regard [131]. The vascular endothelium within a tumor mass also may comprise a barrier for transmigration of inflammatory cells, and the combination of anti-angiogenesis agents plus tumor antigen vaccination may prove to be synergistic. Finally, the observation that tumor cells can express molecules such as Fas-ligand, that have the capability of killing activated T cells that actually succeed in penetrating into the tumor mass [132], illustrates the level of complexity of tumor resistance to immune elimination and another category of obstacle that must be overcome.

Most tumor antigens defined to date have been characterized from melanoma cells, and ongoing work in a number of laboratories is advancing this technology to tumors of other histologies. Once optimal immunization against single epitopes has been achieved, then polyvalent vaccines will be examined, which have a better likelihood of generating CTL that recognize a larger proportion of tumor cells among heterogenous tumor masses. The possibility that antigen-specific CTL can select for tumor cells that have lost expression of tumor antigen or MHC molecules has been demonstrated by recent clinical observations [133]. A better understanding of NK cell biology should allow optimization of NK cell responses against such MHC-loss variants. Finally, it is likely that tumor vaccination approaches will provide maximal benefit in the setting of minimal residual disease following surgical resection of macroscopic tumor. Once vaccine strategies are optimized in patients with metastatic disease, advancing them to the adjuvant setting will be the next logical step.

## References

1. Coley WB (1909) The treatment of inoperable sarcoma by bacterial toxin (the mixed toxins of the Streptococcus erysipelas and the Bacillus prodigious). John Bale, Sons & Banielsson, Ltd. London
2. Gross L (1943) Intradermal immunization of C3H mice against a sarcoma that originated in the same line. Cancer Res 3:326–333
3. Globerson A, Feldman M (1964) Antigen specificity of benzopyrene-induced sarcomas. J Natl Cancer Inst 32:1229–1243
4. Kripke ML (1974) Antigenicity of murine skin tumors induced by ultraviolet light. J Natl Cancer Inst 53:1333–1336
5. Boon T, Kellermann O (1977) Rejection by syngeneic mice of cell variants obtained by mutagenesis of a malignant teratocarcinoma cell line. Proc Natl Acad Sci USA 74:272–275
6. Boon T, Van Snick J, Van Pel A, Uyttenhove C, Marchand M (1980) Immunogenic variants obtained by mutagenesis of mouse mastocytoma P815. II. T lymphocyte-mediated cytolysis. J Exp Med 152:1184–1193
7. Van Pel A, Van der Bruggen P, Coulie PG, Brichard VG, Lethe B, Van den Eynde B, Uyttenhove C, Renauld J-C, Boon T (1995) Genes coding for tumor antigens recognized by cytolytic T lymphocytes. Immunol Rev 145:229–250
8. Uyttenhove C, Van Snick J, Boon T (1980) Immunogenic variants obtained by mutagenesis of mouse mastocytoma P815. I. Rejection by syngeneic mice. J Exp Med 152:1175–1183
9. Sibille C, Chomez P, Wildmann C, Van Pel A, De Plaen E, Maryanski JL, de Bergeyck V, Boon T (1990) Structure of the gene of tum‑transplantation antigen P198: a point mutation generates a new antigenic peptide. J Exp Med 172:35–45
10. De Plaen E, Lurquin C, Van Pel A, Mariame B, Szikora J-P, Wolfel T, Sibille C, Chomez P, Boon T (1988) Immunogenic (tum⁻) variants of mouse tumor P815: Cloning of the gene of tum⁻ antigen P91 A and identification of the tum⁻ mutation. Proc Natl Acad Sci USA 85:2274–2278
11. Van den Eynde B, Lethe B, Van Pel A, De Plaen E, Boon T (1991) The gene coding for a major tumor rejection antigen of tumor P815 is identical to the normal gene of syngeneic DBA/2 mice. J Exp Med 173:1373–1384

12. Lethe B, Van den Eynde B, Van Pel A, Corradin G, Boon T (1992) Mouse tumor rejection antigens P815 A and P815B: two epitopes carried by a single peptide. Eur J Immunol 22:2283–2288
13. Uyttenhove C, Godfraind C, Lethe B, Amar-Costesec A, Renauld J-C, Gajewski TF, Duffour M-T, Warnier G, Boon T, Van den Eynde BJ (1997) The expression of mouse gene P1 A in testis does not prevent safe induction of cytolytic T cells against a P1 A-encoded tumor antigen. Int J Cancer 70:349–356
14. Van der Bruggen P, Traversari C, Chomez P, Lurquin C, De Plaen E, Van den Eynde B, Knuth A, Boon T (1991) A gene encoding an antigen recognized by cytolytic T lymphocytes on a human melanoma. Science 254:1643–1647
15. De Plaen E, Arden K, Traversari C, Gaforio JJ, Szikora J, De Smet C, Brasseur F, Van der Bruggen P, Lethe B, Lurquin C, Brasseur R, Chomez P, De Backer O, Cavenee W, Boon T (1994) Structure, chromosomal location, and expression of 12 genes of the MAGE family. Immunogenetics 40:360–369
16. Rosenberg SA, Yang JC, Topalian SL, Schwartzentruber DJ, Weber JS, Parkinson DR, Seipp CA, Einhorn JH, White DE (1994) Treatment of 283 consecutive patients with metastatic melanoma or renal cell cancer using high-dose bolus interleukin 2. JAMA 271:907–913
17. Kirkwood JM, Strawderman MH, Ernstoff MS, Smith TJ, Borden EC, Blum RH (1996) Interferon alpha-2b adjuvant therapy of high-risk resected cutaneous melanoma: the Eastern Cooperative Oncology Group trial EST 1684. J Clin Oncol 14:7–17
18. Liu CC, Young LH, Young JD (1996) Lymphocyte-mediated cytolysis and disease. N Engl J Med 335:1651–1659
19. Van der Broek ME, Kagi D, Ossendorp F, Toes R, Vamvakas S, Lutz WK, Melief CJ, Zinkernagel RM, Hengartner H (1996) Decreased tumor surveillance in perforin-deficient mice. J Exp Med 184:1781–1790
20. Atkinson EA, Bleackley RC (1995) Mechanisms of lysis by cytotoxic T cells. Crit Rev Immunol 15:359–384
21. Long EO, Wagtmann N (1997) Natural killer cell receptors. Curr Opin Immunol 9:344–350
22. Harding FA, Allison JP (1993) CD28-B7 interactions allow the induction of CD8+ cytotoxic T lymphocytes in the absence of exogenous help. J Exp Med 177:1791–1796
23. Gajewski TF, Renauld J-C, Van Pel A, Boon T (1995) Costimulation with B7-1, IL-6, and IL-12 is sufficient for primary generation of murine anti-tumor cytolytic T lymphocytes in vitro. J Immunol 154:5637–5648
24. Gajewski TF (1996) B7-1 but not B7-2 efficiently costimulates CD8+ T lymphocytes in the P815 tumor system in vitro. J Immunol 156:465–472
25. Tan P, Anasetti C, Hansen JA, Melrose J, Brunvand M, Bradshaw J, Ledbetter JA, Linsley PS (1993) Induction of alloantigen-specific hyporesponsiveness in human T lymphocytes by blocking interaction of CD28 with its natural ligand B7/BB1. J Exp Med 177:165–173
26. Gimmi CD, Freeman GJ, Gribben JG, Gray G, Nadler LM (1993) Human T-cell clonal anergy is induced by antigen presentation in the absence of B7 costimulation. Proc Natl Acad Sci USA 90:6586–6590
27. Schwartz RH (1990) A cell culture model for T lymphocyte clonal anergy. Science 248:1349–1356
28. Hsieh C-S, Macatonia SE, Tripp CS, Wolf SF, O'Garra A, Murphy KM (1993) Development of Th1 CD4+ cells through IL-12 produced by Listeria-infected macrophages. Science 260:547–549

29. Mosmann TR, Coffman RL (1989) TH1 and TH2 cells: Different patterns of lymphokine secretion lead to different functional properties. Annu Rev Immunol 7:145–173

30. Fitch FW, McKisic MD, Lancki DW, Gajewski TF (1993) Differential regulation of murine T lymphocyte subsets. Ann Rev Immunol 11:29–48

31. Sad S, Marcotte R, Mosmann TR (1995) Cytokine-induced differentiation of precursor mouse CD8+ T cells into cytotoxic CD8+ T cells secreting Th1 or Th2 cytokines. Immunity 2:271–279

32. Cronin DC, Stack R, Fitch FW (1995) IL-4-producing CD8+ T cell clones can provide B cell help. J Immunol 154:3118–3127

33. Fallarino F, Uyttenhove C, Boon T, Gajewski TF (1996) Endogenous IL-12 is necessary for rejection of P815 tumor variants in vivo. J Immunol 156:1095–1100

34. Gajewski TF, Fallarino F (1997) Rational development of tumour antigen-specific immunization in melanoma. Therapeutic Immunol 2:211–225

35. Mulé JJ, Shu S, Schwarz SL, Rosenberg SA (1984) Adoptive immunotherapy of established pulmonary metastases with LAK cells and recombinant interleukin-2. Science 225:1487–1489

36. Lefor AT, Rosenberg SA (1991) The specificity of lymphokine-activated killer (LAK) cells in vitro: fresh normal murine tissues are resistant to LAK-mediated lysis. J Surg Res 50:15–23

37. Rosenberg SA, Lotze MT, Yang JC, Topalian SL, Chang AE, Scwartzentruber DJ, Aebersold P, Leitman S, Linehan WM, Seipp CA et al. (1993) Prospective randomized trial of high-dose interleukin-2 alone or in conjunction with lymphokine-activated killer cells for the treatment of patients with advanced cancer. J Natl Cancer Inst 85:622–632

38. Ochoa AC, Longo DL (1995) Alteration of signal transduction in T cells from cancer patients. Important Adv Oncol 43–54

39. Saxton ML, Longo DL, Wetzel HE, Tribble H, Alvord WG, Kwak LW, Leonard AS, Ullmann CD, Curti BD, Ochoa AC (1997) Adoptive transfer of anti-CD3-activated CD4+ T cells plus cyclophosphamide and liposome-encapsulated interleukin-2 cure murine MC-38 and 3LL tumors and establish tumor-specific immunity. Blood 89:2529–2536

40. Curti BD, Longo DL, Ochoa AC, Conlon KC, Smith JW, Alvord WG, Creekmore SP, Fenton RG, Gause BL, Holmlund J et al. (1993) Treatment of cancer patients with ex vivo anti-CD3-activated killer cells and interleukin-2. J Clin Oncol 11:652–660

41. Levine BL, Mosca JD, Riley JL, Carroll RG, Vahey MT, Jagodzinski LL, Wagner KF, Mayers DL, Burke DS, Weislow OS, St.Louis DC, June CH (1996) Antiviral effect of ex vivo CD4+ T cell proliferation in HIV-positive patients as a result of CD28 costimulation. Science 272:1939–1943

42. Boehm U, Klamp T, Groot M, Howard JC (1997) Cellular response to interferon-gamma. Ann Rev Immunol 15:749–795

43. Wadler S (1991) The role of interferons in the treatment of solid tumors. Cancer 70:949–958

44. de Wit R (1992) AIDS-associated Kaposi's sarcoma and the mechanism of interferon alpha's activity: a riddle within a puzzle. J Intern Med 231:321–325

45. Lienard D, Ewalenko P, Delmotte J-J, Renard N, Lejeune FJ (1992) High-dose recombinant tumor necrosis factor alpha in combination with interferon gamma and melphalan in isolation perfusion of the limbs for melanoma and sarcoma. J Clin Oncol 10:52–60

46. Fraker DL, Alexander HR, Andrich M, Rosenberg SA (1996) Treatment of patients with melanoma of the extremity using hyperthermic isolated limb perfusion with melphalan, tumor necrosis factor, and interferon gamma: results of a tumor necrosis factor dose-escalation study. J Clin Oncol 14:479–489

47. Ruegg C, Yilmaz A, Bieler G, Bamat J, Chaubert P, Lejeune FJ (1998) Evidence for the involvement of endothelial cell integrin αVβ3 in the disruption of the tumor vasculature induced by TNF and IFN-γ. Nat Med 4:408–413

48. Brooks PC, Clark RA, Cheresh DA (1998) Requirement of vascular integrin apha v beta 3 for angiogenesis. Science 264:569–571

49. Slamon DJ, Godolphin W, Jones LA, Holt JA, Wong SG, Keith DE, Levin WJ, Stuart SG, Udove J, Ullrich A, Press MF (1989) Studies of the HER-2/neu proto-oncogene in human breast and ovarian cancer. Science 244:707–712

50. Cobleigh MA, Vogel CL, Tripathy D, Robert NJ, Scholl S, Fehrenbacher L, Paton V, Shak S, Lieberman G, Slamon D (1998) Efficacy and safety of Herceptin (humanized anti-HER2 antibody) as a single agent in 222 women with HER2 overexpression who relapsed following chemotherapy for metastatic breast cancer. Proc Am Soc Clin Oncol 17:97a (Abstract)

51. Shak S, Paton V, Bejamonde A, Fleming T, Eirmann W, Wolter J, Baselga J, Norton L (1998) Addition of Herceptin (humanized anti-HER2 antibody) to first line chemotherapy for HER2 overexpressing metastatic breast cancer (HER2+/MBC) markedly increases anticancer activity: a randomized, multinational controlled phase III trial. Proc Am Soc Clin Oncol 17:98a (Abstract)

52. Maloney DG, Grillo-Lopez AJ, White CA, Bodkin D, Schilder RJ, Neidhart JA, Janakiraman N, Foon KA, Liles TM, Dallaire BK, Wey K, Royston I, Davis T, Levy R (1997) IDEC-C2B8 (Rituximab) anti-CD20 monoclonal antibody therapy in patients with relapsed low-grade non-Hodgkin's lymphoma. Blood 90:2188–2195

53. Fisher RI, Czuczman M, Gilman P, Lowe AM, Vose JM (1998) Phase II pilot study of the safety and efficacy of Rituximab in combination with CHOP chemotherapy in patients with previously untreated intermediate- or high-grade NHL. Proc Am Soc Clin Oncol 17:3a (Abstract)

54. Riddell SR, Watanabe KS, Goodrich JM, Li CR, Agha ME, Greenberg PD (1992) Restoration of viral immunity in immunodeficient humans by adoptive transfer of T cell clones. Science 257:238–241

55. Rosenberg SA, Speiss P, Lafreiniere R (1986) A new approach to the adoptive immunotherapy of cancer with tumor-infiltrating lymphocytes. Science 233:1318–1321

56. Costanzi JJ, Al-Sarraf M, Groppe C, Bottomley R, Fabian C, Neidhart J, Dixon D (1982) Combination chemotherapy plus BCG in the treatment of disseminated malignant melanoma: A Southwest Oncology Group study. Med Ped Oncol 10:251–258

57. Veronesi U, Adamus J, Aubert C, Bajetta E, Beretta G, Bonadonna G, Bufalino R, Cascinelli N, Cocconi G, Durand J, De Marsillac J, Ikonopisov RL, Kiss B, Lejeune F, MacKie R, Madej G, Mulder H, Mechl Z, Milton GW, Morabito A, Peter H, Priario J, Paul E, Rumke P, Sertoli R, Tomin R (1982) A randomized trial of adjuvant chemotherapy and immunotherapy in cutaneous melanoma. N Engl J Med 307:913–916

58. Mastrangelo MJ, Sulit HL, Prehn LM, Bornstein RS, Yarbro JW, Prehn RT (1976) Intralesional BCG in the treatment of metastatic malignant melanoma. Cancer 37:684–692

59. Nseyo UO, Lamm DL (1996) Therapy of superficial bladder cancer. Semin Oncol 23:598–604

60. Stover CK, de la Cruz VF, Fuerst TR, Burlein JE, Benson LA, Bennett LT, Bansal GP, Young JF, Lee MH, Hatfull GF, Snapper SB, Barletta RG, Jacobs WRJ, Bloom BR (1991) New use of BCG for recombinant vaccines. Nature 351:456–460

61. Ellenhorn JDI, Hirsch R, Schreiber H, Bluestone JA (1988) In vivo administration of anti-CD3 prevents malignant progressor tumor growth. Science 242:569–571

62. Urba WJ, Ewel C, Kopp W, Smith JW, Steis RG, Ashwell JD, Creekmore SP, Rossio J, Sznol M, Sharfman W et al. (1992) Anti-CD3 monoclonal antibody treatment of patients with CD3-negative tumors: a phase IA/B study. Cancer Res 52:2394–2401

63. Sosman JA, Weiss GR, Marholin KA, Aronson FR, Sznol M, Atkins MB, O'Boyle K, Fisher RI, Boldt DH, Doroshow J, Ernest ML, Fisher SG, Mier J, Vachino G, Caliendo G (1993) Phase IB clinical trial of anti-CD3 followed by high-dose bolus inter-leukin-2 in patients with metastatic melanoma and advanced renal cell carcinoma: clinical and immunologic effects. J Clin Oncol 11:1496–1505

64. Riedle S, Rosel M, Zoller M (1998) In vivo activation and expansion of T cells by a bi-specific antibody abolishes metastasis formation of human melanoma cells in SCID mice. Int J Cancer 75:908–918

65. Philip PA, Flaherty L (1997) Treatment of malignant melanoma with interleukin-2. Semin Oncol 24 (suppl 4):S4–32-S4–38

66. Manetti R, Parronchi P, Giudizi MG, Piccinni M, Maggi E, Trinchieri G, Romagnani S (1993) Natural killer cell stimulatory factor (Interleukin 12 [IL-12]) induces T helper type 1 (Th1)–specific immune responses and inhibits the development of IL-4-producing Th cells. J Exp Med 177:1199–1204

67. Mehrotra PT, Wu D, Crim JA, Mostowski HS, Siegel JP (1993) Effects of IL-12 on the generation of cytotoxic activity in human CD8+ T lymphocytes. J Immunol 151:2444–2452

68. Trinchieri G (1995) Interleukin-12: a proinflammatory cytokine with immunore-gulatory functions that bridge innate resistance and antigen-specific adaptive immunity. Ann Rev Immunol 13:251–276

69. Brunda MJ, Luistro L, Warrier RR, Wright RB, Hubbard BR, Murphy M, Wolf SF, Gately MK (1993) Antitumor and antimetastatic activity of interleukin 12 against murine tumors. J Exp Med 178:1223–1230

70. Zitvogel L, Tahara H, Robbins PD, Storkus WJ, Clarke MR, Nalesnik MA, Lotze MT (1995) Cancer immunotherapy of established tumors with IL-12. Effective delivery by genetically engineered fibroblasts. J Immunol 155:1393–1403

71. Voest EE, Kenyon BM, O'Reilly MS, Truitt G, D'Amato RJ, Folkman J (1995) Inhibition of angiogenesis in vivo by interleukin 12. J Natl Cancer Inst 87:581–586

72. Noguchi Y, Richards EC, Chen YT, Old LJ (1995) Influence of interleukin 12 on p53 peptide vaccination against Meth A sarcoma. Proc Natl Acad Sci USA 92:2219–2223

73. Fallarino F, Ashikari A, Boon T, Gajewski TF (1997) Antigen-specific regression of established tumors induced by active immunization with irradiated IL-12-but not B7–1-transfected tumor cells. Inter Immunol 9:1259–1269

74. Fallarino F, Yttenhove C, Boon T, Gajewski TF (1998) Co-administration of IL-12 obviates the need to use dendritic cells during tumor antigen immunization sche-mes in vivo: successful immunization of mice with peptide-pulsed PBMC plus rmIL-12. Int. J. Cancer. In Press

75. Si Z, Hersey P, Coates AS (1996) Clinical responses and lymphoid infiltrates in metastatic melanoma following treatment with intralesional GM-CSF. Melanoma Res 6:247–255

76. Jager E, Ringhoffer M, Dienes HP, Arand M, Karbach J, Jager D, Ilsemann C, Hegedorn M, Oesch F, Knuth A (1996) Granulocyte-macrophage colony-stimula-ting factor enhances immune response to melanoma-associated peptides in vivo. Int J Cancer 67:54–62

77. Lyman SD, Williams DE (1995) Biology and potential clinical applications of Flt3 ligand. Curr Opin Hematol 2:177–181

78. Esche C, Subbotin VM, Maliszewski C, Lotze MT, Shurin MR (1998) Flt3 ligand administration inhibits tumor growth in murine melanoma and lymphoma. Cancer Res 58:380–383

79. Lynch DH, Andreasen A, Maraskovsky E, Whitmore J, Miller RE, Schuh JC (1997) Flt3 ligand induces tumor regression and antitumor immune responses in vivo. Nat Med 3:625–631

80. Stopeck AT, Hersh EM, Akporiaye ET, Harris DT, Grogan T, Unger E, Warneke J, Schluter SF, Stahl S (1997) Phase I study of direct gene transfer of an allogeneic histocompatibility antigen, HLA-B7, in patients with metastatic melanoma. J Clin Oncol 15:341–349

81. Nabel GJ, Gordon D, Bishop DK, Nickoloff BJ, Yang ZY, Aruga A, Cameron MJ, Nabel EG, Chang AE (1996) Immune response in human melanoma after transfer of an allogeneic class I major histocompatibility complex gene with DNA-liposome complexes. Proc Natl Acad Sci USA 93:15388–15393

82. Mastrangelo MJ, Schultz S, Kane M, Berd D (1988) Newer immunologic approaches to the treatment of patients with melanoma. Semin Oncol 15:589–594

83. Morton DL, Barth A (1996) Vaccine therapy for malignant melanoma. CA Cancer J Clin 46:225–244

84. Berd D, Maguire HCJ, Mastrangelo MJ (1993) Treatment of human melanoma with a hapten-modified autologous vaccine. Ann NY Acad Sci 690:147–152

85. Berd D, Murphy G, Maguire HCJ, Mastrangelo MJ (1991) Immunization with haptenized, autologous tumor cells induces inflammation of human melanoma metastases. Cancer Res 51:2731–2734

86. Berd D, Maguire HC, Schuchter LM, Hamilton R, Hauck WW, Sato T, Mastrangelo MJ (1997) Autologous hapten-modified melanoma vaccine as postsurgical adjuvant treatment after resection of nodal metastasis. J Clin Oncol 15:2359–2370

87. Colombo MP, Forni G (1994) Cytokine gene transfer in tumor inhibition and tumor therapy: where are we now? Immunol Today 15:48–51

88. Pardoll DM (1995) Paracrine cytokine adjuvants in cancer immunotherapy. Ann Rev Immunol 13:399–415

89. Linsley PS, Brady W, Grosmaire L, Aruffo A, Damle NK, Ledbetter JA (1991) Binding of the B cell activation antigen B7 to CD28 costimulates T cell proliferation and Interleukin 2 mRNA accumulation. J Exp Med 173:721–730

90. Lenschow DJ, Walunas TL, Bluestone JA (1996) CD28/B7 system of T cell costimulation. Ann Rev Immunol 14:233–258

91. Townsend SE, Allison JP (1993) Tumor rejection after direct costimulation of CD8+ T cells by B7-transfected melanoma cells. Science 259:368–370

92. Chen L, Linsley PS, Hellstrom KE (1993) Costimulation of T cells for tumor immunity. Immunol Today 14:483–486

93. Chen L, Ashe S, Brady WA, Hellstrom I, Hellstrom KE, Ledbetter JA, μgowan P, Linsley PS (1992) Costimulation of antitumor immunity by the B7 counterreceptor for the T lymphocyte molecules CD28 and CTLA-4. Cell 71:1093–1102

94. Gajewski TF, Uyttenhove C, Fallarino F, Boon T (1996) Tumor rejection requires a CTLA4 ligand provided by the host or expressed on the tumor: Superiority of B7-1 over B7-2 for active tumor immunization. J Immunol 156:2909–2917

95. Dranoff G, Jaffee E, Lazenby A, Golumbek P, Levitsky H, Brose K, Jackson V, Hamada H, Pardoll D, Mulligan RC (1993) Vaccination with irradiated tumor cells engineered to secrete granulocyte-macrophage colony-stimulating factor stimulates potent, specific, and long-lasting anti-tumor immunity. Proc Natl Acad Sci USA 90:3539–3543

96. Huang AYC, Golumbek P, Ahmadzadeh M, Jaffee E, Pardoll D, Levitsky H (1994) Role of bone marrow-derived cells in presenting MHC class I-restricted tumor antigens. Science 264:961–965

97. Zitvogel L, Robbins PD, Storkus WJ, Clarke MR, Maeurer MJ, Campbell RL, Davis CG, Tahara H, Schreiber RD, Lotze MT (1996) Interleukin-12 and B7.1 costimula-

tion cooperate in the induction of effective anti-tumor immunity and therapy of established tumors. Eur J Immunol 26:1335–1341

98. Boon T, Gajewski TF, Coulie PG (1995) From defined human tumor antigens to effective immunization? Immunol Today 16:334–335

99. Feltcamp MC, Smits HL, Vierboom MP, Minnaar RP, de Jongh BM, Drijfhout JW, ter Schegget J, Melief CJ, Kast WM (1993) Vaccination with cytotoxic T lymphocyte epitope-containing peptide protects against a tumor induced by human papillomavirus type 16-transformed cells. Eur J Immunol 23:2242–2249

100. Zhang S, Graeber LA, Helling F, Ragupathi G, Adluri S, Lloyd KO, Livingston PO (1996) Augmenting the immunogenicity of synthetic MUC1 peptide vaccines in mice. Cancer Res 56:3315–3319

101. Mandelboim O, Vadai E, Fridkin M, Katz-Hillel A, Feldman M, Berke G, Eisenbach L (1995) Regression of established murine carcinoma metastases following vaccination with tumor-associated antigen peptides. Nature Med 1:1179–1183

102. Marchand M, Weynants P, Rankin E, Arienti F, Belli F, Parmiani G, Cascinelli N, Bourlond A, Vanwijck R, Humblet Y, Canon J-L, Laurent C, Naeyaert J-M, Plagne R, Deraemaeker R, Knuth A, Jager E, Brasseur F, Herman J, Coulie PG, Boon T (1995) Tumor regression responses in melanoma patients treated with a peptide encoded by gene MAGE-3. Int J Cancer 63:883–885

103. Rosenberg SA, Yang JC, Schwartzentruber DJ, Hwu P, Marincola FM, Topalian SL, Restifo NP, Dudley ME, Schwarz SL, Spiess PJ, Wunderlich JR, Parkhurst MR, Kawakami Y, Seipp CA, Einhorn JH, White DE (1998) Immunologic and therapeutic evaluation of a synthetic peptide vaccine for the treatment of patients with metastatic melanoma. Nature Med 4:321–327

104. Bliss J, Van Cleave V, Murray K, Wiencis A, Ketchum M, Maylor R, Haire T, Resmini C, Abbas AK, Wolf SF (1996) IL-12, as an adjuvant, promotes a T helper 1 cell, but does not suppress a T helper 2 cell recall response. J Immunol 156:887–894

105. Srivastava PK, Udono H, Blachere NE, Zihai L (1994) Heat shock proteins transfer peptides during antigen processing and CTL priming. Immunogenetics 39:93–98

106. Suto R, Srivastava PK (1995) A mechanism for the specific immunogenicity of heat shock protein-chaperoned peptides. Science 269:1585–1588

107. Thomson SA, Elliot SL, Sherritt MA, Sproat KW, Coupar BE, Scalzo AA, Forbes CA, Ladhams AM, Mo XY, Tripp RA, Doherty PC, Moss DJ, Suhrbier A (1996) Recombinant polyepitope vaccines for the delivery of multiple CD8 cytotoxic T cell epitopes. J Immunol 157:822–826

108. Lam JS, Reeves ME, Cowherd R, Rosenberg SA, Hwu P (1995) Anti-tumor activity of cytotoxic T lymphocytes elicited with recombinant and synthetic forms of a model tumor-associated antigen. J Immunother 18:139–146

109. Roth J, Dittmer D, Rea D, Tartaglia J, Paoletti E, Levine AJ (1996) p53 as a target for cancer vaccines: recombinant canarypox virus vectors expressing p53 protect mice against lethal tumor cell challenge. Proc Natl Acad Sci USA 93:4781–4786

110. Wang M, Bronte V, Chen PW, Gritz L, Panicali D, Rosenberg SA, Restifo NP (1995) Active immunotherapy for cancer with a nonreplicating recombinant fowlpox virus encoding a model tumor-associated antigen. J Immunol 154:4685–4692

111. Rao JB, Chamberlain RS, Bronte V, Carroll MW, Irvine KR, Moss B, Rosenberg SA, Restifo NP (1996) IL-12 is an effective adjuvant to recombinant vaccinia virus-based tumor vaccines: enhancement by simultaneous B7-1 expression. J Immunol 156:3357–3365

112. Warnier G, Duffour MT, Uyttenhove C, Gajewski TF, Lurquin C, Haddada H, Perricaudet M, Boon T (1996) Induction of a cytolytic T-cell response in mice with a recombinant adenovirus coding for tumor antigen P815 A. Int J Cancer 67:303–310

113. Pan ZK, Ikonomidis G, Lazenby A, Pardoll D, Paterson Y (1995) A recombinant Listeria monocytogenes vaccine expressing a model tumor antigen protects mice against lethal tumour cell challenge and causes regression of established tumours. Nature Med 1:471–477

114. Tahara H, Zeh HJ, Storkus WJ, Pappo I, Watkins SC, Gubler U, Wolf SF, Robbins PD, Lotze MT (1994) Fibroblasts genetically engineered to secrete interleukin 12 can suppress tumor growth and induce antitumor immunity to a murine melanoma in vivo. Cancer Res 54:182–189

115. Syrengelas AD, Chen TT, Levy R (1996) DNA immunization induces protective immunity against a B-cell lymphoma. Nature Med 2:1038–1041

116. Ciernik IF, Berzofsky JA, Carbone DP (1996) Induction of cytotoxic T lymphocytes and antitumor immunity with DNA vaccines expressing single T cell epitopes. J Immunol 156:2369–2375

117. Corr M, Lee DJ, Carson DA, Tighe H (1996) Gene vaccination with naked plasmid DNA: Mechanism of CTL priming. J Exp Med 184:1555–1560

118. Pisetsky DS (1996) Immune activation by bacterial DNA: A new genetic code. Immunity 5:303–310

119. Mayordomo JI, Loftus DJ, Sakamoto H, De Cesare CM, Appasamy PM, Lotze MT, Storkus WJ, Appella E, DeLeo AB (1996) Therapy of murine tumors with p53 wild-type and mutant sequence peptide-based vaccines. J Exp Med 183: 1357–1365

120. Ossevoort MA, Feltkamp MC, van Veen KJ, Melief CJ, Kast WM (1995) Dendritic cells as carriers for a cytotoxic T-lymphocyte epitope-based peptide vaccine in protection against a human papillomavirus 16-induced tumor. J Immunother 18:86–94

121. Puccetti P, Bianchi R, Fioretti MC, Ayroldi E, Uyttenhove C, Van Pel A, Boon T, Grohmann U (1994) Use of a skin test assay to determine tumor-specific CD8+ T cell reactivity. Eur J Immunol 24:1446–1452

122. Paglia P, Chiodoni C, Rodolfo M, Colombo MP (1996) Murine dendritic cells loaded in vitro with soluble protein prime cytotoxic T lymphocytes against tumor antigen in vivo. J Exp Med 183:317–322

123. Boczkowski D, Nair SK, Snyder D, Gilboa E (1996) Dendritic cells pulsed with RNA are potent antigen-presenting cells in vitro and in vivo. J Exp Med 184:465–472

124. Gabrilovich DI, Cunningham HT, Carbone DP (1997) IL-12 and mutant p53 peptide-pulsed dendritic cells for the specific immunotherapy of cancer. J Immunother 19:414–418

125. Ashley DM, Faiola B, Nair S, Hale LP, Bigner DD, Gilboa E (1997) Bone marrow-derived dendritic cells pulsed with tumor extracts or tumor RNA induce antitumor immunity against central nervous system tumors. J Exp Med 186:1177–1182

126. Condon C, Watkins SC, Celluzzi CM, Thompson K, Falo LD (1996) DNA-based immunization by in vivo transfection of dendritic cells. Nature Med 2:1122–1128

127. Strunk D, Rappersberger K, Egger C, Strobl H, Kromer E, Elbe A, Maurer D, Stingl G (1996) Generation of human dendritic cells/langerhans cells from circulating CD34+ hematopoietic progenitor cells. Blood 87:1292–1302

128. Nestle FO, Alijagic S, Gilliet M, Sun Y, Grabbe S, Dummer R, Burg G, Schadendorf D (1998) Vaccination of melanoma patients with peptide- or tumor lysate-pulsed dendritic cells. Nature Med 4:328–332

129. Livingston PO, Wong GYC, Adluri S, Tao Y, Padavan M, Parente R, Hanlon C, Calves MJ, Helling F, Ritter G, Oettgen HF, Old LJ (1994) Improved survival in stage III melanoma patients with GM2 antibodies: a randomized trial of adjuvant vaccination with GM2 ganglioside. J Clin Oncol 12:1036–1044

202 T.F. Gajewski

130. Reich Z, Boniface JJ, Lyons DS, Borochov N, Wachtel EJ, Davis MM (1997) Ligand-specific oligomerization of T-cell receptor molecules. Nature 387:617–620
131. Laning J, Kawasaki H, Tanaka E, Luo Y, Dorf ME (1994) Inhibition of in vivo tumor growth by the ß chemokine, TCA3. J Immunol 153:4625–4635
132. Hahne M, Rimoldi D, Schroter M, Romero P, Schreier M, French LE, Scheider P, Bornand T, Fontana A, Lienard D, Cerottini J-C, Tschopp J (1996) Melanoma cell expression of Fas (Apo-1/CD95) ligand: Implications for tumor immune escape. Science 274:1363–1366
133. Lehmann F, Marchand M, Hainaut P, Pouillartd P, Sastre X, Ikeda H, Boon T, Coulie P (1995) Differences in the antigens recognized by cytolytic T cells on two successive metastases of a melanoma patient are consistent with immune selection. Eur J Immunol 25:340–347
134. Margolin K, Aronson FR, Sznol M, Atkins MB, Gucalp R, Fisher RI, Sunderland M, Doroshow JH, Ernest ML, Mier JW, Dutcher JP, Gaynor ER, Weiss GR (1994) Phase II studies of recombinant human interleukin-4 in advanced renal cancer and malignant melanoma. J Immunother 15:147–153
135. Weber J, Gunn H, Yang J, Parkinson D, Topalian S, Schwartzentruber D, Ettinghausen S, Levitt D, Rosenberg SA (1994) A phase I trial of intravenous interleukin-6 in patients with advanced cancer. J Immunother 15:292–302
136. Smith JWI, Urba WJ, Clark JW, Longo DL, Farrell M, Creekmore SP, Conlon KC, Jaffe H, Steis RG (1991) Phase I evaluation of recombinant tumor necrosis factor given in combinatin with recombinant interferon-gamma. J Immunother 10:355–362
137. Legha SS (1997) The role of interferon alpha in the treatment of metastatic melanoma. Semin Oncol 24 (suppl 4):S4–24-S4–31
138. Negrier S, Escudier B, Lasset C, Douillard J-Y, Savary J, Chevreau C, Ravaud A, Mercatello A, Peny J, Mosseau M, Philip T, Tursz T (1998) Recombinant human interleukin-2, recombinant interferon alpha-2a, or both in metastatic renal-cell carcinoma. N Engl J Med 338:1272–1278
139. Aulitzky W, Gastl G, Aultzky WE, Herold M, Kemmler J, Mull B, Frick J, Huber C (1989) Successful treatment of metastatic renal cell carcinoma with a biologically active dose of recombinant interferon-gamma. J Clin Oncol 7:1875–1884
140. Kopp WC, Smith JWI, Ewel CH, Alvord WG, Main C, Guyre PM, Steis RG, Longo DL, Urba WJ (1993) Immunomodulatory effects of interferon-γ in patients with metastatic malignant melanoma. J Immunother 13:181–190
141. Sanda MG, Yang JC, Topalian SL, Groves ES, Childs A, Belfort R, de Smet MD, Scwartzentruber DJ, White DE, Lotze MT, Rosenberg SA (1992) Intravenous administration of recombinant human macrophage colony-stimulating factor in patients with metastatic cancer: A phase I study. J Clin Oncol 10:1643–1649
142. Redman BG, Flaherty L, Chou TH, Kraut M, Martino S, Simon M, Valdivieso M, Groves E (1992) Phase I trial of recombinant macrophage colony-stimulating factor by rapid intravenous infusion in patients with cancer. J Immunother 12:50–54
143. Byers VS, Rodvien R, Grant K et al. (1989) Phase I study of monoclonal antibody-ricin A chain immunotoxin XomaZyme-791 in patients with metastatic colon cancer. Cancer Res 49:6153–6160
144. Grossbard ML, Freedman AS, Ritz J et al. (1992) Serotherapy of B-cell neoplasms with anti-B4-blocked ricin: A phase I trial of daily bolus infusion. Blood 79:576–585
145. Nasi LM, Meyers M, Livingston PO, Houghton AN, Chapman PB (1997) Anti-melanoma effects of R24, a monoclonal antibody against GD3 ganglioside. Melanoma Res 7 (suppl 2):S155-S162

146. Dippold W, Bernhard H, Dienes HP, Meyer zum Buschenfelde KH (1988) Treatment of patients with malignant melanoma by monoclonal ganglioside antibodies. Eur J Clin Oncol 24 (suppl 2):S65-S67

147. Boel P, Wildmann C, Sensi ML, Brasseur F, Renauld JC, Coulie P, Boon T, Van der Bruggen P (1995) BAGE: a new gene encoding an antigen recognized on human melanoma by cytolytic T lymphocytes. Immunity 2:167–175

148. Van den Eynde B, Peeters O, De Backer O, Gaugler B, Lucas S, Boon T (1995) A new family of genes coding for an antigen recognized by autologous cytolytic T lymphocytes on a human melanoma. J Exp Med 182:689–698

149. Robbins PF, el Gamil M, Li YF, Kawakami Y, Loftus D, Appella E, Rosenberg SA (1996) A mutated beta-catenin gene encodes a melanoma-specific antigen recognized by tumor infiltrating lymphocytes. J Exp Med 183:1185–1192

150. Mandelboim O, Berke G, Fridkin M, Feldman M, Eisenstein M, Eisenbach L (1994) CTL induction by a tumour-associated antigenic octapeptide derived from a murine lung carcinoma. Nature 369:67–71

151. Monach PA, Meredith SC, Siegel CT, Schreiber H (1995) A unique tumor antigen produced by a single amino acid substitution. Immunity 2:45–59

152. Wang RF, Parkhurst MR, Kawakami Y, Robbins PF, Rosenberg SA (1996) Utilization of an alternative open reading frame of a normal gene in generating a novel human cancer antigen. J Exp Med 183:1131–1140

153. Coulie PG, Lehmann F, Lethe B, Herman J, Lurquin C, Andrawiss M, Boon T (1995) A mutated intron sequence codes for an antigenic peptide recognized by cytolytic T lymphocytes on a human melanoma. Proc Natl Acad Sci USA 92:7976–7980

154. Noguchi Y, Chen YT, Old LJ (1994) A mouse mutant p53 product recognized by CD4+ and CD8+ cells. Proc Natl Acad Sci USA 91:3171–3175

155. Peace DJ, Smith JW, Chen W, You SG, Cosand WL, Blake J, Cheever MA (1994) Lysis of ras oncogene-transformed cells by specific cytotoxic T lymphocytes elicited by primary in vitro immunization with mutated ras peptide. J Exp Med 179:473–479

156. Theobald M, Biggs J, Dittmer D, Levine AJ, Sherman LA (1995) Targeting p53 as a general tumor antigen. Proc Natl Acad Sci USA 92:11993–11997

157. Bosch GJ, Joosten AM, Kessler JH, Melief CJ, Leeksma OC (1996) Recognition of BCR-ABL positive leukemic blasts by human CD4+ T cells elicited by primary in vitro immunization with a BCR-ABL breakpoint peptide. Blood 88:3522–3527

158. Bloom MB, Perry-Lally D, Robbins PF, Li Y, el Gamil M, Rosenberg SA, Yang JC (1997) Identification of tyrosinase-related protein 2 as a tumor rejection antigen for the B16 melanoma. J Exp Med 185:453–459

159. Coulie PG, Brichard V, Van Pel A, Wolfel T, Schneider J, Traversari C, Mattei S, De Plaen E, Lurquin C, Szikora J, Renauld J, Boon T (1994) A new gene coding for a differentiation antigen recognized by autologous cytolytic T lymphocytes on HLA-A2 melanomas. J Exp Med 180:35–42

160. Brichard V, Van Pel A, Wolfel T, Wolfel C, DePlaen E, Lethe B, Coulie P, Boon T (1993) The tyrosinase gene codes for an antigen recognized by autologous cytolytic T lymphocytes on HLA-A2 melanomas. J Exp Med 178:489–495

161. Wang RF, Appella E, Kawakami Y, Kang X, Rosenberg SA (1996) Identification of Trp-2 as a human tumor antigen recognized by cytotoxic T lymphocytes. J Exp Med 184:2207–2216

162. Henderson RA, Nimgaonkar MT, Watkins SC, Robbins PD, Ball ED, Finn OJ (1996) Human dendritic cells genetically engineered to express high levels of the human epithelial tumor antigen mucin (MUC-1). Cancer Res 56:3763–3770

163. Kast WM, Offringa R, Peters PJ, Voordouw AC, Meloen RH, Van der Eb AJ, Melief
     CJM (1989) Eradication of adenovirus E1-induced tumors by E1 A specific cyto-
     toxic T lymphocytes. Cell 59:603–614
164. Disis ML, Bernhard H, Shiota FM, Hand SL, Gralow JR, Huseby ES, Gillis S,
     Cheever MA (1996) Granulocyte-macrophage colony-stimulating factor: an
     effective adjuvant for protein and peptide-based vaccines. Blood 88:202–210
165. Krensky AM, Clayberger C, Reiss CS, Strominger JL, Burakoff SJ (1982) Specificity
     of OKT4+ cytotoxic T lymphocyte clones. J Immunol 129:2001–2003
166. Braciale TJ, Andrew ME, Braciale VL (1981) Simultaneous expression of H-2-
     restricted and alloreactive recognition by a cloned line of influenza virus-speci-
     fic cytotoxic T lymphocytes. J Exp Med 153:1371–1376

# Multimodality Therapy

E.E. Vokes

Multimodality therapy is an important cancer treatment concept. It is frequently utilized in patients with intermediate stage tumors. These patients are distinguished by the presence of large primaries and/or extensive regional lymph node involvement; at the same time, they have no clinically overt distant metastases. They represent a common solid tumor stage and have traditionally been treated with surgery and/or radiation therapy. However, in many solid tumors survival or cure rates achieved with surgery and/or radiotherapy have been low. This is due to the tendency of tumors to recur locoregionally indicating the inability of combined surgery and radiation therapy to reliably extinguish locoregional tumor bulk; in addition, tumors frequently recur outside of the initially involved area indicating the presence of systemic microdissemination at the time of initial diagnosis. Such microscopic tumor cells are not affected by the administration of surgery and radiation. In fact, there is some evidence that micrometastatic tumor deposits may display accelerated growth following removal of a primary or regional tumor mass.

In order to improve cure rates for intermediate stage tumors, multimodality or combined modality treatment concepts have been developed:
- Surgery, XRT
- Surgery, XRT, adjuvant CT
- Induction CT, surgery, XRT
- Concomitant chemoradiotherapy (plus/minus-surgery)
- (Surgery) concomitant chemoradiotherapy

Such approaches can thus involve the sequential administration of multimodality therapy or the concomitant use of chemotherapy and radiation therapy.

Among the sequential approaches, adjuvant chemotherapy is the best defined and most established approach. It is administered following potentially curative surgery and/or radiotherapy. Chemotherapy is administered to individual patients in the absence of known residual disease based on statistical observations derived from large cohorts of patients indicating a significant risk of tumor recurrence. Adjuvant chemotherapy has lead to improved survival and increased cure rates in patients with early and intermediate stage breast cancer as well as intermediate stage colorectal cancer. Its primary target in these diseases is micrometastatic dissemination; an impact on improved locoregional control is not evident.

Another sequentially administered multimodality therapy approach is induction chemotherapy ("neoadjuvant" chemotherapy). Here patients receive initial chemotherapy which may lead to successful eradication of micrometastatic disease; in addition, it is possible to "downstage" the local and regional tumor bulk. The latter might allow for a higher locoregional control rate following subsequent administration of surgery and/or radiotherapy. Alternatively, it might be possible to use less extensive surgical procedures allowing for "organ preservation". A potential downside of induction chemotherapy is the delay of standard surgery or radiotherapy. Delay of surgery or radiotherapy may lead to inability to successfully administer these modalities should the local tumor mass be unresponsive to chemotherapy. One obvious advantage of induction chemotherapy is that it allows clinicians and patients to directly assess for a potential benefit of chemotherapy, i.e., the response of the primary tumor site to the chemotherapy. Induction chemotherapy has been shown to be of clinical benefit in patients with stage III unresectable non-small cell lung cancer. It has also been extensively studied in advanced head and neck cancer and esophageal cancer. In the latter two sites, however, no impact on survival has been demonstrated to date.

Concomitant chemoradiotherapy is conceptually somewhat more complex than the sequential administration of chemotherapy and radiation therapy. Like sequential approaches, concomitant chemoradiotherapy allows for eradication of systemic micrometaseses through the effects of chemotherapy and treatment of locoregional disease via the use of radiotherapy [1–8]. In addition, concomitant chemoradiotherapy allows for a direct intereaction of the two modalities within the irradiated field. The latter might allow chemotherapy to directly increase the cytotoxicity of radiotherapy. This effect is referred to as radiation "sensitization" when inactive chemotherapy drugs are used; when drugs with known single agent activity in a given disease are used this effect is referred to as radiation "enhancement". Sensitization or enhancement may occur as an effect of a variety of interactions which are well-described in preclinical models. For example, hypoxic cells are known to be radiation resistant, but may be eradicated by certain bioreductive alkylating agents. Similarly, rapidly proliferating cells in the S-phase of the cell cycle are less sensitive to radiation therapy but may respond to antimetabolite-based chemotherapy. Cell cycle synchronization in a radiation sensitive cell cycle phase has also been described. For example, paclitaxel is thought to arrest the $G_2$-M phase of the cell cycle, a radiation sensitive cell cycle phase. Radiation exerts its effects through damaging the DNA. DNA can be repaired in the presence of DNA nucleosides. When the latter are depleted through the simultaneous use of antimetabolites, DNA repair may not be able to be implemented. Given these complex interactions, it is clear that concomitant chemoradiotherapy has to be administered with caution. In particular, acute radiation toxicities (within the irradiated field) are usually increased with concomitant chemoradiotherapy. This may require the use of lower doses of chemotherapy or, at times, interruptions of radiation therapy. The latter should be done with great caution, however, since administration of radiation therapy over a more protracted period of time decreases the effects of radiotherapy, at least as a single treatment modality.

In clinical practice, concomitant chemoradiotherapy is frequently successful. In particular, increased locoregional control and survival rates have been demonstrated in advanced head and neck cancer, small cell lung cancer, esophageal cancer, pancreatic cancer, anal cancer, and rectal cancer.

Since combined modality therapy always involves physicians from multiple specialties, it is necessary to initially establish an overall treatment plan that covers all potentially involved treatment modalities. Therefore, if induction chemotherapy is to be administered it is necessary that both the Surgeon and Radiation Oncologist evaluate and stage the patient together with the Medical Oncologist prior to institution of induction chemotherapy since the disease may be significantly decreased in size following chemotherapy. This also applies to concomitant chemoradiotherapy. In almost all cases of combined modality therapy, it is desirable to treat patients on a clinical protocol since an accurate assessment of toxicity and activity of treatment is necessary. Institutions that do not have the logistics to support joint patient evaluations and staging by all involved specialties and do not participate in clinical research, generally, should not engage in multimodality therapy administration.

## References

1. Steel GG, Peckham MJ. Exploitable mechanisms in combined radiotherapy-chemotherapy: the concept of additivity (1979). Int J Radiat Oncol Biol Phys 5:85–91
2. Steel GG. Terminology in the description of drug-radiation interactions (1979). Int J Radiat Oncol Biol Phys 5:1145–1150
3. Vokes EE, Weichselbaum RR. Concomitant chemoradiotherapy: rationale and clinical experience in patients with solid tumors (1990). J Clin Oncol 8:911–934
4. Vokes EE. Concomitant chemoradiotherapy for solid tumors: rationale and clinical experience. Proceedings of a symposium (1992). Vokes EE (Chairman). Semin Oncol 19 (suppl 11):1–102
5. Vokes EE. Drug-Radiation Interactions (1996) In: Principles of Antineoplastic Drug Development and Pharmacology (ed.) Schilsky RL, Milano GA, Ratain MJ. Marcel Dekker, Inc. New York, NY 10:203–222
6. Tannock IF. Treatment of cancer with radiation and drugs (1996). J Clin Oncol 14 (12):3156–3174
7. Perez CA, Brady LW. Principles and Practice of Radiation Oncology (1998), 3rd edn. Philadelphia: JB Lippincott
8. Vokes EE. Combined modality therapy of solid tumours. Lancet (1997), 349 (suppl II):4–6

# Complications

# The Diagnosis and Management of Oncologic Emergencies

E.B. Lamont, P.C. Hoffman

## Introduction

This chapter details the epidemiology, pathophysiology, clinical presentation, diagnosis, and treatment of several of the most common oncologic emergencies (for other oncologic emergencies – hypercalcemia, SIADH, and tumor lysis syndrome – see chapter by Helft and Rudin, this volume). Because of the systemic nature of cancer, these emergencies often affect organ systems remote from the original cancer, making diagnosis challenging. Given the long natural history of many advanced cancers, the successful diagnosis and managment of these emergencies may be rewarded with prolonged patient survival. However, when cancer patients become end-stage, the same invasive diagnostic procedures and aggressive treatments may become onerous. Decisions regarding management of these patients are best made jointly by the patient, the primary oncologist, the family, and the treating physician.

## Cardiovascular Emergencies

### Superior Vena Cava Syndrome

Superior vena cava (SVC) syndrome is the clinical manifestation of SVC obstruction and occurs through external compression, thrombosis, or invasion of the vein. While previously in the realm of non-neoplastic entities like syphilitic aortitis, SVC syndrome is now almost exclusively (>90%) secondary to malignancy [1]. The syndrome complicates 2%–8% of primary thoracic malignancies, most frequently small cell carcinoma of the lung, followed by other lung cancer histologies, non-Hodgkin's lymphoma and mediastinal germ cell tumors [2–5].

Because the venous drainage from the upper extremities, upper thorax and head is obstructed, SVC syndrome presents with symptoms related to engorgement of these areas. Both the degree of SVC compromise and the extent of collateral veins determine the varied clinical presentation, which can be as mild as slight facial and upper extremity edema, or as dire as intracranial swelling, seizure, hemodynamic instability or tracheal obstruction. Table 1 lists the frequency of symptoms in 66 patients admitted with superior vena cava obstruction [2]. Because of the lore of the dire symptomatologies, physicians often react to suspected SVC syndrome with panicked urgency and are tempted to initiate treatment before a pathologic diagnosis can be made. However, some argue convincingly that the SVC syndrome is rarely so urgent as to preclude timely and methodical radiologic and pathologic evaluations prior to therapy [6].

**Table 1.** Presenting symptoms and signs of SVC obstruction in 66 patients (from [1], with kind permission of the publishers)

| Symptoms | % | |
|---|---|---|
| Facial swelling | 83 | |
| Dyspnea | 83 | |
| Cough | 70 | |
| Orthopnea | 64 | |
| Nasal congestion | 35 | |
| Hoarseness | 35 | |
| Stridor | 33 | |
| Dizziness | 29 | |
| Tongue swelling | 24 | |
| Headache | 3 | |
| Syncope | 3 | |
| Dysphagia | 1 | |
| Epistaxis | 1 | |
| | | |
| Signs | | |
| Neck vein distention | 92 | |
| Facial swelling | 86 | |
| Arm vein distention | 68 | |
| Upper extremity swelling | 64 | |
| Mentation changes | 27 | |
| Glossal edema | 24 | |
| Laryngeal edema | 24 | |
| Rhinorrhea | 18 | |
| Stupor | 14 | |
| Coma | 6 | |
| Upper body plethora | 3 | |

When a patient presents with suspected SVC syndrome, the first step is to obtain an imaging study to both confirm the diagnosis and to assist in treatment decisions. Of the several imaging modalities available for diagnosing the syndrome, the best study is the one that can be obtained most expediently. Magnetic resonance imaging (MRI), contrast enhanced computed tomography (CT), radionuclide flow study, or traditional venography are all adequate modalities, but at most centers CT is the most readily available. CT and MRI also provide information regarding possible etiologies and can thereby direct the approach to a tissue diagnosis. The approach to establishing a tissue diagnosis is defined by both the patient's clinical stability and the findings on examination and radiographic studies. Table 2 summarizes the diagnostic yields for several tests, ranging from non-invasive approaches like sputum cytology to the maximally invasive thoracotomy [7].

Tissue diagnoses are important as they guide treatment; specifically, they identify those patients for whom SVC syndrome should be treated with combination chemotherapy, rather than with local measures like radiation therapy or percutaneous vascular procedures. Patients with known thoracic malignancies clearly do not require a further tissue diagnosis.

Treatment of SVC syndrome is divided into supportive and definitive therapy. Acutely, patients should be supported with elevation of the head of their bed and supplemental oxygen. Although dexamethasone is sometimes used, its utility has never been supported by experimental data. The definitive treatment of SVC syndrome depends on the etiology. Studies of small cell lung cancer patients with SVC syndrome reveal systemic combination chemotherapy to be more efficacious than radiation therapy, with 73%–100% of patients experiencing symptomatic relief within 7

**Table 2.** Diagnostic yield of various tests in SVC syndrome (from [7], with kind permission of the publishers)

| Test | % Positive |
|---|---|
| Thoracotomy | 98 |
| Bronchoscopy | 90 |
| Mediastinoscopy | 77 |
| Thoracentesis | 73 |
| Lymph node biopsy | 67 |
| Sputum cytology | 50–90 |
| Bone marrow biopsy | 23 |

days [5, 8, 9]. Conversely, for non-small cell lung cancer and for solid tumors metastatic to the thorax like breast cancer, radiation therapy is the preferred treatment modality and is associated with a 56%–70% success rate within two weeks [2]. Finally, in patients with non-Hodgkin's lymphoma, single modality chemotherapy or radiation therapy appear equally efficacious, with 100% of patients experiencing relief of symptoms within two weeks [3]. For these patients, chemotherapy is argued to be the better modality as it also provides systemic therapy. Patients with recurrent or refractory symptoms may benefit from percutaneous stent placement. Stenting is associated with immediate relief of symptoms in >90% of patients, but reportedly carries a 29% morbidity and 4% mortality rate [10–14]. Vascular bypass surgery is a treatment modality available for similar patients, but the even higher morbidity and mortality in such patients makes it an infrequently employed therapy. Finally, for patients whose SVC syndrome is secondary to venous catheter thrombosis, thrombolytic therapy given within 5 days of the onset of symptoms is associated with an 88% success rate [15]. For thromboses of longer duration, catheter removal in the setting of systemic anticoagulation with heparin and warfarin may be a more successful approach.


## Malignant Pericardial Disease

Pericardial disease in cancer patients can result from a variety of medical conditions including radiation, uremia, infection, or malignancy. Autopsy series have shown that malignant involvement of the pericardium complicates 5% of cancers and is usually clinically silent [16, 17]. However, the series reveal that when malignant pericardial disease is symptomatic, it is often the direct or a supporting cause of death. Thoracic tumors are the most frequent tumors to directly or hematogenously invade the pericardium, with lung cancer first, followed by lymphoma and breast cancer [16, 17]

Malignant pericardial effusion leading to tamponade can be an immediately life-threatening complication of malignant pericardial disease and should be suspected in cancer patients with new cardiopulmonary complaints. Because the right-sided cardiac chambers are compressed by surrounding fluid, signs of both right heart failure and left heart insufficiency result. As Table 3 details, the presenting symptoms reflect these circulatory disruptions and are, in decreasing order of fre-

**Table 3.** Clinical presentation of malignant pericardial effusion in 93 patients (from [18], with kind permission of the publishers)

| Symptoms | % |
| --- | --- |
| Dyspnea | 91 |
| Cough | 42 |
| Orthopnea | 32 |
| Chest pain | 20 |
| Peripheral edema | 17 |
| Nausea | 12 |
| Impaired level of consciousness | 5 |
| Diaphoresis | 4 |
| Dysphagia | 3 |
| Hemoptysis | 2 |
| Syncope | 2 |
| Facial swelling | 2 |
| | |
| Signs | |
| Paradoxical pulse (>10 mmHg) | 62 |
| Elevated jugular venous pressure | 51 |
| Tachycardia (>110 bpm) | 43 |
| Systolic BP (<110 mmHg) | 42 |
| Respiratory rate (>20 breaths/min) | 35 |
| Kussmaul's sign | 14 |
| Pericardial friction rub | 6 |
| Hepatomegaly | 2 |

quency: dyspnea, cough, orthopnea, chest pain and pedal edema [18]. Examination often reveals hypotension, tachycardia, distended jugular veins, and a paradoxical pulse of >10 mmHg. Chest radiographs reveal cardiomegaly in most, and pleural effusions in approximately half of patients. However, patients with prior chest radiotherapy may not have radiographic evidence of cardiomegaly due to radiation-induced fibrosis of the pericardium. EKG abnormalities are protean, usually non-specific and commonly include sinus tachycardia and decreased voltage in the limb leads, but rarely electrical alternans [17–19]. Echocardiography confirms the diagnosis by revealing effusion associated with inspiratory increase in right ventricular dimensions, and right atrial and/or right ventricular collapse. Classically, right heart catheterization reveals equalization of intra pericardial, right atrial, right ventricular, and pulmonary capillary wedge pressures [20]. Since not all pericardial effusions in cancer patients are malignant, both the clinical setting and the results of a diagnostic pericadiocentesis or pericardial biopsy are critical to determining the etiology and therefore the correct treatment for this condition.

Management of malignant pericardial effusions can be challenging and is divided into temporizing and definitive therapies. The immediate management of a hemodynamically significant pericardial effusion is pericardiocentesis. In 97% of patients, the fluid is successfully removed and symptoms resolve immediately [21]. Unfortunately, in approximately 50% of patients, the fluid reaccumulates, requiring subsequent pericardiocenteses. Several more definitive therapies targeted at decreasing the reaccumulation rate have been paired with pericardiocentesis, including radiation therapy, systemic chemotherapy, pericardial sclerotic therapies, and mechanical therapies. When administered following initial pericardiocentesis, these therapies have the following reaccumulation rates: radiation therapy 33%, systemic chemotherapy 30%, pericardial sclerosis with tetracycline 15%–30%, and mechanical therapies like thoracotomy with pericardial window placement or balloon pericardiotomy 0%–15% [21].

Of all the mechanical therapies, balloon pericardiotomy has the best reaccumulation profile with 0%–6% reaccumulation [22–24]. The procedure includes a pericardiocentesis followed by balloon catheter dilation of the pericardial needle entrance site. Typically, a balloon catheter is placed across the pericardial entrance site and inflated two to three times, each for one to two minutes for a total procedure time of 20–40 min. Side effects have been limited to asymptomatic pleural effusions in most patients [22, 23]. Not only is balloon pericardiotomy more successful than other less invasive therapies, but it is the most successful and least morbid of the other mechanical therapies, most of which require general anesthesia and thoracotomies. At centers with staff facile with this technique, patients requiring definitive management of malignant pericardial effusions should be evaluated for this therapy.

## Neurologic Emergencies

### Spinal Cord Compression

Malignant compression of the spinal cord complicates between 5 and 10% of all malignancies and requires emergent initiation of therapy to arrest what is often rapid and irreversible neurologic deterioration [25]. In 85% of patients, the condition results from the hematogenous spread of a previously diagnosed cancer to the vertebral body that then compresses the cord directly or causes vertebral body collapse, compressing the cord [26]. In a small number of patients (10%), the condition results from paraspinal malignancies like lymphoma that compress neural structures traversing the foramina. The most common vertebral levels of spinal cord compression (SCC) are thoracic (70%), lumbosacral (15%), and cervical (15%), and up to 50% of patients have tumor in more than one, often non-contiguous, vertebrae [26, 27]. Clinical series have shown that the tumors most likely to cause SCC are in decreasing order of frequency: breast carcinoma, lung carcinoma, lymphoma, prostate carcinoma, renal cell carcinoma, and myeloma, together accounting for nearly 70% of histologies [26].

The presenting symptoms and signs of malignant SCC in 130 patients are detailed in Table 4 [26]. While back pain is the presenting complaint in almost all patients (96%), the pain can be either localized or radicular, and it can be challenging to distinguish SCC from benign conditions like degenerative joint disease or disk disease. Characteristics suggestive of SCC include a history of pain worsening with Valsalva, cough, or recumbency. Subsequent examination reveals clear, objective weakness (usually bilateral and symmetric) in 87% of patients. Sensory deficits are noted in 78% and autonomic dysfunction (like urinary retention or incontinence) in 57% of patients [26]. Those patients with autonomic dysfunction at the time of diagnosis form an important, poor prognosis subgroup in which 66% lose ambulation [26].

After the suspicion of malignant SCC is raised by history and/or physical examination, dexamethasone should be administered (see details of dosing below) and radiologic evaluation must be obtained quickly. The absence of objective neurologic signs of SCC should not dissuade the clinician from the appropriate diagnostic evaluation. Nearly all patients (80%–84%) with SCC will have abnormal plain films [25, 27–29]. The AP

**Table 4.** Signs and symptoms of epidural spinal cord compression in 130 patients (from [26], with kind permission of the publishers)

| Sign/symptom | % First symptom | % With symptom/ sign at diagnosis |
|---|---|---|
| Pain | 96 | 96 |
| Weakness | 2 | 76 |
| Autonomic dysfunction | 0 | 57 |
| Sensory loss | 0 | 51 |
| Ataxia | 2 | 3 |
| Herpes zoster | 0 | 2 |
| Flexor spasms | 0 | 1 |

view can reveal pedicle pathology like erosion or displacement; the lateral view can reveal vertebral body pathology like collapse; and the oblique view can reveal foramina pathology like encroachment or enlargement [27]. Since plain films are both highly sensitive and specific for malignant SCC, they are preferable to bone scans which, although quite sensitive for malignant bony disease, are less sensitive for SCC [29]. An important exception to this rule occurs in lymphoma patients, 60% of whom will have no abnormalities on plain films [30]. Subsequent imaging with gadolinium enhanced MRI will both confirm the diagnosis and determine the extent of disease for radiation planning [31, 32]. If MRI is unavailable or contraindicated, the more invasive metrizamide myelography with or without CT can confirm the diagnosis.

In most cases, pretreatment neurologic function portends post treatment function, with most ambulatory patients (approximately 80%), fewer paretic patients (<50%) and even fewer paraplegic patients (<10%) ambulatory after therapy [26, 27, 29]. Therapy for SCC is divided into temporizing therapy and definitive therapy. Acutely, patients should be given dexamethasone 10 mg intravenously, followed by 4 mg every 6 h to continue until the completion of definitive therapy. The steroid will decrease cord edema and thereby transiently improve neurologic signs and symptoms in some patients. Radiation therapy (RT) and surgical decompression via laminectomy are the two definitive treatment modalities. Series examining the effect of laminectomy followed by RT compared to RT alone, reveal radiation alone to be equally as efficacious and far less morbid than the more invasive therapy in most patients [26, 33]. However, there are several instances in which surgery with RT is preferable to RT alone, including cases where a tissue diagnosis is needed, where the tumor is radio-refractory such as sarcoma or melanoma, where there is spinal instability requiring surgical stabilization, and where disease occurs in a previously irradiated field.


Cerebral Herniation Syndromes

In cancer patients, cerebral herniation syndromes result from space occupying brain tumors that increase intracranial pressure and thereby compress the brain against rigid cranial elements. Herniation can result from primary central nervous system tumors, or from those metastatic to the central nervous system, with lung cancer, breast cancer, melanoma, renal cell carcinoma, and lymphoma the most common [34]. With increased intracranial pressure, patients initially experience intermittent bilateral frontal or occipital headaches. The headaches often awaken them from sleep or are present on awakening in the morning. They can be accompanied by signs of elevated intracranial pressure like projectile vomiting, unsteady gait, and papilledema. As intracranial pressure increases further, cerebral function decreases, leading to inattention, apathy, psychomotor retardation, and somnolence. Because the brain is compartmentalized by the falx cerebri and tentorium, increased pressure in one compartment is equalized into the other compartments through characteristic herniations. MRI may reveal the herniation as well as the causative tumor and edema.

Management of malignant cerebral herniation syndromes centers around decreasing intracranial pressure through several simultaneous interventions and then initiating definitive antitumor therapy. First, the patient should be loaded with dexamethasone 100 mg intravenously, followed by 25 mg every 6 h to mitigate cerebral edema and thereby reduce intracranial pressure. The patient then should be intubated for both airway protection and hyperventilation to a $PaCO_2$ of 25–30 mmHG. Hypocapnia to this level results in cerebral vasoconstriction which will decrease intracranial volume and thereby reduce intracranial pressure. The effect, however, is of a short duration (48–72 h), as renal bicarbonate wasting will act to normalize cerebral pH and thereby normalize cerebral blood flow [35]. Finally, a loading dose of the osmotic diuretic mannitol 100 g, followed by 25 g as needed may further reduce intracranial edema. The patient should be evaluated emergently by a radiation oncologist for more definitive therapy with cranial RT.

## Carcinomatous Meningitis

Carcinomatous meningitis results from the direct or hematogenous seeding of the meninges by tumor cells and should be suspected in cancer patients presenting with deficits in multiple areas of the neuraxis. Autopsy studies suggest that malignant involvement of the meninges is common, occurring in 8% of cancer patients. These studies reveal that patients with acute leukemias have the highest rates of leptomeningeal disease, followed by patients with non-Hodgkin's lymphoma, small cell lung cancer and breast cancer [34].

The diagnosis of carcinomatous meningitis is often elusive, with symptoms that can be both diffuse and localized. Diffuse symptoms result from decreased brain metabolism that is seen with malignant central nervous system disease, from cerebral spinal fluid (CSF) obstruction causing hydrocephalus and increased intracranial pressure, or from diffuse meningeal irritation. These patients most frequently present with headache and have signs of altered mental status on examination. Localized signs result from spinal and/or cranial nerve root invasion. In cases of spinal nerve root involvement, the most frequent presenting complaint is weakness and the most frequent examination findings are reflex asymmetry and lower motor neuron weakness. Spinal sensory nerves can also be affected, resulting in complaints of paresthesias and findings of sensory loss. Cranial nerves damaged by tumor deposits result in cranial nerve palsies. Among those with cranial nerve involvement, the most frequent presenting complaint is double vision, and the most frequent exam finding is ocular muscle paresis due to compromise of cranial nerves III, IV, and VI [36].

Carcinomatous meningitis is most reliably diagnosed through examination of the CSF, not through neuroimaging. Once a head CT excludes a concomitant mass lesion that could cause herniation during lumbar puncture, the patient should undergo a lumbar puncture followed by CSF examination. Table 5 details the initial CSF results of 90 patients with leptomeningeal metastases. It reveals that ninty seven percent of patients with carcinomatous meningitis have CSF abnormalities with the following distribution: elevated protein (81%), elevated white blood cell count (57%), positive cytology (54%), elevated opening pressure (50%) and depressed glucose (31%). The cytology yield increases to 86% if three lumbar punctures are performed [36]. MRI with gadolinium can

**Table 5.** Leptomeningeal metastases from solid tumors in 90 patients: CSF findings (from [36], with kind permission of the publishers. Copyright: 1982, American Cancer Society))

| Test | % Postive on initial LP |
| --- | --- |
| Protein >50 mg/dl | 81 |
| White blood cells >5 μl | 57 |
| Positive cytology | 54 |
| Opening pressure >160 mm CSF | 50 |
| Glucose <40 mg/dl | 31 |
| Normal | 3 |

identify leptomeningeal deposits as areas of enhancement, but is positive in only 33%–66% of cases [37, 38].

Successful treatment of carcinomatous meningitis can arrest or sometimes reverse neurologic loss, extending patient survival from weeks to months [36]. The treatment modalities are intrathecal chemotherapy and/or radiation therapy. Because the blood brain barrier hinders the passage of systemic chemotherapy into the brain, chemotherapy must be administered intrathecally through a ventricular reservoir (e.g., Ommaya shunt) or through a lumbar puncture. Standard regimens are methotrexate 10–15 mg twice weekly with systemic leucovorin, thiotepa 10–20 mg twice weekly, or cytarabine 50 mg twice weekly until clinical neurologic improvement occurs or until CSF cytology clears of malignant cells. The interval between doses is then increased to weekly or monthly. While acute side effects are transient nausea and vomiting, the late side effects are myelosuppression and mucositis from systemic absorption of chemotherapy. Radiation therapy is a second treatment option for established cranial or cauda equina neuropathies and may be given either singly or in association with intrathecal chemotherapy. Focal areas of disease are irradiated rather than the entire neuraxis, as the latter is associated with substantial myelosuppression. The acute side effect is transient nausea. A rare complication of concomitant methotrexate and radiation therapy is leukoencephalopathy [36]. With these therapies, approximately 50% of patients will experience either improvement or stabilization of their disease [36]. As carcinomatous meningitis is often a late finding in the course of a patient's malignancy and since treatment often has limited success, the decision of whether to treat needs to be carefully considered, taking into account the patient's performance status and the state of his or her systemic cancer.

## Urologic Emergencies

### Uric Acid Nephropathy

Uric acid nephropathy results from intrarenal precipitation of massive amounts of uric acid liberated by tumors with high proliferative indices, either because of their rapid cell turnover or because of their lysis by cytotoxic chemotherapy. This condition is often part of the tumor lysis syndrome, which is discussed in the chapter by Helft and Rudin in this volume. Uric acid crystals in the renal collecting system obstruct urine flow, raising intrarenal pressure and thereby decreasing vascular perfusion. The end result is acute oliguric renal failure. Patients, many of whom will also suffer from fulminant tumor lysis syndrome, may develop lethargy, seizures, nausea, and vomiting, and eventually symptoms and signs of volume overload. Laboratory evaluation typically reveals chemistry values consistent with tumor lysis syndrome (see Chapter #, Metabolic and Electrolyte Complications) including uric acid levels in the range of 25–90 mg/dl. Urine evaluation often reveals serum uric acid concentrations of 150–200 mg/dl and both uric acid and sodium monourate crystals [46].

The management of uric acid nephropathy is primarily preventive, with the goal to decrease uric acid production and increase its urine solubility. Decreased production is achieved through use of allopurinol, a xanthine oxidase inhibitor. Treatment with allopurinol should precede chemotherapy by 2–3 days if possible. The initial dose of 300–800 mg daily should reflect tumor burden. The dose may eventually be decreased to between 100–300 mg daily and should continue through the period of cytoreduction. The dose should be reduced for renal insufficiency. Increased uric acid solubility can be achieved by maximizing urine output, and by making the urine alkaline through the use of sodium bicarbonate or acetazolamide [47, 48]. Urinary output of 3 l/day (125 ml/h) and a urinary pH of >7 are often recommended. For patients in whom uric acid nephropathy develops despite these measures, hemodialysis can both acutely decrease serum uric acid and correct the volume and electrolyte effects of acute renal failure [57].

Hemorrhagic Cystitis

Hemorrhagic cystitis results from inflammation of the bladder and presents with dysuria, hematuria, and urinary frequency. In cancer patients, the condition can result from chemotherapy, radiation therapy, or infections. Cyclophosphamide and ifosfamide are the most frequent chemotherapy agents implicated in hemorrhagic cystitis and act through their metabolite acrolein to damage the bladder mucosa. While previously complicating more than 40% of bone marrow transplants, hemorrhagic cystitis now occurs in less than 5% due to preventive management with hydration and the drug mesna [49–55]. Vigorous intravenous hydration generates high urine output that limits bladder exposure to acrolein. Mesna is a thiol that is activated in the kidney and inactivates acrolein in the bladder. Because its half-life is shorter than that of cyclophosphamide, mesna must be started prior to cyclophosphamide and continued after the completion of the cyclophosphamide infusion. For patients in whom hemorrhagic cystitis develops despite these measures, emergent urologic consultation must be obtained regarding possible bladder irrigation, cystoscopy with clot extraction and fulguration, or chemical hemostasis with formalin. In refractory cases, vascular ligation or even cystectomy may be required.

**Other Emergencies** (see also the chapter by Helft and Rudin, this volume)

Disorders of Blood Viscosity

Hyperviscosity syndrome (HVS) and leukostasis are disorders resulting from a malignant excess of blood components and requiring rapid evaluation for possible emergent apheresis, chemotherapy, and radiotherapy.

HVS results from high levels of serum paraprotein often elaborated by Waldenstrom's macroglobulinemia (IgM) or multiple myeloma (IgA, IgG, and very rarely light chain disease). HVS is characterized by a clinical triad of visual changes, bleeding, and neurologic changes, with patients often presenting with blurred vision, mucosal oozing, and "dizzy headache", [39]. The visual and neurologic symptoms result from sludging of blood through end arterioles, and the bleeding from paraprotein-induced platelet dysfunction, clotting factor inhibition, and fibrin inhibition. Funduscopic examination can reveal tortuous vessels with a sausage-like appearance termed *fundus paraproteinaemicus*, as well as retinal hemorrhage and papilledema. The diagnosis is made by observing a serum paraprotein in the setting of an elevated blood viscosity (usually >4.0 cp). Treatment is plasmapheresis to decrease the paraprotein acutely, followed by chemotherapy to decrease production of the paraprotein. Of note, some IgM paraproteins are cold-reactive, making plasmapheresis with a room-temperature cell separator problematic. These patients should undergo plasmapheresis with pre-warmed equipment in a warm room.

Leukostasis is a rare condition that results from an excess of white blood cells. The signs and symptoms result from end organ ischemia, infarction, and hemorrhage due to microvascular thrombi from leukocyte aggregates. Patients may present with visual changes, confusion, and dyspnea. Evaluation may reveal, papilledema, mental status changes, cardiogenic or non-cardiogenic pulmonary edema, liver dysfunction, renal failure and priapism. Blood rheology studies and clinical reports reveal the risk of leukostasis to be a complex function of white blood cell type, maturity, and number as well as the concurrent hematocrit and platelet count. Patients with acute leukemias or the accelerated phase of CML with blast counts greater than $50,000/\mu l$ are at a far greater risk for leukostasis than patients with chronic lymphocytic leukemias with lymphocyte counts of even $500,000/\mu l$ [40, 41]. Leukemia patients who present with leukostasis should not receive blood product transfusions until their white blood cell count has been substantially decreased through leukapheresis, chemotherapy, or both because additional blood products will exacerbate their condition through increasing blood viscosity. Patients with pulmonary or central nervous system leukostasis may require emergent local radiation therapy to arrest organ compromise.

Lactic Acidosis

Tumor-induced lactic acidosis is an extremely rare condition that occurs in malignancies with exceptionally high proliferative indices, such as Burkitt's lymphoma, small non-cleaved, non-Burkitt's lymphoma, or acute lymphoblastic leukemia. Although the mechanism has not been established definitively, it is likely a function of tumor cell hypoxia that leads to anaerobic metabolism and the production of lactate. Concomitant hepatic impairment by the malignancy may reduce the patient's ability to metabolize the lactate produced. The diagnosis of lactic acidosis should be suspected in cancer patients with large tumor burdens who have anion gap acidoses and no history of toxic ingestion or clinical or laboratory evidence of diabetic ketoacidosis or uremia. The mainstay of treatment of this condition is treatment of the malignant cause of the acidosis with urgent chemotherapy. The malignancies which cause lactic acidosis are typically highly responsive to chemotherapy. The role of exogenous sodium bicarbonate in the management is controversial, with several animal and human studies reporting increased cellular acidosis, increased serum lactate, and higher mortality in subjects treated with bicarbonate [42–45]. Although standard texts recommend supplemental bicarbonate therapy in patients with blood pH <7.1, it is not clear that this improves clinical outcome in this patient population.

### References

1. Lochridge SK, Knibbe WP, Doty DB (1979) Obstruction of the superior vena cava. Surgery, 85:14–24
2. Armstrong BA, Poerez CA, Simpson JR, Hederman MA (1987) Role of irradiation in the management of superior vena cava syndrome. Int J Radiat Oncol Biol Phys 13:531
3. Perez-Soler R, μlaughlin P, Velasquez WS, et al (1984) Clinical features and results of managment of superior vena cava syndrome secondary to lymphoma. J Clin Oncol 2:260
4. Salsali M, Cliffton EE (1969) Superior vena cava obstruction in carcinoma of the lung. NY State J Med 69:2875
5. Sculier JP, Evans WK, Feld R, et al (1986) Superior vena cava syndrome in small-cell lung cancer. Cancer 57:847
6. Ahmann, F (1984) A reassessment of the clinical implications of the superior vena cava syndrome. J Clin Oncology 2:961
7. Gradishar WJ, Hoffman PC (1997) The Oncologic Emergencies. In: J. Hall, G. Schmidt & L.D.H. Wood (eds) Priniciples of Critical Care, 2nd edition. McGraw-Hill Publishers,. New York, pp 1075–1090
8. Dombernowsky P, Hansen HH (1978) Combination chemotherapy in the management of superior vena cava obstruction in small-cell anaplastic cancer of the lung. Acta Med Scand 204:513
9. Maddox AM, Valdivieso M, Lukeman J, et al (1983) Superior vena cava obsturction in small cell bronchogenic carcinoma. Caner 52:2165
10. Gaines PA, Belli AM, Anderson PB, McBride K, Hemingway AP (1994) Superior vena caval obstruction managed by the Gianturco Z stent. Clin Radiol 49:202
11. Hennequin LM, Fade O, Fays JG, et al (1995) Superior vena cava stent placement: results with the Wallstent endoprosthesis. Radiology 196:353
12. Kishi K, Sonomura T, Mitsuzan K, et al (1993) Self-expandable metallic stent therapy for superior vena cava syndrome: clinical observations. Radiology 189:531–535
13. Oudkerk M, Heystraten FM, Stoter G (1993) Stenting in malignant vena caval obstruction. Cancer 71 (1) 142–6
14. Shah R, Sabanathan S, Lowe RA, Mearns AJ (1996) Stenting in malignant obstruction of superior vena cava. J Thorac Cardiovasc Surg 112:335–340
15. Gray BH, Olin JW, Graor RA, et al (1991) Safety and efficacy of thrombolytic therapy for superior vena cava syndrome. Chest 99:54–59
16. Skhvatsabaju LV (1986) Secondary tumors of the heart and pericardium in neoplastic disease. Oncology 43:103
17. Thurber DL, Edwards JE, Achor RW (1962) Secondary malignant tumors of the pericardium. Circulation 26:228–241
18. Maher EA, Shepherd FA, Todd TJR (1996) Pericardial sclerosis as the primary management of malignant pericardial effusion and cardiac tamponade. J Thorac Cardiovasc Surg 112:637–643
19. Laham RJ, Cohen DJ, Kuntz RE, et al (1996) Pericardial effusion in patients with cancer: outcome with contemporary management strategies. Heart 75:67–71

20. Braunwald, E. (1988) Pericardial Disease. In: Braunwald E (ed): Heart Disease (ed 3). Philadelphia, PA, WB Saunders, pp 1492–1498

21. Vaitkus PT, Herrmann HC, LeWinter MM (1994) Treatment of Malignant Pericardial Effusion. JAMA 272 (1):59–64

22. Galli M, Politi A, Fausto P, et al (1995) Percutaneous balloon pericardiotomy for malignant pericardial tamponade. Chest 108 (6):1499–1501

23. Palacios IF, Tuzcu EM, Ziskind AA, et al (1991) Percutaneous balloon pericardial window for patients with malignant pericardial effusion and tamponade. Cathet Cardiovasc Diagn 22 (4):244–249

24. Ziskind AA, Pearce AC, Lemon C, et al (1993) Percutaneous pericardotomy for the treatment of cardiac tamponade and large pericardial effusion: description of technique and report of the first 50 cases. J Am Coll Cardiol 21:1–5

25. Barron KD, Hirano A, Araki S, et al (1959) Experience with metastatic neoplasms involving the spinal cord. Neurology 9:91

26. Gilbert RW, Kim JH, Posner JB (1978) Epidural spinal cord compression from metastatic tumor: diagnosis and treatment. Ann Neurol 3:40

27. Stark RJ, Henson RA, Evans SJW (1982) Spinal metastasis: a retrospective survey from a general hospital. Brain 105:189

28. Portenoy RK, Galer BS, Salamon O et al (1989) Identification of epidural neoplasm: radiography and bone scintigraphy in the symptomatic and asymptomatic spine. Cancer 64:2207

29. Rodichok LD, Ruckdeschel JC, Harper GR, et al (1986) Early detection and treatment of spinal epidural metastases: the role of myelography. Ann Neurol 20:696–702

30. Haddad P, Thaell JF, Kiely JM, et al (1976) Lymphoma of the spinal and extradural space. Cancer 38:1862–1866

31. Koch D, Wakhloo AK, van Velthoven V (1995) Magnetic resonance imaging in spinal emergency. 134:100

32. Pigott KH, Baddeley H, Maher EJ (1994) Pattern of disease in spinal cord compression on MRI scan and implications for treatment. Clin Oncol R Coll Radiol 6 (1):7–10

33. Young RF, Post EM, King GA (1980) Treatment of spinal epidural metastases: randomized prospective comparison of laminectomy and radiotherapy. J Neurosurg 53:741

34. Posner J, Chernick N (1978) Intracranial metasteses from systemic cancer. Adv Neurol 19:575

35. Heffner JE, Sahn SA (1983) Controlled hyperventilation in patients with intracranial hypertension. Arch Int Med 143:765–769

36. Wasserstrom WR, Glass JP, Posner JB (1982) Diagnosis and treatment of leptomeningeal metastases from solid tumors: experience with 90 patients. Cancer 49:759–772

37. Sze G, Soletsky S, Bronen R, Krol G (1989) MR imaging of the meninges with emphasis on contrast enhancement and meningeal carcinomatosis. AJNR 10:965–975

38. Yousem DM, Patrone PM, Grossman RI (1990) Leptomeningeal metastases: MR elevation. J Comput Assist Tomogr 14:255–261

39. Fahey JL, Barth WF, Solomon A (1965) Serum hyperviscosity syndrome. JAMA 192:120–123

40. Baer MR, Stein RS, Dessypris EN (1985) Chronic lymphocytic leukemia with hyperleukocytosis. The hyperviscosity syndrome. Cancer 56 (12):2865–2869

41. Litchman MA and Rowe JM (1982) Hyperleukocytic leukemia: rheologic, clinical, and therapeutic considerations. Blood 60 (2) 279–283

42. Arieff AI, Leach W, Park R, Lazarowitz VC (1982) Systemic effects of NaHCO3 in experimental lactic acidosis in dogs. Am J Physiol 242:F586–591
43. Fields ALA, Wolman SL, Halperin ML (1981) Chronic lactic acidosis in a patient with cancer. Cancer 47:2026–29
44. Fraley DS, Adler S, Bruns FJ, Zett B (1980) Stimulation of lactate production by administration of bicarbonate in a patient with a solid neoplasm and lactic acidosis. N Engl J Med 303 (19):1100–1102
45. Park R, Arieff AI (1982) Treatment of lactic acidosis with dichloroacetate in dogs. J Clin Invest 70:853–862
46. Conger JD (1990) Acute uric acid nephropathy. Medical Clinics of North America. 74 (4):859–87
47. Conger JD, Falk SA (1977) Intrarenal dynamics in the pathogenesis and prevention of acute urate nephropathy. J Clin Invest 59:786–793
48. Kursch ED, Resnick MI (1984) Dissolution of uric acid calculi with systemic alkalinization. J Urol 132:286–287
49. Watson NA, Noteley RG (1973) Urologic complications of cyclophosphamide. Br J Urology 45:606
50. Texter JH, Koontz WW, McWilliams NB (1979) Hemorrhagic cystitis as a complication of the management of pediatric neoplasms. Urol Surv 29:47
51. Antman K, Ryan L, Elias A et al (1989) Response to ifosfamide and mesna: 124 previously treated patients with metastatic or unresectable sarcoma. J Clin Oncol 7:126–131
52. Pratt CB, Horowitz ME, Meyer WH et al (1987) Phase 2 trial of ifosphamide in children with malignant solid tumors. Cancer Treat Rep 71:131
53. Williams SD, Munshi N, Einhorn LH et al (1990) Cyclophosphamide and ifosfamide: role of uroprotective agents. Cancer Invest 8:269
54. Andriole GL, Sandland JI, Miser JS et al (1989) The efficacy of mesna (2-mercaptoethane sodium sulfonate) as a uroprotectant in patients with hemorrhagic cystitis receiving further oxazaphosphorine chemotherapy. J Clin Oncol 5:799–803
55. Brugieres L, Hartmann JP, Travagli E et al (1989) Hemorrhagic cystitis in bone marrow transplantation in children with malignancies: incidence, clinical course, and outcome. J Clin Oncol 7:194–199
56. Shepard JD, Pringle LE, Barnett MJ et al (1991) Mesna versus hyperhydration for the prevention of cyclophosphamide-induced hemorrhagic cystitis in bone marrow transplantation. J Clin Oncol 9:2016–2020
57. Steinberg SM, Galen MA, Lazarus JM et al (1975) Hemodialysis for acute anuric uric acid nephropathy. Am J Dis Child 129:956–958

# Infectious Complications of Oncologic Therapy

J. Flaherty

## Introduction

Infection complicates the treatment of malignancy either as a direct result of the neoplastic process (e.g., post-obstructive pneumonia in a patient with lung cancer) or more commonly, as a result of treatment (e.g., gram-negative sepsis in a neutropenic patient following high dose chemotherapy). As our understanding of the pathogenesis of infection in cancer patients has grown and the availability of effective antimicrobial therapy has improved, cancer treatment has become more intensive and antimicrobial resistance has kept pace with the development of new antimicrobial agents. The management of infectious complications in oncology patients requires continued vigilance for evidence of infection in susceptible patients, an awareness of trends in emerging antimicrobial resistance, and knowledge of the appropriate place for newer antimicrobial agents.

## Neutropenic Febrile Patient

Most febrile neutropenic episodes are assumed to represent infection. At least 50% of neutropenic cancer patients (absolute neutrophil count [ANC] <500/mm$^3$ or <1000/mm$^3$ and expected to soon fall to ≤500/mm$^3$) with fever (a single oral temperature >38.3°C [101°F] or ≥38.0°C [100.4°F] over at least 1 h) prove to have clinically documented infection; half of these can be documented microbiologically [1, 2]. Approximately 15%–20% of patients with fever and profound neutropenia (ANC <100/mm$^3$) have bacteremia. Primary infection is generally caused by aerobic gram-positive cocci (in particular coagulase-negative staphylococci, viridans streptococci, and *Staphylococcus aureus*) and gram-negative bacilli (especially *Escherichia coli, Klebsiella pneumoniae, and Pseudomonas aeruginosa*). Fungi, especially *Candida* and *Aspergillus* species, commonly cause secondary infection in neutropenic patients receiving broad-spectrum antibiotic therapy, but occasionally cause primary infection. Non-infectious causes of fever including blood products, pyrogenic drugs such as amphotericin B, thrombophlebitis or hematoma may be responsible for a substantial proportion of febrile episodes [3]. For example, some physicians interpret a fever developing within 6 h of blood product administration in the absence of a definable clinical focus of infection to be non-infectious. Evaluation of these patients is further complicated as the signs and symptoms of infection may be diminished in the absence of neutrophils. The incidence and magnitude of localizing findings such as exudate and fluctuance are reduced in direct relationship to the ANC [4]. Other findings such as erythema and localized tenderness appear to be unaffected by reductions in the ANC.

Clinically identifiable infection typically involves integument (skin, oropharynx, gastrointestinal tract or respiratory tract) breached by invasive procedures, medical devices or radiation or chemotherapy. Commonly infected sites including the oropharynx, sinuses, lungs, skin (especially intravascular catheter entry sites and bone marrow aspiration sites), and perianal region should be examined carefully for subtle signs and symptoms of inflammation. Two cultures of blood for bacteria and fungi should be obtained from all patients. If a central venous catheter is in place, some authorities recommend that a blood sample for culture be obtained from each catheter lumen as well as from a peripheral vein. If the catheter entry site is inflamed or draining, a gram stain and culture for bacteria and fungi should be performed on draining fluid. Diarrheal stools should be tested for *Clostridium difficile* toxin. Tests for enteric bacterial or protozoan pathogens may be reasonable for patients admitted with diarrhea but rarely identify a pathogen in cases of nosocomial diarrhea. Urine cultures are indicated if the patient has urinary frequency, dysuria or flank pain, a urinary catheter is in place, or the urinalysis is abnormal. Note that pyuria may be may be absent in neutropenic patients with urinary tract infection. A chest X-ray is indicated in any patient with signs or symptoms of respiratory disease. In addition, a baseline chest X-ray may prove valuable for patients who develop persistent or recurrent fever [5]. Suspicious skin lesions should be aspirated or biopsied promptly for gram stain, culture and cytology.

Empiric antibiotic therapy is necessary for febrile neutropenic patients because currently available diagnostic tests are not sufficiently sensitive, specific or rapid enough to identify the infectious cause of a febrile episode. Many antibiotic regimens are effective in the treatment of infection, but careful selection can enhance efficacy and minimize toxicity. When selecting an antibiotic regimen, physicians should consider the frequency and antibiotic susceptibility of individual bacterial pathogens at their local institution and on their inpatient units. Aminoglycosides should be avoided in patients with renal dysfunction, and combinations of drugs such as cisplatin, cyclosporine, aminoglycosides, and amphotericin B should be avoided, if possible, because of potential additive nephrotoxicity. Patients with penicillin allergy should not be given antipseudomonal penicillin or carbapenem antibiotics. The risk of allergic reactions to cephalosporins in patients with penicillin allergy is difficult to quantify. It seems advisable to avoid all beta-lactam antibiotics in a patient with a history of severe IgE-mediated reaction (anaphylaxis or angioedema) or desquamating rash (e.g. Stevens-Johnson syndrome) to any beta-lactam agent. The antimicrobial agents commonly used in cancer therapy-related infections are listed in Table 1.

Three general schemes for empiric antibiotic therapy in febrile neutropenic cancer patients have been recommended by Infectious Diseases Society of America (IDSA) guidelines with the caveat that one may be more appropriate for certain patients and in certain institutions: monotherapy, two-drug therapy and vancomycin plus one or two other drugs (Fig. 1) [2]. Ceftazidime and imipenem-cilastatin are the most extensively studied of the monotherapy regimens [6–9], but cefepime and meropenem appear to be similarly effective [10, 11]. Monotherapy with ciprofloxacin has given both favorable (at higher doses) [12] and unfavorable results [13] and cannot be recommended routinely at this time. Quinolone monotherapy is discouraged in particular for patients and institutions utilizing quinolone prophylactic regimens.

The most commonly used combination antibiotic regimens are an aminoglycoside (gentamicin, tobramycin or amikacin) and an antipseudomonal penicillin (piperacillin±tazobactam, ticarcillin±clavulanate or mezlocillin) [14] or an aminoglycoside plus a third-generation antipseudomonal cephalosporin (ceftazidime or cefipime) [15]. Combination regimens provide potential synergistic activity against some gram-negative bacilli and gram-positive cocci and theoretically lower the risk of emergence of resistant strains during treatment. The disadvantages of

**Table 1.** Commonly used antibiotics for treatment of infections in cancer patients (usual dosage for 70 kg adult with normal renal function)

| Beta-lactam antibiotics | |
|---|---|
| Ceftazidime | 2 g iv q 8h |
| Cefepime | 2 g iv q 8–12h |
| Imipenem-cilastatin | 500 mg iv q 6h |
| Meropenem | 1 g iv q 8h |
| Mezlocillin | 4 g iv q 6h |
| Piperacillin + tazobactam | 3.375–4.5 g q 6h |
| Ticarcillin + clavulanate | 3.1 g q 4–6h |

| Aminoglycosides | |
|---|---|
| Gentamicin | 2–3 mg/kg iv q 12h |
| Tobramycin | 2–3 mg/kg iv q 12h |
| Amikacin | 7.5 mg/kg iv q 12h |

| Fluorquinolones | |
|---|---|
| Ciprofloxacin | 400 mg iv q 8–12h |
| | 500–750 mg po q12 h |
| Ofloxacin | 400 mg po q 12h |

| Miscellaneous | |
|---|---|
| Metronidazole | 500 mg q 8h |
| Clindamycin | 600 mg q 8h |
| Trimethoprim/sulfamethoxazole | 10–20 mg TMP/kg daily in 4 divided doses |
| Erythromycin | 0.5–1 g iv q 6h |
| Azithromycin | 500 mg iv q 24h |
| Vancomycin | 1 g iv q 12h |
| Amphotericin B | 0.5–1.5 mg/kg daily iv |
| Amphotericin B lipid complex | 2.5–5 mg/kg daily iv |
| Fluconazole | 200 mg-800 mg po/iv q 24h |
| Itraconazole | 200 mg po q 12–24 h |
| 5-Flucytosine | 100–150 mg/kg daily po in 4 divided doses |
| Acyclovir | 5–10 mg/kg IV q 8h |
| Ganciclovir | 5 mg/kg q 12h |

combination regimens are largely attributed to the nephrotoxicity and ototoxicity associated with aminoglycosides.

The inclusion of vancomycin in the initial antimicrobial regimen has been a very controversial issue. The increased frequency of infection caused by gram-positive organisms susceptible only to vancomycin has fueled the widespread use of empiric vancomycin in oncology units [16]. Nevertheless, initial vancomycin use has not been shown to improve overall mortality or morbidity [17]. A randomized, controlled trial evaluating the role of empirical vancomycin showed superior initial rates of defervescence among vancomycin recipients (76% vs. 63%, $p<0.001$) but

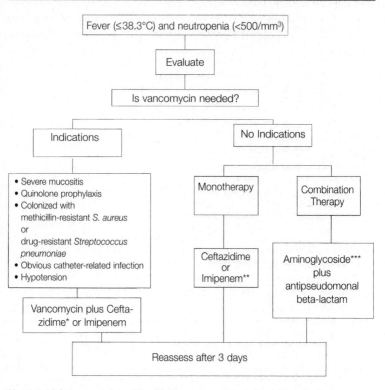

**Fig. 1.** Initial management of the febrile neutropenic patient. *Or cefepime or mero-penem; **or meropenem, cefipime, or aminoglycoside plus antipseudomonal beta-lactam; ***avoid if patient is also receiving nephrotoxic drugs or has renal dysfunc-tion. (Adapted from [2])

no difference in infection-related mortality (6% vs. 7%) because failures in the control arm were effectively managed by the subsequent addition of vancomycin [18]. Furthermore, the overuse of vancomycin has been associated with the emergence of vancomycin-resistant enterococcal infection in oncology units [19]. Selected gram-positive infections, inclu-ding bacteremia caused by viridans streptococci, have been associated with increased mortality when vancomycin was not included in the initi-al regimen [20, 21]. Vancomycin should be included in the initial regimen in patients at high risk for fulminant infection with gram-positive organisms (Fig. 1), but empirical vancomycin should be discontinued if initial cultures are negative for gram-positive organisms after 48 h. Carbapenems (imipenem-cilastatin and meropenem) and selected antipseudomonal penicillins (especially piperacillin-tazobactam and ticarcillin-clavulanate) are active against most gram-positive organisms with the exception of methicillin-resistant staphylococci and vancomycin-resistant enterococci and may be useful in situations where more gram-positive coverage is desired but vancomycin use is discouraged.

The standard practice has been to hospitalize all febrile neutropenic patients for administration of intravenous antibiotics and for monitoring and management of complications. Recent studies suggest that a group of low-risk individuals (controlled or responding cancer and no comorbid conditions such as recent hospitalization, hypotension, altered mental status, respiratory failure, dehydration, inadequate oral intake or gross bleeding) can be managed safely and effectively on an outpatient basis [22]. Both home intravenous antibiotic therapy and oral therapy using antimicrobial agents with very good bioavailability in compliant patients may be appropriate [23, 24].

At least three days are necessary to judge the efficacy of the initial regimen. If an etiologic agent is identified then the antibiotic regimen should be adjusted appropriately. If no etiology is identified and the fever resolves but the patient remains profoundly neutropenic (ANC $<100/mm^3$), the initial regimen should be continued. Patients with less severe neutropenia (ANC $100-500/mm^3$) in the absence of clinically identifiable infection or positive cultures can be switched to an oral antibiotic (cefixime or a quinolone). Antibiotics should be continued for a minimum of 7 days and are generally continued until neutropenia has resolved.

If fever persists and no etiology is identified, changes in therapy should be dictated by the patients' condition. If the patient remains stable, consider stopping vancomycin and continuing empirical gram-negative coverage. If the patient has evidence of progressive disease, consider adding vancomycin and broadening gram-negative coverage. If fever persists through days 5–7 and resolution of neutropenia is not imminent, add amphotericin B [25]. Up to one-third of patients with febrile neutropenia unresponsive to broad-spectrum antibacterial therapy will prove to have fungal infection, [26] and delayed antifungal therapy is associated with decreased survival in patients with filamentous fungal infections [27]. An exception to the routine of adding empiric amphotericin B at day 5–7 might include patients with no clinical suggestion of fungal infection (sinusitis or pulmonary infiltrate), no prior recovery of *Candida* or *Aspergillus* species from any site and anticipated recovery of the neutrophil count in the near future.

Fluconazole may be an acceptable alternative if mold and drug-resistant *Candida* infection is uncommon in the institution, sinusitis and pulmonary infiltrates are absent, and the patient has underlying renal insufficiency or amphtericin B intolerance. This alternative is less attractive if the local rates *C. krusei or C. glabrata* isolation are high or if the patient has been receiving fluconazole prophylaxis. If systemic fungal infection is identified, the duration of antifungal therapy is determined by the causative agent and the extent of disease. For patients who remain febrile and neutropenic, antimicrobial therapy is generally continued for a minimum of two weeks. If despite persistent fever and neutropenia, no fungal infection is identified by clinical evaluation, chest X-ray and CT scanning of the chest and abdomen, antibiotics can be discontinued and the patient monitored carefully. Antimicrobial therapy can usually be discontinued 4–5 days after the neutrophil count reaches $\geq 500/\text{mm}^3$, despite persistent fever, if no clinical evidence of infection is identified. The differential diagnosis of fever persisting beyond neutrophil recovery includes, most notably, fungal infection and drug reactions [28, 29]. The causes of persistent fever following recovery of neutropenia include:
– Fungal infection
  – Aspergillosis
  – Chronic systemic candidiasis
  – Fusariosis
  – Histoplasmosis
  – Mucormycosis
  – Trichosporonosis
– Localized bacterial infection
  – Intravascular catheter-related infection
  – Neutropenic enterocolitis
  – *Clostridium difficile* colitis
  – Intraabdominal abscess
  – Peri-rectal abscess
  – Viral infection
  – Herpes simplex virus
  – Cytomegalovirus
  – Herpes zoster (varicella zoster virus)

- Drug reaction
- Thrombophlebitis
- Hematoma
- Relapsed malignancy

## Oropharyngeal and Esophageal Infection

Cytotoxic chemotherapy-associated mucositis may be exacerbated by superimposed infection by oropharyngeal bacteria (viridans streptococci, anaerobic gram-negative bacilli, and anaerobic gram-positive cocci), fungi (especially *Candida albicans*) and reactivated latent herpes simplex virus (HSV). As the clinical appearance may be atypical, severe episodes of mucositis should be evaluated for evidence of yeast infection (budding yeast or pseudohyphae on gram stain or KOH and culture) or HSV infection (direct herpes antigen detection and viral culture). Culture may identify a non-albicans *Candida* species as the cause of mucositis or esophagitis (eg, *C. glabrata* or *C. krusei*) and predict a greater likelihood of fluconazole resistance. Oropharyngeal candidiasis can be treated with oral nystatin suspension or fluconazole 200–400 mg IV/po qday. Esophageal candidiasis should be treated with fluconazole 400 mg IV/po q24 h or amphotericin B 0.3–0.5 mg/kg per day. Herpes simplex virus infection should be treated with acyclovir 5 mg/kg IV q 8 h.

## *Clostridium difficile* Colitis

*Clostridium difficile* colitis is the major cause of nosocomial infectious diarrhea in the United States. While colonization of healthy, non-hospitalized adults by *C. difficile* is uncommon, the rate of colonization among hospitalized patient may exceed 20% for those hospitalized >1 week [30]. Almost all patients developing *C. difficile* disease have recently been treated with an antimicrobial or occasionally, chemotherapeutic agent. Third-generation cephalosporins such as ceftazidime have been implicated most frequently. The lack of a rapid, sensitive and specific laboratory test complicates diagnosis. The most rapid test, latex agglutination, is neither sensitive nor specific. The most sensitive test, stool culture for C. difficile requires a minimum of 2 days to yield results and fails to distinguish toxigenic from non-toxigenic strains. The most specific test, the cell cytotoxin assay, is labor intensive and also has 2 day turnaround time. The EIA for toxin A and B is rapid (2–4 h), very specific, but less sensitive than the cytotoxin assay. The recommended treatment is metronidazole 250 mg po qid or 500 mg po tid. Vancomycin 125 mg po qid is second-line therapy because of higher cost, the risk of selection of vancomycin-resistant gram-positive organisms, and the absence of proven clinical superiority. The usual treatment course is 10 days, but should probably be continued as long as other antibiotic therapy is continued. No end-of-treatment or follow-up testing is recommended unless diarrhea recurs.

### Neutropenic Enterocolitis

Neutropenic enterocolitis or typhlitis is a syndrome seen most commonly seen in neutropenic leukemia patients following chemotherapy, but is increasingly reported with other malignancies following intensive chemotherapy regimens. Enteric bacteria invade ischemic areas of bowel mucosa. The cecum is favored possibly due to its relatively poor blood supply. The spectrum of disease ranges from mild cecal inflammation to fulminant bowel necrosis with perforation. Patients report abdominal pain and fever and develop abdominal distension, nausea, vomiting, and watery or bloody diarrhea. CT scanning demonstrates thickening and edema of the colonic wall and may show gas in the intestinal wall or inflammatory phlegmon. Treatment is with bowel rest and broad spectrum antibiotic therapy. Surgery should be reserved for patients with perforation, uncontrollable GI bleeding, uncontrollable sepsis or complete bowel obstruction [31]. The mortality for a single episode of neutropenic enterocolitis approaches 50% and patients with one episode have a high risk of recurrence with subsequent cycles of chemotherapy [32].

### Vascular Access Device Infection

Central venous catheters reduce the risk of phlebitis but increase the risk of catheter-related bloodstream infections when compared with peripheral venous catheters. Comparisons between tunneled catheters (eg, Hickman catheter) and totally implantable devices (e.g., Port-a-Cath) have shown both lower infection rates in totally implantable devices [33] and similar infection rates [34]. Peripherally inserted central venous catheters (PICC) are associated with a significant risk of insertion site phlebitis (26% in one study) and a risk of catheter-related bacteremia similar to that seen with Hickman catheters [35].

The different categories of catheter infection reflect differences in pathogenesis of infection [36]:

- Catheter-related bacteremia or fungemia: isolation of the same organism (i.e., identical species, antibiogram) from a semiquantitative or quantitative culture of a catheter segment and from the blood in a patient with clinical symptoms of sepsis and no other apparent source for the infection.
- Catheter colonization: $\geq 15$ CFU (semiquantitative culture) or $\geq 10^3$ CFU (quantitative culture) from a removed catheter tip.
- Exit site infection: inflammation (erythema, tenderness, induration) or purulence within 2 cm of the catheter exit site.
- Tunnel infection: inflammation in the tissues overlying a tunnelled catheter and >2 cm from the exit site.
- Pocket infection: erythema and necrosis of the skin overlying the reservoir of a totally implantable device, or purulent exudate in the subcutaneous pocket containing the reservoir.

Exit-site infection, tunnel infection, and pocket infection result from extraluminal colonization by skin organisms similar to the usual pathogenesis of infection seen in short-term central venous catheters. Eradication of infection is difficult without removal of the catheter except in cases of infection limited to the exit site (extending <2 cm proximally along the catheter). In contrast, catheter-related bacteremia in long-term tunneled catheters or totally implantable devices is generally intraluminal and results from hub contamination during catheter manipulation [37]. It is not surprising then that silver impregnated cuffs failed to decrease the infection risk associated with long-term Hickman catheters in cancer patients [38]. Intraluminal infections can often be eradicated with retention of the catheter. The likelihood of success is increased if antibiotics are infused directly through the colonized lumen. This may be accomplished in multilumen catheters by rotating the lumen used for intravenous antibiotic infusion. In selected circumstances this approach may be augmented by the antibiotic-lock technique whereby catheter lumens not in use are flushed with antibiotic solution rather than heparin or saline.

Approximately 80% of coagulase-negative staphylococcal catheter-related bacteremias may be cured with retention of the catheter [39]. Vancomycin or other anti-staphylococcal therapy given for 7–10 days is ususally effective. Note that the risk of recurrent bacteremia is 20%. *S. aureus* and *Candida* catheter-related infections are much more difficult to treat. In the setting of catheter-related bacteremia or fungemia, each of these pathogens is associated with an 80% risk of failure if the catheter is retained [40, 41]. *S. aureus* bacteremia should be treated with a minimum of 10–14 days of intravenous anti-staphylococcal antibiotics. Patients with cardiac valvular disease or fever and/or bacteremia persisting >3 days after catheter removal and antibiotic initiation require more prolonged treatment (i.e., 4–6 weeks) [42]. Other indications for catheter removal include refractory hypotension, persistently positive cultures, septic emboli, or when the catheter is no longer required.

## Invasive Fungal Infection

The two most frequent invasive fungal infections complicating cancer chemotherapy are disseminated candidiasis and invasive aspergillosis. Protracted neutropenia, broad spectrum antibiotics, corticosteroids, and central venous catheters are the key risk factors for invasive fungal infection. Even a single positive blood culture for *Candida* should be considered significant. In one study, 35% of patients with presumed "transient candidemia" proved to have disseminated infection [41]. If the patient with disseminated candidiasis is stable and has not received prior fluconazole, fluconazole is as effective as amphotericin B and significantly less toxic [43, 44]. Some authorities would recommend fluconazole 800 mg IV qd in this situation [45]. If the patient is unstable or has received prior fluconazole, amphotericin B is recommended at least until the isolate proves to be a *Candida* species likely to respond to fluconazole (i.e., not *C. krusei* or *C. glabrata*). Amphotericin B is usually administered in doses 0.7–1.5 mg/kg per day in this setting. The appropriate duration of fluconazole or total dose of amphotericin B is uncertain, but treatment should probably be continued until all signs and symptoms of infection are resolved and for a minimum of 2 weeks. A number a lipid-based amphotericin preparations have been introduced: amphotericin B colloidal dispersion (Amphotec), amphotericin B lipid complex (Abelcet) and liposomal amphotericin B (AmBisome) [46]. All are less nephrotoxic than the standard amphotericin B deoxycholate preparation and of the three, liposomal amphotericin B appears to associated with less infusion-related toxicity. Nevertheless, none have been yet demonstrated to be more effective than amphotericin B deoxycholate. These agents are best reserved for patients with renal dysfunction, concomitant cyclosporine therapy, amphotericin B intolerance, or progressive disease.

*Aspergillus fumigatus* or *Aspergillus flavus* recovered from the respiratory tract from severely immunosuppressed patients (eg, neutropenic leukemia patients or bone marrow transplant recipients) is strongly suggestive of invasive aspergillosis [47, 48]. Isolates of *Aspergillus niger* or recovery of *Aspergillus* from the rectum can be discounted. Amphotericin B results in overall success rates of approximately 34% and similar rates are attained with itraconazole. Amphotericin B is usually administered at doses 1.0–1.5 mg/kg per day. The recommended dose of itraconazole is 200 mg po tid for 4 days then 200 mg po bid thereafter. Even after a course of "induction therapy" with amphotericin B, "consolidation therapy" with itraconazole is often appropriate, for an extended duration [49]. The lipid-based amphotericin preparations appear to to be equally efficacious, but not more so [50].

Patients with invasive fungal infection have a high risk for recurrence during subsequent episodes of chemotherapy-induced neutropenia [51], but prophylactic antifungal therapy can decrease the risk [52]. Patients with previous disseminated candidiasis can be treated with fluconazole while those with previous invasive aspergillosis can be treated with itraconazole or amphotericin B.

## Infection Prevention and Emerging Antimicrobial Resistance

Antibacterial prophylaxis with quinolones during periods of neutropenia following chemotherapy has shown a substantial decrease in the incidence of gram-negative infection but not death [53]. Furthermore, the reductions in fever and empiric antibiotic use have been small. Augmentation of gram-positive activity in one study reduced the incidence of gram-positive infection, but did not influence the overall incidence of fever episodes or impact on overall mortality [54]. The benefit of prophylactic regimens in preventing infection must be weighed against the lack of effect on mortality and the problem of emerging drug resistance. Widespread quinolone use has led to the emergence of quinolone-resistant gram-negative bacilli [55]. The addition of penicillin to quinolone prophylaxis regimens to cover viridans streptococci has led to the emergence of penicillin-resistant streptococci [56]. Similarly, antifungal prophylaxis with fluconazole has been shown effective in preventing superficial and disseminated fungal infection following bone marrow transplantation but overall mortality was unaffected [57]. Studies in leukemic patients confirmed prevention of oropharyngeal candidiasis but failed to demonstrate prevention of deep fungal infection [58]. In addition, some institutions have noted the emergence of fluconazole-resistant *Candida* species in response to fluconazole prophylaxis [59]. The routine use of quinolone and fluconazole prophylaxis is not recommended. However, in some special cases of profound and prolonged neutropenia quinolone prophylaxis may be indicated if the potential for antimicrobial resistance is appreciated and outweighed [2]. Similarly, in certain circumstances where the incidence of systemic infection due to *C. albicans* is high and non-albicans *Candida* species is low, fluconazole prophylaxis may be considered.

## References

1. Bodey GP, Buckley M, Sathe YS et al. Quantitative relationships between circulating leukocytes and infection in patients with acute leukemia. Ann Intern Med 1966, 64:328–39
2. Hughes WT, Armstrong D, Bodey GP et al. 1997 Guidelines for the use of antimicrobial agents in neutropenic patients with unexplained fever. Clin Infect Dis 1997, 25:551–73
3. Bow EJ, Rayner E, Louie TJ. Comparison of norfloxacin with cotrimoxazole for infection prophylaxis in acute leukemia. Am J Med 1988, 84:847–54
4. Sickles EA, Greene WH, Wiernik PH. Clinical presentation of infection in granulocytopenic patients. Arch Intern Med 1975, 135:715–9
5. Donowitz GR, Harmon C, Pope T, Stewart FM,. The role of the chest roentgenogram in febrile, neutropenic patients. Arch Intern Med 1991, 151:701–704
6. Sanders JW, Powe NR, Moore RD. Ceftazidime monotherapy for empiric treatment of febrile neutropenic patients: a metaanalysis. J Infect Dis 1991, 164:907–16
7. De Pauw BE, Deresinski SC, Feld R et al. Ceftazidime compared with piperacillin and tobramycin for the empiric treatment of fever in neutropenic patients with cancer. Ann Intern Med 1994, 120:834–44
8. Freifeld AG, Walsh T, Marshall D et al. Monotherapy for fever and neutropenia in cancer patients: a randomized comparison of ceftazidime versus imipenem. J Clin Oncol 1995, 13:165–76
9. Yamamura D, Gulcalp R, Carslisle P et al. Open randomized study of cefipime versus piperacillin-gentamicin for treatment of febrile neutropenic cancer patients. Antimicrob Agents Chemother 1997, 41:1704–8
10. Cometta A, Calandra T, Gaya H et al. Monotherapy with meropenem versus combination therapy with ceftazidime plus amikacin as empiric therapy for fever in

granulocytopenic patients with cancer. Antimicrob Agents Chemother 1996, 40:1108–15

11. Rolston KVI, Berkey P, Bodey GP et al. A comparison of imipenem to ceftazidime with or without amikacin as empiric therapy in febrile neutropenic patients. Arch Intern Med 1992, 152:283–91

12. Meunier F, Zimmer SH, Gaya H et al. Prospective randomized evaluation of cipro-floxacin versus piperacillin plus amikacin for empiric antibiotic therapy of febrile granulocytopenic cancer patients with lymphoma and solid tumors. Antimicrob Agents Chemother 1991, 35:873–8

13. Johnson PRE, Lin Yin JA, Tooth JP. A randomized trial of high-dose ciprofloxacin vs. azlocillin plus netilmicin in the empirical therapy of febrile neutropenic pati-nets J Antimicrob Chemother 1992, 30:203–14

14. Cometta A, Zinner S, DeBock R et al. Piperacillin-tazobactam plus amikacin ver-sus ceftazidime plus amikacin as empiric therapy for fever in granulocytopenic patients with cancer. Antimicrob Agents Chemother 1995, 39:445–452

15. Cordonnier C, Herbrecht, R, Pico JL et al. Cefipime/amikacin versus ceftazidi-me/amikacin as empirical therapy for febrile episode in neutropenic patients; a comparative study. Clin Infect Dis 1997, 24:41–51

16. Ena J, Dick RW, Jones RN, Wenzel RP. The epidemiology of intravenous vancomy-cin usage in a University Hospital: a 10 year study. JAMA 1993, 269:598–602

17. Rubin M, Hathorn, Marshall D et al. Gram-positive infections and the use of van-comycin in 550 episodes of fever and neutropenia. Ann Intern Med 1988, 108:30–5

18. EORTC International Antimicrobial Therapy Cooperative Group and NCI-CTG. Vancomycin added to empirical combination antibiotic therapy for fever in gra-nulocytopenic cancer patients. J Infect Dis 1991, 163:951–8

19. Montecalvo MA, Horowits H, Gedris C et al. Outbreak of vancomycin-, ampicillin-, and aminoglycoside-resistant *Enterococcus faecium* in an adult oncology unit. Antimicrob Agents Chemother 1994, 38:1363–7

20. Elting LS, Bodey GP, Keefe BH. Septicemia and shock syndrome due to viridans streptococci: a case-control study of predisposing factors. Clin Infect Dis 1992, 14:1201–7

21. Bochud PY, Eggiman P, Calandra T et al. Bacteremia due to viridans streptococcus in neutropenic patients with cancer: clinical spectrum and risk factors. Clin Infect Dis 1994, 18:25–31

22. Talcott JA, Finberg R, Mayer RJ, Goldman L. The medical course of cancer patients with fever and neutropenia: clinical identification of a low-risk subgroup at pre-sentation. Arch Intern Med 1988, 148:2561–8

23. Talcott JA, Whalen A, Clark J et al. Home antibiotic therapy for low-risk cancer patients with fever and neutropenia: a pilot study of 30 patients based on a valida-ted prediction rule. J Clin Oncol 1994, 12:107–14

24. Malik IA, Khan WA, Karim M et al. Feasibility of outpatient management of fever in cancer patients with low-risk neutropenia: results of a prospective randomized trial. Am J Med 1995, 98:224–231

25. EORTC International Antimicrobial Therapy Cooperative Group. Empiric antifun-gal therapy in febrile granulocytopenic patients. Am J Med 1989, 86:668–72

26. Pizzo PA, Robichard KJ, Gill FA, Witebsky FG. Empiric antibiotic therapy in gra-nulocytopenic patients with cancer. Am J Med 1982, 72:101–11

27. Karp JE, Merz WG, Charache P. Response to empiric amphotericin B during anti-leukemic therapy-induced granulocytopenia. Rev Infect Dis 1991, 13:592–9

28. Talbot GH, Provencher M, Cassileth PA. Persistent fever after recovery from gra-nulocytopenia in acute leukemia. Arch Intern Med 1988, 148:129–35

29. Barton TD, Schuster MG. The cause of fever following resolution of neutropenia in patients with acute leukemia. Clin Infect Dis 1996, 22:1064–8

30. Johnson S, Gerding DN. *Clostridium difficile*-associated diarrhea. Clin Infect Dis 1998, 26:1027–36
31. Moir CR, Scudamore CH, Benny WB. Typhlitis: selective surgical management. Am J Surg 1986, 151:56–6
32. Keidan RD, Fanning J, Gatenby RA, Weese JL. Recurrent typhlitis: a disease resulting from aggressive chemotherapy. Dis Colon Rectum 1989, 32:206–9
33. Groeger JS, Lucas AB, Thaler HT et al. Infectious morbidity associated with long-term use of venous access devices in patients with cancer. Ann Intern Med 1993, 119:1168–74
34. Mueller BU, Callender DPE, Marshall D et al. A prospective randomized trial comparing the infectious and noninfectious complications of an externalized catheter versus a subcutaneously implanted device in cancer patients. J Clin Oncol 1992, 10:1943–8
35. Raad II, Davis S, Becker M et al. Low infection rate and long durability of nontunneled silastic catheters. Arch Intern Med 1993, 153:1791–6
36. Pearson ML, Hospital Infection Control Practices Advisory Committee. Guideline for prevention of intravascular device-related infections. Infect Control Hosp Epidemiol 1996, 17:438–473
37. Raad II, Costerton W, Sabharwal et al. Ultrastructural analysis of indwelling vascular catheters: a quantitative relationship between luminal colonization and duration of placement. J Infect Dis 1993, 168:400–7
38. Groeger JS, Lucas AB, Coit D et al. A prospective, randomized evaluation of the effect of silver impregnated cuffs for preventing tunneled chronic venous access catheter infections in cancer patients. Ann Surg 1993, 218:206–10
39. Raad II, Davis S, Khan A et al. Impact of central venous catheter removal on the recurrence of catheter-related coagulase-negative staphylococcal bacteremia. Infect Control Hosp Epidemiol 1992, 13:215–21
40. Dugdale DC, Ramsey PG. *Staphylococcus aureus* bacteremia in patients with Hickman catheters. Am J Med 1990, 89:137–41
41. Lecciones JA, Lee JW, Navarro EE et al. Vascular catheter-associated fungemia in patients with cancer: analysis of 155 episodes. Clin Infect Dis 1992, 14:875–83
42. Raad II, Sabbagh MF. Optimal duration of therapy for catheter-related *Staphylococcus aureus* bacteremia: a study of 55 cases and review. Clin Infect Dis 1992, 14:75–82
43. Anaissie EJ, Darouchie RO, Abi-Said D et al. Management of invasive candidal infections: results of a prospective, randomized, multicenter study of fluconazole versus amphotericin B and review of the literature. Clin Infect Dis 1996, 23:964–72
44. Nguyen MH, Peacock JE, Tanner DC. Therapeutic approaches in patients with candidemia. Arch Intern Med 1995, 155:2429–35
45. Edwards JE, Bodey GP, Bowden RA et al. International conference for the development of a consensus on the management and prevention of severe candidal infections. Clin Infect Dis 1997, 25:43–59
46. Hiemenz JW, Walsh TJ. Lipid formulations of amphotericin B: recent progress and future directions. Clin Infect Dis 1996, 22 (suppl2):S133–44
47. Nalesnik MA, Myerowitz RL, Jenkins R, Lenkey J, Herbert D. Significance of *Aspergillus* species isolated from respiratory secretions in the diagnosis of invasive pulmonary aspergillosis. J Clin Micro 1980, 11:370–6
48. Wald A, Leisenring W, van Burik JA, Bowden RA. Epidemiology of *Aspergillus* infections in a large cohort of patients undergoing bone marrow transplantation. J Infect Dis 1997, 175:1459–66
49. Denning DW. Invasive aspergillosis. Clin Infect Dis 1998, 26:781–805

50. White MH, Anaissie EJ, Kusne S et al. Amphotericin B colloidal dispersion vs. amphotericin B as therapy for invasive aspergillosis. Clin Infect Dis 1997, 24:635–42

51. Robertson MJ, Larson RA. Recurrent fungal pneumonias in patients with acute nonlymphocytic leukemia undergoing multiple courses of intensive chemotherapy. Am J Med 1988, 84:233–9

52. Martino R, Nomdendeu J, Atles A et al. Successful bone marrow transplantation in patients with previous invasive fungal infections: report of four cases. Bone Marrow Transplant 1994, 13:265–9

53. Engels EA, Lau J, Barza M. Efficacy of quinolone prophylaxis in neutropenic cancer patients: a meta-analysis. J Clin Oncol 1998, 16:1179–87

54. Bow EJ, Mandell LA, Louie TJ et al. Quinolone-based antibacterial chemoprophylaxis in neutropenic patients: effect of augmented gram-positive activity on infectious morbidity. Ann Intern Med 1996, 125:183–90

55. Carratala J, Fernandez-Sevilla A, Tubau F et al. Emergence of quinolone-resistant Escherichia coli bacteremia in neutropenic patients with cancer who have received prophylactic norfloxacin. Clin Infect Dis 1995, 20:557–60

56. Catarrala J, Alcaide F, Fernandez-Sevilla A et al. Bacteremia due to viridans streptococci that are highly resistant to penicillin: increase among neutropenic patients with cancer. Clin Infect Dis 1995, 20:1169–73

57. Goodman JL, Winston DJ, Greenfield RA et al. A controlled trial of fluconazole to prevent fungal infections in patients undergoing bone marrow transplantation. N Engl J Med 1992, 326:845–51

58. Schaffner A, Schaffner M. Effect of prophylactic fluconazole on the frequency of fungal infections, amphotericin B us, and health care costs in patients undergoing intensive chemotherapy for hematologic neoplasias. J Infect Dis 1995, 172:1035–41

59. Wingard JR, Merz WG, Rinaldi et al. Increase in Candida krusei infection among patients with bone marrow transplantation and neutropenia treated prophylactically with fluconazole. N Engl J Med 1991, 325:1274–7

# Metabolic and Electrolyte Complications of Malignancy

P.R. Helft, C.M. Rudin

## Introduction

The paraneoplastic syndromes affecting metabolic and electrolyte homeostasis are important causes of morbidity and mortality in cancer patients. Significant advances have recently been made in our knowledge of both the underlying pathophysiology and therapeutic management of these complex conditions. A basic understanding of these syndromes is critical for any practicing oncologist. Here we provide an overview of recent progress made in the areas of the hypercalcemia of malignancy, the syndrome of inappropriate secretion of antidiuretic hormone, the cancer cachexia syndrome, and the tumor lysis syndrome.

## Hypercalcemia of Malignancy

### Introduction

Hypercalcemia is the most common life-threatening electrolyte disorder associated with malignancy. It has been estimated that between 10% and 20% of cancer patients become hypercalcemic during the course of their disease [1]. Primary hyperparathyroidism and hypercalcemia of malignancy together account for approximately 90% of all cases of hypercalcemia. Their incidences are estimated to be 250 new cases per million per year and 150 new cases per million per year respectively [2]. Cancers commonly associated with hypercalcemia include both solid tumors (breast, non-small cell lung, and head and neck cancer) and hematologic malignancies, in particular multiple myeloma. Although duration of survival in hypercalcemic patients may vary widely depending on the underlying malignancy, the development of clinically significant hypercalcemia is generally a dismal prognostic indicator, with estimates of average survival ranging from one month to six months from presentation. Deaths in some cases are directly attributable to complications of hypercalcemia, but more commonly hypercalcemia appears simply to constitute a marker of advanced metastatic disease.


Pathophysiology

Substantial changes in our understanding of the pathophysiology of hypercalcemia in cancer patients have been made in the past decade. Normal calcium homeostasis is dependent on a regulatory network integrating rates of bone formation, bone resorption, renal excretion and intestinal absorption. Deregulation of bone resorption has been the principal factor implicated in the hypercalcemia of malignancy, although defects in renal clearance and intestinal absorption have also been described.

Hypercalcemia of malignancy was previously thought to be either secondary to direct bony destruction by tumor cells or to "humoral factors" in the case of tumors with no evident bone metastases. However, current evidence suggests that in the majority of both cases increased bone resorption is due to diffusible factors produced in excess by cancer cells. The best characterized of these factors is the parathyroid hormone related peptide, PTHrP.

The gene encoding PTHrP was identified in the late 1980s and several isotypes have been described [3]. This gene is expressed at detectable levels in a variety of tissues, suggesting a normal physiologic function; however, this function has not been clearly delineated. PTHrP is closely related to PTH at the amino-terminal PTH receptor binding domain, and has similar biologic activity, increasing osteoclast activity, renal tubular calcium resorption, and possibly intestinal calcium absorption [4].

PTHrP is not normally detectable in serum. Remarkably, elevated levels of PTHrP have been reported in the sera of up to 80% of hypercalcemic solid tumor patients [5]. In cancers metastatic to bone, the bony destruction that was originally attributed to the tumor cells themselves may in most cases be secondary to high local concentrations of PTHrP resulting in osteoclast activation. One recent study found 92% of bony metastases to be PTHrP positive [6].

Other diffusible factors have also been implicated in tumor-related osteolysis. Notably multiple myeloma cells, which rarely express detect-

able PTHrP, may similarly stimulate osteoclast activity through generation of locally high concentrations of other factors including tumor
necrosis factor-$\alpha$ and interleukin-6 [7, 8].


Differential Diagnosis

There is a wide variety of conditions which can result in hypercalcemia,
but approximately 90% of cases are associated with either primary
hyperparathyroidism or malignancy:

– Primary hyperparathyroidism       (90%)
– Malignant neoplasm

– Vitamin D intoxication             (10%)
– Vitamin A intoxication
– Hyperthyroidism
– Immobilization
– Familial hypocalciuric hypercalcemia
– Chronic renal failure
– Sarcoidosis
– Milk-alkali syndrome
– Paget's disease
– Addison's disease
– Thiazide diuretics

These two conditions can usually be differentiated by limited clinical
and laboratory evaluation. Primary hyperparathyroidism tends to develop slowly, frequently resulting in asymptomatic hypercalcemia. In contrast, hypercalcemia of malignancy is typically associated with nausea,
vomiting, dehydration, and weight loss. Other clinical clues include the
degree and pattern of hypercalcemia, as malignancy tends to cause more
marked and unrelenting increases in serum calcium (see Table 1).
Laboratory tests distinguishing the two major causes of hypercalcemia
have been markedly improved. Older assays for PTH were confounded
by the test's inability to distinguish immunologically reactive from biologically active molecules; the modern immunoradiometric assay
(IRMA) for PTH, however, has reduced cross-reactivity to inactive PTH
fragments [9]. Decreased concentration of PTH in the presence of hypercalcemia excludes primary hyperparathyroidism and is suggestive of

underlying malignancy; conversely, an increased level of PTH is highly suggestive of primary hyperparathyroidism. The relatively rare exceptions include PTH-producing parathyroid carcinomas and co-existing malignancy and primary hyperparathyroidism.

Treatment

The bisphosphonate pamidronate has become the principal agent used in the treatment of the hypercalcemia of malignancy. Pamidronate directly interferes with osteoclast activity and has been reported to decrease PTHrP concentrations. A single 60- to 90-mg dose is sufficient to normalize serum calcium in the majority of patients [10]. Administered as a continuous intravenous infusion over 4–24 h, pamidronate typically corrects serum calcium levels within 3–5 days, with mean duration of normocalcemia of 28 days [11, 12]. Sixty milligrams of IV pamidronate every two weeks has been found to maintain normocalcemia in the majority of hypercalcemic cancer patients.

Other therapeutic measures may be required in acute, symptomatic hypercalcemia. These include the liberal use of intravenous fluids to increase glomerular filtration rate, leading to decreased calcium resorption in the proximal nephron. Calcitonin given at the dose of 200–400 MRC units intramuscularly or subcutaneously every 12 h will rapidly lower serum calcium and, although its effects are short-lived, may be useful in the period before the bisphosphonate effect has occurred. Except in rare circumstances, loop diuretics should be avoided as dehydration is commonly associated with hypercalcemia.

Many cancer patients with osteolytic bone lesions and normal serum calcium levels may nevertheless suffer from pain, pathologic fracture, spinal cord compression, and are at increased risk for developing hyper-

**Table 1.** Clinical clues to differential diagnosis

|  | Primary hyperparathyroidism | Hypercalcemia of malignancy |
|---|---|---|
| Calcium levels | Mildly increased, fluctuating | Markedly increased, progressive |
| Duration of hypercalcemia | >6 months | Recent onset |
| Serum chloride | >103 mmol/l | <100 mmol/l |
| Serum PTH | High | Suppressed |

calcemia. A 1996 study of almost 400 patients with multiple myeloma suggested that pamidronate may also be of significant benefit. Patients were treated with monthly pamidronate administrations, and bony complications such as fracture, the need for radiation, and development of hypercalcemia were reduced [13]. This treatment was also associated with reduced pain and improved quality of life.

## Syndrome of Inappropriate Secretion of Antidiuretic Hormone

Introduction

The syndrome of inappropriate secretion of antidiuretic hormone (SIADH) was first described in 1957 by Schwartz et al., who reported the finding of hyponatremia associated with renal sodium loss and high urine osmolality in two lung cancer patients [14]. The authors theorized that the cancer produced arginine vasopressin, which was responsible for the syndrome. Their postulate has subsequently been confirmed by a large number of studies. The tumor most frequently associated with SIADH is small cell lung cancer, though many other cancers have been reported to cause the syndrome. There has been no correlation between SIADH and tumor mass or pathologic stage. The clinical syndrome is characterized by hyponatremia, hypoosmolality, euvolemia, renal sodium wasting, less than maximally dilute urine (i.e. inappropriately high urine osmolality for a given serum osmolality), and intact renal function. The plasma osmolality is typically less than 280 mmol/kg with urine osmolality greater than 500 mmol/kg and urine sodium concentration greater than 20 mEq/l. The measurement of antidiuretic hormone (ADH) has no current role in the diagnosis of SIADH.

The differential diagnosis of causes of SIADH is large and includes many non-malignant etiologies. Some of the common causes of the syndrome are:
– Malignant tumors
– Infection (tuberculosis, pneumonia and empyema, meningitis)
– Vasculitis
– Head injury
– Intracranial tumors
– Psychosis
– Pain and emotional stress

– Positive pressure ventilation
– Medications

## Pathophysiology

Antidiuretic hormone, also known as arginine vasopressin, is an oligopeptide of eight amino acids. ADH is normally synthesized in the posterior pituitary and functions as a critical physiologic regulator of water balance and blood volume. It acts primarily on the collecting tubules of the nephron to stimulate upregulation of water channels, permitting increased free water resorption. It is controlled by a complex network of signals derived from volume- and osmo-receptors in the hypothalamus, left atrium, and pulmonary veins, and from circulating angiotensin II. Excessive autonomous secretion of ADH leads to excess water resorption out of proportion to sodium, resulting in progressive water intoxication and hyponatremia. This can produce central nervous system toxicity, with headaches and fatigue ultimately progressing to confusion, seizures, coma, and death.

## Treatment

The mainstay of treatment of SIADH caused by tumors is surgery or cytotoxic therapy for the underlying malignancy. When this is not sufficient and in patients with serum sodium less than 130 mEq/l, fluid restriction is recommended. For relatively mild cases restriction of free water to 1 l/day may be adequate to correct serum sodium. Greater fluid restriction may occasionally be required, though it is difficult to accomplish, especially in the outpatient setting. In severe or life-threatening cases, and in light of the devastating neurologic consequences that can accompany severe hyponatremia [15], it has been argued that the disorder should be rapidly corrected [16]. Too rapid correction of the serum sodium, however, may lead to central pontine myelinolysis [17]. Correction with 3% saline via large central vein is indicated only in patients with acute (<48 h), symptomatic hyponatremia. The rate of change in serum sodium should not exceed 1–2 mEq/l per hour and an absolute change of greater than 20 mEq/l in 24 h should be avoided. After serum sodium reaches 120–125 mEq/l, therapy should continue with free water restriction.

For chronic cases of hyponatremia where free water restriction is not feasible, pharmacologic therapy with demeclocycline has proven to be effective. Demeclocycline is the most widely used pharmacologic treatment of SIADH. It specifically inhibits the renal effects of ADH and when used in doses of 600–1200 mg/day usually restores serum sodium to normal in 5–14 days [18].

## Cancer Cachexia

### Introduction

The cancer cachexia syndrome describes the pathologic state characterized by weight loss, anorexia, weakness, fatigue, and tissue wasting seen in more than two-thirds of cancer patients. Sources estimate that the syndrome is responsible for deaths of between 20% and 65% of cancer patients [19]. Weight loss has been associated with adverse psychological consequences and lower quality of life for cancer patients, and is a negative prognostic factor for both survival and response to therapy [20, 21]. The syndrome is often apparent before cancer is actually discovered. Cachexia has been described in nearly every type of cancer and there appears to be no obvious correlation with cell type, tumor size, or stage of malignancy [22].

### Pathophysiology

Since anorexia is often a prominent part of the cancer cachexia syndrome, it was thought to be a primary contributor to wasting. However recent studies suggest that anorexia is primarily an effect of cachexia rather than a cause; cancer patients often lose weight despite adequate caloric intake and do not have lasting weight gain even with the addition of nutritional supplementation. Three factors seem to contribute to this paradox: (a) elevated energy expenditure, (b) disrupted metabolism and, (c) competition between host and tumor for nutrients. The most convincing argument for elevated energy expenditure in cancer patients is that expenditure decreases after tumor resection [23]. Metabolic derangements affect carbohydrate, lipid, and protein pathways [49]:

- Carbohydrate metabolism
  - Glucose intolerance
  - Increased hepatic gluconeogenesis
  - Increased Cori cycle activity
  - Decreased skeletal muscle glucose uptake
- Lipid metabolism
  - Decreased total host lipid
  - Hyperlipidemia
  - Increased lipolysis
  - Decreased white adipose tissue lipolysis
- Protein metabolism
  - Increased whole-body protein turnover
  - Increased hepatic protein synthesis
  - Increased skeletal muscle breakdown
- Main hormonal changes
  - Insulin resistance
  - Decreased insulin secretion
  - Increased counter-regulatory hormones

Frequently documented changes in carbohydrate metabolism include accelerated gluconeogenesis and loss of energy by futile glucose utilization. In addition, uptake of fat is frequently decreased, with a concomitant increase in lipolysis. Protein turnover is typically accelerated by 50% to 70%. Other factors that contribute to wasting may include physical disruptions, as in head and neck and mediastinal tumors, that may cause difficulty ingesting food. Chemotherapy-induced disruptions in the mucosa of the alimentary tract may similarly interfere with feeding. Nausea, vomiting, and alterations in taste and smell perception from the malignancy itself or secondary to chemotherapy, as well as depression, may also cause decreased caloric intake.


Role of Cytokines

Although the exact mechanisms of cancer cachexia are not fully understood, it is clear that multiple humoral factors – of both tumor and host origin – are involved. A number of studies stress the role of host-derived cytokines, in particular, as major mediators of the syndrome. In 1986 Beutler and Cerami postulated that a macrophage-derived cytokine, cachectin or tumor necrosis factor-α, was responsible for the cachexia syndrome [24]. TNF-α inhibits lipoprotein lipase (LPL) [25], increases protein catabolism [26], and may promote anorexia [27]. Interleukin-1 and interferon-γ appear to share similar effects with TNF-α, namely inhibition of LPL and induction of anorexia and weight loss [28–31]. Interleukin-6, which causes weight loss and altered protein metabolism in animal models, has been proposed as a critical factor in cancer cachexia [32, 33]. Finally, the recently defined leukemia inhibitory factor and lipid mobilizing factors have been proposed as contributors to the syndrome via their effects on fat metabolism [34, 35].

## Treatment

Principal therapeutic strategies for the cancer cachexia syndrome have focused on augmenting appetite and increasing caloric intake in an attempt to increase nutritional reserves. Two major questions remain to be answered in the treatment of cancer cachexia:
– Do pharmacologic agents for the stimulation of appetite improve quality of life or survival in patients with cachexia?
– Is nutritional support for cachectic patients beneficial?

Although it is not yet possible to give a full response to our first question, investigations of several pharmacologic agents provide some preliminary information. The most promising of these agents has been megestrol acetate. Megestrol has been found to enhance weight gain, sense of well being, and caloric intake in patients with advanced cancer [36]. Though the optimal dose is not known, a CALGB dose-response study in breast cancer patients suggested that 160 mg per day resulted in optimal quality of life [37]. A 1993 phase III study of patients with anorexia/cachexia evaluated 342 patients and demonstrated a positive dose-response effect on appetite and calorie intake between the doses of 160 mg and 800 mg per day. Higher doses were not shown to increase response [38]. It thus seems reasonable to recommend 160 mg daily as a starting dose and 800 mg daily as a maximum dose of megestrol acetate. Other agents with less convincing support include medroxyprogesterone acetate, corticosteroids, and tetrahydrocannabinol (THC) derivatives, the primary active ingredients in marijuana.

A recent meta-analysis by Klein and Koretz sheds light on our second question about nutritional support. This meta-analysis evaluated 72 prospective randomized controlled trials [39] including more than 4000 patients and concluded that there are no strong indications for nutritional support specific to cancer patients. The authors point out that parenteral nutrition may increase the risk of infection, but may reduce complications in severely malnourished patients and improve long-term survival after bone marrow transplantation. Although enteral nutritional supplementation has a lower risk of infection and may decrease infections in the post-operative period, there is as yet no solid evidence that interventional nutritional support should play a significant role in the management of patients with the cancer cachexia syndrome.

## Tumor Lysis Syndrome

### Introduction

Tumor lysis syndrome (TLS) was first described in 1929 by Bedrna and Polcak [40] in patients with chronic leukemia and by Merrill and Jackson [41] in acute leukemics with hyperuricemia and renal failure. The syndrome is manifest by the combination of hyperkalemia, hyperuricemia, hyperphosphatemia, and hypocalcemia, and can result in fulminant acute renal failure. It is usually provoked by chemotherapy-induced cytoreduction, although it may also occur in the setting of large, bulky, rapidly dividing malignant tumors in the absence of therapy. While of greatest clinical significance in the initial management of rapidly dividing tumors such as Burkitts lymphoma and acute lymphoblastic leukemia, TLS has also been reported in the chronic leukemias [42], small cell lung cancer [43, 44], and breast cancer [45]. Clinical risk factors for the development of TLS include advanced, bulky lymphoproliferative malignancy with abdominal disease, young age, male sex, elevated serum LDH, volume depletion, and acid urine pH. Most of the serious complications of TLS, including renal failure, are reversible and often preventable.

Pathophysiology

Tumor lysis syndrome is caused by the precipitous systemic release of large quantities of cytoplasmic solutes, most notably potassium, uric acid, and inorganic phosphate. The kidneys are primarily responsible for elimination of these products; clearance may become saturated, resulting in elevated serum concentrations, and onset of acute renal failure can lead to sudden and life-threatening electrolyte imbalance. Severe hyperkalemia and hypocalcemia (secondary to hyperphosphatemia) can both contribute to potentially fatal cardiac arrhythmias.

The pathophysiology of renal failure in these patients is complex, with contributing factors including relative volume depletion, uric acid and calcium phosphate precipitation. Many of the patients at risk for TLS have pre-existing hyperuricemia, which is likely to be exacerbated by chemotherapy, and may not be prevented by therapy with allopurinol [46]. Uric acid tends to precipitate in the renal tubules at pH <5.0 and can cause a precipitous decrease in glomerular filtration rate; this mechanism appears to be a principal cause of urate nephropathy in the tumor lysis syndrome. Hyperphosphatemia also contributes to renal failure in TLS. The large quantities of inorganic phosphate released from dying cells can precipitate with calcium, resulting in metastatic calcification in the renal tubules [47, 48].

Treatment

The mainstays of the management of tumor lysis syndrome are hydration and management of electrolyte and renal disturbances. Allopurinol in doses of 600 mg/day should be given along with intravenous fluids with sodium bicarbonate to alkalinize the urine and prevent urate precipitation. Urine output should be kept brisk and urine pH should be maintained above 7.0. These measures should be instituted prior to administration of cytoreductive agents and may need to be continued for several days thereafter. If renal failure does occur, hemodialysis is often necessary and, given the reversibility of the renal failure of TLS, should be strongly considered. Hyperkalemia must be detected early and aggressively treated, with insulin, glucose, and sodium bicarbonate to shift potassium to the intracellular compartment, and kayexelate at doses between 50 and 100 grams to decrease total body potassium load. Severe or refractory cases should be managed with hemodialysis.

## References

1. Burt and Brennan. Incidence of hypercalcemia and malignant neoplasm. Archives of Surgery 1980, 115:704–7
2. Mundy et al. The hypercalcemia of cancer: clinical implications and pathologic mechanisms. New England Journal of Medicine 1984, 310:1718–27
3. Suva et al. A parathyroid hormone-related protein implicated in malignant hypercalcemia cloning and expression. Science 1987, 237:893–6
4. Horiuchi et al. Similarity of synthetic peptide from human tumor to parathyroid hormone in vivo and in vitro. Science 1987, 238:1566–8
5. Burtis et al. Immunochemical characterization of circulating parathyroid hormone-related protein in patients with humoral hypercalcemia of cancer. New England Journal of Medicine 1990, 322 (1106–1112)
6. Powell et al. Localization of parathyroid hormone-related protein in breast cancer metastasis: increased incidence in bone compared with other sites. Cancer Research 1991, 51:3059–61
7. Johnson et al. Tumors producing human tumor necrosis factor induce hypercalcemia and osteoclastic bone resorption in nude mice. Endocrinology 1989, 124:1424–7
8. Black et al. Chinese hamster ovarian cells transfected with murine IL-6 gene causes hypercalcemia as well as cachexia, leukocytosis, and thrombosis in tumor-bearing mice. Endocrinology 1991, 128:2657–60
9. Nussbaum et al. Highly sensitive two-site immunoradiometric asay of parathyrin and its clinical utility in evaluating patients with hypercalcemia. Clinical Chemistry 1987, 33:1364–7
10. Nussbaum et al. Single-dose intravenous therapy with pamidronate for the treatment of hypercalcemia of malignancy: comparison of 30-, 60-, and 90-mg dosages. American Journal of Medicine 1993, 95 (3):297–304
11. Purohit et al. Randomised double-blind comparison of intravenous pamidronate and clodronate in the hypercalcemia of malignancy. British Journal of Cancer 1995, 72 (5):1289–93
12. Wimalawansa WJ. Optimal frequency of administration of pamidronate in patients with hypercalcemia of malignancy. Clinical Endocrinology 1994, 41 (5):591–5
13. Berenson et al. Efficacy of pamidronate in reducing skeletal events in patients with advanced multiple myeloma. New England Journal of Medicine 1996, 334:488–93
14. Schwartz et al. A syndrome of renal sodium loss and hyponatremia probably resulting from inappropriate secretion of antidiuretic hormone. American Journal of Medicine 1957, 23:529–42
15. Ayus et al. Pathogenesis of hyponatremic enaphalopathy. Endocrinology and Metabolism Clinics of North America 1993, 22:425
16. Ayus et al. Rapid correction of severe hyponatremia with intravenous hypertonic saline. American Journal of Medicine 1982, 72:43
17. Sterns RH et al. Osmotic demyelination syndrome follwing correction of hyponatremia. New England Journal of Medicine 1986, 314:1535

18. Forrest et al. Superiority of demeclocycline over lithium in the treatment of chronic syndrome of inappropriate secretion of antidimetric hormone. New England Journal of Medicine 1978, 298:173

19. Lawson et al. Metabolic approaches to cancer cachexia. Annual Review of Nutrition 1982, 2:277–301

20. De Wys et al. Prognostic effect of weight loss prior to chemotherapy in cancer patients. American Journal of Medicine 1980, 69:491–7

21. De Wys WD et al. Diet and Cancer prevention: An overview. Seminars in Oncology 1983, 10:255–6

22. Waterhouse C. Nutritional Disorders in neoplastic disease. Journal of Chronic Disease 1963, 16:637–44

23. Peacock et al. Resting energy expenditure and body cell mass alterations in non-cachectic patients with sarcoma. Surgery 1987, 102:465–72

24. Beutler B, Cerami A. Cachectin and tumor necrosis factor as two sides of the biological coin. Nature 1986, 320:584–8

25. Berg et al. Characterization of differentiation factor/leukemia inhibitory factor effect on lipoprotein lipase activity and mRNA in 3T3-LI adipocytes. Cytokine 1994, 6:425–32

26. Starnes HF. TNF and the acute metabolic response to tissue injury in man. Journal of Clinical Investigation 1982, 82:1321–25

27. Tracey et al. Metabolic effects of cachectin/tumor necrosis factor-secreting tumor in skeletal muscles induces chronic cachexia, while implantation in brain produces predominantly anorexia. Journal of Clinical Investigation 1990, 86:2014–24

28. Gelin et al. The role of endogenous TNFα and interleukin 1 for experimental tumor progression and development of cancer cachexia. Cancer Research 1991, 51:415–21

29. Yasumoto et al. Molecular analysis of the cytokine network involved in cachexia in colon 26 adenocarcinoma-bearing mice. Cancer Research 1995, 55 (921–927)

30. Patton et al. Interferons and tumor necrosis factors have similar catabolic effects on 3T3 L1 cells. Proceedings of the National Academy of Science USA 1986, 83:8313–7

31. Langstein et al. The role of γ-interferon and tumor necrosis factor-α in an experimental rat model of cancer cachexia. Cancer Research 1991, 51:2302–6

32. Strassman et al. Evidence for the involvement of interleukin-6 in experimental cancer cachexia. Journal of Immunology 1992, 148:3674–8

33. Tamura et al. Involvement of human interleukin-6 in experimental cachexia induced by a human uterine carcinoma xenograft. Clinical Cancer Research 1995, 1:1353–8

34. Mori et al. Cancer cachexia syndrome developed in nude mice bearing melanoma cells producing leukemia-inhibitory factor. Cancer Research 1991, 51:6656–9

35. Tisdale and Beck. Inhibition of tumour-induced lipolysis in vitro and cachexia and tumour growth in vivo by eicosapentaenoic acid. Biochemical Pharmacology 1991, 41:103–7

36. Tchekmedyian et al. Megestrol acetate in cancer anorexia and weight loss. Cancer 1992, 69:1268–74

37. Kornblith et al. Effect of megestrol acetate upon the quality of life in advanced breast cancer patients in a dose-response trial. Proceedings of the American Society of Clinical Oncology 1992 (abstract);11:337

38. Loprinzi et al. Phase III evaluation of four doses of megestrol acetate as therapy for patients with cancer anorexia and/or cachexia. Journal of Clinical Oncology 1993, 11:762–7

39. Klein and Koretz. Nutrition support in patients with cancer: What do the data really show? Nutrition in Clinical Practice 1994, 9:91–100

40. Bedrna and Polcak. Akuter harnleiterverschluss nach bestrahlung chronischer leukamien mit rontgenstrahlen. Med Kin 1929, 25:1700–1
41. Merril and Jackson. The renal complications of leukemia. New England Journal of Medicine 1943, 228:27
42. List et al. Tumor lysis syndrome complicating treatment of chronic lymphocytic leukemia with fludarabine phosphate. American Journal of Medicine 1990, 89 (3):388–90
43. Hussein and Feum. Tumor lysis syndrome after induction chemotherapy in small cell lung carcinoma. American Journal of Clinical Oncology 1990, 13 (1):10–3
44. Kalemkerian et al. Tumor lysis syndrome in small cell carcinoma and other solid tumors. American Journal of Medicine 1997, 103:363–7
45. Drakos et al. Tumor lysis syndrome in non-hematologic malignancies. American Journal of Clinical Oncology 1994, 17:502–5
46. Kjellstrand et al. Hyperuricemic acute renal failure. Archives of Internal Medicine 1974, 133:349–59
47. Boles et al. Acute renal failure caused by extreme hyperphosphatemia after chemotherapy of an acute lymphoblastic leukemia. Cancer 1984, 53:2425–9
48. Cadman et al. Hyperphosphatemia and hypocalcemia accompanying rapid cell lysis in a patient with Burkitts lymphoma and Burkitt cell leukemia. American Journal of Medicine 1977, 62:283–90
49. Argilès et al. The metabolic basis of cancer cachexia. Medicinal Research Reviews, 1997, 17 (5):477–98

# Hematologic Malignancies

# Acute Leukemia in Adults

R.A. Larson

The acute leukemias are characterized by aberrant differentiation and proliferation of malignantly transformed hematopoietic stem cells. These cells accumulate within the bone marrow and, once a substantial burden of leukemia cells is present, lead to suppression of the growth and differentiation of normal blood cells. Symptoms result from varying degrees of anemia, neutropenia, and thrombocytopenia or from infiltration into tissues. Although virtually any organ system may become involved once leukemia cells enter the peripheral blood, the lymph nodes, liver, spleen, central nervous system (CNS), and skin are the most common sites detected clinically.

The traditional classification of the acute leukemias has relied most heavily on morphological and cytochemical characteristics. However, recent advances in immunology, molecular biology, and cytogenetics have substantially enhanced our understanding of the biologic markers which distinguish normal hematopoietic cells from their leukemic counterparts. Such technologies have firmly advanced our knowledge of leucocyte differentiation and the cellular origins of acute leukemia. Application of newly available molecular probes capable of identifying rearrangements of immunoglobulin and T-cell receptor genes and highly specific monoclonal antibodies to defined cell surface antigens have greatly facilitated our ability to distinguish a normal cell from a malignant one. Furthermore, these technologies afford the accurate classification of a malignant clone as myeloid, B-lymphoid, T-lymphoid, or biphenotypic in most cases.

Advances in cytogenetics have increased our understanding of the association of certain non-random chromosomal abnormalities with specific morphological subtypes of acute leukemia, providing further evidence that genetic changes play a major role in the transformation of a normal cell to a neoplastic one. A number of recurring chromosomal alterations have been identified which carry important prognostic weight with regard to response to chemotherapy and overall survival. Contemporary characterization of any acute leukemia requires the application of immunologic phenotyping, molecular biologic techniques, and cytogenetic analysis which together complement and expand the more traditional morphological and cytochemical descriptions of these diseases.

## Etiology

While the cause of acute leukemia in humans is unknown, a variety of factors appear to play an etiologic role. It is likely that in most cases leukemia results from the interaction of several factors, both hereditary and environmental [1a]. Much of the evidence is indirect and has been inferred from epidemiological studies. In the past, investigators have relied heavily on animal models of leukemogenesis. For instance, when certain nonhuman species have been exposed to a potential leukemogenic agent such as radiation or a chemical carcinogen, there is an increased likelihood that the disease will develop. From such observations, it seems apparent that the pathogenesis of acute leukemia involves complex interactions between host susceptibility, chromosomal damage secondary to physical or chemical exposure, and possibly the incorporation of genetic information transmitted virally into susceptible progenitor cells.

### Age and Sex

Although acute leukemia can occur at any age, there is a clear increase in incidence as age rises above 50 years. Across the entire age spectrum, acute lymphoblastic leukemia (ALL) and acute myeloid leukemia (AML) are nearly equal in overall incidence, but ALL predominates among children while AML accounts for the majority of cases in adults. Acute leukemia is, in general, more common among men than women. This difference is due in part to a higher incidence in young boys and older men. Factors such as occupational and environmental exposure may account for some of these differences.

## Ethnic and Geographic Differences

Acute leukemia is more common among whites than blacks at all ages. Jews are more commonly affected than non-Jews, but it is unclear if this is due to genetic or environmental factors. Differences in the reported increase among higher social classes may be secondary to greater access to medical care among the upper socioeconomic groups. Geographic variations in incidence are likely related to a number of factors including socioeconomic, ethnic, and urban or rural setting and may account for the higher frequency reported in industrialized countries and urban areas. Some cytogenetic abnormalities have been reported more frequently from some countries than from others.

## Radiation

The leukemogenic potential of ionizing radiation has been well recognized for a number of years. These leukemias generally derive from the myeloid lineage but have features of multi-potential stem cells. Much of the epidemiologic evidence emanates from observations following human exposures to radiation following nuclear explosions, therapeutic or diagnostic radiation, and from occupational radiation. Following the atomic bomb attacks on Hiroshima and Nagasaki, exposed survivors experienced a marked increase in the incidence of leukemia, both acute and chronic [1]. The chance of developing leukemia was related to the intensity of radiation exposure, with relatively little risk observed in those exposed to less than 100 cGy [2].

Patients who have received therapeutic radiation for ankylosing spondylitis, menorrhagia, or $^{32}$P for treatment of polycythemia vera have experienced an increased incidence of acute leukemia [3–5]. Current use of diagnostic X-ray imaging does not appear to result in any increased leukemia risk to patients. However, fetal exposure to intrauterine X-rays increases the risk of subsequent childhood leukemia [6].

The risk of developing leukemia in persons receiving radiation exposure through their work-place was documented from early studies among women employed as radium dial painters and from the increased incidence among radiologists during the early part of this century [7, 8]. Current radiation protection practices appear to have markedly diminished this risk.

Chemicals

Although less clearly established than the evidence implicating ionizing radiation, there is substantial epidemiologic data linking the development of acute leukemia to either therapeutic or industrial chemicals. Exposure to alkylating agents such as melphalan or nitrogen mustard is associated with the development of acute myeloid leukemia, usually within 4–6 years [9, 10]. Therapy-related leukemia (t-AML) is a well recognized complication of Hodgkin's disease and ovarian cancer [11]. The risk is greater in patients receiving both chemotherapy and radiotherapy. Recently, another subtype of t-AML has been observed in patients treated for certain hematologic and solid neoplasms with the epipodophyllotoxin drugs etoposide or teniposide, and with other agents that inhibit topoisomerase II activity [10, 12].

In the early part of this century acute leukemia was noted among workers occupationally exposed to benzene. For example, the incidence of acute leukemia among Turkish cobblers chronically exposed to benzene was two to three times greater than its incidence in the general population [13]. With the advent of stronger occupational safety laws, benzene-associated leukemia has nearly disappeared in Western countries.

Viruses

A number of viruses are known to cause acute leukemia in several non-human species. The potential role of viruses in human leukemogenesis has been explored for decades. There are at present no conclusive data that any of the common types of acute leukemia in humans have a viral origin. However, there is mounting circumstantial evidence that viruses may play a role. African Burkitt's lymphoma has been closely associated with the Epstein-Barr virus. DNA from this virus is integrated into the genome of African (endemic) but not sporadic (American) Burkitt's lymphoma and leukemia cells. In general, however, virologic studies have not confirmed a causal relationship between Epstein-Barr virus infections and acute leukemia. An uncommon form of adult leukemia, adult T-cell leukemia, largely restricted to Southern Japan and the Caribbean regions, is closely linked to infection by a leukemogenic virus, HTLV-1 [14]. However, most individuals expressing antibodies to this virus never manifest evidence of malignancy. Thus, it appears that viral leukemogenesis in both human and non-human species depends on a number of factors interacting together including host age and sex, alterations of host genome and gene expression, and host immune recognition and response to neoplasia.


## Heredity and Genetics

Observations of the increased incidence of acute leukemia among members of certain high-susceptibility families, the high frequency of concordant leukemia in monozygotic twins, and the association of acute leukemia among individuals with genetic disorders have established that hereditary factors play a role in the development of leukemia. Several studies have demonstrated that although leukemia does not often occur within families, there is a significant tendency for leukemia to cluster among certain families.

Identical twins of children with leukemia have an increased risk of developing acute leukemia, often before the age of 8 years [15]. These individuals usually develop the disease within a year of their twin's diagnosis. Non-identical siblings of those affected by leukemia have a lesser risk, but still greater than that observed among the general population [16].

Acute leukemia is increased in patients affected by Down's syndrome, a disease characterized by chromosomal nondisjunction. Further evidence of the relationship between leukemia and chromosomal abnormalities is the increased incidence in patients with Bloom's syndrome and Fanconi's anemia. Both disorders are hereditary conditions characterized by increased chromosomal breakage. Other genetic conditions not normally associated with chromosomal abnormalities, such as ataxia telangiectasia and congenital agammaglobulinemia, are associated with acute leukemia. In these conditions, deficiencies of cellular and humoral immunity exist which may render such hosts more susceptible to leukemogenesis.


## The Morphological Classification of Leukemia

The traditional classification of the acute leukemias has relied on morphological description, reflecting the predominant cell type present within the bone marrow population and relating that cell to its normal hematopoietic counterpart. In 1976, a group of hematopathologists formed the French-American-British (FAB) Co-operative group with the aim to establish a subclassification system for the acute leukemias that would clearly separate ALL and AML into distinct disorders [17]. This system was based solely on light microscopic evaluation of routinely stained blood and marrow smears, supplemented by a limited number of cytochemical procedures. Due to its ease of use and applicability when comparing treatment results among institutions, this system has gained widespread adoption. In addition, the classification system was shown to have independent prognostic significance regarding survival. The system was revised in 1985 to provide clarification and extend to new diagnostic techniques [18].

## Acute Lymphoblastic Leukemia

The FAB classification system described three subtypes of ALL (L1, L2, and L3) defined by individual cytologic features such as cell size, nuclear chromatin pattern, nuclear shape, nucleoli, and amount of basophilia in the cytoplasm. The subtype L1, which accounts for over 80% of the ALL cases in children and approximately 30% in adults, consists of predominantly small cells, up to twice the diameter of a small lymphocyte. The nuclear chromatin is homogenous and the nuclear shape is regular. Nucleoli are often not visible, but when detected are inconspicuous. The cytoplasm is scant in amount and is usually only slightly or moderately basophilic. The majority of adult cases of ALL are L2. These cells are larger than in L1 and are often heterogeneous in size. The nuclear chromatin pattern is heterogenous as well. Nuclear shape is often irregular and nucleoli are more conspicuous than in L1. The amount of cytoplasm is variable but is often moderately abundant and variably basophilic. The least common type of ALL, seen in approximately 3%–4% of both children and adults, is termed L3. This subtype is morphologically identical to the neoplastic cells in Burkitt's lymphoma. These cells are large and uniform with finely stippled chromatin and regular nuclear shape. Nucleoli are often prominent. Cytoplasm is moderately abundant and deeply basophilic.

The FAB group later recognized that the distinction between L1 and L2 was not always straightforward. In order to improve reproducibility among observers, a simplified scoring system was adopted which stressed three key features of the blast cell population: nuclear/cytoplasmic ratio (N/C), nucleoli, and irregular nuclear membrane [19]. Cell size was considered important only if 50% or more of the leukemia cells were large.

Cytochemical evaluations of blast cells in ALL reveal characteristic patterns. By definition, stains for lysosomal enzymes such as myeloperoxidase or the Sudan black reaction must be negative to support a diagnosis of ALL. The periodic acid-Schiff (PAS) reaction will reveal clumpy positivity due to glycogen in ALL blasts (except L3, which reacts negatively) but is a poor discriminator of cell lineage as many AML cells will also react positively. Chloroacetate esterase and lysozyme stains are negative, but alpha-naphthyl acetate esterase may be positive in T-lymphoblasts. ALL blast cells contain the enzyme terminal deoxynucleotidyl transferase (TdT) which when present in the great majority of cells is a fairly reliable marker for ALL. L3 leukemia cells often stain positively with oil red O due to neutral lipid within the cytoplasmic vacuoles.

## Acute Myeloid Leukemia

The blast cells of patients with AML are most often larger than lymphoblasts and display a greater heterogeneity in size and shape. AML blasts have more abundant cytoplasm and usually contain cytoplasmic granules. Auer rods, azurophilic crystalline-like accumulations of abnormal lysosomal granules visible in the cytoplasm with Wright's stain, are detected in about 10% of patients with AML.

A diagnosis of AML is established when 30% or more of all the nucleated marrow cells are blast cells. The FAB group has defined eight variants of AML (Table 1) including three types (M1, M2, and M3) with predominantly granulocytic differentiation, two with at least 20% monocytic precursors (M4, M5), one with a high proportion of erythroblasts (M6), and a more recently recognized and rarely occurring variant with predominance of megakaryoblasts (M7) [18]. In addition, the FAB group has described a form of AML with minimal myeloid differentiation, designated MO, which cannot be diagnosed solely on morphologic or cytochemical grounds but also requires the use of immunohistochemical staining [20]. These cases express myeloid antigens on the blast cell surface but lack myeloperoxidase activity. The FAB classification of AML is summarized in Table 1.

**Table 1.** French-American-British (FAB) classification of AML

| FAB subtype | Morphologic and cytochemical features | Frequency (%) |
|---|---|---|
| M0 | Large, agranular myeloblasts, sometimes resembling lymphoblasts of FAB subtype L2. Stain negative for myeloperoxidase and Sudan black. Express CD13 or CD33 antigens on cell surface. | 2–3 |
| M1 | Acute myeloblastic leukemia without maturation: Large, poorly differentiated myeloblasts represent 90% or more of the non-erythroid cells. At least 3% of the myeloblasts stain positive for myeloperoxidase. | 20 |
| M2 | Acute myeloblastic leukemia with maturation: Between 30 and 89% of the non-erythroid cells are myeloblasts having abundant cytoplasm with moderate to many granules. Auer rods are often visible. | 25–30 |
| M3 | Leukemia cells usually contain heavy azurophilic granulation. Nuclear size varies greatly. Nuclei are often bilobed or kidney-shaped. Some cells contain bundles of Auer rods. Leukemia cells stain strongly positive for myeloperoxidase. There is a micro-granular variant. Usually HLA-DR negative. | 8–15 |
| M4 | Myeloblasts comprise over 30% of the non-erythroid cells but total granulocytic precursors do not exceed 80%. Monocytic cells account for >20% of the non-erythroid cells. Non-specific esterase and chloroacetate stains are often positive. Auer rods may be present. | 20–25 |
| M4Eo | Myelomonoblasts plus morphologically and cytochemically abnormal eosinophils. | 5 |
| M5 | Monoblasts, promonocytes, or monocytes comprise 80% or more of the non-erythroid cells. In one subtype (M5A), 80% or more of all the monocytic cells are monoblasts. In the well-differentiated subtype (M5B), less than 80% are monoblasts. Alpha-naphthyl acetate positivity is extinguished by NaF. | 10 |
| M6 | Greater than 50% of the nucleated marrow cells are erythroid. Erythroblasts are usually strongly PAS positive. Myeloblasts represent 30% or more of the non-erythroid cells. | 5 |
| M7 | Large and small megakaryoblasts with high nuclear/cytoplasm ratio. Cytoplasm is pale and agranular. Standard cytochemical stains are not definitive. Platelet peroxidase and platelet-specific antibodies are often positive. | 1–2 |

**Immunobiology of Acute Leukemia** [21]

Approximately 80% of ALL arise from the B-cell lineage and express B-cell differentiation antigens (CD19 and/or CD20) and have undergone heavy and/or light chain immunoglobulin gene rearrangements. Many of these cases also express the common ALL antigen or CALLA, designated CD10. Progenitor B-cell ALL does not express CD10. CD10-bearing cells can be further divided based on the presence of cytoplasmic immunoglobulin (cIg). Most cases do not express cIg and are termed early B-precursor ALL or common ALL. Approximately 20% of CD10 positive cases express cIg and are designated pre-B ALL. Surface immunoglobulin (SIg) expression occurs in only 2%–5% of ALL cases; these are termed B-cell ALL or Burkitt-type ALL and typically display the FAB L3 morphology.

Between 15%–20% of ALL cases arise from the T-cell lineage. These cells express T-cell antigens such as CD5 and CD7. CD10 may also be present. In the majority of cases, one or more of the T-cell receptor genes is rearranged. Further subclassification of T-cell ALL into early, intermediate, or mature thymocyte types is based on the expression of various T-cell differentiation antigens.

A very small percentage of ALL cases lack either B or T-cell features and are termed acute undifferentiated leukemia (AUL). Certain antigens normally found only on myeloid cells can be expressed by malignant lymphoblasts of either B or T-cell origin. These cases are called myeloid antigen (My) positive ALL [22].

As yet, no AML-specific surface antigens have been identified. Rather, AML cells often express antigens simultaneously on the cell surface that are not normally co-expressed by their normal myeloid counterparts [23, 24]. Efforts to correlate immunologic phenotyping with the FAB classification of AML or with clinical outcome have in general been imprecise. However, the expression of certain antigens such as CD34, an early stem cell marker, may carry important prognostic information [25]. In addition, CD33 which is expressed on most myeloblasts has become an important target for monoclonal antibody directed therapy.

Hybrid Leukemias

Recent application of both immunophenotyping and molecular probes has uncovered a number of cases in which leukemia cells display characteristics of both myeloid and lymphoid cells. In such instances, a single neoplastic cell may co-express features of distinct lineages (biphenotypic) or, alternatively, two distinct sub-populations of leukemia cells may express either myeloid or lymphoid features separately (bilineal). Various theories have been put forward to explain the occurrence of these hybrid leukemias. One hypothesis, termed lineage infidelity, states that the leukemia cell displays aberrant gene expression by virtue of its neoplastic transformation. Another theory, lineage promiscuity, proposes that normally differentiating cells may express characteristics of more than one distinct lineage and that the leukemia cell is merely reflecting that particular phase in a cell's development. Finally, a theory termed lineage switching proposes that in some cases leukemia is a malignancy of a pluripotent stem cell capable of differentiation along either a myeloid or lymphoid lineage. Thus, any individual case may express one or both phenotypes.

## Cytogenetics

Cytogenetic abnormalities occur commonly in the acute leukemias. Since the application of chromosome banding techniques in the early 1970s, cytogenetic analysis has provided the most clinically useful approach to subclassifying the acute leukemias. Syndromes of acute leukemia have been well described in which a particular non-random chromosomal abnormality correlates with a specific morphologic subtype and clinical profile. Such recurring chromosomal abnormalities have provided important independent information regarding response to therapy and overall prognosis [26].

Cytogenetic analysis has furthered our understanding of leukemogenesis [27]. Careful analyses of the chromosomal breakpoints associated with leukemia-specific cytogenetic abnormalities have permitted identification of a number of genes that appear to play an integral role in leukemogenesis [27a, 27b]. The chromosomal location of a large number of these so-called oncogenes has been identified. The functions of these oncogenes are being investigated, but many are involved in intracellular signaling pathways and the control of cellular proliferation and differentiation. Structural chromosomal changes may lead to activation or perturbation of oncogene expression resulting in disturbance of cellular regulation and eventually malignant transformation. Deletions or loss of DNA may eliminate genes that have tumor suppressor functions.

## Cytogenetic Abnormalities in AML

Clonal chromosomal abnormalities can be detected in most cases of AML. These abnormalities include gains or losses of whole chromosomes or the long (q) or short (p) arms of chromosomes (deletions) as well as a variety of structural rearrangements (translocations, inversions, or insertions).

It is strongly recommended that cytogenetic analysis prior to initiation of therapy be performed on every newly diagnosed patient since studies of the prognostic significance of recurring cytogenetic abnormalities in AML have yielded consistently similar results [28]. Cytogenetic characterization has become the strongest predictor of both response to therapy and remission duration. Thus, in many centers plans for post-remission therapy currently rely heavily on cytogenetic analysis at diagnosis [29].

Cytogenetic analysis of an individual patient's leukemia cells has become an increasingly important component of diagnosis prior to treatment in both AML and ALL. An adequate (>2 ml) sample of bone marrow aspirate from a fresh puncture site should be submitted for cytogenetic analysis in all patients suspected of having leukemia. Metaphase cells are stained, and the chromosome number and banding pattern are determined. Specific and well-characterized, recurring chromosomal abnormalities facilitate diagnosis, confirm subtype classification and have major prognostic value for treatment planning (Table 2).

Cytogenetic data have been used to map chromosomal breakpoints at a molecular level, allowing use of probes for fluorescence in situ hybridization (FISH) and of primers for reverse transcriptase polymerase chain reaction (RT-PCR) methods for the detection of tumor cells. FISH and RT-PCR can detect molecular genetic rearrangements not visible when examining chromosomal banding by conventional methods. However, both of the former methods test only for specific, defined genetic mutations and cannot be used initially for general screening or for a comprehensive evaluation. FISH analysis is more sensitive than conventional karyotype analysis and can be performed on both metaphase and interphase cells. The morphology of the positive cells can be determined concurrently, and the proportional involvement by leukemia of all of the hematopoietic cells can be evaluated.

RT-PCR is the most sensitive method available for detecting occult leukemia cells (about 1 in $10^5$ cells). As yet, however, the method is non-

**Table 2.** Cytogenetic subsets in AML, treatment, and outcomes

| Karyotype | Complete remission rate | Remission duration | Treatment approach |
|---|---|---|---|
| t(8,21) | High | Long | Standard induction with an anthracycline. Intensive consolidation chemotherapy with high dose cytarabine (HiDAC). |
| inv(16) (p13q22) or t(16,16) | High | Intermediate to long | Standard induction with an anthracycline. Intensive consolidation chemotherapy with high dose cytarabine |
| t(15,17) | High | Intermediate to long | All-trans retinoic acid (ATRA) together with an anthracycline. |
| t(9,11) | High | Intermediate | Standard induction and intensive consolidation with HiDAC. Reserve BMT for second remission for most t(9,11) patients. |
| del(5q), +13, +8, inv 3, del(12p), t(9,22), or other 11q23 abnormalities, or complex abnormalities | Low | Short | New induction regimens, including use of growth factors during or after chemotherapy, or modulators of drug resistance. Perform BMT in first CR. |

quantitative, and the results do not identify the cell type involved. The clinical significance of a positive result is currently being investigated. A positive assay confirms the presence of cells with the specific genetic abnormality but does not necessarily indicate the neoplastic growth potential of these cells. For example, a positive RT-PCR assay after treatment appears to predict leukemia relapse reliably in patients with APL and a t(15,17), but not in those with AML-M2 and a t(8,21) [30, 31].

## Diagnosis

### Clinical Features of AML

The median age of patients with AML is approximately 60 years. Older patients are clearly under-represented in the literature due to selection of younger adults for clinical trials. The incidence is approximately equal between sexes. Typically, antecedent symptoms such as fatigue are brief. About one third of patients will present with bruising or hemorrhage. One quarter of patients will have a serious infection involving the lung, soft tissues, or skin. Splenomegaly or hepatomegaly are not common and occur in less than 25% of patients. Lymphadenopathy is even less common. Gingival hypertrophy or skin infiltration by leukemia (called leukemia cutis) occurs in half of patients with monocytic leukemia.

The WBC count is elevated in one third of patients, but in recent years counts >100,000/μl occur in less than 10% of patients probably due to earlier diagnoses. The peripheral blood will contain some leukemic blast cells in 85%–90% of cases. The absolute granulocyte count is almost always depressed in AML and is less than 1500/μl in half of patients at diagnosis. A moderate degree of anemia is common, and the platelet count is typically <100,000/μl and often <20,000/μl.

Mild to moderate elevations of serum uric acid levels are common and typically reflect increased cell turn-over. The serum lactate dehydrogenase (LDH) level may be elevated but not as commonly as in ALL. Muramidase (lysozyme) is elevated in the serum or urine of patients with acute myelomonocytic or monoblastic leukemias.

AML is not limited to the bone marrow and peripheral blood. Abnormalities in one or more organ systems may result from leukemia cell infiltration or metabolic complications related to leukemia. Rarely, a patient with AML will develop a solid mass of leukemia cells called a granulocytic sarcoma. The skin and bones, particularly sternum, ribs, or orbit, are most commonly involved, but granulocytic sarcomas can occur in any organ. Respiratory distress in patients with AML is most often due to infection. However, patients with very high numbers of circulating blast cells (>100,000/μl) may develop severe dyspnea and hypoxemia due to leukostasis within the pulmonary capillaries. Cardiac dysfunction, including murmurs, congestive heart failure, and dysrhythmias, are most often secondary to anemia.

Retinal hemorrhages are most often due to thrombocytopenia. However, patients with extreme hyperleukocytosis may develop "cotton wool" spots due to retinal ischemia. Frank CNS involvement and cranial neuropathies are unusual at initial diagnosis of AML.

## Clinical features of ALL

ALL accounts for approximately 20% of adult acute leukemias. The clinical presentation in adults is most often acute. Symptoms are usually present for only a few weeks prior to diagnosis. Malaise, lethargy, weight loss, fever, and night sweats may be present but are typically not severe. Bone pain and arthralgias occur occasionally but much less frequently in adults than in children. Infection and hemorrhage are present in one third of patients at diagnosis but are most often not as severe as in AML. Lymphadenopathy, splenomegaly, and hepatomegaly are more common than in AML, affecting half of adults with ALL. Chest radiographs may reveal a thymic mass in 15% of adults. The majority of these patients have T-cell ALL.

CNS involvement by leukemia occurs in 5%–10% of adult cases but is less frequent at diagnosis. Cranial nerve palsies most often involve the 6th and 7th cranial nerves. Headache and papilledema resulting from meningeal infiltration and obstruction of the outflow of CSF with raised intracranial pressure may be present. Retinal hemorrhages may be the result of thrombocytopenia.

Varying degrees of neutropenia, anemia, and thrombocytopenia are detected on the peripheral blood examination. In one series of over 1200 adult cases, the granulocyte count was below 1500/μl in only one-fifth [32]. Mild to moderate reductions in hemoglobin level were typical, but almost one-third of patients had a hemoglobin level below 8 g/dl. Thrombocytopenia was frequent and over one-half of patients had a platelet count below 50,000/μl. The total WBC was diminished in about one-third of patients and normal or moderately elevated in close to one-half. Sixteen percent of cases had a marked leukocytosis (>100,000/μl) at diagnosis. Characteristic lymphoblasts can be identified in the peripheral blood in over 90% of the cases.

## Prognostic Factors

Several patient factors are known to be important in determining prognosis in acute leukemia [29]. Most risk factors, however, are not independent of advances in treatment nor are they predictive across all of the specific biological subsets of leukemia.

Age is the most important independent patient variable in determining outcome. Treatment results are best in young adults and are considerably poorer in patients older than 60 years. In addition, young or middle-aged adults may benefit from the availability of BMT to rescue patients after suffering a relapse. Elderly patients have a lower response rate to remission induction chemotherapy and increased treatment toxicity, in part due to their high incidence of co-morbid disorders. The poor survival of elderly patients, however, is not fully explained by their lower tolerance for intensive treatment. The disease itself appears to have a different natural history in this group. Elderly patients with AML are more likely to have had a myelodysplastic syndrome (MDS), and are also more likely to have unfavorable cytogenetic features. Similarly, older patients with ALL have a higher incidence of the Philadelphia (Ph) chromosome, and this subgroup has a poor outcome.

Antecedent hematological disorders such as MDS are a major adverse prognostic factor. Therapy-related leukemia (t-AML) following treatment with alkylating agents or topoisomerase II inhibitors or radiotherapy for a prior cancer has been well described and has a similarly poor outcome with conventional chemotherapy programs [10].

## General Principles of Therapy

The goal of remission induction chemotherapy is the rapid restoration of normal bone marrow function. The term complete remission (CR) is reserved for patients who have full recovery of normal peripheral blood counts and bone marrow cellularity with <5% residual blast cells. Induction therapy aims to reduce the total body leukemia cell population from approximately $10^{12}$ to below the cytologically detectable level of about $10^9$ cells. It is generally assumed, however, that a substantial burden of leukemia cells persist undetected, leading to relapse within a few weeks or months if no further therapy were administered. Post-induction or remission consolidation therapy, usually comprising one or more courses of chemotherapy, is designed to eradicate residual leukemia, allowing the possibility of cure. Multiple chemotherapy drugs in high doses are typically used in order to prevent the emergence of resistant subclones, and to limit cumulative and overlapping toxicities. Lower doses of prolonged remission maintenance therapy lasting 1–3 years have been used with some success in ALL, but this adjunctive therapy has uncertain value in AML.

Bone marrow transplantation using an HLA identical sibling donor is an established treatment modality in acute leukemia and is indicated for suitable high risk patients in first remission or for any young or middle-aged patient in first relapse or second remission [33, 34]. Allogeneic BMT (alloBMT) has two therapeutic components. Intensive myeloablative therapy is used to eradicate all tumor cells, if possible. In addition, T-cells in the donor marrow can produce a graft versus leukemia (GvL) immune response which can destroy remaining leukemia cells; this effect has been correlated with improved disease-free survival. Unfortunately, this beneficial immune response is closely associated with acute and chronic graft versus host disease (GvHD), a major cause of morbidity and mortality following alloBMT. GvHD can be reduced by T-cell depletion from the donor marrow, but only at the cost of increased rates of graft failure and leukemia relapse. Because the risk of treatment-related mortality increases with age, most centers restrict BMT to patients <60 years old. The use of alloBMT is also limited in part by donor availability. A patient has a 25%–30% chance that a sibling will be HLA identical. Using siblings mismatched at only one HLA locus results in increased GvHD but may provide equivalent survival. Allogeneic transplantation using a matched unrelated donor (MUD) is an option for younger adults who lack a sibling donor. The likelihood of finding a donor in the National Bone Marrow Donor Registry is related to the ethnic background of the patient compared to the volunteer donor pool; the overall match rate is between 40%–50%. MUD BMT often involves prolonged delays until the transplant can be performed (median time, about 6 months), increased costs, and more severe complications. Non-engraftment and severe GvHD result in increased early mortality.

Autologous BMT allows the use of myeloablative therapy in patients who lack an allogeneic marrow donor as well as in older patients [35]. The appropriate role for this treatment modality is controversial. Treatment-related morbidity and mortality (<5%) are relatively low, thus allowing its use in older patients, but relapse rates are high, and overall outcomes are not clearly better than in patients who receive intensive but non-ablative therapy. The relative contribution to relapse of tumor cell contamination in the reinfused cryopreserved marrow versus the failure of the high dose therapy to eradicate all disease in vivo has not been determined. Purging of leukemia cells from the harvested hematopoietic cells in vitro using monoclonal antibodies or chemotherapy agents has been attempted. Purging techniques considerably delay engraftment without having a proven benefit in decreasing the incidence of disease recurrence. Hematopoietic cells capable of reconstituting bone marrow function can be harvested for autologous transplantation by direct bone marrow aspiration or by apheresis of progenitor cells from peripheral blood. The yield from peripheral blood can be augmented by mobilization following chemotherapy and/or growth factors. The use of peripheral blood stem cells has not been proven to decrease the risk of relapse, but it does accelerate the rate of hematopoietic reconstitution.

## Treatment of Acute Leukemia

### Remission Induction Therapy for AML

The most common remission induction regimen used for patients with AML is cytarabine given by continuous intravenous (IV) infusion daily for 7 days plus daunorubicin given daily for 3 days (7+3 regimen). Depending on age and patient selection, 60%–80% of patients achieve a CR [36, 37]. The outcome in general has not been improved by the substitution of other anthracyclines, increasing the dose of cytarabine, or adding a third or fourth drug (Table 3).

Daunorubicin was the first anthracycline of demonstrated value against AML. It has equivalent efficacy and less toxicity than doxorubicin. Idarubicin is a more lipophilic analogue of daunorubicin, and its

**Table 3.** AML remission induction chemotherapy regimens

| Drugs | Dose | Comment |
|---|---|---|
| Cytarabine + daunorubicin | 100 mg/m$^2$ daily as a continuous infusion for 7 days; 45-60 mg/m$^2$ iv push on each of the first 3 days of treatment | "Standard" induction regimen resulting in approximately 60% to 80% remission rate and acceptable toxicity in patients under 60 years old |
| Cytarabine (HiDAC) + daunorubicin | 3 g/m$^2$ twice daily for a total of 12 doses; 45 mg/m$^2$ iv push for 3 days following cytarabine | Yields a 90% remission rate. However, substantial toxicity precludes postremission therapy in a high proportion of patients |
| Cytarabine + idarubicin | 100 mg/m$^2$ daily as a continuous infusion for 7 days; 13 mg/m$^2$ iv push on each of first 3 days of treatment | Has produced a greater remission rate (88% vs 70%) compared to cytarabine/daunorubicin in younger patients. Appears superior to daunorubicin in patients with hyperleukocytosis. Overall survival not clearly superior to "standard" regimen. |
| Cytarabine + daunorubicin + etoposide | 100 mg/m$^2$ daily as a continuous infusion for 7 days; 50 mg/m$^2$ iv push on each of first 3 days of treatment; 75 mg/m$^2$ daily for 7 days | Remission rate similar to "standard" induction regimen. Remission duration significantly improved but overall survival comparable to "standard" regimen. May prolong survival in patients less than 55 years old but at expense of increased toxicity. |
| Cytarabine (HiDAC) + daunorubicin + etoposide | 3 g/m$^2$ twice daily on days 1, 3, 5, and 7; 50 mg/m$^2$ on each of the first 3 days; 75 mg/m$^2$ daily for 7 days | More toxicity during induction, but longer CR duration. No significant effect in survival. |

active first metabolite, 13-hydroxyidarubicin, has a long half-life. Animal studies demonstrated greater activity against leukemia with less cardiotoxicity than daunorubicin. Evidence of the superiority of idarubicin compared to daunorubicin for AML is not compelling. Randomized trials showed nearly equivalent CR rates, survival, and cardiotoxicity [38–40]. More recent data suggest that idarubicin may have greater cytotoxicity than daunorubicin against leukemia cells that express the multidrug resistance (MDR) phenotype [41].

Mitoxantrone is an anthracenedione, a synthetic anthracycline analogue. It has been useful in combination with conventional and high doses of cytarabine, both for primary treatment and in relapsed disease [42, 43]. Amsacrine is currently under investigation [44, 45].

Cytarabine in conventional doses of 100–200 mg/m$^2$ per day is generally given by continuous IV infusion for 7–10 days [46]. High dose cytarabine (HDAC) regimens typically use 1000–3000 mg/m$^2$ given IV over 1–3 h every 12 h for 8–12 doses. HDAC increases the CR rate to 79%–90% but at the cost of increased toxicity [47]. Treatment mortality, the rate of early relapse, and overall survival are not clearly improved [48].

Attempts have been made to improve the CR rate of induction therapy by adding potentially non-cross-resistant drugs. Etoposide has activity as a single agent in approximately 25% of patients with previously treated AML. In a randomized trial among newly diagnosed patients, the addition of etoposide at 75 mg/m$^2$ per day for 7 days to cytarabine and daunorubicin (7+3+7 regimen) produced increased toxicity but also prolonged remission duration in the etoposide arm [49]. There was no survival benefit. A randomized comparison between cytarabine at standard doses versus high doses, both in combination with daunorubicin and etoposide, showed no improvement in the CR rate or overall survival in the HDAC arm, although disease-free survival was significantly prolonged [50].

Acute promyelocytic leukemia

APL (FAB M3) is a biologically distinct disease with characteristic clinical, morphological, and cytogenetic features [51, 52]. Disseminated intravascular coagulation at presentation or soon after the initiation of cytotoxic chemotherapy can cause pulmonary or cerebrovascular hemorrhage in up to 40% of patients and a high mortality rate. The cytoplasmic granules in the leukemic blasts contain factors with procoagulant as well as fibrinolytic activity.

All-trans retinoic acid (ATRA; tretinoin) was first used in the treatment of APL in China in 1986 and has proved to be a highly effective remission induction agent [52–55]. ATRA accelerates the terminal differentiation of malignant promyelocytes to mature neutrophils, leading to apoptosis and CR without bone marrow hypoplasia. This effect is a unique consequence of the rearranged PML/RAR-α gene resulting from the t(15,17) which defines APL. ATRA induction therapy produces CR rates of 80%–95% in both previously untreated and relapsed patients. Most treatment failure is due to early mortality. Primary resistance is rare. The median time to CR ranges from 38–44 days but may take as long as 90 days. As yet, the drug is only available as an oral preparation. The recommended daily dose is 45 mg/m². Doses from 15–100 mg/m² have been evaluated, and the optimal dose has not yet been determined. The best results have been obtained when ATRA was combined with daunorubicin and cytarabine or with idarubicin alone.

ATRA does not have the usual toxicities associated with cytotoxic chemotherapy. Intrinsic drug toxicity is generally minor. Headache is common; pseudotumor cerebri has been described but is rare. Nasal stuffiness, dry red skin, transient elevations in the transaminase levels and bilirubin, and hypertriglyceridemia are usually not treatment limiting. ATRA is neither immunosuppressive, nor myelosuppressive. The coagulopathy of APL typically improves rapidly with initiation of treatment.

Two serious and specific complications may occur with ATRA treatment of APL [56]. In 25%–40% of patients, the retinoic acid syndrome develops within 2–21 days after initiation of treatment and is characterized by fever, peripheral edema, pulmonary infiltrates and respiratory distress, hypertension, renal and hepatic dysfunction, and serositis resulting in pleural and pericardial effusions. The syndrome is possibly due to tissue infiltration by maturing malignant promyelocytes and the systemic effects of cytokine release. Many cases are associated with hyperleukocytosis, but the retinoic acid syndrome occurs with normal leukocyte counts in a third of cases. Early recognition and aggressive management with high dose dexamethasone therapy (10 mg IV every 12 hr for 6 doses) has been effective. Cessation of ATRA therapy alone does not reverse the syndrome. However, once the complication resolves, ATRA can be restarted in most cases.

Hyperleukocytosis occurs in up to 50% of patients treated with ATRA and is probably secondary to the induction of cellular maturation. This may result in leukostasis, but complications are uncertain, and management is controversial. The European APL 91 group instituted full doses of induction chemotherapy using cytarabine and daunorubicin in all patients showing a rapid rise in the leukocyte count after starting ATRA therapy (70% of patients) [53]. In contrast, investigators at the Memorial Sloan-Kettering Cancer Center have reported that an increased leukocyte count is not intrinsically dangerous, and thus chemotherapy is not usually indicated [56]. The leukocytosis has also been treated successfully with hydroxyurea.

Management of the coagulopathy associated with APL may be difficult and should be managed expectantly. Coagulation parameters, including fibrinogen, D-dimer, and platelet levels, should be monitored closely. Platelet transfusions and cryoprecipitate or fresh frozen plasma are used to maintain the fibrinogen level >100 mg/dl and the platelet count >20,000/μl. The role of heparin is controversial. Continuous infusions of 5–10 U/kg per hour are widely used and appear effective at stopping the consumption of clotting factors. Inhibitors of fibrinolysis should be considered only for life-threatening hemorrhage.

Complete hematological remissions induced by ATRA alone are rarely associated with complete molecular remissions and have had a median duration of only 3.5 months. Thus, remission consolidation using cytotoxic chemotherapy (generally daunorubicin and cytarabine) is required for long term survival. Arsenic trioxide is now under investigation in clinical trials for patients with relapsed APL.

## Post remission therapy for AML

Additional chemotherapy after a successful remission induction is mandatory to cure AML. The median disease-free survival for patients who receive no additional therapy is 4–8 months. When several courses of consolidation chemotherapy are given, survival at 2–3 years is 35%–50% for young and middle-aged adults. For patients under 60 years old, consolidation therapy results in significantly longer survival than maintenance therapy alone [29, 36, 57, 58].

The same induction therapy may be repeated for one or more cycles, with or without dose intensification, or non-cross resistant drugs can be used for consolidation (Table 4). There is increasing evidence that high dose cytarabine (HDAC) provides the best survival for good and inter-

**Table 4.** Options for postremission therapy for adult AML patients in first remission

| Option | Drug | Comment |
|---|---|---|
| High-dose consolidation therapy | Cytarabine 2–3 g/m$^2$ every 12 h for a total of 12 doses; or twice/day on Days 1, 3, and 5 for 6 doses. | Very effective regimen administered monthly for two or more courses. Causes significant toxicity in patients >60 years old |
| Standard consolidation therapy | Cytarabine 100 mg/m$^2$ daily as a continuous infusion for 5–7 days, plus daunorubicin 30–45 mg/m$^2$ intravenous push on each of the first 2–3 days of treatment | Myelosuppressive but has acceptable toxicity even in older patients. Usually given monthly for 2–4 courses. |
| Intensive maintenance therapy over 3 years | Cytarabine 100 mg/m$^2$ IV every 12 h, plus 6-thioguanine 100 mg/m$^2$ orally every 12 h, until severe marrow hypoplasia is achieved. | Less toxic than high-dose consolidation chemotherapy especially in older patients. Bone marrow recovery is relatively rapid. Requires continuous treatment for up to 3 years. |
| Bone marrow or blood stem cell transplantation | High dose busulfan and cyclophosphamide; or total body irradiation and cyclophosphamide. | Effective therapy for younger patients with a suitable donor. Leukemia relapse is less frequent than in other forms of postremission therapy but substantial toxicity results in comparable overall survival. Autologous bone marrow transplantation may be employed in patients up to 60 years old. |

mediate prognosis patients. Cytarabine has a favorable response relationship over a wide dose range. High intracellular drug concentrations saturate the deaminating metabolic enzyme pathway, leading to increased levels of the active agent ara-cytidine triphosphate. HDAC may be effective in eliminating resistant cell populations that survive induction therapy. The Cancer and Leukemia Group B (CALGB) conducted a randomized trial of consolidation therapy using four courses of cytarabine at low (100 mg/m$^2$ per day) or intermediate doses (400 mg/m$^2$ per day) as continuous IV infusions for 5 days or at high doses (3 g/m$^2$ every 12 hr on days 1, 3 and 5) [59]. For patients <60 years old with a good or intermediate prognosis, disease-free survival in the HDAC arm was 46% at 3 years compared to 35% for the intermediate dose and 31% for the low dose group ($p$=0.003). There were relatively few relapses in the HDAC group more than 2 years after attaining CR. HDAC was considerably more toxic, however, and had a 5% treatment-related mortality. Among patients >60 years old, the toxic death rate was even higher and contributed to the overall failure to improve outcome in this group. The age-related occurrence of cerebellar ataxia, which is irreversible in some patients, is of concern. The best results from consolidation therapy in patients over 60 years old is likely to be two cycles of daunorubicin (30–45 mg/m$^2$ for 2 days) and cytarabine (100 mg/m$^2$ per day for 5 days) [60]. Alternating courses of other two-drug combinations (e.g. etoposide/cyclophosphamide, mitoxantrone/etoposide, or mitoxantrone/diaziquone) are being tested [61].

Most studies reporting on allogeneic or autologous BMT for AML patients in first CR are non-randomized, and many are retrospective. Considerable selection bias is generated by the delay between remission induction and transplantation, and by the entry requirements for good performance status for most trials. Prospective randomized studies comparing intensive consolidation therapy and BMT have failed to show a clear survival advantage (Table 5). An EORTC/GIMEMA trial demonstrated increased disease-free survival without improved overall survival [62, 63]. Patients relapsing after consolidation chemotherapy had better survival than those relapsing after BMT. A recent intergroup trial for patients <55 years old showed no significant differences in disease-free survival after allogeneic or autologous BMT or HDAC consolidation chemotherapy [63B]. However, overall survival was better after chemotherapy alone than after allogeneic or autologous transplantation (Table 6). The MRC AML-10 study confirmed the finding that autologous BMT in

**Table 5.** The French randomized trial testing BMT in adults with AML in first CR (from [62])

| Subgroup | Ages (years) | $n^a$ | 4-Year estimates | |
| | | | Disease-free survival | Overall survival |
| --- | --- | --- | --- | --- |
| Allogeneic BMT | <45 | 168 | 55±4% | 59±4% |
| Autologous BMT | <60 | 128 | 48±5% | 56±5% |
| Intensive chemotherapy | <60 | 126 | 30±4% | 46±5% |

[a]Intention-to-treat analysis (No. actually completing assigned treatment: allo=144; auto=95; intensive consolidation chemotherapy=104).

**Table 6.** The American Intergroup Randomized Trial testing BMT in adults with AML in first CR (from [63B])

| Subgroup | Ages (years) | $n^a$ | 4-Year estimates | |
| | | | Disease-free survival | Overall survival |
| --- | --- | --- | --- | --- |
| Allogeneic BMT | <55 | 113 | 43% | 46% |
| Autologous BMT | <55 | 116 | 34% | 43% |
| High-dose cytarabine | <55 | 117 | 34% | 52% |

[a]Intention-to-treat analysis (Number (%) actually completing assigned treatment: allo=92, 81%; auto=63, 54%; high-dose cytarabine=106, 91%).

first CR does not presently confer a survival advantage [64]. Consequently, for patients with AML, autologous BMT is often reserved as salvage therapy after relapse for suitable candidates without an allogeneic donor.

Maintenance therapy with relatively nonmyelosuppressive doses of cytotoxic drugs has no proven benefit in the management of AML. Maintenance chemotherapy with low dose cytarabine has been shown to be less effective than consolidation therapy. Relapses occurring in APL patients receiving ATRA maintenance are resistant to ATRA reinduction.

## Salvage Therapy for Patients With Relapsed or Refractory AML

A limited number of agents are effective in the treatment of AML, and management of patients with resistant or relapsed disease is difficult. Patients with long initial remissions (>1 year) have a 50%–60% reinduction rate with daunorubicin and cytarabine, or with HDAC, but the duration of the second remission is usually shorter than the first. BMT should be considered for any patient who has relapsed after an intensive initial treatment program.

A HDAC regimen may be effective in 35%–40% of patients resistant to conventional dose cytarabine regimens [65]. A regimen using etoposide and cyclophosphamide at high doses has produced CR in 42% of similar patients [66]. Mitoxantrone (10–12 mg/m² per day) and etoposide (100 mg/m² per day) given for 5 days is a commonly used relapse regimen [67, 68]. Mitoxantrone has also been used in combination with diaziquone, a highly lipid soluble aziridinylbenzoquinone [69]. Patients failing all conventional drug protocols may elect to undergo experimental treatment with investigational drugs. Several immunotoxins that bind to myeloblasts are now in clinical trials. Patients who relapse more than one year after alloBMT may benefit from a second alloBMT. Although transplant-related mortality is high (30%–40%), a 4-year disease-free survival of 20%–30% has been reported.

## Elderly Patients with Acute Leukemia

Registry data indicate that the median age for patients with AML is 63–65 years old, nearly a decade older than the median ages of patients reported on in clinical trials. Older patients are clearly under-represented in the literature, and the best treatment for elderly patients with AML (or ALL) remains controversial.

Two factors combine to explain in large part the poor outcome of elderly patients with leukemia. First and most obvious, is the inability of many of these patients to withstand the rigors of intensive chemotherapy and its expected complications. Patients with age-related chronic cardiac, pulmonary, or renal disorders suffer greater acute toxicity from chemotherapy. Older patients may also have lesser bone marrow regenerative capacity, even after successful leukemia cytoreduction. Inability to tolerate long periods of pancytopenia and malnutrition, or the nephrotoxicity of aminoglycosides or amphotericin remain major barriers to successful treatment.

At the same time, the genetic mutations most often associated with treatment failure in young patients (e.g., abnormalities of chromosomes 5 or 7 in AML or t(9;22) in ALL) are more common in older patients.

Conversely, all of the "favorable" cytogenetic abnormalities, such as t(8;21), or t(15;17), or inv(16) in AML, are more common in younger adults, and are responsible in part for the better disease-free survival of young and middle-aged adults [27].

Myelodysplastic syndromes are also more common in older patients, and many cases of AML in elderly patients have presumably evolved through a myelodysplastic phase. The syndrome of myelodysplasia is characterized by the stepwise accumulation of genetic abnormalities, analogous to the evolution of new chromosomal abnormalities that occurs as chronic myelogenous leukemia accelerates into the blast phase. The multi-drug resistant phenotype may also emerge during this evolutionary process. At the same time, normal hematopoiesis is increasingly inhibited, and the normal stem cell compartment may be lost. The net result leads to ineffective hematopoiesis and dysfunctional blood cells. By the time that AML emerges, these patients are often colonized by pathogenic flora, threatened by recurrent bleeding episodes, and dependent on transfusions.

Primum Non Nocere

Not every patient benefits from intensive chemotherapy, and this is particularly true among elderly patients. Well meaning attempts to induce remissions may actually shorten survival. Patients unlikely to survive treatment can be identified by their poor performance status or co-morbid disorders. Case series from large referral institutions suggest that 25%–50% of AML patients older than 60 years are not offered remission induction chemotherapy.

There are a few patients with "acute leukemia" by the usual quantitative criteria of >30% bone marrow blast cells whose disease has a much more smoldering course. These patients suffer from bone marrow failure and pancytopenia more than hyperleukocytosis. Their survival may be equally long and their quality of life better, using transfusion support and antibiotics rather than intensive chemotherapy. This may be particularly true for "hypoplastic" AML.

The EORTC have reported on a randomized clinical trial for patients older than 65 years, comparing daunorubicin, cytarabine and vincristine treatment with a "watch and wait" strategy, using supportive care and only resorting to cytoreductive chemotherapy for relief of AML-related symptoms [70]. The 31 patients receiving remission induction chemotherapy survived significantly longer (median, 21 weeks vs 11 weeks; $p$=0.015) than the "supportive care" group. The latter group first received hydroxyurea and cytarabine within a median of 9 days after diagnosis (range, 0–395 days) and spent a median of 50% of their remaining days in hospital, compared to 54% for the intensively treated cohort.

Many clinical trials have investigated the use of low doses of cytarabine, particularly in the elderly. Investigators in France randomized 46 AML patients older than 65 years to receive intensive chemotherapy with cytarabine and rubidazone (a daunorubicin analogue) and 41 patients to receive subcutaneous cytarabine at 10 mg/m$^2$ per 12 h for 21 days [71]. Although the number of complete remissions was greater with intensive chemotherapy, the early death rate was also higher, so that there were no differences in survival or remission duration between the two groups.

Otherwise healthy, older patients with acute leukemia, especially those with favorable cytogenetic features, should be offered curative chemotherapy. Although pilot studies have used more intensive initial chemotherapy, a reasonable standard regimen for many elderly patients is 7 days of continuous infusion cytarabine (100 mg/m$^2$ per day) plus 3 days of daunorubicin (30 mg/m$^2$ per day) [59]. Using this regimen in 346 patients older than 60 years, the Cancer and Leukemia Group B (CALGB) has reported a CR rate of 47% with three-quarters of remissions occurring after one course. Unfortunately, even with post-remission consolidation chemotherapy, the overall survival for this elderly group was only 9% after 4 years. More recent trials using higher anthracycline doses have reported CR rates of 55%–65%, but the impact on overall survival is not yet known.

## Hematopoietic Growth Factors

Improvements in supportive care, especially transfusions and antibiotics, have enhanced the outlook for both young and elderly leukemia patients. Uncontrolled trials using GM-CSF or G-CSF suggested that the duration of neutropenia was decreased when growth factors were given after remission induction chemotherapy, and thus more intensive and effective chemotherapy could be given [72, 73]. At the same time, stimulation of leukemia regrowth by myeloid growth factors appears to be uncommon in vivo.

Data from several large controlled trials have recently been reported, but the issue remains unsettled. Differences in dose and schedule, and the specific growth factor and chemotherapy agents used, as well as the particular disease (i.e., AML or ALL) and the age group studied prevent firm conclusions. Even though a more rapid recovery of neutrophils has been observed in some trials, the nadir has not been affected, and thus, the incidence of severe infection remains high. There may be greater benefit from using growth factors following consolidation chemotherapy when patients are already in remission than there is earlier during remission induction [74]. As yet, growth factors have not had a marked impact on survival or remission duration for patients with AML.

Prognostic Factors for ALL

Important adverse prognostic factors in ALL have a major influence on complete remission rates, and on remission durations and survivals [22, 75–77]. In multivariate analyses, patients presenting with white blood cell (WBC) counts >30,000/μl have had significantly shorter durations of remission compared with patients with lower leukocyte counts. However, among patients with T-cell ALL, extreme leukocytosis does not negatively affect outcome [22]. Older age (>60 years) is another adverse characteristic. Remission duration and overall survival have decreased in almost every adult ALL trial as the ages of the patient groups have increased. Minor factors or those that have had some significance with certain treatment regimens are the percentage of circulating blast cells, the degree of bone marrow involvement, the presence of hepatomegaly, splenomegaly, or lymphadenopathy, lactate dehydrogenase (LDH) levels, central nervous system (CNS) involvement at presentation, and the time required to achieve complete remission (e.g. >4–6 weeks).

Treatment of ALL

The aims of modern ALL treatment regimens are: the rapid restoration of bone marrow function, using multiple chemotherapy drugs at acceptable toxicities, in order to prevent the emergence of resistant subclones; the use of adequate prophylactic treatment of sanctuary sites such as the CNS; and post-remission consolidation therapies to eliminate minimal (undetectable) residual disease. Post-remission therapy has traditionally been categorized as intensification or consolidation treatment, and prolonged maintenance.

Four or five drugs are typically used for remission induction followed by similar agents plus antimetabolites for remission consolidation treatment [22, 75–78]. There are data suggesting that high doses of cytarabine or cyclophosphamide may be particularly beneficial for patients with T-cell ALL and some high-risk subsets, and that high dose methotrexate may be particularly useful in B-lineage ALL. CNS prophylaxis is most often administered with intrathecal methotrexate plus either systemic methotrexate or cranial irradiation. Since some of the agents used systemically in the more intensive remission induction and consolidation programs do penetrate the leptomeninges, the need for additional CNS treatment may have diminished. The likelihood of an isolated CNS relapse for adults with ALL appears to be about 5%. For late intensification therapy, many approaches have been used, including bone marrow transplantation. Some period of maintenance chemotherapy has traditionally been given for 1–3 years, using 6-mercaptopurine and methotrexate, often with monthly pulses of vincristine and prednisone.

Critical appraisal of the impact of each component of post-remission therapy on disease-free survival in any given trial is difficult for many reasons. There are few well-controlled randomized studies analyzing the importance of individual treatment components on outcome. Changes in treatment protocols have rarely been made in a stepwise fashion. Rather, changes in post-remission therapy are often made simultaneously with new induction regimens. New drugs have been introduced along with other changes, making their impact on outcome difficult to discern. At present, the benefit of newer drugs such as etoposide or teniposide, high-dose cytarabine, or mitoxantrone cannot be critically evaluated.

Remission Induction in ALL

The use of vincristine and corticosteroids (prednisone or dexamethasone) plus an anthracycline (either doxorubicin or daunorubicin) form the cornerstone of most modern induction regimens. The additional benefit of adding daunorubicin to vincristine, prednisone and L-asparaginase was proven in a randomized trial conducted by the CALGB (study

7612) when patients who also received daunorubicin had a CR rate of 83% versus 47% for those who did not [79].

L-asparaginase improves the CR rate when added as a third drug to vincristine and prednisone, but its value in improving either the CR rate or disease-free survival (DFS) when daunorubicin is included in the induction regimen is unclear. In childhood ALL, L-asparaginase appears to prolong DFS when given during consolidation.

Other agents that have been incorporated into induction regimens include: cyclophosphamide, conventional and high dose cytarabine, mercaptopurine, conventional and high dose methotrexate, and mitoxantrone. The relative importance of individual drugs and drug schedules is difficult to discern given the lack of randomized comparative trials. As yet, none of the modifications involving the addition of a fourth or fifth drug to a three drug regimen have demonstrated reliably higher cure rates, although considerable benefit may accrue to certain subsets of patients.

Remission Consolidation Treatment of ALL

Post-remission consolidation therapy is designed to eradicate the rapidly proliferating neoplastic cells that are thought to be responsible for early relapses. In general, drugs given during this period are cell-cycle phase specific. The need for intensive consolidation therapy in achieving cure, unlike that of remission induction therapy, is, however, controversial. The relative benefit of any particularly consolidation therapy is likely to be inversely proportional to the intensity of the initial induction therapy and its efficacy in rapidly reducing the leukemia cell mass.

Maintenance Therapy

A prolonged period of treatment with low doses of chemotherapy drugs, called remission maintenance therapy, is still standard in ALL. This approach stands in marked contrast to most other "curable cancers", such as Hodgkin's disease, large cell lymphoma, or testicular cancer, where cure follows the initial intensive cytoreductive therapy, and low-dose maintenance chemotherapy provides no additional benefit. The necessity for prolonged maintenance therapy for adults with ALL may also be a function of the intensity and the success of initial chemotherapy. As yet, the need for maintenance therapy has not been proven in adults.

The experience in childhood ALL has led to the use of methotrexate and 6-mercaptopurine in most maintenance regimens. Most adult trials have also used these two drugs, either alone or in combination with others. The duration of therapy has been derived empirically, and programs lasting 1–3 years are commonly used. The uncertainties regarding duration and even the necessity of maintenance therapy are due in part to our lack of knowledge about its mechanism of action. The continuous presence of low doses of anti-metabolite drugs may kill drug-resistant leukemia cells or slowly dividing leukemia cells. Alternatively, maintenance therapy may modify the host immune response so that residual leukemia cells are destroyed, or it may suppress the proliferation of residual leukemia cells until senescence or apoptosis occurs, that is, until reinstitution of the normal regulation of lymphocyte survival. One or more of these mechanisms may be active in any individual patient. Clearly much additional work remains to be done in this area.

CNS Prophylaxis

The CNS is an important site of involvement by ALL. Although uncommonly found at diagnosis, CNS involvement is common at the time of relapse. The meninges may harbor leukemia cells, and the blood-brain barrier may shelter them from systemic chemotherapy. Recurrence within the CNS usually coincides with systemic relapse. Preventive treatment of the CNS during post-remission therapy, termed CNS prophylaxis, has become an integral part of virtually all current adult ALL treatment protocols. Although the true value of CNS prophylaxis in adults is controversial, studies in which adult patients either refused or could not receive CNS prophylaxis have demonstrated a higher rate of CNS relapse compared with those receiving prophylaxis. CNS leukemia is more easily prevented than treated; once overt CNS leukemia has developed, there is a high likelihood of subsequent CNS relapse despite treatment.

CNS prophylaxis typically consists of cranial irradiation plus intrathecal methotrexate. Cytarabine and hydrocortisone are occasionally added to the methotrexate for "triple intrathecal therapy." In lieu of cranial irradiation, some investigators have substituted high-dose systemic chemotherapy with either methotrexate or cytarabine, since therapeutic levels of these drugs can be achieved in the cerebrospinal fluid when they are administered intravenously in high doses. Overall, the superiority of any one prophylactic therapy has not been established.

## Modern Multiagent Clinical Trials

What is the expected outcome for patients with ALL treated with one of the modern multi-agent chemotherapy regimens? The CALGB has recently reported on their 8811 trial which evaluated 197 adults from 16–80 years old (median, 32 years) and used a dose-intense, multicourse two year treatment program [22]. The CR rate was 85%, the median remission duration was 29 months, and the median survival overall was 36 months. The five drug induction regimen used a single dose of cyclophosphamide, 3 days of daunorubicin, and four weeks of vincristine, prednisone and L-asparaginase. The two myelosuppressive drugs were given within the first three days, and the doses were reduced by one-third for patients over the age of 60. This was followed by early and late intensification courses. The first included two months of treatment using cyclophosphamide, intrathecal methotrexate, subcutaneous cytarabine, oral 6-mercaptopurine, intravenous vincristine, and more L-asparaginase. CNS prophylaxis was then completed with cranial irradiation and five weekly doses of intrathecal methotrexate together with daily 6-mercaptopurine. The late intensification course lasted six weeks, followed by prolonged maintenance treatment with daily 6-mercaptopurine and weekly oral methotrexate plus monthly pulses of vincristine and prednisone until two years after diagnosis.

More recently, the CALGB has completed a trial (study 9111) using the same chemotherapy program but randomizing patients in a double-blind fashion to receive either filgrastim (G-CSF) or a placebo during the induction and early intensification courses [80]. The CR rate among the patients who received G-CSF was 91% compared to 83% for the placebo group, but this difference was not statistically significant. There was a significant shortening in the time to recover >1000 neutrophils/μl during the induction course from 22 days to 16 days. The shortening in the duration of neutropenia was more apparent in patients >60 years old (16 days with G-CSF versus 29 days on the placebo arm). Data from two other randomized trials suggest that concurrent use of G-CSF may improve the ability to deliver intensive chemotherapy more safely [81, 82].

## Burkitt cell ALL

The first of the high risk subsets that warrants special attention is Burkitt cell ALL, also known as FAB L3 or mature B-cell ALL. This subset makes up 3%–5% of adult ALL cases. The ubiquitous biological features are the presence of monoclonal surface immunoglobulin and the 8; 14 translocation or one of its two variants. It is relatively easily recognized at diagnosis from the characteristic clinical findings of hepatosplenomegaly and lymphadenopathy. The LDH and uric acid levels are usually markedly elevated, and there is often leptomeningeal involvement. The lymphoblasts usually lack TdT reactivity. In the past, few if any of these patients survived following standard ALL treatment regimens of the type just reviewed.

More recently, there have been several reports using short intensive chemotherapy programs for B-cell ALL that yield a high CR rate and a survival plateau in the range of 50% [83]. These regimens which may only require as few as 16–18 weeks of treatment use high doses of methotrexate, cytarabine, and cyclophosphamide or ifosfamide together with other ALL drugs. The CALGB has tested a similar regimen and has confirmed these encouraging results [84].

## Elderly Patients With ALL

A review of the annual age-specific leukemia incidence in the United States underscores the observation that ALL is relatively uncommon in the middle adult years, but increases rapidly in incidence over the age of 60. These patients have only rarely been included in clinical trials, and as yet, there are no optimal treatment programs available (Table 7).

In a recent report from the northern counties of England, approximately one-third of ALL cases in adults occurred in patients over the age of 60 [85]. Various treatment approaches have been taken in this elderly group of patients, but the outcomes are uniformly poor. Investigators at the M.D. Anderson Hospital have reported on 52 patients treated with infusional vincristine, adriamycin and dexamethasone (VAD). This regi-

**Table 7.** Acute lymphoblastic leukemia in patients >60 years old

|  | $n$ | Median age (years) (range) | Complete remissions (%) | Median survival (months) (range) | 3-Year survival (%) |
|---|---|---|---|---|---|
| Newcastle, 1994 [85] |  |  |  |  |  |
| No treatment | 9 | 83 (67–91) | – | <1 (0–2) | 0 |
| Palliative | 25 | 74 (63–88) | 4 (16) | 3 (0–27) | 0 |
| Curative | 28 | 67 (60–80) | 10 (36) | 3 (0–84+) | 20 |
| MD Anderson, 1993 [86] |  |  |  |  |  |
| VAD | 52 | (>60) | 30 (58) | 10 (0–48+) | <10 |
| CALGB, 1994 [22, 80] |  |  |  |  |  |
| 8811/9111 | 55 | 65 (60–80) | 36 (65) | 10 (0–48+) | 20 |

men produced a high CR rate with relatively low toxicity in elderly patients [86]. In the most recent CALGB trials, a CR rate of 65% was observed in elderly patients (60–80 years old, with a median age of 65) [22, 80]. Nevertheless, the three-year survival in all three of these reports remains quite poor. The low tolerance of elderly patients for intensive chemotherapy remains one of the obstacles to increasing the overall cure rate in adults.

Philadelphia Chromosome-Positive ALL

Ph+ ALL is currently the major challenge in curing ALL since it makes up approximately one-third of all adult cases and perhaps one-half of all B-lineage ALL [87]. Some progress has been made. Ph+ ALL has a high initial response rate but a short duration of remission [22]. Shown in Table 8 are the outcomes of a group of 30 patients prospectively identified in a CALGB study (8811) to have a t(9;22) or the BCR/ABL rearrangement compared to 83 patients known not to have this mutation. Although the complete remission rates were similar (70% vs 84%), the remission durations were markedly shorter: 7 months (median) for the Ph+ cases versus >33 months for those known not to have a Ph chromosome ($p<0.001$). This was also reflected in the median survival which was 11 months versus 44 months ($p<0.001$). As yet, no chemotherapy regimen alone appears to have the potential to cure this group of patients.

**Table 8.** Ph$^+$ ALL has a high response rate but short duration of remission (CALGB 8811 study; from [22])

|                                  | Ph$^+$ or BCR-ABL$^+$ ($n$=30) | Not Ph$^+$ ALL ($n$=83) |           |
| -------------------------------- | ------------------------------ | ----------------------- | --------- |
| Complete remission rate          | 70%                            | 84%                     | $p$=0.11  |
| Remission                        |                                |                         |           |
| Median remission duration        | 7 mos                          | >33 mos                 | $p$<0.001 |
| 3-Year remission rate            | 11%                            | 56%                     |           |
| Survival                         |                                |                         |           |
| Median survival duration         | 11 mos                         | 44 mos                  | $p$<0.001 |
| 3-Year survival rate             | 16%                            | 56%                     |           |

In contrast, the International Bone Marrow Transplant Registry has reported on the outcome after HLA-identical sibling marrow transplants for Ph$^+$ ALL, either in first CR or with more advanced disease, and for a small number of Ph$^+$ ALL patients with primary induction failure [88]. The leukemia-free survival was approximately 35% for all three groups. The probability of relapse after transplantation was approximately 30%–50% for the group overall, attesting in part to the therapy-resistant nature of this disease.

Thus, at this time, the treatment for Ph$^+$ ALL should include an intensive remission induction chemotherapy program, followed by allogeneic bone marrow transplantation in the first CR if a donor were available. Alternatively, intensive post-remission chemotherapy is being explored using high dose cytarabine or methotrexate. There are preliminary data suggesting a possible benefit from the use of alfa interferon during maintenance therapy. Considerable interest exists to investigate new agents including immunotoxins, modulators of multi-drug resistance, and anti-sense molecules in this high-risk group of patients.

Salvage Treatment for Patients With Relapsed or Refractory ALL

More than half of adult patients with ALL relapse despite modern chemotherapy [77]. Most relapse within the first two years. Over 80% of relapses occur first in the bone marrow, while the remainder occur in extramedullary sites, primarily the CNS. Relapses in other sites such as lymph nodes, skin, or testes occur much less frequently. Patients with an isolated extramedullary relapse have a very high risk for subsequent

**Table 9.** A randomized trial testing BMT in adults with ALL in first CR (from [89])

| Subgroup | Ages (years) (median) | $n^a$ | 3-Year estimates | |
| --- | --- | --- | --- | --- |
| | | | Disease-free survival | Overall survival |
| Allogeneic BMT | <40 (26) | 116 | 43%±5% | 55%±5% |
| Autologous BMT (purged, 81%) | <50 (25) | 95 | 39%±5% | 49%±5% |
| Chemotherapy | <50 (28) | 96 | 32%±5% | 42%±6% |

Intention-to-treat analysis (actually transplanted: allo=92, auto=63).

bone marrow relapse and should receive systemic chemotherapy following local treatment (Table 9).

A variety of treatment protocols have been employed in relapsed or refractory patients. High-dose cytarabine with or without additional agents produces complete remissions in about 50% of adult patients. However, in almost every instance, the median remission duration has been <6 months, and only a small fraction of these patients become long-term survivors. The best results for such patients have been obtained with allogeneic BMT in second remission.

## Future Directions

Despite major advances in the treatment of adults with acute leukemia in the past decade, many patients continue to die either from their disease or from complications of its treatment. However, a number of novel experimental and clinical approaches hold promise for improving cure rates.

In recent years, the biologic heterogeneity of these diseases has been further defined. A variety of clinical and laboratory parameters convey useful prognostic information. The most consistently observed prognostic factors have been age and karyotype. Currently, detection of chromosomal abnormalities at the time of initial diagnosis provides the most useful means of identifying patients at risk of failing induction therapy as well as those likely to have short, intermediate, or prolonged remissions after achieving CR. In the future, such prognostic information will become valuable for assigning risk categories and in individualizing post-remission therapy for a given patient.

Application of modern molecular technologies designed to detect minimal residual leukemia may aid clinicians in monitoring disease during and after chemotherapy. It could, therefore, lead to the early detection of patients likely to relapse and for whom further therapy may be necessary. Novel methods of circumventing multi-drug resistance, exploiting immune mechanisms, or altering the control of malignant cell growth need to be investigated.

## References

1a. Sandler DP, Ross JA: Epidemiology of acute leukemia in children and adults. Semin Oncol 24:3–16, 1997
 1. Brill AB, Tomonoga M, Heyssel RM: Leukemia in man following exposure to ionizing irradiation: Summary of findings in Hiroshima and Nagasaki and comparison to other human experience. Ann Intern Med 56:590, 1962
 2. Kato H, Schull WJ: Studies of the mortality of A-bomb survivors. 7. Mortality, 1950–1978: Part I. Cancer Mortality. Radiat Res 90:395, 1982
 3. Smith PG, Doll R: Mortality among patients with ankylosing spondylitis after a single treatment course with X-rays. Br Med J 284:449, 1982
 4. Smith PG: Leukemia and other concerns following radiation treatment of pelvic disease. Cancer 39 (Suppl):1901, 1977
 5. Modan B, Lilienfeld AM: Polycythemia vera and leukemia – the role of radiation treatment. Medicine 44:305, 1965
 6. Graham S, Levin ML, Lilienfeld AM, et al. Preconception, intrauterine, and postnatal irradiation as related to leukemia. Natl Cancer Inst Monagraph 19:347, 1966
 7. Polednak AP, Stehney AF, Rowland RE: Mortality among women first employed before 1930 in the U.S. radium dial painting industry. Am J Epidemiol 107:179, 1978
 8. March HC: Leukemia in radiologists. Radiology 43:275, 1944
 9. Rosner F, Grunwald HW: Cytotoxic drugs and leukemogenesis. Clin Hematol 9:663, 1980
10. Thirman MJ, Larson RA: Therapy-related myeloid leukemia. Hem/Oncol Clinics No Amer 10:293–320, 1996
11. Tucker MA, Coleman CN, Cox RS, et al. Risk of second cancers after treatment for Hodgkin's disease. N Engl J Med 318:76, 1988
12. Pui CH, Ribeiro RC, Hancock ML, et al. Acute myeloid leukemia in children treated with epipodophyllotoxins for acute lymphoblastic leukemia. N Engl J Med 325:1682, 1991
13. Aksoy M, Erdem S, Din Col G: Leukemia in shoeworkers chronically exposed to benzene. Blood 44:837, 1974
14. Robert-Guroff M, Nakao Y, Natake K, et al. Natural antibodies to human retrovirus HTLV in a cluster of Japanese patients with adult T-cell leukemia. Science 215:975, 1982
15. Miller RW: Deaths from childhood leukemia and solid tumors among twins and other sibs in the United States, 1960–67. J Natl Cancer Inst 46:203, 1971
16. Drapner GF, Heaf MM, Kinnear Wilson LM: Occurrence of childhood cancers among sibs and estimation of familial risks. J Med Genet 14:81, 1977

17. Bennett JM, Catovsky D, Daniel MT, et al. Proposals for the classification of the acute leukemias. Br J Haematol 33:451, 1976
18. Bennett JM, Catovsky D, Daniel MT, et al. Proposed revised criteria for the classification of acute myeloid leukemia. A report of the French-American-British cooperative group. Ann Intern Med; 103:620–625, 1985
19. Bennett JM, Catovsky D, Daniel MT, et al. The morphologic classification of acute lymphoblastic leukemia: Concordance among observers and clinical correlations. Br J Haematol 47:553, 1981
20. Bennett JM, Catovsky D, Daniel MT, et al. Proposal for the recognition of minimally differentiated acute myeloid leukemia (AML-M0). Br J Haematol 78 (3):325, 1991
21. Terstappen LWMM: Cell differntiation and maturation in normal bone marrow and acute leukemia. In: Macey MG, ed. Flow cytometry clinical applications. Oxford: Blackwell Scientific Publications, 1995:101
22. Larson RA, Dodge RK, Burns CP, et al. A five-drug remission induction regimen with intensive consolidation for adults with acute lymphoblastic leukemia: Cancer and Leukemia Group B study 8811. Blood 85:2025–2037, 1995
23. Ball ED, Davis RB, Griffin JD et al. Prognostic value of lymphocyte surface markers in acute myeloid leukemia. Blood 77:2242, 1991
24. Parrera A, Pombo de Olivera MS, Matutes E et al. Terminal deoxynucleotidyl transferase positive acute myeloid leukemia: An association with immature myeloblastic leukemia. Br J Haematol 69:219, 1987
25. Geller RB, Zahurak M, Hurwitz CA et al. Prognostic importance of immunophenotyping in adults with acute myelocytic leukaemia: The significance of the stem-cell glycoprotein CD34 (My10). Br J Haematol 76 (3):340, 1990
26. The Fourth International Workshop on Chromosomes in Leukemia: a prospective study of acute nonlymphocytic leukemia, Chicago, Illinois, September 2–7, 1982. Cancer Genet Cytogenet 11:249, 1984
27a. Caligiuri MA, Strout MP, Gilliland DG: Molecular biology of acute myeloid leukemia. Semin Oncol 24:32–44, 1997
27b. Thandla S, Aplan PD: Molecular biology of acute lymphocytic leukemia. Semin Oncol 24:45–56, 1997
27. LeBeau MM, Larson RA: Cytogenetics and neoplasia. In: Hematology Basic Principles and Practice, Second Edition. Hoffman R, Benz Jr EJ, Shattil SJ, Furie B, Cohen HJ, Silberstein LE, eds. Churchill Livingstone, New York 1995, pp 878–898
28. Mrozek K, Heinonen K, de la Chapelle A, Bloomfield CD: Clinical significance of cytogenetics in acute myeloid leukemia. Semin Oncol 24:17–31, 1997
29. Devine SM, Larson RA: Acute leukemia in adults: Recent developments in diagnosis and treatment. CA-A cancer journal for clinicians 44 (6):326–352, 1994
30. Miller WH, Levine K, DeBlasio A, et al. Detection of minimal residual disease in acute promyelocytic leukemia by a reverse transcription polymerase chain reaction assay for the PML/RAR fusion mRNA. Blood 82:1689–1694, 1993
31. Nucifora G, Larson RA, Rowley JD: Persistence of the 8, 21 translocation in patients with acute myeloid leukemia type M2 in long-term remission. Blood 82:712–715, 1993
32. Hoelzer DF: Diagnosis and treatment of adult acute lymphocytic leukemia. In: Weirnik PH, Canellos GP, Kyle RA, Schiffer CA, eds. Neoplastic diseases of the blood. New York; Churchill Livingstone, 1991
33. Christiansen NP: Allogeneic bone marrow transplantation for the treatment of adult acute leukemias. Hematol/Oncol Clinics North Am 7:177–200, 1993
34. Appelbaum FR: Allogeneic hematopoietic stem cell transplantation for acute leukemia. Semin Oncol 24:114–123, 1997

35. Ball ED, Rybka WB: Autologous bone marrow transplantation for adult acute leukemia. Hematol/Oncol Clinics North Am 7:201–231, 1993
36. Stone RM, Mayer RJ: Treatment of the newly diagnosed adult with de novo acute myeloid leukemia. Hematol/Oncol Clinics North Am 7:47–64, 1993
37. Bishop JF: The treatment of adult acute myeloid leukemia. Semin Oncol 24:57–69, 1997
38. Vogler WR, Velez-Garcia E, Weiner RS, et al. A phase III trial comparing idarubicin and daunorubicin in acute myelogenous leukemia: A Southeastern Cancer Study Group study. J Clin Oncol 10:1103, 1992
39. Berman E, Heller G, Santorsa J, et al. Results of a randomized trial comparing idarubicin and cytosine arabinoside with daunorubicin and cytosine arabinoside in adult patients with newly diagnosed acute myelogenous leukemia. Blood 77:1666–1674, 1991
40. Wiernik PH, Banks PLC, Case Jr DC, et al. Cytarabine plus idarubicin or daunorubicin as induction and consolidation therapy for previously untreated adult patients with acute myeloid leukemia. Blood 79:313–319, 1992
41. Berman E, McBride M. Comparative cellular pharmacology of daunorubicin and idarubicin in human multidrug-resistant leukemia cells. Blood 79:3267, 1992
42. Arlin ZA, Case Jr DC, Moore J, et al. Randomized multicenter trial of cytosine arabinoside with mitoxantrone or daunorubicin in previously untreated adults with acute nonlymphocytic leukemia. Leukemia 4:177–183, 1990
43. MacCallum PK, Davis CL, Rohatiner AZS et al. Mitoxantrone and cytosine arabinoside as treatment for acute myelogenous leukemia at first recurrence. Leukemia 7:1496–1499, 1993
44. Larson RA, Day RS, Azarnia N et al. The selective use of AMSA following high-dose cytarabine in patients with acute myeloid leukemia in relapse: a Leukemia Intergroup Study. Br J Haematol 82:337–346, 1992
45. Berman E, Arlin ZA, Gaynor J, et al. Comparative trial of cytarabine and thioguanine in combination with amsacrine or daunorubicin in patients with untreated acute nonlymphocytic leukemia: Results of the L-16 M protocol. Leukemia 3:115–121, 1989
46. Dillman RO, Davis RB, Green MR, et al. A comparative study of two different doses of cytarabine for acute myeloid leukemia: A phase III trial of Cancer and Leukemia Group B. Blood 78:2520–2526, 1991
47. Phillips GL, Reece DE, Shepherd JD, et al. High-dose cytarabine and daunorubicin induction and postremission chemotherapy for the treatment of acute myelogenous leukemia in adults. Blood 77:1429–1435, 1991
48. Schiller G, Gajewski J, Nimer S, et al. A randomized study of intermediate versus conventional-dose cytarabine as intensive induction for acute myelogenous leukemia. Br J Haematol 81:170, 1992
49. Bishop JF, Lowenthal RM, Joshua D, et al for the Australian Leukemia Study Group: Etoposide in acute nonlymphocytic leukemia. Blood 75:27–32, 1990
50. Bishop JF, Matthews JP, Young GA, et al. A randomized study of high dose cytarabine in induction in acute myeloid leukemia. Blood 87:1710–1717, 1996
51. Fenaux P, Chomienne C, Degos L: Acute promyelocytic leukemia: Biology and treatment. Semin Oncol 24:92–102, 1997
52. Warrell RP, De The H, Wang Z, Degos L: Acute promyelocytic leukemia. N Engl J Med 329:177–189, 1993
53. Fenaux P, Le Deley MC, Castaigne S, et al. Effect of all trans retinoic acid in newly diagnosed acute promyelocytic leukemia. Results of a multicenter randomized trial. Blood 82:3241–3249, 1993

54. Warrell RP, Maslak P, Eardley A, et al. Treatment of acute promyelocytic leukemia with all-trans retinoic acid: An update of the New York experience. Leukemia 8:929–933, 1994

55. Tallman MS, Andersen JW, Schiffer CA, et al. All-trans-retinoic acid in acute promyelocytic leukemia. N Engl J Med 337:1021–1028, 1997

56. Vandat L, Maslak P, Miller WH, et al. Early mortality and the retinoic acid syndrome in acute promyelocytic leukemia: Impact of leukocytosis, low-dose chemotherapy, PML/RAR-a isoform, and CD13 expression in patients treated with all-trans retinoic acid. Blood 84:3843–3849, 1994

57. Cassileth PA, Lynch E, Hines JD, et al. Varying intensity of postremission therapy in acute myeloid leukemia. Blood 79:1924–1930, 1992

58. Bishop, JF: Intensified therapy for acute myeloid leukemia. N Engl J Med 331:941–942, 1994

59. Mayer RJ, Davis RB, Schiffer CA, et al. Intensive postremission chemotherapy in adults with acute myeloid leukemia. N Engl J Med 331:896–903, 1994

60. Stone RM, Mayer RJ: The approach to the elderly patient with acute myeloid leukemia. Hematol/Oncol Clinics North Am 7:65–79, 1993

61. Moore JO, Dodge RK, Amrein PC, et al. Granulocyte-colony stimulating factor (filgrastim) accelerates granulocyte recovery after intensive postremision chemotherapy for acute myeloid leukemia with aziridinyl benzoquinone and mitoxantrone: Cancer and Leukemia Group B study 9022. Blood 89:780–788, 1997

62. Zittoun RA, Mandelli F, Willemze R, et al. Autologous or allogeneic bone marrow transplantation compared with intensive chemotherapy in acute myelogenous leukemia. N Engl J Med 332:217–223, 1995

63. Lowenberg B. Post-remission treatment of acute myelogenous leukemia. N Engl J Med 332:260–262, 1995

63b. Cassileth P, Harrington D, Paietta E, et al. Comparison of autologous bone marrow transplant with high dose cytarabine in adult acute myeloid leukemia in first remission: an ECOG intergroup study. Proc Am Soc Clin Oncol 16:89a (#311), 1997

64. Burnett AK, Goldstone AH, Stevens RF et al. The role of BMT in addition to intense chemotherapy in AML in first CR – results of the MRC AML-10 trial. Blood 89 (1) 2311, 1997

65. Herzig RH, Lazarus HM, Wolff SN, et al. High-dose cytosine arabinoside therapy with and without anthracycline antibiotics for remission reinduction of acute nonlymphoblastic leukemia. J Clin Oncol 3:992, 1985

66. Brown RA, Herzig RH, Wolff SN, et al. High-dose etoposide and cyclophosphamide without bone marrow transplantation for resistant hematologic malignancy. Blood 76:473–479, 1990

67. Ho AD, Lipp T, Ehninger G, et al. Combination of mitoxantrone and etoposide in refractory acute myelogenous leukemia – an active and well tolerated regimen. J Clin Oncol 6:213–217, 1988

68. Daenen S, Lowenberg B, Sonneveld P, et al. Efficacy of etoposide and mitoxantrone in patients with acute myelogenous leukemia refractory to standard induction therapy and intermediate-dose cytarabine with amsidine. Leukemia 8:6–10, 1994

69. Amrein PC, Davis RB, Mayer RJ, Schiffer CA: Treatment of relapsed and refractory acute myeloid leukemia with diaziquone and mitoxantrone: A CALGB phase I study. Am J Hematol 35:80–83, 1990

70. Lowenberg B, Zittoun R, Kerkhofs H, et al. On the value of intensive remission-induction chemotherapy in elderly patients of 65 + years with acute myeloid leukemia: A randomized phase III study of the European Organization for Research and Treatment of Cancer Leukemia Group. J Clin Oncol 7:1268–1274, 1989

71. Tilly H, Castaigne S, Bordessoule D, et al. Low-dose cytarabine versus intensive chemotherapy in the treatment of acute nonlymphocytic leukemia in the elderly. J Clin Oncol 8:272–279, 1990

72. Stone RM: Hematopoietic growth factors and leukemia. Curr Opinion Oncol 4:33–44, 1992

73. Schiffer CA: Hematopoietic growth factors as adjuncts to the treatment of acute myeloid leukemia. Blood 88:3675–3685, 1996

74. Heil G, Hoelzer D, Sanz MA et al. A randomized, double-blind, placebo-controlled, phase III study of filgrastim in remission induction and consolidation therapy for adults with de novo acute myeloid leukemia. Blood 90:4710–4718, 1997

75. Hoelzer D: Treatment of acute lymphoblastic leukemia. Semin Hematol 31:1–15, 1994

76. Hoelzer D, Thiel E, Loffler H, et al. Prognostic factors in a multicenter study for treatment of acute lymphoblastic leukemia in adults. Blood 71:123–131, 1988

77. Laport GF, Larson RA: Treatment of adult acute lymphoblastic leukemia. Semin Oncol 24:70–82, 1997

78. Linker CA, Levitt LJ, O'Donnell M, et al. Treatment of adult acute lymphoblastic leukemia with intensive cyclical chemotherapy: A follow-up report. Blood 78:2814–2822, 1991

79. Gottlieb AJ, Weinberg V, Ellison RR, et al. Efficacy of daunorubicin in the therapy of acute adult lymphocytic leukemia: A prospective randomized trial by the Cancer and Leukemia Group B. Blood 64:267–274, 1984

80. Larson RA, Dodge RK, Linker CA, et al. A randomized controlled trial of filgrastim during remission induction and consolidation chemotherapy for adults with acute lymphoblastic leukemia: Cancer and Leukemia Group B Study 9111. Blood 92:1556–1564, 1998

81. Ohno R, Tomonaga M, Kobayashi T, et al. Effect of granulocytic colony-stimulating factor after intensive induction therapy in relapsed or refractory acute leukemia. N Engl J Med 323:871–877, 1990

82. Ottmann OG, Hoelzer D, Gracien E, et al. Concomitant granulocyte colony-stimulating factor and induction chemoradiotherapy in adult acute lymphoblastic leukemia: a randomized phase III trial. Blood 86:444–450, 1995

83. Hoelzer D, Ludwig WD, Thiel D, et al. Improved outcome in adult B-cell acute lymphoblastic leukemia. Blood 87:495–508, 1996

84. Lee EJ, Pettoni GR, Freter CE, et al. Brief duration high intensity chemotherapy for patients with small non-cleaved lymphoma (IWF J) and FAB L3 acute lymphocytic leukemia in adults: preliminary results of CALGB 9251. Proc Am Soc Clin Oncol 16:24 A (#85), 1997

85. Taylor PRA, Reid MM, and Proctor SJ: Acute lymphoblastic leukemia in the elderly. Leukemia Lymphoma 13:373–380, 1994

86. Kantarjian HM, Walters RS, Keating MJ, et al. Results of the vincristine, doxorubicin, and dexamethasone regimen in adults with standard- and high-risk acute lymphocytic leukemia. J Clin Oncol 8:994–1004, 1990

87. Westbrook CA, Hooberman AL, Spino C, et al. Clinical significance of the BCR-ABL fusion gene in adult acute lymphoblastic leukemia: A Cancer and Leukemia Group B Study (8762). Blood 80:2983–2990, 1992

88. Barrett AJ, Horowitz MM, Ash RC, et al. Bone marrow transplantation for Philadelphia chromosome-positive acute lymphoblastic leukemia. Blood 79:3067–3070, 1992

89. Fiere D, Lepage E, Sebban C, et al. Adult acute lymphoblastic leukemia: A multicentric randomized trial testing bone marrow transplantation as postremission therapy. J Clin Oncol 11:1990–2001, 1993

# Chronic Myelogenous Leukemia (CML)

K. J. Finiewicz, Chr. K. Daugherty

## I Introduction

The first cases of CML were described in 1845 by Bennett [1] and subsequently by Craigie and Virchow [2,3]. This was followed by decades of studies detailing the histologic and clinical features of CML. The discovery of the Philadelphia (Ph) chromosome by Nowell and Hungerford in 1960 marked the beginning of a new era in studying cancer pathogenesis [4]. The significance of this finding was that, for the first time, a consistent chromosomal abnormality was linked to a specific type of human neoplasm. After chromosome banding techniques became available, Rowley demonstrated that the shortening of chromosome 22 observed by Nowell is not a result of deletion but, rather, a translocation between chromosomes 9 and 22, t(9;22)[5]. More recently, the chimeric gene encoded by t(9;22), bcr-abl, has been defined [6,7]. As a result of these events, the leukemogenesis of CML has become one of the most studied models for cancer pathogenesis, both on a cytogenetic and molecular level.

## II Epidemiology/Risk Factors

CML is a rare hematologic malignancy, which accounts for 7–15% of all cases of leukemia in adults. The annual incidence of CML is approximately 1 per 100,000, with little variation in geographic distribution and no association with race or social class. CML is uncommon in children and the incidence of the disease continues to rise with age; most patients are diagnosed between the age of 30–50 years. There is slight male predominance, with a male to female ratio 1.4 to 1 [8,9].

The etiology of CML is unknown, and no specific hewtable predisposing factors for the development of CML have been identified. Several observations suggest that the genetic defects implicated in the pathogenesis of CML are acquired. Although rare examples of multiple cases of CML occurring in one family have been described [10], they are thought to be a result of chance clustering rather than familial inheritance. Studies on monozygotic twins have revealed a lack of concordance [11]. Furthermore, offspring of patients with CML do not appear to be at a higher risk of developing CML. Finally, the presence of the Ph chromosome in hematopoietic cells alone, strongly argues that it is an acquired condition [12,13].

High dose radiation exposure is the best established and the only potential environmental risk factor for the development of CML, with data acquired from epidemiological studies of populations exposed to radiation after the atomic bombings in Hiroshima and Nagasaki [14] and from long term follow-up of patients receiving therapeutic radiation [15, 16].

## III  Biological Characteristics

CML is a clonal disorder of the primitive hematopoietic stem cell. CML develops through the accumulation of abnormally maturing cells of myeloid origin. The Ph chromosome can be found in neutrophil, eosinophil, basophil, monocyte, macrophage and erythroid precursors, as well as in B-lymphocytes (involvement of T-lymphocytes is still controversial) [17]. The neoplastic clone eventually grows to dominate the entire hematopoietic compartment.

The presence of the Ph chromosome appears necessary for the development of CML and is considered a hallmark for diagnosis. However, the finding of the Ph chromosome is not by any means diagnostic of CML as it is found in several other phenotypically and biologically distinct hematologic malignancies. Approximately 90–95% of patients with CML are Ph chromosome-positive, with 10% lacking evidence for the Ph chromosome. In a few cases, the failure to detect the Ph chromosome may be attributed to technical difficulties. Several complex aberrations, involving bcr and abl on chromosomes 22 and 9 respectively, have been described. These so called variant translocations are present in up to 5 % of cases and occasionally may result in a "masked" Ph chromosome. In one third of Ph-negative CML, the bcr-abl protein can be detected by molecular studies. These patients have CML which is morphologically and clinically indistinguishable from Ph-positive CML [18]. A subset of Ph-negative and bcr-abl-negative patients, appears to have a biologically different disease; these patients typically have monocytosis, anemia, a higher percentage of blasts in the bone marrow and a higher LAP score than Ph-positive or bcr-abl-positive patients. They tend to be older and their prognosis is poorer, with a median survival of only 12-14 months [19]. Whether these patients should actually be classified as CML remains a matter of controversy. Many of these patients are closer in their manifestation to chronic myelomonocytic leukemia. In summary, the existence of Ph-negative CML has been seriously questioned in recent years. It is currently accepted that the presence of bcr-abl fusion gene defines the disease. Bcr-abl is created by a reciprocal translocation of genetic material between the long arm of chromosome 9 (containing the oncogene c-abl) and the long arm of chromosome 22 (containing the bcr gene), correctly annotated t(9;22)(q34.1;q11.21). The chimeric protein encoded by bcr-abl has potent tyrosine kinase activity. The break on chromosome 22 may occur in different locations within the breakpoint cluster region, resulting in different fusion protein products. CML is primarily associated (99% cases) with the major breakpoint cluster region of the bcr gene (M-bcr) encoding a p210 fusion protein. Only in a small minority of patients do the translocation breakpoints occur in the minor breakpoint cluster region (m-bcr), translated into a smaller p190 protein product.

The natural course of CML is one of inevitable progression from an initial chronic phase (CML-CP) to a more aggressive accelerated phase (CML-AP), and then to a rapidly fatal blast phase (CML-BP). It is thought that these transformation steps result from the accumulation of additional molecular changes in genetically unstable cells that already contain the bcr-abl rearrangement. The blasts in CML-BP may co-express multiple hematopoietic lineage markers and their exact phenotype may be difficult to characterize. In approximately 70–75% of patients developing BP, blasts express myeloid markers (myeloid BP), while the remaining patients in CML-BP have blasts showing lymphoid differentiation (lymphoid BP). The type of blastic transformation seems to correlate with cytogenetic abnormalities acquired in the process of transfromation. Patients with myeloid blast crisis commonly harbor +8, +19, +21, i(17) or +Ph [20]. The structural abnormalities in patients with lymphoid blast crisis are often random in nature and present in a small percentage of cells; the clonal aberrations, if observed in lymphoid BP, usually result from the loss of genetic material and hypodiploidy.

## IV  Clinical features of the three phases of CML

CML has a biphasic or triphasic clinical course. The duration of chronic phase may last from a few months to several years, with the median time to the development of BP being 3–5 years. Ultimately, the disease progresses either through abrupt transformation to BP or through slower evolution into an accelerated phase (AP) and then BP. The criteria for the diagnosis of BP are well defined. However, criteria for defining AP are imprecise, and detecting the change in the pace of the disease may sometimes be difficult. The list of signs and symptoms strongly suggestive of transformation includes:

– Rapid doubling of WBC count or loss of control of WBC count with conventional chemotherapy (Hydrea)
– Anemia or thrombocytopenia
– ≥10% Blasts in blood or bone marrow
– ≥20% Blasts plus promyelocytes in blood or bone marrow
– ≥20% Basophils plus eosinophils in blood
– Increasing splenomegaly
– Development of granulocytic sarcomas (chloromas) or myelofibrosis
– Karyotypic evolution

*Chronic phase (CML-CP)* is often referred to as the "benign" phase. Patients with CML-CP have less than 5% blasts and promyelocytes in the peripheral blood or bone marrow. Patients in CML-CP are often asymptomatic. In more than half of initially presenting patients, the diagnosis is established following the incidental discovery of an elevated WBC count on routine screening tests. The list of symptoms, if they occur, in patients diagnosed with CML-CP include: asthenia (46%), abdominal discomfort and increasing abdominal girth due to splenomegaly (28%), significant weight loss (26%), fever (17%), bone or muscle pain (9%), and sweats (8%). In a small number of patients, presenting features are related to platelet dysfunction, i.e., easy bruising or epistaxis. Patients with a very high WBC count may present with symptoms of hyperviscosity, such as visual disturbances or priapism.

The main sign on physical examination is splenomegaly, which can be detected in 50–70% of cases (70% in older series). Hepatomegaly is found 10-40% of patients. Lymphadenopathy is rarely a feature of chronic phase, and it's appearance often heralds AP or BP.

*Accelerated phase (CML-AP):* Patients with CML-AP have greater than 5%, but less than 30%, blasts in the bone marrow or peripheral blood. In many patients the disease accelerates "silently" and the change in the activity of the disease can be detected only by careful analysis of peripheral blood and bone marrow biopsy (see above).

*Blast phase (CML-BP):* Patients with CML-BP have greater than 30% blasts in the bone marrow or peripheral blood. Blast phase is often associated with the onset of symptoms typical for acute leukemia including fatique, weight loss, fever, sweats, bone pain, bruising, bleeding or thrombosis. Sometimes patients develop lymphadenopathy and/or skin nodules. Central nervous system involvement may occur, particularly in patients in lymphoid blast crisis.

## V  Work-up of newly diagnosed CML

In the majority of cases, the diagnosis of CML can be made with reasonable certainty based on the results of peripheral blood cell counts and examination of the peripheral blood smear.

*Laboratory tests:*
Peripheral blood:
– Elevated WBC count, frequently above 100,000/µl
– WBC differential classically shows granulocytes in all stages of differentiation, with two peaks involving neutrophils and myelocytes, absolute basophilia and low percentage of monocytes
– Eosinophilia and thrombocytosis are frequently seen
Other changes in laboratory tests:
– Low leukocyte alkaline phosphatase acivity (LAP score) in more than 90% of patients with CML (it should be noted that low LAP scores are not specific for CML and may be seen in other hematologic disorders such as acute leukemia, idiopathic myelofibrosis, paroxysmal nocturnal hemoglobinuria)
– Increased serum vitamin $B_{12}$ levels
– Hyperuricemia and hyperuricosuria
– Elevated LDH

*Bone marrow biopsy:* The bone marrow biopsy is done to assess cellularity, the degree of collagen and reticulin fibrosis and cytogenetics. The bone marrow is usually hypercellular, with a greatly elevated M:E ratio. Examination of the bone marrow aspirate shows a shift in myeloid series towards immaturity. Increased numbers of basophils and eosinophils are often found. Fibrosis may be seen at the time of diagnosis and increases with disease progression. Megakaryocytic hyperplasia is also frequently seen.

*Cytogenetic examination:* In the absence of molecular testing, cytogenetic analysis is mandatory for confirming the diagnosis of CML. Overall, 90-95% of patients with typical CML have the standard t(9;22). This test is usually performed on a diagnostic sample of the bone marrow aspirate, although using peripheral blood for this purpose may be a reasonable alternative if the WBC is sufficiently elevated. The Ph chromosome remains the sole cytogenetic abnormality for the duration of the chronic phase, with additional aberrations detectable in only 10-30% of cases. In most cases the appearance of secondary cytogenetic abnormalities usually precedes the onset of the acelerated and blast phases of the disease, with up to 80% of patients with CML-AP and CML-BP having secondary cytogenetic abnormalities [20,21].

*Molecular analysis:* Molecular analysis is necessary for confirming the diagnosis of Ph-negative CML [18]. The two type of molecular studies available for this purpose are,
1. Southern blot analysis, and,
2. Reverse transcription PCR (RT-PCR).
Southern blot analysis appears of no advantage over standard cytogenetic analysis in Ph-chromosome positive CML.

*Fluorescence in situ hybridization (FISH):* This form of analysis can be employed for studying the karyotype of non-dividing cells, which can be particularly useful when insufficient number of metaphase cells are available for routine karyotyping.

## VI Prognosis

Patients in chronic phase often enjoy relatively good health until they enter BP, which is rapidly fatal in the vast majority of cases. Thus, survival is determined by the duration of chronic phase and the time to transformation.

Prior to the development of effective therapies, the expected median survival of patients with CML was 3 years, with less than 20% surviving longer than 5 years. The prognosis reported in more recent cohorts appears much improved, with a median survival 60–65 months, and survival rates of 75–85% and 50–60% at 3 and 5 years respectively. It is thought that the improvement in prognosis has occurred as a result of a variety of factors, including earlier diagnosis, improved treatment and improved methods of supportive care.

CML can run a highly variable course. Several predictive models using multivariate analysis of clinical and laboratory features at presentation have been proposed. The list of poor prognostic factors in CML usually includes the clinical presence of constitutional symptoms at diagnosis, male sex and splenomegaly. With regard to poor prognositc laboratory features, these include cytogenetic abnormalities in addition to the Ph chromosome, a higher proportion of marrow or peripheral blood blasts and/or basophils, anemia, thrombocytopenia, and grade 3-4 collagen or reticulin fibrosis.

Five different staging systems derived from these analyses have been developed for assigning patients to different risk groups [22-27]. They are generally based on the number of unfavorable prognostic features. Survival expectations for patients classified into good, intermediate and poor risk are 5-6 years, 3-4 years and 2 years respectively. One of the staging systems utilizing observations from earlier studies of prognostic factors in CML is presented in Table 1 [22].

In addition to clinical and laboratory features at presentation, treatment-associated prognostic factors have also been recognized. The poor prognostic factors associated with conventional chemotherapy

**Table 1.** Staging System for CML (adapted from reference 22]

|  | Stage | Definition |
|---|---|---|
| For chronic phase: | | |
| Age ≥60 years | 1 | 0 or 1 characteristic |
| Spleen ≥ 10 cm below costal margin | | |
| Blasts ≥ 3% in blood or ≥5% in marrow | 2 | 2 characteristics |
| Basophils ≥7% in blood or ≥3% in marrow | | |
| Platelets ≥ 700 x $10^3$ μl | 3 | ≥ 3 characteristics |
| For acelerated phase: | | |
| Cytogenetic clonal evolution | 4 | ≥ 1 characteristic |
| Blasts ≥ 15% in blood | | (regardless of |
| Blasts + promyelocytes ≥30% in blood | | characteristics for |
| Basophils ≥ 20% in blood | | chronic phase) |
| Platelets <100 x $10^3$ μl | | |

(Hydrea or Busulfan) include longer time to achieve hematologic remission, short remission duration, and a high total dose of the therapeutic agent required to control the disease in the first year since diagnosis.

For those treated with IFN-α the response to treatment has emerged as a dominant treatment-associated prognostic factor. Patients' pretreatment features that seem to correlate with response to IFN-α therapy are the percent of blasts and the degree of thrombocytosis. The two pre-treatment features that correlate with survival of patients treated with IFN-α are splenomegaly and marrow basophilia (from multivariate analysis) [22, 28]. The probability of achieving a major cytogenetic response to IFN-α is much higher in patients who have criteria for good risk CML, 50% versus 14–26% for poor risk patients. The expected median survival of all patients treated with IFN-α also varies by prognostic group and is greater than 8 years (102 months) for good-risk CML, 82–90 months for intermediate risk CML and 47–56 months for poor risk CML [29]. However, the expected survival of patients who achieved a major cytogenetic response is equivalent, irrespective of their pre-treatment assignment to a prognostic group. Thus, response to IFN-α is an overriding prognostic factor. However, a response often takes months, and a cytogenetic response may take up to 12–24 months. Mahon et al described the occurrence of either a complete hematologic response at 3–8 months, cytogenetic response at 12 months or a major cytogenetic response at 24 months is associated with a significant prolongation in survival [30,31]. It should be noted that IFN therapy can be costly and is associated with significant side effects. Therefore, early selection of patients who benefit from prolonged therapy with IFN-α would be of great value as the remaining patients could be considered for other treatment options.

## VII Differential Diagnosis

CML may sometimes be difficult to differentiate from other myeloproliferative disorders (Essential Thrombocythemia, Polycythemia Vera, and Agnogenic Myeloid Metaplasia). In addition, leukemoid reaction can closely mimic CML. In these cases, the cytogenetic examination demonstrating the presence of the Ph chromosome and a low LAP score are usually sufficient to make the distinction.

Other diseases that can occasionally be confused with CML include juvenile chronic myeloid leukemia, eosinophilic leukemia, chronic neutrophilic leukemia, chronic myelomonocytic leukemia and Ph-positive acute lymphoblastic leukemia. Many of these diseases are believed to be related to CML, but making the exact diagnosis and differentiating them from CML is absolutely necessary.

## VIII  Treatment: Non-Transplant related Therapies

Treatment for CML is usually initiated at the time of diagnosis. The majority of patients with a high WBC count have symptoms related to their anemia and/or splenomegaly. The initial goal of treatment should be to either alleviate symptoms or delay the onset of symptoms, which can be achieved by controlling the WBC count. It should be noted that treatment is not urgent, and may even be unnecessary, in asymptomatic patients.

No curative approach is available for treatment of CML, short of allogeneic stem cell transplantation. Conventional chemotherapy for CML appears to be beneficial, yet there is no convincing data that it can affect the natural course of the disease. Conventional chemotherapy does not prevent transformation to BP.

Unlike treatment with conventional chemotherapy, IFN-α appears to be able to modify the course of the disease. The single most important finding to emerge from the published clinical trials of the past 5–7 years has been the prolonged survival of patients treated with IFN-α. However, many questions remain unanswered regarding the optimal dose, schedule, and duration of treatment with IFN-α for this disease.

Treatment of chronic myelogenous leukemia
in chronic phase (CML-CP)

1. *Conventional chemotherapy* with either hydroxyurea or busulfan produces hematologic remissions in up to 70% of patients. However, cytogenetic responses are rare, and if they occur, are usually minor and transient.

In the past, both drugs were used with similar frequency for controlling CML-CP. A large randomized trial comparing hydroxyurea to busulfan for treatment of CML-CP demonstrated a significantly longer median survival for patients treated with hydroxyurea (56 vs 44 months, p=0.01) [32]. Additionally, approximately 5% of patients treated in the busulfan arm experienced serious treatment-related side-effects, while there were none on the hydroxyurea arm. This study, together with earlier reports[216], established the role of hydroxyurea as first line treatment for newly diagnosed patients with CML-CP. This is especially true for patients who are candidates for allogeneic bone marrow transplantation, as a history of treatment with busulfan appears to increase transplant-related mortality [33]. Busulfan can be considered an alternative for patients who are not able to tolerate Hydrea, or who become resistant to Hydrea.

At the present time, the standard practice is to treat newly diagnosed patients with **hydroxyurea (Hydrea)**, with the goals of therapy being to control the proliferation of cells in the chronic phase. An initial dose of 1-3 gm/day given by mouth, will usually result in a fall in WBC count within 48 hours. The dose of Hydrea is usually reduced by 50% following a WBC count decrease by 50%. Patients should be closely followed, and the dose of Hydrea should be titrated aiming for a target WBC count of 5,000-20,000/µl. Indirect evidence exists that aggressive treatment with Hydrea, with the goal of normalizing WBC count, may be beneficial [34]. The usual maintenance dose is 1–1.5 gm/day. Treatment may need to be continued indefinitely, as the white blood cell count may begin to rise within a few days of stopping chemotherapy. Hydrea is generally well tolerated and most patients experience minimal side effects. Rare patients develop skin rashes or aphthous mucosal ulcers. Gastrointestinal symptoms such as nausea, vomiting or diarrhea may be seen with higher doses.

**Busulfan (Myleran)** is administered orally; the starting dose is 4–6 mg/day, and the usual maintenance dose is 1-3mg/day (titrated to WBC). Peripheral blood should be checked weekly. Since busulfan-induced myelosuppresion is more durable than that from hydroxyurea, it can be administered in 2-4 week courses. Unfortunately, the myelosuppression from busulfan can be quite unpredictable and patients require close monitoring. Other side effects of busulfan are organ fibrosis (mainly pulmonary) and an Addisonian-like disease.

2. *Interferon-alpha (IFN-α)* has a direct, selective antiproliferative effect on leukemic cells. Little is known, however, about the basis of this select-

ivity or the general mechanism of action of IFN-α. For patients in early CML-CP treatet with IFN-α-2a at a dosage of $5 \times 10^6$ U/m²/day, MD Anderson reported complete hematologic responses (CHR) in 70–80% and cytogenetic responses in up to 40–60%, with major cytogenetic responses in 30–40% of cases [29]. Table 2 defines the criteria of response to IFN-α in CML-CP.

Several single-arm studies of IFN-α for CML-CP have been published up to date, some reporting significantly lower response rates than that observed by the investigators at MD Anderson, with CHR rates varing from 46% to 84%, and cytogenetic response rates from 19% to 63%. The difference in response results may be related to patient selection, the timing of starting treatment with IFN-α, different dose and schedule of IFN-α (actual dose of IFN-α delivered), as well as patient and physician motivation. The influence of pre-treatment characteristics on the probability of response to IFN-α is discussed above. In regard to time from diagnosis to starting therapy with IFN-α, the best results have been reported in patients who started treatment within 1 year of diagnosis [35].

The goal of the treatment with IFN-α should be to achieve a complete hematologic and major cytogenetic response (see Table 2 for definition).

**Table 2.** The criteria of response to IFN-α for treatment of CML-CP

---

Hematologic response:
– Complete hematologic response (CHR):
   normalization of peripheral blood counts (WBC<10,000/µl, platelet count
   <450,000/µl)
   no immature cells
   no systemic symptoms
   no splenomegaly
– Partial hematologic response:
   normalization of peripheral blood counts (WBC<10,000/µl) with persistence of
   thrombocytosis, immature cells or splenomegaly

Cytogenetic subsets of complete hematologic response:
– Complete cytogenetic response (CCR): Ph 0%
– Partial cytogenetic response: Ph 1%–34%
– Minor cytogenetic response: Ph 35%–90%

---

*Major cytogenetic response = complete cytogenetic response +partial cytogenetic response
*Ph-Philadelphia chromosome

There are four randomized trials published to date comparing standard chemotherapy to IFN-α [34,36–38]. All four trials demonstrated a significantly higher rate of achieving a major cytogenetic response with IFN-α than with conventional chemotherapy. Three of these trials reported that patients who achieved major cytogenetic response survived longer than those who did not [36–38]. The largest single arm study concurred with this observation [29]. Two other studies, however, have failed to show a survival benefit [34–39], possibly because of lower IFN-α doses. Overall, the improved survival found in these studies is mainly, if not exclusively, accounted for by patients who achieved a cytogenetic remission. Interestingly, one study suggested longer survival duration even for patients with a poor cytogenetic response, although those who achieved cytogenetic response lived longer than those who did not [36].

**Dose of IFN-α:** There appears to be a close correlation between response and dose intensity. An indirect comparison of $5 \times 10^6$ U/m² daily to lower doses ($5 \times 10^6$ U/m² three times a week and $\leq 2 \times 10^6$ U/m² three times a week) strongly suggests higher response rates with higher doses. A randomized Italian trial designed to answer this question confirmed the superiority of higher doses [40]. This was later confirmed by Freund et al [41]. The dose-response relationship for IFN-α in CML has been observed in another study in which the initial dose of $2 \times 10^6$ U/m² five times weekly had to be increaed to $5 \times 10^6$ U/m² daily after poor response rates was noted among the first 16 patients entered[39]. One recent trial, however, has revealed conflicting data, with low doses of IFN-α appearing to be as effective as higher doses [42]. Randomized trials comparing $5 \times 10^6$ U/m² daily to lower doses are pending. Until the results from these studies become available, the goal of therapy should be a dose of $5 \times 10^6$ U/m² daily, or at (least) the lower maximally tolerated individual dose.

**Side effects of treatment with IFN-α:** Treatment with IFN-α is associated with significant side effects, which may necessitate dose reduction or even discontinuation. Initially, most patients complain of flu-like symptoms (fever, chills, myalgias, arthralgias, fatigue and headaches), which tend to improve or entirely resolve after 1–2 weeks. Gastrointestinal symptoms (nausea, diarrhea, anorexia, weight loss) and elevated transaminases can occur at any time in the course of treatment. Neurologic toxicities can be wide ranging and severe, including impairment of con-

**Table 3.** Practical guidelines of IFN-α therapy [adapted from reference 83].

**Therapy Initiation**

    Hydroxyurea to reduce WBC to less than 10–20,000/µl, may continue later or taper off Slow dose escalation: 3 x $10^6$ U daily for a week; then 5 mlnU daily for a week: then 5 x $10^6$ U/$m^2$ daily or maximally tolerated individual dose

    Improve Tolerance

    Premedicate with acetaminophen

    Evening dose

    Tricyclic antidepressants for neurologic side effects (insomnia, depression, fatigue)

**Therapeutic Monitoring**

    Complete blood counts weekly until counts stable

    Maintain WBC $\geq$ 2 to 4,000/µl and platelets > 50,000/µl

    Chemistries monthly

    Cytogenetic evaluation on bone marrow aspirate or peripheral blood Southern blot testing every 3 months in the first year, then every 6 months

**Dose Modifications**

    Interrupt IFN-α for grade 3 to 4 toxicities, then resume at 50%

    Reduce IFN-α dose by 25% for grade 2 persistent toxicities

    Reduce IFN-α dose by 25% for cytopenias WBC<2,000/µl and platelets <60,000/µl

    Hold IFN-α for moderate acute intercurrent disease

    Immune mediated-complications may necessitate treatment with steroids and/or discontinuation of treatment

**Efficacy Assessment**

    Hematologic remission at 3 to 6 months

    Cytogenetic response by 12 months

    Major cytogenetic response by 18 months

**Cessation of Therapy**

After achievement of major cytogenetic remission, IFN-α should be continued for at least 3 years, with cytogenetic (or molecular based) monitoring every 6 months

centration and other cognitive functions, as well as more serious disturbances such as a frontal lobe syndrome manifested by severe apathy, Parkinsonian syndrome, depression and psychotic reactions. Rare patients develop late immune-mediated complications such as hypothyroidism, immune-mediated nephrotic syndrome, hemolysis or thrombocytopenia and connective tissue diseases. Cases of heart dysfunction have been reported. Late side effects can be dose-limiting in 10–25% of patients. See Table 3 for guidlines of management of side effects from IFN-α therapy.

**Assesing a response and follow-up of treatment with IFN-α (see Table 2):** Achieving a cytogenetic response may take up to 12 months, and a major cytogenetic response up to 18 months. The two most significant factors predicting for achievement of a major cytogenetic response are complete hematologic response and minor cytogenetic response at 3 months [31].

The optimal duration of treatment with IFN-$\alpha$ remains unknown. Many investigators recommend that treatment with IFN-$\alpha$ should be continued indefinitely, or until relapse, for all patients who achieve a major cytogenetic response. However, some major cytogenetic responses appear to be durable even with discontinuation of IFN-$\alpha$. In one study of 34 patients in CCR, 16 patients were taken off therapy, and 7 remained in remission 18+ to 62+ months. The remaining 9 patients had cytogenetic relapse; 3/9 were described as being in continued hematologic remission without treatment and 6/9 were re-challanged with IFN-$\alpha$ and achieved a second major cytogenetic response (3 CCR and 3 PCR) [83]. This aspect of treatment with IFN-$\alpha$ needs further investigation. Treatment with IFN-$\alpha$ does not appear to be curative, with most patients in CCR having detectable bcr-abl transcript by RT-PCR [42-45]. The quantitative assessment of minimal residual disease in patients in CCR and it's correlation with both cytogenetic examination as well as clinical behaviour remain significant areas of ongoing interest.

3. *Combination of IFN-$\alpha$ with conventional chemotherapy:* In an attempt to improve upon results of treatment with IFN-$\alpha$ as a single agent, IFN-$\alpha$ has been combined with either hydroxyurea or low dose Ara-C. The rationale behind combining IFN-$\alpha$ and Ara-C lies in the fact that Ara-C is known to selectively suppress the growth of leukemic cells in vitro, in additive (or even synergistic) fashion with IFN-$\alpha$ [46]. With regard to hydroxyurea, it is often used prior to starting IFN-$\alpha$, in order to lower the WBC count, which in addition to decreasing symptoms related to catabolic leukocyte products leads to better and faster hematological response. The results of earlier trials with combination chemotherapy seemed promising in patients with CML in late chronic phase (seemed to prolong late chronic phase)[47,48]. Following this experience, further studies of combination treatments were conducted on patients who had suboptimal responses to IFN-$\alpha$, or became refractory to IFN-$\alpha$ administered as a single agent [49-53]. More recently, combination treatments were tried in newly diagnosed patients . The French have demonstrated the superiority of the IFN-$\alpha$ at a dose of $5 \times 10^6$ U/m$^2$ daily plus Ara-C 20mg/m$^2$/day for 10days administered in monthly courses over IFN-$\alpha$ alone [34]. Although a confirmatory study would be desired, the above

mentioned regimen may be considered an alternative front line therapy for newly diagnosed patients with CML-CP. The predominant Ara-C related side effects were: thrombocytopenia and gastrointestinal disturbances. The regimen is otherwise well tolerated, although the compliance with multiple daily subcutaneous injections may be a problem.

Treatment of chronic myelogenous leukemia in acute phase:
CML-AP and CML-BP

The prognosis of patients with CML-AP and CML-BP is poor, with median survival of 6-18 months and 3-4 months respectively [54]. No effective therapies for CML in acute phase, short of allogeneic stem cell transplantation, exist. Patients may be treated with intensive cytoreductive chemotherapy. However, at this stage, the disease tends to be highly resistant to chemotherapy and remissions, if observed, are very short-lived [54-58]. The type of chemotherapy is dictated by the phenotype of the blast cells in the CML-BP. Patients with myeloid phenotypes are more likely to respond to regimens similar to that used for acute myelogenous leukemia, i.e., containing anthracyclines, high/intermediate dose Ara-C and etoposide. Patients with lymphoid phenotypes usually respond to the combination of corticosteroid and vincristine with or without anthracycline or asparaginase. If a second chronic phase is achieved, treatment with regimens similar to those used for acute lymphoblastic leukemia may be of benefit in a highly selected subset of patients. This should include CNS prophylaxis with intrathecal methotraxate or Ara-C.

## IX  Treatment: Allogeneic stem cell Trasplantation (allo-SCT)

*Allogeneic stem cell transplantation using HLA-identical sibling donor:*
Allogeneic stem cell transplantation is the only currently available curative treatment modality for CML.

Outcome of patients transplanted in chronic phase is significantly better than that of patients transplanted in accelerated or blast phase. Long-term survival can be achieved in 50%–60% of recipients of HLA-identical sibling transplants for CML in chronic phase, with greater than 80% cure rates for those under the age of 40. Based on the most recent report by IBMTR, the 3-year probabilities of leukemia-free survival

(LFS) were 59% +/– 2% for patients treated in chronic phase, 37% +/–5% for patients treated in accelerated phase and 17% +/– 7% for patients treated in blast phase [59]. For patients transplanted in chronic phase, complications of transplant, usually directly or indirectly related to graft-versus-host disease (GVHD), account for up to 30–35% of the failures, and relapse for the remaining 15–20%. The relapse rate is much higher for patients transplanted in accelerated phase or blast phase and is largely responsible for the poor results associated with transplants in the late stages of the disease. The IBMTR reported 3-year probabilities of relapse: 16% +/–2% for CML-CP, 36% +/–5% for CML-AP and 61% +/–11% for CML-BP [59]. These numbers are generally in concurrence with the results reported by other investigators [60-66].

Thus, the timing of transplant appears crucial. Although it is readily agreed upon that transplant should be carried out, the optimal timing in chronic phase has been a controversial issue. Several facts suggest that transplant should be performed sooner rather than later. Firstly, delaying transplant can be hazardous, as the transformation to blast phase can occur rapidly. Secondly, evidence exists that patients who receive transplant within a year of diagnosis have a significantly better outcome than patients transplanted later in the course of chronic phase [61,62].

The major prognostic factors affecting transplant outcome are the stage of the disease, interval from the diagnosis to bone marrow transplant (as mentioned above), age and prior therapy. Age appears to be a constant variable. Prior therapy with busulfan (versus hydroxyurea) has been shown to compromise the outcome [60,61]. Beelen et al suggested that prolonged therapy with IFN-$\alpha$ prior to transplant might have an adverse impact on post-transplant survival [67]. Other investigators, however, have not found a correlation between prior therapy with IFN-$\alpha$ and the outcome among patients receiving HLA-idetical sibling allo-SCT [67-70]. This issue seems yet unresolved, as prior therapy with IFN-$\alpha$ also emerged as an independent poor predictor of outcome of HLA-identical matched unrelated SCT for CML-CP [71].

The analysis of the prognostic features allows characterization of certain subgroups of patients with an excellent prognosis with allo-SCT. The updated data from Seattle report 90% survival at 1 year and 80% survival at 8 years in patients transplanted within 1 year from diagnosis [72]. In light of this evidence, there is very little to be gained by delaying the transplant for patients with newly diagnosed CML-CP who have a suitable HLA-identical sibling donor available, and are otherwise candidates for transplant.

*Allogeneic stem cell transplant using matched unrelated donors (MUD-SCT):* HLA-identical sibling transplant can cure a significant proportion of patients with CML. However, approximately 70% of patients with CML are without a suitable matched sibling donor. Matched unrelated donor transplant remains an option for younger patients without an HLA-identical sibling donor. To date, such transplants have often been delayed because of the time required to identify an unrelated donor and because of reluctance to risk the high transplant-related mortality associated with this procedure (significantly higher than that with sibling transplant). The median time from the start of search to an unrelated transplant has been reported as 8.4 months. Over the past several years the steady improvement in the outcome of patients undergoing MUD-SCT, largely due to improvement in HLA-matching using molecular methods instead serology alone. IBMTR recently reported 3 year LFS of 51% +/–3% for MUD-SCT for CML-CP performed less than 1 year from diagnosis and 35% +/–13% for transplants performed more than 1 year from diagnosis [59].

The Seattle group recently summarized their experience with MUD-SCT for CML [73]. The estimate of survival at 5 years was comparable with that reported by IBMTR, i.e. 57% for all patients with CML-CP who were 55 years old or younger. A subgroup of patients with a particularly favorable outcome was identified: 50 years or younger, matched for HLA-A, B, and DRB1, and transplanted within first year after diagnosis. The estimated 5-year survival for these patients was 74%.

*Follow up of allo-SCT recipients/predicting relapse:* The long term follow-up of patients after allo-SCT has demonstrated a small number of patients at risk of late relapses. The three methods for detection of minimal residual disease can be employed in this clinical setting: standard cytogenetic examination, Southern blot analysis, and polymerase chain reaction studies (PCR) (both qualitative and quantitative). Attainment and then preservation of Ph-negative status after allo-SCT for CML correlates with good prognosis. The sensitivity of Southern blot analysis in patients with CML in complete cytogenetic remission does not appear improved over that of standard cytogenetic examination [36]. Interestingly, quantitative molecular monitoring by Southern blot analysis of peripheral blood samples was found to be equivalent to marrow monitoring at all time points, suggesting that the analysis of the peripheral blood samples can be substituted for bone marrow samples [74]. Approximately 40%-50% of patients after allo-SCT will be PCR-positive at 12 months. These patients, as well as patients who convert to PCR-positivity after being known to be negative, are at a higher risk of relapse [75,76]. However, it should be noted that the predictive value of PCR-positivity is limited, as only minority of PCR-positive patients are actually known to relapse. Although, in contrast, nearly all long-term survivors are PCR-negative. Quantitative PCR methods to improve the reliability of this method are under investigation.

*Treatment of relapse after allo-SCT for CML:* A significant proportion of patients relapsing after an HLA-identical sibling SCT for CML may achieve another durable hematologic or even cytogenetic remission. This stresses the need for close follow-up after SCT. The treatment options that can be considered in this setting are: withrawal of immunosuppresion for patients who are still on immunosuppresive therapy for prophylaxis or treatment of GVHD, infusion of donor lymphocytes, and a trial of treatment with IFN-$\alpha$. A significant number of patients relapsing in CP are still sensitive to IFN-$\alpha$ [77].

The antileukemia effect of allo-SCT depends both on the high intensity cytotoxic regimen used in the preparative regimen as well as on the immune-mediated reaction of donor lymphocytes directed against residual CML cells in the recipient, called the graft-versus-leukemia (GVL) effect. Indirect evidence of existence of a GVL effect was provided by the observation of higher relapse rates after syngeneic and T-cell depleted grafts compared to nonsyngeneic and unmanipulated grafts respectively[78–80]. Subsequently, the GVL effect was linked to GVHD. For patients who are still on immunosuppresive therapy for prophylaxis or treatment of GVHD, regression of leukemia can occur following discontinuation of immunosuppression. Many patients may achieve a durable remission with infusion of donor lymphocytes. Both options are associated with the considerable risk of prolonged marrow hypoplasia and flare of GVHD. Lastly, a second allo-SCT can be performed successfully in some cases [77]. It deserves mention that the known clinical effects of the immunologic-based benefits for allo-SCT were first and best described in the setting of mild to moderate GVHD and relapse after transplant. It this information that has become a cornerstone on which both future immunotherapies and stem cell transplants will continue to be based.

## X  Summary: The treatment of CML-CP

Decisions regarding the optimal treatment strategy for CML-CP, parti-cularly for patients between the ages of 40–60 years have become very complex. A proposed algorithm is presented in Figure 1.

In the absence of any contraindications, all patients younger than 60 years, who have an HLA-identical sibling donor should undergo allo-SCT within the first year of diagnosis. The remaining patients should receive a trial of treatment with IFN-α, with or without Ara-C. Patients who achieve any cytogenetic response at 6 months or major cytogenetic response at 12 months should continue with IFN-α until the response is lost, or patients find further therapy intolerable. Non-responders can be offered MUD-SCT or investigational regimens, depending on their age. In lieu of the newer data regarding the negative impact of the prolonged

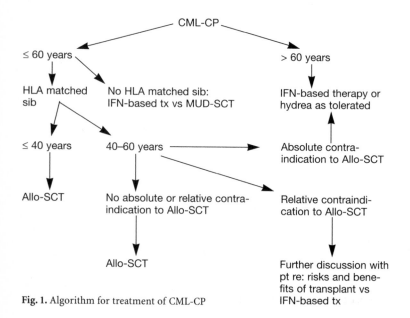

**Fig. 1.** Algorithm for treatment of CML-CP

treatment with IFN-α (>6months) on the outcome of MUD-SCT, MUD-SCT may be considered for patients who belong to the good prognostic category [71] early in the course of chronic phase.

## XI Current and future investigational approches/key questions

As discussed above, several unanswered questions remain regarding the best therapeutic approaches for patients with CML. These include identifying those patients most likely to greatly benefit from IFN therapy, establishing the optimal dose and schedule (including duration) of INF therapy, expanding the ability to perform potentially curative allogeneic stem cell therapies for greater numbers of patients, and reducing the morbidity and mortality associated with IFN and allogeneic transplant respectively. In addition, continued study of new therapeutic agents remains important. One such agent, homoharringtonine, has shown promising response rates in early studies [82]. Further studies of this agent, particularly in combination with standard therapies need to be conducted before any firm recommendation can be made regarding it's appropriate place in the therapeutic arsenal for CML.

## References

1. Bennett JH: Case of hypertrophy of the spleen and liver, in which death took place from suppuration of the blood. Edinb Med Surg J, 64: 413, 1845
2. Craigie D: Case of disease of the spleen, in which death took place in consequence of the presence of purulent matter in the blood. Edinb Med Surg J, 64: 400, 1845
3. Virchow R: Weisses blut. Froriep's Notizen, 36:151, 1845
4. Nowell, P.C., Incidence: and Hungerford, D.A.: Chromosome studies in normal and leukemic human leukocytes. J Nat Canc Inst, 25:85, 1960
5. Rowley, J.D.: A new consistent chromosomal abnormality in chronic myelogenous leukemia identified by quinacrine fluorescence and Giemsa staining. Nature, 243:290, 1973
6. Heisterkamp N, Stam K, Groffen J, et al: Structural organization of the bcr gene and its role in the Ph translocation. Nature 315:758, 1985
7. Daley GQ, van Etten RA, Baltimore D: Induction of chronic myelogenous leukemia in mice by the P210 bcr/abl gene of the Philadelphia chromosome. Science 247:824, 1990
8. Cartwright RA, Alexander FE, McKinney PA, et al: Leukaemia research fund data collection survey: descriptive epidemiology of chronic myeloid leukaemia. Leukemia 5:138, 1991
9. Prospective confirmation of a prognostic classification for Ph+ chronic myelogenous leukemia. The Italian Cooperative Study Group of Chronic Myelogenous leukemia. Br J Haematol 69:463, 1988

10. Eglin RP, Swann RA, Isaacs D, et al: Chronic leukaemia in siblings. Lancet 2:984, 1984
11. Goh K, Swisher SN, Herman EC Jr: Chronic myelocytic leukemia and identical twins: Additional evidence of the Philadelphia chromosome as postzygotic abnormality. Arch Intern Med 120:214, 1967
12. Nowell PC, Hungerford DA: Chromosome studies in human leukemia. II. Chronic granulocytic leukemia. J Natl Cancer Inst, 27:1013, 1961
13. Tough IM, Court Brown WM, Baikie AG, et al: Cytogenetic studies in chronic myeloid leukaemia and acute leukaemia associated with mongolism. Lancet 1;411, 1961
14. Ichimaru M, Ishimaru T, Mikami M, et al: Incidence of Leukemia in a Fixed Cohort of Atomic Bomb Survivors and Controls, Hiroshima and Nagasaki October 1950-December 1978. Technical Report RERF TR 13-81. Hiroshima, Radiation Effects Research Foundation, 1981.
15. Darby SC, Doll R, Gill SK, et al: Long term mortality after a single treatment course with X-rays in patients treated for ankylosing spondylitis. Br J Cancer 55:179, 1987
16. Boice JD Jr, Blettner M, Kleinerman RA, et al: Radiation dose and leukemia risk in patients treated for cancer of cervix. J Natl Cancer Inst 79:1295, 1987
17. Martin PJ, Najfeld V, Fialkow PJ: B-lymphoid cell involvement in chronic myelogenous leukemia:implications for the pathogenesis of the disease. Cancer Genet Cytogenet 6:359, 1982
18. Wiedemann LM, Karhi KK, Shivji M, et al: The correlation of breakpoint cluster region rearrangement and P210Ph1/abl expression with morphological analysis of Ph-negative chronic myeloid leukemia and other myeloproliferative diseases. Blood 71:349, 1988
19. Cortes J, Talpaz M, O'Brien et al: Philadelphia chromosome-negative chronic myelogenous leukemia with rearrangement of the breakpoint cluster region: Long term follow-up results. Cancer 75:464, 1995
20. Bernstein R: Cytogenetics of chronic myelogenous leukemia. Semin Hematol 25:20, 1988
21. Watmore AE, Potter AM, Sokal RJ, et al: Value of cytogenetic studies in prediction of acute phase of CML. Cancer Genet Cytogenet 14:293, 1985
22. Kantarjian H, Keating M, Smith T, et al: Proposal for a simple synthesis prognostic staging system in chronic myelogenous leukemia. Am J Med 88:1, 1990
23. Sokal JE, Cox EB, Baccarani M, et al: Prognostic dyscrimination in good risk chronic granulocytic leukemia. Blood 63:789, 1984
24. Sokal JE, Baccarani M, Russo D, et al: Staging and prognosis in chronic myelogenous leukemia. Seminars in Hematology 25(1):49, 1988
25. Tura S, Baccarani M, Corbell G: Staging of chronic myeloid leukemia. Br J Haematol 47:105, 1981
26. Cervantes F, Rozman C. A multivariate analysis of prognostic factors in chronic myeloid leukemia. Blood 60:1298, 1982
27. Kantarjian H, Smith TL, Mc Credie KB, et al: Chronic myelogenous leukemia: a multivariate analysis of the association of patient characteristics and therapy with survival. Blood 66:1326, 1985
28 . Kantarjian H, Smith T, O'Brien S: Prognostic factors for response and survival with alpha interferon therapy in early chronic phase of chronic myelogenous leukemia. Blood 80 (suppl 1):378a, 1993 [Abstract]
29. Kantarjian HM, Smith TL, O'Brian S, et al: Prolonged survival in chronic myelogenous leukemia after cytogenetic response to IFN-a therapy. Ann Intern Med 122:254, 1995

30. Mahon F, Montastruc M, Faberes C, et al: Predicting complete cytogenetic response in chronic myelogenous leukemia patients treated with recombinant interferon. Blood 84:3592, 1994

31. Mahon F, Faberes C, Boiron J, et al: High response rates using recombinant alpha interferon in patients with newly diagnosed chronic myeloid leukemia – analysis of predictive factors. Blood 88(suppl 1):638a, 1994

32. Hehlmann R, Heimpel H, Hasford J, et al: Randomized comparison of busulfan and hydroxyurea in chronic myelogenous leukemia. Prolongation of survival by hydroxyurea. Blood 82:398, 1993

33. Goldman J, Szydlo R, Horowitz M, et al: Choice of pre-transplant treatment and timing of transplants for chronic myelogenous leukemia in chronic phase. Blood 82:2235, 1993

34. Hehlmann R, Heimpel H, Hasford J, et al: Randomized comparison of interferon-alfa with busulfan and hydroxyurea in chronic myelogenous leukemia. Blood 84:4064, 1994

35. Sacchi S, Kantarjian H, O'Brien S, et al: Long-term follow-up results of alpha-interferon-based regimens in patients with late chronic phase chronic myelogenous leukemia [abstract]. Blood 88(suppl 1):201b, 1996

36. Allen NC, Richards SM, Shepherd PC, et al: UK Medical Research Council randomized multicenter trial of interferon-an1 for chronic myeloid leukemia: Improved survival irrespective of cytogenetic response. Lancet 345:1392, 1995

37. Italian Cooperative Study Group on Chronic Myeloid Leukemia: Interferon alfa-2a as compared with conventional chemotherapy for the treatment of chronic myeloid leukaemia. N Engl J Med 330:820, 1994

38. Ohnishi K, Ohno R, Tomonaga M, et al: (The Kouseisho Leukemia Study Group): A randomized trial comparing interferon-a with busulfan for newly diagnosed chronic myelogenous leukemia in chronic phase. Blood 86:906, 1995

39. Ozer H, George S, Schiffer C, et al: Prolonged subcutaneous administration of recombinant alpha-2b interferon in patients with previously untreated Philadelphia chromosome positive chronic phase chronic myelogenous leukemia: Effect on remission duration and survival: Cancer and Leukemia Group B Study

40. Alimena G, Morra E, Lazzarino M, et al: Interferon alpha-2b as therapy for Ph-positive chronic myelogenous leukemia. A study of 82 patients treated with intermittent or daily administration. Blood 72:642, 1988

41. Freund M, von Wussow P, Dietrich H, et al: Recombinant human interferon alpha-2b in chronic myelogenous leukaemia: Dose dependency of response and frequency of neutralizing anti-interferon antibodies. Br J Haematol 72:350, 1989 8583. Blood 82:2975, 1993

42. Schofield JR, Robinson WA, Murphy JR, et al: Low doses of interferon-alpha are as effective as higher doses in inducing remissions and prolonging survival in chronic myeloid leukemia. Ann Intern Med 121:736, 1994

43. Dhingra K, Kurzrock R, Kantarjian HM, et al: Polymerase chain reaction (PCR) for minimal residual disease in 20 CML patients in complete cytogenetic remission by interferon therapy. Blood 74(suppl 1):235a, 1989

44. Lee M-S, Kantarjian HM, Talpaz M, et al: Detection of minimal residual disease by polymerase chain reaction in Philadelphia chromosome-positive chronic myelogenous leukemia following interferon therapy. Blood 79:1920, 1992

45. Malinge M-C, Mahon FX, Delfau MH, et al: Quantitative determination of the hybrid Bcr-Abl RNA in patients with chronic myelogenous leukemia under interferon therapy. Br J Haematol 82:701, 1992

46. Sokal JE, Leong SS, Gomez GA: Preferential inhibition by cytarabine of CFU-GM from patients with chronic granulocytic leukemia. Cancer 59:197, 1987

47. Giles F, Aitchison R, Syndercombe-Court D, et al: Recombinant alpha 2B interferon in combination with oral chemotherapy in late chronic phase chronic myeloid leukemia. Leuk Lymphoma 7:99, 1992

48. Kantarjian HM, Keating M, Estey E, et al: Treatment of advanced stages of Philadelphia chromosome-positive chronic myelogenous leukemia with interferon-a and low dose cytarabine. J Clin Oncol 10:772, 1992

49. Guilhot F, Chastang C, Machallet M, et al: Interferon-alpha 2b combined with cytarabine versus interferon alone in chronic myeloid leukemia. N Engl J Med 337:223, 1997

50. Arthur C, Ma D: Combined interferon alfa-2b and cytosine arabinoside as first line treatment for chronic myeloid leukemia. Acta Haematol 89(suppl 1):15,1993

51. Kantarjian H, O'Brian S, Keating M, et al: Interferon alpha and low dose cytosine arabinoside therapy in Philadelphia chromosome-positive chronic myeloid leukemia. Proc Am Soc Clin Oncol 16:13a, 1997

52. Thaler J, Hilbe W, Apfebeck U, et al: Interferon-alpha-2c and low dose ara-c for the treatment of patients with CML.: Results of the Austrian multicenter phase II study. Leukemia Res 21:75, 1997

53. Silver R, Szatrowski T, Peterson B, et al: Combined a-interferon and low dose cytosine arabinoside for Ph+ chronic phase chronic myeloid leukemia. Blood 88 (suppl 1):638a, 1996

54. Kantarjian HM, Keating MJ, Talpaz, et al: Chronic myelogenous leukemia in blast crisis: analysis of 242 patients. Am J Med 83:445, 1987

55. Kantarjian HM, Talpaz, Kontoyiannis D, et al: Treatment of chronic myelogenous leukemia in accelerated and blast phases with daunorubicin, high dose cytarabine, and granulocyte-macrophage colony-stimulating factor. J Clin Oncol 10:398, 1992

56. Walters RS, Kantarjian HM, Keating MJ, et al: Therapy of lymphoid and undifferentiated chronic myelogenous leukemia in blast crisis with continuos vincristine and adriamycin infusions plus high dose decadron. Cancer 60:1708, 1987

57. Kantarjian HM, Walters RS, Keating MJ, et al: Treatment of the blastic phase of chronic myelogenous leukemia with mitoxantrone and high dose cytosine arabinoside. Cancer 62:672, 1988

58. Dann EJ, Anastasi J, Larson RA: High-dose cladribine therapy for chronic myelogenous leukemia in the accelerated or blast phase. J Clin Oncol 16:1498, 1998

59. Rowlings PA: 1996 IBMTR/ABMTR summary slides. ABMTR Newsletter, November 1996

60. Thomas ED, ED, Clift RA, Fefer A, et al: Marrow transplantation for the treatment fo chronic myelogenous leukemia. Ann Intern Med 104:155, 1986

61. Goldman JM, Szydlo P, Horowitz MM, et al: Choice of pre-transplant treatment and timing of transplants for chronic myelogenous leukemia in chronic phase. Blood 82:2235, 1993

62. Biggs JC, Szer J, Crilley P, et al: Treatment of chronic myeloid leukemia with allogeneic bone marrow transplantation after preparation with BuCy2. Blood 80:1352, 1992

63. Goldman JM, Apperley JF, Jones L, et al: Bone marrow transplantation for patients with chronic myelogenous leukemia. N Engl J Med 314:202, 1986

64. Snyder DS, Mc Glave PB: Treatment of chronic myelogenous leukemia with bone marrow transplantation. Bone Marrow Transplant 4:535, 1990

65. Delage R, Ritz J, Anderson KC: The evolving role of bone marrow transplantation in the treatment of chronic myelogenous leukemia. Hematol Oncol Clin North Am 4:369, 1990

66. Grathwohl A: Bone marrow transplantation for chronic myelogenous leukemia.. The European Bone Marrow Transplantation Experience in Chronic Myelogenous Leukemia. 2nd International Conference. Bologna, Italy, 1992

67. Beelen D, Graeven U, Elmaagacli A, et al: Prolonged administration of interferon-a in patients with chronic-phase Philadelphia chromosome-positive chronic myelogenous leukemia before allogeneic bone marrow transplantation may adversely affect the treatment outcome. Blood 85:2981, 1996

68. Giralt S, Kantarjian H, Talpaz M, et al: Effect of prior interferon therapy on the outcome of allogeneic bone marrow transplantation for chronic myelogenous leukemia. J Clin Oncol 11:1055, 1993

69. Horowitz MM, Giralt S, Szydlo R, et al: Effect of prior interferon therapy on outcome of HLA-identical sibling bone marrow transplants for chronic myelogenous leukemia in first chronic phase. Blood 88(suppl 1):682a, 1996

70. Sheperd O, Richards S, Allan N: Survival after allogeneic bone marrow transplantation in patients randomized into a trial of IFN-a versus chemotherapy: No significant adverse effect of prolonged IFN-a administration. Blood 86 (suppl 1):94, 1995

71. Morton AJ, Gooley T, Hansen JA, et al: Impact of pre-transplant interferon-alpha (INFa) on outcome of unrelated donor marrow transplants for chronic myeloid leukemia (CML) in first chronic phase. Blood 90 (suppl 1):536a, 1997

72. Clift RA, Storb R: Marrow transplantation for CML: the Seattle experience. Bone Marrow Transpl 17 (suppl 3): S1-S3, 1996

73. Bone marrow transplants from unrelated donors for patients with chronic myeloid leukemia. N Engl J Med 338:962, 1998

74. Stock W, Westbrook CA, Peterson B, et al: Value of molecular monitoring during the treatment of chronic myeloid leukemia: a Cancer and Leukemia Group B study. J Clin Oncol 15:26, 1997

75. Hughes T, Gareth JM, Martiat P, et al: Detection of residual leukemia after bone marrow transplant for chronic myeloid leukemia: Role of polymerase chain reaction in predicting relapse. Blood 77:874, 1991

76. Negrin RS, Blume KG: The use of polymerase chain reaction for the detection of minimal residual disease. Blood 78:225, 1991

77. Arcese W, Goldman JM, D'Arcangelo E, et al: Outcome for patients who relapse after allogeneic bone marrow transplantation for chronic myeloid leukemia. Chronic Leukemia Working Party. European Bone Marrow Transplantation Group. Blood 15:3211, 1993

78. Gale RP, Horowitz MM, Ash RC, et al: Identical twin bone marrow transplants for leukemia. Ann Intern Med 120:646, 1994

79. Goldman JM, Gale RP, Horowitz MM, et al: Bone marrow transplantation for chronic myelogenous leukemia in chronic phase: increased risk for relapse associated with T-cell delpletion. Ann Intern Med 108:806, 1988

80. Butturini A, Gale RP: The role of T-cells in preventing relapse in chronic myelogenous leukemia. Bone Marrow Transplant 2:351, 1987

81. Bolin RW, Robinson WA, Sutherland J, et al: Busulfan versus hydroxyurea in long therapy for chronic myelogenous leukemia. Cancer 50:1683, 1982

82. O'Brien S, Kantarjian H, Keating M, et al: Homoharringtonine therapy induces responses in patients with chronic myelogenous leukemia in late chronic phase. Blood 86: 3322, 1995

83. Kantarjian HM, Giles FJ, O'Brien SM, et al: Clinical course and therapy of chronic myelogenous leukemia with interferon-alpha and chemotherapy. Hematol Oncol Clin North Am 12: 31–80

# Therapy of Chronic Myelogenous Leukemia

F. J. Giles, H. M. Kantarjian

## Introduction

The therapy of chronic myelogenous leukemia (CML) has markedly evolved since 1856 when the use of arsenicals was first advocated in this condition. [154] In the early 1900s, systemic and/or splenic irradiation therapy began to be used to control the signs and symptoms of CML, and was the standard of care for the next 50 years [178, 185]. In the 1950 s, chemotherapy with oral alkylating agents was proven to be more effective than radiation therapy, and busulfan (BU) became a mainstay of treatment [83, 84, 190]. Hydroxyurea (HU) was introduced in the 1970s, and replaced BU as the preferred agent for CML because of its more predictable and manageable marrow suppression and lack of pulmonary and other organ toxicities [135]. In the 1980s, interferon alpha (IFN-$\alpha$) was studied in CML patients and, over the past decade, IFN-$\alpha$-containing regimens have become optimal first-line therapy for the majority of CML patients [211]. Younger patients who have a matched sibling donor available for allogeneic stem cell transplantation (AlloSCT) benefit from this strategy as first-line therapy in preference to IFN-$\alpha$-containing regimens [34, 40, 41, 97, 133, 165, 180]. This chapter will discuss (1) the natural history of CML with an emphasis on prognostic features, (2) the standard therapy of CML with IFN-$\alpha$ as a single agent and in combination with other agents, and (3) the role of additional agents in CML.

## Natural History and Prognostic Features

### Epidemiology

CML accounts for 7% to 15% of adult leukemias, with approximately 1 to 1.5 cases per 100,000 population [28, 30] with a male to female ratio of

1.4–2.2 to 1. The incidence of CML has remained steady for the last 50 years. The median age at presentation is 50 to 60 years, but the disease occurs in all age groups [90]. In earlier reports, 54% to 63% of patients were age 60 years and older, but this incidence has decreased in more recent reports to as low as 12% [120]. This may be a consequence of earlier detection, referral of younger patients to large centers, or the exclusion of patients with CML-like tumors (other myeloproliferative disorders, Philadelphia chromosome [Ph]-negative CML, chronic myelomonocytic leukemia [CMML]) [31, 46, 65, 67, 76, 86, 118, 141, 146, 147].

## Etiology

The etiology of CML is unknown. There is little evidence for genetic factors linked to CML. There may be however some correlation with HLA antigens CW3 and CW4 [26]. Offspring of parents with CML do not have a higher incidence of CML than the general population. There is also no correlation in monozygotic twins, suggesting that CML is an acquired disorder. Chemicals have not been associated with increased risk for CML. Survivors of the Nagasaki and Hiroshima atomic explosions were reported to have a significantly higher incidence of CML although this was not confirmed by cytogenetic studies since the reports preceded the discovery of the Ph chromosome, and thus many patients may have had CMML or myelodysplastic syndromes (MDS) [150]. Therapeutic radiation has also been associated with increased risk of CML as observed in some patients with ankylosing spondylitis given spinal radiation and women with uterine cervical cancer treated with radiation therapy [23, 29].

## Pathophysiology

CML usually has a biphasic, and sometimes triphasic course. Disease heterogeneity makes precise definitions of the different phases of disease and of prognostic subgroups important to the analysis of therapeutic results [120]. The disease presents in an indolent or chronic phase, which, after 2 to 6 years of conventional therapy, evolves into an accelerated phase that lasts for less than 1 to 1.5 years. Accelerated phase is followed by blastic phase disease which usually results in the patient's death within 3 to 6 months. Twenty percent to 25% of patients die during the

**Table 1.** Definitions of Accelerated and Blastic Phases of CML

A. Blastic phase CML
   30% or more blasts in the marrow or peripheral blood
   Extramedullary disease with localized immature blasts

B. Accelerated phase CML
   1. Multivariate analysis-derived criteria
      Peripheral blasts 15% or more
      Peripheral blasts plus promyelocytes 30% or more
      Peripheral basophils 20% or more
      Thrombocytopenia <100 x 10⁹/L unrelated to therapy
      Cytogenetic clonal evolution
   2. Other criteria used in common practice
      Increasing drug dosage requirement
      Splenomegaly unresponsive to therapy
      Marrow reticulin or collagen fibrosis
      Marrow or peripheral blasts ≥10%
      Marrow or peripheral basophils ± eosinophils ≥10%
      Triad of WBC >50 x 10⁹/L, hematocrit <25% and platelets <100 x 10⁹/L not
      controlled with therapy
      Persistent unexplained fever or bone pains

accelerated phase while another 20% to 25% progress directly from chronic to blastic phase without a discernable intermediate accelerated phase [159]. Standard definitions of the accelerated and blastic phases of CML are needed and have been proposed (Table 1) [120,123,124].

CML is characterized by increased proliferation and accumulation of a myeloid population with variable functional abnormalities, and the presence of a chromosomal marker in the leukemic cells. 95% to 100% of metaphases in the marrow of 90% to 95% of untreated CML patients have the Ph [173,196]. The reciprocal translocation represented by the Ph chromosome may precede overt CML disease by several years. Quantitative analysis of this chromosomal abnormality, and its molecular consequences is the major surrogate marker for therapeutic success in CML [21, 22, 27, 49, 51, 59, 61, 63, 64, 72, 81, 93, 100, 101, 109, 114, 125, 126, 129, 132, 139, 145, 151–153, 155–158, 230]. In CML patients, the Ph chromosome can be found in metaphases of neutrophil, eosinophil, basophil, erythroblast, platelet, B cell, monocyte and macrophage precursors [78]. Occasional PHA-stimulated T cells but neither marrow nor skin fibroblasts display the Ph chromosome [98]. The Ph chromosome is an abbreviated chromosome 22 (22q-) resulting from a reciprocal translocation (9;22) in which most of the distal end of 22 is exchanged for a small terminal piece of the long arm of chromosome 9 (9q+) [196]. Five to ten percent of Ph-positive CML patients show variant cytogenetic changes of which half are 3-way translocations involving chromosome 9, 22, and another chromosome.[58] The breakpoints in chromosomes 9 and 22 are at bands q34 and q11, respectively, resulting in a t(9;22),(q34;q11) which transposes the *c-sis* proto-oncogene from chromosome 22 to chromosome 9 and the cellular Abelson (*c-abl*) proto-oncogene from chromosome 9 to chromosome 22, in proximity to the breakpoint cluster region gene (*bcr*) [13, 57, 137, 145, 167–169]. This latter hybrid *bcr-abl* oncogene produces an abnormal 8.5 kb RNA in contrast to the normal *abl* transcripts of 6.8 and 7.4 kb [82]. The abnormal mRNA produced by *bcr-abl* encodes for a 210 Kd (P210) fusion protein which exhibits tyrosine kinase activity and shows considerable homology to the catalytic subunit of 3',5'-cAMP [16].

Using high-resolution cytogenetic analysis the critical translocation in CML is usually defined as t(9;22)(q34.1;1.21).Although usually located in the intron 5' of exon 2, the breakpoint on chromosome 9 may range over a 200 kb region upstream of the 5' end of the v-*abl* homologous region. *Abl* exons 1a and 1b are sometimes also translocated to chromosome 22, but their transcripts are spliced out of the mature mRNA. Ph-positive CML patients and some 50% of Ph-positive acute lymphoblastic leukemia (ALL) and acute nonlymphoblastic leukemia (ANLL) have breakpoints on chromosome 22 which cluster in a region about 5.8 kb long, termed the major BCR (M-bcr) [145, 167]. M-bcr encompasses four exons (exons 12 through 15, but usually referred to as exons b1 through b4). The breakpoint on chromosome 22 is located 3' of the Cl gene, thus the l chain coding region usually remains on the Ph in a 5' orientation to the translocated c-*abl* gene. In Ph-positive CML, the breakpoints within M-bcr have been assigned to 3' or 5' locations. Depending on whether the hybrid oncogene involves exon 3 or exon 2 of the M-bcr and exon 2 of *abl*, two distinct RNA messages are produced: b3a2 or b2a2. While the 3' *bcr* breakpoints often result in b3a2 and 5' breakpoints in b2a2 messages, some patients with 5' breakpoints produce b3a2 message. The hybrid b3a2 mRNA and the protein for which it codes differ in size by 75 bases and 25 amino acids respectively from b2a2 and its product. This spectrum of abnormalities at the DNA and RNA levels have been variably associated with different disease features (e.g., thrombocytosis or distinct prognostic groups), but not confirmed in most recent studies [72, 81, 114, 167, 169]. The diagnosis of CML is made on the basis of the findings of leukocytosis with basophilia and the presence of the *bcr-abl* rearrangement. In Ph-negative patients with a clinical diagnosis of CML, Southern blot analysis for *bcr* rearrangement will identify Ph-negative, *bcr*-positive CML patients [46].

The mechanisms conferring a growth advantage on CML cells over normal hematopoietic cells are unknown. A reduced duration of stroma-CML hematopoietic cell interaction has been documented and attributed to abnormalities in the patterns of adherence of CML cells to the stromal matrix [19, 69, 96, 223]. Reduced or abnormal contact with stromal elements in CML may abrogate the normal maturation of cell surface moieties such as cytoadhesion molecules (CAM), HLA-DR, required for a normal proliferation-maturation sequence [19, 223]. IFN-α has been shown in vitro to reverse some of these adhesion abnormalities [19, 69, 223]. Discordant nuclear:cytoplasmic maturation in CML may also confer a growth advantage over normal hematopoietic cells. A causal association between the Ph chromosome and the initiation and perpetuation of CML has been established in a number of models. In one study c-DNA encoding for P210 was introduced into mouse marrow cells, which were reinfused into lethally irradiated mice [55]. After 2 to 8 weeks, some mice developed CML-like disorders, including leukocytosis, splenomegaly and monocyte /macrophage extramedullary tumors and ALL. A murine model of blastic-phase CML has also been described [56]. This spectrum of disorders are similar to the pathogenesis of human CML and suggest that *bcr-abl* rearrangement may be sufficient, not only for development of chronic phase CML, but also for its transformation into blastic phase disease.

About 20% of adults and 5% of children with acute lymphocytic leukemia (ALL) have the Ph in their blast cells [184]. These children are usually older than Ph-negative ALL patients (median eight years) and frequently have a higher median white cell count (WBC), more frequent L2 blast cell morphology, and a high incidence of pre-B CALLA-positive disease. Their prognosis is inferior to that of Ph-negative ALL patients. In Ph-positive acute leukemia, 50%–80% of patients have a breakpoint within the m-bcr region, proximal to the M-bcr region, which results in a 7.5 kb mRNA encoding for a 190 Kd (P190) protein. In contrast to P190 acute leukemia, chronic phase disease may follow induction therapy in some patients with P210 Ph-positive acute leukemia. However, the clinical features and prognoses are similar in P210 and P190 acute leukemias.

About 10% of "CML" patients lack the Ph [31]. These patients are usually older, have a lower leukocyte count, have a higher leukocyte alkaline phosphatase (LAP) score, respond poorly to therapy, and have traditionally been described as having a shorter survival time than patients with Ph-positive CML. In 35% of Ph-negative CML patients, the *bcr-abl* rearrangement is detectable and these Ph-negative, *bcr-abl* positive patients have a clinical course and prognosis similar to that of Ph-positive patients. G6PD isozyme studies indicate that Ph-negative, *bcr-abl* negative "CML" is also a clonal disease originating in a neoplastic multipotential stem cell. These patients usually have myeloproliferative disorders other than CML, often clonal myelodysplastic syndromes, most commonly CMML or refractory anemia with excess blasts.[118] While basophilia serves as a marker for Ph-positive CML, this rarely occurs in Ph-negative, *bcr-abl* negative "CML". True Ph-negative, *bcr-abl* negative CML patients may have a lower propensity for blastic transformation than *bcr-abl* positive patients and an intermediate prognosis between CMML and *bcr-abl* positive CML [46, 147]. CML in children may either be a Ph-positive disorder which behaves like adult Ph-positive CML or may occur as juvenile CML which is Ph-negative.[85] The peak incidence of this latter disorder is at age one or two years. These patients usually have a marked elevation of fetal hemoglobin. No consistent associated cytogenetic abnormalities occur. Relative to those with Ph-positive childhood disease, juvenile CML patients tend to have lower WBC and platelet counts at diagnosis, higher LAP scores and to have splenic sequestration crises as a clinical feature. The response to cytotoxic therapy in juvenile CML is poor, and median survival from time of diagnosis is less than one year.

## Clinical Presentation

In chronic phase, CML is frequently asymptomatic. The incidence of asymptomatic cases has increased over the last decade from 15% to about 45% of all cases, possibly from widespread use of routine blood testing (Table 2) [103, 89, 120]. Patients with symptoms usually have a gradual onset of fatigue, anorexia, weight loss, increased sweating, left upper quadrant discomfort, and early satiety because of splenomegaly. The magnitude of splenomegaly correlates well with the total body granulocyte mass and the blood granulocyte count. The enlarged spleen is firm and not tender (unless splenic infarction has occurred). The degree of splenomegaly may be an indication of chronic phase duration, thus

**Table 2.** Clinical characteristics of patients with different phases of CML. Comparison between patients presenting before or after 1983.

| Characteristics | Category | Percentage with Characteristics | | | | | | | | |
| --- | --- | --- | --- | --- | --- | --- | --- | --- | --- | --- |
| | | Chronic Phase | | | Accelerated Phase | | | Blast Phase | | |
| | | Before 1983 (N=336) | Since 1983 (N=494) | p value | Before 1983 (N=51) | Since 1983 (N=139) | p value | Before 1983 (N=48) | Since 1983 (N=61) | p value |
| Age (years) | ≥60 | 18 | 12 | .03 | 16 | 11 | NS | 13 | 21 | NS |
| Asymptomatic | Yes | 15 | 37 | <.01 | 4 | 20 | .02 | 8 | 24 | NS |
| Hepatomegaly | Yes | 46 | 18 | <.01 | 51 | 19 | <.01 | 60 | 22 | .01 |
| Splenomegaly | Yes | 76 | 54 | <.01 | 84 | 70 | NS | 91 | 56 | .01 |
| Hemoglobin (g/dL) | <12 | 58 | 48 | .01 | 50 | 55 | NS | 79 | 50 | .05 |
| WBC count (x10$^9$/L) | ≥100 | 69 | 56 | <.01 | 67 | 64 | .84 | 45 | 46 | NS |
| Platelet (x10$^9$/L) | >700 | 28 | 19 | <.01 | 20 | 14 | NS | 8 | 17 | NS |
| Peripheral blasts | Yes | 65 | 56 | .03 | 48 | 41 | NS | 83 | 50 | .03 |
| Peripheral basophils (%) | ≥7 | 17 | 14 | NS | 17 | 27 | NS | 14 | 13 | NS |
| Marrow blasts (%) | ≥5 | 16 | 9 | <.01 | 35 | 34 | NS | 95 | 91 | NS |
| Marrow basophils (%) | ≥3 | 40 | 35 | NS | 57 | 52 | NS | 33 | 19 | NS |

NS=Not significant

gross splenomegaly predicts a shorter time to blastic phase. Spleno-megaly was documented in approximately 70% of patients in older reports but has decreased to 50% in more recent studies (Table 2). Hepatomegaly is less common (10% to 40% of patients) and less spectacularly present. Lymphadenopathy is uncommon in chronic phase CML, and its appearance suggests either accelerated or blastic phase disease [123, 124]. Rare patients with very high WBC counts may have manifestations of hyperviscosity, including priapism, tinnitus, stupor, visual changes from retinal hemorrhages, and cerebro-vascular accidents [208, 209]. There are few case reports of CML presenting as diabetes insipidus [116]. The accelerated phase is a somewhat ill defined transitional phase [124]. It is occasionally asymptomatic and the diagnosis made based on peripheral blood and/or bone marrow findings. Some patients may have fever and night sweats, and progressive enlargement of the spleen (Table 2) [124]. At least 20% of chronic phase patients develop a blastic phase without evidence of an accelerated phase. Patients in blastic phase are more likely to have symptoms, including weight loss, fever, night sweats and bone pains (Table 2) [123]. Symptoms of anemia, infectious complications and bleeding are common. Subcutaneous nodules or hemorrhagic tender skin lesions and lymphadenopathy are more common in blastic phase and signs of central nervous system (CNS) leukemia may be seen, particularly with lymphoid blastic transformation (30% cumulative incidence of CNS leukemia). Tissue infiltration can occur in the blastic phase, frequently in the lymph nodes, skin, subcutaneous tissues, and bone [112, 123].

Bleeding and thrombosis are uncommon in the chronic phase of CML but patients with extreme thrombocythemia tend to have both thrombotic and hemorrhagic problems, whereas those with marked leukocytosis are prone to thrombotic complications. Disseminated intravascular coagulation may occasionally be seen in blastic phase disease.

Laboratory Features

The most common peripheral blood feature of CML is an elevated WBC count, usually above 25 x $10^9$/l, and frequently above 100 x $10^9$/l [208]. Some patients have wide cyclic variations in the WBC count of up to an order of magnitude in 50 to 70 days cycles [110]. At diagnosis, circulating BFU-E and CFU-GM progenitor numbers in CML may be increased up to 180-fold and 9,000-fold, respectively. Intravascular plugs of leukemic cells are a serious hazard in CML particularly in patients less than 20 years of age at diagnosis, 50% of whom present with WBC in excess of 300 x 10⁹/l. Leukostasis is also a particular problem in 60% of childhood cases, reflecting the very high WBC in children with Ph-positive CML. Consequences of severe leukostasis may include CNS hemorrhage, headache, dizziness, mental confusion, central or peripheral neuropathy, digital gangrene, cardio-respiratory failure, priapism, and marrow necrosis. Intra-ocular visible manifestations include papilledema, retinal hemorrhages and venous engorgement. CML marrow hyperplasia of all myeloid stages is caused by progenitor cell expansion, a slower cell cycle, prolonged maturation-division times, and delayed compartmental transit. The WBC differential usually shows granulocytes in all stages of maturation, from blasts to mature granulocytes which look morphologically normal. Basophils are usually elevated, but only 10%–15% have $\geq 7\%$ basophils in peripheral blood; a very high proportion of basophils in the peripheral blood (i.e., $\geq 20\%$) is usually associated with accelerated phase disease [124]. Eosinophils are also frequently elevated, although to a lesser degree. The absolute lymphocyte count is usually elevated, mostly representing an expansion of T-lymphocytes. The platelet count is elevated in 30%–50% of the patients, and may be greater than 1000x10⁹/l in some patients [162, 211]. Thrombocytopenia is rarely seen in CML at diagnosis and usually is associated with poor prognosis or with accelerated or blastic phase. Most patients have mild anemia at diagnosis, but untreated patients may be severely anemic.

Patients in chronic phase do not have an increased risk for infections although in vitro neutrophil function abnormalities are common [50, 229]. Granulocyte abnormalities including subnormal adhesiveness to bone marrow stromal surfaces, delayed migration to extravascular sites, reduction in phagocytic and bacteriocidal activities, and subnormal lactoferrin and lysozyme content are frequent. The CML granulocytes capable of extravascular migration (as determined by the skin window technique) are more active in phagocytosis and show higher LAP activities than do kindred cells trapped in the circulation. Phagocytic activity, release of lactoferrin, adhesion to endothelium and extravascular migration capability appear to be linked granulocyte properties involving CAM, all of which are depressed in CML. Natural killer cell (NK) activity is also impaired due to defective maturation of these cells [80]. Platelet function is frequently abnormal in vitro, most frequently with a decreased secondary aggregation with epinephrine, but this usually is not associated with bleeding. The bone marrow is hypercellular with cellularity of 75%–90%, and very scarce fat [141]. The myeloid to erythroid ratio is 10:1 to 30:1 rather than the normal 2:1 to 5:1. Bands plus segmented neutrophils, metamyelocytes, and the combined numbers of myeloblasts, promyelocytes, and myelocytes occur in three equivalent proportions, denoting a marked shift toward myeloid immaturity. Megakaryocytic hyperplasia is common, and dysplastic changes variably affect all cell lines. Cells mimicking Gaucher cells can be seen in the marrow and spleen of 10%–20% of patients, reflecting consumption by mononuclear phagocytes of leukocyte sphingolipids released by leukemic granulocytes [68]. Gaucher's disease results from the absence of sphingolipid hydrolase; in CML the Gaucher-like cells have active hydrolase but are overwhelmed by the substrate load. Fibrosis may be evident at diagnosis and increases with disease progression [60]. About 30% of CML patients acquire focal or diffuse increases in marrow reticulin fibers (reticulin fibrosis) early in the disease, and some 20% develop extensive new collagen formation (collagen fibrosis). Minor degrees of marrow fibrosis occur in many CML patients and appear not to necessarily imply a poor prognosis, but the a rapid rate or development of extensive (grade 3–4) myelofibrosis is a poor prognostic feature [60, 228]. Fibroblasts are not derived from the leukemic clone but represent a secondary reaction to leukemic infiltration.

Leukocyte alkaline phosphatase (LAP) activity is reduced in nearly all patients at diagnosis [193]. The significance of this finding is unclear. LAP activity can be restored after transfusing leukocytes from patients with CML to neutropenic patients, suggesting extrinsic regulation [198]. G-CSF can induce synthesis of LAP in vitro [36]. With infection, inflammation, secondary malignancy, pregnancy, splenectomy, progression to blastic phase or peripheral blood remission as a consequence of therapy, the LAP score can rise to either normal or abnormally high levels. Low LAP scores are not specific for CML and may be seen in paroxysmal nocturnal hemoglobinuria, congenital hypophosphatasia, and some cases of either idiopathic myelofibrosis or AML. Serum vitamin $B_{12}$ levels are increased, up to 10 times normal levels, in proportion to the amounts of transcobalamin I and III released during breakdown of CML granulocytes. Serum vitamin $B_{12}$ levels rise in proportion to the WBC but may remain high in hematologic remission. Transcobalamin II, the physiologic $B_{12}$ carrier, is not increased, and may be decreased in CML.

Increased production of uric acid, with hyperuricemia and hyperuricosuria, is common in untreated CML. If cytolytic therapy causes a heavy
additional burden of filtered purines, urate nephropathy or urinary tract
blockage may ensue. Formation of urate stones is common in CML, and
some patients with latent gout may develop overt gouty arthritis or
nephropathy. Serum levels of lactic dehydrogenase are also frequently
elevated.

## CML Transformation

Blastic phase CML resembles acute leukemia [99, 123, 144, 225]. Its diagnosis requires the presence of at least 30% of blasts in the bone marrow or peripheral blood. In some patients the blastic phase is characterized by extramedullary deposits of leukemia called myeloblastomas
[112, 219]. These usually appear in the CNS, lymph nodes or bones, and
occasionally occur in the absence of blood or bone marrow evidence of
blastic transformation. Most of these patients develop hematologic
manifestations within a few months [219]. Patients in blastic phase
usually die within 3 to 6 months. Approximately 50% of patients have a
myeloid blastic phase, 25% lymphoid, and 25% undifferentiated.
Patients with lymphoid blastic phase respond to ALL therapy (CR rate
50% to 60%) and their median survival is better compared to myeloid
or undifferentiated cases (9 months versus 3 months). However, the prognosis for all patients with blastic phase CML is still very poor [62, 71,
112, 113, 119, 123, 133, 159, 163, 170, 225]. Specific criteria associated with a
survival shorter than 18 months by multivariate analysis have been proposed, including the presence of $\geq$ 15% blasts in peripheral blood, or
$\geq$ 30% blasts and promyelocytes in the blood, or $\geq$ 20% basophils in the
blood, or platelet count < 100 x $10^9$/l [124]. A cytogenetic clonal evolution has been considered a criteria for acceleration. Recent analysis suggests its prognostic effect depends on the specific abnormality, its predominance in marrow metaphases, and the time of appearance [157].
Patients with chromosome 17 abnormalities, $\geq$ 24% abnormal metaphases, clonal evolution >24 months after diagnosis, and no prior
therapy with IFN-$\alpha$ have the worst outcome. The median survival for
patients with none of the pretreatment features is 51 months, compared
to 24, 14, and 7 months when 1, 2, or 3 or 4 features are present.

Prognostic Factors and Models

A number of poor prognostic features have been identified (Table 3) and prognostic systems have been developed in CML [32, 33, 111, 117, 130, 194, 206, 222]. These have allowed the categorization of patients into good, intermediate and poor risk groups with respective median survivals of 6, 3–4, and 2 years in patients receiving conventional therapy. Based on the previous prognostic scoring systems, a synthesis staging and prognostic model has been proposed and applied to IFN-α-treated populations (Table 4) [130]. A feature of more recent large clinical studies in CML is a significant increase in the percentage of good prognosis patients (Table 2) and an improved prognosis in each of the risk groups. The median survivals in the good, intermediate and poor risk groups are 9, 7.5 and 4 to 5 years respectively [104, 125]. Good prognosis patients now account for 45% to 50% of newly diagnosed cohorts, possibly reflecting more readily available screening tests in asymptomatic patients [89, 101, 103, 104]. Any apparent improvement in overall survival in modern CML studies must be judged in the light of this significant change in patient distribution among prognostic subgroups (Table 2). To date, IFN-α therapy has not been associated with significantly different prognostic

**Table 3.** Poor Prognostic Factors in CML

A  Clinical
   Older age
   Symptoms at diagnosis
   Significant weight loss
   Hepatomegaly
   Splenomegaly
   Poor performance
   Black race

B  Laboratory
   Anemia
   Thrombocytosis, thrombocytopenia, megakaryocytopenia
   Increased blasts, or blasts + promyelocytes in blood or marrow
   Increased basophils in blood or marrow
   Collagen or reticulin fibrosis grade 3-4

C  Treatment-associated
   Longer time to achieve hematologic remission with busulfan chemotherapy
   Short remission duration
   High total dose of busulfan or hydroxyurea therapy required in the first year to
   control the disease
   Poor initial hematologic or cytogenetic response to IFN-A therapy

**Table 4.** Staging system for chronic myelogenous leukemia.

| For chronic phase: | Stage | Definition |
|---|---|---|
| Age ≥60 years | 1 | 0 or 1 characteristics |
| Spleen ≥10 cm below costal margin | | |
| Blasts ≥3% in blood or ≥5% in marrow | 2 | 2 characteristics |
| Basophils ≥7% in blood or ≥3% in marrow | | |
| Platelets ≥700x10⁹/L | 3 | ≥3 characteristics |

| For accelerated phase: | 4 | ≥1 characteristic (regardless of characteristics for chronic phase) |
|---|---|---|
| Cytogenetic clonal evolution | | |
| Blasts ≥15% in blood | | |
| Blasts + promyelocytes ≥30% in blood | | |
| Basophils ≥20% in blood | | |
| Platelets <100x10⁹/L | | |

**Table 5.** Response to IFN-A and survival by prognostic groups.

| Prognostic Group* | Cytogenetic Response | No. of patients | Survival (%) | | p value |
|---|---|---|---|---|---|
| | | | 3 years | 5 years | |
| Good | Yes | 73 | 93 | 79 | <0.01 |
| | No | 68 | 86 | 62 | |
| Intermediate | Yes | 25 | 95 | 82 | <0.01 |
| | No | 31 | 76 | 35 | |
| Poor | Yes | 9 | 100 | 83 | <0.01 |
| | No | 31 | 68 | 39 | |

\* According to the Prognostic Synthesis Model

**Table 6.** Response to IFN-A by CML phase.

| Phase | Percent | | |
|---|---|---|---|
| | CHR | Cytogenetic Response | |
| | | Any | Major |
| Early Chronic | 60–80 | 40–50 | 20–30 |
| Late Chronic | 50–60 | 10–20 | <10 |
| Accelerated | 30–40 | <10 | 0 |
| Blastic | 20–30 | <10 | 0 |

CHR=Complete hematologic remission

**Table 7.** Prognostic Factors for Cytogenetic Response and Survival with IFN-A Therapy

| Prognostic Factor | Correlation with: | |
|---|---|---|
| | Major Cytogenetic Response | Survival |
| Symptoms | < 0.01* | NS |
| Splenomegaly | < 0.01* | < 0.01** |
| anemia | < 0.01* | 0.01* |
| WBC > 100 x $10^9$/µl | < 0.01* | 0.02* |
| Marrow Basophilia | NS* | < 0.01** |
| Peripheral Blasts | < 0.01* | 0.01* |

*Selected by univariate analysis.
**Selected by multivariate analysis.
NS = not significant.

factors than those derived in CML patients receiving conventional chemotherapy (Tables 5, 6) [126]. However, major cytogenetic responses are observed among patients in the poor risk category and carry the same import of prolonged chronic phase and survival in this group. (Table 5). A combination of pretreatment risk groups with response to IFN-α therapy at pre-determined endpoints e.g. 3 or 12 months may be the current optimal way to stratify CML patients into prognostic groups [155, 156]. In multivariate analyses, the percent of blasts and degree of thrombocytosis have been correlated with response to IFN-α therapy; splenomegaly, marrow basophilia, anemia and percent of blasts have been associated with survival (Table 7) [126, 130]. Patients with good-risk CML who receive adequate IFN-α therapy have an expected major cytogenetic response rate of about 50% and an expected median survival of greater than 8 years. In contrast, those with poor-risk disease have an expected major cytogenetic response rate of 14% to 26% and an expected median survival of 4 to 5 years.

The in vivo response to IFN-α is the dominant treatment-associated prognostic factor. Achieving a complete hematologic remission (CHR) at 3 to 8 months, a cytogenetic response at 12 months, or a major cytogenetic response at 24 months is associated with a significant prolongation in survival [48, 91, 155, 156]. Combining the patient pretreatment features (risk group) with response to IFN-α may allow early selection of patients who benefit from continued IFN-α therapy, while other patients should proceed with AlloSCT or investigational therapy. Patients who do not achieve a CHR after 6–8 months, or a cytogenetic response after 12 months of IFN-α therapy may be taken off IFN-α, if the sole aim of IFN-α therapy is the achievement of durable cytogenetic response. However the Medical Research Council (MRC) trial suggests that continued IFN-α therapy may still be the optimal approach for patients who do not have an AlloSCT option, even if cytogenetic remission is not achieved [2].

## Chemotherapy

As experience with AlloSCT and IFN-α has evolved, the goals of therapy in CML have changed markedly. In more than 80% of chronic phase CML patients HU and other cytotoxic agents have the ability to control of the signs and symptoms of CML caused by the myeloid hyperplasia, leukocytosis and organomegaly [90, 104]. These agents have little or no effect on progression of the disease into its terminal phase as characterized by blastic transformation or, more rarely, myelofibrosis with marrow failure. All patients receiving traditional cytotoxic therapy will eventually evolve into blastic phase and succumb to their disease after a median survival of 3 to 6 years.

The first successful treatment of CML was achieved with radiotherapy. Until the 1950s radiotherapy, either total body or splenic, was the mainstay of therapy. It caused a reduction in white cell and platelet counts, allowed a rise in hemoglobin, reduced the size of the spleen and improved the patient's well-being but did not improve survival. The benefit typically lasted about 6 months after which re-treatment was required. Radiotherapy is now almost solely used in the therapy of CML in the form of total body irradiation pre-AlloSCT [34, 40, 97]. Radiotherapy is also valuable for treating certain CML complications such as extramedullary disease and massive splenomegaly when splenectomy is not possible [97, 166].

BU, introduced into CML therapy by Galton in 1953, allows long periods of hematologic control and is inexpensive [84]. Fifteen years later the results of an MRC randomized controlled trial comparing radiotherapy with busulfan established that busulfan therapy was superior, since it produced better disease control for longer periods. Subsequent comparisons with dibromomannitol, chlorambucil, 6-mercaptopurine, 6-thioguanine, cyclophosphamide, melphalan and combination cytotoxic therapy, documented BU superiority or equivalence to these agents [84, 134, 189, 204]. In up to 10% of patients, BU can cause severe myelo-suppression which can prove fatal, although survival after aplasia is often associated with very long remissions [66, 77]. Peripheral blood counts may continue to fall after BU is stopped and the period of aplasia may continue for many months. In a small minority of patients a severe idiosyncratic pulmonary reaction, interstitial fibrosis associated with constitutional symptoms, known as BU lung, occurs and may be lethal [177, 181]. Marrow fibrosis may also be caused by BU. An increase in skin pigmentation is found with prolonged use. In women disorders of men-struation occur and infertility is usual in both sexes. An Addisons-like disease, cataract, sicca syndrome, myasthenia gravis and endocardial fibrosis have been reported [149, 182]. The dose of BU is usually 0.1 mg/kg daily until the WBC decrease by 50%, and then the dose is reduced by 50%. Therapy is discontinued when the WBC drops below 20 x $10^9$/l, and restarted when it increases above 50 x $10^9$/l.

HU, a cycle specific inhibitor of DNA synthesis, was introduced into CML therapy in 1972, and has a much better toxicity profile than BU [197]. HU gives rapid but more transient control of hematologic manifestations and thus requires more frequent follow-ups. It is usually given at a dose of 40 mg/kg daily, and reduced by 50% when the WBC dropped below 20 x $10^9$ per liter. The dose is then adjusted individually to keep the WBC at 5 to 10 x $10^9$ per liter. One study has used higher doses of HU, at 2 g/m$^2$ per day until the absolute neutrophil count reached < 1 x $10^9$/l [143]. Patients achieving a cytogenetic response were given additio-nal cycles until maximal response. Fourteen of 25 cycles administered to 14 patients in chronic phase resulted in $\geq$ 25% Ph negative cells. In one patient a complete cytogenetic response (CCR) was achieved. In all cases however, the responses were transient. HU is very well tolerated by most patients with very few side effects including nausea and anorexia, which are usually transient. Skin changes, such as atrophy and scaling, and partial alopecia may occur. HU causes marked red cell macrocytosis and megaloblastic changes in the marrow.

Both BU and HU can control the hematologic manifestations of the disease in more than 80% of CML patients. A recent large randomized study has prospectively compared these two agents in chronic phase CML [104]. On this German/Swiss protocol, between July 1983 and January 1991, 458 patients were randomized to HU or BU. All previous-ly untreated patients with proven CML in early chronic phase were eligible. The 232 patients randomized to HU therapy had a significantly longer median survival (56 versus 44 months, $p = 0.01$), than the 226 patients who received BU. The survival advantage conferred by HU was evident in all prognostic subgroups. The median duration of chronic phase in the HU cohort was significantly longer (47 versus 37 months, $p = 0.04$), than in the BU cohort. No patient achieved a CCR to either agent. There were no serious HU-related adverse events in contrast to serious adverse events including prolonged marrow aplasia or pulmonary toxicity in 6% of patients receiving BU. Therefore, while disease control is clearly better with less toxicity and prolonged survival with HU therapy, rather than BU, neither agent as routinely used achieves cytogenetic remissions or significantly delays time to development of blastic phase.

A recent report documented the use of a continuous infusion of low-dose ara-C in patients with chronic phase CML [191]. Five patients received 15 to 30 mg/m²/day of ara-C. The hematologic manifestations of the disease were controlled in all, and all patients achieved some cytogenetic response, including one CCR and one partial. Other chemotherapeutic agents such as 6-mercaptopurine, melphalan, 6-thioguanine, dibromomannitol and thiotepa have been used infrequently, either alone or in combination with BU [189, 204]. None of these latter agents have an obvious advantage over HU. BU therapy prior to AlloSCT has been shown to have an adverse impact on post transplant survival, [94]. in contrast to data on IFN-$\alpha$ [92]. Data from Beelen et al. suggesting that IFN-$\alpha$ therapy prior to AlloSCT might compromise outcome has not been reproduced in other larger patient cohorts [15, 92, 107]. An analysis of IBMTR data on 882 AlloSCT CML patients showed that IFN-$\alpha$ therapy prior to transplantation had no adverse impact on outcome [107].

Myeloablative chemotherapy, followed by syngeneic or AlloSCT is able, in a subset of patients, to achieve persistent and durable disappearance of Ph positive cells and to prevent progression to the blastic phase, and thus cure the disease [4, 5, 20, 25, 34, 40, 41, 92, 94]. Data on AlloSCT in CML indicates that the most important factor in obtaining long-term disease control is the development and persistence of durable cytogenetic CR (CCR) [12, 22, 24, 35, 51, 97, 109, 153, 171, 195]. Any other potentially-curative therapy in CML would thus probably be required to achieve a significant CCR rate.

## Alpha Interferon Therapy

In 1986, the MD Anderson group reported that IFN-α was able induce CCR in CML patients and it was thus identified as the first agent capable of doing so without causing marrow ablation [214]. In analyzing current data on IFN-α studies of CML, uniform criteria for hematologic and cytogenetic responses, as proposed originally, will be used (Table 8) [210]. A CHR refers to a complete normalization of the peripheral counts

**Table 8.** Criteria for response to IFN-A in CML.

| Response | Category | Criteria |
|---|---|---|
| Hematologic Remission | Complete | Normalization of WBC counts to <9x10⁹/L with normal differential<br>Normalization of platelet counts to <450x10⁹/L<br>Disappearance of all signs and symptoms of disease |
| | Partial | Normalization of WBC with persistent immature peripheral cells, or splenomegaly or thrombocytosis at <50% pretreatment level. |
| Cytogenetic Remission | Complete* | No evidence of Ph-positive cells |
| | Partial* | 1% to 34% of metaphases Ph-positive |
| | Minor | 35% to 90% of metaphases Ph-positive |
| | None | All analyzable cells Ph-positive |

*Major cytogenetic response includes complete and partial cytogenetic responses.

**Table 9.** Results of Treatment with IFN-A in 274 Patients in Early Chronic Phase CML at M.D. Anderson

| Response | Category | No (%) |
|---|---|---|
| Complete hematologic response | | 219 (80) |
| Cytogenetic response | Any* | 159 (58) |
| | Complete | 72 (26) |
| | Partial | 32 (12) |
| | Minor | 55 (20) |
| Partial hematologic response | | 19 (7) |
| Resistant | | 36 (13) |

Includes patients treated with IFN-A, alone or combined with IFN-gamma or hydroxyurea.
*All with complete hematologic response.

**Table 10.** Response to IFN-A based therapy in CML by Phase and Time From Diagnosis

| Time From Diagnosis (mos) | No. Of Patients | No. (%) | |
|---|---|---|---|
| | | CHR | Major Cytogenetic Response |
| Chronic | | | |
| <12 | 274 | 219 (80) | 104 (38) |
| >12 to <36 | 72 | 47 (62) | 6 (8) |
| >36 | 42 | 23 (49) | 4 (8) |
| Accelerated | 61 | 32 (52) | 4 (7) |
| Blastic | 5 | 1 (20) | 0 (0) |

(WBC < $10 \times 10^9$/l), platelets < $450 \times 10^9$/l, absence of immature cells and all signs and symptoms of disease including palpable organomegaly. Patients in CHR are further classified by the degree of Ph suppression (cytogenetic response): 1) CCR (Ph = 0%), partial cytogenetic response (Ph 1% to 34%), and minor cytogenetic response (Ph 35% to 90%). A major cytogenetic response includes CCR and partial cytogenetic responses (Ph < 35%). Long-term follow-up data on patients with early chronic phase CML treated at MD Anderson with IFN-α alone or combined with IFN-γ or HU are now available (Tables 9, 10) [133]. Among 274 patients treated from 1982 through 1990 with IFN-α programs using IFN-α at 5 million units (MU)/$m^2$ daily or the maximally tolerated lower dose schedule, 80% achieved CHR, and 58% had a cytogenetic response (complete 26%, major 38%). The median survival was 89 months (confidence interval 66 to 102 months). Achieving a cytogenetic response after 12 months of therapy was associated with a statistically longer survival by landmark analysis: the 5-year survival rates dated from 12 months into therapy were 90% for CCR, 88% for partial cytogenetic response, 76% for minor cytogenetic response, and 38% for other response categories. A multivariate analysis incorporating major cytogenetic response as a time-dependent variable showed it to be an independent prognostic factor for survival: patients achieving a major cytogenetic response had a 0.21 risk of death per unit time compared with the total study group [125]. Thus the favorable outcome among patients achieving a cytogenetic response was not from identification of "an intrinsically more favorable group" that would live longer regardless of therapy as the benefit of cytogenetic response was observed after accounting for the prognostic effect of known pretreatment variables by multivariate analysis. Confirming this finding is the observation of the favorable impact of cytogenetic response within prognostic risk groups by landmark analysis (Table 5). Survival improvement is due to a delay in progression to the blastic phase and is independent of the pretreatment characteristics.

Studies from many single institutions and cooperative groups have confirmed the efficacy of IFN-α in CML. (Table 11) [1-3, 6, 9, 21, 24, 38, 45, 47, 79, 87, 101–103, 106, 122, 125, 127, 131, 138–140, 171, 172, 175, 179, 199, 202, 205, 211, 213, 214, 217, 218, 220, 221, 226]. Patients treated in early chronic phase CML by Alimena et al., had a CHR rate of 46% and a cytogenetic response rate of 55% (major 12%) [1]. Analysis of patients randomized to IFN-α 5 million units (MU)/m$^2$ or 2 MU/m$^2$ three times weekly, showed a statistically better CHR rate with the higher dose schedule (57% versus 38%), and led to subsequent use of IFN-α 5 MU/m$^2$ daily – a dose-response relationship for IFN-α in CML later confirmed by Freund et al [79]. In another study, the Cancer and Leukemia Group B (CALGB) increased the intended dose of IFN-α from 2 MU/m$^2$ 5 times weekly to 5 MU/m$^2$ daily, after observing poor responses among the first 16 patients on study (excluded from subsequent analysis) [179]. In this study, the hematologic response rate was 59% (CHR 22%, partial 36%), the cytogenetic response rate was 29% (CCR 18% among 78 evaluable patients, 13% among the total 107 study patients), and the median survival was 66 months. The median dose schedule of IFN-α delivered was 3.2 MU/m$^2$ daily; 38% of patients had their dose reduced by 50% or more. The authors did not find a positive relationship between achieving a cytogenetic response and survival, but the number of patients with major (and complete) cytogenetic response was low. In a study by Mahon et al., 101 patients were treated in a single institution with IFN-α 5 MU/m$^2$ daily. [156]. The CHR rate was 79%, and the major cytogenetic response rate was 42% (CCR 32%). Estimated 5-year survival of the 101 patients was 72% and was significantly influenced by the CHR rate at three months ($p = 0.01$) and the achievement of major or CCR ($p < 0.0003$ and $p = 0.0001$, respectively). The most significant factor predicting for achievement of a major cytogenetic remission was the achievement of CHR within three months ($p < 0.0001$). Minor cytogenetic response at three month was also a strong predictive factor ($p = 0.0014$).

Recently four randomized trials comparing IFN-α versus conventional chemotherapy have been reported [2, 103, 111, 176]. Table 11 summari-

**Table 11.** Results of IFN-A Therapy in Early Chronic-Phase CML

| Study | Therapy | No. of Patients | Median Daily Dose IFN-A (MU/m²) | | CHR (%) | CG Response (%) | | | Median Survival (mo) |
|---|---|---|---|---|---|---|---|---|---|
| | | | Planned | Delivered | | Any | Major | Complete | |
| Alimena [1] | IFN-A | 65 | 1 to 2.5 | – | 46 | 55 | 12 | – | – |
| Ohnishi [176] | IFN-A | 80 | 5 | 4.0 | 39 | 44 | 7.5 | 9 | 65+ |
| Mahon [156] | IFN-A | 101 | 5 | 5 | 78 | – | 42 | 32 | 60+ |
| Ozer [179] | IFN-A | 107 | 5 | 3.2 | 59 | – | 29 | 13 | 66 |
| Hehlmann [103] | IFN-A | 133 | 5 | 3 | 31 | 18 | 10 | 7 | 66 |
| ICSG-CML [111] | IFN-A | 218 | 5 | 4.3 | 62 | 55 | 19 | 8 | 72 |
| MDACC [133] | IFN-A | 274 | 5 | 5 | 80 | 56 | 38 | 26 | 89 |
| Allan [2] | IFN-A | 293 | 3 to 12 | 2 (3.2) | 68 | 22 | 11 | 6 | 61 |
| Guilhot [101] | IFN-A | 324 | 5 | 5 | 54 | – | 22 | 7 | 60+ |

zes the results of large IFN-α studies in terms of study design, patient numbers, IFN-α dose intended and delivered, CHR and cytogenetic response profiles, and survival results. In three of the prospective randomized studies IFN-α therapy prolonged survival and delayed progression to the blastic phase when compared with conventional therapy with HU or BU [2, 111, 176]. In a German/Swiss CML study, IFN-α was superior to BU therapy, but did not demonstrate a survival advantage over HU [103]. In all four randomized trials, IFN-α therapy produced a higher rate of major and CCR than conventional chemotherapy.

**Italian Study.** In the Italian Cooperative Study Group on CML (ICSG-CML) patients were randomized to receive IFN-α 5 MU/m² daily or therapy with HU or BU [111]. Between July 1986 and July 1988, 322 patients, representing 25% of the estimated number of available newly-presenting CML patients, were randomized on a 2:1 ratio IFN-α to conventional therapy. Patients under 70 years of age with proven CML in early chronic phase were eligible. The 218 patients randomized to IFN-α therapy had a significantly higher incidence of major cytogenetic response (19% vs 1%, $p < .01$), although the CCR rate was only 8%. Patients receiving IFN-α also had a significantly longer survival (median survival 72 vs 52 months; $p = 0.002$), and a significantly prolonged time to development of accelerated or blastic phase (median time >72 vs 45 months; $p < .001$). Six year survival rate was 50% in the IFN-α cohort, versus 29% in the chemotherapy cohort; $p = 0.002$. The median dose of IFN-α delivered was 4.3 MU/m² daily. Thirty-one percent of patients had IFN-α treatment discontinued, 16% had it discontinued for IFN-α-related adverse events (predominantly influenza-like, gastrointestinal, neurologic) and 18% of patients had IFN-α dose reductions of greater than 50%. By landmark analysis, patients who had achieved at least a CHR after 8 months of therapy had a significantly better survival (5-year survival rate 78% vs 48%; $p < .001$), as did those who had a cytogenetic response after 24 months of therapy (5-year survival rate 88% vs 65% months; $p < .001$).

**German/Swiss Studies.** In the German/Swiss CML studies patients were randomized to receive IFN-α or HU or BU.[103] These cohorts involved 133, 194 and 186 patients respectively. Patients treated with either IFN-α or HU had significantly better survivals than those receiving BU therapy with median survivals of 66, 56, and 45 months respectively ($p < .01$), with no evident survival difference between the IFN-α and HU arms

($p$ = .44). The median IFN-α dose delivered after the first four weeks was 3 MU/m² daily. Twenty-five percent of patients had IFN-α therapy discontinued. Karyotypic analysis was carried out in only 63% of patients receiving IFN-α therapy and overall only 15 patients (7%) had a CCR. The estimated 3 year survival rates were 100% for cytogenetic responders versus 72% for non-responders ($p$ = .20). Possible reasons for the lack of a demonstrable survival advantage in the IFN-α cohort may be (1) the lower dose of IFN-α therapy actually delivered with a consequent lower percentage of patients achieving a significant cytogenetic response; (2) different entry criteria i.e., treating only symptomatic disease (more advanced patients); (3) a higher percentage of poor-risk patients on study, as well as of patients with advanced/accelerated disease; and (4) early IFN-α discontinuation in about 20% of patients, half of whom went on to receive BU, a clearly inferior therapy.

**MRC Study.** The MRC study involved the randomization of patients to receive maintenance therapy with IFN-α or cytotoxic therapy, usually HU.[2] All patients underwent a cytoreductive induction phase in which they received HU, BU or BU plus thioguanine. Maintenance therapy began as per randomization when patients had maintained a low normal WBC count for at least a four week period. Between September 1986 and April 1994, 587 patients were randomized. Patients under 75 years of age with proven CML in early chronic phase were eligible. The 293 patients randomized to IFN-α had a significantly prolonged survival than the 294 patients who received either HU or BU (median survivals 61 and 41 months, respectively; $p$ = 0.0009). Only 59 patients (22%) had any cytogenetic response (complete 5%; partial 6%), and they had a significantly better survival compared with the other patients. The 5-year survival rates were 100% in patients with a CCR, 92% in those with a partial cytogenetic response, 59% in those with a minor cytogenetic response, and 47% in those with no cytogenetic response. Five year survival rates were 52% in the IFN-α cohort, 34% in the chemotherapy cohort; ($p$ = 0.004). The median daily dose of IFN-α actually received was 3.2 MU or about 1.9 MU/m². Patients achieving CHR did significantly better than those who had lesser degrees of hematologic response ($p$ = .01). Patients treated with IFN-α survived longer than those treated with conventional therapy even if they had not demonstrably achieved a cytogenetic response.

**Japanese Study.** On a multicenter Japanese study patients were randomized to receive IFN-$\alpha$ 5 MU/m$^2$ daily or therapy with BU [176]. Between October 1988 and October 1991, 159 patients who could be evaluated were randomized. Patients under 70 years of age with proven CML in early chronic phase were eligible. The 80 patients randomized to IFN-$\alpha$ therapy had a significantly higher incidence of major cytogenetic response than the 79 patients who received BU therapy (16% vs 5%; $p = .046$). The predicted five year survival rate was 54% in the IFN-$\alpha$ cohort, 32% in the BU cohort; ($p = 0.03$). Patients achieving any cytogenetic response with either IFN-$\alpha$ or BU therapy survived significantly longer than patients who did not. In this study, the median daily IFN-$\alpha$ dose delivered was approximately 4 MU/m$^2$.

In summary, cytogenetic response to IFN-$\alpha$ is generally correlated with survival and in two studies that failed to show this prognostic association, both had a low rate of major cytogenetic responses possibly because of low actual doses of IFN-$\alpha$ administered (Table 12) [103, 179]. Two other studies showing a correlation between cytogenetic response and survival also reported that patients on IFN-$\alpha$ therapy who did not achieve a cytogenetic response had survivals equivalent to patients receiving conventional chemotherapy [111, 125]. The MRC study showed a survival advantage for patients receiving IFN-$\alpha$ even without achieving

**Table 12.** Summary of Response and Survival Results With IFN-$\alpha$ Therapy

|  | Design | Survival Advantage with | | |
|---|---|---|---|---|
|  |  | IFN-A Therapy | CHR | Cytogenetic Response |
| MDACC [133] | Single arm | NA | + | + |
| Ozer [179] | Single arm | NA | ND | − |
| Mahon [156] | Single arm | NA | + | + |
| ICSG-CML [111] | Randomized | + | + | + |
| Hehlmann [103] | Randomized | + v busulfan − v hydroxyurea | + | trend |
| Allan [2] | Randomized | + | + | + |
| Ohnishi [176] | Randomized | + | ND | + |
| Guilhot [101] | Randomized (INF-$\alpha$±ara-C) | + | + | + |

NA = not applicable; ND = not done

a cytogenetic response; still, patients achieving a cytogenetic response also had a better survival than those who did not [2].

As shown in Table 11, CHR rates in similar study populations (i.e., early chronic phase CML) have ranged from 31% to 80%. Some of variability in the CHR rates may be due to different response criteria or protocol treatment designs. The use of IFN-α monotherapy in the German/Swiss and CALGB studies, as opposed to allowing the addition of chemotherapy in others, may have produced a lower CHR rate. This would not explain the large differences in the cytogenetic (18% to 58%), major cytogenetic (10% to 38%) and complete cytogenetic (6% to 26%) response rates. Differences in cytogenetic response results may be due to (1) different risk group distributions; (2) patient and physician motivation; (3) the actual dose of IFN-α delivered; (4) the frequency of cytogenetic studies; (5) inclusion of advanced or accelerated phase patients and (6) IFN-α monotherapy as induction with consequent higher early dropout rates. When patients were analyzed for response to IFN-α and for survival within risk groups, current data still showed an IFN-α-associated advantage in each risk group [133], suggesting the value of IFN-α dose-intensity to increase the quality of cytogenetic response and to prolong survival. As with any new anti-cancer therapy, a "learning curve" may exist which improves the results as experience is gained. The CCR rate in the first MD Anderson IFN-α CML study was 14%, similar to some current multi center results, and may be in part due to unfamiliarity with IFN-α-related toxicities [175] and consequent excess dose reductions.

Comparing the median dose of IFN-α delivered among responders versus non-responders is misleading since many studies have, in the treatment design, built-in dose reductions after achieving a response, and dose escalations with resistant disease [2, 103, 111]. Such an approach (higher dosages for resistant disease, lower dosages for responsive disease) would preclude meaningful analyses of the relationship of IFN-α dose-intensity with response within a particular study. However, comparison of the actual median dose of IFN-α delivered versus response rate among different studies may help demonstrating the dose-response phenomenon. Table 11 summarizes the response rates in different studies by the median actual dose of IFN-α delivered. Table 13 shows the dose-response relationship in studies intended to deliver lower versus higher IFN-α doses, and suggests a relationship between IFN-α dose intensity and hematologic and cytogenetic response rates. The extent to which

**Table 13.** Response with IFN-A therapy with different dose schedules.

| Study | IFN-A dose | Schedule | No. Patients | CHR (%) | Cytogenetic responses (%) | | |
|---|---|---|---|---|---|---|---|
| | | | | | Any | Major | Complete |
| MDACC [133] | 5 MU/m$^2$ | Daily | 274 | 80 | 58 | 38 | 26 |
| Schofield et al [202] | 2 MU/m$^2$ | Daily$_{28}$/TIW | 27 | 70 | 33 | 22 | 7 |
| Alimena et al [1] | 5 MU/m$^2$ | TIW | 30 | 63 | NS | NS | NS |
| | 2 MU/m$^2$ | TIW | 30 | 24 | NS | NS | NS |
| Freund et al [79] | 5 MU/m$^2$ | TIW | 10 | 33 | 0 | 0 | 0 |
| Anger et al [3] | 3 MU/m$^2$ | Daily$_{14}$/TIW | 9 | 22 | 20 | 0 | 0 |

TIW=three times a week; NS=Not stated. Daily$_n$/TIW=Daily for n days followed by TIW

variability in the frequency of cytogenetic studies impacts on the documented incidence of cytogenetic response remains to be documented.

A recent study by Schofield et al. suggested that a lower dose schedule of IFN-$\alpha$ i.e., 2 MU/m$^2$ 3 times weekly was as effective as the higher dose schedules of 5 MU/m$^2$ daily recommended for CML (weekly dose 6 MU/m$^2$ versus 35 MU/m$^2$) [202]. The former regimen would certainly be less toxic and less expensive. This report was based on a comparative analysis of 27 patients treated in early chronic phase CML with published data. Comparison of an MD Anderson cohort of 274 patients equivalent to those in the Denver cohort indicates similar overall hematologic response rates, but the incidences and quality of cytogenetic responses was significantly better with the higher IFN-$\alpha$ dose schedules (Table 13). This is an important issue if achievement of minimal residual disease at the cytogenetic level (as discussed later) is associated with a survival benefit. This is further supported by the initial CALGB experience with the lower IFN-$\alpha$ dose schedule, by the comparative study of Alimena et al. with the 2 dose schedules of IFN-$\alpha$, and by other studies of low-dose IFN-$\alpha$ schedules (Table 13) [1, 79]. Another important issue is the relationship between response of to IFN-$\alpha$ and risk groups as outlined in Table 5. The 27 patients reported on by the Denver group predominantly belonged to a good-risk subgroup, in whom the expected major cytogenetic response rate would be 46% to 52% (rather than the reported 22% rate) and the resultant median survival would be expected to be 8 to 9 years [133, 202]. While current data in CML suggest a benefit from higher or maximally tolerated dose schedule of IFN-$\alpha$, the optimal IFN-$\alpha$ dose schedule is controversial, and randomized studies of low versus high dose IFN-$\alpha$ schedules are currently ongoing.


Importance of Achieving Minimal Tumor Burden in CML

In human malignancies, achieving a minimal tumor burden is a prerequisite for improvement of survival or for achieving cures. The causal association between Ph-related molecular events and development of CML encourages the acceptance of Ph reduction as indicative of a reduced CML tumor burden. Reduction in tumor burden as reflected by achieving CHR has been associated with significant survival prolongation in all studies in which it has been examined [2, 103, 111, 156].

Achieving a minimal cytogenetic tumor burden was also associated with a significant survival or remission duration advantage by landmark and/or multivariate analysis in six of eight studies; with a positive trend being observed in a seventh study [2, 111, 125, 155, 176]. In the Japanese study discussed above achieving any cytogenetic response was associated with a significantly better duration of chronic phase CML (5-year rates 79% vs 22%; $p = .0017$) but only a trend for better survival ($p = .10$) [176]. The recent study by Guilhot et al. also showed a significant independent survival advantage with IFN-$\alpha$ alone, or with IFN-$\alpha$ plus ara-C, among patients achieving CHR or cytogenetic response [101]. Thus, most current data suggest that achieving a minimal CML tumor burden as reflected by hematologic and cytogenetic remissions will impact outcome favorably, and should be pursued as a therapeutic objective in future investigations.

## Management of IFN-a-Related Problems

IFN-$\alpha$ requires subcutaneous injection, is relatively expensive and its administration requires knowledge of its potential adverse events, and motivation on the part of both the patient and physician. Clear goals and end points need to be determined at the start of therapy to avoid early discouragement, and to ensure an adequate therapeutic trial of IFN-$\alpha$. Tachyphylaxis to the acute adverse-effects of IFN-$\alpha$ develops within 1 to 2 weeks. Early adverse events such as fever, chills, postnasal drip, and anorexia are usually not dose limiting [186, 213]. The severity of these initial effects is increased with increasing WBC. This may be related to the release of cytokines from the circulating hematopoietic cells, with high tumor burden resulting in more acute side effects. CML cells have been found to have high levels of leukotriene C4, which may induce an inflammatory response. Thus, IFN-$\alpha$ therapy should not be initiated immediately at diagnosis when WBC counts are elevated, often to >100x10$^9$/l. These may be avoided by initial cytoreduction with HU (until the leukocyte count is < 20x10$^9$/l) before instituting IFN-$\alpha$ therapy, by premedication with acetaminophen, nighttime injections, and by starting therapy at 25% to 50% of the recommended dose for the first week, and increasing dosage as tachyphylaxis occurs during the first weeks of therapy. Delayed adverse-effects are dose-limiting in some 10% to 20% of patients, and include persistent fatigue, weight loss, neurotoxicity, depression, insomnia, alopecia, marrow hypoplasia and occasional immune-mediated complications [186, 200, 216]. Autoimmune disorders are noted in 5% of patients [43, 88, 186, 192, 200]. These have included immune-mediated hemolysis or thrombocytopenia, collagen vascular disorders such as rheumatoid arthritis and systemic lupus erythematosus, nephrotic syndrome and hypothyroidism. Rare cases of cardiac dysfunction (arrhythmias, congestive heart failure) have been reported. Severe auto-immune phenomena, cardiac dysfunction, refractory depression or severe neurotoxicity necessitate discontinuation of IFN-α therapy. Immune-mediated thyroid disease does not require IFN-α discontinuation and may be managed by standard therapy. A particularly challenging issue is the therapy of pregnant CML patients – some patients treated successfully with IFN-α while pregnant have been reported [7, 9].

Patients experiencing fatigue shortly after the daily injection may benefit from receiving their IFN-α dose at bedtime. A triad of depression, fatigue, and insomnia (which resembles "jet-lag") is common and can be improved with amitriptyline 25–50 mg at bedtime. Patients sleep excessively in the first few days after this therapy is started, before the response is noted, and beginning this treatment on weekends may allow the patient to continue normal week-time activities. Some patients respond better to other antidepressants (e.g.. fluoxetine, sertraline) if one component of the symptom triad is more prominent; in such cases a neuropsychiatric consult is helpful. Patient education is essential to maintain compliance. Some practical recommendations are included in Table 14 [175].

The actual dose of IFN-α received may be important for obtaining cytogenetic response (Table 13). Patients receiving less than 5 MU/m² three times a week have less than 10% incidence of major cytogenetic remissions as opposed to a 40% likelihood of a major cytogenetic response if receiving 5 MU/m² daily. IFN-α toxicity increases with dose, and efforts should be made to improve the tolerance to IFN-α and optimize compliance. Patients who develop serious toxicities should discontinue IFN-α until these toxicities resolve. Therapy may then be reinstituted with a 50% dose reduction. Moderate chronic toxicities may be alleviated by a 25% reduction of IFN-α. IFN-α should not be discontinued for moderate leukopenia (WBC count between 3 and 5x10⁹/l) – this practice is counterproductive and does allow optimal IFN-α therapy. The dose of IFN-α need not be reduced unless the WBC count is less than 2.0x10⁹/l or the platelet count is less than 50x10⁹/l, in which case a 25% dose reduction of IFN-α is required [175].

**Table 14.** Practical Guidelines on IFN-A Therapy

| |
|---|
| Therapy Initiation |
|         Hydroxyurea to obtain initial cytoreduction (WBC: 10-20 x $10^9$/L). |
|         Slow dose escalation: 3 MU daily for a week; then 5 MU daily for a week; |
|             then 5 MU/m$^2$ daily or maximally tolerated individual dose. |
|         Educate patients and family members. |
| Improve Tolerance |
|         Premedicate with acetaminophen. |
|         Evening self-injection. |
|         Tricyclic antidepressants for neurologic side effects (insomnia, depression, |
|         fatigue) |
| Therapeutic Monitoring |
|         Complete blood counts weekly until counts stable then biweekly. |
|         Maintain WBC between 2 to 4 x $10^9$/L and platelets > 50 x $10^9$/L |
|         Chemistries monthly. |
|         Cytogenetic evaluation on bone marrow aspirate every 3 months in the first |
|              year then every 4 to 6 months. |
| Dose Modifications |
|         Interrupt IFN-A for grade 3 to 4 toxicities then resume at 50% |
|         Reduce IFN-A dose by 25% for grade 2 persistent toxicities. |
|         Do not reduce IFN-A dose schedule for "low counts" unless WBC |
|           is < 2 x $10^9$/L.  25% dose reduction is then appropriate. |
|         Hold IFN-A for moderate acute intercurrent disease. |
| Efficacy Assessment |
|         Hematologic remission at 3 to 6 months. |
|         Cytogenetic response by 12 months. |
|         Major cytogenetic response by 18 months. |

Patients on long-term IFN-$\alpha$ therapy may have cytogenetic analyses showing insufficient metaphases resulting from a poor quality sample. This phenomenon is often associated with difficulty in aspirating the bone marrow and may preclude efficient decision-making regarding further therapy. In addition, poor aspirations may be thought to be due to "marrow fibrosis". Colony-forming cells from patients with CML are defective in their attachment to bone marrow stromal cells. In vitro IFN-$\alpha$ can increase the adherence of primitive CML cells to bone marrow stroma by reducing the amount of neuraminic acid on the stromal cells [69]. Thus, IFN-$\alpha$ may change the marrow microenvironment so that CML progenitors are brought back under local control and produce changes in the extracellular matrix that make aspiration of the marrow more difficult.

To investigate the influence of IFN-$\alpha$ on marrow fibrosis associated with CML, the MD Anderson group recently conducted a study in which 82 marrow biopsies from 41 patients in chronic phase CML were stained with Snook's reticulin stain for argyrophilic fibers [227]. Grading of reticulin fibrosis (scale of 1 to 4) was according to the quantity and pattern of distribution of reticulin. The interval between biopsies was a median of 25 months (range, 12–40). Patients had been treated with IFN-α for at least 12 months, were still on IFN-α during the study, and had achieved at least a CHR. Before the start of IFN-α therapy, reticulin fibrosis was grade 1 in 23 patients (56%) and grade 3 in 18 (44%). During IFN-α therapy, marrow reticulin fibrosis did not increase or was reduced in 33 patients (80%), and increased by one grade in 8 patients (20%). Only 5 patients (12%) with limited fibrosis (grade 1) before start of IFN-α therapy showed an increase towards significant fibrosis (grade 3), while 8 of the 18 (44%) patients with grade 3 fibrosis decreased their grade of fibrosis. Thus, IFN-α therapy was not associated with an enhancing effect on myelofibrosis in patients with CML, and may have prevented increasing fibrosis in patients who responded to therapy. The lack of significant fibrosis in IFN-α treated patients is corroborated by the fact that patients receiving AlloSCT after prior IFN-α therapy showed no significant difference in the time to neutrophil or platelet recovery, or in survival, when compared with similar patients who had not received IFN-α treatment [92]. Stopping IFN-α therapy 1 week before obtaining the bone marrow sample may increase the yield of adequate cytogenetic studies. Patients with long-standing remissions show no change in WBC counts over this period of time. Reinitiation of IFN-α after such a short interval is not associated with significant toxicities. Planning a bone marrow harvest in these patients necessitates prior discontinuation of IFN-α for 1 month in order to obtain adequate cells for subsequent engraftment.

## Duration of IFN-a Therapy and Monitoring of Response

Though major cytogenetic remissions induced by IFN-α therapy are durable, it is uncertain how long they can last after IFN-α therapy is stopped. One approach is to continue IFN-α therapy until a CCR had been documented for 3 years. At that point the decision whether to continue treatment is left to the individual investigator and patient team. In an M.D Anderson group of 34 patients, 18 were continued on IFN-α therapy, sometimes with a dose reduction. All of these patients continue in CCR. Sixteen patients had their therapy discontinued because of toxicity (5 patients) or patient or physician choice (11 patients). Seven patients continue in CR at a median of 40 months off therapy (range, 18+ to 62+ months); nine patients showed increase in Ph-positive cells. IFN-$\alpha$ therapy was reinitiated in six patients, three of whom showed only normal diploid cells after reinstitution of therapy and three of whom showed reduction of Ph-positive cells to < 35%. Three patients with recurrent Ph-positive cells remain without treatment in continued hematologic remission.

More sensitive techniques such as the polymerase chain reaction (PCR) detect rare cells with a BCR rearrangement in most patients with CML in remission after IFN-$\alpha$ therapy.[67,151] However, these patients may remain in remission (sometimes even after discontinuing therapy), do not develop blastic phase CML, and have prolonged survival. The PCR technique may be detecting non-clonogenic cells; alternatively, the immune system may be able to control such minimal residual disease and prevent relapse. The PCR procedure is not useful for making treatment decisions since its results are not easily quantifiable and since, more importantly, the clinical relevance of PCR positivity is unknown. A new technique may be more useful for deciding if patients in remission may discontinue therapy. Hypermetaphase fluorescent in situ hybridization (FISH) allows a large number of cells (500) to be rapidly screened for the presence of the Ph using a fluorescent probe that overlaps the region of the translocation at chromosome 9q34 [203, 230]. In individuals with normal chromosomes, only two fluorescent spots will be seen, corresponding to two normal 9 chromosomes. However, translocations between chromosomes 9 and 22 will allow detection of a third signal representing a small piece of chromosome 9 now present on chromosome 22. This method may allow more informed decisions on the need to continue therapy. Patients in CCR for 3 years and with no evidence of Ph-positive cells by hypermetaphase FISH may have their treatment tapered or discontinued. Reappearance of even $\geq$ 4% Ph-positive cells (10 of 500) would be a significant change and such data may help in therapeutic decisions.

Currently the options of continuous IFN-$\alpha$ treatment, lowering the dose for patients with significant side effects, or stopping therapy are all possibilities. If therapy is stopped, this would require careful follow-up and regular cytogenetic analysis to ensure that IFN-$\alpha$ is restarted immediately if evidence of disease recurrence is documented. A current common practice of stopping IFN-$\alpha$ therapy as soon as a CCR is achieved may jeopardize the treatment goals.

## Alpha Interferon / Cytotoxic Combinations

Initial studies of IFN-α plus cytotoxic agents were conducted in order to investigate whether (1) patients who failed to achieve a CHR or cytogenetic remission on IFN-α alone might do so with combined therapy and (2) whether cytogenetic remission rates might be improve by increased myelosuppression associated with combination therapy. IFN-α combinations with HU and ara-C were initially investigated in patients with late chronic phase disease [87, 122]. Ara-C selectively suppresses the growth of CML cells over that of normal hematopoietic cells in vitro [207].

Data from a UK group indicated that IFN-α/HU seemed to prolong late chronic phase in contrast to patients treated with IFN-α or cytotoxics alone [87]. The initial MD Anderson study of IFN-α and ara-C used a regimen of IFN-A 5 MU/m$^2$ daily plus ara-C 15 mg/m$^2$ daily for 7 days, repeated every 28 days [122]. Forty patients in late chronic phase and 20 patients in accelerated phase received this regimen. Patients who received the combination regimen had a higher CHR (55% vs 28%; $p = .02$) and 3 year survival rates (75% vs 48%; $p < .01$) than patients who received IFN-α alone. Guilhot et al. reported in 1993 on a pilot study of 24 patients, 12 previously untreated, who received a IFN-α/HU induction regimen followed by IFN-α/ara-C maintenance [102]. The ara-C regimen used consisted of 10–20 mg/m$^2$ daily for 10–15 days, repeated every 28 days and was only given to 10 patients who either did not get a CHR (5 patients) or who did not achieve a durable cytogenetic remission (5 patients). Although the regimen was well tolerated, it was not effective in achieving cytogenetic remissions in these resistant patients.

Other investigators began to study IFN-α/cytotoxic combinations in patients with early chronic phase disease (Table 15). Anger et al. documented the efficacy of a IFN-α/HU combination in a small cohort of newly diagnosed CML patients.[3] Elliott et al. reported on this combination in a larger cohort of 31 patients in early chronic phase and documented a major cytogenetic response in 39% of patients with CCR in 29% [72]. Arthur et al. reported on a cohort of 30 patients treated in early chronic phase CML with IFN-α and low dose ara-C [6]. All patients underwent a cytoreductive induction phase in which they received HU with IFN-α. Maintenance therapy began when patients had reached the maximum tolerated dose of IFN-α or four weeks, whichever was shorter. The ara-C regimen used consisted of 20 mg/m$^2$ daily for 21 days, repeated every 42 days. Repeated cycles of ara-C were given for 12 months after

**Table 15.** Summary of Response and Survival Results With IFN-A/Ara-C Therapy In Early Chronic Phase CML

| Study | Patient Number | (Regimen) IFN/day | Ara-C/28days | CHR (%) | Major CR (%) | Complete CR (%) | Survival (%) – (yr) |
|---|---|---|---|---|---|---|---|
| Arthur et al [6] | 30 | 5 MU/m² | 280 mg/m² | 93 | 53 | 33 | 76 – (6) |
| MDACC [127] | 45 | 5 MU/m² | 105 mg/m² | 84 | 38 | 20 | 78 – (5) |
| Thaler et al [220] | 84 | 3.5 MU | 100 mg/m² | 54 | 25 | 18 | 74 – (3) |
| CALGB [205] | 88 | 5 MU/m² | 10 mg/m² BID as required | 72 | 51 | 15 | 72 – (4) |
| MDACC [127] | 93 | 5 MU/m² | 280 mg/m² | 95 | 53 | 30 | 84 – (5) |
| Guilhot et al [101] | 322 | 5 MU/m² | 200 mg/m² | 67 | 39 | 15 | 88 – (3) |

which IFN-$\alpha$ alone was continued. Patients achieved a CHR rate of 93%, and a cytogenetic response rate of 67%, which was major in 53% and complete in 33%. In a recent update, at a median follow-up of 6 years, the projected survival is 76% with median survival not yet reached. (C. Arthur, personal communication). Of the initial cohort, 9 patients are dead – 6 from AlloSCT-related complications, 3 from CML progression. Only one patient discontinued the study regimen because of adverse events.

Following the initial positive M.D. Anderson experience in late chronic phase patients, subsequent studies in a cohort of 148 early chronic phase patients also used IFN-$\alpha$/ara-C combination regimens.[127] All patients received IFN-$\alpha$ 5MU/m$^2$ daily plus Regimen A – ara-C 15 mg/m$^2$ daily for 7 days, repeated every 28 days (47 patients treated between 1989 and 1992) or Regimen B – ara-C 10 mg daily (101 patients treated between 1993 to 1997). 52% of these patients were in the good prognosis category, 15% in the poor prognosis group. With Regimen A, patients achieved a CHR rate of 84%, and a cytogenetic response rate of 64%, which was major in 38% and complete in 20%. The projected 5 year survival in this cohort is 78% with median survival not yet reached. With Regimen B, patients achieved a CHR rate of 95%, and a cytogenetic response rate of 78%, which was major in 53% and complete in 30%. Significant toxicities were: fatigue grade $\geq$ 2%–45%, grade 3–4, 11%; headache, muscle aches grade $\geq$ 2%–29%, grade 3–4, 10%; weight-loss grade $\geq$ 2%–16%; diarrhea grade $\geq$ 2%–6%; depression grade $\geq$ 2%–14%, grade 3–4, 8%; other neurotoxicities grade $\geq$ 2%–4%, thrombocytopenia, anemia grade $\geq$ 2%–16%. The daily ara-C schedule (Regimen B) appears superior to the 7 days every month ara-C (regimen A) in terms of cytogenetic remissions. This data suggests that the IFN-$\alpha$/ara-C combinations may be superior to IFN-$\alpha$ alone.

A CALGB study of an IFN-A/ara-C regimen (5 MU/m$^2$ daily s.c. and ara-C, 15 mg/m$^2$ bid, s.c. in chronic phase CML has also generated positive data in a cohort accrued between November 1990 and August 1993 [205]. Treatment consisted of cycles of therapy of sufficient duration to cause either a WBC < 2 x 10$^9$/l or platelets < 50 x 10$^9$/l. Therapy was discontinued and then resumed when the WBC was >5 x 10$^9$/l and platelets were >100 x 10$^9$/l. Of the first 35 patients, 6 exhibited grade 3 gastrointestinal toxicity; subsequently the dose of ara-C was reduced to 10 mg/m$^2$ bid, which was well tolerated. Among 88 evaluable patients, 63 (72%) had a CHR. At least one post-treatment karyotype was available from 61 patients. Of these 61, 9 (15%) achieved CCR – 6 of these patients were also bcr/abl negative by Southern blot; 3 had no bcr/abl follow up data. There was a 51% major cytogenetic response rate. Median time to major cytogenetic response was 9 months. For all 88 patients, estimated overall survival at 30, 48, and 60 months was 79%, 72%, and 58% respectively. One patient died of rhabdomyolysis. One patient developed grade 4 ARDS.

Thaler et al. reported in 1993 on the achievement of cytogenetic responses in 4 of 10 IFN-α resistant patients when ara-C was added to the IFN-α therapy [220]. This Austrian group has also recently reported their data on an IFN-α/ara-C regimen (3.5 MU flat dose daily s.c. and ara-C, 10 mg/m$^2$ s.c. for 10 days of a 28 day cycle) in chronic phase CML in a cohort accrued between April 1991 and June 1994 [221]. All patients received HU until they had a WBC < 20x10$^9$/l at which time IFN-α/ara-C maintenance therapy began. Among 84 patients who could be evaluated, 45 (54%) had a CHR. Twenty one patients (25%) achieved a major cytogenetic response ( 18% CCR). For all 84 patients, estimated overall survival at 12, 24, 36, and 48 months was 96%, 85%, 74% and 65%, respectively. Sixteen patients (19%) discontinued therapy due to adverse events – myelosuppression (7), gastrointestinal (2), depression (2), muscle and bone pain (2), injection site reaction (1), sepsis (1), and neurotoxicity (1).

In a recently reported randomized study of newly diagnosed CML patients, the combination of IFN-α and ara-C, after initial cyto-reduction with IFN-α and HU, showed a superior cytogenetic response and survival than IFN-α alone [101]. In this French study patients were randomized to receive IFN-α 5 MU/m$^2$ daily either alone or combined with monthly courses of ara-C 20 mg/m$^2$ per day for 10 days. All patients underwent a cytoreductive induction phase in which they received HU with IFN-α. Maintenance therapy began as per randomization when patients achieved a CHR. Between January 1991 and May 1996, 745 patients were randomized – 646 patients who could be evaluated were discussed in the recent report. Patients under 70 years of age with proven CML in early chronic phase were eligible. The 324 patients randomized to IFN-α/ara-C therapy had a significantly higher incidence of CHR than those patients receiving IFN-α alone (67% vs 54%, $p = 0.002$). At 12 months minimum follow-up, a major cytogenetic response was demonstrable in 39% of patients in the IFN-α/ara-C cohort in contrast to 22% in the IFN-α alone cohort; $p < 0.001$) A CCR was demonstrable in 15% of patients in the IFN-α/ara-C cohort in contrast to a 7% rate in the IFN-α alone cohort; $p < 0.001$) The IFN-α/ara-C patients also had a

significantly longer survival and a significantly prolonged time to development of accelerated or blastic phase. Three year survival rate was 88%
in the IFN-α/ara-C cohort, 76% in the IFN-α only cohort; $p$ = 0.006. The
median dose of IFN-α delivered was 5 MU/m$^2$ daily in both cohorts over
the initial 12 months therapy. Predominant ara-C-related adverse events
were gastrointestinal upset and thrombocytopenia. Approximately 22% of
patients in both arms discontinued therapy because of adverse events.
The current frontline approach for the treatment of CML in community
practice may consist of a combination of daily IFN-α (5 MU/m$^2$) and low-
dose ara-C in different schedules (10 mg/d or 10–20 mg/m$^2$ per day x7–10
days). This combination is well tolerated and associated with cytogenetic
and clinical results at least as good as those seen in our equivalent CML
patients who received therapy with IFN-α alone. As suggested by the summary in Table 15, lowering the dose of IFN-α in IFN-α/ara-C regimens
may be associated with a lower major cytogenetic response rate as is seen
with IFN-α only regimens (Table 13). A current International Oncology
Study Group (IOSG) randomized study comparing IFN-α/HU with IFN-
α/ara-C in early chronic phase CML indicates that patient compliance
with twice daily s.c. injections can be a problem [89]. Treatment with IFN-
α/ara-C may thus become more broadly applicable with the availability of
a new oral formulation of ara-C, YNK01 [105].

Current possibilities for combination with IFN-α are novel agents
such as homoharringtonine (HHT), aziothymidine (AZT), decitabine,
topotecan, all-trans retinoic acid (ATRA), tallimustine, IFN-γ, IL-1 receptor antagonists, and GM-CSF [17, 18, 44, 47, 73–75, 119, 121, 138, 148, 174, 218,
224]. In vitro data suggests a possible synergistic anti-CML interaction
between AZT and IFN-α, clinical data is not yet available [74]. HHT, a
synthetic derivative of a Chinese plant alkaloid, has been shown to be
effective in CML. An initial study of HHT alone or in combination with
ara-C in late chronic phase is encouraging [121]. Thirty-six patients with
late chronic phase CML who were resistant to IFN-α therapy received
HHT at a dose of 2.5 mg/m$^2$ daily by continuous infusion for 5 day combined with ara-C 15 mg/m$^2$ per day for 5 days divided into 2 daily s.c.
doses. The combination was given at 28 day intervals. 66% of patients
achieved a CHR and 17% had a major cytogenetic response. Adverse
events noted in 243 courses of therapy included headache (16%),
diarrhea (13%), febrile episodes (8%), fatigue (7%), and mucositis (1%).
Promising results were also reported by the Dana Farber group on a
HHT/ara-C combination in 20 patients who had received prior IFN-α

therapy [73]. Ninety-four percent of patients who could be evaluated achieved a CHR and 50% had a major cytogenetic response. These data compare favorably with those achieved with IFN-α/ara-C combination therapies and thus data on IFN-α/HHT combinations in early chronic phase are eagerly awaited.

Hypermethylation of DNA is a property of tumor progression and aggressiveness, and is found in 50% of patients with chronic phase CML, and in 100% with CML blastic phase. Decitabine is a potent hypomethylating agent which has been recently investigated in patients in accelerated and blastic phases [119]. Of an initial cohort of 37 patients treated, 20 were in blastic phase and 17 in accelerated phase. Decitabine was given as 100 mg/m² IV over 6 h at 12 hourly intervals for 10 doses (1000 mg/m² per course) in 13 patients and 75 mg/m² IV over 6 h at 12 hourly intervals for 10 doses (750 mg/m² per course) in 24 patients. In the accelerated phase group, 29% achieved a CHR, while 10% did so in blastic phase. Two patients achieved a cytogenetic response. Prolonged myelosuppression was the most significant side-effect; the median time to platelet recovery >30 x 10⁹/l was 31 days, and to granulocyte recovery >0.5 x 10⁹/l was 48 days. Febrile episodes were noted in 25 patients (62%) including documented infections in 17 (42%). Other side-effects were nausea and vomiting (12%), diarrhea (17%) and mucositis (7%). Studies of lower doses e.g., (500 mg/m² per course) of decitabine plus IFN-α in CML should be considered.

The activity of topotecan in acute myeloid leukemia and myelodysplastic syndromes has been recently reported [18]. This agent also warrants further study in CML, both in combination with IFN-α in early phase patients and in combination with other cytotoxic agents in patients who have failed or are intolerant to IFN-α. In a pilot study of ATRA in 13 patients, (7 late chronic phase, 5 accelerated phase, 1 blastic phase), significant anti-CML activity has been observed [44]. All patients were extensively pre-treated; 12 had failed IFN-α therapy. Patients received ATRA 175 mg/m² orally in two divided doses daily until evident disease progression. Four of five accelerated phase patients and one of seven late chronic phase patients showed a transient decrease in marrow and/or peripheral blood blast counts and promyelocytes and/or basophil percentages. ATRA was well tolerated with major adverse events headache, nausea, dry skin, and dry mucosal membranes. While ATRA alone is ineffective in these advanced IFN-α refractory patients, it seems worthwhile to examine IFN-α/ATRA combinations.

A potential problem in achieving major cytogenetic responses in patients who shown hematologic or minor cytogenetic response to IFN-$\alpha$ might be that the normal stem cell population has been suppressed to a point where they cannot respond once the growth advantage of the leukemic clone is partially controlled by IFN-$\alpha$. This hypothesis has been addressed by investigating the effect of adding GM-CSF to the therapy of CML patients who had a hematologic response but failed to achieve or lost a major cytogenetic response to IFN-$\alpha$ [47]. There are currently ten patients who can be evaluated for response. Patients received GM-CSF 30 mg/m² daily s.c. GM-CSF was held when WBC increased above 10 x 10⁹/l, and restarted once counts decreased. If tolerated, the dose was escalated to 60 mg/m². Patients showing an improved cytogenetic response continued on maintenance therapy at the same dose for two years after achievement of CCR. IFN-$\alpha$ was continued throughout the study at the same dose the patient was receiving prior to the start of therapy, and dose escalation was allowed as tolerated. Three patients (30%) achieved a major cytogenetic remission with the combination therapy. A fourth patient had a partial cytogenetic remission while on protocol therapy, with 90% diploid cells, which evolved to a CCR shortly after discontinuation of therapy, which has been maintained for over 4 years. Two other patients had minor responses (although one was significant, from 4% diploid to 50% diploid). Therapy was well tolerated in all cases, with no GM-CSF attributable adverse events. The addition of GM-CSF to IFN-$\alpha$ therapy seems beneficial in some patients with IFN-$\alpha$ sensitive CML in whom less than a major cytogenetic response has been achieved with IFN-$\alpha$ alone. Since achieving a major cytogenetic response translates into prolonged survival, this combination therapy should be further investigated.

## Alpha Interferon and Allogeneic Stem Cell Transplantation

AlloSCT is the an effective option for long-term disease control of younger patients with newly diagnosed CML and seems curative in some [5, 8, 20, 25, 34, 40, 41, 51, 91, 94, 97, 107, 133, 160]. However, this treatment is only available to 15% to 25% of CML patients because of age limitations and HLA compatible donor availability. AlloSCT is associated with a significant risk of early mortality and morbidity due to graft-versus-host disease (GVHD) and other SCT-related complications, which contribute to a 30% early SCT-related mortality rate. AlloSCT for CML in chronic phase results in a 3- to 5-year survival rate of 40% to 80%. Mortality is higher with older age, and many transplant centers limit AlloSCT to patients younger than 55 years of age, although recently selected elderly patients have been successfully treated. Other adverse pretransplant prognostic factors include prior therapy with BU, male recipient-female donor pair, and greater length of time from diagnosis to transplantation.[20] In general, AlloSCT is recommended for the younger patients with CML as soon as an HLA-identical-related donor is identified. For older patients, or for patients without an HLA-identical related donor, an initial trial of IFN-α-based therapy is appropriate. Patients achieving a cytogenetic response within 12 months should continue on IFN-α therapy unless they lose the cytogenetic response or develop disease progression. Patients who do not obtain a cytogenetic response within 12 months of initiation of IFN-α therapy should proceed to AlloSCT if an HLA-compatible donor is identified, and they are eligible for this procedure. If this is not available, patients may continue on IFN-α-based therapy because at least one trial has shown a survival advantage regardless of cytogenetic response.[2] Alternatively, patients may be offered investigational approaches aimed at Ph-positive cell suppression such as HHT or intensive chemotherapy with purged AutoSCT [11, 108, 128, 132, 136, 164, 188, 212, 215]. IFN-α may also be effective in patients with cytogenetic relapse post AlloSCT if retransplantation (possibly with donor lymphocytes) is not an option [8, 10, 14, 42, 52, 53, 70, 85, 93, 106, 107, 115, 142, 160, 163, 183, 201]. Higano et al. found that patients who relapsed after AlloSCT for chronic phase CML are often very responsive to treatment with IFN-α [106]. Among the first 29 such patients treated, nine (31%) achieved a CCR with IFN-α, and seven of these remained Ph negative 4–7 years after treatment. In addition, 11 patients in CHR but in cytogenetic relapse were treated with IFN-α and nine achieved a CCR. An exciting approach recently described is the use of infusions of unirradiated donor buffy coat cells, often with IFN-α, to treat recurrent CML. This therapy was developed with the hope that such infusions would augment a graft-versus-leukemia effect. In one series, results on 84 patients were reported of whom 54 (72%) of evaluable patients achieved a CCR [142]. Most patients had a flare of acute GVHD with the buffy coat infusions, approximately half had at least transient pancytopenia, and the one year mortality was 18%. Many of these patients were treated with very high numbers of buffy coat cells and current studies are establishing whether lower buffy coat doses may be as effective and less toxic and whether growth factor mobilized buffy coat can reduce the period of pancytopenia. Recent data on the use of anti-*bcr-abl* oligonucleotide and the use of CML dendritic cells, whose proliferation is selectively enhanced by GM-CSF and other cytokines, to generate enhanced cellular cytotoxicity against the malignant clone may further enhance the use of immunemodulatory therapy [37, 161, 187].

## Late Chronic and Accelerated Phase

Late chronic phase CML is defined by the diagnosis of CML for greater than 1 year. This was based on the early experience with IFN-α showing a decrease in responsiveness with increasing time from diagnosis. Recently, data on 137 patients in late chronic phase treated at MD Anderson from 1982 through 1990 with a series of IFN-α based regimens – human leukocyte IFN-α (7 patients), recombinant IFN-α alone (15 patients), IFN-α plus IFN-γ (29 patients), IFN-α/HU (19 patients), or IFN-α/ara-C (67 patients) has been reported [199]. The duration of disease from diagnosis was greater than 1 year in 39% of patients, greater than 2 years in 22%, and greater than 3 years in 39%. The overall CHR rate was 57%–62% in those less than 36 months from initial diagnosis and 49% in those with a diagnosis to IFN-α treatment interval of more than 36 months. Ten patients (8%) had a major cytogenetic response; 8 of whom were treated with IFN-α/ ara-C. The estimated median overall survival was 49 months, with an estimated 5-years survival rate of 41%. The results of this analysis confirm that IFN-α has modest activity in late chronic phase CML.

Because of relatively low cytogenetic response rate to IFN-α, patients in late chronic phase CML should undergo AlloSCT as soon as a donor is identified. Patients without an HLA-compatible related donor should be considered for investigational approaches.

Patients in late chronic phase CML are potential candidates for investigational strategies aimed at defining new active agents in CML or improving the results of IFN-α therapy. Patients ineligible or unwilling to explore investigational strategies may benefit from combination therapy with IFN-α, e.g., addition of ara-C, HU.

Patients in accelerated phase should receive AlloSCT as first treatment approach if an HLA-identical donor is available [39]. This approach can produce long-term disease control in 10% to 30% of patients treated, and in up to 60% of patients with clonal evolution as the sole manifestation of disease acceleration. Patients without an HLA-compatible related donor should be considered for investigational therapies. IFN-α/ara-C can induce a CHR in 50% of patients with clonal evolution as the sole diagnostic criterion for accelerated phase disease with 20% of these patients achieving a cytogenetic response [122]. These responses are transient and CCR are not obtained.

## Future Directions

Comparative trials of IFN-α versus conventional therapy have clearly shown that an IFN-α-based regimen is current optimal therapy for CML and no further investment in randomized studies involving single agent IFN-α are justified. A series of studies of IFN-α combinations aimed at improving the major cytogenetic remission rates to above 50%, and/or ameliorating treatment-related toxicity are indicated. As survival advantage is most evident with major cytogenetic response, increasing this response rate to significant levels may become the key objective of further pilot studies. This may translate into an evident survival benefit in the overall population, which can be detected when such cytogenetic response rates are achieved in cooperative (rather than single institution) trials with acceptable toxicity. At that time randomized studies of novel IFN-α-based regimens versus IFN-α/ara-C may be indicated.

## Summary

AlloSCT and IFN-α-based therapy have undoubtedly changed the natural history of CML. Despite these advances, most CML patients still die from their disease. Most patients do not qualify for an AlloSCT either because of age or lack of an appropriate donor, and only a fraction of patients achieve a CCR with IFN-α-based therapy. The timing of AlloSCT and treatment sequences of IFN-α and SCT have been discussed. Prognostic factors for response to IFN-A therapy and for survival appear to be similar to those with conventional therapy. Prior treatment with IFN-α does not adversely affect AlloSCT outcome. The issue of optimal timing of AlloSCT remains controversial and will depend on maturing

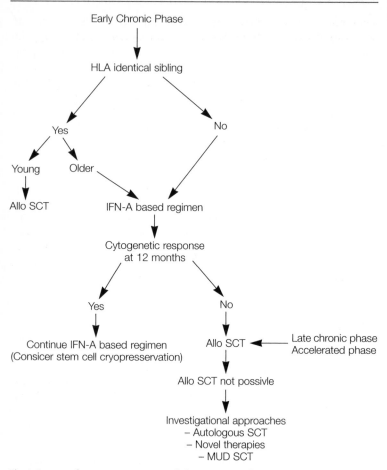

Fig. 1. Suggested management approach for patients with CML

experience with IFN-α combination regimens in different age groups, improvements in supportive care, reductions in AlloSCT-related toxicities and data on matched-unrelated donor SCT. The use of alternative donors may extend the option of AlloSCT to younger patients; however, for older patients AlloSCT may continue to have an unacceptably high incidence of morbidity and mortality until less toxic myeloablative regimens are discovered. Peripheral blood stem cell AlloSCT may also decrease the toxicity of this procedure in CML patients. CML therapy can now move beyond mere symptomatic disease control as achieved by HU and other conventional cytotoxic agents. The optimal choice of therapy for an individual CML patients depends on age, disease stage, availability of a HLA compatible donor, patient preference, and tolerance of IFN-α therapy. IFN-α/ara-C combinations are superior to IFN-α alone and the continuous use of ara-C may be a more effective method of combining it with IFN-α than intermittent administration.

For the majority of patients with CML, investigational strategies seeking to improve the proportion achieving CCR with IFN-α-based therapy are needed. These may involve novel agents (e.g., HHT, GM-CSF, decitabine, topotecan) or new modalities such as intensive chemotherapy followed by autologous SCT with in vitro purging. Further understanding of the molecular biology of CML and of the molecular basis for the anti-CML effect of IFN-α should help provide the rationale for strategies to achieve the goal of obtaining long-term disease control and cures in the majority of CML patients with the least attendant morbidity.

## References

1. Alimena G, Morra E, Lazzarino M, et al: Interferon alpha-2b as therapy for Ph'-positive chronic myelogenous leukemia: A study of 82 patients treated with intermittent or daily administration. Blood 72: 642, 1988
2. Allan N, Richards S, Shepherd P, et al: UK Medical Research Council randomized multicenter trial of interferon-αn1 for chronic myeloid leukemia: improved survival irrespective of cytogenetic response. Lancet 345: 1392, 1995
3. Anger B, Porzsolt F, Leichtle R, et al: A phase I/II study of recombinant interferon alpha 2a and hydroxyurea for chronic myelocytic leukemia. Blut 58: 275, 1989.
4. Antin SH: Graft-versus-leukemia: No longer an epiphenomenon. Blood 82:2273, 1993
5. Apperley JF, Mauro F, Goldman JM et al: Bone marrow transplantation for chronic myeloid leukaemia in chronic phase: importance of graft-versus-leukaemia effect. Br J Haematol 69:239, 1988
6. Arthur C, Ma D: Combined interferon alfa-2a and cytosine arabinoside as first-line treatment for chronic myeloid leukemia. Acta Haematol 89(Suppl 1): 15, 1993
7. Arthur CK. Mijovic A. Dannie E et al: Management of chronic myeloid leukaemia in pregnancy. J Obstet Gynaecol 11:396, 1991
8. Atkinson K. Biggs J, Concannon A et al: Second marrow transplants for recurrence of haematological malignancy. Bone Marrow Transplant 1:159, 1986
9. Baer MR. Ozer H. Foon FA: Interferon-α therapy during pregnancy in chronic myelogenous leukaemia and hairy cell leukaemia. Br J Haematol 81:167, 1992
10. Bär B, Schattenberg A, Mensink E, et al: Donor leukocyte infusions for chronic myeloid leukemia relapsed after allogeneic bone marrow transplantation. J Clin Oncol 11: 513, 1993

11. Barnett M, Eaves C, Phillips G, et al: Autografting with cultured marrow in chronic myeloid leukemia: Results of a pilot study. Blood 84: 724, 1994
12. Barrett A, Jiang Y: Immune responses to chronic myeloid leukemia. Bone Marrow Transplant 9: 305, 1992
13. Bartram C, de Klein A, Hagemeijer A, et al: Translocation of c-abl oncogene correlates with the presence of a Philadelphia chromosome in chronic myelocytic leukemia. Nature 306: 277, 1983
14. Beatty P, Anasetti C, Hansen J, et al: Marrow transplantation from unrelated donors for treatment of hematologic malignancies: Effect of mismatching for one HLA locus. Blood 81: 249, 1993
15. Beelen D, Graeven U, Elmaagacli A, et al: Prolonged administration of interferon-α in patients with chronic-phase Philadelphia chromosome-positive chronic myelogenous leukemia before allogeneic bone marrow transplantation may adversely affect transplant outcome. Blood 85: 2981, 1995
16. Ben-Neriah Y, Daley GQ, Mes-Masson AM et al: The chronic myelogenous leukemia specific p210 protein is the product of the bcr/abl hybrid gene. Science 223:212, 1986
17. Beran M, Jeha S, O'Brien S, et al: Tallimustine, an effective antileukemic agent in a SCID mouse model of adult myelogenous leukemia induces remissions in a phase I study. Blood 88 (Suppl 1): 220a, 1996 (abstr)
18. Beran M, Kantarjian H, O'Brien S, et al: Topotecan, a topoisomerase I inhibitor, is active in the treatment of myelodysplastic syndrome and chronic myelomonocytic leukemia Blood 88: 2473, 1996
19. Bhatia R, Wayner E, McGlave P, et al: Interferon-α restores normal adhesion of chronic myelogenous leukemia hematopoietic progenitors to bone marrow stroma by correcting impaired b1 integrin receptor function. J Clin Invest 94: 384, 1994
20. Biggs S, Szer J, Crilley P, et al Treatment of chronic myeloid leukemia with allogeneic bone marrow transplantation after preparation with BuCy2. Blood 80: 1090, 1992
21. Bilhou-Nabera C, Viard F, Marit G, et al: Complete cytogenetic conversion in chronic myelocytic leukemia patients undergoing Interferon a therapy: follow-up with reverse polymerase chain reaction. Leukemia 6: 595, 1992
22. Bilhou-Nabera C, Bernard P, Marit G, et al: Serial cytogenetic studies in allografted patients with chronic myeloid leukemia. Bone Marrow Transplant 9: 263, 1992
23. Boice J, Day N, Andersen A, et al: Second cancer following radiation treatment for cervical cancer. An international collaboration among cancer registries. J Natl Cancer Inst 74: 955, 1985
24. Borgies P, Ferrant A, Delannoy A, et al: Interferon alpha induced and maintained complete remission in chronic granulocytic leukaemia in relapse after bone marrow transplantation. Bone Marrow Transplant 4:127, 1988
25. Bortin M, Horowitz M, Rowlings P, et al: Report from the International Bone Marrow Transplant Registry. Bone Marrow Transplant 12: 97, 1993
26. Bortin M, D'Amaro J, Bach F, et al: HLA associations with leukemia. Blood 70: 227, 1987
27. Brandwein J, Dube I, Laraya P, et al: Maintenance of Philadelphia-chromosome-positive progenitors in long-term marrow cultures from patients with advanced chronic myeloid leukemia. Leukemia 6: 556, 1992
28. Brincker H: Population-based age- and sex-specific incidence rates in the 4 main types of leukaemia. Scand J Haematol 29: 241, 1982
29. Brown W, Doll R: Mortality from cancer and other causes after radiotherapy for ankylosing spondylitis. Br Med J 2: 1327, 1965

30. Call T, Noel P, Habermann T, et al: Incidence of leukemia in Olmsted County, Minnesota, 1975 through 1989. Mayo Clin Proc 69:315, 1994

31. Canellos G, Whang-Peng J, DaVita V: Chronic granulocytic leukemia without the Philadelphia chromosome. Am J Clin Pathol 65:467, 1976

32. Cervantes F, Robertson J, Rozman C, et al: Long-term survivors in chronic granulocytic leukaemia: a study by the International CGL Prognosis Study Group. Br J Haematol 87: 293, 1994

33. Cervantes F, Rozman C: A multivariate analysis of prognostic factors in chronic myeloid leukemia. Blood 60: 1298, 1982

34. Champlin R, McGlave P: Allogeneic bone marrow transplantation for chronic myeloid leukemia. In: Forman SJ, Blume KG, Thomas ED: Bone marrow transplantation. Boston, MA, Blackwell Scientific Publications, pp. 595, 1994

35. Chen W, Peace D, Rovira K, et al: T-cell immunity and the joining region of p210 bcr-abl protein. Proc Natl Acad Sci USA 89: 1468, 1992

36. Chikkapa G, Wang G, Santella D et al: Granulocyte colony-stimulating factor induces synthesis of alkaline phosphatase in neutrophilic granulocytes of chronic myelogenous leukemia patients. Leuk Res 12:491, 1988

37. Choundhury A, Gajewski J, Liang J, et al: Use of leukemic dendritic cells for the generation of antileukemic cellular cytotoxicity against Philadelphia chromosome-positive chronic myelogenous leukemia. Blood 89: 1133, 1997

38. Claxton D, Deisseroth A, Talpaz M, et al: Polyclonal hematopoiesis in interferon-induced cytogenetic remissions of chronic myelogenous leukemia. Blood 79: 997, 1992

39. Clift R, Buckner C, Thomas E, et al: Marrow transplantation for patients in accelerated phase of chronic myeloid leukemia. Blood 84: 4368, 1994

40. Clift R, Buckner C, Thomas E, et al: Marrow transplantation for chronic myeloid leukemia: a randomized study comparing cyclophosphamide and total body irradiation with busulfan and cyclophosphamide. Blood 84: 2036, 1994

41. Clift R, Appelbaum F, Thomas E: Bone marrow transplantation for chronic myelogenous leukemia. Blood 83: 2752, 1994

42. Collins R, Shpilberg O, Drobyski W, et al: Donor leukocyte infusions in 140 patients with relapsed malignancy after allogeneic bone marrow transplantation. J Clin Oncol 15: 433, 1997

43. Conlon K, Urba W, Smith J, et al: Exacerbation of symptoms of autoimmune disease in patients receiving alpha interferon therapy for malignant carcinoid tumors. Cancer 65: 2237, 1990

44. Cortes J, Kantarjian H, O'Brien S, et al: A pilot study of all-trans retinoic acid in patients with Philadelphia chromosome-positive chronic myelogenous leukemia. Leukemia. In Press, 1997

45. Cortes J, Kantarjian H, O'Brien S, et al: Results of interferon-alpha therapy in patients with chronic myelogenous leukemia 60 years of age and older. Am J Med 100: 452, 1996

46. Cortes J, Talpaz M, O'Brien S, et al: Philadelphia-chromosome negative chronic myelogenous leukemia with rearrangement of the breakpoint cluster region: long-term follow-up results. Cancer 75: 464, 1995

47. Cortes J, Kantarjian H, O'Brien S, et al: GM-CSF can improve the cytogenetic response obtained with interferon-alpha therapy in patients with chronic myelogenous leukemia. Blood 88 (Suppl 1): 232a, 1996 (abstr)

48. Cortes J, Talpaz M, Kantarjian H: Chronic myelogenous leukemia: A review. Am J Med 100: 555, 1996

49. Coulombel L, Kalousek D, Eaves C et al: Long term marrow culture reveals chromosomally normal hemopoietic progenitor cells in patients with Philadelphia-positive chronic myelogenous leukemia. N Engl J Med 308:1493, 1983

50. Cramer E, Auclair C, Hakim J, et al: Metabolic activity of phagocytosing granulocytes in chronic granulocytic leukemia: ultrastructural observation of a degranulation defect. Blood 50: 93, 1977

51. Cross N, Hughes T, Mackinnon S, et al: Minimal residual disease after allogeneic bone marrow transplantation for chronic myeloid leukaemia in chronic phase: correlations with probability of relapse. Br J Haematol 84: 67, 1993

52. Cullis J, Jiang Y, Scwarer A, et al: Donor leukocyte infusions for chronic myeloid leukemia in relapse after allogeneic bone marrow transplantation. Blood 79: 1379, 1992

53. Cullis J, Scwarer A, Hughes T, et al: Second transplants for patients with chronic myeloid leukemia in relapse after original transplant with T-depleted donor marrow: feasibility of using busulfan alone for re-conditioning. Br J Haematol 80: 33, 1992

54. Cunningham I. Gee T, Dowling M et al: Results of treatment of Ph' + chronic myelogenous leukemia with an intensive treatment regimen (L–5 protocol). Blood 53: 375. 1979

55. Daley G, Van Etten R, Baltimore D: Induction of chronic myelogenous leukemia in mice by the $P210^{bcr/abl}$ gene of the Philadelphia chromosome. Science 247: 824, 1990

56. Daley G, Van Etten R, Baltimore D: Blast crisis in a murine model of chronic myelogenous leukemia. PNAS 88: 11335, 1991

57. De Klein A, Geurts van Kessel A, Grosfeld G et al: A cellular oncogene is translocated to the Philadelphia chromosome in chronic myelocytic leukaemia. Nature 300: 765, 1982

58. De Braekeleer D: Variant Philadelphia translocations in chronic myeloid leukemia. Cytogenet Cell Genet 44: 215. 1987

59. Deisseroth A, Zu Z, Claxton D, et al: Genetic marking shows that Ph+ cells present in autologous transplants of chronic myelogenous leukemia contribute to relapse after autologous bone marrow transplant in CML. Blood 83: 3068, 1994

60. Dekmezian R, Kantarjian H, Keating M, et al: The relevance of reticulin stain-measured fibrosis at diagnosis in chronic myelogenous leukemia. Cancer 59: 1739, 1987

61. DeLage R, Soiffer R, Dear K, et al: Clinical significance of bcr-abl rearrangement detected by polymerase chain reaction after allogeneic bone marrow transplantation in chronic myelogenous leukemia. Blood 78: 2759, 1991

62. Derderian P, Kantarjian H, Talpaz M, et al: Chronic myelogenous leukemia in the lymphoid blastic phase: characteristics, treatment response, and prognosis. Am J Med 94: 69, 1993

63. Dhingra K, Kurzrock R, Kantarjian H, et al: Polymerase chain reaction for minimal residual disease in 20 CML patients in complete cytogenetic remission induced by interferon therapy. Blood 74 (Suppl 1): 235a, 1989(abstr)

64. Dhingra, K, Kurzrock R, Kantarjian H, et al: Minimal residual disease in interferon-treated chronic myelogenous leukemia: results and pitfalls of analysis based on polymerase chain reaction Leukemia, 6: 754, 1992

65. Dickstein JI, Vardiman JW: Issues in the pathology and diagnosis of the chronic myeloproliferative disorders and the myelodysplastic syndromes. Am J Clin Pathol 99: 513, 1993

66. Djaldetti M, Padeh B, Pinkhas J, et al: Prolonged remission in chronic myeloid leukemia after one course of busulfan. Blood 27: 103, 1966

67. Dobrovic A, Morley A, Seshadri R, et al: Molecular diagnosis of Philadelphia negative CML using the polymerase chain reaction and DNA analysis: clinical features and course of M-bcr negative and M-bcr-positive CML. Leukemia 5: 187, 1991

68. Dosik H, Rosner F, Sawitsky A: Acquired lipidosis: Gaucher-like cells and "blue cells" in chronic granulocytic leukemia. Semin Hematol 9: 309, 1972

69. Dowding C, Guo AP, Osterholz J, et al. Interferon-α overrides the deficient adhesion of chronic myeloid leukemia primitive progenitor cells to bone marrow stromal cells. Blood 78: 499, 1991

70. Drobyski W, Keevr C, Roth M, et al: Donor leukocyte infusions as treatment for relapsed chronic myelogenous leukemia after allogeneic bone marrow transplantation. Blood 82: 2310, 1993

71. Dutcher J, Eudey L, Wiernik P, et al: Phase II study of mitoxantrone and 5-azacytidine for accelerated and blast crisis of chronic myelogenous leukemia: a study of the Eastern Cooperative Oncology Group. Leukemia 6: 770, 1992

72. Elliott S, Taylor K, Taylor D, et al: Cytogenetic response to α-interferon is predicted in early chronic phase chronic myeloid leukemia by M-bcr breakpoint location. Leukemia 9: 946, 1995

73. Ernst T, Shuman L, Grossbard M. Treatment of the chronic phase of CML with a combined continuous infusion of homoharringtonine and cytarabine. Blood 86 (Suppl 1): 529a, 1995 (abstr)

74. Estrov Z, Talpaz M, Chou T, et al: Synergistic antiproliferative effects of interferon alpha and azidothymidine in chronic myelogenous leukemia. Leukemia 5: 101, 1991

75. Estrov Z, Kurzrock R, Wetzler M, et al: Suppression of chronic myelogenous leukemia colony growth by IL-1 receptor antagonist and soluble IL-1 receptors: a novel application for inhibitors of IL-1 activity. Blood 78: 1476, 1991

76. Ezdinli EZ. Sokal JE. Crosswhite L et al: Philadelphia chromosome-positive and -negative chronic myelocytic leukemia. Ann Intern Med 72: 175, 1970

77. Finney R, McDonald G, Baikie A, et al: Chronic granulocytic leukaemia with Ph¹ cells in bone marrow and 10 year remission after busulphan hypoplasia. Br J Haematol 23: 283, 1972

78. First International Workshop on Chromosomes in Leukaemia: Chromosomes in Ph¹ positive chronic granulocytic leukaemia. Br J Haematol 39: 305, 1978

79. Freund M, von Wussow P, Diedrich H, et al: Recombinant human interferon alpha-2b in chronic myelogenous leukaemia: Dose dependency of response and frequency of neutralizing anti-interferon antibodies. Br J Haematol 72: 350, 1989

80. Fujimiya Y, Chang W, Bakke A, et al: Natural killer (NK) cell immunodeficiency in patients with chronic myelogenous leukemia. Cancer Immunol Immunother 24: 213, 1987

81. Futaki M, Inokuchi K, Matsuoka H, et al: Relationship of the type of bcr-abl hybrid mRNA to clinical course and transforming activity in Philadelphia-positive chronic myelogenous leukemia. Leukemia Res 16: 1071, 1992

82. Gale R, Canaani E: An 8-kilobase abl RNA transcript in chronic myelogenous leukemia. Proc Natl Acad Sci USA 81: 5648, 1984

83. Galton DAG: Busulphan (1,4 dimethanesulphonyloxybutane): summary of clinical results. Ann NY Acad Sci 68: 967, 1958

84. Galton D: Myeleran in chronic myeloid leukemia. Lancet 1: 208, 1953

85. Gamis A, Haake R, McGlave P, et al: Unrelated-donor bone marrow transplantation for Philadelphia chromosome-positive chronic myelogenous leukemia in children. J Clin Oncol 11: 834, 1993

86. Ganesan TS, Rassool F, Guo A-P, et al: Rearrangement of the BCR gene in Philadelphia chromosome negative chronic myeloid leukemia. Blood 68: 957, 1986

87. Giles F, Aitchison R, Syndercombe-Court D, et al: Recombinant alpha 2B interferon in combination with oral chemotherapy in late chronic phase chronic myeloid leukaemia. Leukaemia Lymphoma 7: 99, 1992

88. Giles F, Jewell A, Worman C, et al: Recombinant alpha interferons, thyroid irradiation and thyroid disease. Acta Haematologica 85: 160, 1991

89. Giles F, Salim K, Rapoport B, et al: Presenting features of chronic-phase chronic myelogenous leukemia: A comparison between Asian and French patients on the International Oncology study Group CML1 and French CML88 studies. Br J Haematol 93 (Suppl 2): 273a, 1996 (abstr)

90. Giles F, Koeffler P: Chronic myelogenous leukaemia *in* Cancer Treatment IVth Edition *ed* Haskell, W.B. Saunders, Philadelphia, 933, 1995

91. Giralt S, Kantarjian H, Talpaz M: Treatment of chronic myelogenous leukemia. Semin Oncol 22: 396, 1995

92. Giralt S, Kantarjian H, Talpaz M, et al: Effect of prior interferon alfa therapy on the outcome of allogeneic bone marrow transplantation for chronic myelogenous leukemia. J Clin Oncol 11: 1055, 1993

93. Giralt S, Champlin R: Leukemia relapse after allogeneic bone marrow transplant: A review. Blood 83: 3603, 1994

94. Goldman JM, Szydlo R, Horowitz MM et al: Choice of pretransplant treatment and timing of transplants for chronic myelogenous leukemia in chronic phase. Blood 82: 2235, 1993

95. Gomez G, Sokal J, Mittelman A, et al: Splenectomy for palliation of chronic myeloid leukemia. Am J Med 61: 14, 1976

96. Gordon M, Dowding C, Riley G, et al: Altered adhesive interactions with marrow stroma of hematopoietic progenitor cells in chronic myeloid leukemia. Nature 328: 342, 1987

97. Gratwohl A, Hermans J, Niederwieser D, et al: Bone marrow transplantation for chronic myeloid leukemia: Long-term results. Bone Marrow Transplant 12: 509, 1993

98. Greenberg B, Wilson F, Woo L, et al: Cytogenetics of fibroblastic colonies in Ph[1]-positive chronic myelogenous leukemia. Blood 51: 1039, 1978

99. Griffen JD, Todd RF, Ritz J, et al: Differentiation patterns in the blastic phase of chronic myeloid leukemia. Blood 61: 85, 1983

100. Guerrasio A, Martinelli G, Saglio G, et al: Minimal residual disease status in transplanted chronic myelogenous leukemia patients: Low incidence of polymerase chain reaction positive cases among 48 long disease-free subjects who received unmanipulated allogeneic bone marrow transplants. Leukemia 6: 507, 1992

101. Guilhot F, Chastang C, Michallet M, et al: Interferon-alpha 2b combined with cytarabine versus interferon alone in chronic myelogenous leukemia. N Engl J Med 337: 223, 1997

102. Guilhot F, Abgrall J, Harousseau J, et al: A multicenter randomized study of alfa 2b interferon and hydroxyurea with or without cytosine-arabinoside in previously untreated patients with Ph+ chronic myelocytic leukemia: Preliminary cytogenetic results. Leukemia Lymphoma 11 (Suppl 1): 181, 1993

103. Hehlmann R, Heimpel H, Hasford J, et al: Randomized comparison of interferon-$\alpha$ with busulfan and hydroxyurea in chronic myelogenous leukemia. Blood 84: 4064, 1994

104. Hehlmann R, Heimpel H, Hasford J, et al: Randomized comparison of busulfan and hydroxyurea in chronic myelogenous leukemia: Prolongation of survival by hydroxyurea. Blood 82: 398, 1993

105. Heubner P, Willemze R, Ganser A, et al: YNKO1, an oral ara-C derivative in patients with AML, MDS, low-grade NHL and CML. Blood 81(Suppl 1): 302a, 1994 (abstr)

106. Higano C, Raskind W, Singer J: Use of a Interferon for the treatment of relapse of chronic myelogenous leukemia in chronic phase after allogeneic bone marrow transplantation. Blood 80: 1437, 1992

107. Horowitz MM, Giralt S, Szydlo R, et al: Effect of prior interferon therapy on outcome of HLA-identical sibling bone marrow transplants for chronic myelogenous leukemia in first chronic phase. Blood 88 (Supp 1): 682a, 1996 (abstr)

108. Hoyle C, Gray R, Goldman J: Autografting for patients with CML in chronic phase: An update. Br J Haematol 86: 76, 1994

109. Hughes T, Morgan G, Martiat P, et al: Detection of residual leukemia after bone marrow transplant for chronic myeloid leukemia: role of polymerase chain reaction in predicting relapse. Blood 77: 874, 1991

110. Inbal A, Akstein E, Barak I, et al: Cyclic leukocytosis and long survival in chronic myeloid leukemia. Acta Haematol 69: 353, 1983

111. Italian Cooperative Study Group on Chronic Myeloid Leukaemia: Interferon alfa-2a as compared with conventional chemotherapy for the treatment of chronic myeloid leukaemia. N Engl J Med 330: 820, 1994

112. Jacknow G, Frizzera G, Gajl-Peczalska K, et al: Extramedullary presentation of the blast crisis of chronic myelogenous leukemia. Br J Haematol 61: 225, 1985

113. Janossy G. Woodruff RK. Pippard MJ et al: Relation of "lymphoid" phenotype and response to chemotherapy incorporating vincristine- prednisolone in the acute phase of Ph' positive leukemia. Cancer 43: 426, 1979

114. Jaubert J, Martiat P, Dowding C, et al: The position of the M-BCR breakpoint does not predict the duration of chronic phase or survival in chronic myeloid leukaemia. Br J Haematol 74: 30, 1990

115. Jiang Y, Cullis J, Kanfer E, et al: T cell and NK cell mediated graft-versus-leukaemia reactivity following donor buffy coat transfusions to treat relapse after marrow transplantation for chronic myeloid leukaemia. Bone Marrow Transplant 11: 133, 1993

116. Juan D, Hsu S, Hunter J: Case report of vasopressin-responsive diabetes insipidus associated with chronic myelogenous leukemia. Cancer 56: 1468, 1985

117. Kantarjian H, Smith T, McCredie K, et al: Chronic myelogenous leukemia: A multivariate analysis of the association of patient characteristics and therapy with survival. Blood. 66, 1326, 1985

118. Kantarjian H, Kurzrock R, Talpaz M: Philadelphia chromosome-negative chronic myelogenous leukemia and chronic myelomonocytic leukemia. Hematol Oncol Clin North Am 4: 389, 1990

119. Kantarjian H, O'Brien S, Beran M, et al: Results with decitabine, a hypomethylating agent, in the treatment of chronic myelogenous leukemia in accelerated or blastic phases. Blood 88 (Suppl 2): 199b, 1996 (abstr)

120. Kantarjian H, Deisseroth A, Kurzrock R, et al: Chronic myelogenous leukemia: a concise update. Blood 82: 691, 1993

121. Kantarjian H, O'Brien S, Keating M, et al: Hommoharringtonine and low-dose cytosine arabinoside combination therapy has significant activity in patients with late phase Philadelphia chromosome positive chronic myelogenous leukemia.Blood 88 (Suppl 1): 578a, 1996 (abstr)

122. Kantarjian H, Keating M, Estey E, et al: Treatment of advanced stages of Philadelphia chromosome-positive chronic myelogenous leukemia with Interferon-$\alpha$ and low-dose cytarabine. J Clin Oncol 10: 772, 1992

123. Kantarjian H, Keating M, Talpaz M, et al: Chronic myelogenous leukemia in blast crisis. Analysis of 242 patients. Am J Med 83: 445, 1987

124. Kantarjian H, Dixon D, Keating M, et al: Characteristics of accelerated disease in chronic myelogenous leukemia. Cancer 61: 1441, 1988

125. Kantarjian H, Smith T, O'Brien S, et al: Prolonged survival following achievement of cytogenetic response with alpha interferon therapy in chronic myelogenous leukemia. Ann Intern Med 122: 254, 1995

126. Kantarjian H, Smith T, O'Brien S: Prognostic factors for response and survival with alpha interferon therapy in early chronic phase chronic myelogenous leukemia. Blood 80 (Suppl 1): 378a, 1993 (abstr)

127. Kantarjian H, O'Brien S, Keating M, et al: Interferon alpha and low-dose cytosine arabinoside therapy in Philadelphia chromosome-positive chronic myelogenous leukemia. Proc ASCO 16 : 47a, 1997 (abstr)

128. Kantarjian H, Talpaz M, Andersson B, et al: High doses of cyclophosphamide, etoposide, and total body irradiation followed by autologous stem cell transplantation in the management of patients with chronic myelogenous leukemia. Bone MarrowTransplant 14: 57, 1994

129. Kantarjian H, Talpaz M, LeMaistre C, et al: Intensive combination chemotherapy and autologous bone marrow transplantation leads to the reappearance of Philadelphia chromosome-negative cells in chronic myelogenous leukemia. Cancer 67: 2959, 1991

130. Kantarjian H, Keating M, Smith T, et al: Proposal for a simple synthesis prognostic staging system in chronic myelogenous leukemia. Am J Med 88: 1, 1990

131. Kantarjian H, Talpaz M, Keating M, et al: Intensive chemotherapy induction followed by interferon-alpha maintenance in patients with Philadelphia chromosome-positive chronic myelogenous leukemia. Cancer 68: 1201, 1991

132. Kantarjian H, Talpaz M, Hester J, et al: Collection of peripheral blood diploid cells from chronic myelogenous leukemia patients early in the recovery phase from myelosuppression induced by intensive-dose chemotherapy. J Clin Oncol 13: 553, 1995

133. Kantarjian H, O'Brien S, Anderlini P, et al: Treatment of chronic myelogenous leukemia: Current status and investigational options. Blood 87: 3069, 1996

134. Kenis Y, Dustin P, Henry J, et al: Action du myleran dans 22 cas de leucemie myeloide chronique. Rev Fr Etudes Clin Biol 1: 435, 1956

135. Kennedy B, Yarbro K: Metabolic and therapeutic effects of hydroxyurea in chronic myeloid leukemia. JAMA 195: 1038, 1966

136. Khouri I, Kantarjian H, Talpaz M, et al: High-dose chemotherapy and unpurged autologous stem cell transplantation in 73 patients with chronic myelogenous leukemia : The M.D. Anderson experience. Bone Marrow Transplant 17: 775, 1996

137. Klein A, van Kessel A, Grosveld G, et al: A cellular oncogene is translocated to the Philadelphia chromosome in chronic myelocytic leukemia. Nature 300: 765, 1982

138. Kloke O, Wandl U, Opalka B, et al: A prospective randomized comparison of single-agent interferon-alpha with the combination of IFN-alpha and low-dose IFN-gamma in chronic myelogenous leukaemia. Eur J Haematol 48: 93, 1992

139. Kloke O, Niederle N, Qiu J, et al: Impact of interferon alpha-induced cytogenetic improvement on survival in chronic myelogenous leukemia. Br J Haematol 83: 399, 1993

140. Kluin-Nelemans J, Lowagie A, Delannoy A, et al: CML treated by interferon alfa-2b vs hydroxyurea alone: preliminary report of a large multicenter randomized trial. Blood 80 (Suppl 1): 358a, 1992 (abstr)

141. Knox W, Bhavnani M, Davson J, et al: Histological classification of chronic granulocytic leukaemia. Clin Lab Haematol 6: 171, 1984

142. Kolb H, Schattenberg A, Goldman J, et al: Graft-versus-leukemia effect of donor lymphocyte in marrow grafted patients. Blood 86: 2041, 1995

143. Kolitz J, Kempin S, Schluger A, et al: A phase II pilot trial of high-dose hydroxyurea in chronic myelogenous leukemia. Semin Oncol 19 (Suppl 9): 27, 1992

144. Koller C, Miller D: Preliminary observations in the therapy of myeloid blast phase of chronic granulocytic leukemia with plicamycin and hydroxyurea. N Engl J Med 315: 1433, 1986

145. Kurzrock R, Gutterman J, Talpaz M: The molecular genetics of Philadelphia chromosome-positive leukemias. N Engl J Med 319: 990, 1988

146. Kurzrock R, Blick M, Talpaz M, et al: Rearrangement of the breakpoint cluster region in Philadelphia-negative chronic myelogenous leukemia. Ann Intern Med 105: 673, 1986

147. Kurzrock R, Kantarjian H, Shtalrid M, et al: Philadelphia chromosome-negative chronic myelogenous leukemia without breakpoint cluster region rearrangement: a chronic myeloid leukemia with a distinct clinical course. Blood 75: 445, 1990

148. Kurzrock R, Talpaz M, Kantarjian H, et al: Therapy of chronic myelogenous leukemia with recombinant interferon-γ. Blood 70: 943, 1987

149. Kyle R, Schwartz R, Oliner H, et al: A syndrome resembling adrenal cortical insufficiency associated with long term busulfan therapy. Blood 18: 497, 1961

150. Lange R, Moloney W, Yamawaki T: Leukemia in atomic bomb survivors. 1. General observations. Blood 9:514, 1954

151. Lee M, Kantarjian H, Talpaz M, et al: Detection of minimal residual disease by polymerase chain reaction in Philadelphia chromosome-positive chronic myelogenous leukemia following interferon therapy. Blood 79: 1920, 1992

152. Leemhuis T, Leibowitz D, Cox G, et al: Identification of BCR/ABL-negative primitive hematopoietic progenitor cells within chronic myeloid leukemia marrow. Blood 81: 801, 1993

153. Lion T, Henn T, Gaiger A, et al: Early detection of relapse after bone marrow transplantation in patients with chronic myelogenous leukaemia. Lancet 341: 275, 1993

154. Lissauer H: Zwei Fälle von leucaemie. Klin Wochenschr 2: 403, 1865

155. Mahon F, Montastruc M, Faberes C, et al: Predicting complete cytogenetic response in chronic myelogenous leukemia patients treated with recombinant interferon. Blood 84: 3592, 1994

156. Mahon F, Fabères C, Boiron J, et al. High response rate using recombinant alpha interferon in patients with newly diagnosed chronic myeloid leukemia – analysis of predictive factors. Blood 88 (Suppl 1): 638a, 1996 (abstr)

157. Majlis A, Kantarjian H, Smith T, et al: What is the significance of cytogenetic clonal evolution in patients with Philadelphia chromosome-positive chronic myelogenous leukemia? Blood 84 (Suppl 1): 150a, 1994 (abstr)

158. Malinge M, Mahon F, Delfau M, et al: Quantitative determination of the hybrid bcr-abl RNA in patients with chronic myelogenous leukemia under interferon therapy. Br J Haematol 82: 701, 1992

159. Marks S, McCaffrey R, Rosenthal D, et al: Blastic transformation in chronic myelogenous leukemia: experience with 50 patients. Med Pediatr Oncol 4: 15, 1978

160. Marks D, Cullis J, Ward K, et al: Allogeneic bone marrow transplantation for chronic myeloid leukemia using sibling and volunteer unrelated donors: a comparison of complications in the first two years. Ann Intern Med 119: 207, 1993

161. Martiat P, Lewalle P, Taj A, et al: Retrovirally transduced antisense sequences stably suppress P210$^{BCR/ABL}$ and inhibit the proliferation of bcr/abl-containing cell lines. Blood 81: 502, 1993

162. Mason J, DeVita V, Cannelos G: Thrombocytosis in chronic granulocytic leukemia. Incidence and clinical significance. Blood 44: 183. 1974

163. McGlave P, Arthur D, Weisdorf D, et al: Allogeneic bone marrow transplantation as treatment for accelerating chronic myelogenous leukemia. Blood 63: 219, 1984

164. McGlave P, De Fabritis P, Deisseroth A, et al: Autologous transplants for chronic myelogenous leukemia: Results from eight transplant groups. Lancet 343: 1486, 1994

165. McGlave P: Bone marrow transplants in chronic myelogenous leukemia: an overview of determinants of survival. Sem Hematol (Suppl 4) 27: 23, 1990

166. Medical Research Council: Randomised trial of splenectomy in Ph positive chronic granulocytic leukaemia including an analysis of prognostic features. Br J Haematol 54: 415. 1983

167. Melo JV: The diversity of bcr-abl fusion proteins and their relationship to leukemia phenotype. Blood 88: 2375, 1996

168. Melo J, Gordon D, Cross N, et al: The abl-bcr fusion gene is expressed in chronic myeloid leukemia. Blood 81: 158, 1993

169. Mills K, Benn P, Birnie G: Does the breakpoint within the major cluster region influence the duration of the chronic phase in chronic myeloid leukemia? An analytical comparison of current literature. Blood 78: 1155, 1991

170. Nathwani A, Goldman J: The management of chronic myeloid leukemia in lymphoid blast crisis. Haematologica 78: 162, 1993

171. Newland A, Jones L, Mir M, et al: Alpha 2 interferon in chronic myeloid leukaemia following relapse post-allogeneic transplant. Br J Haematol 66: 141, 1987

172. Niederle N, Kloke O, Osieka R, et al: Interferon alfa-2b in the treatment of chronic myelogenous leukemia. Semin Oncol 14: 29, 1987

173. Nowell PC, Hungerford D: A minute chromosome in human chronic granulocytic leukemia. Science 132: 1497, 1960

174. O'Brien S, Kantarjian H, Keating M, et al: Homoharringtonine therapy induces responses in patients with chronic myelogenous leukemia in late chronic phase. Blood 86: 3322, 1995

175. O'Brien S, Guidelines for chronic myelogenous leukemia treatment with alpha interferon. Leukaemia Lymphoma 23: 247, 1996

176. Ohnishi K, Ohno R, Tomonaga M, et al: A randomized trial comparing interferon-$\alpha$ with busulfan for newly diagnosed chronic myelogenous leukemia in chronic phase. Blood 86: 906, 1995

177. Oliner H, Schwartz R, Rubio F, et al: Interstitial pulmonary fibrosis following busulfan therapy. Am J Med 31: 134, 1961

178. Ordway T: Remission in leukemia produced by radium in cases completely resistant to x-ray and benzol treatment. Boston Med Surg J 176: 490, 1917

179. Ozer H, George S, Schiffer C, et al: Prolonged subcutaneous administration of recombinant alfa-2b interferon in patients with previously untreated Philadelphia chromosome-positive chronic-phase chronic myelogenous leukemia: Effect on remission duration and survival: Cancer and Leukemia Group B Study 8583. Blood 82: 2975, 1993

180. Pap G, Arcese W, Mauro F, et al: Standard conditioning regimens and T-cell depleted donor marrow for transplantation in chronic myeloid leukemia. Leuk Res 10: 1469, 1986

181. Podoll L, Winkler S: Busulfan lung. Report of two cases and review of the literature. Am J Roentgenol Radium Ther Nucl Med 120: 151, 1974

182. Podos SM, Canellos GP: Lens changes in chronic granulocytic leukemia: possible relationship to chemotherapy. Am J Ophthalmol 68: 500, 1969

183. Porter D, Roth M, McGarigle C, et al: Induction of graft-versus-host disease as immunotherapy for relapsed chronic myeloid leukemia. N Engl J Med 330: 100, 1994

184. Preti H, O'Brien S, Giralt S, et al: Philadelphia-chromosome-positive adult acute lymphocytic leukemia: characteristics, treatment results, and prognosis in 41 patients. Am J Med 97: 60, 1994

185. Pusey W: Report of cases treated with roentgen rays. JAMA 38: 911, 1902

186. Quesada J, Talpaz M, Rios A, et al: Clinical toxicity of interferons in cancer patients: a review. J Clin Oncol 4: 234, 1986

187. Ratajczak M, Hijiya N, Catani L, et al: Acute- and chronic-phase chronic myelogenous leukemia colony-forming units are highly sensitive to the growth inhibitory effects of c-myb antisense oligodeoxynucleotides. Blood 79: 1956, 1992

188. Reiffers J, Trouette R, Marit G, et al: Autologous blood stem cell transplantation for chronic granulocytic leukaemia in transformation: a report of 47 cases. Br J Haematol 77: 339, 1991

189. Renner D, Queisser U, Martinez C, et al: Treatment of excessive thrombocytosis in chronic myeloid leukemia by thombocytopheresis and intravenous thiotepa. Onkologie 10: 324, 1987

190. Report of the MRC Working Party: Comparison of radiotherapy and busulfan therapy in chronic granulocyric leukemia. Br Med J 1: 201, 1968

191. Robertson M, Tantravahi R, Griffin J, et al: Hematologic remission and cytogenetic improvement after treatment of stable-phase chronic myelogenous leukemia with continuous infusion of low-dose cytarabine. Am J Hematol 43: 95, 1993

192. Ronnblom L, Alm F, Oberg K: Autoimmunity after alpha-interferon therapy for malignant carcinoid tumors. Ann Intern Med 115: 178, 1991

193. Rosner F, Schreiber Z, Parise F: Leukocyte alkaline phosphatase. Arch Intern Med 130: 892, 1972

194. Ross D, Brunning R, Kantarjian H, et al. A proposed staging system for chronic myeloid leukemia. Cancer 71: 3788, 1993

195. Roth M, Antin J, Ash R, et al: Prognostic significance of Philadelphia chromosome-positive cells detected by the polymerase chain reaction after allogeneic bone marrow transplant for chronic myelogenous leukemia. Blood 79: 276, 1992

196. Rowley JD: A new consistent chromosomal abnormality in chronic myelogenous leukaemia identified by quinacrine fluorescence and Giemsa banding. Nature 243: 290, 1973

197. Rushing D, Goldman A, Gibbs G, et al: Hydroxyurea versus busulfan in the treatment of chronic myelogenous leukemia. Am J Clin Oncol 5: 307, 1982

198. Rustin G, Goldman J, McCarthy D, et al: An extrinsic factor controls neutrophil alkaline phosphatase synthesis in chronic granulocytic leukaemia. Br J Haematol 45: 381, 1980

199. Sacchi S, Kantarjian H, O'Brien S, et al: Long-term follow-up results of alpha-interferon-based regimens in patients with late chronic phase chronic myelogenous leukemia.Blood 88 (Suppl 1): 201b, 1996 (abstr)

200. Sacchi S, Kantarjian H, Cohen P, et al: Immune-mediated and unusual complications during alpha-interferon therapy in chronic myelogenous leukemia. Blood 84 (Suppl 1): 150a, 1994 (abstrt)

201. Sanders J, Buckner C, Clift R, et al: Second marrow transplants in patients with leukemia who relapse after allogeneic marrow transplantation. Bone Marrow Transplant 3: 11, 1988

202. Schofield J, Robinson W, Murphy J, et al: Low doses of interferon a are as effective as higher doses in inducing remissions and prolonging survival in chronic myeloid leukemia. Ann Intern Med 121: 736, 1994

203. Seong D, Kantarjian H, Ro J, et al: Hypermetaphase fluorescence in situ hybridization for quantitative monitoring of Philadelphia chromosome-positive cells in patients with chronic myelogenous leukemia during treatment. Blood 86: 2343, 1995

204. Shepherd P, Fooks J, Gray R, et al: Thioguanine used in maintenance therapy of chronic myeloid leukemia causes non-cirrhotic portal hypertension. Br J Haematol 79: 185, 1991

205. Silver R, Szatrowski T, Peterson B, et al: Combined α-interferon and low dose cytosine arabinoside for Ph+ chronic phase chronic myeloid leukemia. Blood 88 (Suppl 1): 638a, 1996 (abstr)

206. Sokal J, Cox E, Baccarani M, et al: Prognostic discrimination in "good risk" chronic granulocytic leukemia. Blood 63: 789, 1984

207. Sokal J, Leong S, Gomez G: Preferential inhibition by cytarabine of CFU-GM from patients with chronic granulocytic leukemia.Cancer 59: 197, 1987

208. Spiers A, Bain B, Turner J: The peripheral blood in chronic granulocytic leukaemia: study of 50 untreated Philadelphia positive cases. Scand J Haematol 18: 25, 1977

209. Suri R, Goldman J, Catovsky D, et al: Priapism complicating chronic granulocytic leukemia. Am J Hematol 9: 295, 1980

210. Talpaz M, Kantarjian H, Kurzrock R, et al. Interferon-alpha produces sustained cytogenetic responses in chronic myelogenous leukemia. Ann Inter Med 114: 532, 1991

211. Talpaz M, Mavligit G, Keating M, et al: Human leukocyte interferon to control thrombocytosis in chronic myelogenous leukemia. Ann Med Intern 99: 789. 1983

212. Talpaz M, Kantarjian H, Liang J, et al: Percentage of Philadelphia chromosome-negative and Ph-positive cells found after autologous transplantation for chronic myelogenous leukemia depends on percentage of diploid cells induced by conventional-dose chemotherapy before collection of autologous cells. Blood 85: 3257, 1995

213. Talpaz M, Kantarjian H, McCredie K et al: Clinical investigation of human alpha interferon in chronic myelogenous leukemia. Blood 69: 1280, 1987

214. Talpaz M, Kantarjian H, McCredie K, et al: Hematologic remission and cytogenetic improvement induced by recombinant human interferon alpha A in chronic myelogenous leukemia. N Engl J Med 314: 1065, 1986

215. Talpaz M, Kantarjian H, Khouri I, et al: Diploid cells collected from chronic myelogenous leukemia patients during recovery from conventional dose induced myelosuppression generate complete cytogenetic remissions after autologous transplantation. Blood 84 (Suppl 1): 537a, 1994 (abstr)

216. Talpaz M, Kantarjian H, Kurzrock R, et al: Bone marrow hypoplasia and aplasia complicating interferon therapy for chronic myelogenous leukemia. Cancer 69: 410, 1992

217. Talpaz M, Estrov Z, Kantarjian H, et al: Persistence of dormant leukemic progenitors during interferon-induced remission in chronic myelogenous leukemia. J Clin Invest 94: 1383, 1994

218. Talpaz M, Kurzrock R, Kantarjian H, et al: A phase II study alternating alpha-2a-interferon and gamma-interferon therapy in patients with chronic myelogenous leukemia. Cancer 68: 2125, 1991

219. Terjanian T, Kantarjian H, Keating M, et al: Clinical and prognostic features of patients with Philadelphia chromosome-positive chronic myelogenous leukemia and extramedullary disease. Cancer 59: 297, 1987

220. Thaler J, Fluckinger T, Huber H et al: Treatment of 11 patients with chronic myelogenous leukemia with interferon-alpha-2c and low dose ara-C. Leukemia Res 17: 711, 1993

221. Thaler J, Hilbe W, Apfelbeck U, et al: Interferon-alpha-2c and low dose ara-C for the treatment of patients with CML: Results of the Austrian multi-center phase II study. Leukemia Res 21: 75, 1997

222. Tura S, Baccarani M, Corbelli G, et al: Staging of chronic myeloid leukaemia. Br J Haematol 47:105, 1981

223. Upadhyaya G, Guba S, Sih S, et al: Interferon-alpha restores the deficient expression of the cytoadhesion molecule lymphocyte function antigen-3 by chronic myelogenous leukemia progenitor cells. J Clin Invest 88: 2131, 1991

224. Vey N, Baume D, Lafage M, et al: Recombinant interleukin-2 induces cytogenetic responses in patients with chronic myelogenous leukemia in chronic phase. Blood 88 (Supp 1): 202b, 1996 (abstr)

225. Walters R, Kantarjian H, Keating M, et al: Therapy of lymphoid and undifferentiated chronic myelogenous leukemia in blast crisis with continuous vincristine and adriamycin infusions plus high dose decadron. Cancer 60: 1708, 1987

226. Wandl U, Kloke O, Nagel-Hiemke M, et al: Combination therapy with interferon alpha-2b plus low-dose interferon gamma in pretreated patients with Ph-positive chronic myelogenous leukemia. Br J Haematol 81: 516, 1992

227. Wilhelm M, Ramos C, O'Brien S, et al: Effect of interferon-alpha therapy on bone marrow fibrosis in chronic myelogenous leukemia. Blood 88 (Supp 1): 202b, 1996 (abstr)

228. Winfield D, Polacarz S: Bone marrow histology. 3: Value of bone marrow core biopsy in acute leukaemia, myelodysplastic syndromes, and chronic myeloid leukaemia. J Clin Pathol 45: 855, 1992

229. Yuo A, Kitagawa S, Okabe T, et al: Recombinant human granulocyte colony-stimulating factor repairs the abnormalities of neutrophils in patients with myelodysplastic syndromes and chronic myelogenous leukemia. Blood 70: 404, 1987

230. Zhao L, Kantarjian H, Van Oort J, et al: Detection of residual proliferating leukemic cells by fluorescence in situ hybridization in CML patients in complete remission after interferon treatment. Leukemia 7: 168, 1993

# Myelodysplastic Syndromes

R.A. Larson

## Introduction

Myelodysplastic syndromes (MDS) are a heterogeneous group of hematopoietic stem cells disorders, characterized by cytologic dysplasia in the bone marrow and blood and by various combinations of anemia, neutropenia, and thrombocytopenia. These disorders have in common the progressive evolution of a monoclonal population of hematopoietic cells, usually involving multiple lineages, generally with accompanying suppression of normal hematopoiesis. The natural history of these syndromes varies widely, ranging from chronic anemias with a low propensity for leukemic conversion to syndromes with severe hematologic disturbances and a high risk of progression to acute myeloid leukemia (AML).

A variety of terms, including preleukemia, smoldering or sub-acute leukemia, dysmyelopoietic syndrome, and myelodysplasia, have all been used to describe this group of patients. There is considerable evidence that these disorders are clonal and neoplastic from their earliest detection. Thus, the term "preleukemia" seems inappropriate as it implies a premalignant condition. Rather, these disorders are better considered as a chronic or "smoldering" leukemia. Unfortunately, our diagnostic abilities and nomenclature are not yet adequate to discriminate between clinically distinct subsets within this syndrome, with rare exceptions. There are considerable overlaps with other morphologically determined diseases, particularly those categorized as chronic myeloproliferative disorders (CMPD). Whereas the latter diseases have qualitatively unimpaired differentiation of hematopoiesis, at least in their early stages, MDS is characterized chiefly by impaired differentiation. Thus, one can speculate that MDS results from alterations of genes controlling transcription and cellular differentiation rather than those regulating cell proliferation or survival.

In 1982, the French-American-British (FAB) Cooperative Group attempted to standardize the classification of MDS patients using criteria based on cytology and the number of blast cells in the marrow and peripheral blood (Table 1) [1]. More recently, another important subset has been described, refractory cytopenia with multilineage dysplasia (RCMD) [2]. In some patients there is a natural progression of disease between categories as cellular maturation becomes more arrested and blast cells accumulate. In other patients, however, the diagnostic category does not change during the patient's lifespan.

Increased use of cytogenetic analysis and the development of new techniques for assessing clonality are proving useful not only for diagnosis (Table 2), but also for providing insights into pathogenesis and patterns of responsiveness to growth factors and possible differentiation-inducing agents [3–5]. Considerable data suggest that MDS results from combined defects of both stroma and hematopoietic stem cells. Several clinical syndromes that may have a more predictable natural history can now be defined. For example, a deletion of the long arm of chromsome-5 can be detected in some older patients, especially females, with a macrocytic, refractory anemia [6]. The platelet count is typically normal or elevated. The bone marrow (BM) picture in the "refractory anemia (RA) with 5q minus" syndrome is characterized by the presence of monolobulated and bilobulated micromegakaryocytes. Two-thirds of

**Table 1.** The subtypes of primary MDS [1, 2]

| Subtype | Peripheral blood | Bone marrow |
|---|---|---|
| Refractory anemia | <1% blasts; reticulocytopena, macrocyosis or normochromic/normocytic | Usually erythroid hyperplasia with dyserythropoiesis; <5% blasts |
| RA with ringed sideroblasts | <1% blasts; dimorphic red cell morphology | As in RA, but type III sideroblasts >15% of erythroid prercursors |
| RA with excess of blasts | <5% blasts; cytopenias in 2 or 3 cell lines | 5%–20% blasts; dyspoiesis in 2 or 3 cell lines |
| RAEB in transformation | 5%–29% blasts, or any Auer rods | 20%–30% blasts; any Auer rods; otherwise as RAEB |
| Chronic myelomonocytic leukemia | <5% blasts; >1x10$^9$/l monocytes | 1%–20% blasts; monocytosis |
| Refractory cytopenia with multilineage dysplasia | <1% blasts; cytopenia; multilineage dysplasia | <5% blasts; multilineage dysplasia |

**Table 2.** Recurring chromosome abnormalities in primary and therapy-related MDS (from (5))

| Abnormality | Approximate incidence (%) | |
|---|---|---|
| | Primary MDS | t-MDS |
| Partial chromosomal deletion | | |
| del (5q) | 20 | 20 |
| del (20q) | 3 or 4 | <1 |
| del (7q) | 1 or 2 | 10 |
| del (3p) or t(3p) | | |
| der or del (11q) | 2 or 3 | <1 |
| der or del (12p) | 1 or 2 | 3 or 4 |
| del (13q) | 1 | <1 |
| Chromosome loss | | |
| Monosomy 5 | | |
| Monosomy 7 | 10–15 | 50 |
| Loss of Y chromosome | 3 or 4 | 10 |
| Monosomy 17 | 3 | 5–7 |
| Chromosome gain | | |
| Trisomy 8 | 10–15 | 10 |
| Trisomy 11 | 3 | 1 |
| Trisomy 21 or iso (21q) | 2 | 1 |
| Translocations | | |
| t(1;3) (p36;q21.2) | | |
| t(3;3) (q21;q26) | 1 or 2 | 3 |
| t(2;11) (p21;q23) | | |
| t(1;7) (p11;p11) | <1 | 4 or 5 |
| t(3;21) (q21;q26) | | |
| t(5;17) (p11;p11) | 1 or 2 | 4–5 |
| t(7;17) (p11;p11) | 1 or 2 | 2–3 |
| t(5;7) (q11;p11) | <1 | 2 |
| t(9;11) (p22;q23) | | |
| t(11;19) (q23;p13) | | |
| Other findings | | |
| iso(17q) | <1 | 3 or 4 |
| inv(3) (q21q26) | <1 | 3 |
| Complex findings (>3 chromosome abnormalities) | 15–20 | 50 |

these patients have RA or RARS, and the remainder have RAEB (RA with excess of blasts). Those patients who have a del (5q) as their sole cytogenetic abnormality tend to have a relatively benign course that seldom progresses to AML. Although MDS is not commonly seen in patients less than 50 years old, there are two distinct pediatric syndromes of importance: juvenile chronic myelogenous leukemia (JCML) and the monosomy 7 syndrome.

## Morphology and Diagnostic Issues

MDS should be suspected whenever there is anemia, neutropenia, thrombocytopenia and/or monocytosis without any known cause for bone marrow failure. The diagnosis can usually be confirmed by the examination of well-prepared peripheral blood smears (PB), BM aspirate smears and BM biopsy specimens. The BM should be at least normocellular for the patient's age, and cytologic evaluation of the blood and aspirate smear should reveal some of the morphologic abnormalities described below in at least one cell line. It should be emphasized that none of the abnormalities described are specific for MDS but can be seen in a variety of other inherited and acquired hematologic disorders. Care must be taken to exclude these other processes before making a diagnosis of MDS.

Morphologic Characteristics of MDS

*Dyserythropoiesis*

In the PB the anemia may be normochromic, normocytic or, commonly, macrocytic. Basophilic stippling, fragmented red cells and spiculated red cells can be observed. In the BM, morphologic abnormalities of the erythroid precursors include nuclear-cytoplasmic asynchrony, frequently with megaloblastic changes, nuclear budding, karyorrhexis, multinuclearity, and vacuolation of the cytoplasm in acidophilic normoblasts. Ringed sideroblasts (Type III sideroblasts) may be identified with the Prussian blue reaction as erythroid precursors with numerous granules of iron forming a characteristic ring around the nucleus.

*Dysgranulopoiesis*

Morphologic abnormalities of the granulocytes may be seen in the PB and BM specimens. Nuclei of the neutrophils may be hypolobated (pseudo-Pelger-Huet change), hypersegmented, or demonstrate multiple nuclear excrescences. Abnormalities in the granulation of the cytoplasm are common. In the BM, abnormal staining of the primary granules is common, resulting in promyelocytes that appear devoid of granules.

Secondary granules may also be absent or reduced, resulting in hypo-granular cytoplasm in the myelocytes and more mature forms, including the neutrophils in the PB. Care should be taken to assure that the slides are well-stained, since a poor quality Romanowsky stain may cause even normal neutrophils to appear hypogranular.

A careful analysis of early granulocytic precursors will permit the recognition of two forms: Type I blasts – a primitive cell without gran-ules, containing 1–2 nucleoli. The chromatin is uncondensed. Type II blasts – usually slightly larger with a lower nuclear:cytoplasmic ratio than Type I blasts. They have a few (5–6) primary granules. The nucleus is still centrally placed, and there is uncondensed chromatin.

## Dysmegakaryocytopoiesis

Platelet production and function are often abnormal. In the BM, the number of megakaryocytes is usually normal or increased, but they may be present in decreased numbers as well. Micromegakaryocytes, large mononuclear forms, or megakaryocytes with widely separated nuclei may be found. Hypogranularity of megakaryocyte cytoplasm has also been reported.

## Bone Marrow Biopsy

The most accurate estimate of bone marrow cellularity is established from biopsy specimens. In patients with MDS, significant discrepancies between estimates of cellularity made from the biopsy specimens and from aspirate smears have been reported to occur in up to 20% of pa-tients [7].

Biopsy specimens may provide information that is useful in confirm-ing a diagnosis of MDS. For example, in MDS there is disruption of the normal bone marrow architecture that is characterized by a displace-ment of the site of granulopoiesis from its normal, paratrabecular loca-tion toward the central intertrabecular regions of the marrow [8]. In con-trast, erythropoiesis and megakaryocytopoiesis are shifted from their normal location in the central regions of the marrow toward the bony trabecular surface. The dislocation of immature granulocytic cells, refer-red to as abnormal localization of immature precursors (ALIP), has been reported by some to have prognostic significance [8, 9]. Although more recent studies have failed to confirm this clinical significance [3, 7, 10], the finding of ALIP may be helpful in some cases in substantiating the diagnosis of MDS, because it signifies an abnormal pattern of hematopoiesis in the marrow.

## Chronic Myelomonocytic Leukemia

The criteria for CMMoL include a peripheral monocytosis of $>1\times10^9/l$, increased numbers of monocytic cells in the BM, dysplasia in either the erythroid, megakaryocytic or granulocytic series, and $<5\%$ circulating blasts and $<20\%$ marrow blasts. CMMoL was placed in the MDS category primarily because of the striking dysplasia, and because cytopenias of one or more PB elements are not uncommon [1, 11]. The clinical course (reported median survivals range from 8–36 months), the rate (20%–40%) and pattern of leukemic transformation, and the high incidence of point mutations in the *RAS* oncogene family are also most in keeping with a myelodysplastic process [3, 11–13]. However, the nosologic position of CMMoL as a subtype of MDS is not accepted by all investigators, because myeloproliferative features predominate in a substantial number of patients [12, 14]. These latter features include marked monocytosis or neutrophilic leukocytosis in nearly one-half of all patients, the finding of tissue infiltration by monocytes, and splenomegaly in 50% and hepatomegaly in up to 20% of patients. In addition, the culture pattern of CMMoL in vitro resembles that of the myeloproliferative disorders with increased numbers of colonies and clusters, rather than the pattern of MDS in which progenitor cells do not grow well in short term cultures. Therefore, CMMoL may be considered as a disorder that encompasses features of both the CMPD and MDS.

## Therapy-Related MDS

Although in most cases MDS arises de novo, patients who have been treated with cytotoxic chemotherapy, radiotherapy or both are at an increased risk of developing MDS (t-MDS) or AML (t-AML). In 75% or more of patients with t-AML, a myelodysplastic phase is present prior to development of overt leukemia [15, 16]. In general, the features of t-MDS are similar to those of MDS arising de novo, although hypocel-lularity and reticulin fibrosis are more commonly present. Additionally, many cases of t-MDS do not readily fit into the FAB clas-sification scheme because of the finding of severe trilineage dysplasia but fewer than 5% blasts in the BM at presentation (thus lacking the criteria for any of the FAB subtypes). t-MDS is most often discovered 5–7 years following the initial therapy (15). The time frame for evoluti-on of t-MDS to t-AML is usually brief, and often the ensuing t-AML is difficult to classify [16].

Diagnostic issues in MDS

Problems in establishing the diagnosis of MDS may be due to a number of causes. Occasionally, these are related to failure to obtain adequate BM aspirate smears for evaluation of cytology, either because of BM hypo-cellularity or because of reticulin fibrosis. In the first case, the unexpect-ed finding of marrow hypocellularity, and thus, the lack of cells for detailed cytologic assessment, may make the distinction between "hypo-cellular MDS" and aplastic anemia quite difficult [17, 18]. In the second case, MDS with fibrosis of the marrow can not be readily separable from a variety of acute and chronic myeloid disorders that are also associated with marrow fibrosis and an inaspirable bone marrow [19, 20]. Some chronic myeloproliferative disorders (CMPD) may mimic MDS because they often demonstrate dyspoiesis as they transform to more accelerated stages. Confusion between MDS and CMPD may be further confounded in those cases of MDS, in which there is leukocytosis rather than leuko-penia. Diagnostic and classification problems may also be caused by blast cell counts that lie at either end of the spectrum of MDS. RCMD encompasses unclassifiable cases of MDS that have BM specimens with severe trilineage dysplasia but too few blasts for a diagnosis of RAEB. These patients generally follow a course more typical of RAEB than of RA. Even more concern exists for those cases in which the percentage of blasts is borderline between RAEB in transformation (RAEB-T) and overt AML [20]. The evolution of MDS to AML clearly follows a contin-um and the use of a sharp boundary is clearly unsatisfactory both diag-nostically and conceptually.

## Management of Adults With MDS

Survival is unfortunately short for the majority of patients with MDS. MDS is a life-threatening disorder due to persistent and profound cytopenias regardless of whether transformation to leukemia occurs. Morphologic classification has been limited in its ability to predict the natural history of the disease. Several scoring systems including the Bournemouth score and the FAB classification are based on the severity of cytopenia in conjunction with the BM blast count and the degree of granulocytic and megakaryocytic dysplasia [22–24]. Multi-lineage dysplasia and higher blast cell count are associated with more rapid development of AML and thus decreased survival, but most patients die from infection or bleeding or transfusion-related complications prior to developing AML.

Cytogenetic abnormalities are an important prognostic factor in MDS and are included in the International Prognostic Scoring System (Tables 3, 4) [3–6, 18, 24]. Certainly, the detection of clonal abnormalities in a patient's BM cells clearly establishes a neoplastic diagnosis and removes any doubt about a possible nutritional deficiency or drug toxicity as the cause for cytopenia. Half of patients with MDS have detectable

**Table 3.** International prognostic scoring system for evolution to AML and survival with MDS (from (24))

| Variable | Score value | | | | |
|---|---|---|---|---|---|
| | 0 | 0.5 | 1.0 | 1.5 | 2.0 |
| BM blasts (%) | <5 | 5–10 | – | 11–20 | 21–30 |
| Karyotype[a] | Good | Intermediate | Poor | | |
| PB cytopenias | 0 or 1 | 2 or 3 | | | |

[a] Good cytogenetics: normal, -Y, del (5q), del (20q); poor: complex (>3 abnormalities), abnormalities of no. 7; intermediate: all other abnormalities.

**Table 4.** Outcomes of 816 patients with primary MDS according to IPSS risk group (from 24)

| Risk groups | Score | Median survival (years) | 25% Evolution to AML (years) |
|---|---|---|---|
| Low | 0 | 5.7 | 9.4 |
| Low-intermediate | 0.5–1.0 | 3.5 | 3.3 |
| High-intermediate | 1.5–2.0 | 1.2 | 1.1 |
| High | >2.5 | 0.4 | 0.2 |

karyotypic abnormalities, most commonly a del (5q), monosomy 7 or del (7q), trisomy 8, and del (20q). These chromosomal abnormalities are also common in AML. The specific structural rearrangements that are closely associated with distinct morphologic subsets of AML de novo, such as t(15;17) in AML-M3, are almost never seen in MDS. Sometimes, however, patients will present with cytopenia and 10%–20% BM blasts, and a t(8;21) will be found in a cytogenetic analysis. These patients are best considered "evolving acute leukemia" [25]. Their outcome appears to be very good when managed with usual AML therapies. Complex cytogenetic abnormalities correlate with short survival. Abnormalities of chromosomes 5 and/or 7 are extremely common in therapy-related MDS (t-MDS) and have been linked with the poor prognosis of this disorder [15].

Supportive Care

No specific, uniformly effective therapy currently exists for MDS. Clinical prognostic factors, including BM morphology and cytogenetics, should be evaluated at diagnosis. A period of observation with close follow-up of serial PB counts is recommended for initial management, and a second BM examination after several months is useful to assess the rapidity of disease progression.

Patients with RA or RARS often have a clinically indolent course and may need no treatment for variable lengths of time. However, patients who are severely anemic (hemoglobin <7–8 g/dl), should receive red blood cell (RBC) transfusions. Washed RBC units are rarely necessary. Patients with peripheral vascular or coronary artery disease who are symptomatic should also receive red cell transfusions to ameliorate their symptoms. Commonly, the recurrence of fatigue or angina is a more useful indicator of the need for the next RBC transfusion than any particular hemoglobin level. Transfusion requirements increase as MDS progresses, and iron overload and hemochromatosis may occur when the cumulative transfusion burden exceeds 80–100 RBC units. This is not a common problem since most MDS patients are elderly and die first of intercurrent illnesses or from other complications of MDS. In younger patients, however, iron overload can lead to cardiac, hepatic, or endocrine disease. In these patients, iron stores can be estimated by measurement of serum iron concentration, transferrin saturation, and serum ferritin. Chronic chelation therapy with subcutaneously administered deferoxamine can delay the development of hemochromatosis.

Prophylactic platelet transfusions should not routinely be administered to thrombocytopenic patients with MDS because of the expense, inconvenience, and risk of alloimmunization. This risk increases with the frequency of platelet transfusion and may limit future treatment options. Platelet support should be reserved for treatment of acute hemorrhage or for prophylaxis prior to surgery. MDS patients with thrombocytopenia should be carefully instructed to avoid aspirin-containing products and other non-steroidal anti-inflammatory agents which interfere with platelet function.

Infections are a common problem in patients with MDS and can be life-threatening. The utility of vaccinations (Pneumovax, influenza, hepatitis B) should not be overlooked. Fever, localized infections, or even general malaise should be seriously evaluated in these patients who have both quantitative as well as functional neutropenia. Prompt institution of broad spectrum antibiotic coverage while trying to locate the source of infection is critical, and therapy should continue for 7–10 days even without an obvious source or positive blood cultures. Chronic outpatient antibacterial suppression with a quinolone derivative or another broad spectrum oral antibiotic can be considered for those patients who have required frequent hospitalizations for fevers presumed to be due to bacterial infections. If a neutropenic patient fails to respond to antibacterial agents or has repeated episodes of fever without an obvious source, a fungal infection should be suspected and treatment with amphotericin B or fluconazole or itraconazole should be initiated.

## Hematinics, Corticosteroids, Immunosuppressive Therapy, and Androgens

In the absence of evidence that a vitamin deficiency exists, supplementation with folic acid, vitamin $B_{12}$, pyridoxine, or iron is rarely helpful. Glucocorticoids at varying dosages have not been helpful in most patients with MDS and may lead to further immunosuppression [26]. The syndromes of autoimmune aplastic anemia and MDS overlap, and both can cause marked pancytopenia. Perhaps for that reason, improvements in blood counts have been reported from selected patients who received T-cell immunosuppression with antithymocyte globulin or cyclosporin.

Although androgens may stimulate erythropoiesis in patients with aplastic anemia or myelofibrosis, the evidence that androgens are beneficial in the treatment of MDS is largely anecdotal. Clinical trials including all FAB subtypes have demonstrated their lack of efficacy. A possible exception to these failures is the synthetic attenuated androgen danazol, which may prove useful in some thrombocytopenic patients with platelet-associated immunoglobulin [26].

### Cytotoxic Chemotherapy

The role of cytotoxic drugs in the treatment of MDS is uncertain for the majority of patients but should be considered for the younger and healthier patients with more aggressive forms of disease, such as those with RAEB, RAEB-T, and t-MDS. It is important to recognize patients presenting with "evolving" AML de novo, that is, AML with fewer than 30% blasts in the marrow but lacking significant dysplasia or an antecedent hematologic disorder. These patients respond to chemotherapy in the same fashion as do patients presenting with overt AML de novo [25]. In general, cytotoxic therapy with standard regimens used in the treatment of AML (containing daunorubicin and standard or high doses of cytarabine, for example) have had limited success in extending survival for the majority of MDS patients [26, 27]. This is not surprising for a number of reasons: (1) most MDS patients are elderly and poorly able to tolerate aggressive treatment, (2) the number of normal hematopoietic stem cells available to regenerate the marrow following therapy-induced hypoplasia is probably reduced, and (3) since the majority of effective antileukemia drugs act primarily during cell division, they may be relatively ineffective in the low proliferative states seen in MDS. For these reasons, intensive chemotherapy has been associated with complete response rates of only 10–40 percent with durations of remissions generally lasting less than one year. In older patients, the toxicity of the therapy and the prolonged marrow hypoplasia and cytopenia that it produces may actually shorten their lives. It is, therefore, important to direct this treatment option primarily to the younger group of MDS patients who are better able to tolerate it.

More recently, allogeneic bone marrow transplantation (BMT) has been tested as curative therapy in the small group of MDS patients who are younger than 60 years of age (approximately 10%–20% of all MDS patients) and who have a histocompatible donor [27, 28–30]. Several clinical trials have been published describing a variety of preparative regimens using combinations of busulfan and cyclophosphamide, etoposide, or cytarabine, or with total body irradiation. Results show disease-free survivals in approximately 45% of patients transplanted. Patients with favorable or intermediate cytogenetic factors have better outcomes than those with poor risk factors. These data suggest that appropriately chosen patients can respond to BMT with prolonged remissions and can probably be cured.

## Differentiating Agents

Since the vast majority of patients with MDS are not candidates for BMT, and the outcome with conventional cytotoxic therapy has generally been poor, attention has been focused on a variety of agents which can induce differentiation of acute leukemia cell lines in vitro, slowing proliferation and restoring apparently normal maturation and function. Several such "differentiating agents" have been tested in clinical trials of MDS [31].

Low doses of cytarabine can induce differentiation of leukemia cell lines in vitro together with inhibition of proliferation. Treatment has consisted of an average cytarabine dose of 20 mg/m$^2$/day, given subcutaneously over 14–21 days in single or divided doses or by continuous intravenous infusion. A large retrospective review of 170 MDS patients treated with low dose cytarabine revealed an overall response rate of 37%; the median duration of response was 10.5 months [32]. A randomized prospective trial, however, compared low dose cytarabine to supportive care and found no difference in overall survival in the two groups [33]. In addition low dose cytarabine therapy does have significant toxicity, particularly in elderly patients, and treatment related deaths are reported in about 15% of patients. In view of these results, low doses of cytarabine can not be broadly recommended for general use.

Clinical trials are continuing with polar-planar compounds such as HMBA, protein kinase C inhibitors such as bryostatin, and nucleoside analogues such as 5-azacytidine and 5-aza-2'-deoxycytidine. 5-Azacytidine is incorporated into newly synthesized DNA, leading to a reduction in DNA methyltransferase activity and to DNA hypomethylation.

13-Cis-retinoic acid (isotretinoin) has been reported to improve hematopoiesis in up to 30% of MDS patients in small series [34]. No significant hematologic responses were noted, however, in a larger random-ized trial comparing 13-cis retinoic acid at 100 mg/m$^2$ daily to oral place-bo [35]. Similarly disappointing results have been obtained when an-other differentiating agent, 1, 25-dihydroxy vitamin D3, was tested in MDS patients [36]. Attempts to increase the therapeutic benefit by escalating the vitamin D3 dose have been limited by hypercalcemia which occurs in most patients receiving more than 4 µg/day. All-trans retinoic acid (tret-inoin), which can produce marked and rapid differentiation in acute promyelocytic leukemia, is now being tested in MDS.

Part of the difficulty in evaluating benefit from treatment in patients with MDS is that the same criteria for assessing response in AML have generally been used. However, a "complete remission" may not be such an important goal in MDS. It may be more appropriate to evaluate the ability of specific therapy to palliate the symptoms of these chronic BM failure disorders in elderly patients, that is, to improve blood cell pro-duction and reduce transfusion requirements without necessarily eradi-cating the disease. The Cancer and Leukemia Group B (CALGB) has reanalyzed response data from two consecutive Phase II trials using low doses of 5-azacytidine either IV or SC in patients with MDS [37]. Trilineage responses were noted in 42% of the combined series with restitution of >50% of the deficit in all three peripheral blood cell lines. A significant reduction in RBC transfusions occurred in many patients. In a recently completed phase III trial, the CALGB showed significant improvements in quality of life as well as clinical outcome when patients received 5-azacytidine compared to supportive care alone [38].

## Hematopoietic Growth Factors

Recombinant human hematopoietic growth factors have recently become available for use in clinical trials in patients with various states of BM failure, including those with MDS [39]. Both recombinant human GM-CSF (granulocyte-CSF) and G-CSF (granulocyte colony stimulating fac-tor) have demonstrated potent stimulation of hematopoiesis in patients with MDS [40]. As yet, there are little data to suggest any specificity of response (i.e., normal or neoplastic) to the growth factors. Prolonged intravenous infusions or daily subcutaneous injections of GM-CSF elicit dose-related increases in peripheral neutrophils, eosinophils and mono-cytes in almost all patients. A GM-CSF dose of 3 ug/kg per day is sufficient to produce a granulocyte count of 5000–10,000/µl in most RA and RAEB patients. The useful dose range of G-CSF is also about 1–3 ug/kg per day. These drugs have been generally well tolerated even in elderly patients, and tachyphylaxis or neutralizing antibodies have not yet been observed with repeated administration. A multi-institutional clinical trial demonstrated that MDS patients receiving GM-CSF for 3 months had fewer infections than a matched control group [41]. Unfortunately, despite the multi-lineage potency of GM-CSF in vitro, improvements in anemia or thrombocytopenia have only occasionally been observed in treated patients. The use of G-CSF together with antibiotics is justifiable in neutropenic MDS patients with severe infections.

Other recombinant growth factors with potential for multi-lineage stimulation are IL-3 (interleukin 3 or multi-CSF), IL-1, c-kit ligand (stem cell factor, SCF), and FLT3 ligand, and these, too, have recently entered clinical trials. IL-3 has demonstrated the ability to augment leukocytes (neutrophils, eosinophils, basophils, monocytes, and lymphocytes) but improvements in platelet counts were transient and disappointing [42].

Anemic MDS patients who have normal renal function usually have very high, physiological levels of endogenous erythropoietin. As yet, there are few data that additional erythropoietin in pharmacological doses will provide any clinical benefit for these patients. Patients with suboptimal serum erythropoietin levels, however, may benefit from moderate or high doses of recombinant erythropoietin [43]. Recent trials that have combined erythropoietin with G-CSF have demonstrated that the dosage, timing, and duration of administration of these 2 cytokines are important and need further investigation [44].

One mechanism that might explain the central paradox of MDS, namely a hypercellular marrow with severe PB cytopenia, is increased apoptosis. Higher than normal levels of inhibitory cytokines such as TNF-$\alpha$, TGF-$\beta$, and IL1-$\beta$ have been measured in MDS marrows. Anti-cytokine therapies have produced clinical responses [45]. Amifostine has proliferative effects on normal hematopoiesis and has been used in pilot studies in MDS [46].

## Summary and Future Directions

The myelodysplastic syndromes are biologically heterogeneous and differ with respect to clinical features and prognosis. Good supportive care

remains the mainstay of management for most patients. Complete eradication of the abnormal clone is a possibility for those MDS patients who
are younger, with advanced disease, and who can tolerate aggressive
cytotoxic chemotherapy or who are candidates for allogeneic BMT. Some
patients have had clinical benefit after treatment with 5-azacytidine.
Occasional patients may benefit from treatment with low dose cytarabine, cyclosporin, cis-retinoic acid, corticosteroids, danazol, or amifostine, but empiric therapy with these agents cannot be generally
recommended.

Enrollment of MDS patients into clinical trials testing new therapeutic approaches should be given high priority. Use of new retinoids or
vitamin D analogues with a higher therapeutic index or low doses of
chemotherapy agents that alter gene expression merit further investigation. The early results of treatment with recombinant hematopoietic
growth factors indicate that, either alone or in combination, they are
likely to prove useful in reducing the infectious and hemorrhagic complications that are currently the major cause of morbidity and mortality
in MDS. CSF's may also decrease morbidity after chemotherapy by
shortening the interval to hematologic recovery. Thirdly, CSF's that have
primarily differentiating activity with less proliferative activity may be
useful in slowing the progression of MDS to leukemia. Major advances in
the treatment of MDS may depend on the application of these concepts
in future investigations.

## References

1. Bennett JM, Catovsky D, Daniel MT, et al. Proposals for the classification of the
   myelodysplastic syndromes. Br J Haematol 51:189–199, 1982
2. Rosati S, Mick R, Xu F, et al. Refractory anemia with multilineage dysplasia: further
   characterization of an "unclassifiable" myelodysplastic syndrome. Leukemia
   10:20–26, 1996
3. Jacobs RH, Cornbleet MA, Vardiman JW, et al. Prognostic implications of morphology and karyotype in primary myelodysplastic syndromes. Blood 67:1765–1772,
   1986
4. List AF, Garewal HS, and Sandberg AA: The myelodysplastic syndromes: Biology
   and implications for management. J Clin Oncol 8:1424–1441, 1990
5. Fenaux P, Morel P, Lai JL. Cytogenetics of myelodysplastic syndromes. Semin
   Hematol 33:127–138, 1996
6. Van den Berghe H, Vermaelen K, Mecurri C, et al. The 5q- anomaly. Cancer Genet
   Cytogenet 17:189–255, 1985
7. Delacretaz F, Schmidt PM, Piguet D, et al. Histopathology of myelodysplastic syndromes: The FAB classification (proposals) applied to bone marrow biopsy. Am J
   Clin Pathol 87:180–186, 1987

8. Tricot G, De Wolf-Peeters C, Hendricks B, et al. Bone marrow histology in myelo-dysplastic syndromes. I. Histological findings in myelodysplastic syndromes and comparison with bone marrow smears. Br J Haematol 57:423–430, 1984

9. Tricot G, De Wolf-Peeters C, Vlietinck R, et al. Bone marrow histology in myelo-dysplastic syndromes. II. Prognostic value of abnormal localization of immature precursors in MDS. Br J Haematol 58:217–225, 1984

10. Rios A, Canizo MC, Sanz MA, et al. Bone marrow biopsy in myelodysplastic syn-dromes: Morphological characteristics and contribution to the study of prognostic factors. Br J Haematol 75:26–33, 1990

11. Storniolo AM, Moloney WC, Rosenthal DS, et al. Chronic myelomonocytic leuke-mia. Leukemia 4:766–770, 1990

12. Tefferi A, Hoagland HC, Therneau TM, et al. Chronic myelomonocytic leukemia: Natural history and prognostic determinants. Mayo Clin Proc 64:1246–1254, 1989

13. Hirsch-Ginsberg C, LeMaistre AC, Kantarjian H, et al. RAS mutations are rare events in Philadelphia chromosome-negative/bcr gene rearrangement-negative chronic myelogenous leukemia, but are prevalent in chronic myelomonocytic leu-kemia. Blood 76:1214–1219, 1990

14. Hamblin TJ, Oscier DG: The myelodysplastic syndrome: A practical guide. Hematol Oncol 5:19–34, 1987

15. Thirman MJ, Larson RA: Therapy-related myeloid leukemia. Hem/Oncol Clinics No Am 10:293–320, 1996

16. Vardiman JW, Le Beau MM, Albain K, et al. Myelodysplasia: A comparison of thera-py-related and primary forms. Ann Biol Clin 43:369–387, 1985

17. Yoshida Y, Oguma S, Uchino H, et al. Refractory myelodysplastic anaemias with hypocellular bone marrow. J Clin Pathol 41:763–767, 1988

18. Appelbaum FR, Barrall J, Storb R, et al. Clonal cytogenetic abnormalities in pati-ents with otherwise typical aplastic anemia. Exp Hematol 15:1134–1139, 1987

19. Kampmeier P, Anastasi J, Vardiman JW. Issues in the pathology of myelodysplastic syndromes. Hemato Oncol Clinic North Am 6:501–22, 1992

20. Rosati S, Anastasi J, Vardiman JW. Recurring diagnostic problems in the patholo-gy of the myelodysplastic syndromes. Semin Hematol 33:111–126, 1996

22. Mufti GJ, Stevens JR, Oscier DG, et al. Myelodysplastic syndromes: A scoring system with prognostic significance. Br J Haematol 59:425–33, 1985

23. Sanz GF, Sanz MA, Vallespi T, et al. Two regression models and a scoring system for predicting survival and planning treatment in myelodysplastic syndromes: A mul-tivariate analysis of prognostic factors in 370 patients. Blood 74:395–408, 1989

24. Greenberg P, Cox C, LeBeau MM et al. International scoring system for evaluating prognosis in myelodysplastic syndromes. Blood 89:2079–2088, 1996

25. Bernstein SH, Brunetto VL, Davey FR et al. Acute myeloid leukemia-type chemo-therapy for newly diagnosed patients without antecedent cytopenias having myelodysplastic syndrome as defined by French-American-British Criteria: A Cancer and Leukemia Group B Study. J Clin Oncol 14:2486, 1996

26. Cheson BD: The myelodysplastic syndromes: Current approaches to therapy. Ann Intern Med 112:932–941, 1990

27. Gassmann W, Schmitz N, Loffler H, DeWitte T. Intensive chemotherapy and bone marrow transplantation for myelodysplastic syndromes. Semin Hemal 33:196–205, 1996

28. Anderson JE, Appelbaum FR, Fisher LD, et al. Allogeneic bone marrow transplan-tation for 93 patients with myelodysplastic syndrome. Blood 82:677–681, 1993

29. O'Donnell MR, Nademanee AP, Snyder DS, et al. Bone marrow transplantation for myelodysplastic and myeloproliferative syndromes. J Clin Oncol 5:1822, 1987

30. Bunin NJ, Casper JT, Chitambar C, et al. Partially matched bone marrow transplantation using T-cell depletion in patients with myelodysplastic syndrome. J Clin Oncol 6:1851, 1988
31. Morosetti R, Koeffler HP. Differentiation therapy in myelodysplastic syndromes. Semin Hematol 33:236–245, 1996
32. Cheson BD, Jasperse DM, Simon R, and Friedman MA: A critical appraisal of low-dose cytosine arabinoside in patients with acute non-lymphocytic leukemia and myelodysplastic syndromes. J Clin Oncol 4:1857–64, 1986
33. Miller KB, Kim K, Morrison FS, et al. The evaluation of low-dose cytarabine in the treatment of myelodysplastic syndromes: a phase III intergroup study. Ann Hematol 65:162–168, 1992
34. Clark RE, Ismail SA, Jacobs A, et al. A randomized trial of 13-cis retinoic acid with or without cytosine arabinoside in patients with the myelodysplastic syndrome. Br J Haematol 66:77–83, 1987
35. Koeffler HP, Heitjan D, Mertelsmann R, et al. Randomized study of 13-cis retinoic acid vs placebo in the myelodysplastic disorders. Blood 71:703–8, 1988
36. Koeffler HP, Hirji K, Itri L: 1, 25-Dihydroxyvitamin D3: in vivo and in vitro effects on human preleukemic and leukemic cells. Cancer Treat Rep 69:1399–1407, 1985
37. Silverman LR, Holland JF, Nelson D, et al. Trilineage response of myelodysplastic syndromes to subcutaneous azacytidine. Proc Am Soc Clin Oncol 10:222 (#747), 1991
38. Silberman LR, Demakos EP, Peterson B et al. A randomized controlled trial of subcutaneous azacitidine in patients with the myelodysplastic syndrome: A study of the Cancer and Leukemia Group B. Proc Am Soc Clin Oncol, 1998 (in press)
39. Greenburg PL, Negrin R, Nagler A: The use of hematopoietic growth factors in the treatment of myelodysplastic syndromes. Cancer Surveys 9:199–212, 1990
40. Ganser A, Hoelzer D. Clinical use of hematopoietic growth factors in the myelodysplastic syndromes. Semin Hematol 33:186–195, 1996
41. Schuster MW, Larson RA, Thompson JA, et al. Granulocyte-macrophage colony-stimulating factor for myelodysplastic syndrome: Results of a multi-center randomized controlled trial. Blood 76 (Suppl 1) 318a (#1263), 1990
42. Ganser A, Seipelt G, Lindermann A, et al. Effects of recombinant human interleukin-3 in patients with myelodysplastic syndromes. Blood 76:455–462, 1990
43. Stein RS, Abels RI, Krantz SB: Pharmacologic doses of recombinant human erythropoietin in the treatment of myelodysplastic syndromes. Blood 78: 1658–1663, 1991
44. Negrin RS, Stein R, Vardiman J et al. Treatment of the anemia of myelodysplastic syndromes using recombinant human granulocyte colony-stimulating factor in combination with erythropoietin. Blood 82:737–743, 1993
45. Raza A, Gezer S, Mundle S et al. Apoptosis in bone marrow biopsy samples involving stromal and hematopoietic cells in 50 patients with myelodysplastic syndromes. Blood 86:268–276, 1995
46. List AF, Brasfield F, Heaton R et al. Stimulation of hematopoiesis by amifostine in patients with myelodysplastic syndrome. Blood 90:3364–3369, 1997

# Myeloproliferative Syndromes

T.P. Szatrowski

## Introduction

The name "myeloproliferative disorders" was coined by William Dameshek in 1951 [1], and these include four sub-diseases: polycythemia vera (PV), essential thrombocythemia (ET), agnogenic myeloid metaplasia (AMM), and chronic myelogenous leukemia (CML). CML can also be considered a form of chronic leukemia, and hence is discussed in the chapter by that name. The myeloproliferative disorders (MPD) often share many features in common and may be difficult to distinguish one from another. This heterogeneous group of chronic hematopoietic neoplasms is characterized by proliferation of one or more cell lines in the bone marrow and one or more elevated peripheral blood counts. Other frequent clinical features include splenomegaly, fibrosis of the bone marrow, eosinophilia and basophilia, and alterations in certain biochemical parameters such as vitamin $B_{12}$, $B_{12}$-binding capacity, and leukocyte alkaline phosphatase. The myeloproliferative disorders are characterized by the frequent occurrence of chromosomal abnormalities. These cytogenetic characteristics, as well as glucose-6-phosphate dehydrogenase studies and molecular genetic methods have served to establish the clonal origin of the MPD [2].

## Polycythemia Vera

Polycythemia vera is a disease whose clinical picture is dominated by an elevated hemoglobin concentration, that is neither spurious nor secondary – whence the name. It is characterized by the occurrence of spenomegaly and an increased production of all myeloid elements. Its course is chronic and usually slowly progressive.

Epidemiology/Risk Factors

Polycythemia vera is a rare entity, with an annual incidence rate that varies worldwide somewhat from about 0.2 to about 50 per million. PV may be slightly more common in men than women, and occurs most commonly in the sixth and seventh decades of life. It may occur with increased frequency in Jews of Eastern European ancestry, and with decreased frequency in African-Americans.

No etiologic agent has been clearly identified for the vast majority of patients with polycythemia vera. A few instances of the familial occurrence of PV have been reported, while a relatively higher incidence of PV has been reported in survivors of the atomic bomb explosion in Hiroshima, in United States military personnel involved in the detonation of a nuclear device in 1957, and anecdotally in patients occupationally exposed to chemical toxins.

Pathology and Staging of PV

Most patients with PV present in the early stages of the disease, manifesting plethora, splenomegaly, and pancytosis. It is not uncommon however for relatively asymptomatic patients to have an elevated hemoglobin level on a routine complete blood count. Patients also frequently have an elevated leukocyte alkaline phosphatase (LAP) level, hyperuricemia from increased production and destruction of myeloid cells, basophilia, and hepatomegaly. Bone marrow examination is non-specific, and shows erythroid hyperplasia or panhyperplasia. An abnormal karyotype is seen in 12% to 31% of patients with PV. While patients typically experience nonspecific symptoms such as headache, dizziness, visual changes, pruritus, upper gastrointestinal symptoms, dyspnea, pleuritic chest pain, and paresthesias, the major source of morbidity and mortality in PV patients is arterial and venous thromboembolic disease. Hemorrhagic manifestations are also common. The abnormal platelet function seen in this and other myeloproliferative disorders does not clearly correlate with the occurrence of thrombohemorrhagic phenomena, which occur more frequently in the presence of thrombocytosis [3] and erythrocytosis [4]. Finally it may be important to consider a diagnosis of polycythemia vera in the patient with a hemoglobin or hematocrit in the upper normal range who also has microcytosis and iron deficiency.

The median survival in patients with polycythemia vera from the time of diagnosis currently stands at approximately 15 years [5]; survival may depend on age at diagnosis, younger patients experiencing a considerably better prognosis than older patients. Though there is the appearance of an increasing trend in the reports of overall survival estimates for patients with PV over time [6], this may be due to lead time bias in diagnosis as asymptomatic patients have blood counts performed more routinely.

Though life expectancy in the first 10 years following diagnosis for patients with PV is not greatly different than age-matched controls [7], subsequently they may develop advanced fatal manifestations of PV, including postpolycythemia myeloid metaplasia ("spent phase"), fatal thromboembolic events, and acute leukemia. Postpolycythemia myeloid metaplasia is characterized by extensive bone marrow fibrosis resulting in a leukoerythroblastic peripheral blood picture, worsening splenomegaly with extramedullary hematopoiesis, and anemia unrelated to myelosuppressive treatment. Most patients die within 3 years of the onset of spent phase PV. Acute leukemia with or without prior myelodysplasia can occur in 1% to 2% of patients treated without myelosuppressive agents, and it is usually refractory to remission induction attempts.

## Work-up and Staging of PV

The most important consideration in the work-up of a patient with suspected polycythemia vera is the definitive exclusion of spurious and secondary erythrocytosis. Spurious erythrocytosis, which is not associated with an increased red cell mass, may be seen in the presence of dehydration, hypertension, and tobacco use. Secondary erythrocytosis, accompanied by an increased red cell mass, is, unlike polycythemia vera, non-clonal and most often associated with augmented erythropoietin production as in chronic hypoxic states (most commonly chronic lung disease and high altitudes) and in the case of pathologic production of erythropoietin by certain tumors and in kidney disorders.

Given the rarity of PV and the considerable clinical judgement needed in its accurate diagnosis, it may be reasonable to appeal early to the expertise of experienced academic medical centers to expedite diagnosis of the patient with an elevated hematocrit. The recommendations of the Polycythemia Vera Study Group [8] for the diagnosis of polycythemia vera were empirically derived, but have been widely followed. Largely based on the measurement of the red blood cell mass by isotope dilution of $^{51}Cr$-labeled autologous red blood cells, these guidelines suggested a diagnosis of polycythemia vera whenever (a) an increased red cell mass was accompanied by (b) normal arterial oxygen saturation and (c) splenomegaly – three major criteria; a PV diagnosis was also suggested in the presence of the first two major criteria and any two of the following five minor criteria: thrombocytosis, leukocytosis, elevated LAP score, increased serum vitamin $B_{12}$ level, or increased serum vitamin $B_{12}$ binding capacity. Subsequently it has been recognized that a simpler algorithm that takes advantage of the availablity of reliable serum erythropoietin assays may be more appropriate [9]. Since it is unlikely that spurious erythrocytosis could account for a hematocrit above 58 in men or 52 in women, measurement of the red cell mass may be superfluous, and one may proceed directly to measurement of the serum erythropoietin. For hematocrit values that are abnormally high but below the aforementioned values, polycythemia vera is unlikely in the absence of spenomegaly or microcytosis, and patients should have a repeat blood count in 90 days; a higher value should prompt serum erythropoietin testing. Patients with borderline elevations in hematocrit as well as splenomegaly or microcytosis should have an erythropoietin level drawn. Since splenomegaly may increase plasma volume and make the hematocrit an inaccurate reflection of red cell mass, in patients with a large spleen, the direct measurment of the red cell mass is diagnostically helpful. In all instances, of course, the presence of other manifestations of PV may help confirm a diagnosis.

The serum erythropoietin level is usually below the lower limits of normal in patients with polycythemia vera, and normal in spurious erythropoietin. Secondary erythrocytosis is by definition associated with elevated erythropoietin levels. Interpreted in the appropriate clinical setting, reliable serum erythropoietin levels may therefore be very helpful in the differential diagnosis of PV [10].

Specific Treatment Options for PV

Although much has been learned in recent decades about the treatment of PV, the optimal therapy for individual patients cannot be readily described. It is generally agreed that untreated polycythemia vera carries a very high two-year mortality. At the same time, patients vary widely in age, and may develop a variety of comorbid conditions in the course of this chronic disease. Moreover it has been shown that patients whose hematocrit is controlled with phlebotomy are still at an increased risk of thrombosis [11].

Phlebotomy, which is safe and conveniently performed, remains the mainstay of treatment for all patients. Newly diagnosed patients should have their hematocrit reduced into the gender-specific normal range, typically less than 45 for men, and less than 40 for women. In the absence of other vascular risk factors, younger patients can initially undergo phlebotomy without vascular instability as often as every other day. Those patients who may need to avoid rapid fluctuations in blood volume, such as those undergoing emergency surgery, can undergo exchange phlebotomy with an appropriate plasma expander; it is important to realize that peri-operative morbidity and mortality are approximately fivefold increased in the patient with uncontrolled erythrocytosis from PV.

The strategy for longer-term management of the patient with PV is less clear-cut. The results of a series of clinical trials carried out by the Polycythemia Vera Study Group [12] have been widely quoted. In one study 431 patients were initially phlebotomized to a normal hematocrit and then randomly assigned to either continued phlebotomy alone, treatment with the radioisotope $^{32}$P, or treatment with the alkylating agent chlorambucil. Treatment with either chlorambucil or $^{32}$P was associated with an increased incidence of secondary hematopoietic (chiefly acute leukemia) and nonhematopoietic malignancies, and a diminished overall survival compared to those treated with phlebotomy alone. Consequently, alkylating agents and radioisotopes are rarely any longer used in the treatment of polycythemia vera.

Results from the same study indicated, however, that treatment with phlebotomy alone was associated with a somewhat elevated risk of thrombosis in the first three years following initiation of treatment; this finding has led to a search for an optimal therapeutic regimen, minimizing the risk of both leukemogenesis and thrombosis. Subsequent Polycythemia Vera Study Group trials have suggested that nonleukemogenic myelosuppression may be achieved with the combined use of phlebotomy and hydroxyurea, which acts by inhibiting DNA synthesis. A reasonable starting dose is 1000 mg p.o. q.day, which can then be adjusted to keep the patient's platelet count under 400,000/µl. Sometimes the platelet count cannot be controlled without leukopenia or anemia, in which case the platelet-lowering agent anagrelide may be useful [13]; a starting dose is 0.5 mg p.o. q.i.d.. In general patients with PV should receive thromboreductive treatment when their platelet counts exceed 600,000/µl. Patients who have an acute thrombohemorragic event in the setting of thrombocytosis may need immediate platelet apheresis in additon to a platelet lowering agent.

Though platelet antiaggregating agents such as aspirin and dipyrida-mole augmented the risk of hemorrhage without decreasing the risk of thrombosis in a Polycythemia Vera Study Group clinical trial, these agents may be indicated in patients with erythromelalgia and other vasomotor symptoms, and in patients with a prior history of thrombosis.

An alternative, recently elucidated, therapeutic option in patients whose disease is difficult to control with the modalities discussed above is the use of interferon-$\alpha$, a biological response modifier that has controlled myeloproliferation and splenomegaly in small numbers of patients [14]. The starting dose is $3 \times 10^6$ U/m$^2$ administered subcutaneously three times per week. Again this dose may be adjusted according to blood counts and side effects, the latter frequently being not insignificant. Given these complexities in the therapy of PV and the considerable clinical judgement therein required, it may be reasonable to appeal early to experienced academic medical centers to obtain expert guidance.

Other useful adjunctive agents in the treatment of polycythemia vera include $H_1$ and $H_2$ blockers for pruritus, and allopurinol for clinically important hyperuricemia associated with myeloproliferation.

## Essential Thrombocythemia

Essential thrombocythemia is a myeloproliferative disorder whose dominant characteristic is an abnormally elevated platelet count. Though ET is felt to be a disorder of a multipotent stem cell, like PV and AMM it has no pathognomonic feature. It must therefore be distinguished diagnostically from the other myeloproliferative disorders and from so-called reactive forms of thrombocytosis. The major source of morbidity in patients with ET is the occurrence of thrombohemorrhagic complications.

## Epidemiology/Risk Factors of ET

ET is the least frequent of the myeloproliferative disorders, occurring with an estimated annual incidence of about 1 per million. The median age at the time of diagnosis is 60 years, and reported cases range from infancy to the tenth decade. The female-to-male ratio is about 1.3:1. The etiology of ET remains obscure. Surprisingly, early studies attempting to evaluate the role of thrombopoietin and its receptor (c-mpl) in ET have not shown clear correlations between serum thrombopoietin levels and the presence or absence of various types of thrombocytosis [15]. Nevertheless it appears that the proto-oncogene c-mpl is involved in spontaneous megakaryopoiesis in myeloproliferative disorders [16].

## Pathology and Staging of ET

Examination of the peripheral blood usually shows giant platelets and platelet aggregates, while the marrow is hyperproliferative and often has large numbers of megakaryocytes, with variable amounts of fibrosis. Neither these findings nor theabsolute platelet count has been found to predict prognosis or overall survival, which is probably not vastly different from a control population. Similarly, while platelet function testing sometimes reveals an abnormality in response to agonists, particularly epinephrine, these do not predict the occurance of bleeding or thrombosis.

Cytogenetic abnormalities are quite rare in ET. Moderate splenomegaly may be seen in up to two-thirds of patients with ET.

While most patients with ET are asymptomatic at presentation, typically a time of routine blood count, some will have manifested a hemorrhagic or thrombotic episode. The latter are often arterial such as transient ischemic attacks or frank strokes.

## Work-up and Staging of ET

Analogous to the setting of polycythemia vera, the work-up of the patient with marked thrombocytosis focuses on the exclusion of reactive – secondary – thrombocytosis and the other myeloproliferative disorders. This may be aided clinically by the recognition of obvious conditions that are know to be associated with reactive thrombocytosis: infectious or inflammatory states, tissue damage (including post-surgery), post-splenectomy, non-hematologic malignancy, and iron deficiency and acute blood loss anemia. Reactive thrombocytosis is not otherwise associated with thrombosis, hemorrhage, splenomegaly, or bone marrow fibrosis. The Polycythemia Vera Study Group has proposed the following diagnostic criteria [17], whose utility has not however been verified: (a) platelet count greater than 600,000/μl, (b) absence of conditions associated with thrombocytosis, (c) normal red blood cell mass, (d) no Philadelphia chromosome, and (e) absent bone marrow fibrosis, or, in the absence of both splenomegaly and leukoerythroblastosis, fibrosis less than one-third the cross-sectional area of the bone marrow biopsy.

It may in fact be most difficult to distinguish between ET with considerable marrow fibrosis on the one hand, and early (relatively cellular) agnogenic myeloid metaplasia with myelofibrosis on the other. The absence of the Philadelphia chromosome and of an elevated red cell mass effectively rule out CML and PV respectively.


Specific Treatment Options for ET

It is generally agreed that patients with ET require treatment of their elevated platelet count because of the risk, which may reach 20%, of major thrombohemorrhagic complications. Nonetheless, the overall benefit to such patients has not been demonstrated in a randomized clinical trials. ET patients with extreme thrombocytosis of more than 2,000,000 platelets per μl carry a particulaly high risk of hemorrhage [18] and may be appropriate for immediate thromboreductive measures. Agents with anti-platelet effects such as non-steroidal anti-inflammatory drugs are likely to precipitate hemorrhage and are best avoided.Special consideration may be accorded the patient who is pregnant or under the age of 40 (see below).

Since anagrelide, whose mechanism of action may be at the level of megakaryocyte maturation, is not thought to be leukemogenic, this agent may be the drug of choice for patients with ET [19]. The response rate in patients with ET is over 90%, and the median time to response is approximately three weeks. A starting dose is 0.5 mg p.o. q.i.d.. The side effect profile includes palpitations, headaches, fluid retention, anemia, nausea, diarrhea, dizziness, and occasionally heart failure; overall most side effects are mild to moderate.

Interferon-α has also been used in the treatment of ET [20], but has cost and side effect considerations.

The treatment of young patients with ET is an area of considerable controversy. The five-year risk of thrombohemorrhagic complications in this demographic subgroup may be as low as 10% [21]. Similarly, it has been difficult to demonstrate a benefit to any particular form of treatment for the pregnant patient. Therefore, it may be prudent to consider observation only in good-risk, young patients who are pregnant or are asymptomatic and free of cardiovascular risk factors.

**Agnogenic Myeloid Metaplasia**

Agnogenic myeloid metaplasia is a clonal hematopoietic stem cell disorder, which shares many of the clinical features of myeloproliferative disorders. It is characterized by bone marrow fibrosis and extramedullary hematopoiesis; these in turn give rise to pancytopenia, leukoerythroblastosis, dacrocytosis, and hepatosplenomegaly. It is thought that myelofibrosis is mediated by certain megakaryocyte-derived growth factors, notably TGF-β [22], PDGF, and EGF, which augment the proliferation and synthetic activity of nonclonal fibroblasts and inhibit the the degradation of excess collagen, especially types I and III.

Epidemiology/Risk Factors of AMM

The annual incidence of AMM is about 5 per million. The median age is 60, and there is a slight male preponderance.

Pathology and Staging of AMM

The five- and ten-year overall survival rates are about 50% and 20% respectively. One study of prognosis in AMM identified the presence of more than 10% white cell precursors myeloblasts, promyelocytes, or myelocytes) in the peripheral white blood cell count and a hemoglobin of less than 10 g/dl as predictors of inferior outcome; in this study, leukemic transformation was responsible for up to 27% of the observed deaths [23]. About one-third of AMM patients will have cytogenetic abnormalities at the time of diagnosis, and these may connote poorer prognosis [24].

## Work-up and Staging of AMM

Patients typically present with normocytic anemia and splenomegaly, but may frequently have other hematologic abnormalities typical of myeloproliferative disorders, including leukocytosis, thrombocytosis, or thrombocytopenia. Since an important precipitant of surgical bleeding in these patients is occult disseminated intravascular coagulation, a careful screening for this entity should be made prior to any operative procedure [25]. Hypermetabolism and constitutional symptoms often occur in AMM patients. Extramedullary hematopoiesis may occur in the small bowel, spinal cord, brain, lungs, peritoneal cavity, and urinary tract, in addition to the liver and spleen, leading to sometimes painful symptoms. Bone radiographs show osteosclerosis and increased bone density.

The hallmark of AMM is bone marrow fibrosis, which is readily identified on stain for either collagen or reticulin. However it is a non-specific finding, occurring in at least 10% of other myeloproliferative disorders, and several other important hematologic malignancies including myelodysplasia (chronic myelomonocytic leukemia), acute megakaryoblastic leukemia (acute myeloid leukemia FAB M-7), hairy cell leukemia, Hodgkin's disease and non-Hodgkin's lymphoma; occasionally myelofibrosis is seen in benign disorders and in metastatic carcinoma.

## Specific Treatment Options for AMM

No curative therapy is currently available for patients with agnogenic myeloid metaplasia. Moreover it has been difficult to establish a clear benefit to most treatment modalities. Presently available treatment is aimed at alleviation of symptoms and optimization of quality of life.

Splenectomy may be useful in the patient with symptomatic splenomegaly, which can be massive, who has an otherwise good performance status. Low-dose splenic irradiation (200 cGy delivered in 10–15 daily fractions) may be useful in poor surgical candidates but the benefit is usually short-lived.

Androgens (oxymethalone) have been given for anemia, and anagrelide (vide supra) may be useful in the AMM patient manifesting thrombocytosis.

Attempts to use chemotherapy, high-dose chemotherapy with bone marrow support, and interferon have not been successful. New treatments for agnogenic myeloid metaplasia are clearly urgently needed, and patients with this rare disorder may be candidates for referral to experienced academic medical centers, particularly where protocol-based therapy may be available.

## References

1. Dameshak W (1951) Some speculations on the myeloproliferative syndromes. Blood 6:372–375
2. Adamson JW et al. (1978) Polycythemia vera: Stem cell and probable clonal origin of the disease. N Engl J Med 295:913–916
3. Najean Y, Dresch C, Rain JD (1994) The very-long-term course of polycythaemia: a complement to the previously published data of the Polycythemia Vera Study Group. Br J Haematol 86:233–235
4. Wade JP (1983) Transport of oxygen to the brain in patients with elevated haematocrit values before and after venesection. Brain 106:513–523
5. Gruppo Italiano Studio Policitemia (1995) Polycythemia vera: the natural history of 1213 patients followed for 20 years. Ann Intern Med 123:656–664
6. Berk et al. (1986) Therapeutic recommendations in polycythemia vera based on PVSG protocols. Semin Hematol 23:132–143
7. Rozman C et al. (1991) Life expectancy of patients with chronic nonleukemic myeloproliferative disorders. Cancer 67:2658–2663
8. Berk PD et al. (1986) Therapeutic recommendations in polycythemia vera based on polycythemia vera study group protocols. Semin Hematol 23:132–143
9. Tefferi A, Silverstein MN (1996) Diagnosis and treatment of polycythemia vera, agnogenic myeloid metaplasia, and essential thrombocythemia. In: Wiernik PH et al. (eds) Neoplastic diseases of the blood (3rd edition). Churchill Livingstone, New York, pp 137–139
10. Birgegard G, Wide L (1992) Serum erythropoietin in the diagnosis of polycythemias and after phlebotomy treatment. Br J Haematol 81:603–606
11. Najean Y, Dresch C, Rain JD (1994) The very-long-term course of polycythaemia: a complement to the previously published data of the Polycythemia Vera Study Group. Br J Haematol 86:233–235
12. Berk PD et al. (1995) Treatment of polycythemia vera: a summary of clinical trials conducted by the Polycythemia Vera Study Group. In: Wasserman LR et al. (eds) Polycythemia vera and myeloproliferative disorders. WB Saunders, Philadelphia, pp 166–194
13. Silverstein MN et al. (1988) Anagrelide: a new drug for treating thrombocytosis. N Engl J Med 318:1292–1294
14. Silver RT (1993) Interferon-a2b: a new treatment for polycythemia vera. Ann Intern Med 119:1091–1092
15. Cerutti A et al. (1997) Thrombopoietin levels in patients with primary and reactive thrombocytosis. Br J Haematol 99:281–284
16. Griesshammer M et al. (1997) A possible role for thrombopoietin and its receptor c-mpl in the pathobiology of essential thrombocythemia. Semin Thromb Hemostas 23:419–423

17. Tefferi A, Hoagland HC (1994) Issues in the diagnosis and management of essential thrombocythemia. Mayo Clin Proc 69:651–655
18. Fenaux P et al. (1990) Clinical course of essential thrombocythemia in 147 cases. Cancer 66:549–556
19. Anagrelide study group (1992) Anagrelide, a therapy for thrombocythemic states: experience in 577 patients. Am J Med 92:69–76
20. Middlehoff G, Boll I (1992) A long-term clinical trial of interferon alpha therapy in essential thrombocythemia. Ann Hematol 64:207–209
21. McIntyre KJ et al. (1991) Essential thrombocythemia in young adults. Mayo Clin Proc 66:149–154
22. Terui T et al. (1990) The production of transforming growth factor-beta in acute megakaryoblastic leukemia and its possible implications in myelofibrosis. Blood 57:1540–1548
23. Visani G et al. (1990) Myelofibrosis with myeloid metaplasia: clinical and haematological parameters predicting survival in a series of 133 patients. Br J Haematol 75:4–9
24. Demory JL et al. (1988) Cytogenetic studies and their prognostic significance in agnogenic myeloid metaplasia: a report on 47 cases. Blood 72:855–859
25. Silverstein MN, ReMine WH (1979) Splenectomy in myeloid metaplasia. Blood 53:515–518

# Hairy Cell Leukemia

H.M. Golomb

## Epidemiology, Risk Factors

Hairy cell leukemia (HCL) is a rare disease, involving approximately 600 new patients each year in the U.S.A. The median age at the time of diagnosis is approximately 52 years, and about one-half of the cases occur between 40 and 60 years of age, but have occurred as young as 22 and as old as 86 years of age. Men are affected more often than women by a ratio of approximately 4 to 1. There is a familial inheritance pattern in approximately 1% of the cases with clear parent and child diagnoses of HCL. Other suggested environmental associations such as radiation, or benzene exposures have been repudiated.

## Pathology and Staging

Diagnosis is based on the finding of lymphocytes with the characteristic irregular cytoplasmic projections on blood and bone marrow smears by conventional light microscopy. Transmission electron microscopy can confirm the presence of the cytoplasm projections and also demonstrate a ribosome-lamellae complex in hairy cells in about 50% of cases. The hairy cell is considered to be of B-cell lineage and reacts with monoclonal antibodies in a pattern that supports its B cell origin such as CD11C, CD19, CD20, CD22, and CD25 (interleukin-2 receptor). The bone marrow biopsy usually shows a replacement by a monomorphic mononuclear infiltrate in which the cells have round or oval nuclei and abundant pale cytoplasm; normal hematopoietic cells are reduced in number. Bone marrow aspirates tend to be difficult to collect because of increased reticulin in the marrow. Tartrate-resistant acid phosphatase (TRAP) staining is almost always positive, but this finding is not pathognomonic for

HCL. Staining for reticulin shows increased fibers, accounting in part for the dry tap found in approximately two-thirds of patients when bone marrow aspiration is attempted. No specific staging system has proven useful as is the case for many leukemias.

## Work-up and Staging

The clinical manifestations at presentation are related to cytopenias (fatigue, easy bruising, infection) and splenomegaly (abdominal fullness or discomfort). Splenomegaly is found in the initial physical examination in approximately 85% of the patients, but only causes symptoms in about 20% of patients. Peripheral adenopathy is uncommon, but retroperitoneal adenopathy may be detected by radiological evaluation. Approximately two-thirds of patients have a pancytopenia while only 15%–20% of patients have the leukemic phase of the disease (wbc count >10,000/µl with >50% hairy cells in the peripheral blood) [1]. The cytopenias usually result from a combination of splenic sequestration and bone marrow underproduction as a result of leukemic infiltration. The exact role which cytokines such as tumor necrosis factor alpha and B-cell growth factor play on the hypofunction of the bone marrow remain to be fully determined.

There is no specific tumor marker, but CD 25 is released by hairy cells and can be used as a marker in the course of the disease [2]. However, the expense of the IL-2 receptor kit probably outweighs its clinical usefulness as the blood counts and percentage of circulating hairy cells provide easy markers to follow.

Although it had been customary to not treat approximately 10% of HCL patients as they were not symptomatic at presentation and would not become so for many years, it has now become acceptable to consider treating almost all patients at the time of diagnosis. Regardless, patients should be treated if they have one of the following conditions or clinical signs: (a) cytopenia (hemoglobin <10 g/dl, granulocyte count <1000/µl, and platelet count <100,000/µl); (b) symptomatic splenomegaly; (c) leukemic phase of HCL; (d) recurrent bacterial or opportunistic infections; (e) tissue infiltration; or (f) autoimmune complications. It is a rare patient that does not have any one of the six conditions or clinical signs noted above.

## Specific Treatment Options

Splenectomy

The treatment for HCL has evolved over the last 25 years. The rarity of the disease resulted in an accumulation of case reports in the 1960s and 1970s until the publication in 1974 by Burke and Rappaport [3] demonstrated that splenectomy appeared to be of benefit in a series of patients they had consulted on pathologically. The benefits of splenectomy were confirmed in a study by Golomb et al. [4] which showed that splenectomy normalized blood counts in approximately two-thirds of cases. However, it only corrected one cause of cytopenia, splenic sequestration, and did not lead to any improvement in the bone marrow. They found that the response rate was independent of spleen size. Complications were rare and the surgical mortality ranged from 0% to 2% in various series. However, eventually HCL progresses in 65% of patients after splenectomy, with a median time to failure of approximately 19 months. Splenectomy was clearly the first effective treatment for HCL, but now only remains of value in the management of symptomatic splenic infarction or splenic rupture. However, it should be noted that if a patient is severely infected with a profound pancytopenia that emergency splenectomy will result in the quickest return of the necessary blood counts to reverse the dire clinical situation.

Immunotherapy: Interferon

Interferon was first reported to be active against HCL only in 1984 by Quesada et al. [5]. They showed in the initial report that not only could the blood counts be reversed, but the bone marrow involvement by hairy cells could be decreased and, possibly eradicated. This was a major improvement over the benefits of splenectomy. Treatment with Interferon-Alpha 2b may induce lasting unmaintained remission; approximately 10% of patients obtain a complete response and 80% obtain a partial response (normalization of blood counts, but >5% hairy cells in bone marrow) [6]. Cytopenia and immune function begin to improve within 1–2 months of starting therapy, and improvement continues for up to 6 months. Fever and myalgia, common at the start of treatment, respond well to acetaminophen therapy. Fatigue may be a persistent side effect.

**Table 1.** Summary of responses and response durations

| Drug | Complete response (%) | Overall response (%) | Relapse at 2 years (%) |
|------|------------------------|----------------------|-------------------------|
| Interferon | <10 | 80–90 | ~50 |
| Pentostatin | 60–90 | 90–95 | ~15 |
| Cladribine | 75–85 | 85–100 | ~15 |

Therapy requires at least one year of 3 times weekly self-administered subcutaneous injections using $2 \times 10^6$ U/m$^2$ per day. Lower doses were shown to be less effective. Optimal treatment duration is at least 12 months with some reports suggesting three years if tolerated. However, the treatment is not curative as at least 50% of patients will require retreatment within 2.5 years (Table 1). As a result, Interferon-alpha 2β has been superceded in most cases by more definitive chemotherapy. However, interferon use may be indicated in the initial treatment of elderly patients who cannot tolerate any chemotherapy or significant worsening of their cytopenia(s), and in retreatment of patients who have failed single-agent chemotherapy.

Chemotherapy

Low-grade lymphoproliferative diseases are very slow growing, and most cells are in the resting phase. HCL was shown to have the lowest labeling index of any of the low-grade lymphoproliferative diseases by Braylan et al [7]. Conventional chemotherapy agents are selectively toxic to rapidly growing cells and are ineffective in the low grade lymphoproliferative disease. Effective chemotherapy requires lymphocyte-targeted drugs active against both resting and dividing cells. The purine deoxyribnucleoinide metabolism of lymphocytes has been found to be susceptible to pharmacologic manipulation, which is the basis for the use of pentostatin (Nipent) and cladribine (Leustatin). Adenosine deaminase (ADA) activity is normally high and 5'nucleotidase activity is low. Inhibition of ADA thus allows the accumulation of high concentrations of deoxyribonucleotides and their analogs. Pentostatin is a purine analog and competitive inhibitor of ADA that causes cell death by allowing the accumulation of lethal intracellular concentrations of deoxyribonucleotides. The cytotoxic effect is non-cell cycle specific, it occurs in both resting and active cells. Cladribine is a purine analog resistant to deamination by ADA. Metabolism by the adenosine phosphorylation pathway results in the accumulation of nucleotide analogs that are incorporated into DNA. This incorporation inhibits DNA repair mechanisms, resulting in accumulation of single strands of DNA that activate poly (ADP-ribose) synthetase, causing depletion of intracellular nicotinamide adenine dinucleotide (NAD) and cell death. Cladribine is equally cytotoxic for dividing and resting cells.

Pentostatin (Table 1) emerged as a positive treatment with the first report on 2 patients by Spiers et al. in 1984 [8]. Both patients had normalization of their blood counts, and, apparently, complete clearing of hairy cells from their bone marrow. A follow-up study performed by ECOG and reported by Spiers et al. in 1987 [9] documented 27 patients treated with a dose that was eventually determined to be almost twice which was needed. They showed that all but one patient responded, and, more importantly, 59% of patients had a complete response. The Ohio State group reported by Kraut et al. in 1986 [10], used the lower dose of Pentostatin which has become the dosage of choice (4 mg/m² every other week) to treat 10 HCL patients and reported that 4 patients obtained a complete remission. A second report by Kraut et al. in 1989 [11] updated the original experience with 20 of 23 patients obtaining a complete response. Of importance, they discontinued treatment when CR was achieved at an average time of 5.5 months and found that 15 of those patients remained in remission with an average duration of 12–1/2 months. Various trials have shown that pentostatin leads to a complete response in approximately two-thirds of patients and to an overall response rate of 90%–95%. It is noteworthy that those patients considered to be refractory to interferon-alpha, either because they never responded to it or because the disease progressed shortly after therapy was completed, had response rates similar to those of patients not previously treated with interferon-alpha. In a more recent study sponsored by the NCI and reported by Grever et al [12], previously untreated patients were randomized to receive pentostatin or interferon-alpha. Of the 159 patients receiving interferon-alpha, 11% had a complete response, whereas 79% of 154 patients receiving Pentostatin had a complete response (p<.0001). Crossover was allowed, and 66% of 86 evaluable patients who crossed to receive Pentostatin achieved a complete response. Although several schedules and dosages have been published, the currently recommended dosage of Pentostatin is 4 mg/m² every other week until complete remission is obtained. In the CALGB study reported by Golomb et al. [13] median time to best response was 6.5 months in patients who had previously been treated with IFN.

Cladribine (Table 1) emerged as a successful treatment for HCL with the report by Piro et al. in 1990 in 12 patients [14]. They treated patients with a single seven-day continuous infusion of cladribine at a dosage of 0.1 mg/kg per day. Eleven of the first 12 patients obtained a complete remission and had almost no side effects usually associated with chemotherapy. Subsequently, they updated their results in 1991 on 148 patients and reported an 85% CR rate and a 12% partial response rate; only 2 patients had relapses subsequently [15]. Estey et al. in 1991 [16] reported on 46 patients treated with the same dosages of cladribine and found a CR rate of 78% and a PR rate of 11%. They had 3 resistant patients and 1 patient with a relapse. In 1994, Saven and Piro reviewed all the published patients treated with cladribine [17]. They showed a CR rate of 82% for 245 cladribine treated patients. They noted that fever was the principal adverse effect of treatment (occurring in 44% of patients) and felt it was related to the rapid disappearance of circulating hairy cells and shrinkage of the spleen. Febrile episodes occurred by day 6 (range, 4–10 days), in half the patients and lasted for a median of 3 days (range, 1–13 days). They noted the fever tended to resolve with granulocyte recovery. Although Saven and Piro noted that 6 months after treatment, 58 of 59 patients who had a CR had no circulating hairy cells detected, they did state that it has been demonstrated that "some patients in complete remission have evidence of minimal residual disease on immunohisto-chemical staining of bone marrow." Overall, complete clinical remission rates of 75%–95% have been achieved after a single cycle of cladribine therapy. Complete remissions are durable, with a relapse rate ranging from less than 2% reported at median follow-up of 14 months in one study to 8% at 25 months median follow-up in another. Recently, Tallman et al in 1996 [18] reported a progression-free survival of 72% at 4 years. Relapse rates are higher when more sensitive means of assessment are used. Ellison et al [19]. in 1994 used monoclonal antibodies to identify residual hairy cells in 154 bone marrow biopsies performed between 3 months and 25 months after therapy. Hairy cells were detected in 50% of samples, but generally comprised fewer than 1% of cells, and the patients experienced a stable clinical course. Filleul et al [20]. in 1994 investigated minimal residual disease using PCR and heavy chain immunoglobulin gene rearrangements or TCRd receptors. Of their 10 patients, 8 achieved a clinical CR, and 7 were still in CR at a median follow-up period of 12 months. All of the patients had evidence of minimal residual disease using PCR.

Severe toxicities associated with cladribine therapy are relatively uncommon. Only a rare death has been reported directly attributable to the drug. Approximately 30% of patients have infections, and approximately 20% have nausea and vomiting which is only mild to moderate in seventy. An occasional patient has been reported with prolonged myelosuppression and an opportunistic infection as well as an occasional patient with neurotoxicity.

Cladribine can be administered with comparable activity as a 2 hour infusion for 5–7 days and is readily bioavailable by both the subcutaneous and oral routes. For the 5 day infusion at 2 h per day, the dosage is 0.14 mg/kg per day.

## Summary

Almost all hairy cell leukemia patients should now be treated at the time of diagnosis with one of the purine analogs; either cladribine or pentostatin. Cladribine requires only 5 days of treatment and is probably less toxic.

## References

1. Golomb HM, Catovsky D, Golde DW (1978) Hairy cell leukemia: a clinical review based on 71 cases. Ann Intern Med 89:677–683
2. Richards JM, Mick R, Latta JM et al. (1990) Serum soluble interleukin-2 receptor is associated with clinical and pathological disease status in hairy cell leukemia. Blood 76:1941–1945
3. Burke JS, Byrne GE, Jr., Rappaport H (1974) Hairy cell leukemia (leukemic reticuloendotheliosis). I. A clinical pathologic study of 21 patients. Cancer 33:1399–1410
4. Mintz U, Golomb HM (1979) Splenectomy as initial therapy in twenty-six patients with leukemic reticuloendotheliosis (hairy cell leukemia). Cancer Research 39:2366–2370
5. Quesada JR, Reuben J, Manning JT et al. (1984) Alpha interferon for the induction of remission in hairy cell leukemia. N Engl J Med 310:15–18
6. Ratain MJ, Golomb HM, Bardawil RG et al. (1987) Durability of responses to interferon alfa-2b in advanced hairy cell leukemia. Blood 69:872–877
7. Braylan RC, Jaffe ES, Triche TJ, Nanba K, Fowlkes BJ, Metzger H, Frank MM, Dulan MS, Yee CL, Green I, Bernard C (1978) Structural and functional properties of the "hairy" cells of leukemic reticuloendotheliosis. Cancer 41:210–227

8. Spiers ASD, Parekh SJ, Bishop MD (1984) Hairy cell leukemia: Induction of complete remission with Pentostatin (2'-deoxycoformycin). J Clin Oncol 2:1336–1342

9. Spiers ASD, Moore D, Cassileth PA et al (1987) Remissions in hairy cell leukemia with Pentostatin (2'-deoxycoformycin). N Engl J Med 316:825–30

10. Kraut EH, Bouroncle BA, Grever MR (1986) Low-dose deoxycoformycin in the treatment of hairy cell leukemia. Blood 68:1119–1122

11. Kraut EH, Bouroncle BA, Grever MR (1989) Pentostatin in the treatment of advanced hairy cell leukemia. J Clin Oncol 7:168–172

12. Grever MR, Kopecky K, Foucar, MK et al. (1995) Randomized comparison of pentostatin versus alpha 2a-interferon in previously untreated patients with hairy cell leukemia. An Intergroup study. J. Clin Oncol 13:974–981

13. Golomb HM, Dodge R, Mick R, Budman D, Hutchison R, Horning S, Schiffer CA (1994) Pentostatin treatment for hairy cell leukemia patients who failed initial therapy with recombinant alpha-interferon: A report of CALGB study 8515. Leukemia 8:2037–2040

14. Piro LD, Carrera CJ, Carson DA et al. (1990) Lasting remission in hairy cell leukemia induced by a single infusion of 2'-chlorodeoxyadenosine. N Engl J Med 322:1117–1121

15. Beutler E, Piro LD, Saven A et al. (1991) 2-chlorodeoxyadenosine: a potent chemotherapeutic and immunosuppressive nucleoside. Leukemia Lymph 5:1–8

16. Estey EH, Kurzrock R, Kantarjian HM et al. (1991) 2-chlorodeoxyadenosine: a new anticancer agent in lymphoid malignancies. Cancer Bull 43:253–258

17. Saven A, Piro L (1994) Newer purine analogues for the treatment of hairy cell leukemia. N Engl J Med 10:691–697

18. Tallman MS, Hakimian D, Rademaker AW et al. (1996) Relapse of hairy cell leukemia after 2-chlorodeoxyadenosine: long-term follow-up of the Northwestern University experience. Blood 88:1954–1959

19. Ellison DJ, Sharpe RW, Robbins BA et al. (1994) Immunomorphologic analysis of bone marrow biopsies after treatment with 2-chlorodeoxyadenosine for hairy cell leukemia. Blood 84:4310–4315

20. Filleul B, Delannoy A, Ferrant A et al. (1994) A single course of 2-chlorodeoxyadenosine does not eradicate leukemic cells in hairy cell leukemia patients in complete remission. Leukemia 8, 1153–1156

# Cutaneous T-Cell Lymphomas

T. Kuzel, J. Guitart, S.T. Rosen

## Introduction

The cutaneous T-cell lymphomas (CTCL) have been recognized to include a wide variety of clinical disorders with differing prognosis (Table 1). The most common subtypes of CTCL are the epidermotropic variants mycosis fungoides (MF) and the Sezary syndrome (SS). This chapter will focus on the biology and treatment of these two entities, however characteristic features of the other CTCL variants will be described.

**Table 1.** Cutaneous T-cell lymphomas (from [5])

| |
|---|
| Primary |
|  Indolent |
|   Mycosis fungoides |
|   Mycosis fungoides + follicular mucinosis |
|   Pagetoid reticulosis (Woringer-Kolopp disease) |
|   Large Cell CTCL, CD30$^+$ |
|    Anaplastic |
|    Immunoblastic |
|    Pleomorphic |
|   Lymphomatoid papulosis |
|  Aggressive |
|   Sézary syndrome |
|   Large cell CTCL, CD30$^-$ |
|    Immunoblastic |
|    Pleomorphic |
|  Provisional |
|   Granulomatous slack skin |
|   CTCL, Pleomorphic small/medium size |
|   Subcutaneous panniculitis-like T-cell lymphoma |
| Systemic T-cell disorders with skin manifestations |
|  Angioimmunoblastic lymphodenopathy |
|  Lymphomatoid granulomatosis |
|  Adult T-cell leukemia and lymphoma |

Alibert reported the first case of MF in 1806 [1]. His patient developed a skin eruption that progressed into mushroom-like tumors, prompting the term mycosis fungoides. Later in the nineteenth century, Bazin defined the three classic cutaneous phases (patch, plaque, and tumor stage) of the disease [2]. The recognition of the clinical triad of intensely pruritic erythroderma, lymphadenopathy, and abnormal hyperconvoluted "monstrous" cells in the peripheral blood led to the description of SS [3].

## Epidemiology, Risk Factors

### Incidence

MF and SS are the most frequent primary lymphomas involving the skin [4, 5]. Data collected from the Surveillance, Epidemiology, and End Results (SEER) program showed a rapidly increasing incidence from 0.2 cases per 100,000 population in 1973 to 0.4 cases per 100,000 population in 1984. This corresponds to approximately 1000 new cases each year in the United States. Whether this represents a true increase in incidence or is attributable to a better awareness and therefore more frequent recognition of this disease is not resolved.

The incidence of MF/SS increases with advancing age, as does the incidence of non-Hodgkin's lymphomas in general. The average age at presentation is approximately 50 years. Although very young patients have been reported, most patients are at least 30 years of age [6, 7]. MF/SS is seen in all racial groups. There is a 2:1 ratio of black people to white people and a 2.2:1 ratio of men to women with this disorder.

### Etiology and Pathogenesis

The etiology of MF/SS is unknown. It is considered to be a sporadic disease without compelling evidence of transmissibility. Several viruses have been implicated in the pathogenesis of MF/SS including Human T-cell Lymphotropic Virus (HTLV)-I/II, HTLV-V Herpes simplex virus, Herpes virus-6, and the Espstein-Barr virus [8]. However, a viral cause of MF/SS has not been proven.

Investigators have suggested that prolonged exposure to contact allergens may lead to enhanced immune responses leading directly or indirectly to the development of MF/SS. In addition, several reports sugge-sted that exposure to metals or their salts, pesticides or herbicides, and organic solvents (halogenated or aromatic hydrocarbons) could be rela-ted to the development of MF/SS [9]. However, two well-designed case-control studies failed to support these observations [10, 11].

## Genetic Aspects

Clusters of cases of MF/SS within families have been reported [12]. Furthermore, an association with histocompatability antigens AW31, AW32, B8, BW35, and DR5 has been described [13]. However, a solid gene-tic predisposition or inherited genetic defect has not been demonstra-ted.

## Pathology and Staging

The diagnosis of MF/SS is based on light microscopic evidence of a band-like infiltrate involving the papillary dermis containing small, medium-sized, and occasionally large mononuclear cells with hyper-chromatic, hyperconvoluted (cerebriform) nuclei and variable numbers of admixed inflammatory cells. Epidermal exocytosis of single or small clusters of neoplastic cells is a characteristic finding. The presence of Pautrier microabscesses is classic, but seen only in a minority of cases. Tumor stage lesions demonstrate a more diffuse superficial and deep, dermal infiltrate with fewer reactive cells, and an absence of epider-motropism. The malignant T-cell clone often evolves into large cell mor-phology during tumor progression, although rare cases show large cell morphology from the early patch lesions [14]. The histologic features in SS may be similar to those of MF. However, the cellular infiltrates in SS are more often monotonous, and epidermotropism may be absent.

Various theories have been advanced to explain the epidermotropism of malignant T cells in MF/SS. Organ-specific affinity to skin and other organs has been recognized in subsets of normal T cells. Homing of CTCL cells to the skin is probably mediated by more than one adhesion receptor mechanism. For example, CTCL cells express cutaneous lym-phocyte antigen (CLA), a skin homing receptor which interacts with e-selectin on cutaneous endothelium [15].

Lymph node involvement initially involves the paracortical regions. Progression is associated with small to large clusters of atypical cells with preserved nodal architecture, followed by partial or total effacement of the node by neoplastic cells. Visceral involvement is a late clinical feature. Peripheral blood involvement can be demonstrated in all stages of skin disease, though most prevalent in patients with tumor or erthrodermic presentations. Patients with SS may have circulating neoplastic cells, but be lymphopenic. Bone marrow involvement can often be demonstrated in patients with SS or advanced tumor or plaque stage MF but rarely influences management outside of an investigational setting.

The malignant cells are typically $CD3^+$, $CD4^+$, $CD45RO^+$, $CD8^-$, and $CD30^-$ by immunohistochemistry. CD7 is often deleted from the early stages. More aggressive variants and advanced CTCL may have multiple pan-T cell antigen deletions, especially CD2, CD5, and even CD4. T-cell receptor genes are clonally rearranged, and can be demonstrated in most cases by Southern blotting or PCR (polymerase chain reaction) assays when a sufficient malignant infiltrate exists.

In 1979, the staging committee at an international workshop on MF proposed a staging system based on the international tumor-node-metastasis (TNM) system (Table 2) [16]. This classification was based on the evaluation of 347 patients and a multivariate analysis of potential prognostic factors. This group identified several independent prognostic factors: extent of skin disease at diagnosis (T), type of lymph node (N) involvement, presence or absence of peripheral blood (PB) involvement, and finally, presence or absence of visceral (M) involvement. The group also translated the above staging into a recommended clinical staging system (see Table 2).

More recently, investigators at the National Cancer Institute retrospectively analyzed 152 patients who underwent uniform pathologic staging [17]. They were able to identify three distinct prognostic groups. Good-risk patients had plaque-only skin disease without lymph node, blood, or visceral involvement, and a median survival of more than 12 years. Intermediate-risk patients had skin tumors, erythroderma, or plaque disease with lymph node or blood involvement (but no visceral disease), and a median survival of 5 years. Poor-risk patients had visceral disease or complete effacement of lymph nodes by lymphoma, and a median survival of 2.5 years.

**Table 2.** TNM classification of cutaneous T-cell lymphomas

| Classification | Description |
|---|---|
| T skin | |
| T0 | Clinically or histopathologically suspicious lesions |
| T1 | Limited plaques, papules or eczematous patches covering 10% of the skin surface |
| T2 | Generalized plaques, papules or erythematous patches covering 10% of the skin surface |
| T3 | Tumors (one or more) |
| T4 | Generalized erythroderma. Pathology of T1–4 is diagnostic of a cutaneous T-cell lymphoma. When more than one T stage exists, both are recorded and highest is used for staging. Record other features if appropriate (ulcers, poikiloderma, scale, etc.) |
| N lymph nodes | |
| N0 | No clinically abnormal peripheral lymph nodes |
| N1 | Clinically abnormal peripheral lymph nodes (record no. of sites) |
| NP0 | Biopsy performed, not CTCL |
| NP1 | Biopsy performed, CTCL |
| PB peripheral blood | |
| PB0 | Atypical circulating cells not present (£5%) |
| PB1 | Atypical circulating cells not present (>5%), record total WBC, total lymphocyte count, and% of abnormal cells |
| M visceral organs | |
| M0 | No visceral organ involvement |
| M1 | Visceral involvement (must have pathologic confirmation), record organ involved |

Staging classification: stage Ia: T1, N0NP0, M0; Ib: T2, N0NP0, M0; IIa: T1–2, N1NP0, M0; IIb: T3, N0NP0, M0; III: T4, N0NP0, M0; IVa: T1–4, N0, 1NP1, M0; IVb: T1–4, N0, 1NP0, 1, M1.

## Differential Diagnosis of Clinical Variants

### Poilikoderma Vasculare Atrophicans [18]

Poilikoderma Vasculare Atrophicans is characterized by reticulate hyperpigmentation and hypopigmentation, telangiectasia, and skin atrophy. The classic presentation includes multiple skin lesions of variable size, affecting covered areas such as the breasts, buttocks, and flexures in a symmetric distribution. A small percentage of patients will evolve into MF.

## Large Plaque Parapsoriasis [19]

Large plaque parapsoriasis is the classic premalignant lesion of MF. It most commonly consists of a few scattered, erythematous to brown, plaques that are usually greater than 6 cm in size. Histologic examination shows a superficial lymphocytic infiltrate with minimal nuclear atypia. Plaques can persist for decades before a frank evolution to MF occurs. Approximately 10%–30% of patients ultimately develop an overt malignant transformation.

## Alopecia Mucinosa [20]

Alopecia mucinosa presents with grouped erythematous follicular papules or boggy or indurated nodular plaques, notably devoid of hair. There is a predilection for the head and neck area, especially the forehead which has the highest density of pilosebaceous units. Histopathologic evaluation reveals follicular mucinosis and mucinous degeneration of epithelial cells in sebaceous glands and hair follicles, associated with lymphocytic infiltration. Most patients have a benign course, but lymphoma associated with follicular mucinosis has been reported in the literature to range from 9% to 67% [21].

## Lymphomatoid Papulosis [22]

Lymphomatoid Papulosis is characterized by recurrent crops of self-healing, red-brown, centrally necrotic, asymptomatic papules and nodules. Patients may have a few lesions or more than 100 at a time. Histologic evaluation reveals an atypical $CD4^+$ lymphocytic infiltrate with a variable mixed inflammatory infiltrate. T cell receptor gene rearrangement studies demonstrate a clonal origin. Though the typical course is usually indolent spanning decades, approximately 30% of patients develop MF, Hodgkin's or non-Hodgkin's lymphoma during their lifetime. However, the cumulative risk of developing a lymphoma approaches 80% at 15 years, with negligible risk of transformation during the first five years [23].

## Pagetoid Reticulosis (Woringer-Kolopp Disease) [24]

This rare condition affecting young adults presents with hyperkeratotic, often verrucous plaques on the lower limb [25]. Biopsies show atypical cerebriform lymphocytes with a perinuclear halo almost exclusively localized within the intraepidermal compartment [26]. This is a localized form of CTCL.

## Granulomatous Slack Skin [27]

In granulomatous slack-skin syndrome, clonal $CD4^+$ T cells elicit a reactive granulomatous response that destroys the elastic fibers, rendering skin slack, fibrotic and inelastic. The differential diagnosis for such cases includes sarcoidosis and tuberculoid leprosy.

## CD-30⁺ Cutaneous Large T-Cell Lymphoma [28]

Primary cutaneous $CD30^+$ large cell lymphoma (CD30+LCL) typically occurs in adults presenting with solitary or localized (ulcerating) nodules or tumors. Histopathology consists of diffuse nonepidermotropic infiltrates with cohesive sheets of large CD30-positive tumor cells. In most instances the tumor cells have an anaplastic morphology, showing round, oval, or irregularly shaped nuclei, prominent (eosinophilic) nucleoli, and abundant cytoplasm. In contrast to the poor outcome of MF that has transformed to a $CD30^+$ large cell variant, primary CD-30-Positive Cutaneous Large T-Cell Lymphomas are associated with an excellent prognosis. Radiotherapy is the preferred treatment for solitary or localized disease, with combination chemotherapy reserved for patients with generalized skin lesions or extracutaneous dissemination.

## CD-30⁻ Cutaneous Large T-Cell Lymphoma [29]

These lymphomas tend to have an aggressive clinical course. Patients present with localized or generalized plaques, nodules or tumors. Histopathology demonstrates non-epidermotropic infiltrates with variable numbers of medium-sized to large pleomorphic T cells with or without cerebriform nuclei, and immunoblasts. Multiagent chemotherapy is used in most instances, with radiation therapy reserved for patients with localized disease. The five year survival rate is less than 20%.

## Pleomorphic Small/Medium-Sized CTCL [30]

This is an uncommon entity. Patients typically present with red-purplish nodules or tumors. Histopathology shows a dense, diffuse, or nodular infiltrate with small/medium pleomorphic neoplastic cells within the dermis often with extension into the subcutis. Localized disease is typically treated with radiation therapy. Patients with more generalized disease have been treated with regimens utilized for indolent non-Hodgkins lymphomas.

## Subcutaneous Panniculitis-like T-Cell Lymphoma [31, 32]

An extremely rare entity. Patients present with subcutaneous nodules and plaques. Systemic symptoms are common including fevers, fatigue and anorexia. Histopathology reveals a subcutaneous infiltrate with pleomorphic T cells of variable size and mixed with benign macrophages. Tumor cell necrosis, karyorrhexis, and erythrophagocytosis are common findings. The prognosis is in general poor despite aggressive chemotherapy.

## Systemic T-Cell Disorders With Skin Manifestations

### Angioimmunoblastic Lymphadenopathy [33]

Angioimmunoblastic lymphadenopathy is a rare lymphoproliferative disorder frequently accompanied by hepatosplenomegaly, fever, skin rash, and generalized malaise. Approximately 50% of patients have skin involvement at presentation. Common laboratory features include anemia (often Coombs-positive hemolytic), thrombocytopenia, leukocytosis with lymphopenia, and polyclonal hypergammaglobulinemia. Histologic features of lymph node biopsies include complete architectural effacement with replacement by a diffuse polymorphous cellular infiltrate composed of lymphocytes, immunoblasts, and plasma cells, with or without histiocytes and eosinophils. Prominent arborization of postcapillary venules and atrophic germinal centers are seen.

The median survival is approximately 1.5 years, and only 30% of patients survive 2 years. Treatment with corticosteroids and/or chemotherapy rarely provides durable control.

## *Lymphomatoid Granulomatosis* [34]

Lymphomatoid Granulomatosis is a rare multiorgan disease of the lungs, nasopharynx, joints, peripheral and central nervous system. Cutaneous involvement occurs in 25%–50% of patients. Though nodules are most common, some patients have nonspecific macules, papules, or ulceration. Histologic evaluation reveals an angiocentric, polymorphous infiltrate of both atypical lymphocytes and histiocytes surrounding and invading blood vessels within the dermis.

Though the clinical course is variable, the prognosis for patients with diffuse pulmonary involvement or the appearance of high-grade lymphoma is poor, with a median survival of less than 2 years. Treatment which depends on histologic findings and extent and location of disease, may include corticosteroids, radiotherapy, and/or chemotherapy. Recently interferon has been demonstrated to have significant activity against this disease [35].

## *Adult T Cell Leukemia and Lymphoma (ATLL)* [36, 37]

ATLL is in most instances a rapidly progressive T-cell neoplasm expressing a helper phenotype. It is endemic in southern Japan and the Caribbean islands and is associated with the retrovirus HTLV-1. However, most HTLV-l infected patients remain asymptomatic and only 2%–4% develop ATLL. The clinical presentation is polymorphous and can resemble MF or SS. Advanced stages of the disease, which affects a younger population than seen with MF, are characterized by visceral involvement, immunodeficiency, elevated LDH and hypercalcemia. For purposes of treatment and prognosis it is wise to view ATLL as a spectrum with two subgroups, acute and all others, with treatment though inadequate, reserved for those with acute ATLL. Therapeutic options include multiagent chemotherapy and antibody or recombinant toxins directed against the IL-2 receptor. Patients with acute ATLL have poor survival rates, with median duration of 4–6 months.

## Work-up and Staging

The work-up and staging of MF and SS involves a comprehensive history and physical exam, documentation (e.g. photographs) of type and extent of skin lesions, and a skin biopsy for histologic review. Palpable lymph nodes should be biopsied. Immunophenotyping and molecular studies remain in general investigative procedures. SS patients should have a Sezary evaluation performed on peripheral blood.

Analysis of serum may reveal an elevated LDH (lactate dehydrogenase) in a small percentage of patients with advanced disease or an aggressive tempo. Eosinophilia and hypergammaglobulinemia is not uncommon is SS patients. A limited number of patients will have an associated monoclonal gammopathy. Elevated serum $B_2$ microglobulin and IL-2 receptor levels have also been noted in advanced cases.

Imaging studies for classic MF/SS are generally of modest utility. CT scans of the chest, abdomen or pelvis should be reserved for patients with SS, nodal involvement or CTCL variants. In an investigational setting electron microscopy, cytogenetics, and molecular analyses have shown that a higher percentage of patients will have occult internal involvement.

## Treatment

The goals of treatment in MF are the relief of symptoms and improvement in cosmetics. The therapeutic options are:
– Topical
  – Ultra-violet light A with psoralen (PUVA)
  – Ultra-violet light B (UVB)
  – Total skin electron beam radiation
  – Topical chemotherapy
  – Topical retinoids
– Systemic
  – Photophoresis

– Interferon alpha
– Single agent chemotherapy
– Combination chemotherapy
– Oral retinoids
– Investigational agents

Despite some uncontrolled clinical trial results which have been reported to suggest "cures" in this disease, the general perception remains that this disease is not curable with standard therapies available today. The disease behaves much as other low-grade lymphomas, with periods of remission gradually becoming shorter with subsequent therapeutic interventions. Unlike B-cell low grade lymphomas, however, advanced stage MF is associated with a relatively short median life expectancy. Patients with either significant nodal involvement (LN3 or LN4) or extensive skin involvement (T4) have median life expectancies of 30–55 months [38, 39]. Thus, a driving force in the development of treatments for this disease is the goal of altering the natural history for this group of poor prognosis patients. No clinical trial has yet determined that aggressive early therapy is better than sequential palliative approaches or investigational approaches, [40] and thus new treatments continue to be developed and tested for these patients.

Therapy can be conveniently divided into two approaches: (a) topical (skin directed), such as psoralens with ultraviolet light A (PUVA), topical chemotherapy application (nitrogen mustard or carmustine), and total skin electron beam radiotherapy, and (b) systemic (skin and viscera directed), such as interferons, oral or parenteral chemotherapy, photopheresis, retinoids, and investigational new compounds. No studies have demonstrated that one topical therapy is more effective than another, and patient and investigator preference remain the most important discriminating factor governing choice. However, as the biology of the neoplastic cell has become better understood, [41] it has become clear that some therapies may actually have topical and systemic effects through alterations in the body's cytokine milieu and ability to mount a host response against the neoplastic cell [42]. Finally, investigational approaches combining therapies remains an active research strategy. An algorithim for the management of patients with MF or SS is provided in Figure 1.

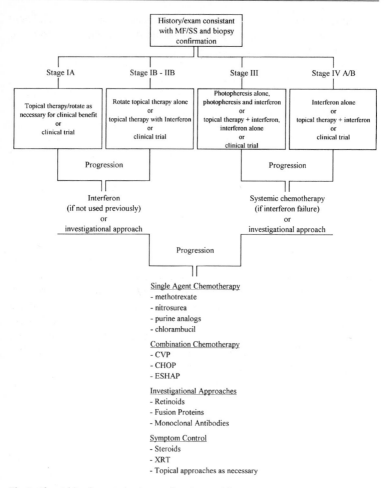

**Fig. 1.** Algorithim for managed care of patients with MF/SS

PUVA

8-Methoxypsoralen (8-MOP) is a member of a family of photoactivated compounds (furocoumarin derivatives), which may inhibit both DNA and RNA synthesis through formation of mono- or bifunctional thymine adducts, gene mutations, or sister chromatid exchanges [43, 44]. These drugs are only active if the tissue containing the psoralen compound is exposed to ultraviolet A rays (UVA).

Photochemotherapy units with UVA lamps emit a continuous spectrum of long UVA in the range of 320–400 nm with peak emission between 350 and 380 nm. Initial exposure times of patients to high output UVA are based on the degree of pigmentation before therapy, history of ability to tan, and the output of the photochemotherapy units. Exposure times are increased with each treatment depending upon the patient's response, and evidence of erythema. The initial UVA dose is 1.0–2.0 J/cm², and can be increased by approximately 0.5 J/cm² per treatment as tolerated. UV light-blocking glasses should be worn for 24 h after administration of 8-MOP. Therapy is typically given three times weekly until complete clearing occurs. The frequency of treatments can then be reduced, but some maintenance therapy (once every two to four weeks) may prolong the duration of remission.

Side effects with PUVA are quite tolerable. Occasional nausea or vomiting due to the psoralen ingestion is observed, and erythema, pruritus, and chronic dry skin is an effect of the UVA light damage to the skin. Long-term PUVA exposure has been associated with a number of late effects. These include dry skin, lichenification, keratosis and rarely amyloid deposition in the skin [45]. Most importantly is the late development of iatrogenic (both basal and squamous) carcinomas, [46] secondary malignant melanomas of the skin, [47] and rarely cataract formation.

Radiation Therapy

The non-Hodgkin's lymphomas in general, and the CTCL in particular, have been shown to be radiosensitive [48]. External-beam radiation has been shown to adequately control local areas of otherwise resistant MF, or provide palliation in cases of bulky tumor lesions [49, 50]. Unfortunately, the cumulative dosage that can be given to patients over time is limited due to normal organ toxicity.

The limitations of external-beam radiation led to increasing use of electron-beam radiotherapy for cases of MF confined to the skin. Linear accelerator-generated electron beams are scattered by a penetrable plate placed at the collimator site. The energy of the electrons is reduced to 4–7 MeV and allows adequate field distribution. Because of this low energy level, the beam only penetrates the surface several millimeters to 1 cm (into the dermis). Patients may be treated using six-field or rotational treatments [51, 52]. Thus, the total skin surface can be treated without significant internal organ toxicity [53]. Most patients are able to tolerate total doses of approximately 3000–3600 cGy over an 8–10 week period [54].

Patients with tumor lesions, generalized erythroderma, peripheral blood or nodal involvement, and even visceral spread can be successfully palliated with electron beam radiation therapy, as well. Side effects, however, can be occasionally extreme, including scaling, dryness of skin, erythema, extremity edema, telangiectasia formation, skin ulceration, and hair or sweat gland loss (frequently permanent).

Topical Chemotherapy

Mechlorethamine hydrochloride was the first topical agent evaluated to demonstrate efficacy in MF [55]. The solution used for topical application contains 10–20 mg of mechlorethamine dissolved in 50–100 mL of tap water (no vesicant activity at this low concentration). Although several methods may be used for administration, self-administration at home to the entire skin surface is preferred. The concentration may need to be varied depending on patient tolerance and sensitivity [56]. The time to initial response is usually short, approximately 1–2 weeks, but long-term application is usually required to obtain the maximum response.

Side effects consist of delayed hypersensitivity in approximately 35% of patients, although ointment-based solutions appeared to offer a reduced risk of allergic contact dermatitis. Once hypersensitivity develops, patients can be desensitized by either injecting minute daily doses of mechlorethamine over a period of several weeks [57] or diluting the preparation and gradually increasing the strength based on tolerance. Some clinicians, however, believe that a mild hypersensitivity reaction may have beneficial antitumor effects.

There has been an increased risk of secondary skin cancers in patients receiving long-term mechlorethamine. Of recent concern is the safety of family members or health care workers secondarily exposed to the topical solutions. However, we are unaware of any documented adverse outcomes, and believe this to be a theoretical concern more than practical.

Several other topical agents have been tested and show to be of benefit in the treatment of MF, including corticosteroids, cytarabine, dianhydrogalactitol, dacarbazine, quanazole, teniposide, hyroxyurea, thiotepa, and methotrexate [58]. However, topical carmustine is the only agent that has demonstrated clinical use [59].

Systemic Chemotherapy

Systemic chemotherapy should be reserved for those patients with relapsed or refractory disease after topical interventions, or for those patients with advanced nodal or visceral disease at presentation. Single-agent chemotherapy with alkylating agents, cisplatin, etoposide, bleomycin, doxorubicin, methotrexate, nitrosoureas, vincristine, vinblastine have been used for the treatment of MF or the Sezary syndrome [60, 61, 62, 63].

A new family of compounds, the purine anti-metabolites, has been developed and shown to be active in the treatment of MF. These compounds do not have a single mechanism of action, but all ultimately interfere with intracellular regulation of deoxyribonucleotide pools and this imbalance partially explains their cytotoxicity. This family of drugs includes 2-deoxycoformycin (DCF), fludarabine phosphate, and 2-chlorodeoxyadenosine (2-CdA) [64].

Combination chemotherapy has often been employed for patients with advanced disease, either at presentation or with progression. Usually alkylator agents are used, in combination with doxorubicin, or vinca alkaloids [65, 66]. Response rates of 80%–100% have been achieved, with longer duration of remission than those seen with single agent therapy. However, no trial has demonstrated survival benefits in patients treated with more aggressive regimens versus milder palliative therapies alone.

The natural evolution of combination chemotherapy has been to utilize dose-intensified approaches with hematopoietic reconstitution with autologous [67] or allogeneic bone marrow [68]. There are few reports in the literature of such treatment programs and therefore at the present time transplantation remains investigational.

Photopheresis

An adaptation of the use of psoralens with UVA light called photopheresis has been described by Edelson [69]. Patients ingest 0.6 mg/kg of oral 8-methoxypsoralen before a treatment. The treatment consists of routine leukopheresis with isolation of the mononuclear cell fraction. The cells are then exposed to UVA light ex vivo within a special chamber within the pheresis device and subsequently reinfused into the patient. The mechanism reaction is not thought to be direct cytotoxicity, but rather the induction of a host immune response to the reinfused altered Sezary cells.

Toxicity is mild and includes occasional nausea, erythematous flares, and temperature elevations. Patients may develop hypotension during leukapheresis, which usually responds to saline infusion.

## Interferons

It is now recognized that the most active agent for the treatment of MF is interferon alpha [70–74]. Dosages and routes of administration have differed between studies.

From all these studies it appears that a reasonable and tolerable single agent dose is approximately 12 million IU administered subcutaneously daily. We recommend starting at 3 million IU and gradually increase to 12 million IU as tolerated.

Side effects are dose dependent. Most common, constitutional symptoms of fever, chills, myalgias, malaise, and anorexia are experienced. Rarely, cytopenias, elevations of liver function tests, renal dysfunction, cardiac dysfunction, or changes in mental status can be seen. Patients need to be monitored closely on interferon.

## Investigational Approaches

Because of the chronic relapsing nature of MF, new therapies with different mechanisms of action are needed to circumvent tumor resistance. A variety of such approaches are under investigation. These include the development of existing or new retinoid compounds [75] or combinations of retinoids with interferons [76]. The combination of interferon and topical therapy is now being tested against topical therapy alone in a national cooperative group trial.

Another approach to the therapy of this disease has involved new drugs to exploit the biology of these neoplastic cells. Targeted therapies against unique tumor antigens continue to be tested [77], for a review of such agents as monoclonal antibodies and ligand-toxin fusion proteins. Knowledge of the unique cytokine milieu associated with these neoplastic T-cells has led to trials testing cytokines which may inhibit the growth of these cells, such as IL-12 [78] or IL-2 [79]. Finally, vaccine approaches may be practical [80].

## References

1. Alibert JLM: Description des Maladies de la Peau Observées a l'Hôpital St. Louis. Barrois L'aine et Fils, Paris, 1806
2. Bazin PAE: Maladies de la Peau Observées a l'H"pital St. Louis. Paris, 1876
3. Besnier E, Hallopeau H: On the erythrodermia of mycosis fungoides. Journal of Cutaneous and Genitourinary Diseases 10:453, 1892
4. Weinstock MA: Epidemiology of mycosis fungoides. Semin Dermatol 12:154, 1994
5. Willemze R, Kerl H, Sterry W et al. EORTC classification for primary cutaneous lymphomas: a proposal from the Cuatneous Lymphoma Study Group of the European Organization for Research and Treatment of Cancer. Blood 90:354, 1972
6. Epstein EH, Levine DL, Croft JD et al. Mycosis fungoides: survival, prognostic features, response to therapy and autopsy findings. Medicine 51:61, 1972
7. Levi JA, Wiernik PH: Management of mycosis fungoides: current status and future prospects. Medicine 54:73, 1974
8. Manzari V, Gismondi A, Barillari G et al. HTLV-V: A now human retrovirus isolated in a tac-negative T-cell lymphoma/leukemia. Science 238:1581, 1987
9. Fischmann AB, Bunn PA Jr, Guccion JG et al. Exposure to chemicals, physical agents, and biologic agents in mycosis fungoides and the Sézary syndrom. Cancer Treat Rep 63:591, 1979
10. Tuyp E, Burgoyne A, Aitchison T et al. A case-control study of possible causative factors in mycosis fungoides. Arch Dermatol 123:196, 1987
11. Whittemore AS, Holly EA, Lee IM et al. Mycosis fungoides in relation to environmental exposures and immune response: A case-control study. J Natl Cancer Inst 81:1560, 1989
12. Sandbank M, Katzenellenbogen I: Mycosis fungoides of prolongs duration in siblings. Arch Dermatol 98:620, 1968
13. Rosen ST, Radvany R, Roenigk HH Jr et al. Human leukocyte antigens in cutaneous T-cell lymphoma. J Am Acad Dermatol 12:531, 1985
14. Wood GS, Bahler DW, Hoppe RT, et al. Transformation of mycosis fungoides: T-cell receptor beta gene analysis demonstrates a common clonal origin for plaque-type mycosis fungoides and CD30+ large-cell lymphoma. Journal of Investigative Dermatology 101 (3):296, 1993
15. Drillenburg P, Bronkhorst CA, Van Der Wall AC et al. Expression of adhesion locules in paxetoid reticulosis. Br J Dermatol, 136:613, 1997
16. Bunn PA, Lamberg SI: Report of the committee on staging and classification of cutaneous T-clell lymphomas. Cancer Treat Rep 63:725, 1979
17. Sausville EA, Eddy JL, Makuch RW et al. Histopathologic staging at initial diagnosis of mycosis fungoides and the Sézary syndrome: Definition of the three distinctive prognostic groups. Ann Intern Med 109:372, 1988
18. Samman PD: The natural history of parapsoriasis en plaques (chronic superficial dermatitis) and prereticulotic poikiloderma. Br J Dermatol 87:405, 1972

19. Lambert CW, Everett MA: The nosology of parapsoriasis. J Am Acad Dermatol 5:373, 1985
20. Mehregan DA, Gibson LE, Muller SA: Follicular mucinosis: Histopathologic review of 33 cases. Mayo Clin Proc 66:387, 1991
21. Sentis HJ, Willemze R, Scheffer E. Alopecia mucinosa progressing into mycosis fungoides. Am J Dermpath, 10 (6):478, 1988
22. Karp DL, Horn TD: Lymphomatoid papulosis. J Am Acad Dermatol 30:379, 1994
23. Cabanillas F, Armitage J, Pugh WC et al. Lymphomatoid papulosis: A T-cell dyscrasia with a propensity to transform into malignant lymphoma. Ann Intern Med 122:210, 1995
24. Worringer F, Kolopp P: Lesion erythemato-squameuse polycyclique de l'avant-bras evoluant dupuis 6 ans ches un garconnet de 13 ans: Histologiquement infiltrant intraepidermique d'apparence tumorale. Annales de Dermatologie et de Syphiligraphie 10:945, 1939
25. Davis TH, Morton CC, Miller-Cassman R, Balk SP, Kadin ME: Hodgkin's disease, lymphomatoid papulosis and cutaneous T-cell lymphoma derived from a common T-cell clone. New Engl J of Med. 326:1115, 1992
26. Deneau DG, Wood GS, Beckstead J, et al. Woringer-Kolopp disease (pagetoid reticulosis). Four cases with histopathologic, ultrastructural, and immunohistologic observations. Arch Derm 120 (8):1045, 1984
27. Balus L, Bassetti F, Gentili G: Granulomatous slack skin. Arch Dermatol 121:250, 1985
28. Beljaards RC, Kaudewitz P, Berti E et al. Primary cutaneous CD30-positive large cell lymphoma: Definition of a new type cutaneous lymphoma with a favorable prognosis. A European multicenter study on 47 cases. Cancer 71:2097, 1993
29. Beljaards RC, Meijer CJLM, van der Putte SCJ et al. Primary cutaneous T-cell lymphomas. Clinicopathologic features and prognostic parameters of 35 cases other than mycosis fungoides and CD30-positive large cell lymphoma. J Pathol 172:53, 1994
30. Friedmann D, Wechsler J, Delfau MH et al. Primary cutaneous pleomorphic small T-cell lymphoma. Arch Dermatol 131:1009, 1995
31. Gonzalez CL, Medeiros LJ, Braziel RM Jaffe ES: T-cell lymphoma involving subcutaneous tissue. A clinicopathologic entity commonly associated with hemophagocytic syndrome. Am J Surg Pathol 15:17, 1991
32. Wang CE, Su WPD, Kurtin PJ: Subcutaneous panniculitic T-cell lymphoma. Int J Dermatol 35:1, 1996
33. Steinberg AD, Seldin MF, Jaffe ES et al. Angioimmunoblastic lymphadenopathy with dysproteinemia. Ann Intern Med 108:575, 1988
34. Carlson KC, Gibson LE: Cutaneous signs of lymphomatoid granulomatosis. Arch Dermatol 127:1693, 1991
35. Wilson WH, Kingma DW, Raffeld M et al. Association of lymphomatoid granulomatosis with Epstein-Barr viral infection of B lymphocytes and response to interferon-alpha 2b. Blood 87:4531, 1996
36. Bunn PA Jr, Schechter GP, Jaffe E et al. Clinical course of retrovirus-associated adult T-cell lymphoma in the United States. N Engl J Med 309:257, 1983
37. Hollsberg P, Hafler DA: Pathogenesis of diseases induced by human lymphotropic virus type I infection. N Engl J Med 328:1173, 1993
38. Sausville EA, Worsham GF, Matthews MJ et al. Histopathologic assessment of lymph nodes in mycosis fungoides/Sezary syndrome (cutaneous T-cell lymphoma): Clinical correlations and prognostic import of a new classification system. Hum Pathol 16:1098, 1985

39. Kim YH, Bishop K, Varghese A, Hoppe RT: Prognostic factors in erythrodermic mycosis fungoides and the Sezary syndrome. Arch Dermatol 131:1003, 1995
40. Kaye FJ, Bunn PA Jr., Steinberg SM et al. A randomized trial comparing combination electron-beam radiation and chemotherapy with topical therapy in the initial treatment of mycosis fungoides. N Engl J Med 321:1784, 1989
41. Rook AH, Gottlieb SL, Wolfe JT et al. Pathogenesis of cutaneous T-cell lymphoma: implications for the use of recombinant cytokines and photopheresis. Clin Exp Immunol 107 (suppl 1):16, 1997
42. Berger C, Liu W, Heald P et al. Anti-tumor response in cutaneous T-cell lymphoma. Proc of SID, J Invest Dermatol 102:566, 1994
43. Czech T, Pathak MA, Biswas RK: An electron microscopic study of the photochemical cross-linking of DNA in guinea pig epidermis by psoralen derivatives. Biochim Biophys Acta 562:342, 1979
44. Loveday KS, Donahue BA. Induction of sister chromatid exchanges and gene mutations in Chinese hamster ovary cells by psoralens. NCI Monograph 66:149, 1984
45. Greene I, Cox AJ: Amyloid deposition after psoriasis therapy with psoralen and long wave ultraviolet light. Arch Dermatol 115:1200, 1979
46. Stern RS, Members of the Photochemotherapy Follow-up study: Genital tumors among men with psoriasis exposed to psoralens and ultraviolet A radiation (PUVA) and ultraviolet B radiation. N Engl J Med 322:1093, 1990
47. Stern RS, Nichols KT, Vakeva LH et al. Malignant melanoma in patients treated for psoriasis with methoxsalen (psoralen) and ultraviolet A radiation (PUVA). N Engl J Med 336:1041, 1997
48. Trowel OA. The sensitivity of lymphocytes to ionizing irradiation. J Pathol Bacteriol 64:687, 1952
49. Levin OL, Behrman HT: Roentgen ray therapy of mycosis fungoides. Arch Dermatol Syphilol 21:307, 1945
50. Trump JG, Wright KA, Evans WW et al. High energy electrons for the treatment of extensive superficial malignant lesions. Am j Roent 69:623, 1953
51. Hoppe RT, Cox RS, Fuks Z et al. Electron beam therapy for mycosis fungoides: The Stanford University experience. Cancer Treat Rep 63:691, 1979
52. Nisce LA, Safai B, Kim JH: Effectiveness of once-weekly total skin electron beam therapy in mycosis fungoides and Sezary syndrome. Cancer 47:870, 1981
53. Nisce LA, Safai B, Kim JH: Effectiveness of once-weekly total skin electron beam therapy in mycosis fungoides and Sezary syndrome. Cancer 47:870, 1981
54. Jones GW, Hoppe RT, Glatstein E: Electron beam treatment for cutaneous T-cell lymphoma. Hematol/Oncol Clin of North Amer 9 (5):1057, 1995
55. Kierland RR, Watkins CH, Schullenberger CC: The use of nitrogen mustard in the treatment of mycosis fungoides. J Invest Dermatol 9:195, 1947
56. Vonderheid EC: Topical mechlorethamine chemotherapy-considerations on its use in mycosis fungoides. Int J Dermatol 23:180, 1984
57. Van Scott EJ, Kalmanson JD. Complete remissions of mycosis fungoides lymphoma induced by topical nitrogen mustard. Cancer 32:18, 1973
58. Argyropoulos CL, Lamberg SI, Clendenning WE et al. Preliminary evaluation of 15 chemotherapeutic agents applied topically in the treatment of mycosis fungoides. Cancer Treat Rep 63:623, 1979
59. Ramsay DJ, Meller JA, and Zackheim HS: Topical treatment of early cutaneous T-cell lymphoma. Hematol/Oncology Clin of North Amer 9:1031, 1995
60. Levi JA, Wiernik PH. Management of mycosis fungoides: Current status and future prospects. Medicine 54:73, 1974

61. Holmes RC, μgibbon DH, Black MM: Mycosis fungoides: Progression towards Sezary syndrome reversed with chlorambucil. Clin Exp Dermatol 8:429, 1983

62. Wiman G, Cadman E, Braverman I: Cisplatin treatment of cutaneous T-cell lymphoma. Cancer Treat Rep 65:920 (letter), 1981

63. Molin L, Thomsen K, Volden G, et al. Epipodophylotoxin (VP-16–23) in mycosis fungoides: a report for the Scandanavian Mycosis Fungoides Study Group. Acta Derm Venereol 59:84, 1979

64. Saven A, and Piro LW: The newer purine analogs. Cancer 72:3470, 1993

65. Winkelman RK, Buechner SA, Diaz-Perez JL: Pre Sezary syndrome. J Am Acad Dermatol 10:992, 1984

66. Grozea PN, Jones SE, McKelvey EM, et al. Combination chemotherapy for mycosis fungoides: A Southwest Oncology Group Study. Cancer Treat Rep 63:647, 1979

67. Sterling JC, Marcus R, Burrows NP, and Roberts SO: Erythrodermic mycosis fungoides treated witih total body irradiation and autologous bone marrow transplantation. Clin and Exp Dermatol 20:73, 1995

68. Koppel MC, Stoppa AM, Resbeut M, et al. Mycosis fungoides and allogeneic bone marrow transplanation. Acta Derm Venereol (Stockh) 74:331, 1994

69. Edelson RL, Berger C, Gasparro F, et al. Treatment of cutaneous T-cell lymphoma by extracorporeal photochemotherapy. N Engl J Med 316:297, 1987

70. Bunn PA Jr., Foon KA, Ihde DC, et al. Recombinant leukocyte A interferon: an active agent in advanced cutaneous T-cell lymphomas. Ann Intern Med 101:484, 1984

71. Bunn PA Jr., Ihde DC, Foon KA: The role of recombinant interferon alfa-2a in the therapy of cutaneous T-cell lymphomas. Cancer 57:1689, 1986

72. Olsen EA, Rosen ST, Vollmer RT, et al. Interferon alfa-2a in the treatment of cutaneous T-cell lymphoma. J Amer Acad Dermatol 20:395, 1989

73. Covelli A, Cavalieri R, Coppla G, et al. Recombinant leukocyte A interferon as initial therapy in mycosis fungoides and Sezary syndrome. Proc Am Soc Clin Oncol 6:189 (abst), 1987

74. Tura S, Mazza P, Ainzani PL, et al. Alpha recombinant interferon in the treatment of mycosis fungoides. Haematologica 72:337, 1987

75. Foss FM, Kuzel TM: Experiemental therapies in the treatment of cutaneous T-cell lymphoma. Hematol/Oncol Clin North Amer 9:1127, 1995

76. Torii H, Kaneko T, Matsuyama T et al. Interferon alpha and etretinate in the treatment of mycosis fungoides. J of Dermatol 21:767, 1994

77. Kuzel TM, Rosen ST: Monoclonal antibody based therapy of cutaneous T-cell non-Hodgkin's lymphoma (in) Monoclonal antibody based therapy of cancer. (Ed) Grossbard ML (in press)

78. Rook AH, Kubin M, Fox FE et al. The potential therapeutic role of interleukin-12 in cutaneous T-cell lymphoma. Annals NY Acad Sci 132:310, 1995

79. Marolleau JP, Baccard M, Flageul B et al. High-dose recombinant interleukin-2 in advanced cutaneous T-cell lymphoma. Arch Dermatol 131:574, 1995

80. Berger C, Liu W, Heald P, Christensen I, Edelson R: Anti-tumor response in cutaneous T-cell lymphoma. J Invest Dermatol suppl 1:566 (abst 253), 1995

# Hodgkin's Disease

J.M. Shammo, H.M. Golomb

## Epidemiology, Risk Factors

Incidence: Approximately 9000 new cases of Hodgkin's disease (HD) will be diagnosed in North America in 1998. HD is less common in African-Americans (1.6 cases per 100,000 person years) compared to caucasians (2.9 per 100,000 person years). HD is a diagnosis made more often in men with a male to female ratio of 1.3:1.0. Its age-specific incidence has been repeatedly reported as bimodal, with the greatest pool in the third decade of life and a second, smaller pool in the 50–60 decade.

The cause of HD remains unknown, and there are no well-defined risk factors for its development. However, certain associations have been noted and may provide clues to possible etiologic factors. Familial factors are most interesting with same-sex siblings of patients with HD having a 10 times higher risk for the disease. A study of twins of patients effected by HD showed that a homozygotic twin of a patient with HD has a risk of developing the disease that is 99 times higher than that of a dizygotic twin. The risk of a dizygotic twin developing HD does not differ from that of the general population. This information reported by Mack et al [1] demonstrates a strong genetic component in the etiology of HD A second concern for the cause of HD could be an abnormal response to an infective agent. The Epstein-Barr virus (EBV) has been implicated in the etiology of HD by both epidemiologic and serologic studies, as well as by the detection of the EBV genome in 20%–80% of tumor specimens. Although there have been no conclusive studies regarding the possible increased frequency of HD in patients with HIV infection, the HD in HIV positive patients is associated with advanced stage and poor therapeutic response. In a group of 114 patients reported by the Italian Cooperative Group in AIDS and tumors, there was a high prevalence of stage IV disease, B symptoms, and extra-nodal involvement [2].

## Clinical Features

Hodgkin's disease usually presents as an asymptomatic lymphadenopathy and subsequently spreads to contiguous lymphoid structures. More than 80% of patients present with lymphadenopathy above the diaphragm, commonly involving mediastinal, supraclavicular and axillary lymph nodes. About 10%–20% of all patients present with infradiaphragmatic lymphadenopathy. Extranodal involvement can occur by direct invasion or by hematogenous spread to lung, liver and bone marrow. The majority of patients have few or no symptoms related to this disease; however, about 25%–30% may develop constitutional symptoms of fever and night sweats.

## Pathology

The diagnosis of HD is usually made by microscopic examination of resected lymph nodes from patients with lymphadenopathy. Disruption of nodal architecture and the unequivocal demonstration of Reed-Sternberg cells is essential.

- Reed-Sternberg (RS) cells are binucleated giant cells with ample eosinophilic cytoplasm and multiple nucleoli. They are commonly CD15 and CD30 positive. Several variants of RS cells exists:
  - The lacunar cell variant is a giant cell with multilobated nucleus and a clear cytoplasm, and is commonly seen in the nodular sclerosing subtype.
  - The lymphocytic-histiocytic or L and H cell variant, is a large cell with multilobulated nucleus and several small basophilic nucleoli. It is typically associated with lymphocyte predominant subtype.
- According to the Rye classifications four histologic subtypes exist.

**Nodular Sclerosis.** The most common subtype accounting for 40%–60% of all cases of HD with a modest female predominance. It most frequently involves the mediastinum and the supraclavicular areas. It's distinct features are the presence of broad bands of collegen that divide the lymph node into cellular nodules and interspersed lacunar cells.

**Mixed Cellularity.** The second most frequent histology accounting for 15%–30% of all cases of HD, male predominance and retroperitoneal involvement is characteristic. Microscopically the nodal architecture is effaced by a pleomorphic cellular infiltrate composed of a mixture of histocytes, neutrophils, eosinophils and lymphocytes with abundant RS cells.

**Lymphocyte-Depletion.** Diagnosed in fewer than 5% of cases, typically occurring in an elderly male presenting with advanced stage disease, it may also be associated with HIV infection. The major characteristic feature is profound depletion of lymphocytes in the stroma of the involved nodes, with diffuse fibrosis and abundance of RS cells. This subtype can be difficult to distinguish from Non-Hodgkin's lymphoma (NHL) particularly peripheral T-cell and anaplastic large cell (Ki-1) lymphomas.

**Lymphocyte Predominance.** This is an infrequent form of HD with two-third of cases affecting men of all ages. It is often clinically localized to cervical, axillary, or inguinal nodes and almost never involves the mediastinum. It tends to run an indolent course even when left untreated. Microscopically the cellular background is primarily lymphocytes in a diffuse or nodular pattern with numerous L and H cells.

Staging

Precise delineation of the extent of nodal involvement in patients with newly diagnosed HD has been essential in the recent past because choice of treatment, results of treatment and natural history are all affected by stage of disease at the time of diagnosis. The universally accepted Ann Arbor anatomic and clinical staging classification has been modified in 1989 by a group of pathologists, radiologists, medical and radiation oncologists who convened in Cotswolds, UK [3].

The updated Cotswold staging classification recognizes the prognostic significance of bulky disease and the use of CT scanning for detection of intra-abdominal disease (Table 1). Clinical staging refers to information obtained by history, physical examination, laboratory and imaging studies, whereas pathologic staging is determined by surgical assessment of potentially involved sites e.g. laparotomy.

Pre-treatment Evaluation

– A careful history with special emphasis on recognizing B-symptoms should always be obtained. The presence of B symptoms is considerd a poor prognostic indicator. They are carefully defined in the staging system. Pruritus is no longer considered a B symptom. However, the presence of generalized itching is considered an adverse prognostic symptom [4].
– A complete physical exam with special attention to evaluation of lymphadenopathy including Waldeyer's ring, with measurements of nodal size in each area and assessment of hepatomegaly and splenomegaly.

**Table 1.** Cotswold's modification of the Ann Arbor staging classification

| | |
|---|---|
| Stage I | Involvement of a single lymph node region or lymphoid structure (e.g. spleen, thymus, Waldeyer's ring). |
| Stage II | Involvement of two or more lymph node regions on the same side of). The diaphragm (the mediastinum is single site: hilar lymph nodes should be considered to be lateralized and when involved on both sides constitute stage II disease). The number of anatomical regions involved should be indicated by a subscript (e.g. $II_3$). |
| Stage III | Involvement of lymph node regions or lymphoid structures on both sides of the diaphragm. |
| Stage $III_1$ | subdiaphragmatic involvement limited to spleen. Splenic hilar nodes, celiac nodes, or portal nodes. |
| Stage $III_2$ | subdiaphragmatic involvement includes paraaortic, iliac, or mesenteric nodes plus structures in $III_1$. |
| Stage IV | Involvement of extranodal site(s) beyond that designated as E. Involvement of liver or bone marrow. |
| A | No symptoms. |
| B | Unexplained weight loss of more than 10% of the body weight during the 6 months before staging investigation. |
| X | Bulky disease: >10 cm maximum dimension of nodal mass Mediastinal mass maximum width >1/3 the internal transverse diameter of the thorax at the level of T5/6 on PA CXR. |
| E | Localized involvement of extralymphatic tissue, alone as the only site of disease ($I_E$), or by limited direct extension from (contiguous with) a known nodal site or proximal to a know nodal site (excluding liver and bone marrow). |
| CS | Clinical stage |
| PS | Pathological stage, indicating staging biopsies |

CS or PS subscript designations for identified extranodal sites: M, bone marrow; H, liver; L, lung; O, bone; P, pleura; D, skin.

- Laboratory studies should include a complete blood count, tests for liver and kidney function, lactate dehydrogenase (LDH), and serum alkaline phosphatase.
  - Abnormalities in liver function tests should prompt further evaluations of that organ to rule out involvement with HD
  - An elevated alkaline phosphatase may indicate bone involvement and mandates proper evaluation with bone scan.
  - An elevated LDH has been associated with poor prognosis.
  - Bilateral bone marrow biopsy and aspirates should always be performed. Bone marrow biopsy may be eliminated in patients with CSIA-IIA who have less than 1% likelihood of marrow involvement. Recently position emission tomography (PET) has been shown to detect bone marrow involvement with lymphoma. This method in addition to being noninvasive is also more sensitive than bone marrow biopsy in detecting disease involvement [5].

**Imaging Studies.** These should include CT scans of the chest, abdomen and pelvis with IV contrast. Bipedal lymphangiogram (LAN) can be useful in detecting infrarenal paraoartic involvement with a 95% overall accuracy [6] compared with 87% overall accuracy for abdominal CT scan [7]; the limitations of LAN is its insensitivity for detecting disease above the renal veins. We no longer recommend (LAN). Gallium radionuclide scan can provide valuable information and is particularly useful in the post treatment evaluation; a negative gallium scan implies the absence of active disease even in the presence of apparent residual adenopathy noted on CT scan.

Staging Laparotomy

Imaging studies are only 50% accurate in predicting splenic involvement [6–7]. Furthermore, one third of patients with an enlarged spleen are found to have no splenic involvement at laparotomy. Laparotomy is the most definitive method for detecting occult infradiaphragmatic involvement, approximately one-third of clinical stage (CS) I or II patients will be upstaged after laparotomy. It is generally considered in patients with CS I or II for whom radiation would be indicated if they prove to be PS I or II after laparotomy. It involves splenectomy, a wedge or needle biopsy of the liver, sampling of the celiac, splenic, hilar, portahepatic, paraortic, paracaval and iliac nodes and bilateral bone marrow biopsies if not already done.

Several factors enter the decision making process regarding laparotomy including the short and long term risks of splenectomy, the probability of relapse in understaged patients and the impact of upgrading the stage on choice of treatment. We no longer recommend laparotomy (see treatment of early stage disease).


Treatment of Early Stage Disease

Most patients with early stage (defined as nonbulky stage I-II) can be cured. However, the choice of the most effective therapeutic approach with the least risk of treatment complications continues to represent a major challenge in the treatment of early stage HD. Radiotherapy with subtotal lymphoid irradiation is known to result in improved outcome when compared with involved field radiation in pathologically and clinically staged patients [9, 10]. Radiotherapy is associated with short-term acute complications including nausea, esophagitis and trachietis which could be controlled with symptomatic means and is usually reversible. Long-term complications occur several months to several years after irradiation and include cardiovascular disease and secondary neoplasms arising in the breast, lung, gastrointestinal tract and connective tissue [11].

The results of a prospective randomized study comparing RT vs chemotherapy with MOPP showed that MOPP was at least as effective as RT in the treatment of patients with early stage HD and as a result exploratory laparatomy could be eliminated from the staging workup [13, 14]. In 1975 ABVD chemotherapy was designed to treat MOPP resistant patients, [15] and was found to be as effective as MOPP alone or MOPP alternating with ABVD in advanced stage disease, [16]. It is less myelotoxic, not associated with sterility or secondary leukemia which has been associated with MOPP chemotherapy. Two trials have reported the results of using brief ABVD and irradiation for clinical stage IA or IIA nonbulky HD; disease free survival was 94% and 100%, overall survival was 100% and 96% with a median follow-up of 38 and 31 months respectively [17, 18].

A cooperative trial comparing chemotherapy alone vs combined modality therapy for early stage HD is being conducted by the National Cancer Institute in Canada and the Eastern Cooperative Oncology Group (ECOG). We await the results of this study with great anticipation, in the meantime, our current approach is that once the diagnosis of HD is made and the extent of disease is determined, the patient should begin systemic chemotherapy with ABVD. This approach eliminates the role of staging laparotomy with splenectomy. The only remaining role for radiation therapy in the initial treatment of HD is in patients with bulky mediastinal disease who require combined modality therapy.

Treatment of Advanced Stage Disease

Prior to using MOPP chemotherapy by DeVita et al. at the National Cancer Institute in the 1960s, the median survival for patients with advanced disease was 2 years or less. It is currently believed that about two-thirds of patients with unfavorable or advanced stage HD will be cured with chemotherapy alone or combined with radiotherapy [31]. Over the last several years ABVD has been shown to be more effective and less toxic than MOPP. The mature results of clinical trials comparing ABVD to MOPP as single agents [16] or in combination with radiotherapy [19] demonstrate the superiority of ABVD. The difference between MOPP and ABVD in the cancer and leukemia group B (CALGB) trial has become more impressive with longer follow-up [20]. It would appear that ABVD should be considered an acceptable standard regimen for advanced stage HD. Promising early results have been reported using a seven drug regimen, Stanford V, which is completed in 12 weeks and contains reduced doses of Doxorubicin and Bleomycin, radiotherapy is given to patients with initial bulky disease. A 3 year overall survival rate of 96% and failure free survival rate of 87% were reported. Long term follow-up is not yet available [21].

The German HD study group designed a regimen utilizing intensified Bleomycin, Etoposide, Doxorubicin, Cyclophosphamide, Vincristine, Prednisone and Procarbazine (BEACOPP) plus granulocyte colony stimulating factor. At 30 months 93% of 60 patients treated as such were disease free [22].

The role of radiotherapy as consolidation to chemotherapy in advanced stage disease remains controversial. Radiation is usually considered in patients with bulky disease. In a randomized clinical trial conducted by the South West Oncology Group (SWOG), 278 patients with stage III and IV who achieved complete response after chemotherapy were randomized to either no further treatment or low dose radiation to initial sites of disease. Remission duration was better in the irradiated group (85% vs 67% 5 year free survival), however, no survival differences were observed [23].

## Posttreatment Evaluation

After completion of chemotherapy, imaging studies should be repeated including chest, abdominal and pelvic CT Scan and gallium scan. Bone marrow biopsy and aspirates should be done only if the marrow was involved with HD at the time of diagnosis. If complete remission is documented, no further therapy is indicated except for patients who initially present with bulky mediastinal disease in whom involved field radiotherapy is indicated. A positive gallium scan in patients whose disease has been previously found to be gallium avid may indicate the need for additional or more aggressive chemotherapy. A biopsy of residual masses may also be indicated. Maintenance therapy after the achievement of complete remission does not prolong remission or survival [32], thus it is not indicated.

Patients in CR should be seen every three months in the first two years, every 4–6 months for the next 3 years and annually thereafter. Visits should include a complete physical exam, CBC, a chemistry profile with LDH, and imaging studies.

## Treatment of Relapsed Disease

More than 40% of patients with advanced stage disease and a fraction of patients with early stage disease treated with radiotherapy alone will relapse and require salvage therapy. Several poor prognostic indicators have been identified for early stage HD and include: the presence of B symptoms, age over 45 years, bulky mediastinal disease and extranodal involvement [4].

## Relapse After Radiation Therapy

Patients with early stage HD who relapse after radiation therapy have an excellent response to chemotherapy (listed in Table 2) with expectant

**Table 2.** Commonly used chemotherapeutic regimens

| | |
|---|---|
| ABVD | (Repeat cycle every 28 days for 6 cycles) |
| | Doxorubicin, I.V., 25 mg/m$^2$, days 1 and 15 |
| | Bleomycin, I.V. 10/U/m$^2$, days 1 and 15 |
| | Vinblastine, I.V., 6 mg/m$^2$, days 1 and 15 |
| | Dacarbazine, I.V., 375 mg/m$^2$, days 1 and 15 |
| | Or: dacarbazine, I.V. 150 mg/m$^2$, days 1–5 |
| MOPP | (Repeat cycle every 28 days for 6 cycles) |
| | Mechlorethamine, I.V., 6 mg/m$^2$, days 1 and 8 |
| | Vincristine, I.V. 1.4 mg/m$^2$ (max 2.5 mg), days 1 and 8 |
| | Procarbazine, P.O., 100 mg/m$^2$, days 1–14 |
| | Prednisone, P.O., 40 mg/m$^2$, days 1–14 |
| MOPP/ABV hybrid | (Repeat cycle every 28 days for 6 cycles) |
| | Mechlorethamine, I.V. 6 mg/m$^2$, days 1 |
| | Vincristine, I.V., 1.4 mg/m$^2$, days 1 |
| | Procarbazine, P.O., 100 mg/m$^2$, days 1–7 |
| | Prednisone, P.O., 40 mg/m$^2$, days 1–14 |
| | Doxorubicin, I.V., 35 mg/m$^2$, day 8 |
| | Bleomycin, I.V., 10/U/m$^2$, days 8 |
| | Vinblastine, I.V., 6 mg/m$^2$, days 8 |
| Stanford V[a] | (Repeat cycle every 28 days) |
| | Mechlorethamine, I.V., 6 mg/m$^2$, days 1 |
| | Doxorubicin, I.V., 25 mg/m$^2$, days 1, 15 |
| | Vinblastine, I.V., 6 mg/m$^2$, days 1, 15[b] |
| | Vincristine, I.V., 5/U/m$^2$, days 8, 22[b] |
| | Bleomycin, I.V., 60 mg/m$^2$, days 8, 22 |
| | Etoposide, I.V., 60 mg/m$^2$, days 15, 16 |
| | Prednisone, P.O., 40 mg/m$^2$, every other day[c] |

[a] Total of 3 cycles.
[b] Vinblastine dose decreased to 4 mg/m$^2$, and vincristine dose decreased to 1 mg/m$^2$ during cycle 3 for patients >50 years of age.
[c] Taper by 10 mg qod starting at week 10.

complete remission rates between 75%–90% and long-term survival ranging from 45%–70%. Patients who have previously received mediastinal irradiation are at increased risk of cardiac and pulmonary toxicity following chemotherapy with ABVD. Thus a hybrid regimen (e.g. MOPP/ABV hybrid or MOPP alternating with ABVD) is preferred as delivery of fewer cycles of ABVD should lead to a decrease in the cardiac and pulmonary toxicity caused by the synergy of radiation with doxorubicin and bleomycin.

Relapse After Chemotherapy

The likelihood of response to salvage chemotherapy depends on the response to initial therapy and the duration of remission. Three different groups exist in this category:
– Induction failures includes patients who fail to enter complete remission.
– Relapse within 12 months after achieving CR
– Relapse greater than 12 months after achieving CR

The last group has an excellent response to salvage chemotherapy even when the same regimen initially used to induce remission is utilized with a complete response rate of about 79% and an actuarial 22-year disease free survival of 45% [24].

The first two groups (nonresponders and patients with short initial remission) do less well with salvage chemotherapy with reported remission rates of 49% and 5-year disease free survival of 14%. Those patients should be considered for high dose chemotherapy with hematopoietic rescue.

A variety of chemotherapeutic regimens other than MOPP and ABVD are used in the salvage setting (Table 3) with response rates ranging from 13% to 72% and remissions lasting 12–24 months.


High-Dose Chemotherapy

Since its introduction more than 15 years ago, high-dose chemotherapy with autologous hematopoietic support (HDC/HS) has become the treatment of choice for patients with HD who failed or relapsed after induction chemotherapy [25]. The rational for using HDC stems from trials that proved the existence of a steep dose-tumor kill curve for lymphoma cell lines and suggested that chemothearpy dose escalation in humans might result in higher response rates [26].

Several controversies exist in regard to the ideal timing of transplantation, the choice of preparative regimen, and the definition of poor prognostic features [25]. It is important to point out that there are no prospective trials directly comparing salvage chemotherapy to HDC/HS. Recently, a group of investigators at Stanford compared the outcome of 60 patients with HD treated with HDC/HS with a matched historical

**Table 3.** Salvage chemotherapeutic regimens

| | |
|---|---|
| DHAP | (Repeat cycle every 21–28 days[a]) |
| | Dexamethasone, I.V., 10 mg q6 h, days 1–4, or 40 mg days 1–4 |
| | Cytarabine, I.V., 2 g/m$^2$ q12 hx2 doses, day 2 |
| | Cisplatin, I.V., 100 mg/m$^2$ per 24 h continuous infusion, day 1 |
| ESHAP | (Repeat cycle every 21–28 days[a]) |
| | Etoposide, I.V., 60 mg/m$^2$, days 1–4 |
| | Cisplatin, I.V., 25 mg/m$^2$ continous infusion, days 1–4 |
| | Cytarabine, I.V., 2 g/m$^2$, immediately following completion of etoposide and cisplatin therapy |
| | Methylprednisolone, I.V., 500 mg/d, days 1–4 |
| IMVP-16 | (Repeat cycle every 21–28 days[a]) |
| | Ifosfamide, I.V., 5 g/m$^2$ continous infusion over 24 h, day 1 |
| | Mesna, I.V. 800 mg/m$^2$ bolus prior to ifosfamide, then 4 g/m$^2$ continuous infusion over 24 h concurrent w/ifosfamide; then 2.4 g/m$^2$ continuous infusion over 12 h after ifosfamide infuson, day 2 |
| | Methotrexate, I.V., 30 mg/m$^2$ days 3 and 10 |
| | Etoposide, I.V., 100 mg/m$^2$ days 1–3 |
| MINE | (Repeat cycle every 28 days[a]) |
| | Mesna, I.V., 1.33 g/m$^2$ per day concurrent with ifosfamie dose, then 500 mg I.V. 4 hours and 8 h after each ifosfamide dose, days 1–3 |
| | Ifosfamide, I.V., 1.33 g/m$^2$ per day, days 1–3 |
| | Mitoxantrone, I.V. 8 mg/m$^2$, day 1 |
| | Etoposide, I.V., 65 mg/m$^2$ per day, days 1–3 |

[a]For two cycles then re-evaluate to assess response.

control group consisting of 109 patients who received salvage chemotherapy at first relapse. Overall survival, event free survival, and freedom from progression at 4 years favored patients who received HDC/HS [27]. The benefit of HDC is particularly pronounced among patients with less favorable prognostic factors, in particular those with the least impressive responses to induction chemotherapy [28].

Several studies suggest that HDC/HS performed early after relapse while the disease is more likely chemosensitive and less bulky, may improve outcome compared with transplantation later in the disease course [27, 33]. Furthermore, it has been suggested that certain patients especially those with minimal disease may benefit by proceeding directly to HDC/HS after relapse without first receiving conventional-dose salvage chemotherapy with a reported failure-free survival of 90% [33]. However, salvage chemotherapy and local radiotherapy prior to HDC may also improve outcome by decreasing tumor burden in patients with bulky disease [27]. A variety of preparative regimens have been used for

HDC with autologous hematopoietic support including BEAC, BEAM, Cy/TBI and MBE (B=BCNU, E=etoposide, A=Ara-C, C/Cy=cyclophosphamide, M=melphalan, TBI=total body irradiation).

The use of either chemotherapy mobilized or chemotherapy and growth factor mobilized stem cells has improved both neutrophil and platelet recovery thus reducing the hematologic toxicity of the chemotherapy used and resulting in decreased length of hospitalization and cost. It also offers the potential for use in the outpatient setting.

Allogeneic transplantation does not offer a survival advantage over autologous stem cell transplantation [29], however, HLA/matched allogeneic transplant may be useful in patients with relapsed HD and concomitant myelodysplasia.

Complications of HDC include myelosuppression, pulmonary toxicity, and veno-occulsive disease. Long term complications include myelodysplasia or frank acute leukemia occurring between 1–3 years after transplant [30]. Currently it is believed the transplant related mortality represents less than 10% compared to mortality rates of 20% or greater in the early transplant literature [25]. Longer followup is required to determine the overall effectivenss of HDC and impact on survival in HD

## References

1. Mack TM, Cozen W, Shibata DK, Weiss LM, Nathwani BN, Hernadez AM, Taylor CR, Hamilton AS, Deapen DM, Rappaport EB.Deapen DM, Rappaport EB. (1995) Concordance for Hodgkin's disease in identical twins suggesting genetic susceptibility to the young-adult form of the disease. NEJM 332:413–8
2. Tirelli U, Errante D, Dolcetti R, Gloghini A, Serraino D, Vaccer E, Franceschi S, Boiocchi M, Carbone A. (1995) Hodgkin's disease and human immunodeficiency virus infection: Clinicopathologic and virologic features of 114 patients from the Italian Cooperative Group on AIDS and Tumors. JCO 13:1758–1767, 1995
3. Lister TA, Crowther D, Sutcliffe SB, Glatstein E, Canellos G, Young RC, Rosenberg SA, Coltman CA, Tubiana M (1989) Report on a committee convened to discuss the evaluation and staging of patients with Hodgkin's disease: Cotwswolds meeting. J Clin Oncology 7:1630
4. Yahalom J, Straus D (1996) Hodgkin's Disease, Chapter 11, Cancer Management, a multidisciplinary approach, pp 217–237
5. Bogart JA, Chung Ct, Mariados NF, Vermont AI, Lemke SM, Grethlein S, Graziano SL (1998) the value of gallium imaging after therapy for Hodgkin's Disease. Cancer 15:82 (4):754–9
6. Castellino RA, Dunnick NR, Goffinet Dr, Rosenberg SR, Kaplan HS (1983) Predictive value of lymphography for sites of subdiaphragmatic disease encountered at staging laparotomy in newly diagnosed Hodgkin's disease and non-Hodgkin's lymphoma. J Clin Oncol 1:532

7. Castellino RA, Hoppe RT, lank N, Young SW, Newmann C, Rosenberg SA, Kaplan HS (1984) Computer tomography, lymphography, and staging laparotomy: correlations in initial staging of Hodgkin's disease. Am J Roentgenol 143:37

8. Glatstein E, Trueblood HW, Enright LP, Rosenberg SA, Kaplan HS (1970) Surgical staging of abdominal involvement in unselected patients with Hodgkin's disease. Radiology 97:425–432

9. Rosenberg S, Kaplan H (1985) The evolution and summary results of the Stanford randomized clinical trials of the management of Hodgkin's disease. Int J Radiat Oncol Biol Phys 11:5

10. Fuller L, Hutchison G (1982) Collaborative clincial trial for stage I and II Hodgkin's disease: Significant of mediastinal and nonmediastinal disease in laparotomy-and non-laparotomy-staged patients. Cancer Treatment Rep 66:775

11. Wolden SL, Lamborn KR, Cleary SF, Tate DJ, Donaldson SS (1998) Second cancers following pediatric Hodgkin's disease. J Clin Oncol 16 (2):536–44

12. Valagussa P, Santoro A, Fossati-Bellani F. et al. (1986) Second acute leukemia and other malignancies following treatment for Hodgkin's disease. J Clin Oncol 4:830–837

13. Cimino G, Biti GP, Anselmo AP, et al (1989) MOPP chemotherapy versus extended-field radiotherapy in the management of pathological stages I-IIA Hodgkin's diease. J Clin Oncol 7:732–737

14. Longo DL, Glatstein E, Duffey PL, et al (1991) Radiation therapy versus combination chemothearpy in the treatment of early-stage Hodgkin's disease

15. Bonadonna G, Zucali R, Monfardini S, DeLewa M, Uslenghi C (1975) Combination chemotherapy of Hodgkin's disease with adriamycin, bleomycin vinblastine, and imidazole carboxmide versus MOPP. Cancer 36:252–259

16. Canellos GP, Anderson JR, Propert KJ et al. (1992) Chemotherapy of advanced Hodgkin's disease with MOPP, ABVD, or MOPP alternating with ABVD. N Engl J Med 327, 1478–1484

17. Santoro A, Bonfante V, Viviani S et al. (1996) Subtotal nodal versus involved field irradiation after 4 cycles of ABVD in early stage Hodgkin's disease. Proc Am Soc Clin Oncol 15:415, (abstr 1271)

18. Klasa R, Connors JM, Fairey R, et al (1996) Treatment of early stage Hodgkin's disease: Improved outcome with brief chemotherapy and radiotherapy without staging lapatomy. Ann Oncol 7, 10 (abstr 67)

19. Bonfante V, Santoro A, Viviani S, et al (1996) ABVD in the treatment of Hodgkin' disease. Semin Oncol 19:5:38–45

20. Canellos GP (1996) Is ABVD the standard regimen for Hodgkin's disease based on randomized CALGB comparison of MOPP, ABVD and MOPP alternating with ABVD? Leukemia 2:s68, 1996

21. Bartlett NL, Rosenberg SA, Hoppe RT, et al (1995) Brief chemothearpy, Stanford V, and adjuvant radiotherapy for bulky or advanced-stage Hodgkin's disease: A preliminary reprot. J Clin Oncol 13:1080–1088

22. Tesch H, Lathan B, Rüffer U, et al (1996) Escalation of dose intensity for advanced Hodgkin's disesae using the BEACOPP scheme–Studies of the German Hodgkin's Study Group. Blood 81:673a (suppl 1, abstr)

23. Fabian CJ, Mansfield CM, Dahlberg S, et al (1994) Low-dose involved field radiation after chemotherapy in advanced Hodgkin's disease. A Southwest Oncology Group randomized study. Ann Intern Med 120:903–912

24. Longo DL, Duffey PL, Young RC, Hubbard SM, Ihde DC, Glatstein E, Phares JC, Jaffe ES, Urba WJ, DeVita VT (1992) Conventional-dose salvage combination chemotherapy in patients relapsing with Hodgkin's disease after combination chemotherapy: the low probability for cure. J Clin Oncol 10:210

25. Horning SJ, Chao NJ, Negrin RS, Hoppe RT, LonG GW, Hu WW, Wong RM, Brown BW, Blume KG (1997) High-dose therapy and autologous hematopoietic progenitor cell transplantation for recurrent or refractory Hodgkin's disease: Analysis of the Stanford University results and prognostic indices. Blood 801–813

26. Rapoport AP, Rowe JM, Kouides PA, Duerst RA, Abboud CN, Liesveld JL, Packman CH, Eberly S, Sherman M, Tanner MA, Constine LS, DiPersio JF (1993) One hundred autotransplants for relapsed or refractory Hodgkin's disease and lymphoma: Value of pretranslant disease status for predicting outcome. JCO 11:2351–2361

27. Anderson JE, Litzow MR, Appelbaum FR, Schoch G, Fisher LD, Buckner CD, Petersen FB, Crawford SW, Press OW, Sanders JE, Besinger WI, Martin PJ, Storb R, Sullivan KM, Hansen JA, Thomas ED (1993) Allogeneic, syngeneic, and autologous marrow transplantation for Hodgkin's disease: The 21-year Seattle experience. JCO 11:2342–2350

28. Yuen AR, Rosenberg SA, Hoppe RT, Halpern JD, Horning SJ (1997) Comparison between conventional salvage therapy and high-dose therapy with autografting for recurrent or refractory Hodgkin's disease. Blood 89:814–822

29. Milpied N, Fielding AK, Pearce RM, Ernst P, Gladstone AH (1996) Allogeneic bone marrow transplant is not better than autologous transplant for patients with relapsed Hodgkin's disease. JCO 14:1291–1296

30. Forman JS (1997) Role of high dose chemotherapy and stem cell transplantation in the management of Hodgkin's disease. American Society of Clin Onc Educational Book 244–247

31. Horning SJ (1997) Treatment of unfavorable and advanced-stage Hodgkin's disease. American Society of Clinical Oncology Educational Book 235–239

32. Young RC, Canellos GP, Chabner BA, Schein PS, DeVita VT (1973) Maintenance chemotherapy for advanced Hodgkin's disease in remission. Lancet I:1339

33. Bierman PJ, Anderson JR, Freeman MB, Vose JM, Kessinger A, Bishop MR, Armitage JO (1996) High dose chemotherapy followed by autologous hematopoietic rescue for Hodgkin's disease patients following first relapse after chemotherapy. Annals of Oncology 7:151–156

# Non-Hodgkin's Lymphoma

K.J. Finiewicz, J.E. Ultmann

## Epidemiology, Risk Factors

Incidence

Non-Hodgkin's lymphomas (NHL) account for approximately 4.0% of newly diagnosed cancer cases in adult population. Based on estimates by American Cancer Society 53,600 new cases of NHL will be diagnosed in the United Stated in 1997, and 23,800 Americans will die of NHL, placing NHL among the leading causes of cancer mortality [1]. Interestingly, for reasons not entirely clear, the incidence of NHL is continuously rising at the rate of 7% per year, representing one of the largest increases in a cancer incidence, that is an increase of approximately 60% in years 1973–1989 [2, 3]. Up to 1987, the age adjusted increases in incidence rates were highest in older population, lower among middle-age adults i.e. 35–64 year old and lowest, though still appreciative, among young adults. This was thought to reflect the increasing life expectancy and to some extend improvement in diagnostic technics and wide access to medical care rather than a true increase in morbidity. However, the increasing exposure to an unknown carcinogen cannot be excluded as the possible explanation for this phenomenon. The AIDS epidemics emerged in 1980s as a new risk factor responsible for a significant increase in NHL incidence, particularly in young men.

Race, Sex, Age, Geographic Distribution

**Race.** The incidence of NHL in general as well as the incidence of certain histologic subtypes varies by race. In the United States NHL is more common in Caucasians than in Afro-Americans, Native-Americans or Asian-Americans [1].

**Sex.** NHL is more common among men than women; among 53,600 new NHL cases estimated for 1997, 30,300 are men and 23,300 are women.

**Age.** The overall incidence of NHL increases steadily throughout life. However certain pathologic subtypes are more prevalent in specific age groups. Low and intermediate grade lymphomas predominate in adults, while high grade lymphomas are more common in children. After excluding high grade lymphomas, the median age of presentation for NHL is over 50 years.

**Distribution.** The geographic differences in incidence of certain subtypes of NHL are significant and reflect endemic areas of the viruses thought to be implicated in pathogenesis of those subtypes. Thus HTLV-1 associated NHL is prevalent in Japan and the Caribbean, where approximately 1% of population are carriers of HTLV-1 as opposed to the United States with only 0.025% HTLV-1 seropositivity. The EBV-associated Burkitt's lymphoma accounts for approximately 80% of childhood cancers in endemic areas of equatorial Africa. The non-endemic type of Burkitt's lymphoma however, so called sporadic Burkitt's lymphoma, is infrequently seen in other parts of the world, including the United States. Follicular lymphomas are most common in Europe and the United States, bur relatively uncommon in Latin America.

## Localization

Lymphoma is a neoplasm of lymphoid tissue and as such most commonly originates in one of the lymphatic tissue organs i.e. lymph nodes, spleen and bone marrow. However NHL may involve and spread to almost any organ of the body. The site of origin, the pattern of spread and the involvement of specific extranodal sites are mostly dependent on the histologic subtype of NHL.

## Risk Factors

Multiple risk factors and pathogenic mechanisms have been described in lymphomagenesis. Epidemiologic studies have identified several environmental factors linked to the development of NHL such as exposure to petroleum products, pesticides and herbicides, ionizing radiation as well as drugs, including chemotherapeutic agents. Other less well established risk factors may also be implicated as lymphoma has been identified as an occupational hazard in association with various working environments and chemicals.

## Etiology

The new remarkable advances in molecular biology have permitted combination of the concepts from the field of cytogenetics, virology and immunology, and have resulted in a dramatic increase of our understanding of the process of lymphomagenesis. The development of lymphoid neoplasm is thought to be a result of a multistep process that involves: 1) clonal expansion of the cells at a certain level of differentiation, 2) acquisition of genetic aberration resulting in the uncontrolled growth or immortalization, and 3) modification of the tumor growth by the immune system.

The recognized histologic subtypes of lymphoma can be traced to the normal lymphocyte counterpart in the immune system arrested at the certain stage of maturation. The immune system under normal conditions is in a state of dynamic equilibrium. The normal function of the system depends on the precisely regulated expansion and longevity of particular subsets of lymphocytes. Neoplastic transformation of the immune system, viewed in the broader aspect of oncogenesis, involves the poorly controlled growth of a single clone of cells with either higher proliferative potential or greater longevity or both.

Chromosomal analyses reveal that cytogenetic abnormalities are present in almost all cases of NHL. The nonrandom genetic aberrations seen in NHL seem to correlate closely with histology and immunophenotype underlying their role in pathogenesis. The predominant molecular event behind the cytogenetic aberrations recognized in NHL is thought to be the activation of various cellular proto-oncogenes through somatic mutation, chromosomal translocation or incorporation of viral oncogenes or viral enhancers of host oncogenes into the host genome. The most common translocation in NHL, t (14, 18) (q32;q21), found in 85% of follicular lymphomas, juxtaposes the bcl-2 oncogene next to the heavy chain immunoglobulin gene on 14q32, which results in altered bcl-2 expression. The overexpression of bcl-2, the apoptotic inhibitor gene, results in development of a neoplasm through accumulation of cells characterized by increased longevity. The overexpression of bcl-1 gene, resulting from t (11, 14) (q13;q32) is associated with mantle cell lymphoma. Translocations involving band 8q24 lead to c-myc dysregulation and are consistently seen in high grade small non-cleaved cell lymphomas, Burkitt's and non-Burkitt's type.

Immunodeficiency state is one of the well established predisposing factors for NHL. Patients with congenital immunodeficiency states like ataxia-telangiectasia, Wiskott-Aldrich syndrome, severe combined immunodeficiency have long been known to have high risk of developing NHL. The incidence of cancer in patients with congenital immune deficiency is approximately 100 times higher than expected, with NHL comprising the majority of the tumors. Increased incidence of lymphoma has also been noted in association with acquired immunodeficiency states: HIV infection, iatrogenic immunosuppression (in post-transplant setting and in long-term survivors of Hodgkin's disease) and in the setting of collagen vascular and other autoimmune diseases, especially following therapy with cytotoxic agents. The overall incidence of malignancies in HIV-infected individuals is estimated to be 40%, with B-cell NHL being the most common.

It is not known what triggers the initial expansion and then drives the selection of a clone that eventually will give rise to a neoplasm. The chronic antigenic stimulation by an infectious agent may be implicated in this process, especially in its early stage. There is strong evidence suggesting that Helicobacter pylori may play a role in the development of primary gastric lymphoma. Viruses are able to induce various tumors in animals. Their role in human tumorigenesis appears to be less important, however there are three examples of a very strong association between viruses and human NHLs: EBV has been reported in association with lymphoma seen in the setting of immune suppression, HHV-8 with primary effusion lymphoma, and HTLV-1 with adult T-cell lymphoma. The exact contribution of viral infection to lymphomagenesis has yet to be established. The cooperation of other environmental and genetic factors in the setting of the disruption of the balance between the virus and the host immune response seem to be required in all cases and the long latency period usually separates the initial viral infection and the presentation of the malignant phenotype.

**Pathology**

Classification

The broad entity of NHL can be categorized based on pathologic, immunologic, cytogenetic, molecular and clinical features. Several classification systems have been proposed for NHL. Historically the Rappaport classification (1956), and later Lukes-Collins classification (1974) and Kiel classification (1975) were all used in different parts of the world, being the source of confusion and creating difficulties in comparing the results of clinical trials. Each system had its advantages and contributed to our understanding of pathogenesis of lymphoma. However it was not until The Working Formulation (WF) was developed by an international collaborative group in 1982 [11], that a uniform language was established. The WF categorized NHL based on morphologic and clinical features, mainly the natural history of the disease and survival of patients treated for lymphoma in 1960s and 1970s.

The three prognostic categories within the WF are as follows:
– Low-grade
    – A. Small lymphocytic, consistent with chronic lymphocytic leukemia (SL)
    – B. Follicular, predominant small cleaved cell (FSC)
    – C. Follicular, mixed small cleaved and large cell (FM)
– Intermediate-grade
    – D. Follicular, predominantly large cell (FL)
    – E. Diffuse, small cleaved cell (DSC)
    – F. Diffuse mixed, small and large cell (DM)
    – G. Diffuse, large cell cleaved or noncleaved cell (DL)
– High-grade
    – H. Immunoblastic, large cell (IBL)
    – I. Lymphoblastic, convoluted or nonconvoluted cell (lymphocytic leukemia)
    – J. Small noncleaved cell, Burkitt's or non-Burkitt's (SNC)

The natural history of untreated low grade lymphoma is measured in years, intermediate grade lymphoma in months and high grade lymphoma in weeks. The main virtue of WF is simplicity, which facilitated the wide acceptance by pathologists and clinicians. Oncologists learned to

**Table 1.** REAL classification schema

B-cell neoplasms
  I. Precursor B-cell neoplasm: precursor B-lymphoblastic leukemia/lymphoma
 II. Peripheral B-cell neoplasms
    A. B-cell chronic lymphocytic leukemia/prolymphocytic leukemia/small lym-
       phocytic lymphoma
    B. Lymphoplasmacytoid lymphoma/immunocytoma
    C. Mantel cell lymphoma
    D. Follicle center cell lymphoma, follicular
       1. Provisional cytologic grades: I (small cell), II (mixed small and large cell),
          III (large cell)
       2. Provisional subtype: diffuse, predominantly small cell type
    E. Marginal zone B-cell lymphoma
       1. Extranodal (MALT-type±monocytoid B cells)
       2. Provisional subtype: nodal (±monocytoid B cells)
    F. Provisional entity: splenic marginal zone lymphoma (±villous lymphocytes)
    G. Hairy cell leukemia
    H. Plasmacytoma/plasma cell myeloma
    I. Diffuse large B-cell lymphoma
       1. Subtype: primary mediastinal (thymic) B-cell lymphoma
    J. Burkitt's lymphoma
    K. Provisional entity: high-grade B-cell lymphoma, Burkitt-like

T-cell and putative NK-cell neoplasms
  I. Precursor T-cell neoplasm: precursor T-lymphoblastic ymphoma/leukemia
 II. Peripheral T-cell and NK-cell neoplasms
    A. T-cell chronic lymphocytic leukemia/prolymphocytic leukemia
    B. Large granular lymphocyte leukemia
       1. T-cell type
       2. NK-cell type
    C. Mycosis fungoides/Sezary's syndrome
    D. Peripheral T-cell lymphoma, unspecified
       1. Provisional cytologic categories: medium-sized cell, mixed medium and
          large cell, large cell, lymphoepitheloid cell
       2. Provisional subtype: hepatosplenic gamma/delta T-cell lymphoma
       3. Provisional subtype: subcutaneous panniculitic T-cell lymphoma
    E. Angioimmunoblastic T-cell lymphoma
    F. Angiocentric lymphoma
    G. Intestinal T-cell lymphoma (±enteropathy associated)
    H. Adult T-cell lymphoma/leukemia
    I. Anaplastic large cell lymphoma
       1. CD30+ -cell type
       2. T-cell type
       3. Null-cell types
    J. Provisional entity: anaplastic large cell lymphoma, Hodgkin's-like

make therapeutic decisions based on the grade of the lymphoma with
little or no attention to specific subtypes of the disease.

With advances in understanding of lymphoma biology it became
obvious that the subgroups broadly defined by the WF often consist of

several distinct entities, that may be characterized using the modern immunohistochemical, cytogenetic and molecular methods. The recognition and definition of the new lymphoma entities, as well as, the more concise description of "old" entities was the ambitious goal of the "Revised European-American Lymphoma" classification schema (REAL) proposed in 1994 (Table 1) [4, 9]. The REAL schema classifies lymphoid malignancies into B-cell, NK/T-cell and Hodgkin's disease, which are further traced to their presumed cell of origin and thus divided into central and peripheral. The NHL subtypes recognized by the REAL schema are both homogeneous and reproducible and likely represent the "real" biologic entities. Several new B-cell lymphoma subtypes with indolent course, previously "hidden" in A-E WF subcategories have been characterized by the new REAL classification such as: marginal zone lymphoma (MZL), mantle cell lymphoma (MCL), immunocytoma. The peripheral T-cell lymphoma (PTL) has become an immunologically defined category under the REAL classification with a few specified and provisional subtypes, among others Ki1 anaplastic large cell lymphoma (ALCL), HTLV-1-associated Japanese T-cell lymphoma/leukemia, enteropathy-associated T-cell lymphoma (EATL), hepatosplenic T gamma/delta cell lymphoma. As opposed to indolent lymphomas and T-cell lymphomas, the REAL classification did not subdivide, but compressed several more aggressive lymphoma subtypes previously described in WF (E, F, G, H, J categories) into one category i.e. diffuse large cell lymphoma, recognizing perhaps limitations in the current diagnostic technics that would prevent the elucidation of the biologically or clinically meaningful entities.

The initial impression was that the emphasis on pathologic description of lymphoma by the REAL proposal did not translate to clinically relevant groupings and several reservations, mainly in regard to practicality, were reported [10]. The reproducibility and distinct clinical behavior of many entities defined by the REAL classification have been validated since then. The data from the first clinical trials based on the REAL classification have been reported and strongly imply that the recognition of the new REAL entities may be clinically highly relevant [5–7]. The best examples are MCL and MALT lymphoma. One more evidence was supplied by the results of the recent large French study, which recognized the peripheral T-cell phenotype as an independent adverse prognostic factor in patients with aggressive lymphoma [8].

The REAL classification is probably best understood as the excellent summary of known entities and should be considered a foundation for future schemas that will satisfy both requirements: pathologic precision as well as practical applicability. The World Health Organization project on lymphoma classification, currently in progress, will hopefully result in a widely acceptable, simple and clinically relevant classification that should satisfy both pathologists and clinicians. Table 2 illustrates one of the most recent WHO proposals.

**Table 2.** World Health Organization classification of neoplastic diseases of the hematopoietic and lymphoid tissues (personal communication E.S. Jaffe)

B-cell neoplasms
  *Precursor B cell lymphoblastic leukemia*/lymphoma (*B-lineage ALL*/lBL)
  Mature B-Cell Neoplasms
  *B-cell chronic lymphocytic leukemia*/small lymphocytic lymphoma
  B-cell prolymphocytic leukemia
  Lymphoplasmacytic lymphoma
  Splenic marginal zone B-cell lymphoma
  Hairy cell leukemia
  *Extranodal marginal Zone B-cell Lymphoma of mucosa-associated lymphoid tissue (MALT) type*
  *Mantle cell lymphoma*
  *Follicular lymphoma*
  Nodal marginal zone lymphoma±monocytoid B-cells
  *Diffuse large B-cell lymphoma*
  *Burkitt lymphoma*
  Plasmacytoma
  *Plasma cell myeloma*

T-cell neoplasms
  *Precursor T cell lymphoblastic lymphoma/leukemia (T-lineage LBL/ALL)*
  Mature T-cell and NK-cell neoplasms
  T-cell prolymphocytic leukemia
  T-cell large granular lymphocytic leukemia
  Sezary syndrome
  NK cell leukemia
  *Extranodal NK/T cell lymphoma, nasal and nasal-type*
  *Mycosis fungoides*
  Primary cutaneous anaplastic large cell lymphoma
  Subcutaneous panniculitis-like T-cell lymphoma
  Enteropathy-type intestinal T-cell lymphoma
  Hepatosplenic?/d T-cell lymphoma
  *Angioimmunoblastic T-cell lymphoma*
  *Peripheral T-cell lymphoma (unspecified)*
  *Anaplastic large cell lymphoma, primary systemic type*
  *Adult T-cell lymphoma/leukemia (HTLV1+)*[a]

Most common lymphoid neoplasms are shown in italics.

[a] Significant variations in incidence are found in different parts of the world. These diseases are rare in Europe and the United States but are common in certain parts of Asia.

Histologic Subtypes and Clinical Presentation

The immunophenotypic, genetic, molecular and clinical features characteristic for each type of NHL discussed in this chapter are summarized in Table 3.

Laboratory Methods for Diagnosis and Classification of NHL:

1. Traditional hematopathologic examination of all slides with at least one paraffin block representative of the tumor.
2. Immunophenotyping using specific monoclonal antibodies which can be applied to viable cell suspensions, frozen sections or paraffin-embedded sections to establish lineage and clonality. Flow cytometry is the rapid tool which allows detection of monoclonal population of lymphoid cells in blood or other body fluids. Monoclonality in B-cell lymphoma is demonstrated by detecting of a uniform population of cells expressing aberrant, malignant phenotype or light chain restriction. Malignant phenotype of T-cell lymphomas is often characterized by the lack of one or more of the pan-T-cell antigens. Immunophenotyping is necessary for diagnosing of certain new lymphoma entities recognized under the REAL classification.
3. Cytogenetic studies are performed on fresh tissue and allow recognition of specific chromosomal abnormalities.
4. Molecular studies i.e. polymerase chain reaction (PCR) and Southern blott analysis, are routinely done on fresh, unfixed tissue, although fixed tissue may be also used in certain cases. Generally these studies aid in recognition of monoclonal population of lymphocytes by detection of immunoglobulin gene rearrangement in B-cell lymphoma or T-cell receptor gene rearrangement in T-cell lymphoma.

**Work-Up and Staging**

The mainstay of the diagnosis of NHL is the histopathologic examination of the tumor. Thus the definitive diagnosis of NHL can be established only by an adequate biopsy of neoplastic lymphoid tissue, usually a peripheral lymph node. One cannot overestimate the importance of this step in evaluation and if the obtained sample is considered inadequate, the

**Table 3.** The immunophenotypic, genetic, molecular-and clinical features of NHL

| Natural course of disease | NHL subtype | Presumptive cell of origin | Immuno-phenotype | Genetic and molecular features | Typical clinical features at presentation | Common extranodal sites | Potential for cure |
|---|---|---|---|---|---|---|---|
| Indolent lymphoma | SLL/CLL | Recirculating naive B-cells (?) | Pan B-cell CD19(+), faint CD20(+) CD23(+), CD5(+) faint sIgM(+), cIgM(-) | +12; 13q14; 14q+ | Older adults with generalized lymphadenopathy; hypogammaglobulinemia and auto-immune phenomena i.e. thrombocytopenia and hemolytic anemia | Liver, spleen, marrow | No |
| | FC | Germinal center B-cells, both centrocytes and centroblasts | Pan B-cell CD19(+), CD20(+)CD5(-) CD10(+) sIg(+)(M>G>A) | T(14;18) (bcl-2) | The most common lymphoma in Caucasian population; most patients present with wide-spread disease | Liver, spleen, marrow | No, in grade 1 Probable, in grade |
| | MZL (provisional group) | Postgerminal center B memory cell with the capacity to differentiate into marginal zone, monocytoid and plasma cells | Pan B-cell CD19(+), CD20(+) CD5(-), CD10(-) sIg(+)(M>G>A) | +3, t(11;18) | Older adults, often with a history of auto-immune disease: 50–80% present with stage I | Extranodal type i.e. MALTOMAs can be found in the stomach, orbit, lungs, thyroid, salivary gland | Uncertain |

**Table 3.** Continued

| Natural course of disease | NHL subtype | Presumptive cell of origin | Immuno-phenotype | Genetic and molecular features | Typical clinical features at presentation | Common extranodal sites | Potential for cure |
|---|---|---|---|---|---|---|---|
| | MCL | Naive B-Cell of follicle mantle or germinal center origin | Pan B-cell CD19(+), CD20(+), CD23(-),CD5(+) CD10(-) sIgM(+) and sIgD(+). Often γ | T(11; 14) (cyclin D1) | Wide-spread disease at diagnosis | Waldeyer's ring, bone marrow or/and other extranodal sites involvement; multiple GI sites involvement (lymphomatous polyposis) | No |
| | Immuno-cytoma | Postgerminal center cells that have undergon e somatic mutation | Pan B-cell CD19(+), CD20(+), CD23(-), CD5(-), CD10(-), sIgM(+), cIgM(+) | ? t(9; 14) | Older adults; IgM paraprotein +/- hyperviscosity; Auto-antibodies or cryoglo-bulin (in most cases assoc. with hepatitis C) | Common bone marrow involvement | No |
| Aggressive lymphoma | DLC lymphoma | Proliferating peripheral B-cells (centro-blasts or immunoblasts) | Pan B-cell CD19(+) CD20(+) CD5(+/-), CD10(+/-) sIg(+) | T(14;18) (bcl-2); 3q27(bcl-6) | All ages; most patients present with rapidly enlarging masses; common extranodal presentation | Liver, spleen, Waldeyer's ring/GI tract, skin, bone marrow | Yes |
| | Primary mediastinal DLC lym-phoma with | | Pan B-cell CD19(+) CD20(+) often sIg(-) | ? | Female predominance, median age 40 yr; patients present with rapidly enlarging | Very invasive locally, may invade pericar-dium, lungs, | Yes |

**Table 3.** Continued

| Natural course of disease | NHL subtype | Presumptive cell of origin | Immuno-phenotype | Genetic and molecular features | Typical clinical features at presentation | Common extranodal sites | Potential for cure |
|---|---|---|---|---|---|---|---|
| | sclerosis | | | | mediastinal mass originating in the thymus | pleura, chest wall. Relapses tend to be wide spread and involve multiple extranodal sites. | |
| Highly aggressive lymphoma | Lympho-blastic lymphoma | Precursor T-cell (antigen independent) | CD3(+), CD7(+) TdT(+) CD4,8 often double positive or double negative | Variable | Adolescent or young adults presenting with a large mediastinal mass | Liver, spleen, lung/pleura, skin, bone marrow | Yes |
| | Small non-cleaved cell lymphoma | Peripheral B-cells of unknown stages, possibly B blasts of the early germinal center | Pan B-cell CD19(+), CD20(+), CD23(-), CD5(-), CD10(+), sIg(+)(M>G) | T(2;8); t(8;14); t(8;22)(c-myc) | Adolescent or young adults with head and neck masses(endemic) or abdominal masses (non-endemic) | GI tract, lung/pleura, bone marrow | Yes |

procedure should be repeated. As mentioned above the fresh tissue should be collected and frozen for molecular analysis and/or immuno-phenotyping, which may be necessary for identification of specific lymphoma subtype. Bilateral bone marrow biopsy and aspirate is considered a part of routine staging procedure for NHL.

The complete physical examination and history, with attention to the node-bearing areas and the presence of B symptoms respectively, are important in assessment of the extend of the disease and are used to guide further diagnostic work-up.

The extensive panel of laboratory tests is considered an indispensable part of initial evaluation and should include CBC with differential count and platelet count, as well as, chemistry profile with LDH and $\beta_2$-microglobulin. Peripheral blood may be examined for the presence of circulating malignant cells by molecular analysis or immunophenotyping although the practical value of this information is not well established. HIV serology should be checked in all patients with diffuse large cell, immunoblastic and small noncleaved lymphoma. Serum protein electrophoresis and immunoelectrophoresis is indicated in all cases of small lymphocytic lymphoma.

Radiologic tests routinely performed in the staging of NHL are: chest X-ray and CT scan of the neck, chest, abdomen and pelvis. This is usually sufficient for evaluation of lymphadenopathy, organomegaly and other organ involvement by lymphoma. Gallium scans are valuable, especially in detection and follow-up of aggressive NHL. They are less sensitive in low grade NHL. The results of gallium scan tend to correlate very well with disease activity.

Other diagnostic studies may be required for completion of initial evaluation based on the signs or symptoms elucidated during history or physical examination. The best imaging test and/or diagnostic procedures should be chosen for specific sites of lymphomatous involvement to allow proper follow-up and assessment of the response to treatment. For example MRI/CT scan or bone scan may be needed in lymphoma associated with bone involvement, EGD and/or upper GI series with small bowel follow-through in patients with primary GI lymphoma.

The extent of clinical investigation prior to therapy beyond the above outlined routine evaluation often depends on the histology (see Table 3). Involvement of Waldeyer's ring warrants a subsequent evaluation of GI tract. The CT scan of the head and spine (or MRI) as well as lumbar puncture with cytologic examination of CSF should be performed whenever

**Table 4.** Ann Arbor staging system

| Stage | Description in regard to nodal NHL | Description in regard to extranodal NHL |
|-------|-----------------------------------|------------------------------------------|
| I | Involvement of a single lymph node region | Involvement of a single extralymphatic organ or site (IE) |
| II | Involvement of two or more lymph node regions on the same site of the diaphragm | Localized involvement of a single associated extralymphatic organ or site and its regional lymph nodes with or without other lymph node regions on the same side of the dia-phragm (IIE) |
| III | Involvement of lymph nodes on the both sides of the diaphragm | Involvement of lymph nodes on the both sides of the diaphragm accompanied by localized involvement of an extralymphatic organ or site (IIIE), or spleen (IIIS), or both (IIISE) |
| IV | Disseminated involvement of one or more extralymphatic sites with or without associated lymph node involvement or isolated extralymphatic organ involvement with distant nodal involvement | |

CNS involvement is suspected. In fact it should be a part of routine eva-luation in all settings known to be associated with high incidence of CNS involvement i.e. aggressive lymphoma with extranodal involvement (especially bone marrow or bone involvement), high grade lymphoblastic lymphoma, Burkitt's and non-Burkitt's type or HIV-related lymphoma.

In general, histologic subtype predicts the stage quite reliably and as indicated above may be used to direct the staging work-up. The Ann Arbor staging system (Table 4) originally developed for Hodgkin's disease, has been adapted and traditionally used in NHL, although it's accuracy in predicting prognosis and survival is limited [12]. The capital letter is added to the Roman number designating the stage: "A" for the absence and "B" for the presence of so called "B symptoms" i.e. unex-plained weight loss >10% of body weight in the 6 months prior to diagnosis, unexplained fevers above 38°C or night sweats. The letter "E" is sometimes used to denote extranodal involvement.

## Treatment

The histologic subtype is the most significant, but not the only predictor of the course and the final outcome of NHL. It should be recognized that

NHL is a highly heretogenous group of diseases. Several prognostic factors valid across the entire spectrum of lymphoma have been identified. They may be divided into the two groups: patient-related factors such as age or general health of the patient, and the tumor-related factors such as bulkiness, high rate of tumor growth, LDH level, β2-microglobulin level or the number and the specific sites of tumor involvement. The chemosensitivity of the disease as measured by the rapidity of the response to treatment is also highly predictive of outcome. Considering the different biology of the disease and different treatment goals in indolent and aggressive lymphoma, the risk estimates in these two major subgroups of NHL have different consequences.

The prognostic groups in indolent NHL are not well defined and a reliable widely accepted stratification system does not exist [15]. The International Prognostic Index (IPI), described below, primarily developed for aggressive NHL, has been occasionally successfully applied to indolent lymphoma. In a recent interesting analysis, Denham et al demonstrated that a new staging system taking into account three criteria: the number of involved sites, presence of constitutional symptoms and splenomegaly, may be superior to the Ann Arbor classification system and highly accurate in follicular lymphoma [13].

The situation appears better in regard to aggressive NHL, where the risk assessment has a high bearing on treatment. The International Non-Hodgkin's Lymphoma Prognostic Factors Project has identified four risk groups among patients with aggressive NHL treated with modern anthracyclin-based chemotherapy regimen (Table 5) [14]. The risk factors used in the model were: age (> 60 yo), LDH level (>normal), performance status (> 2), Ann Arbor stage (I-II v/s III-IV) and extranodal involvement (>than one site). The variant of this model has been developed for younger, <60 yo patients, and is referred to as Age Adjusted International Index. The age-adjusted model recognizes the three pro-

**Table 5.** International Prognostic Index for aggressive NHL

| Risk group | Number of adverse risk factors | Predicted 5-year survival for patients <60 years of age | Predicted 5-year survival for patients of all ages |
|---|---|---|---|
| 1 | 0–1 | 85% | 73% |
| 2 | 2 | 69% | 51% |
| 3 | 3 | 46% | 43% |
| 4 | 4–5 | 32% | 26% |

gnostic features: LDH (>normal), performance status (> 1), and stage (I-II v/s III-IV). IPI may be even further modified by measuring $\beta_2$-microglobulin serum level in every IPI category. The ability to tolerate the recommended treatment (all cycles delivered as scheduled) as well as the time to complete remission are very important treatment-related prognostic factors in aggressive NHL. Thus every attempt should be made to administer all cycles of treatment on schedule.

Identifying high risk patients within each histologic subtype has several important implications, especially for young patients, who are not likely to benefit from conventional treatment and thus may be offered an alternative to participate in investigational trials.

The therapeutic approach to the NHL is generally based on the histologic subtype, the prognostic profile and the physiologic status of the patient. Chemotherapy is the mainstay treatment modality for NHL. Radiation therapy has a limited application and is used mainly for treatment of localized disease, as consolidation or as palliation. Surgery in general has no role in therapy of NHL except for the rare cases of life-threatening situations caused by a mass effect. Another possible application of surgery is in localized MALT lymphoma.

For the purpose of this chapter we will discuss the approach to treatment of B-cell NHL using the modified REAL schema, which classifies the pathologic entities into the three prognostic categories defined by WF: low-, intermediate- and high-grade lymphoma (indolent, aggressive and highly aggressive lymphoma respectively). This is difficult to avoid as WF has been of great help in development of uniform approach to treatment of NHL and many of the multiagent chemotherapy regimens, now commonly used, have been developed based on WF. However, delineation of the new entities defined by the REAL classification allowed better understanding of the biology of NHL. The new treatment approaches individualizing management for the each newly described subtype of NHL have begun to emerge and will be discussed briefly in regard to each entity. The management of peripheral T-cell NHL is discussed elsewhere in this book.

Low-Grade, Indolent Lymphoma

The approach to the treatment of indolent lymphoma is generally determined by the lack of convincing evidence that this subtype of NHL can be cured with any currently known therapy. Indolent lymphomas are highly responsive to a variety of therapeutic options; however, it appears that the response rate does not translate into any significant long-term benefit; up to date no study has demonstrated any significant impact of aggressive treatment of low-grade lymphoma on overall survival (OS). The main obstacle is, in fact, the indolent course of the disease, which makes comparative studies of various treatment modalities very difficult due to a very long follow-up, beyond 10–20 years, required to measure the survival benefit. Until the surrogate markers measuring the efficacy of treatment become available, significant progress in designing new treatment strategies in indolent lymphoma is very unlikely.

Since the treatment does not appear to affect the natural history of the disease, it should be generally considered **palliative in nature**. Initiating treatment early in the course of the disease or choosing more intensive regimen may unnecessarily subject the patient to treatment-related morbidities and impair quality of life. This should always be remembered before the decision regarding initiation of therapy for an otherwise asymptomatic patient is made.

Stage I and contiguous stage II of the disease account for approximately 10%–20% of cases at the time of presentation. Local irradiation is the generally accepted treatment recommendation for newly diagnosed stage I and contiguous stage II indolent NHL. The dose usually ranges from 3000 to 4000 cGy applied to the involved sites. The radiation field can be extended to cover the adjacent nodal sites. This type of regional radiation results in a very high rate of sustained remission and 50%–85% 5–10 years survival [16–19]. It has been postulated that radiation may be able to cure truly localized indolent lymphoma, although this has never been convincingly demonstrated. Stanford University recently published an update of their 177 patients with stage I and II indolent lymphoma [16]. The median time to relapse/progression in 79 evaluable patients was 3.3 years. The survival and freedom from relapse (FFR) curves do not appear to plateau even with the adequately long follow up, although the likelihood of relapse for patients who are disease free at 10 years (44% of patients) is very small. A "watchful waiting" approach is still recommended for asymptomatic patients with localized indolent NHL if radiotherapy is contraindicated. The attempts to improve upon the results of local irradiation by intensification of treatment have been generally unsuccessful. The addition of chemotherapy to irradiation does not appear to be of any benefit. The earlier studies employing the

CVP regimen showed no difference in outcome [19–21]. In two more recent studies, the adjuvant CHOP significantly improved disease free survival (DFS) but not OS [22, 23]. The value of extended field radiation or subtotal nodal irradiation has not been proven and thus is not recommended. The randomized study which addressed this issue concluded that the patients treated with total lymphoid irradiation had significantly better FFR than the patients treated with more limited radiation, however following the well known pattern in indolent lymphoma, the overall survival was no different at 10 years [24].

Non-contiguous stage II, stage III and IV indolent lymphoma comprise approximately 90%–80% of cases at the time of presentation. The complete response rate with chemotherapy of previously untreated patients ranges from 50% to 88%, with median remission duration of 2 years and overall survival approaching 10 years. Regardless of the therapy a continuous pattern of relapses beyond 10 years has been observed. Several clinical trials evaluating the optimal therapy for advanced stage indolent lymphoma are in progress and until their results become available, the issue will remain controversial [31–33]. The randomized studies addressing the early aggressive treatment versus conservative approach i.e. no initial treatment for asymptomatic patients failed to demonstrate survival advantage for the treatment arm [25, 26]. Based on their results, a "watchful waiting" approach, first introduced by investigators at Stanford University [27] is now recommended for all asymptomatic patients with advanced indolent NHL. It should be remembered that this approach requires a close follow up and cooperation of a compliant patient in order to allow timely intervention once the patient becomes symptomatic. The list of symptoms warranting initiation of treatment includes: high tumor growth rate or steady progression over at least 6 months, bulky lymphadenopathy, splenomegaly, threatened end-organ dysfunction, cytopenias including autoimmune cytopenia, recurrent infections and/or other systemic symptoms.

Upon appearance of symptoms a few chemotherapeutic regimens may be considered (Table 6). Their efficacy in inducing a response is generally comparable and quality of life issues as well as the desired rapidity of the response are often used in choosing the most appropriate regimen in each individual case. The anthracycline-containing regimen i.e. CHOP has been commonly used although its advantage over CVP in the setting of indolent NHL has never been shown [34]. As chemotherapy does not appear to be curative, the goal is to induce comple-

**Table 6.** Chemotherapy used in treatment of indolent NHL

| Clinical setting | Regimen | Chemotherapy regimen | Dose | Route and frequency | Comments |
|---|---|---|---|---|---|
| Primary or Secondary treatment | Purine analogs | Fludarabine | 25–30 mg/m² | IV on days 1–5 *Repeat cycle every 21-28 days* | New class of agents with not fully explored potential. Emerging evidence of high effectiveness in certain subtypes of indolent lymphoma. |
| | | 2-CDA (cladribine) | 0.1 mg/kg | IV on days 1–7 (continuous infusion) *Repeat cycle every 21-28 days* | |
| | Oral alkylating agents +/- steroids | Cyclophosphamide | 1.5–2.5 mg/kg | PO, daily | A few months of treatment may be needed to induce a response. |
| | | Chlorambucil | 0.1–0.2 mg/kg | PO, daily *Continue until CR achieved* | |
| | | Prednisone | 30–50 mg/m² | PO for 4 weeks May be started with a single drug | |
| | Combination chemotherapy | **CVP:** | | | Combination regimens are recommended if a rapid response is desired. The role of anthracyclins in indolent lymphoma is unproven. |
| | | Cyclophosphamide | 400 mg/m² | PO, on days 1–5 | |
| | | Vincristine | 1.4 mg/m² (max. 2 mg) | IV on day 1 | |
| | | Prednisone | 100 mg | PO, on days 1–5 *Repeat cycle every, 21 days* | |
| | | **CHOP:** | | | |
| | | Cyclophosphamide | 750 mg/m² | IV, on day 1 | |
| | | Doxorubicin | 50 mg/m² | IV, on day 1 | |
| | | Vincristine | 1.4 mg/m² (max. 2 mg) | IV, on day 1 | |
| | | Prednisone | 100 mg | PO, on days 1–5 *Repeat cycle every 21 days* | |
| Secondary (salvage) treatment | Combination chemotherapy containing purine analogs | Fludarabine | 25 mg/m² | IV, on days 1–3 | Not recommended for fludarabine-refractory patients. |
| | | Mitoxantrone | 10 mg/m² | IV, on day 1 | |
| | | +/-Dexamethasone | 20 mg | IV or PO, on days 1–5 | |
| | | Fludarabine | 30 mg/m² | IV on days 1–3 | May be considered for patients refractory to fludarabine. |
| | | Cyclophosphamide | 300 mg/m² | IV on days 1–3 *Repeat cycle every 21–28 days* | |

te remission or stable partial remission and once the goal has been reached the treatment should be discontinued. Local irradiation may be a useful alternative to systemic therapy. The addition of total lymphoid irradiation, low dose total body irradiation or involved field irradiation to chemotherapy has been investigated and was found to be of no benefit. Likewise, central lymphatic irradiation for non-contiguous stage II and stage III is not recommended [29, 30].

**Relapsed Indolent Lymphoma.** The overall response rate for indolent NHL in the first relapse is quite high, in the range of 70%–80% with the median second remission duration of 13 months and median survival of 53 months [35]. Re-treatment with the same agent at the time of relapse is often effective. If there is no response, the more intensive regimen like CHOP may be warranted. Irradiation also remains an option for relapsed disease, especially when chemotherapy is contraindicated or only local control of the growth is desired. The salvage combination regimen consisting of fludarabine, mitoxantrone and dexamethasone has been reported to induce a CR in 47% and PR in 47% of patients with indolent lymphoma which has recurred or has become refractory to other chemotherapeutic agents [36].

In the Stanford series, 76% of patients with localized indolent lymphoma at the time of the initial diagnosis, had localized disease at relapse [35]. In 79% of cases relapse occurred entirely outside the radiation field. The main predictors of freedom from progression and overall survival at the time of relapse were the stage of disease and the presence of symptoms. Interestingly, the duration of the first complete remission was not significant.

**New Directions in Treatment of Indolent Lymphoma.** The recommendations for therapy of indolent NHL have been based on the management of the disease in elderly. The conservative approach outlined above may be difficult to accept for younger patients with advanced indolent NHL. We believe that those patients whose disease exhibits unfavorable clinical features should be presented with an option of participating in one of the many ongoing investigative trials. The novel approaches tested for indolent lymphoma include new chemotherapy regimens employing the purine nucleoside analogs, immune modulation therapy (interferon alpha), monoclonal antibodies, and high dose chemotherapy with stem cell transplantation. As maintaining remission seems to be more of an issue in indolent NHL than obtaining remission, various strategies designed to prolong remission duration have been considered. The use of interferon alpha concomitantly with anthracycline-containing regimen [39] or as a long-term maintenance treatment of follicular lymphoma [40] appears to prolong disease-free survival when given in adequate doses and duration. However, similarly to all the other treatment modalities in indolent NHL, its impact on overall survival has not been demonstrated. Impressive response rates have been reported following the treatment with monoclonal antibodies, either alone or radiolabeled, to target B-cell surface antigens in NHL resistant to conventional therapy. Rituximab, the chimeric murine/human monoclonal antibody has been recently approved for the treatment of patients with relapsed or refractory low-grade or follicular B-cell lymphoma. The application of this new agent in other clinical settings awaits evaluation. The role of high dose chemotherapy and autologous bone marrow or stem cell transplantation in low grade lymphoma has not yet been defined and remains investigational.

## Special Considerations in Treatment of Certain Histologic Subtypes of Indolent NHL

**Small Lymphocytic Lymphoma** (SLL) is treated like chronic lymphocytic leukemia and in many aspects both entities represent continuum of the same disease. Purine nucleoside analogs are the new, promising agents with exceptionally high activity in this particular subtype of NHL [41]. Fludarabine as a single agent is able to induce a response of 70%–80% of untreated patients and 20%–70% in previously treated patients. MD Anderson reported 79% response rate in previously untreated patients, 54% in patients treated with alkylators only and 37% in patients treated with alkylators and fludarabine (but not refractory). Randomized studies comparing fludarabine with other regimens including alkylating agents, demonstrated the superiority of fludarabine as the first-line agent with the higher response rate and disease-free survival, but no influence on overall survival [42, 43]. New combination regimens containing fludarabine are being explored. The use of mitoxantrone with fludarabine did not increase the efficacy over fludarabine alone in CLL. The preliminary data suggests that combination of fludarabine and cyclophosphamide may be able to improve the response rate over that expected with single-agent fludarabine in previously treated patients but not in untreated patients. Interestingly this combination may be effective in a subgroup of patients refractory to fludarabine alone.

**Follicular Center Cell Lymphomas** (FL) are divided into three cytologic grades: 1 (small cell), 2 (mixed cell), 3 (large cell) based on the relative proportions of small cleaved follicle center cells (centrocytes) and larger noncleaved cells (centroblasts). FL is clearly a biologically heterogenous disease; approximately 20% of patients with follicular lymphoma die within 2 years from diagnosis, but also approximately 20% survive more than 15 years. Under WF grade 1 and 2 are considered low-grade lymphomas while grade 3 has more aggressive features and is being treated like diffuse large B-cell lymphoma. While most studies agree that patients with FL comprised of predominantly small cleaved cells have a better overall survival than those with FL comprised primarily of large cells, the significance of assigning the particular grade seems less convincing and the results are often not reproducible [44]. Additionally, the believe that long-term survival and possibly cure may be achieved with anthracycline-containing regimen in a subgroup of patients with grade 3 follicular center cell lymphoma has recently gained many critical opponents [45]. The recent analysis of 389 patients with follicular lymphoma uniformly staged and treated with CHOP chemotherapy on the three SWOG protocols strongly suggests that the three histologic subtypes may in fact represent one biologic entity [46]. The survival curves were nearly superimposable and more importantly there was no evidence of potential cure for any subtype. This interesting analysis questions the currently accepted aggressive treatment for grade 3 follicular lymphoma with curative intent. However, until this observation becomes validated by other studies, an anthracycline-containing chemotherapy regimen i.e. CHOP remains a standard of care for grade 3 follicular lymphoma.

**Marginal Zone B-Cell Lymphoma** generally encompasses two major subtypes: primarily extranodal MALT lymphoma (MALTOMA) and its morphologically identical counterpart in patients with no extranodal disease called nodal marginal zone B-cell lymphoma. MALTOMA remains localized long before systemic spread and for this reason local treatment, mainly surgery and/or irradiation are especially effective for patients who present with an early stage of the disease. An excellent 5 year survival, in the range of 80%–100%, has been reported for localized forms of the disease with any of the above mentioned treatment modalities [47]. The stomach is the relatively common site of involvement by MALTOMA. The causative relationship between Helicobacter pylori gastritis and the development of gastric MALTOMA has lead to the new treatment approaches in the management of biopsy-proven, localized (i.e. stage IE), H. pylori-associated MALT lymphoma. The multiagent antibiotic regimen consisting of amoxicillin, metronidazole and Pepto Bismol or Omeprazole ("triple therapy"), results in eradication of H. pylori infection in the majority of patients and is followed by regression of malignancy in 60%–70% of cases [47, 48]. The complete regression of lymphoma may take up to several months. Patients who do not respond to this treatment or respond slowly having residual lymphoma after 6 months of treatment should receive more conventional therapy. They should also undergo re-evaluation at that time to rule out the coexistence of large cell lymphoma, which is often associated with refractoriness to triple therapy in face of successful eradication of H. pylori by antibiotic therapy. Low-intensity chemotherapy with chlorambucil or cyclophosphamide, followed by locoregional irradiation seems to be sufficient treatment of limited stage gastric lymphoma and generally yields 70%–80% cure rate. The prognosis of patients with more advanced disease, bulky disease or B symptoms is relatively poor with median survival of 4.5 years in comparison to 7.0 years for other indolent lymphoma categories [5]. Therefore they should be treated with six-eight cycles of chemotherapy±consolidative irradiation. In face of the excellent results of chemotherapy, the role of surgery, historically recommended to prevent perforation or hemorrhage remains unresolved and seems to be more of an issue in gastric lymphoma with higher grade histology as the serious complications are rarely seen with low grade histology. The long-term results of the newer approaches including an antibiotic treatment are unknown and will have to be determined. It seems prudent to recommend close follow up with serial endoscopies for all responders to this new treatment modality. Non-gastric MALTOMAs are generally treated according to general guidelines for indolent lymphoma.

**Mantle Cell Lymphoma** (MCL) is an incurable lymphoma entity with relatively aggressive clinical course. For this reason it stands out from other indolent lymphomas although it is often grouped with this category. MCL usually responds to initial chemotherapy, however the disease-free survival as well as the overall survival are significantly shorter than that of other indolent NHL. The prognosis is uniformly fatal although a small subgroup of cases manifests an indolent course. Prognostic factors are poorly defined and those patients are difficult to recognize. Several centers reported encouraging results with using very aggressive chemotherapy regimens like hyper-CVAD [53]. There is not much data however to support early intensive treatment of MCL. CHOP, i.e. an anthracycline-containing regimen, does not seem to be superior to CVP [49, 50]. In the two recent small studies fludarabine was reported to have some activity but this data still awaits validation [51, 52]. Preliminary data suggests that high dose chemotherapy with ABMT/PSCR does not seem to offer any advantage over a conventional approach, but this also needs further investigation. In summary the currently available treatments options for MCL are quite disappointing.

**Lymphoplasmacytoid Lymphoma/Immunocytoma** is often associated with the presence of a monoclonal protein in the patient's serum. The subtype of lymphoplasmacytoid lymphoma secreting IgM is known as Waldenström's macroglobulinemia. An interesting association between lymphoplasmacytoid lymphoma and hepatitis C has been noted recently [54]. Generally the approach to treatment of lymphoplasmacytoid lymphoma is similar to that of other low-grade lymphomas. Purine analogs appear to be quite promising. The specific management of paraproteinemia is discussed elsewhere in this book.

Intermediate Grade, Aggressive Lymphoma,
Diffuse Large Cell Lymphoma

Diffuse large B-cell lymphoma is the most common B-cell NHL in adults. The management of aggressive NHL generally depends on the stage of the disease and the prognostic category according to the International Index (Table 4). As opposed to indolent lymphoma as many as 50% of patients with large cell lymphoma may be cured with conventional chemotherapy. Anthracyclin-containing multiagent chemotherapy is the mainstay of treatment for aggressive NHL. The randomized trials have revealed no advantage of the second and third generation chemotherapy regimens over CHOP (Table 6) and thus established this relatively simple regimen as the treatment of choice for aggressive NHL [55] (Table 7).

**Table 7.** The most commonly used chemotherapy regimens for aggressive NHL

| Clinical setting | Chemotherapy regimen | Dose | Route and frequency | Comments |
|---|---|---|---|---|
| Primary treatment | **CHOP** | | | All four and many more first-line regimens are still being used. Based on the results of large randomized trial, CHOP appears equally effective and at the same time better tolerated than other listed here regimens. Thus CHOP is especially recommended for treatment of older patients who may have difficulty tolerating more intensive regimens [55] |
| | Cyclophosphamide | 750 mg/m$^2$ | IV, on day 1 | |
| | Doxorubicin | 50 mg/m$^2$ | IV, on day 1 | |
| | Vincristine | 1.4 mg/m$^2$ (max 2 mg) | IV, on day 1 | |
| | Prednisone | 100 mg | PO, on days 1–5 *Repeat cycle every 21 days* | |
| | **m-BACOD** | | | |
| | Methotrexate | 200 mg/m$^2$ | IV, on days 8 and 15 | |
| | Leucovorin calcium | 10 mg/m$^2$ | PO, 8 doses q 6 h, beginning 24 h after each MTX dose, on days 8 and 15 | |
| | Bleomycin | 4 U/m$^2$ | IV, on day 1 | |
| | Doxorubicin | 45 mg/m$^2$ | IV, on day 1 | |
| | Cyclophosphamide | 600 mg/m$^2$ | IV, on day 1 | |
| | Vincristine | 1 mg/m$^2$ | IV, on day 1 | |
| | Dexamethasone | 6 mg/m$^2$ | PO, on days 1–5 *Repeat cycle every 21 days* | |
| | **ProMACE-CytaBOM** | | | |
| | Prednisone | 60 mg/m$^2$ | PO, on days –14 | |
| | Doxorubicin | 25 mg/m$^2$ | IV, on day 1 | |
| | Cyclophosphamide | 650 mg/m$^2$ | IV, on day 1 | |
| | Etoposide | 120 mg/m$^2$ | IV, on day 1 | |
| | Cytarabine | 300 mg/m$^2$ | IV, on day 8 | |
| | Bleomycin | 5 U/m$^2$ | IV, on day 8 | |
| | Vincristine | 1.4 mg/m$^2$ (max 2 mg) | IV, on day 8 | |
| | Methotrexate | 120 mg/m$^2$ | IV, on day 8 | |
| | Leucovorin calcium | 25 mg/m$^2$ | PO, 6 doses q 6 h, on days 9, 10 *Repeat cycle every 28 days* | |
| | **MACOP-B** | | | |
| | Methotrexate | 400 mg/m$^2$ | IV, weeks 2, 6, 10 | |
| | Doxorubicin | 50 mg/m$^2$ | IV, weeks 1, 3, 5, 7, 9, 11 | |
| | Cyclophosphamide | 350 mg/m$^2$ | IV, weeks 1, 3, 5, 7, 9, 11 | |
| | Vincristine | 1.4 mg/m$^2$ (max 2 mg) | IV, weeks 2, 4, 8, 10, 12 | |
| | Bleomycin | 10 U/m$^2$ | IV, weeks 4, 8, 12 | |
| | Prednisone | 75 mg | daily over 12 weeks, taper during last 15 days | |
| | Leucovorin calcium | 25 mg | PO, 6 doses q 6 h, beginning 24 h after each MTX dose, weeks 2, 6, 10 | |

**Table 7.** Continued

| Clinical setting | Chemotherapy regimen | Dose | Route and frequency | Comments |
|---|---|---|---|---|
| Secondary (salvage) treatment | **DHAP** [63] | | | Cisplatin/ cytarabine-based regimens |
| | Dexamethasone | 10 mg | PO, p 6 h, days 1–4 | |
| | Cytarabine | 2 g/m$^2$ | IV, q 12 h x 2 doses, on day 2 | |
| | Cisplatin | 100 mg/m$^2$ | IV, 24 h continuous infusion on day 1 *Repeat cycle every 21–28 days* | |
| | **ESHAP** [64, 65] | | | |
| | Etoposide | 60 mg/m$^2$ | IV, on days 1–4 | |
| | Cisplatin | 25 mg/m$^2$ | IV, 24-h continuous infusion on days 1–4 | |
| | Cytarabine | 2 g/m$^2$ | IV, on day 5, immediately following completion of etoposide and cisplatin therapy | |
| | Methylprednisolone | 500 mg | IV, on days 1–4 *Repeat cycle every 21–28 days* | |
| | **IMVP-16** [76] | | | Regimens utilizing high dose ifosfamide |
| | Ifosfamide | 5 g/m$^2$ | IV, 24-h continuous infusion on day 1 | |
| | Mesna | 800 mg/m$^2$ | IV, bolus prior to Ifosfamide | |
| | | 4 g/m$^2$ | IV, 24-h continuous infusion concurrent with ifosfamide on day 1 | |
| | | 2.4 g/m$^2$ | IV, 12-h continuous infusion after fosfamide on day 2 | |
| | Methotrexate | 30 mg/m$^2$ | IV, on days 3 and 10 | |
| | Etoposide | 100 mg/m$^2$ | IV, on days 1–3 *Repeat cycle every 21–28 days* | |
| | **MINE** [77, 78] | | | |
| | Mesna | 1.33 g/m$^2$ | IV, on days 1–3 concurrent with fosfamide | |
| | | 500 mg | IV 4 and 8 h after each ifosfamide dose | |
| | Ifosfamide | 1.33 g/m$^2$ | IV on days 1–3 | |
| | Mitoxantrone | 8 mg/m$^2$ | IV day 1 | |
| | Etoposide | 65 mg/m$^2$ | IV days 1–3 *Repeat cycle every 28 days* | |

**Table 7.** Continued

| Clinical setting | Chemotherapy regimen | Dose | Route and frequency | Comments |
|---|---|---|---|---|
| | **MINE/ESHAP** [75] (see above for the exact description of MINE and ESHAP) | | Repeat MINE every 21 days for 6 courses, then start ESHAP. If complete response is achieved with MINE, consolidate with 3 courses of ESHAP. If there is only a partial MINE response, then give up to 6 courses of ESHAP (see original study [75] for details) | MINE consolidated by ESHAP |
| | **EPOCH** [79] | | | Regimen utilizing continuous infusion of drugs as a mean to overcome resistance |
| | Etoposide | 50 mg/m$^2$ | IV, 24-h continuous infusion on days 1–4 | |
| | Vincristine | 0.4 mg/m$^2$ | IV, 24-h continuous infusion on days 1–4 | |
| | Doxorubicin | 10 mg/m$^2$ | IV, 24-h continuous infusion on days 1–4 | |
| | Cyclophosphamide | 750 mg/m$^2$ | IV. on day 6 | |
| | Prednisone | 60 mg/m$^2$ | PO, daily on days 1–6 *Repeat cycle every 21 days* | |

Patients with non-bulky stage I or contiguous stage II of disease can be successfully treated with six–eight cycles of combination chemotherapy or brief course of chemotherapy (three-four cycles of CHOP) followed by involved field radiation. Traditionally radiation has been the primary treatment in this setting however the long-term disease free survival appears to be somewhat inferior when compared to any of the two above mentioned alternatives (60%–70% vs 80%–90% at 5 years). The small benefit of combined modality treatment over chemotherapy alone has been suggested by the two large randomized trials. The SWOG trial compared three cycles of CHOP plus radiation therapy with eight cycles of CHOP, demonstrating better overall survival on combined modality arm. Interestingly progression free survival was comparable between the two study arms and the difference in overall survival was attributed to the excess of cardiotoxic deaths on chemotherapy alone arm. It has been suggested that six cycles of CHOP may be equivalent to three cycles plus radiation therapy. The ECOG trial evaluated eight cycles of CHOP vs eight cycles of CHOP plus adjuvant radiation also favoring combined modality treatment arm. Both studies were published in the abstract form only and longer follow up as well as more detailed analysis would be needed before definitive conclusions are drawn. Patients with bulky disease (>10 cm) and extranodal disease should be treated with full course of chemotherapy consisting of six-eight cycles of CHOP followed by irradiation.

Patients with non-contiguous stage II, stage III or IV should receive six-eight cycles of CHOP. A randomized clinical trial revealed no added benefit of irradiation to chemotherapy [58]. The outcome of low or low-intermediate risk patients with advanced aggressive NHL with this type of conventional treatment is relatively good, however patients who belong to poor-intermediate prognostic category i.e. have more than two risk factors at the time of diagnosis have less than 50% chance of being cured. Various investigational approaches are being tested for these patients, mainly the different ways of chemotherapy dose intensification with autologous bone marrow or peripheral stem cell reinfusion (ABMT/PSCR) [59]. This is based on the evidence for the dose-response effect observed with chemotherapy and radiation therapy in aggressive NHL. Promising results were reported by French investigators who randomized patients with aggressive NHL in first complete remission and with at least one adverse prognostic factor to additional treatment with either non-cross resistant conventional dose chemotherapy or high dose therapy with PSCR [60, 61]. A significantly improved disease-free survival and overall survival was demonstrated in a subgroup of patients with high-intermediate/high-risk features. No difference was seen in patients with low and low-intermediate risk. Other randomized trials designed to reproduce this observation are in progress; until their results become available, the issue of high dose chemotherapy with PSCR in aggressive NHL in first complete remission remains unresolved.

The chemosensitivity of the disease at any stage of the treatment is the overall strongest predictor of long-term survival. In addition, the rapidity of response to the primary treatment has been reported to correlate strongly with the final outcome. Interestingly the intensification of the primary chemotherapy followed by ABMT/PSCR for "slow responders" does not improve the overall survival and therefore cannot be recommended in this setting [62].

**Primary Refractory and Relapsed Aggressive NHL.** A small number of patients with primary refractory disease or relapsed disease may be rescued with non-cross resistant standard dose chemotherapy regimen containing different drugs such as: cisplatin, etoposide, cytarabine or ifosfamide. The examples of regimens are presented in Table 6. The remission duration following treatment with such salvage regimen is usually short and translates into relatively few, if any, cures. The recently published long-term follow-up of platinum-based regimens indicated that ESHAP appears superior to DHAP, however less than 6% of patients can be cured with this treatment modality and most of the patients progress or relapse within 6 months [63–65].

Primary refractory disease is defined as no response, only partial response or relapse within 6 months following attainment of complete remission. Although it generally predicts poor prognosis, fine differences between the three subgroups can be appreciated. Patients who have failed to demonstrate any response to primary induction chemotherapy have a rapidly fatal outcome and in general are very unlikely to respond to any rescue treatment. A subset of patients with partial remission or early relapse, may respond to a salvage regimen and/or dose intensification with ABMT/PSCR.

In the setting of primary refractory/relapsed disease, the chemosensitivity of the disease is the strongest predictor of the response to treatment with high dose chemotherapy with ABMT/PSCR. There is no significant difference in outcome between primary refractory disease and relapsed disease as long as the patient demonstrates good response to a salvage regimen. IPI score assessed at the time of starting of the rescue protocol seems to be another good predictor of outcome. The PARMA randomized trial established the role of high dose chemotherapy with transplantation as the gold standard for patients with chemosensitive relapsed aggressive NHL [66]. On this study, patients with relapsed chemosensitive disease were randomized to treatment with conventional salvage regimen (DHAP) or high dose chemotherapy with autologous bone marrow reinfusion, clearly demonstrating the superiority of autologous bone marrow reinfusion arm in disease-free survival and overall survival, 46% and 53% at 5 years respectively. Smaller studies also confirmed the long-term disease-free survival in this setting. Of note, bone marrow reinfusion was not beneficial for patients who relapsed on a conventional salvage chemotherapy arm. There is no evidence that patients with chemotherapy-resistant aggressive NHL benefit from high dose chemotherapy with ABMT/PSCR, which should be offered to those patients only within a clinical trial.

Special sites of extranodal presentation of aggressive NHL may require specific condideration. Orbital and sinus as well as testicular NHL are often associated with a high rate of CNS involvement, therefore all patients should receive CNS prophylaxis in addition to systemic chemotherapy and involved field radiation [80, 81]. In localized testicular lymphoma, irradiation should involve the entire testicular bed to prevent relapse in the opposite site.

## Special Considerations in Treatment of Certain Histologic Subtypes of Aggressive NHL

**Primary Mediastinal Large Cell Lymphoma with Sclerosis** has been recognized recently as a distinct clinicopathologic entity within the larger group of large B-cell lymphomas [67, 68]. The presenting symptoms are most often attributable to a large mediastinal mass invading the surrounding tissue: superior vena cava syndrome, pericardium, lungs, pleura and chest wall. The aggressive nature of this neoplasm requires prompt diagnosis which should be followed by administration of uninterrupted treatment with a full dose anthracycline-based regimen [70, 71]. Several investigators advocate the use of more intensive anthracycline-containing regimens rather than CHOP although their superiority in the treatment of this particular subtype of aggressive NHL has not been demonstrated adequately. The role of radiation therapy in treatment of primary mediastinal lymphoma is still being disputed. The tumor is definitely very radiosensitive and considering the bulkiness of the disease, the irradiation to the chest for all patients with locally advanced disease, limited to the thorax in consolidative fashion seems to be a reasonable recommendation. The lack of recognition of rapidly and relentlessly progressive course of this entity likely accounts for many primary treatment failures and may be responsible for poor treatment outcomes reported by some investigators. Our experience is that this disease should be managed on a semi-emergent basis from the very beginning. Delays in administering the treatment may result in loss of control over this rapidly progressing malignancy, which once spread, portends extremely poor prognosis. Patients who achieve complete remission should be followed closely. The vast majority of relapses occur within the first few months following completion of treatment. Salvage chemotherapy for primary refractory or relapsed disease is generally ineffective [69]. The role of high dose chemotherapy with peripheral stem cell rescue in improving upon the more standard treatment results is unproven and remains investigational.

## High Grade, Highly Aggressive, Lymphoblastic Lymphoma and Small Non-Cleaved Cell Lymphoma

High grade NHLs are rapidly growing tumors, much more common in the pediatric population than in adults. Expeditious diagnosis is essential and should be followed by prompt initiation of treatment. Prolonged staging procedures should be avoided. Due to the propensity of high grade lymphoma to spread to CNS and bone marrow, a lumbar puncture should be a part of the routine work-up in each case. Both Ann Arbor staging system and International Index are largely suboptimal in estimating the prognosis of these patients. CNS, bone marrow involvement or other stage IV involvement is considered a reflection of a high tumor burden and together with high serum LDH are the most significant predictors of poor outcome. Complex multiagent chemotherapeutic regimens are responsible for dramatic improvement in survival and cure rate in this rapidly fatal subtype of NHL. The treatment protocols used for high grade lymphomas are modified from childhood regimens; no uniformly accepted Astandard of care for high grade lymphoma exists. Many protocols adhering to the general guidelines described below appear to have comparable efficacy.

Lymphoblastic lymphoma is morphologically indistiguishable from acute lymphoblastic leukemia (ALL). Most cases are of T-cell phenotype. Intensive chemotherapy derived from ALL-type regimens with intrathecal therapy and 2–3 years long maintenance, employed in treatment of lymphoblastic lymphoma result in high complete response rate of approximately 80% with long-term survival up to 45%. Patients with adverse prognostic factors may be considered for consolidation with high dose chemotherapy with ABMT/PSCR or allogeneic bone marrow transplant.

Small non-cleaved cell lymphoma, Burkitt's and Burkitt's-likeis best treated with a CHOP-like regimen with high dose antimetabolite (methotrexate) and intrathecal prophylaxis. A few regimens based on these guidelines have been developed [72, 73]. A brief duration, high intensity regimen incorporating high doses of cyclophosphamide, devised by Vanderbilt University has been reported to result in approximately 50% long-term survival among patients with this particular histology [74]. High dose chemotherapy with peripheral stem cell rescue as consolidation is sometimes offered but remains an experimental approach.

## References

1. Parker SL, Tong T, Bolden S, et al (1997) Cancer statistics. CA 47:5–21
2. Rabkin C, Devesa SS, Zahm SH, et al (1993) Increasing incidence of non-Hodgkin's lymphoma. Semin Hematol 30:286
3. Devesa SS, Fears T (1992) Non-Hodgkin's lymphoma time trends: United States and international data. Cancer Res 52:5432 s
4. Harris NL, Jaffe ES, Stein H, et al (1994) A Revised European-American Classification of lymphoid neoplasms: a proposal from the International Lymphoma Study Group. Blood 84:1361–1392
5. Fisher RI, Dahlberg S, Nathwani BN, et al (1995) A clinical analysis of two indolent lymphoma entities: mantle cell lymphoma and marginal zone lymphoma (including the mucosa-associated lymphoid tissue and monocytoid B-cell subcategories): a Southwest Oncology Group Study. Blood 85:1075–1082
6. The Non-Hodgkin's Lymphoma Classification project. A clinical evaluation of the International Lymphoma Study Group. (1997) Blood 89:3909–3918
7. Grogan TM, Miller TP, Dahlberg S, et al (1996) REAL classification of lymphoma allows improved delineation of histologic risk groups: A Southwest Oncology Group (SWOG) study [abstract]. ASCO
8. Coiffier B, Brouse N, Peuchmaur M, et al for the GELA (1990) Peripheral T-cell lymphomas have a worse prognosis than B-cell lymphomas: A prospective study of 361 immunophenotyped patients treated with the LNH-84 regimen. Ann Oncol 1:45–50
9. Chan JKC, Banks PM, Clearly ML, et al (1995) A revised European-American classification of lymphoid neoplasms proposed by the International Lymphoma Study Group. A summary version. Am J Clin Pathol 103:543–560
10. O'Connor N: New classification for lymphomas 1995) Lancet 345:1521
11. Non-Hodgkin's lymphoma pathologic classification project (1982) National Cancer Institute sponsored study of classification of non-Hodgkin's lymphomas: Summary and description of a Working Formulation for clinical usage. Cancer 49:2112
12. Rosenberg SA (1977) Validity of the Ann Arbor staging classification for the non-Hodgkin's lymphomas. Cancer Treat Rep 61:1023
13. Denham JW, Denham E, Dear KB, et al (1996) The follicular lymphomas. II. Prognostic factors: What do they mean? Eur J Cancer 32 A:470
14. The International Non-Hodgkin's Lymphoma prognostic Factors Project (1993) A predictive model for aggressive non-Hodgkin's lymphoma. N Engl J Med 329:987
15. Coiffier B, Bastion Y, Berger F, et al (1993) Prognostic factors in follicular lymphomas. Semin Oncol 20 (suppl 5) 89–95

16. Mac Manus MP, Hoppe RT (1996) Is radiotherapy curative for stage I and II low grade follicular lymphoma?: Reslts of long term follow up of patients treated at Stanford University. J Clin Oncol 14:1282

17. Hudson BV, Hudson GV, MacLennan KA, et al (1994) Clinical stage 1 non-Hodgkin's lymphoma: long-term follow-up patients treated by the British National Lymphoma Investigation with radiotherapy alone as initial therapy. British Journal of Cancer 69 (6):1088

18. Denham JW, Denham E, Dear KB, et al (1996) The follicular non-Hodgkin's lymphomas. I. The possibility of cure. European Journal of Cancer 32 A (3):470

19. Monfardini S, Banfi A, Bonadonna G, et al (1980) Improved five year survival after combined radiotherapy-chemotherapy for stage I-II non-Hodgkin's lymphoma. Int J Rad Oncol Biol Phys 6:125

20. Landberg T, Hakansson L, Moller T, et al (1979) CVP remission maintenance in stage I or II non-Hodgkin's lymphomas: preliminary results of randomized study. Cancer 44:831

21. Toonkel L, Fuller L, Gamble J et al (1980) Laparotomy staged I and II non-Hodgkin's lymphomas: preliminary results of radiotherapy and adjunctive chemotherapy. Cancer 45, 249

22. MCLaughlin P, Fuller L, RedmanJ, et al (1991) Stage I-II low-grade lymphomas: a prospective trial of combination chemotherapy and radiotherapy. Ann Oncol (Suppl2)2:137

23. Yahalom J, Varsos G, Fuks Z, et al (1993) Adjuvant cyclophosphamide, doxorubicin, vincristine, and prednisone chemotherapy after radiation therapy in stage I low-grade and intermediate-grade non-Hodgkin's lymphoma. Cancer 71:2342

24. Paryani SB, Hoppe RT, Cox RS, et al (1983) Analysis of non-Hodgkin's lymphomas with nodular and favorable histologies, stages I and II. Cancer 52:2300

25. Young RC, Longo DL, Glatstein E, et al (1988) The treatment of indolent lymphomas: Watchful waiting vs. Aggressive combined modality treatment. Semin Hematol 25 (Suppl):11

26. Brice P, Solal-Celigny P, Lepage E, et al (1995) A randomized study in low tumor burden follicular lymphoma between no treatment, prednimustine and interferon. Am Soc Clin Oncol 14:394

27. Horning S, Rosenberg S (1984) The natural history of initially untreated low-grade non-Hodgkin's lymphomas. N Engl J Med 311:1471

28. Rosenberg S (1985) The low-grade non-Hodgkin's lymphomas: challenges and opportunities. J Clin Oncol 3:299

29. Jacobs JP, Murray KJ, Schultz CJ, et al (1993) Central lymphatic irradiation for stage III nodular malignant lymphoma: long-term results. J Clin Oncol 11 (2):233

30. Mendenhall NP, Million RR (1989) Comprehensive lymphatic irradiation for stage II-III non-Hodgkin's lymphoma. Am J Clin Oncol 12 (3):190

31. Lister T (1991) The management of follicular lymphoma. Ann Oncol 2:131

32. Coiffier B (1995) Towards a cure in indolent lymphoproliferative diseases? Eur J Cancer 31 A:2135

33. Longo D (1993) What's the deal with follicular lymphomas? J Clin Oncol 11:202

34. Dana BW, Dahlberg S, Nathwani BN, et al (1993) Long-term follow-up of patients with low-grade malignant lymphomas treated with doxorubicin-based chemotherapy or chemoimmunotherapy. J Clin Oncol 11:644

35. Johnson PWM, Rohatiner AZ, Whelan JS, et al (1995) Patterns of survival in patients with recurrent follicular lymphoma: A 20 year study from a single center. J Clin Oncol 13:140

36. MCLaughlin P, Hagemeister FB, Romaguera JE, et al (1996) Fludarabine, Mitoxantrone, and dexamethasone: an effective new regimen for indolent lymphoma. J Clin Oncol 14:1262

37. Kaminski MS, Zasadny KR, Francis IR, et al (1993) Radioimmunotherapy of B-cell lymphoma with [131]I anti-B1 (anti-CD20) antibody. N Engl J Med 329:459
38. Press OW, Eary JF, Frederick R, et al (1993) Radiolabeled-antibody therapy of B-cell lymphoma with autologous bone marrow support. N Engl J Med 329:1219
39. Solal-Celigny P, Lepage E, Brousse N, et al (1993) Recombinant Interferon alfa-2b combined with a regimen containing doxorubicin in patients with advanced follicular lymphoma. N Engl J Med 329:1608
40. Hagenbeek A, Carde P, Somers R, et al (1995) Interferon-alfa-2a vs control as a maintenance therapy for low grade non-Hodgkin's lymphoma: results from a prospective randomized clinical trial. Proc Am Soc Clin Oncol 14:386 (Abstract)
41. Tallman M, Hakimian D (1995) Purine nucleoside analogs: Emerging roles in indolent lymphoproliferative disorders. Blood 86:2463–2474
42. French Cooperative Group on CLL, Johnson S, Smith AG, et al (1996) Multicenter prospective randomized trial of fludarabine versus cyclophosphamide, doxorubicin and prednisone (CAP) for treatment of advanced-stage chronic lymphocytic leukemia. Lancet 347:1432
43. Rai KR, Peterson B, Elias L, et al (1996) A randomized caparison of fludarabine and chlorambucil for patients with previously untreated chronic lymphocytic leukemia. A CALGB, SWOG, CTC/NCI-C and ECOG inter-group study. Blood 88 (Suppl 1):141 A. Abstract 552
44. Metter GE, Nathwani BN, Burke JS, et al (1985) Morphological subclassification of follicular lymphoma: Variability of diagnosis among hematopathologists: Collaborative study between the repository center and pathology panel for lymphoma clinical studies. J Clin Oncol 3
45. Bartlett NL, Dorfman RF, Helpern J et al (1994) Follicular large-cell lymphoma: Intermediate or low grade? J Clin Oncol 12:1349
46. Miller TP, LeBlanc M, Grogan TM, et al (1997) Follicular lymphomas: Do histologic subtypes predict outcome? Hematol Oncol Clin North Am 11 (5)
47. Pinotti G, Roggero E, Zucca E, et al (1995) Primary low grade gastric MALT lymphoma. Proc Am Soc Clin Oncol 14:393
48. Bayerdorffer E, Neubauer A, Rudolph B, et al (1995) Regression of primary gastric lymphoma of mucosa -associated lymphoid tissue type after cure of Helicobacter pylori infection. MALT lymphoma study group. Lancet 345:1591
49. Meusers P, Engelhard M, Bartels H, et al (1989) Multicenter randomized therapeutic trial for advanced centrocytic lymphoma: Anthracycline does not improve the prognosis. Hematol Oncol 7:365
50. Teodorovic I, Pittaluga JC, Kluin-Nelemans J, et al (1995) Efficacy of four different regimens in 64 mantle-cell lymphoma cases: Clinicopathologic comparison with 498 other non-Hodgkin's lymphoma subtypes. European Organization for the Research and Treatment of Cancer Group. J Clin Oncol 13:2819
51. Decaudin D, Munck J, Nedellec G, et al (1996) Is fludarabine efficient in mantle cell lymphomas? Blood 88 (Suppl 1):568 A, Abstract 2262
52. Kaufmann T, Coleman M, Pasmantier M (1996) Purine analogue therapy for untreated mantle cell and monocytoid lymhpomas: Immunophenotype does not predict response to fludarabine and cladribine (2-CdA). Proc Am Soc Clin Oncol 15:427, Abstract 474
53. Khouri I, Kantarjian JR, Pugh W, et al (1997) Preliminary report of an active regimen for mantle cell lymphoma (MCL). Blood90 (10) (Suppl. 1) 248a, Abstract 1092
54. Silvestri F, Pipan C, Barillari G, et al (1996) Prevalence of hepatitis C virus infection in patients with lymphoproliferative disorders. Blood 87:4296–4301
55. Fisher RI, Gaynor ER, Dahlberg S, et al. Comparison of a standard regimen (CHOP) with three intensive chemotherapy regimens for advanced non-Hodgkin's lymphoma. N Engl J Med 327 (19) (1992) 1342

56. Miller TP, Dahlberg S, Cassady JR, et al (1996) Three cycles of CHOP (3) plus radiotherapy (RT) is superior to eight cycles of CHOP (8) alone for localized intermediate and high grade non-Hodgkin's lymphoma (NHL): A Southwest Oncology Group. Proc Am Soc Clin Oncol 15:411, Abstract 1257

57. Glick JH, Kim K, Earle J, et al (1996) An ECOG randomized phase III trial of CHOP vs CHOP + radiotherapy (XRT) for intermediate grade early stage non-Hodgkin's lymphoma. Proc Am Soc Clin Oncol 14:391, Abstract 1221

58. O'Connell MJ, Harrington DP, Earle JD, et al (1987) Prospectively randomized clinical trial of three intensive chemotherapy regimens for the treatment of advanced unfavorable histology non-Hodgkin's lymphoma. J Clin Oncol 5 (9):1329

59. Canellos GP (1997) CHOP may have been part of the beginning but certainly not the end: issues in risk-related therapy of large-cell lymphoma. J Clin Oncol 15950:1713

60. Haioun C, Lepage E, Gisselbrecht C, et al (1994) Comparison of autologous bone marrow transplantation over sequential chemotherapy for intermediate-grade and high-grade non- Hodgkin's lymphoma in first complete remission: a study of 464 patients. J Clin Oncol 12 (12):2543

61. Haioun C, Lepage E, Gisselbrecht C, et al (1997) Benefit of autologous bone marrow transplantation over sequential chemotherapy in poor risk aggressive non-Hodgkin's lymphoma: updated results of the prospective study LNH87–2. J Clin Oncol 15 (3):1131

62. Vrdonck LF, Van Putten WL, Hagenbeek A, et al (1995) Comparison of CHOP chemotherapy with autologous bone marrow transplantation for slowly responding patients with aggressive non-Hodgkin's lymphoma. N Engl J Med 332 (16) 1045

63. Velazquez WS, Cabanillas F, Salvador P, et al (1988) Effective salvage therapy for lymphomas with cisplatin in combination with high dose Ara-C and dexamethasone (DHAP). Blood 71:117

64. Velazquez WS, MCLaughlin, Tucker S, et al (1994) ESHAP – an effective chemotherapy regimen in refractory and relapsing lymphoma: A 4-year follow-up study. J Clin Oncol 12:1169

65. Rodriguez-Monge EJ, Cabanillas F (1997) Long-term follow-up of platinum-based lymphoma salvage regimens. Hematol Oncol Clin North Am 11 (5):937

66. Philip T, Gugliemi C, Hagenbeek A, et al (1995) Autologous bone marrow transplantation as compared with salvage chemotherapy in relapses of chemosensitive non-Hodgkin's lymphoma. N Engl J Med 333:1540

67. Rodriguez J, Pugh WC, Romaguera JE, et al (1994) Primary mediastinal large cell lymphoma (review). Hematol Oncol 94:175

68. Aisenberg AC (1993) Primary large-cell lymphoma of the mediastinum. J Clin Oncol 11:2291

69. Kirn D, Mauch P, Shaffer K, et al (1993) Large-cell and immunoblastic lymphoma of the mediastinum: prognostic features and treatment outcome in 57 patients. J Clin Oncol 11:1336

70. Lazzarino M, Orlandi E, Pauli M, et al. Treatment outcome and prognostic factors for primary mediastinal (thymic) B-cell lymphoma: A multicenter study of 106 patients. J Clin Oncol 15:1646

71. Cazals-Hatem D, Lepage E, Brice P, et al (1996) Primary mediastinal large B-cell lymphoma. A clinicopathologic study of 141 cases compared with 916 nonmediastinal large B-cell lymhpomas, a GELA study. Am J Surg Pathol 20:877

72. Soussain C, Patte C, Ostronoff M, et al (1995) Small noncleaved cell lymphoma and leukemia in adults: A retrospective study of 65 adults treated with the LMB pediatric protocols. Blood 85:664

73. Magrath I, Adde M, Shad A, et al (1996) Adults and children with small non-clea-ved-cell lymphoma have a similar excellent outcome when treated with the same chemotherapy regimen. J Clin Oncol 14:925

74. Waits TM, Greco FA, Greer JP, et al (1993) Effective chemotherapy for poor-pro-gnosis non-Hodgkin's lymphoma with 8 weeks of high-dose-intensity combinati-on chemotherapy. J Clin Oncol 11:943

75. Rodriguez MA, Cabanillas FC, Velasquez W, et al (1995) Results of a salvage treat-ment program for relapsing lymphoma: MINE consolidated with ESHAP. J Clin Oncol 13:1734

76. Cabanillas F, Hagemeister FB, Bodey GP, et al (1982) An effective regimen for pati-ents with lymphoma who have relapsed after initial combination chemotherapy. Blood 60:693

77. Cabanillas F, Hagemeister FB, MCLaughlin P et al (1987) Results of MIME salvage regimen for recurrent of refractory lymphoma. J Clin Oncol 5:407

78. Cabanillas F (1991) Experience with salvage regimens at M.D.Anderson Hospital. Ann Oncol (Suppl. 1) 2:31

79. Wilson WH, Bryant G, Bates S, et al (1993) EPOCH chemotherapy: Toxicity and efficacy in relapsed and refractory non-Hodgkin's lymphoma. J Clin Oncol 11:1573

80. Cooper DL, Ginsberg SS (1992) Brief chemotherapy, involved field radiation thera-py, and central nervous system prophylaxis for paranasal sinus lymphoma. Cancer 69:2888

81. Tourouglou N, Dimopoulos MA, Younes A, et al (1995) Testicular lymphoma: Late relapses and poor outcome despite doxorubicin-based therapy. J Clin Oncol 13:1361.

# Multiple Myeloma
# and Other Plasma Cell Dyscrasias

T. M. Zimmerman

Plasma cell dyscrasias are a heterogenous group of disorders characterized by the accumulation of monoclonal cells that resemble mature or immature plasma cells or plasmacytoid B-lymphocytes. Furthermore, these disorders are characterized by the overproduction of a monoclonal immunoglobulin product, the M-protein, with only a small fraction of plasma cell neoplasms being non-secretory. Although several plasma cell dyscrasias exist, multiple myeloma is the most common malignant disorder and as such, will be the focus of this chapter.

## Epidemiology, Risk Factors

### Incidence, Distribution

The average age-adjusted annual incidence for myeloma in whites is 4.3 of 100,000 men and 3.0 of 100,000 women [1]. In blacks, the incidence is higher: 9.6 of 100,000 men and 6.7 of 100,000 women. The incidence of myeloma increases with age with fewer than 2% of the patients younger than 40 years of age at diagnosis [2]. In the United States, the median age of onset is 68 years for men and 70 for women, and mortality patterns closely parallel the incidence with the median age at death of 70 years for men and 71 for women [3]. In 1983 and 1984, the mortality rate for the United States white population with multiple myeloma was 8.7 of 100,000 men and 5.1 of 100,000 women. From the late 1940s to the late 1970s, the incidence and mortality rates for myeloma have risen considerably for both sexes, with net increases of 145% or more [4]. However, the data supporting this trend suggest that this apparent increase may reflect prior underdiagnosis, rather than a true increase in incidence.

Risk Factors, Etiology

Although the cause of multiple myeloma is unknown, both genetic and environmental have been implicated. With regards to genetic factors, the incidence of both multiple myeloma [5] and monoclonal gammopathy [6] is increased in the first-degree relatives of patients with myeloma. In addition, the higher incidence in blacks supports a genetic susceptiblity, albeit this may be consistent with environmental differences. Numerous environmental or occupational factors have been implicated in the etiology of myeloma including agricultural, food processing and chemical products, with a strong association noted with petroleum product exposure [7]. In myeloma as in other hematologic malignancies, there is as an association between exposure to radiation and the development of myeloma. The increased incidence of myeloma among survivors of the atomic bomb in Hiroshima and Nagasaki has been well documented [8], and the finding of excessive rates of myeloma documented in radiologists and nuclear power plant workers implicates the risk of low-level radiation exposure [9, 10]. Chronic antigenic stimulation has also been implicated in several studies as a predisposing state to myeloma [11], supporting a two hit-hypothesis in the genesis of myeloma.

## Pathology, Clinical Features, and Staging

Pathology

**Morphology.** The morphologic appearance of malignant and benign plasma cells is frequently quite similar [12]. The plasma cell contains a highly, differentiated cytoplasm, which is rich in rough endoplasmic reticulum necessary for the production of immunoglobulin. Although the cytoplasm of most cells stains blue with Wright's stain, some plasma cells, called flame cells, stain red-orange; these are typically seen in plasma cell dyscrasias containing an immunoglobulin with a high carbohydrate content such as IgA myeloma [13]. The nucleus of the plasma cell is typically eccentrically placed with clumped or diffuse chromatin with a perinuclear clear zone – the site of the Golgi apparatus, which is involved in the packaging and secretion of immunoglobulin.

**Immunophenotyping.** Several cell surface molecules have been identified on malignant plasma cells including CD19, CD38 and CD56 [14]. In addition, several studies have demonstrated occasional expression of myeloid, megakaryocytic and erythroid surface markers, which are not expressed on normal plasma cells [15]. Controversy persists regarding the expression of the CD34 antigen on malignant plasma cells, an important issue with regard to autologous stem cell transplantation; most studies, however, suggest no expression or only low level expression of CD34 in the malignant clone [16, 17].

**Cytogenetics.** Conventional cytogenetics in multiple myeloma are limited because of the low rate of tumor cell proliferation. Aneuploidy in myeloma, as assessed by cytogenetics or FISH (fluorescent in situ hybridization) studies, is common [18], but specific chromosomal abnormalities remain poorly defined. Recurring trisomies for chromosomes 3, 5, 7, 9, 11, 15, 19, and 21 have been reported and monosomy 13 is the most commonly reported chromosomal loss; the most commonly involved breakpoint band is 14q32 [19]. Similar abnormalities have been described in monoclonal gammopathy of unknown significance [20].

## Clinical Features

**Hematologic.** Anemia is frequently encountered at presentation in patients with multiple myeloma often resulting from direct infiltration of the bone marrow by the malignant plasma cells [21]. Moreover, the anemia may be exaggerated by expansion of the plasma volume secondary to hyperviscosity [22]. In more advanced cases, neutropenia and thrombocytopenia may also result from bone marrow infiltration or as a result of prior stem cell injury from alkylating agents or radiation therapy.

**Skeletal.** Skeletal complications, a common feature of multiple myeloma, manifest as lytic lesions which may result in bone pain, pathologic fractures, and hypercalcemia. Adjacent to the areas of bone reabsorption in the lytic lesions, are osteoclasts, which are separated from the myeloma cells by a thin membrane. Osteoclast activating factor, most likely interleukin (IL)-1 and IL-6, is important in the genesis of these bony lesions

[23]. In addition to pain and risk for fracture, hypercalcemia is a common feature of multiple myeloma at diagnosis and a significant number of patients will develop hypercalcemia as the disease becomes refractory [24].

**Renal Failure.** Renal failure in multiple myeloma is associated with a poor prognosis [25] and the etiology is frequently multi-factorial, often secondary to Bence-Jones proteinuria, hypercalcemia, or both. The presence of lambda light chain is more often associated with renal failure than kappa light chain disease. Dense tubular casts are a characteristic finding in myeloma kidney, and the proteinuria is compromised mostly of monoclonal light chain [26]. Amyloid kidney, on the other hand, is characterized by generalized proteinuria. It is also important to recognize that renal insufficiency in myeloma may be secondary to analgesics such as non-steroidal anti-inflammatory agents or acetaminophen, making microscopic examination of the urine sediment essential.

**M-Protein.** The physical and immunologic effects of the M-protein may also contribute to the clinical picture of myeloma. Although more common in macroglobulinemia, hyperviscosity may result in a variety of symptoms including neurologic findings and spontaneous bleeding [27]. The syndrome, seen in less than 5% of patients with myeloma, is rarely manifested clinically until the viscosity exceeds 4.0 c.p. units. The M-protein also may exhibit immunologic properties, resulting in autoimmune phenomenon such acquired deficiencies of Factor VIII causing bleeding disorders or thrombocytopenia [28]. Cryoglobulins are M-proteins with low thermal amplitudes and are usually of the IgM class. They result in acrocyanosis and Raynaud's phenomenon and are particularly evident after cold exposure [29].

**Immunodeficiencies.** Despite the elevated total globulin fraction, suppression of polyclonal immunoglobulins is a common feature of myeloma [30]. Malignant plasma cells have been demonstrated to suppress normal antigen-stimulated B-cell proliferation after antibody production as a result of plasmacytoma-induced macrophage substance (PIMS) [31]. As a result, patients with multiple myeloma are at an increased risk of bacterial infections [32], which is exacerbated by the frequent use of glucocorticoids.

## Staging

The most common staging system for multiple myeloma, developed by Durie and Salmon, is detailed in Table 1 [33]. This staging system, which correlates with the overall tumor burden as measured by metabolic techniques, offers important prognostic information. Stage III, indicative of high tumor cell mass, is associated with a median survival of >24 months. Stage II, indicative of intermediate tumor cell mass has a median survival of 50 months, and stage I, indicative of low tumor cell mass, has a median survival of 60 months. In addition, renal insufficiency has been documented to independently impact on outcome and has been added as a subclassification [34].

## Prognosis

Although disease stage is the most important prognostic factor for patients with multiple myeloma, several other factors have been identified. If

Table 1. Myeloma staging system

| Stage | Criteria | Measured myeloma cell mass (cells $\times 10^{12}/m^2$) |
| --- | --- | --- |
| I | All of the following:<br>　Hemoglobin >10 g/dl<br>　Normal Serum Calcium<br>　Normal Bone Structure<br>　Low M-Component production<br>　　IgG <5 g/dl<br>　　IgA <3 g/dl<br>　　Urinary light chain <4 g/24 h | <0.6 |
| II | Fitting neither stage I or Stage II | >0.6–1.20 |
| III | One or more of the following:<br>　Hemoglobin <8.5 g/dl<br>　Serum calcium >12 mg/dl<br>　Advanced lytic bone lesions<br>　High M-component production<br>　　IgG >7 g/dl<br>　　IgA >5 g/dl<br>　　Urinary light chain >12 g/24 h | >1.20 |

Subclassifications: A, creatinine <2.0 mg/dl; B, creatinine >2.0 mg/dl.

renal function is normal, the serum beta-2 microglobulin (b2 M) closely reflects tumor burden and correlates with survival [35]. In addition, it may be utilized to assess disease response in patients who have non-secretory myeloma. The plasma cell labeling index (LI) is a measurement of the number of dividing cells in a population of myeloma cells [36]. Most patients have a LI between 1%–5% at presentation and a LI >3% is associated with a poor prognosis, especially if associated with a high-tumor burden. Patients who have an elevated LI respond more rapidly to chemotherapy, but the remissions are often short-lived and relapse tends to occur rapidly. Conversely, disease with a low LI responds slowly to therapy, often with longer remissions and slow regrowth upon relapse. Because LI is not readily available at many institutions, C-reactive protein (CRP) has been demonstrated to correlate with LI and may be measured as a surrogate [37].

## Work-up and Staging

### Diagnostic Criteria

Patients with suspected myeloma should undergo evaluation of the M-protein by serum protein electrophoresis and immunoelectrophoresis. In addition, a 24-h urine should be collected and tested for the presence and quantification of light chain. Quantification of immunoglobulins should be obtained by nephelometry to not only assess the affected immunoglobulin, but also document suppression of the other immuno-globulin classes. A skeletal survey including both long bones and axial skeleton should be obtained. Bone scans are of little to no benefit since rarely are myelomatous lesions osteoblastic in nature. Finally, a bone marrow aspiration and core biopsy and/or biopsy of a suspected plasmacytoma should be performed. To complete the staging evaluation, a complete blood count and differential, and serum chemistries including urea nitrogen, creatinine, electrolytes, calcium and liver function tests are necessary as shown in Table 1. In addition, b2-M, LI, and CRP offer important prognostic information. Additional tests that should be considered in special circumstances include serum viscosity and abdominal fat pad biopsy.

## Therapy

Patients with asymptomatic, stable myeloma (smoldering or indolent myeloma) do not benefit from early treatment. As such, those patients should be followed closely without therapy. Therapy should not be started unless signs of progression or other significant disease manifestations such as bone pain, anemia or renal insufficiency become evident.

### Radiotherapy

Radiation therapy is a rapid and highly effective palliative therapy for the treatment of multiple myeloma, and most patients will eventually require some form of irradiation during the course of their disease [38]. Multiple myeloma is usually quite sensitive to radiation therapy and tumor doses of 20–24 Gy in five to seven fractions are usually sufficient to treat painful bone lesions. The delivery of higher doses is most often not required, and may result in the delay of systemic therapy. This allows for a more rapid return to normal use of the involved bone and prevents further demineralization from disuse. The rapid response also prevents further tumor progression, making this effective for preventing pathologic fracture in large lytic lesions. In patients who present with evidence of spinal cord compression, emergent radiation therapy plays a crucial role in preventing the development or progression of debilitating neurologic symptoms.

### Chemotherapy

Assessing the response to systemic therapy in myeloma depends heavily on quantifying the M-protein. Quantification of the involved immunoglobulin by nephelometry allows for accurate assessment of response to therapy. Serum protein electrophoresis may be beneficial however, once the immunoglobulin level approaches the normal range. In myeloma, marrow involvement is patchy, making this an unreliable method to assess response; repeat marrow aspiration and biopsy, however, are useful in verifying a remission or defining unexplained cytopenias. In light chain disease, serial quantification of the urinary M-protein is often required, and for non-secretors with stable renal function, b2 M may be beneficial to assess response.

**Remission Induction.** Melphalan was first introduced as an effective agent in the treatment of multiple myeloma nearly thirty years ago, and intermittent courses of melphalan and prednisone has been the mainstay of initial therapy for years [39]. The two drugs are given orally for four days; melphalan at 8 mg/m$^2$ and prednisone at 60 mg/m$^2$. Because the absorption of melphalan from the gastrointestinal tract is erratic [40], it is important to monitor the patient for mild neutropenia after oral therapy. If mild neutropenia (ANC 1000–1500/µl) or mild thrombocytopenia (platelet <100,000/µl) is not achieved, the dose should be increased by 20% increments with each subsequent cycle until this occurs. Failure to follow this guideline may result in significant underdosing of the melphalan. In approximately 40% of newly diagnosed myeloma patients receiving melphalan and prednisone, a partial or complete response may be achieved, and the median length of remission is 2 years; the median survival is approximately three years. Less than 10 percent of patients live longer than 10 years and there is no evidence that even a small subset of patients can be cured with standard therapy.

Several combinations of alkylating agents have been tested in untreated multiple myeloma with selected regimens shown in Table 2 [41–43]. In spite of the more intensive nature of many of these treatment regimens, most randomized trials and meta-analyses have found no benefit of these regimens when compared to melphalan and prednisone [44]. One commonly utilized regimen is the combination of vincristine, doxorubicin and dexamethasone (VAD). This regimen has the advantage over melphalan and prednisone in resulting in a more rapid reduction in the tumor cell burden and paraprotein; neither time to progression or overall survival, however is prolonged with this regimen. In spite of this, earlier remissions are beneficial in patients with complications related to high tumor burden such as renal failure. The VAD regimen is also safer in patients with renal failure because none of the drugs are excreted by the kidney.

High-dose dexamethasone is the most active single agent in the treatment of multiple myeloma [45], and because glucocorticoids do not contribute to the potential myelosuppression of radiotherapy, they are useful when concominant therapy is required. In addition, the use of single agent dexamethasone avoids the interactions between radiotherapy and doxorubicin in the VAD regimen.

**Table 2.** Commonly utilized combination chemotherapy regimens for multiple myeloma.

| Drug regimen | VCR | Melphalan | CTX | BCNU | DOX | GC |
|---|---|---|---|---|---|---|
| M2 | 0.03 mg/kg, d1 | .25 mg/kg daily, d 1–7 | 10 mg/kg, d1 | 0.5 mg/kg, d1 | | Pred 1 mg/kg daily, d 1–7 |
| VMCP | 1 mg, d1 | 6 mg/m² daily d 1–4 | 125 mg/m² daily d 1–4 | | | Pred 60 mg/m² daily, d 1–4 |
| VBAP | 1 mg, d1 | | | 30 mg/m², d1 | 30 mg/m², d1 | Pred 100 mg d1–4 |
| VAD | 0.4 mg, d1–4 CI | | | | 9 mg/m², d1–4 CI | Dex 40 mg daily d1–4, 9–12, 17–20 |

VCR, Vincristine; CTX, cyclophosphamide; Pred, prednisone; BCNU, carmustine; DOX, doxorubicin; GC, glucocorticoids; Dex, dexamethasone; CI, continuous infusion.

**Remission Maintenance.** Once a patient has achieved a response to chemotherapy, the goal is to maintain the remission for as long as possible with the fewest possible side effects. In one trial of responders to melphalan and prednisone, patients were randomized to receive either no further therapy, or monthly melphalan and prednisone or carmustine and prednisone [46]. Although patients who did not receive maintenance therapy relapsed sooner, they responded to second-line therapy and there was no difference in overall survival. As such, remission induction therapy should be discontinued once a plateau has been achieved.

Interferon-alpha 2b (IFN-a) has been evaluated extensively as remission maintenance therapy. In a randomized trial of patients who had responded to induction chemotherapy, the remission was prolonged in the treatment arm; unfortunately, there was no improvement in survival [47, 48]. Despite this potential advantage, interferon therapy is costly and has significant side effect including fatigue, fevers, myalgias and mental depression. Many of these effects may be exaggerated in elderly patients. As such, there is no consensus regarding the role of IFN-a for remission maintenance.

**Relapsed/Refractory Myeloma.** Patients who have relapsed after an unmaintained remission may respond once more to the primary regimen. For those who do not respond initially or fail to respond to re-induction therapy, combination regimens such as VAD may induce remissions in 25% of patients. In VAD resistant patients, resistance may be due in part to enhancement of the multi-drug resistant (MDR) gene [49]; randomized, placebo controlled trials are currently underway to assess the potential benefit of MDR modulation in resistant myeloma. In primary refractory and relapsed refractory patients, the use of combinations of alkylating agents has been associated with disappointing results and non-cross resistant regimens, such as EDAP, may be beneficial for a small number of patients with VAD-resistant myeloma [50]. The single agent activity of high-dose glucocorticoids has been well established in relapsed and refractory myeloma [51] and because glucocorticoids are non-myelosuppressive, they are particularly beneficial in patients with poor bone marrow reserves.

**High-Dose Chemotherapy.** A growing body of literature has supported the role of high-dose chemotherapy with autologous stem cell support in the treatment of multiple myeloma. High-dose melphalan has been reported to have activity in patients refractory to standard dose alkylating agents [52] and in minimally pretreated, or untreated patients, several phase II trials have demonstrated high response rates and favorable survival with high-dose chemotherapy [53, 54]. The absence of a tail on the survival curves, however, suggests that this approach is not curative. Recently, a randomized intent-to-treat trial demonstrated superior response rates, progression-free and overall survival for patients receiving high-dose, as opposed to standard dose chemotherapy [55]. Multivariate analysis has identified several favorable prognostic factors, including chemotherapy responsive disease, low tumor burden and less than two years prior therapy. Autologous transplantation is also well tolerated may be safely offered to healthy patients greater than 60 years old.

Several questions remain to be answered regarding the role of high-dose chemoradiotherapy in multiple myeloma, including the role of tandem v single transplants, the optimal timing of transplant in the course of the disease and the role of tumor cell purging, such as CD34 selected autografts. For patients who are being considered for high-dose chemotherapy and autologous stem cell rescue, a regimen such as VAD should be used to spare the stem cells from the toxic effects of alkylating agents.

Allogeneic stem cell transplantation holds several potential advantages over autologous transplantation including the infusion of a tumor free stem cell source and possible graft-versus-myeloma effect [56]. The toxicity of allogeneic transplantation, however, limits this treatment to only a small fraction of patients – those who are younger, in good health and have an HLA-identical sibling. In series with allogeneic transplantation, considerable mortality has been reported despite patient selection. Despite this high mortality, there is a subset of patients who achieve long-term disease free survival. In a multivariate analysis of 162 patients undergoing allogeneic transplantation, female sex, stage I disease at diagnosis, one line of prior therapy, a complete response at the time of transplant were identified as favorable prognostic factors [57]. There was also a trend towards improved survival with IgA myeloma and a low b2 M. In patients who relapse after allogeneic transplantation, remissions may once again be obtained through the infusion of donor lymphocytes [56]. Even in light of potential for cure with allogeneic transplantation, this modality should be considered for only a select group of patients until the supportive care measures are improved.

## Osseus Complications

Bone pain is the most common symptom of multiple myeloma, often resulting in pathologic fractures and debilitating pain. Such patients should be considered for early radiotherapy. In addition to debilitating bone lesions, lytic lesions in long bones in which the diameter of the lesion is one-half of the bone's diameters or involve a significant component of the cortex should undergo radiotherapy to prevent further progression and pathologic fracture. Moreover, skeletal strength is enhanced by ambulation and should be encouraged for all patients with myeloma. Internal fixation may be required for certain patients, but this again must be followed by radiotherapy.

The bisphosphonates, such as pamidronate, inhibit osteoclastic activity and have been tested extensively in myeloma [58]. In a randomized, placebo-controlled trial, there was a decrease in skeletal events, defined as bone pain, pathologic fractures and hypercalcemia in patients receiving monthly pamidronate [59]. For all patients with significant bone involvement, pamidronate 90 mg intravenously should be given monthly and continued up to 21 months [60].

## Miscellaneous

Complications arising from the immunologic or physical effects of the M-protein, such as hyperviscosity or auto-antibody phenomenon, respond well to plasma exchange therapy which results in rapid removal of the paraprotein [61]. Although plasma exchange may relieve the symptoms temporarily, systemic therapy is required to result in satisfactory long-term control. Patients with renal failure often benefit as well from plasmapheresis along with aggressive systemic therapy to reduce the overall tumor burden and potentially reverse the renal insufficiency [62].

## Other Plasma Cell Dyscrasias

### Monoclonal Gammopathy of Unknown Significance

Approximately 1% of patients over 50 have an M-protein, the incidence of which increases with age to >3% in patients over 70 years [63]. In one large longitudinal series of patients with isolated M-proteins, 24% experienced no significant increase in the M-protein, 22% developed multiple myeloma or a related plasma cell dyscrasia and the remaining patients died of unrelated causes. Because of the uncertainty of the clinical course of the M-protein at the time of diagnosis, these isolated M-proteins in the absence of plasma cell neoplasms are termed monoclonal gammopathies of unknown significance or MGUS. The criteria for the diagnosis of MGUS are detailed in Table 3. Because patients with MGUS have no symptoms or physical findings related, the diagnosis of MGUS is made typically as an incidental finding and no therapy is required. If the serum M-protein is less than 2.0 g/dl, the level should be repeated in 6 months and annually thereafter if stable. If the M-protein is greater than 2.0 g/dl, the level should be repeated at 3 and 6 months and annually thereafter if stable.

**Table 3.** Diagnostic criteria for multiple myeloma and monoclonal gammopathy of unknown significance

Multiple myeloma
  Major criteria
    Plasmacytoma on biopsy
    BM plasmacytosis >30% plasma cells
    Monoclonal spike on SPEP
      IgG >3.5 g/dl
      IgA >2.0 g/dl
    Urinary light chain >1.0 g/24 h
  Minor criteria
    BM plasmacytosis 10%–30%
    M-component <above
    Lytic bone lesions
    Hypogammaglobulinemia
The diagnosis of myeloma requires a minimum of one major and one minor criteria, or three minor criteria which must include both a and b

Monoclonal gammopathy of unknown significance
  Monoclonal gammopathy
  M-component level
    IgG <3.5 g/dl
    IgA <2 g/dl
    Urinary light chain <1 g/24 h
  BM plasmacytosis <10%
  No bone lesions
  No symptoms

## Amyloidosis

Amyloidosis is a general term for the deposition of amyloid fibrils in tissues. The modern classification [64] of amyloidosis is based on the nature of the precursor plasma proteins that form the fibril deposits, a betafibrillar structure that stains red with Congo red stain. Systemic amyloidosis occurs in approximately 15% of patients with multiple myeloma and contains light chains in the fibrils (AL Amyloid). The distinction of amyloid secondary to myeloma from primary amyloid is artificial because the amyloid is of a similar genesis. The tissues most subject to amyloid deposition are the tongue, gastrointestinal tract, heart, skin and skeletal muscle. Although amyloid deposition is most often ubiquitous (excluding the central nervous system) in affected patients, the symptoms reflect the organ or organs most prominently involved. Commonly the symptoms include weakness, weight loss, dyspnea, and syncope. Symptoms related to carpal tunnel syndrome and other peripheral neuropathies are also frequently encountered.

The diagnosis of amyloidosis is contingent upon the demonstration of amyloid deposition on biopsy. When a biopsy has not been obtained, an abdominal fat pad biopsy will establish the diagnosis in more than 80% of affected patients [65]. Patients with AL Amyloid have a poor prognosis with a median survival of only 1–2 years [66]; those with cardiac involvement have an even worse prognosis with median survival of only six months. The treatment for systemic amyloidosis should be directed towards the causative plasma protein and supportive therapy of the affected organs [67]. In AL amyloid, the treatment is similar to myeloma with similar effectiveness in reducing the M-protein [68]. As therapy does not reverse the amyloid deposition, it is effective only in preventing progression, and not reversing, organ damage.

## Macroglobulinemia

Waldenstrom's macroglobulinemia is a distinct disorder characterized by the accumulation of malignant plasmacytoid B cells and the production of a high molecular weight M-protein. Patients present with symptoms more similar to non-Hodgkin's lymphoma, commonly exhibiting lymphadenopathy, hepatosplenomegaly and hematologic manifestations such as anemia and some degree of thrombocytopenia. The hyperviscosity syndrome is common (occurring in 15% of patients with macroglobulinemia), but other M-protein complications such as cryoglobulinemia and peripheral neuropathy are less common. The treatment of macroglobulinemia is similar to that of low grade lymphoproliferative disorders with control of the disease often achieved with oral alkylating agents and glucocorticoids [69]. Therapy with nucleoside analogues such as fludarabine and 2-chlorodeoxyadenosine has been demonstrated to be equally effective [70, 71]. Plasmapheresis plays a crucial role for patients who exhibit symptoms of hyperviscosity and can be utilized to maintain chemotherapy refractory patients with a low proliferative rate. In addition, plasmapheresis may be used concomitantly with chemotherapy to decrease the requirements for cytostatic therapy [72].

Solitary Plasmacytoma

Approximately five percent of patients with plasma cell malignancies have only one bone lesion and no evidence of bone marrow plasmacytosis. The age of presentation tends to be younger than myeloma, and there is an increased incidence in males. The diagnosis is based on histologic evidence of a tumor consisting of plasma cell, in the absence of additional lytic lesions on skeletal survey and no evidence of myeloma on bone marrow biopsy and aspirate. Fifty percent of patients will have low concentrations of monoclonal immunoglobulin in serum or urine [73], and magnetic image resonance imaging of the thoracic and lumbar spine shows no intramedullary defects that are characteristic of myeloma [74]. Intensive radiation therapy with at least 45–50 Gy eradicates the tumor in virtually all patients [75]. After radiotherapy, patients should be screened with serum and protein electrophoresis as generalized myeloma will develop in two thirds, usually within three years after the initial diagnosis. In the other one third of patients any myeloma protein that was present disappears, suggesting that the disease has been completely eradicated by radiotherapy.

Solitary plasmacytomas that arise outside of the bone marrow cavity, extramedullary plasmacytomas, most frequently occur in the upper respiratory tract. Treatment again consists of intensive radiotherapy, and the prognosis is overall more favorable than patients with solitary bone plasmacytomas.

## Plasma Cell Leukemia

Patients with plasma cell leukemia have more than 20% plasma cell in the peripheral blood and an absolute plasma cell count greater than 2000/µl. This disorder may be classified as primary or secondary, arising out of a previous diagnosis of multiple myeloma. The treatment, while quite unsatisfactory, is similar to the treatment of multiple myeloma, and higher response rates have been associated with combination regimens [76]. Unfortunately, response duration, as is survival, is typically brief. The prognosis is even worse for those with secondary plasma cell leukemia, as they are most often refractory.

## References

1. Young JL, Percy CL, Asire AJ (1981) Surveillance, epidemiology and end results: Incidence and mortality data. NCI Monograph 57. Bethesda: Department of Health and Human Services, NIH ZS81
2. Hewell GM, Alexanian R (1976) Myeloma in young persons. Ann Intern Med 84:441–414
3. Blattner WA, Blair A, Mason TJ (1981) Multiple myeloma in the United States. 1950–1975. Cancer 48:2547–2556
4. Devesa SS, Sliverman DT, Young JL, et al (1987) Cancer incidence and mortality trends among whites in the United States. J Nat Cancer Inst 79:701–706
5. Maldonado JE, Kyle RA (1974) Familial myeloma. Report of eight families and a study of serum proteins in their relatives. Am J Med 57:875–878
6. Meijers KAE, Leeuw B, Voormolen-Kalova M (1972) The multiple occurrence of myeloma and asymptomatic paraproteinemia within one family. Clin Exp Immunol 12:185–192
7. Cuzick J, DeStavola B (1988) Multiple myeloma. A case-control study. Br J Cancer 57:516–520
8. Cuzik J (1981) Radiation-induced myelomatosis. N Engl J Med 304:204–211
9. Lewis EB (1963) Leukemia, multiple myeloma, and aplastic anemia in American radiologists. Science 142:1492–1503
10. Mancuso TE, Stewart A, Kneale G (1977) Radiation exposures of Hanford workers dying from cancer and other causes. Health Phys 33:369–371
11. Penny R, Hughes S (1970) Repeated stimulation of the reticuloendothelial system and the development of plasma cell dyscrasias. Lancet 1:77–83
12. Robbins SL, Cotran RS, Kumar V (1984) Diseases of white cells, lymph nodes and spleen, In *Pathologic Basis of Disease* WB Saunders: Philadelphia p. 690
13. Maldonado JE, Bayrd ED, Brown AL (1965) The flaming cell in multiple myeloma: A light and electron microscopy study. Am J Clin Path 44:605–610
14. Pilarski LM, Jensen GS (1992) Monoclonal circulating B cells in multiple myeloma. Hem Oncol Clin N Amer 6:297–322
15. Epstein J, Xiao H, Xiao-Yan, H (1990) Markers of multiple hematopoietic-cell lineage in multiple myeloma. N Eng J Med 322:664–668
16. Fruehauf S, Haas R, Zeller WJ, Hunstein W (1994) CD34 selection for purging in multiple myeloma and analysis of CD34+ B cell precursors. Stem Cells 12:95–102

17. Gazitt Y, Reading C, Hoffman R, et al (1995) Purified CD34+/THY-1+/lIN- stem cells do not contain clonal myeloma cells. Blood 86:381–389
18. Huber H (1995) High-incidence of chromosomal aneuploidy as detected by interphase fluorescense in-situ hybridization. Cancer Res 55:3854–3859
19. Sawyer JR, Waldron A, Jagannath S, Barlogie B (1995) Cytogenetic findings in 200 patients with multiple myeloma. Cancer Genet Cytogenet 82:41–47
20. Zandecki M, Obein V, Bernardi F et al (1995) Monoclonal gammapathy of undetermined significance-chromosome changes are a common finding within bone-marrow plasma-cells. Br J Haematol 901:693–696
21. Kyle RA (1975) Multiple myeloma: Review of 869 cases. Mayo Clin Proc 50:29–40
22. MacKenzie MR, Brown E, Fudenberg HH et al (1970) Waldenstrom's macroglobulinemia correlation between expanded plasma volume and increased serum viscosity. Blood 35:934–938
23. Bataille R (1995) The mechanisms of bone lesions in human plasmacytomas. Stem Cells 13:40–47
24. Payne R, Little A, Williams R et al (1973) Interpretation of serum calcium in patients with abnormal serum proteins. Br Med J 4:643–649
25. Alexanian R, Barlogie B, Dixon D (1990) Renal failure in multiple myeloma. Ann Inter Med 150:1693–1695
26. Solomon A, Weiss DT, Kattine AA (1991) Nephrotoxic potential of Bence-Jones proteinuria. N Eng J Med 324:1845–1851
27. Crawford J, Cox EB, Cohen HJ (1985) Evaluation of hyperviscosity in monoclonal gammopathies. Am J Med 79:13–22
28. Bovill EG, Ershler WB, Golden EA et al (1986) A human myeloma-produced monoclonal protein directed against the active subpopulatoin von Willebrand factor. Am J Path 85:115–123
29. Liss M, Fudenberg HH, Kritzman J (1967) A Bence-Jones cryoglobulin: clinical physical and immunologic properties. Clin Exp Immunol 2:467–471
30. Pruzanski W, Gidon MS, Roy RA (1980) Suppression of polyclonal immunoglobulins in multiple myeloma: relationship to the staging and other manifestations at diagnosis. Clin Innumol Immunopath 17:280–283
31. Quesada S, Leo R, Dercher H, Peest D (1995) Functional and biochemical characteristics of a soluble B-lymphocyte proliferation inhibiting activity produced by bone marrow cells from multiple-myeloma patients. Cell Immunol 162:275–281
32. Jacobson DR, Zolla-Pazner S (1986) Immunosuppression and infection in multiple myeloma. Semin Oncol 13:282–290
33. Durie BGM, Salmon SE (1975) A clinical staging system for multiple myeloma. Correlation of measured myeloma cell mass with presenting clinical features, response to treatment and failure.Cancer 36:842–849
34. Durie B, Salmon S, Moon T (1980) Pretreatment tumor mass, cell kinetics and prognosis in multiple myeloma. Blood 55:364–372
35. Norfolk D, Child JA, Cooper EH, et al (1980) Serum beta (2) –microglobulin in myelomatosis: potential value in stratification and monitoring. Br J Cancer 42:510–515
36. Greipp PR, Katzman JA, O'Fallen Wm et al (1988) Value of beta-2-microglobulin level and plasma cell labeling indices as prognostic factors in patients with newly diagnosed myeloma. Blood 72:219–223
37. Bataillie R, Boccadoro M, Klein B et al (1992) C-reactive protein and beta-2-microglobulin produce a simple and powerful myeloma staging system. Blood 80:733–737
38. Bosch A, Frias Z (1988) Radiotherapy in the treatment of multiple myeloma. Int J Radat Oncol Biol Phys 15:1363–1369

39. Alexanian R, Dimopoulos M (1994) The treatment of multiple myeloma. N Eng J Med 330:484–489
40. Albert DS, Chang FY, Chen HSG et al (1979) Oral melphalan kinetics. Clin Pharmacol Ther 6:737–741
41. Case DC, Lee BJ, Clarkson BD (1977) Improved survival times in multiple myeloma treated with melphalan, prednisone, cyclophosphamide, vincristine and BCNU: M2 protocol. Am J Med 63:897–901
42. Salmon SE, Haut A, Bonnet J et al (1983) Alternating combination chemotherapy improves survival in multiple myeloma: A Southwest Oncology Group study. J Clin Oncol 1:453–461
43. Barlogie B, Smith L, Alexanian R (1984) Effective treatment of advanced multiple myeloma refractory to alkylating agents. N Eng J Med 310:1353–1356
44. Gregory WM, Richards MA, Malpas JS (1992) Combination chemotherapy versus melphalan and prednisone in the treatment of multiple myeloma: An overview of published trials. J Clin Oncol 10:334–342
45. Alexanian R, Dimonopoulos MA, Delasalle K, Barlogie B (1992) Primary dexamethasone treatment of mutliple myeloma. Blood 80:887–890
46. Alexanian R, Gehan E, Haut A, Saiki J, Weick J (1978) Unmaintained remissions in multiple myeloma. Blood 51:1005–1011
47. Mandelli F, Avvisati G, Amadori S et al (1990) Maintenance treatment with recombinant interferon alpha-2b in patients with multiple myeloma responding to conventional induction chemotherapy. N Eng J Med 320:1430–1434
48. The Nordic Myeloma Study Group (1996) Interferon-α2b added to melphalan-prednisone for initial and maintenance therapy in multiple myeloma. Ann Int Med 124:212–222
49. Dalton WS, Grogan TM, Meltzer PS et al (1989) Resistance in multiple myeloma and non-Hodgkin's lymphoma: detection of P-glycoprotein and potential circumvention by addition of verapamil to chemotherapy. J Clin Oncol 7:415–424
50. Barlogie B, Alexanian R, Cabanillas F (1989) Etoposide, dexamethasone, cytosine-arabinoside and cisplatin (EDAP) in VAD refractory myeloma. J Clin Oncol 7:1514–1517
51. Alexanian R, Barlogie B, Dixon D (1986) High-dose glucocorticoid treatment of resistant myeloma. Ann Int Med 105:8–11
52. McElwain TJ, Powles RL (1983) High-dose intravenous melphalan for plasma cell leukemia and myeloma. Lancet 1:822–823
53. Bensinger WI, Rowley SD, Demirer T et al (1996) High-dose therapy followed by autologous hematopoietic stem-cell infusion for patients with multiple myeloms. J Clin Oncol 14:1447–1456
54. Barlogie B, Jagannath S, Vesole DH et al (1997) Superiority of tandem autologous transplantation over standard therapy for previously untreated multiple myeloma. Blood 89:789–793
55. Attal M, Harousseau JL, Stoppa AM et al (1996) A prospective, randomized trial of autologous bone marrow transplantation and chemotherapy in multiple myeloma. N Eng J Med 335:91–97
56. Verdonck LF, Lokhurst HM, Dekker AW, Niewenhuis HK, Petersen EJ (1996) Graft-versus-myeloma effect in two cases. Lancet 347:800–801
57. Gahrton G, Tura S, Ljungman P et al (1995) Prognostic factors in allogeneic bone marrow transplantation for mutliple myeloma. J Clin Oncol 13:1312–1322
58. Belch AR, Bergsagel DE, Wilson K et al (1991) Effect of daily etidronate on the oestolysis of myeloma. J Clin Oncol 9:1397–1402
59. Berenson JR, Lichtenstein A, Porter L et al (1996) Efficacy of pamidronate in reducing skeletal events in patients with advanced myeloma. N Engl J Med 334:488–493

60. Berenson JR, Lichtenstein A, Porter L et al (1998) Long-term pamidronate of advanced multiple myeloma patients reduces skeletal events. 16:593–602
61. Avnstorp C, Nielsen H, Drachmann O, et al (1985) Plasmapheresis in hyperviscosity syndrome. Acta Med Scand 217:133–137
62. Pasquali S, Cagnoli L, Rovinetti C et al (1984) Plasma exchange therapy in rapidly progressive renal failure due to multiple myeloma. Int J Artif Organs 8:27–31
63. Kyle RA, Finkelstein S, Elveback LR, Kurtland LT (1972) Incidence of monoclonal proteins in a Minnesota county with a cluster of multiple myeloma. Blood 40:719–724
64. WHO-IUIS Nomenclature Sub Committee (1993) Nomenclature of amyloid and amyloidosis. Bull World Health Org 71:105–112
65. Libbey CA, Skinner M, Cohen AS (1983) Use of abdominal fat tissue aspirate in the diagnosis of systemtic amyloidosis. Arch Int Med 143:1549–1552
66. Kyle RA, Gertz MA (1995) Primary systemic amyloidosis: Clinical and laboratory features in 474 cases. Semin Hematol 32:45–59
67. Skinner N (1996) Amyloidosis. In Lichtentsein LM, Fauci AS eds. Current therapy in allergy, immunology and rheumatology. St.Louis:Mosby-Year Book 235–240
68. Kyle RA, Gertz MA, Greipp PR et al (1997) A trial of three regimens for primary amyloidosis: colchicine alone, melaphalan and prednisone, and melphalan, prednisone and colchicine. Ne Eng J Med 336:1202–1207
69. Kyle RA, Garton JP (1987) The spectrum of IgM monoclonal gammopathies in 430 cases. Mayo Clin Proc 62:719–731
70. Dimopoulos MA, O'Brien S, Kantarjian H et al (1993) Fludarabine therapy in Waldenstorm's macroglobulinemia. Am J Med 95:49–52
71. Dimopoulos MA, Kantarjian SA, Estey EH et al (1993) Treatment of Waldenstrom's macroglobulinemia with 2-chlorodeoxyadenosine. Ann Int Med 118:195–198
72. Busnach G, DalCol A, Brando B et al (1986) Efficacy of combined treatment with plasma exchange and cytostatics in macroglobulinemia. Int J Artif Organs 9:267–270
73. Bataille R, Saney J (1981) Solitary myeloma: Clinical and prognostic features of a review of 114 cases. Cancer 48:845–850
74. Mouloupoulos LA, Dimopoulos MA Weber D et al (1993) Magnetic resonance imaging in the staging of solitary plasmacytoma of the bone. J Clin Oncol 11:1311–1315
75. Dimopoulos MA, Goldstein J, Fuller L, Delasalle K, Alexanian R (1992) Curability of solitary bone plasmacytomas. J Clin Oncol 10:587–590
76. Noel P, Kyle RA (1987) Plasma cell leukemia: an evaluation of response to therapy. Am J Med 83:1062–1068

# Breast Cancer

# Early Breast Cancer

T. Dragovich, O. Olopade

## Introduction

Breast cancer remains a major health problem in the United States and other industrialized nations in spite of recent advances in its early detection and treatment. Significant progress has been made through decades of basic research and clinical trials, but many questions remain unanswered. In this chapter we will summarize current information on the treatment of early breast cancer (i.e., breast cancer in which all clinically apparent disease can be removed surgically). The other, related topics will be covered as much as they are relevant to therapeutic decision making. The treatment of locally advanced and metastatic breast cancer will be addressed in the next chapter.

## Epidemiology

Breast cancer is the second leading cause of cancer mortality among women in the majority of industrialized nations. The age-adjusted incidence of breast cancer varies geographically with rates being higher in Western countries than in Asia or Africa [1]. In 1998, it is estimated that about 178,000 women will be diagnosed with breast cancer in the U.S. accounting for 30% of all new cancers in women [2]. It is also estimated that some 1400 men will develop breast cancer in 1997 in the U.S. However, the overall breast cancer mortality has been declining since 1989. This likely reflects an impact of both, improved screening programs and better therapy. A larger proportion of breast cancers are now diagnosed at an earlier stage.

The incidence of breast cancer increases with age. It is rare before age 25 and peaks at age 75 years. The lifetime risk of breast cancer has changed over the past several decades reflecting increased incidence and increasing longevity in industrialized nations. It is currently estimated that the lifetime risk of breast cancer in U.S. women is about 1 in 8, calculated to age of 85 years.


## Risk Factors and Etiology

A better understanding of the etiology and risk factors for breast cancer is important in order to identify women who might benefit from increased surveillance and preventive therapy. Unfortunately the cause of breast cancer remains unknown in the majority of patients in spite of numerous risk factors identified by epidemiologic studies. A family history of breast cancer is one of the strongest risk factors, particularly when the diagnosis was made in multiple first degree relatives and at young ages [3]. About 5%–10% of breast cancer cases are thought to be due to inheritance of highly penetrant mutations in breast cancer susceptibility genes. These include recently described mutations in *BRCA-1*, *BRCA-2* genes and *TP53* mutations in the Li-Fraumeni syndrome [4]. Considering the high prevalence of breast cancer, screening for cancer susceptibility genes may translate into a decrease in mortality for a significant number of women. Early menarche and late menopause are weak risk factors. However, induced abortions do not appear to have an effect [5]. Recent data suggest that fat intake does not strongly correlate with breast cancer incidence but physical activity may reduce the risk [6–7]. Moderate alcohol consumption [8] and smoking in women with genetic defects in the aromatic amine metabolism appear to confer an increased breast cancer risk [9]. Previous exposure to radiation, especially in survivors of Hodgkin's disease is another significant risk factor. In addition, lobular carcinoma in situ has been categorized as a risk factor for subsequent development of invasive breast cancer.

In summary, there are not many readily preventable environmental or genetic risk factors for breast cancer. However, most of the patients affected with breast cancer will have at least one risk factor in addition to gender and age (Table 1). Considering the high prevalence of breast cancer, it is important to screen for known risk factors so that women at high risk can be offered appropriate surveillance. Every woman with a family history of breast cancer requires a careful risk assessment and calculation of their lifetime risk of breast cancer. Genetic counseling and

**Table 1.** Number of breast cancer risk factors in patients aged 55–84 (from [49])

| No. of risk factors | No. of women | % of cases |
|---|---|---|
| 0 | 25.4 | 17.8 |
| 1 | 36.9 | 33.7 |
| 2 | 24.8 | 28.2 |
| 3 | 9.9 | 15.5 |
| >4 | 3.0 | 4.8 |
| 1 or more | 74.6 | 82.2 |

testing, when appropriate, should be offered and provided [3]. Survivors of Hodgkin's disease, especially those treated with radiation therapy should be routinely screened for breast cancer, starting from age 25.

## Pathology, Staging, and Prognostic Factors

Noninvasive Breast Cancer

*Ductal carcinoma in situ* (DCIS) is a non-invasive growth characterized by the proliferation of cancer cells within the lactiferous ducts. It accounts for about 10% of breast cancers but the numbers are increasing due to increased mammographic detection. It represents a continuum that begins with atypical intraductal hyperplasia, with progression to DCIS and finally to invasive cancer. Untreated DCIS usually develops into invasive cancer after a 5- to 10-year delay.

*Lobular carcinoma in situ* (LCIS) is a non-invasive cancerous lesion contained within the borders of breast lobules. It is difficult to diagnose clinically or by mammography. Incidence ranges from 1% to 3% of all breast biopsy specimens. It is commonly multicentric and is considered as a risk factor for invasive breast cancer and not necessarily a component of invasive disease. It identifies women who are at high risk for subsequent development of invasive cancer which is more often invasive ductal carcinoma.

Invasive Breast Cancer

*Infiltrative ductal carcinoma* is the most common histologic type of breast cancer. It accounts for 75% of all breast cancers.

*Infiltrating lobular carcinoma* is relatively uncommon, accounting for only 5%–10% of cases. It has a similar prognosis to that of ductal carcinoma but tends to metastasize to unusual sites.

*Tubular carcinoma* constitutes only 2% of all breast cancers and carries a better prognosis.

*Medullary carcinoma* is another rare form with better prognosis when compared to ductal cancer.

*Mucinous carcinoma* accounts for 3% of all breast cancers, grows slowly with a bulky appearance and generally has a good prognosis. There appears to be excess of medullary carcinoma in BRCA, carriers. Other rare and special types of breast cancers include *papillary, adenoid cystic, secretory* and *apocrine* carcinomas.

Paget's Disease of the Breast

Paget's disease is clinically characterized by eczematoid lesion of the nipple and areola. It is almost always associated with an underlying cancer infiltrating the epidermis. Prognosis is dependent on the size and dissemination of the original cancer.

Inflammatory Carcinoma

This is a distinct clinicopathological entity which is usually characterized by sudden onset of breast erythema, edema and often tenderness. Histologically it is characterized by cancerous invasion of dermal lymphatics. It has a poor prognosis due to high incidence of metastases at presentation. It is regarded as locally advanced cancer in the absence of distant metastases.

**Staging**

Breast cancer is staged on a clinical and pathological basis. The staging is important because it reflects on the prognosis and the choice of therapy. An international TNM staging system has been widely adopted (UICC and AJCCS Tables 2, 3). It is based on the size and extension of the primary tumor, involvement of lymph nodes and presence of metastases.

**Table 2.** AJCC staging of breast cancer (from [50])

Primary
tumor (T)

| | |
|---|---|
| TX | Primary tumor cannot be assessed |
| T0 | No evidence of primary tumor |
| Tis | Carcinoma in situ: Intraductal carcinoma, lobular carcinoma in situ, or Paget's disease of the nipple with no tumor |
| T1 | Tumor 2 cm or less in greatest dimension |
| pT1mic | Microinvasion 0.1 cm or less in greatest dimension |
| T1a | Tumor more than 0.1 cm but not more than 0.5 cm in greatest dimension |
| T1b | More than 0.5 cm but not more than 1 cm in greatest dimension |
| T1c | More than 1 cm but not more than 2 cm in greatest dimension |
| T2 | Tumor more than 2 cm but not more than 5 cm in greatest dimension |
| T3 | Tumor more than 5 cm in greatest dimension |
| T4 | Tumor of any size with direction extension to (a) chest wall or (b) skin, only as described below |
| T4a | Extension to chest wall |
| T4b | Edema (including peau d?orange) or ulceration of the skin of breast or satellite skin nodules confined to same breast |
| T4c | Both (T4a and T4b) |
| T4d | Inflammatory carcinoma |
| | (Paget's disease associated with a tumor is classified according to the size of the tumor.) |

Regional
lymph
nodes (N)

| | |
|---|---|
| NX | Regional lymph nodes cannot be assessed (e.g., previously removed) |
| N0 | No regional lymph node metastasis |
| N1 | Spread to movable ipsilateral axillary lymph node(s) |
| N2 | Spread to ipsilateral axillary lymph node(s)fixed to one another or to other structures |
| N3 | Spread to epsilateral internal mammary lymph node(s) |

Pathologic
classification
(pN)

| | |
|---|---|
| pNX | Resional lymph nodes cannot be assessed (e.g., previously removed, or not removed for pathologic study) |
| pN0 | No regional lymph node metastasis |
| pN1 | Metastasis to movable ipsilateral axillary lymph node(s) |
| pN1a | Only micrometastasis (none larger than 0.2 cm) |
| pN1b | Metastasis to lymph nodes, any larger than 0.2 cm |
| pN1bi | Metastasis in 1–3 lymph nodes, an more than 0.2 cm and all less than 2 cm in greatest dimension |
| pN1bii | Metastasis to 4 or more lymph nodes, any more than 0.2 cm and all less than 2 cm in greatest dimension |
| pN1biii | Extension of tumor beyond the capsule of a lymph node metastasis less than 2 cm in greatest dimension |
| pN1biv | Metastasis to a lymph node 2 cm or more in greatest dimension |

**Table 2.** Continued

| | |
|---|---|
| pN2 | Metastasis to ipsilateral axillary lymph nodes that are fixed to one another or to other structures |
| pN3 | Metastasis to ipsilateral internal mammary lymph node(s) |
| Distant Metastasis (M) | |
| MX | Distant metastasis cannot be assessed |
| M0 | No distant metastasis |
| M1 | Distant metastasis (includes metastasis to ipsilateral superclavicular lymph node(s)) |

**Table 3.** Stage grouping and 5-year survival rates (from [50])

| | | | | 5-year survival |
|---|---|---|---|---|
| Stage 0 | Tis | N0 | M0 | 0.92 |
| Stage I | T1 | N0 | M0 | 0.87 |
| Stage IIA | T0 | N1 | M0 | 0.78 |
| | T1 | N1 | M0 | |
| | T2 | N0 | M0 | |
| Stage IIB | T2 | N1 | M0 | 0.68 |
| | T3 | N0 | M0 | |
| Stage IIIA | T0 | N2 | M0 | 0.51 |
| | T1 | N2 | M0 | |
| | T2 | N2 | M0 | |
| | T3 | N1 | M0 | |
| | T3 | N2 | M0 | |
| Stage IIIB | T4 | Any N | M0 | 0.42 |
| | Any T | N3 | M0 | |
| Stage IV | Any T | Any N | M1 | 0.13 |

For practical purposes, early breast cancer is often regarded as node-negative or node-positive. Node-positive cancers are further divided into those with 1–3, 4–9 or more than 10 positive lymph nodes.

## Work-up

*Physical examination* should include careful assessment of primary tumor and lymph node status. *Mammmograms* can be used to rule out multicentricity and define the extension of tumor to chest wall or skin. *Excisional biopsy* is diagnostic procedure of choice for all palpable masses and mammographically detected tumors. *Fine needle aspiration*

*(FNA)* is less reliable but can be done to quickly establish a diagnosis. If negative, *FNA* should be followed by excisional biopsy. In many centers a *core needle biopsy* after needle localization is replacing excisional biopsy as diagnostic procedure of choice. Excisional biopsy and final breast conserving surgery should be done as a single step procedure when possible.

*Routine studies* should include chest X-ray, complete blood count and liver profile in all newly diagnosed patients with breast cancer. Bone scans and liver imaging are low yield diagnostic tests unless the patient has bone pain or abnormal liver function tests. ER and PR receptor status, histologic/nuclear grade and S-phase fraction should be determined in all biopsy or surgical specimens. Other prognostic factors such as cathepsin-D, p53 and Her-2/neu are optional and ideally should be done in the context of controlled trial. A thorough family history and genetic counseling is indicated, especially in young patients with strong family history of breast cancer.

## Prognostic Factors

Breast cancer often has a long and unpredictable course. The challenge is to identify the patients that would benefit from adjuvant therapy and tailor the treatment based on the risk/benefit ratio for an individual patient. A number of prognostic factors have emerged over the past two decades. They have limitations and should at best complement clinical judgement.

### Axillary Lymph Node Involvement

The involvement of axillary lymph nodes by breast cancer is the single most influential predictor of cancer recurrence and survival. The most important prognostic information is the number of involved nodes. However, a total number of nodes dissected or percentage of positive nodes does not seem to add prognostically to the absolute number of involved nodes [10].

### Tumor Size

The prognostic importance of tumor size is second only to lymph node involvement. It also impacts on the prognosis of node-positive cancers

[11]. Node-negative tumors smaller than 1 cm in size have excellent 5-year disease free survival of about 95%. These patients may only get a marginal benefit from adjuvant therapy.

Estrogen and Progesterone Receptor Status

About 50%–80% of breast cancers are ER positive, more commonly in elderly, postmenopausal patients, and majority of them show a good response to antiestrogen therapy. A co-existence of a positive assay for progesterone receptors indicates an even better response to antiestrogen therapy. Patients with positive receptor status have better survival following adjuvant therapy but it is unclear if this is due to their better response to hormonal therapy. The pS2 protein is a newly discovered estrogen regulated protein that appears to be expressed by a subset of ER positive tumors with favorable outcome [10, 12].

Histologic and Nuclear Grade

Histologic grade is based on the degree of tubule formation, number of mitoses and nuclear pleomorphism in tissue sections. It is graded from 1–3, with 1 indicating well differentiated tumors (low or good grade). In node-negative patients the prognostic role of histologic and nuclear grade becomes important. As with other descriptive diagnostic tests there is a problem of interobserver variability. Most pathologists now use a grading system developed by Richardson and Bloom [13].

Ploidy and S-Phase Fraction

This is determined by flow cytometry and relates to the DNA content of tumor cells (diploid vs. aneuploid) and number of cells in each phase of the cell cycle including the S-Phase. Low DNA index/diploidy and low S-phase fraction are good prognostic features. The S-phase fraction has more utility than a ploidy status as an independent prognostic factor [10, 12].

## Other Prognostic Factors

*Her-2/neu* (c-erb b-2) is a proto-oncogene overexpressed in about 25% of breast cancers. It encodes for a membrane protein similar to epidermal growth factor receptor (EGFR). High expression of this marker may be a determinant of chemoresponsiveness to Adriamycin in node positive patients [41]. Cathepsin D is an estrogen dependent lysosomal protease that is secreted by some breast cancers and is associated with high risk of recurrence and poor survival [14].

Prognostic factors provide additional guidance for treatment decisions. Based on combination of prognostic factors, it is possible to identify patients with good prognosis and less than a 10% risk of recurrence. Since adjuvant therapy reduces that risk by 30%, the absolute risk reduction of 2%–3% may not justify the risks associated with treatments. On the other hand, patients with tumors >2 cm in size and/or involvement of axillary lymph nodes have risk of recurrence high enough to justify adjuvant therapy.

### Therapy of Early Breast Cancer

Noninvasive Cancer

*Ductal Carcinoma In Situ*

Ductal carcinoma in situ (DCIS) is becoming more common with the widespread use of mammography (15). More than two thirds are less than 1 cm in size. DCIS is frequently multifocal and has a potential to progress into invasive cancer. A traditional treatment for DCIS was mastectomy. A more recent data from NSABP protocol B-06 established the efficacy of lumpectomy followed by radiation in preventing recurrences [16]. Only patients presenting with extensive, multifocal DCIS should now be treated with simple mastectomy. The role of systemic adjuvant therapy for extensive DCIS is unclear and is awaiting data from recently completed NSABP B-24 trial. In NSABP B-24, patients were randomized to tamoxifen vs. placebo after primary treatment that included breast conserving surgery and radiation therapy.

*Lobular Carcinoma In Situ*

Due to relative insensitivity of mammography to detect LCIS, frequent multicentricity and bilateral involvement, the recommended treatment for LCIS until recently involved bilateral mastectomy or mastectomy with a biopsy of the opposite breast. New data indicates that not all of LCIS necessarily transform into invasive cancer. However there is a 30% risk of subsequent development of invasive breast cancer over the period of 15–20 years from the time of LCIS diagnosis. When LCIS transforms into invasive cancer, it is more often as a ductal invasive carcinoma which is detectable by mammography [17]. Therefore, patients with biopsy -proven LCIS could be spared extensive surgery but need intense surveillance as their risk of developing invasive breast cancer is higher than in general population. Recert data from the Tamoxifen NSABP-PI prevention trial suggest that Tamoxifen reduced the risk of breast cancer in patients with LCIS.

Invasive Breast Cancer

*Surgical Treatment*

Surgical approach to breast cancer has evolved significantly over the past 2 decades. Historically a primary treatment mode, surgery is now regarded as a component of multimodality treatment for early breast cancer. Radical and modified radical mastectomy are largely replaced by breast conservation surgery. While mastectomies involved en block resection of breast tissue, lymphatics and contiguous structures, breast conservation surgery only involves the resection of primary tumor with tumor-free margin. It is also referred to as a lumpectomy or segmental mastectomy. The NSABP B-06 trial showed that patients treated by lumpectomy with or without radiation, had disease free and overall survival comparable to those treated by simple mastectomy [18]. The trial included patients with primary tumors less than 4 cm in size regardless of their lymph node status. Women with positive lymph nodes received appropriate adjuvant therapy. Another, earlier study, from Milan, had demonstrated the efficacy of limited surgery in early breast cancer [19]. This study included only node-negative patients and compared quadrantectomy (which is more extensive than lumpectomy) to radical mastectomy. Based on these studies, it is recommended that patients with stages I and II breast cancer (less than 4 cm in size) should have breast conserving surgery because it provides survival equivalent to mastectomy and gives better cosmetic result. There are relatively few contraindications to breast conserving surgery and these include presence of diffuse or multifocal disease, tumors large to relative breast size and coexistence of collagen vascular disease (poor cosmetic results).

Axillary node dissection is still done as a part of breast conservation surgery. The role of axillary node dissection is to assure accurate pathological staging and serve as a guide for adjuvant therapy. It is regarded as an indicator of the presence of systemic micrometastatic dissemination [20].

Until better prognostic indicators are developed, lymph node dissection is indicated for majority of patients. The only subgroup of patients that could be spared dissection are elderly patients with favorable prognostic factors who are not candidates for chemotherapy and will therefore only receive tamoxifen. The role of sentinel node dissection as a substitute of complete axillary node dissection is under investigation and will be discussed below.

*Radiation Therapy*

Radiation therapy is used as an adjunct to surgery with intention to prevent or delay local and regional recurrence in women with early breast cancer. There is a number of studies that have confirmed the efficacy of adjuvant radiation therapy in reducing locoregional recurrence by a factor of 2–3 [21]. However, until recently there was no evidence that adjuvant radiation therapy had an impact on survival. Two recent reports, from Canada and Denmark, found that addition of radiotherapy to mastectomy improves not only local control but also overall survival [22, 23]. The Canadian study found almost 30% reduction of death from breast cancer at 15 years of follow-up in women treated with adjuvant radiation after mastectomy. Both studies included patients with stage III, node-positive cancer who had mastectomy as a primary treatment. It is unclear if survival benefit will also extend to women with smaller tumors or the ones treated with breast conserving surgery. Nevertheless, this data supports the role of adjuvant radiation therapy in some women with early breast cancer.

*Chemotherapy*

Chemotherapy steadily gained a bigger role in the treatment of breast cancer. Initially considered experimental, it is now standard adjuvant therapy for majority of patients and may even become the primary mode of therapy in the future. This evolution reflects the change in our understanding of the biology of breast cancer. Once regarded as a local and "surgical" disease, breast cancer is now widely accepted as a systemic disease even et early stages.

The initial results with single agent adjuvant chemotherapy (thiotepa, cyclophosphamide, L-PAM) were modest but encouraging [24]. A randomized trial from Milan, Italy, was the first one to establish the role of combination chemotherapy (cyclophosphamide, methotrexate, 5-fluorouracil-CMF) [25]. The Early Breast Cancer Trialist's Group data further confirmed the benefit of adjuvant chemotherapy in early breast cancer [26]. They reported data on 75,000 women and found a 26% risk reduction of recurrence and 16% reduction in mortality in patients treated with postoperative adjuvant combination chemotherapy. The benefit in reduced recurrence and improved survival was greater in node-positive than in node-negative women.

Although adjuvant chemotherapy demonstrated effectiveness in early breast cancer, we are still in search for better combination regimens, optimal dosing and scheduling, and sequencing of chemotherapy in respect to surgery and radiation therapy.

Data from the Early Breast Cancer Trialists' Collaborative group demonstrated the superiority of combination regimens to single agent chemotherapy (Table 4). The combination of Cytoxan, methotrexate and 5-fluorouracil (CMF) was shown to be more effective than methotrexate,

**Table 4.** Data from Early Breast Cancer Trialists' Collaborative Group: efficacy of adjuvant therapies (from [51])

|  | % Reduction in annual odds of | |
|  | Recurrence | Death from any cause |
|---|---|---|
| Patients aged <50 years | | |
|   Tamoxifen vs. no tx | 27 | 17 |
|   Chemotx vs. no tx | 37 | 27 |
|   ovarian ablation vs. no tx | 30 | 28 |
| Patients aged >50 years | | |
|   Tamoxifen vs. no tx | 30 | 19 |
|   Chemotx vs. no tx | 22 | 14 |

5-fluorouracil (M-F) alone [27]. While CMF was tested in node- negative patients with early breast cancer, antracycline based combinations sho- wed efficacy in node- positive patients (NSABP-15 and -16). Although doxorubicin remains one of the most active single agents in breast can- cer, the overall efficacy of doxorubicin containing regimens (AC, CAF) is marginally better that CMF [28]. There is however a difference in the toxicity profile and administration sequence for each of the standard regimens now in use (Table 5).

**Table 5.** Standard adjuvant chemotherapy regimens for early breast cancer

| AC | Adriamycin I.V. 60 mg/m$^2$, day 1 Cyclophosphamide I.V. 600 mg/m$^2$, day 1 | Repeat every 21 days for 4 cycles |
|---|---|---|
| CAF | Cyclophosphamide I.V. 500 mg/m$^2$, day 1 Adriamycin I.V. 50 mg/m$^2$, day 1 Fluorouracil I.V. 500 mg/m$^2$, day 1 | Repeat every 21 days for 6 cycles |
| CMF | Cyclophosphamide P.O. 100 mg/m$^2$, days 1–14 Methotrexate I.V. 40 mg/m$^2$, days 1 and 8 Fluorouracil I.V. 600 mg/m$^2$, days 1 and 8, or Cyclophosphamide I.V. 600 mg/m$^2$, days 1 and 8 Methotrexate I.V. 40 mg/m$^2$, days 1 and 8 Fluorouracil I.V. 600 mg/m$^2$, days 1 and 8 | Repeat every 28 days for 6 cycles |
| AC/CMF sequential (>3 nodes involved) | Adriamycin I.V. 60 mg/m$^2$, day 1 + Cyclophosphamide I.V. 600 mg/m$^2$, day 1, plus Cyclophosphamide I.V. 600 mg/m$^2$, days 1 and 8 Methotrexate I.V. 40 mg/m$^2$, days 1 and 8 Fluorouracil I.V. 600 mg/m$^2$, days 1 and 8 | Repeat every 21 days for 4 cycles Repeat every 21 days for 8 cycles) |

*Hormonal Therapy*

In addition to chemotherapy, Early Breast Cancer Trialist's Collaborative Group evaluated the efficacy of hormonal therapy from the large number of randomized trials. This overview demonstrated that tamoxifen reduced the annual odds of recurrence by 25% and of death by 17% (Table 4). It also decreased the risk of contralateral breast cancer by almost 40% [26]. It was more effective in postmenopausal women and women with ER positive tumors. Tamoxifen was discovered in 1962 as a potential contraceptive and fertility drug but was shown to be equal to or better than other endocrine therapies such as aminogluthetimide, androgens or high dose progesterone in breast cancer [29]. Tamoxifen is very well tolerated and has favorable toxicity profile. Most common side effects are hot flashes, nausea and vomiting. A modest increase in the risk of endometrial cancer is counterbalanced by favorable effect on lipid profile and reduction of fatal cardiovascular events [30, 31]. The optimal duration of tamoxifen therapy is unclear but the 5-year course appears to be better than the 2-year at least in regard to risk of recurrence [32]. Whether chemotherapy should be used in conjunction to tamoxifen in postmenopausal women is unclear although recent data suggest small but real benefit of combined chemotherapy followed by tamoxifen [33].

Ovarian ablation, another mode of hormonal therapy, is comparable in efficacy to tamoxifen and chemotherapy in premenopausal women [34]. However, this approach is rarely used in developed countries. New hormonal agents such as new antiestrogens and aromatase inhibitors have been investigated in a setting of advanced and metastatic breast cancer but there is no data on their role in adjuvant therapy.

Adjuvant Therapy for Node-Negative Breast Cancer. Even in the absence of lymph node involvement, between 10% and 30% of patients with early breast cancer will have recurrence within the 10 years following surgery. Adjuvant therapy reduces that risk by about 30%. Therefore it is reasonable to offer adjuvant therapy to women with high-risk, node-negative disease. Both premenopausal and postmenopausal women with ER/PR negative tumors larger than 2.0 cm should be offered adjuvant chemotherapy (CA, CAF or CMF). In our institution we recommend adjuvant therapy to everyone with tumors >1 cm (Fig. 1). Postmenopausal patients with ER/PR positive tumors larger then 1 cm should be offered tamoxi-

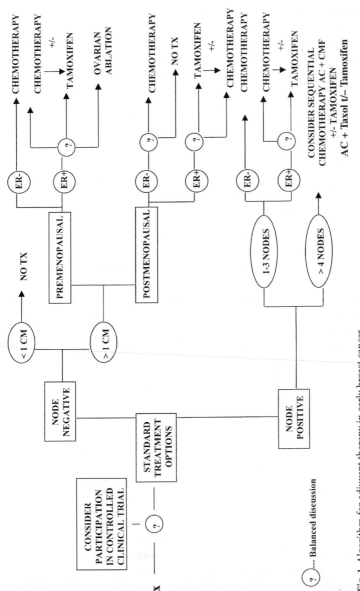

Fig. 1. Algorithm for adjuvant therapy in early breast cancer

fen, and if premenopausal chemotherapy followed by tamoxifen. The justification for adjuvant chemotherapy in node-negative cancers less than 1 cm in size is less clear. The decision should be based on calculated risk of recurrence (additional prognostic factors may be helpful), life expectancy of the patient and individual wishes. Women with node-negative tumors smaller than 1 cm have a favorable prognosis (less than 10% recurrence at 10 years) and may only derive marginal benefit from any adjuvant therapy.

Adjuvant Therapy in Node-Positive Early Breast Cancer. Patients with a node-positive breast cancer have a high risk of recurrence and cancer related death and should be offered a proven benefit of adjuvant therapy. Premenopausal women should be treated with adjuvant chemotherapy followed by optional tamoxifen if ER/PR positive. The side effects of tamoxifen in younger women always need to be balanced with the potential benefits. Postmenopausal and ER/PR positive patients should be offered tamoxifen and optional chemotherapy. Postmenopausal women with ER/PR negative cancers should receive adjuvant chemotherapy. Breast cancer patients with 4 and more lymph nodes involved have >50% risk of recurrence and even with standard adjuvant therapy their risk of recurrence remains high. They should be offered a more intense chemotherapy regimens such as sequential AC plus CMF (4+8 cycles) [35], or referral to specialized centers for participation in clinical trials involving new drug combinations, or high dose chemotherapy with autologous stem cell rescue. New chemotherapeutic agents such as paclitaxel, docetaxel and navelbine demonstrated good activity in metastatic breast cancer and are now being evaluated in high risk patients with early breast cancer [36, 37]. Further advances in the treatment of this group of patients will likely come from ongoing or planned trials evaluating dose intensification of known agents, combinations involving new drugs and role of autologous stem cell rescue in conjunction with high dose chemotherapy.

**Early Breast Cancer in Men**

Carcinoma of the male breast is a rare malignancy. It occurs in middle-aged and elderly men and is associated with hyperestrogenism, hypogonadism and Klinefelter syndrome. Men from families with BRCA-2 mutation have 6% lifetime risk of developing breast cancer. Histology and staging are similar to those in women but it tends to be detected at more advanced stage. Surgery and radiation are the major modes of therapy for early cancer. There is no firm data on the role of adjuvant therapy but the same principles that are applied for women also apply to men with breast cancer.

## Surveillance of Patients with Early Breast Cancer

Surveillance of patients with early breast cancer is implemented with a goal of detecting early recurrences and improving survival with early treatment. Unfortunately data analysis shows that intense surveillance does not affect the survival of patients who are destined to develop recurrent breast cancer. The most recent guidelines by ASCO [39] recommend complete physical and breast exams every 3–6 mo for 3 years, then every 6–12 mo thereafter; monthly breast self-exams; ipsilateral mammogram 6 months after radiotherapy and then annual bilateral mammograms; annual pelvic exam and patient education. Extensive chemistry panels, ultrasound of the liver and bone scans are not recommended in the absence of symptoms.

## Current Key Questions

### Chemoprevention of Breast Cancer

Based on its efficacy in preventing carcinogenesis in preclinical studies and favorable toxicity profile from the clinical experience, tamoxifen was considered as a potentially ideal chemopreventive agent for breast cancer. Recently released NCI data from Breast Cancer Prevention Trial (BCPT) is in support of that. The trial was initiated 6 years ago and it randomized women with high risk for breast cancer to tamoxifen or placebo. Investigators reported a 45% reduction in breast cancer incidence among the women taking tamoxifen. This is the first trial that demonstrated efficacy of tamoxifen for secondary prevention of the breast cancer. Based on the BCPT data tamoxifen becomes an option for women with high risk for breast cancer. It remains to be determined which subsets of patients with increased risk for breast cancer will derive the most benefit from tamoxifen prevention. The BCPT also reported an increased risk of endometrial cancer and thromboembolism in women taking tamoxifen. It is possible that some of the newer antiestrogens investigated, such as raloxifen may have the same chemoprevention efficacy but with less side effects.

## Molecular Markers of Drug Responsiveness

There is still a search for molecular predictors of the tumor sensitivity to various chemotherapeutic agents. New insights into the biology of breast cancer have identified a number of potential markers associated with tumor responsiveness to chemotherapy. Expression of pS2 correlates with sensitivity to hormonal therapy while expression of P-glycoprotein and p53 identifies cancers more resistant to chemotherapeutic agents [40]. More specifically, overexpression of c-erb b-2 may identify the patients who are likely to benefit from higher doses of FAC adjuvant therapy [41]. These investigations are still in experimental phase but may prove to be helpful for therapeutic decision making in the near future.

## Role of Sentinel Node Biopsy

Axillary lymph node dissection and pathologic staging are the most important prognostic factors in breast cancer. This involves a surgical procedure which carries small but significant morbidity, mostly in the form of chronic lymphedema. The question is whether all women with invasive breast cancer require lymph node dissection and how to identify those who do not. Sentinel lymph node mapping and a biopsy relies on identification of the first node (sentinel node) in the lymphatic basin that drains the lymph from the cancerous site [42]. The status of the sentinel node is expected to be an accurate predictor of regional node metastases. If so, this would decrease the need for complete axillary node dissection and decrease overall surgical morbidity in women with breast cancer. Procedure consists of the lymphatic mapping with dye and/or radioisotope and sample biopsy of the labeled node. It is technically feasible but remains to be confirmed as a reliable staging procedure [43].

Neoadjuvant Chemotherapy for Early Breast Cancer

The rationale for the use of pre-operative chemotherapy relates to recent advances in treatment of head and neck cancer and sarcoma where pre-operative chemotherapy reduces the need for extensive surgery without compromising response and survival. The pre-operative chemotherapy would potentially provide additional prognostic stratification of breast cancer patients (i.e. responders vs. non-responders) and increase the number of patients suitable for breast conserving surgery. Two recent studies demonstrated good response rates to pre-operative chemotherapy but it remains to be seen if this will translate into better disease free and overall survival [44, 45].

Sequencing of Radiation Therapy and Chemotherapy

The optimal timing of adjuvant radiation therapy and chemotherapy is another controversial issue. There is no evidence to suggest that delay of radiation therapy to allow for chemotherapy administration decreases survival of breast cancer patients. It does however result in a small increase in local recurrence. On the other hand delay in chemotherapy may have adverse effect on survival [46]. Until a more definitive answer is obtained (NSABP B-28 trial) it is prudent to initiate chemotherapy within 4–6 weeks after surgery and keep the delay in radiation therapy as short as reasonably achievable [47]. For node-negative women, we recommend radiation therapy before chemotherapy while node-positive patients should have chemotherapy before radiation therapy.

**Future Investigational Approaches**

Breast cancer remains a major health problem. Further advancement in therapy for early breast cancer is likely to evolve from better understanding of its etiology and pathogenesis. The role of newly discovered *BRCA1* and *2* genes and their relation to cause and progression of the disease is on the horizon [48]. Agents such as tamoxifen and other hormonal therapies appear promising in breast cancer prevention. New drugs, effective in the treatment of metastatic cancer will likely find their role in adjuvant chemotherapy of early breast cancer. Also, the role for immunotherapy and cancer vaccines using known antigens such as *Her-2/neu* is of great interest.

## References

1. Forbes JF (1997) The incidence of breast cancer: The global burden, public health considerations. Sem Oncol 24:SI20-SI35
2. Landis SH, Murray T, Bolden S, Wingo P (1998) Cancer Statistics. CA Cancer J Clin 48:6–9
3. Olopade OI (1997) Genetics in clinical cancer care: The example of breast cancer. ASCO Education Book 33rd Annual Meeting, 311–316
4. ASCO Public Issues Committee, Subcommittee on Genetic Testing for Cancer Susceptibility (1996) Statement of the American Society of Clinical Oncology: Genetic testing for cancer susceptibility. J Clin Oncol 14:1730–1736
5. Melbye M, Wohlfahrt J, Olsen JH, et al (1997) Induced abortion and the risk of breast cancer. N Engl J Med 336:81–85
6. Hunter DJ, Spiegelman D, Adami HO, et al (1996) Cohort studies of fat intake and the risk of breast cancer-a pooled analysis. N Engl J Med 334:356–361
7. Thun F, et al (1997) Physical activity and the risk of breast cancer. N Engl J Med 36:1276–1282
8. Willett WC, Stampfer MJ, Colditz GA, et al (1987) Moderate alcohol consumption and the risk of breast cancer. N Engl J Med 316:1174–1179
9. Ambrosone CB, Freudenheim JL, Graham S, et al (1996) Cigarette smoking, N-Acetyltransferase 2 genetic polymorphisms, and breast cancer risk. JAMA 276:1494–1501
10. Donegan WL (1997) Tumor-related prognostic factors for breast cancer. CA Cancer J Clin 47:28–51
11. Rosen PP, Groshen S, Saigo PE, et al (1989) Pathological prognostic factors in stage I (T1 N0 M0) and stage II (T1 $N_1$ $M_0$) breast carcinomas: A study of 644 patients with median follow-up of 18 years. J Clin Oncol 7:1239–1251
12. Wong WW, Vijayakumar S, Weichselbaum RR (1992) Prognostic indicators in node-negative early stage breast cancer. Amer J Med 92:539–548
13. Page DL, Ellis IO, Elston CW (1945) Histologic grading of breast cancer: Let's do it (editorial) Am J Clin Pathol 103:123–124
14. Tandon AK, Clark GM, Chamness GC, et al (1990) Cathepsin D and prognosis in breast cancer. N Engl J Med 322:297–302
15. Ernster VL, Barclay J, Kerlikowske, et al (1996) Incidence of and treatment of ductal carcinoma in situ of the breast. JAMA 275:913–918
16. Fisher B, Anderson S (1994) Conservative surgery for the management of invasive and noninvasive carcinoma of the breast: NSABP trials. World J Surg 18:63–69
17. Harris JR, Lippman ME, Veronesi U, et al (1992) Medical progress-breast cancer. N Engl J Med 327:319–479
18. Fisher B, Anderson S, Redmond CK, et al (1995) Reanalysis and results after 12 years of follow-up in a randomized clinical trial comparing total mastectomy with lumpectomy with or without irradiation in the treatment of breast cancer. N Engl J Med 333:1456–1461
19. Veronesi U, Saccozzi R, Del Vecchio M, et al (1981) Comparing radical mastectomy with quadrantectomy, axillary dissection, and radiotherapy in patients with small cancers of the breast. N Engl J Med 305:6–11

20. Moore MP, Kinne DW (1997) Axillary lymphadenectomy: A diagnostic and therapeutic procedure. J Surg Oncol 66:2–6
21. Early Breast Cancer Trialists? Collaborative Group (1995) Effects of radiotherapy and surgery in early breast cancer: An overview of randomized trials. N Engl J Med 333:1444–1455
22. Overgaard M, Hansen PS, Overgaard J, et al (1997) Postoperative radiotherapy in high-risk premenopausal women with breast cancer who receive adjuvant chemotherapy. N Engl J Med 337:949–955
23. Ragaz J, Jackson SM, Le N, et al (1997) Adjuvant radiotherapy and chemotherapy in node-positive premenopausal women with breast cancer. N Engl J Med 337 (14):956–962
24. Fisher B, Fisher ER, Redmond C, et al (1986) Ten-year results from the National Surgical Adjuvant Breast and Bowel Project (NSABP) clinical trial evaluating the use of L-Phenylalanine mustard (L-PAM) in the management of primary breast cancer. J Clin Oncol 4:929–941
25. Bonnadonna G, Rossi A, Valagussa P (1985) Adjuvant CMF chemotherapy in operable breast cancer: Ten years later. World J Surg 9:707–713
26. Early Breast Cancer Trialists? Collaborative Group (1992) systemic treatment of early breast cancer by hormonal, cytotoxic, or immune therapy. Lancet 339:71–85
27. Fisher B, Dignam J, Mamounas E, et al (1996) Sequential methotrexate and fluorouracil for the treatment of node-negative breast cancer patients with estrogen receptor-negative tumors: Eight-year results from the National Surgical Adjuvant Breast and Bowel Project (NSABP) B-13 and first report of findings from NSABP B-19 comparing methotrexate and fluorouracil with conventional cyclophosphamide, methotrexate, and fluorouracil. J Clin Oncol 14:1982–1992
28. Fisher B et al (1990) Two months of doxorubicin-cyclophosphamide with and without interval reinduction therapy compared with 6 months of cyclophosphamide, methotrexate and fluozouracle in positive breast cancer patients with tamoxifen-nonreponsive tumors: Results from (NSABP) B-15. J Clin Oncol 8 (9):1483–1496
29. Goldhirsch A, Gelber RD (1996) Endocrine therapies of breast cancer. Sem Oncol 23:494–505
30. Carcangiu ML (1994) RE: Endometrial cancer in tamoxifen-treated breast cancer patients: Findings from the National Surgical Adjuvant Breast and Bowel Project (NSABP) B-14. J Natl Can Inst 86:1251–1252
31. Thangaraju M, Kumar K, Gandhirajan R, et al (1994) Effect of tamoxifen on plasma lipids and lipoproteins in postmenopausal women in breast cancer. Cancer 73:659–663
32. Swedish Breast Cancer Cooperative Group (1996) Randomized trial of 2 versus 5 years of adjuvant tamoxifen in postmenopausal women with early-stage breast cancer. J Natl Cancer Inst 88:1543–1549
33. International Breast Cancer Study Group (1997) Effectiveness of adjuvant chemotherapy in combination with tamoxifen for node-positive postmenopausal breast cancer patients. J Clin Oncol 15:1385–1394
34. Ovarian ablation in early breast cancer: phoenix arisen? Editorials (1992) Lancet 339:95–96
35. Bonnadonna G, Zambetti M, Valagussa P (1995) Sequential or alternative doxorubicin and CMF regimens in breast cancer with more than three positive nodes. Ten year results. JAMA 273:542–547
36. D'Andrea G, Seidman AD (1997) Docetaxel and paclitaxel in breast cancer therapy: Present status and future prospects. Sem Oncol 24:SI13–27-SI13–44
37. de Valeriola D, Awada A, Roy JA, et al (1997) Breast cancer therapies in development: A review of their pharmacology and clinical potential. Drugs 54:385–413

38. Crichlow RW (1974) Breast cancer in men. Sem Oncol 1:145–152
39. Breast Cancer Surveillance Expert Panel (1997) Recommended breast cancer surveillance guidelines. J Clin Oncol 15:2149–2156
40. Piccart MJ, Hortobagyi GN (1997) Conclusions: Future strategies in the treatment of breast cancer. Sem Oncol 24:S3–34-S3–40
41. Muss HB, Thor AD, Berry DA, et al (1994) c-erbB-2 expression and response to adjuvant therapy in women with node-positive early breast cancer. N Engl J Med 330:1260–1266
42. Albertini JJ, Lyman GH, Cox C, et al (1996) Lymphatic mapping and sentinel node biopsy in the patient with breast cancer. JAMA 276:1818–1822
43. Giuliano AE, Jones RC, Brennan M, et al (1997) Sentinel lymphadenectomy in breast cancer. J Clin Oncol 15:2345–2350
44. Smith IE (1997) Patient benefits from new treatment options and schedules for breast cancer. Sem Oncol 24:S10–22-S10–26
45. Fisher B, Brown A, Mamounas E, et al (1997) Effect of preoperative chemotherapy on local-regional disease in women with operable breast cancer: Findings from National Surgical Adjuvant Breast and Bowel Project B-18. J Clin Oncol 15:2483–2493
46. Recht A, Come SE, Henderson C, et al (1996) The sequencing of chemotherapy and radiation therapy after conservative surgery for early-stage breast cancer. N Engl J Med 334:1356–1361
47. Ellerbroek NA (1996) Sequencing of chemotherapy and radiation therapy in the treatment of early breast cancer: The devil is in the details. Radiology 201:605–607
48. Olopade OI (1996) Genetics in clinical cancer care: The future is now. The N Engl J Med 335:1455–1456
49. Seidman H, Stellman SD, Mushinski MH (1982) A different perspective on breast cancer risk factors: some implications of nonattributable risk. CA Cancer I Clin; 32:301–313
50. American Joint Committee on Cancer (AJCC) Cancer Staging Manual, 5th Edition Lippincott-Raven, 1997
51. Gelber RD, Goldhirsh A, and Coates AS (1992) Meta-analysis: The fashion of summing-up evidence. J Clin Oncol 3:683–693

# Locally Advanced, Locally Recurrent, and Metastatic Breast Cancer

G. Fleming

## Tumor Markers and Recurrent Breast Cancer

Early Detection of Recurrence

Two tumor markers are approved by the Food and Drug Administration for the early detection of recurrent disease in breast cancer patients who have stage II and III disease: CA27.29 and CA15-3. The marketed assays use antibodies which recognize similar but not equivalent epitopes on a mucin-like membrane glycoprotein (the product of the MUC-1 gene) which is shed from tumor cells into the serum. These tests are not suitable for screening, as they are rarely positive in early stage disease. CA15-3 levels, for example, are elevated in only 9% of woman with stage I disease, 19% of women with stage II disease, 38% of women with stage III disease, and 75% of women with stage IV disease. They may be elevated in other malignancies, such as ovarian or pancreatic cancer, as well in as patients with benign conditions, particularly kidney and liver disease. (American Society of Clinical Oncology 1996).

In patients with stage II and III disease the CA27.29 assay has been reported to have a sensitivity of 57.7% and specificity of 97.9% for detection of recurrence with a lead time of 5.3 months between first positive value and clinical diagnosis of relapse. The lead time for detecting locoregional recurrence was 2.3 months (Chan 1997). Routine use of markers to monitor patients following primary treatment of their breast cancer was discouraged in the 1996 and 1997 ASCO guidelines (American Society of Clinical Oncology 1996, 1997), and should be tempered by the following considerations:

– Use of a marker to monitor populations at lower risk of relapse (e.g. stage I patients) will increase the number of false-positive assays.

– The clinician must be prepared to deal with the circumstance in which a marker is rising, but clinical and radiologic exam do not show evidence of disease.
– Metastatic breast cancer is not generally curable, and earlier treatment has not yet been shown to prolong overall or symptom-free survival.

Markers for Monitoring Response to Therapy

Tumor markers are also sometimes used to help monitor response to therapy in patients whose disease is difficult to evaluate, such as those with metastases to bone only. CEA is somewhat less sensitive than CA15-3. An overview of trials suggests that 66% of patients show decreasing CA15-3 levels in the presence of responding disease, 73% show stable levels in the presence of stable disease, and 80% show increasing levels in the presence of increasing disease. It has also been noted that a transient increase (flare) in markers may be observed shortly after initiation of effective treatment. The 1996 ASCO guidelines do not recommend routine use of markers for monitoring disease response. However, they suggest that rising levels may be used to suggest treatment failure in the absence of readily measurable disease (American Society of Clinical Onocology 1996). In general, when using a tumor marker to suggest treatment failure, the marker should have increased by at least 25%, should be persistently rising on at least two measurements, and should not be relied on in the first few weeks following initiation of therapy.

**Locoregionally Recurrent Breast Cancer**

Isolated In-Breast Recurrence after Breast-Conserving Surgery

*Incidence, Presentation and Evaluation*

In most series, about 8% to 20% of patients treated with breast-conserving surgery and radiation experience a local recurrence (Fourquet 1989; Kurtz 1989). Unlike the risk of chest wall recurrence after mastectomy, the risk for in-breast recurrence does not seem to be associated with lymph node status or tumor size. Rates of local recurrence are significantly increased in patients who do not receive post-operative radiation, those with tumor extending to the surgical margins, and those under the age of 35 (Veronesi 1995; Heimann 1996).

At least 30% of in-breast recurrences will be detected by mammographic evaluation alone (Orel 1992). Histologic confirmation of recurrent disease is essential. In one series, 28% of patients with both suspicious radiologic findings and palpable masses had no evidence of recurrence on biopsy (Solin 1990). The most common confounding condition is probably fat necrosis, which may both mimic carcinoma radiologically and create a palpable mass (Boyages 1988).

Five to ten percent of patients who present with an in-breast recurrence will have concurrent distant metastases. Restaging, including evaluation of bones, lung, and liver is appropriate. Another 5%–10% of patients will have locally extensive unresectable disease (Fowble 1991; Recht 1989).

## Prognosis

Prognosis for patients who suffer an isolated in-breast recurrence is worse than for those who do not, and their relative risk of developing distant disease is about 3.4 (Fisher 1991; Haffty 1996). It is debatable to what extent local recurrence might further spread and cause metastatic disease versus merely being a marker for more aggressive malignancy. However, those patients whose recurrence is purely noninvasive or only focally invasive do well. Those whose recurrence is inoperable or inflammatory do poorly (Kurtz 1989; Veronesi 1995; Gage 1998). There are no other commonly accepted prognostic factors for survival in patients with a breast recurrence. Axillary node status at the time of recurrence has not usually been assessed, since dissection was performed as part of primary therapy in most series. Most authors (Fourquet 1989; Kurtz 1989; Haffty 1996) though not all (Fowble 1991; Abner 1993) have reported that early recurrence carries a worse prognosis than late recurrence, and it has been speculated that later recurrences, which occur more frequently at sites distant from the original tumor, often represent new primary cancers.

## Therapy

For operable patients, salvage mastectomy is standard therapy, and yields a long-term disease-free survival of 30%–50% (Kurtz 1989; Abner

1993; Haffty 1996). There are limited data on attempts at a second breast-conserving operation, but this approach may yield inferior locoregional control (Kurtz 1989). The role of systemic adjuvant therapy after an in-breast recurrence is unknown, but it is a reasonable option if the patient has not had previous adjuvant treatment, and if characteristics of the recurrence would warrant treatment if it were a de novo cancer (Recht 1996).

## Isolated Chest Wall Recurrence After Mastectomy

### *Incidence, Presentation, and Evaluation*

Local recurrence after mastectomy usually presents as painless nodules in or under the skin of the chest wall. About 30% of patients will present with simultaneous locoregional and distant failure (Beck 1983), a much higher percentage than in the case of in-breast recurrence after breast-conserving surgery. Evaluation of the patient with chest wall disease should include a search for distant metastases.

The term carcinoma en cuirasse describes a diffuse infiltration of the skin which may encase the entire chest wall and abdomen. Older reports state that it is often poorly controlled by chemotherapy and irradiation, but may nonetheless have an indolent course (Kumar 1989).

The frequency of chest wall recurrences following mastectomy appears to be predicted by the same factors which predict the frequency of distant metastatic disease. The most powerful of these is lymph node status. In one large series of premenopausal women with stage II or III breast cancer, the chance of eventually recurring in the chest wall (with or without distant disease) or regional lymph nodes after mastectomy was 17% in patients with node-negative disease and 42% in patients with > 4 involved axillary nodes (Overgaard 1997). This was reduced by the use of chest wall and nodal irradiation to 3% and 14%, respectively. The use of adjuvant tamoxifen has also been noted to reduce the incidence of local failure by about one-half; adjuvant chemotherapy has a less consistent effect (Nolvadex Adjuvant Trial Organization 1988).

## Prognosis

In most series all or the vast majority of patients with isolated chest wall recurrence eventually die of their disease (Aberizk 1986; Gilliland 1983; Kamby 1997). However, many have several years of disease-free survival. There are no universally accepted prognostic factors for survival after chest wall recurrence and analyses are somewhat complicated since most series include both patients with chest wall recurrences and regional nodal recurrences. Indicators which have been suggested to be favorable include prolonged time between initial surgery and local recurrence (Aberizk 1986), fewer involved axillary nodes at the time of initial surgery (Kamby 1997), and smaller volume of recurrent disease (Fentiman 1985). Conflicting results are reported as to whether patients who recur locally after adjuvant chest wall irradiation have a worse prognosis than those who recur without having been irradiated (Baral 1985; Tennvall-Nittby 1993).

## Treatment

Standard therapy consists of excision, where feasible, and radiation therapy for those patients who have not already received chest wall irradiation. This yields a 5-year survival of 30% to 50% (Fentiman 1985; Aberizk 1986; Halverson 1992). One randomized study including only "good risk" patients (3 or fewer nodules, with a maximal diameter of 3 cm and ER+) noted a 5-year overall survival of 76% and a 5-year disease-free survival of 36% after excision and irradiation (Borner 1994). Disease-free survival was increased to 59% by the use of tamoxifen, but overall survival was unaffected. The use of systemic therapy in patients whose local disease is controlled remains controversial, and neither chemotherapy nor hormonal therapy have been shown to affect survival.

Regional Lymph Node Recurrence

This includes failure in the axillae, infra- and supraclavicular areas, and internal mammary node chains. Most post-mastectomy series lump these together with chest wall recurrences. Survival after supraclavicular node recurrence does appear to be about the same as after chest wall recurrence (Fentiman 1986). Axillary recurrences, however, may have a better prognosis than other nodal recurrences (Recht 1991; Fowble 1989). An axillary node recurrence may also occur after breast-conserving surgery, either in isolation or along with a breast recurrence. The likelihood of an axillary node recurrence appears to be related to the extent of initial node dissection and/or regional node irradiation. In one series of 365 patients with clinically negative axillae undergoing a total mastectomy with no or limited axillary dissection (and no axillary irradiation) 18% developed an isolated axillary failure while those with >5 axillary nodes removed had a <1% axillary recurrence rate (Fisher 1981, 1985). Gross total excision and/or irradiation represent standard therapy for an axillary recurrence.

High Dose Chemotherapy for Locoregional Recurrence

Patients with isolated locoregional failures are often included in autologous marrow transplant series, but their results are not always separately reported. In most series the follow up time is short relative to the natural history of locoregional disease; one noted a 2-year survival of 70% in women with an isolated local recurrence or development of a contralateral breast cancer (Ayash 1995). Transplant is clearly not curative for the majority of patients with locoregional failure; whether it represents any improvement over standard local therapy cannot yet be determined. It is unlikely that any randomized trials of high dose chemotherapy will be undertaken in this small subgroup of patients. However, results from randomized clinical trials of transplant vs. non-transplant chemotherapy in the adjuvant setting will soon be available; if these show a benefit to transplant it may be reasonable to extrapolate to other relatively chemotherapy naive patients with a small tumor burden. One report noted that irradiation after high dose chemotherapy decreased the locoregional failure rate and increased the time to any failure in patients undergoing transplant for locoregionally recurrent breast cancer (Mundt 1994).

**Locally Advanced and Inflammatory Breast Cancer**

Locally advanced breast cancer (LABC) encompasses a broad spectrum of disease, including both indolent tumors that have been neglected and cancers that are rapidly progressive. In economically developed parts of the world, LABC makes up only a small fraction of breast cancer cases, amounting to about 5% of patients seen at major University centers (Seidman 1987). In other parts of the world, however, it accounts for half or more of the cases. This may reflect differences in public awareness and medical resources such as screening mammography; however, there may also be biological differences. In Tunesia, for example, up to 55% of patients seen at one center between 1969 and 1974 were reported to have inflammatory breast cancer (Mourali 1980).

## Definition: LABC

Historically, Haagensen and Stout (1943) listed a group of characteristics which classified a tumor as "inoperable" because of the high rates of both local and distant recurrence when radical surgery alone was used. These included skin ulceration, edema, and fixation of tumor to the chest wall. This group of tumors still forms the base of what all authors would consider LABC. However, different trials in LABC admit varying groups of patients. Some include IIIa disease (large primary tumors) which is clearly operable, and has a better prognosis. Some include stage IVa disease when the only site of metastatic disease is the supraclavicular lymph nodes. Inflammatory breast cancer, which can have a particularly fulminant course, may or may not be included. This heterogeneity makes results of phase II trials in LABC difficult to compare.

## Definition: Inflammatory Breast Cancer

Inflammatory breast cancer (staged T4d) typically presents as a sudden onset of increased breast size, with firmness, tenderness, redness, and warmth of the skin, often without a well-defined tumor. It is frequently initially mistaken for mastitis. Mastitis, however, usually occurs in lactating women. In the current (1998) American Joint Committee on Cancer (AJCC) staging system, both the clinical presentation and the pathologic correlate of tumor embolizaton of dermal lymphatics are required for a tumor to be classified as IBC (American Joint Committee on Cancer 1998). In practice, a clinical inflammatory picture may sometimes be seen without the characteristic histologic findings, and carcinomatous emboli may be found in dermal lymphatics of patients without clinical IBC. The prognosis in any case is poor, although patients with only the histologic finding or only the clinical picture may have slightly less aggressive disease (Lucas 1978, Levine 1985). IBC may be of any histologic type; it is more often ER and PR negative than other types of breast cancer (Jaiyesimi 1992).

Evaluation

Patients who present with LABC should be evaluated for the presence of distant metastases in lung, liver, and bone. A core biopsy of the tumor will confirm the diagnosis and allow sufficient tissue for determination of estrogen and progesterone receptor status. Mammography of the opposite breast is indicated to evaluate any possible synchronous primary cancers prior to induction chemotherapy.

Treatment

Treatment of LABC usually involves a multi-modality algorithm. Induction chemotherapy is followed by some combination of surgery, radiation therapy, more chemotherapy, and in appropriate patients, hormonal therapy. Details tend to be dictated by institutional preference and individualized according to patient response; there are few large randomized trials to guide therapy in this patient population. Close multidisciplinary coordination is important for optimal treatment planning.

A typical algorithm has been reported by investigators at the M.D. Anderson Cancer Center. Three to four cycles of FAC (5-fluorouracil, doxorubicin, cyclophosphamide) -based induction therapy was followed, in responders, by surgery (usually mastectomy), further FAC chemotherapy, and radiation therapy. Patients with inadequate response to induction chemotherapy received radiation, second-line chemotherapy, and then surgery if possible (Hortobagyi 1996). This approach, was reported to yield a 28% disease-free survival at 15 years in patients with inflammatory breast cancer (Ueno 1997). Historical results only using local therapy alone for IBC consistently showed local recurrence rates of 50%, and 5-year survival rates of less than 5% (Hortobagyi 1996).

The benefits of systemic chemotherapy are less dramatic in non-IBC LABC which includes a subset of indolent, hormone-responsive tumors. One study demonstrated a survival benefit to hormonal treatment (Bartelink 1997); several randomized trials in LABC have failed to show any survival benefit to the addition of chemotherapy to local therapy (Schaake-Koning 1985; Rodger 1991; Derman 1989). However, these latter trials can be criticized on the basis that few patients were enrolled, the local therapy was not maximized, and the chemotherapy was suboptimal. For most patients, optimization of all treatment modalities remains the preferred approach.

Prognostic Factors

In most phase II studies using a multimodality approach the median overall survival for LABC ranges from 30–60 months, and is not clearly related to the rate of response to induction chemotherapy. Response rates of 50%–90% can be achieved with a variety of doxorubicin or taxane-based regimens. Generally, initial disease bulk (whether assessed by stage, IIIa versus IIIb, or tumor size) and number of involved lymph nodes after induction chemotherapy are the most powerful prognostic factors in multivariate analysis. Patients with inflammatory disease have a worse outcome. Good response to induction therapy is also generally, though not always, found to be a significant positive predictive factor (Hortobagyi 1996, Valagussa 1990).

Breast-Conserving Therapy

Modern multimodality therapy results in adequate local control for the majority of patients with LABC, although for those with inflammatory breast cancer locoregional recurrence as the only component of first failure is still seen in about 20% of patients undergoing mastectomy and chest wall RT (Ueno 1997). As breast-conserving surgery becomes more widely used in early-stage breast cancer, there has been interest in applying it to LABC as well. Historically patients were treated with irradiation alone, but the doses of radiation needed to control bulk disease do not produce good cosmetic results, and lead to high rates of complications, such as brachial plexopathy.

The need to treat the skin in IBC patients precludes any optimal cosmetic outcome after breast conservation, even in patients with a CR after induction chemotherapy. In other LABC patients the issues are less clear. One difficulty is that clinical assessment of response is not very accurate. It has been suggested that MRI may be superior (Abraham 1996), but this remains an expensive, investigational approach. One typical algorithm is to allow breast-conservation in patients with a negative breast biopsy after induction chemotherapy; this may, however, still result in inferior local control rates. For example, Pierce et al (Pierce 1992) found that 5/31 (16%) of LABC patients with a pathologic CR who were treated with radiation only developed local regional failure versus only 2/53 (4%) of those with a PR to induction chemotherapy who were treated with mastectomy and chest wall RT. Similarly, Merajver et al. (1997) permitted LABC patients with a pathologic complete response (who constituted 28% of their series) to be treated with RT only. Fourteen percent of these had an isolated local failure, compared with 13% of these who had only a PR and received mastectomy and radiotherapy. Only one of their three local failures after breast conservation was salvaged with mastectomy. Both of the trials cited above included inflammatory breast cancer patients, which may have contributed to the poor results.

It can be argued that local recurrence is not the major source of mortality in LABC patients, and that some decrease in local control rates will not affect overall survival. However, uncontrolled locoregional disease is distressing and difficult to treat. For most patients with initially unresectable LABC, mastectomy plus chest wall radiation represents appropriate therapy.

Transplant for LABC

Because even the best results in LABC remain poor, consolidation with high-dose chemotherapy has been used to try to improve outcomes. As in other adjuvant settings, there are no randomized data at the time of this writing comparing high dose to conventional dose chemotherapy. Ayash et al (Ayash 1998) treated 50 women, most of whom had inflammatory breast cancer, with four two week cycles of doxorubicin (90 mg/m2), followed by high dose chemotherapy (cyclophosphamide, thiotepa, carboplatin) with peripheral blood progenitor cell support, followed by mastectomy, radiotherapy, and tamoxifen in ER positive patients.

They reported an estimated 30-month disease free survival of 64%. The North American Marrow Transplant Registry (Antman 1997) noted a 42% estimated 3-year disease-free survival DFS and a 52% estimated 3-year overall survival in patients transplanted for inflammatory breast cancer.

## Metastatic Breast Cancer

### Presentation

In the United States fewer than 10% of women diagnosed with breast cancer have distant metastases at the time of presentation (6% of cases among white women and 9% of cases among African American women between 1986 and 1992; Parker 1997). The time from initial presentation to development of metastatic disease varies widely. Recurrences from small node-negative tumors are more likely to be far out from diagnosis than recurrences from large node-positive tumors (Heimann 1996; Saphner 1996), though the peak hazard remains 1–2 years postsurgery in all subgroups.

The most common clinically evident sites of metastatic disease are bone, lung, liver, and soft tissue (usually chest wall or regional lymph nodes). However, breast cancer can involve many other sites as well, including pleura, brain and/or meninges, and endocrine organs (Valagussa 1978). Lobular cancers are much more likely than infiltrating ductal cancers to spread to the peritoneum and/or involve ovaries, uterus, ureters, bladder and intestines (Lamovec 1991).

### Evaluation

Histologic confirmation of recurrent disease is advisable in most cases. A wide variety of conditions, including new primary tumors, can mimic metastatic breast cancer, and it is best to be certain of the diagnosis before administering toxic therapies and telling the patient she has an incurable disease. Standard evaluation should also include bone scan and either chest X-ray plus abdominal CT scan or chest CT extended to the upper abdomen (including liver and adrenal glands). Further testing should be guided by physical exam and patient symptoms. Measurement of serum tumor markers, such as CEA or CA15-3 may, as discussed above, be useful in patients whose disease is otherwise difficult to evaluate.

## Prognosis

Metastatic breast cancer is essentially incurable, and the median survival after diagnosis of metastases is about 2 years (Vogel 1992). However, pace of the disease varies widely. One review of 1581 patients treated between 1973 and 1982 with standard-dose doxorubicin-containing regimens noted that 263 patients (16.6%) achieved a complete response (CR) and that 49 (3.9%) remained in complete remission for over 5 years; over half of these 49 remained disease-free for over 20 years (Greenberg 1996). Obtaining a CR to induction chemotherapy was the most important factor predicting prolonged survival. Factors which have generally been shown to be predictive of longer survival after diagnosis of metastases include ER positivity, and small disease burden (particularly locoregional disease only). Longer disease-free interval and lack of prior adjuvant therapy have been shown to improve outcome in some, but not all series (Vogel 1992; Greenberg 1996; Rubens 1994).

## Hormonal Therapy

For a very few patients with low tumor burden and chemosensitive disease, long-term disease free survival may be possible. For the vast majority of women therapy is palliative, and a standard approach is to try hormonal therapy, which is relatively nontoxic, prior to using cytotoxic drugs in patients with receptor positive disease. Most clinicians will, however, start treatment with chemotherapy when rapid tumor response is needed (for example, lymphangitic spread of tumor to the lungs).

### Predictive Factors

A variety of characteristics are routinely stated to predict for good response to hormonal therapy, including ER and PR positivity, older age and nonvisceral disease (Buzdar 1998). Older age is likely a surrogate for greater likelihood of receptor positivity, which is the most important fac-

**Table 1.** Proportion of patients with metastatic disease not treated with adjuvant hormones who respond to first-line hormone theraapy (from Wittliff 1984)

| Receptor status | Response rate |
| --- | --- |
| ER+/PR+ | 78% |
| ER+/PR– | 34% |
| ER–/PR+ | 45% |
| ER–/PR– | 10% |

tor (Table 1). Incidence of response increase with increasing ER levels (Wittiff 1994). Immunohistochemical and biochemical quantitations of ER and PR correlate both with each other and with the likelihood of response to hormonal therapy, and either may be used (Allred 1990). HER-2/neu positivity has been suggested to predict for resistance to hormonal therapy (Leitzel 1995). However, at least one analysis suggests that while ER-negative tumors are more likely to have high HER-2/neu levels, those HER-2 positive patients who are ER positive are not less likely to respond to tamoxifen, and should not be denied a trial of hormone therapy (Elledge 1998).

Patients who intially respond to hormones and subsequently progress are likely to have a response to further hormonal treatments. Usually those who do not respond to first-line hormone therapy are given chemotherapy. However, the newer generation aromatase inhibitors may prove an exception to this rule. Letrozole, for example, has been reported to produce a 29% response rate in receptor positive or unknown patients who failed initial hormone therapy (Dombernowsky 1998).

*Nonsteroidal Antiestrogens*

The agents in this class of drugs commercially available in the United States are tamoxifen and toremifene. They are inhibitors of estrogen which bind to the estrogen receptor. Tamoxifen and toremifene appear similar in efficacy and side-effect profile and will likely exhibit substantial cross-resistance (Buzdar 1998). The most common troublesome side effect is hot flashes. Both premenopausal and post-menopausal women will respond to tamoxifen; in premenopausal women it has efficacy equal to oophorectomy (Buchanan 1986).

Occasional patients will experience a tumor response when tamoxifen is discontinued without initiation of further therapy. One report noted 5 objective responses to tamoxifen withdrawal among 28 patients who had previously benefitted from tamoxifen. This has been attributed to the fact that tamoxifen has estrogen agonist properties. In-vitro studies have shown that tamoxifen stimulated the growth of cells from some patients whose tumors originally reponded to tamoxifen, and then relapsed (Canney 1987).

## Aromatase Inhibitors

These drugs block the peripheral conversion of androgens produced by the adrenal gland to estrogens. They are not effective in premenopausal women. Anastrazole and letrozole are commercially available in the United States at the time of this writing. They represent a significant advance over the first generation aromatase inhibitor, aminoglutethimide, which, while active, had significant side effects, including skin rash, orthostatic hypotension and lethargy. Both anastrazole and letrozole have shown superiority in efficacy and side effect profile to progestational therapies, such as megestrol acetate, which had been a common second-line hormone therapy in the United States. Hot flashes and mild anorexia are occasional side effects (Buzdar 1998).

## Luteinizing Hormone-Releasing Agonists

These agents suppress ovarian estradiol production by desensitizing pituitary LHRH receptors. They are effective only for premenopausal women, and represent an alternative to surgical or radiation-induced oophorectomy (Taylor 1998). Goserelin and leuprolide are commercially available in the United States, and are administered by monthly injection. Side effects are generally limited to injection-site reactions and menopausal symptoms, such as hot flashes. One interesting small study compared the combination of a LHRH-agonist (buserelin) to tamoxifen to the combination of both in receptor postive premenopausal women with metastatic disease. The combination produced a superior response rate, progression free survival and overall survival compared with either agent alone. Actuarial survival at 5 years was 42% after combined treatment vs. 10% for single agent treatment (Klijn 1996). If confirmed, this would represent an exception to the usual rule that combined endocrine therapies are not superior to sequential treatments.

## Other Hormonal Therapies

Progestational agents are clearly active, although their mechanism of action is not known. The only one with an approved indication for the treatment of postmenopausal advanced breast cancer in the United States is megestrol acetate. Its activity is similar to that of tamoxifen, but it has a higher incidence of side effects, particularly weight gain and thromboembolism. Androgens are usually relegated to fourth-line therapy because of their side effects, and because they appear to be somewhat less active than other categories of hormones. Estrogens, such as DES, are also active, but are now rarely used because of side effects such as nausea, vomiting, uterine bleeding, and edema (Flamm-Honig 1996).

## Chemotherapy

Breast cancer patients whose tumors are receptor negative or who have become refractory to hormone therapy can often be palliated by chemotherapy. There are a number of drugs and drug combinations which produce clinically important response rates as first-line therapy for metastatic disease (40%–60% in multi-institution trials with CRs in the range of 10% and response durations approximating 8 months). These include CMF (cytoxan + methotrexate + 5-FU), CA + F (cyclophosphamide + doxorubicin + 5 fluorouracil) and the taxanes (docetaxel or paclitaxel). Choice of regimen will frequently be influenced by considerations of toxicity and what (if any) adjuvant chemotherapy was given. One report noted that 0/8 patients who had been treated with adjuvant CMF and relapsed within 12 months responded to further CMF. However, 13/27 (48%) patients who received adjuvant CMF and relapsed more than 12 months after surgery responded to further CMF (Valagussa 1989). In the case of doxorubicin, cardiac toxicity limits the total dose which can be administered, although in responding patients the cardioprotectant dexrazoxane can allow doxorubicin doses beyond the usual total of 450 mg/m2 to be given with reasonable safety (Swain 1997). Doxorubicin and the taxanes are generally considered to be the most active agents in the treatment of breast cancer. Combinations of these have been somewhat hampered to date by cardiac toxicity and myelosuppression, and multiple permutations altering choice of taxane, schedule of taxane, or adding cardioprotectants are being explored (Gianni 1995).

Vinorelbine is a vinca alkaloid which has produced response rates of 16%–46% when used as a single agent for second or third line therapy. 5-FU given with leucovorin or as a continuous infusion has consistently produced response rates in the rage of 20% when used for heavily pretreated patients who have received prior 5-FU, and the oral 5-FU analog, capecitabine, appears to have similar activity. Multiple other agents, including gemcitabine and etoposide have been reported to have some activity in the salvage setting, but their role remains to be confirmed. Cisplatin and carboplatin have activity in chemotherapy-naive breast cancer, but in pretreated patients their activity is low and their toxicities substantial (Flamm Honig 1996). Although single-institution series may report higher rates, overall response rates to second and third line therapies are generally in the range of 10%–20%; patients with a response to a previous chemotherapy are more likely to respond to subsequent treatments (Gregory 1993).

## Duration of Therapy

When maximal tumor response appears to have been attained with a salvage regimen, the question arises as to how long to continue treatment. Several small studies suggest that continuous therapy will prolong time to disease progression (which may improve quality of life) but does not have any impact on survival. Decisions about duration of therapy are therefore often based on how much toxicity patients are experiencing (Muss 1991; Coates 1987).

## Intensity of Therapy

In most cases, the goal of salvage therapy is palliation. There is little correlation between response rate and survival in studies of cytotoxic therapies for breast cancer. Nonetheless, it is generally believed that within the "standard" (non-growth factor requiring) dose range, administering full doses results in better response rates, and better quality of life (Tannock 1988; Mouridsen 1992). Attempts to escalate further with growth factor support, while sometimes improving response rates, have led increased toxicity, no evidence of improved quality of life, and no differences in survival (Brufman 1997; Flamm-Honig 1996).

## High Dose Chemotherapy

Reports of long-term survival after treatment with high dose chemotherapy followed by autologous marrow or stem cell reinfusion have led to widespread use of this treatment for young patients with metastatic breast cancer in the United States. Because it is clear that patients with a CR or good PR after standard-dose induction chemotherapy do better, these are the patients now most often referred for transplant. Typical results of a phase II series are those from the Dana Farber Cancer Institute (Ayash 1995), showing a 5 year progression-free survival of 21%; progression-free survival was 31% in patients with a complete response to induction therapy. The North American Transplant Registry reported a median survival of 19 months in women transplanted for metastatic breast cancer. Three year progression-free survival was 18% overall and 32% for those transplanted in complete remission (Antman 1997).

Randomized studies in this area have been slow to accrue. One small (n=90) trial from South Africa has been published (Bezwoda 1995). Patients in this study were not selected on the basis of response to induction chemotherapy, but were randomized directly to standard chemotherapy or transplant. Standard therapy produced a median survival of 45 weeks compared to 90 weeks for the high dose therapy arm. Survival at 140 weeks was under 20% for the transplant group. This trial has been criticized on a number of grounds, including the poor results in the standard arm and the fact only that responders were treated with maintenance tamoxifen and there were many more responders on high-dose therapy.

## Combinations of Chemotherapy and Hormonal Therapy

In general, strategies combining chemotherapy with hormonal therapy in the setting of metastatic disease, while sometimes improving response rates, have not produced differences in duration of remission or survival when compared with single-modality sequential treatment. One interesting exception might be a small ECOG study in which 70 ER positive premenopausal women who had not received prior adjuvant chemotherapy were randomized to either chemotherapy with cyclophosphamide, doxorubicin, and fluorouracil (CAF) or CAF plus oophorectomy. Median survival for CAF was 26 months; for CAF plus oophorectomy it was 59 months (Falkson 1995). Oophorectomy alone, however, was not tested in that trial.

## New Therapies

A variety of antiangiogenic and immune-modulatory therapies are being tested in breast cancer. Among the most developed agents is anti-HER2 monoclonal antibody. Preliminary results demonstrated a 12% response rate to antibody alone in patients with heavily pretreated breast cancer (Baselga 1996). In addition, a randomized trial of chemotherapy (paclitaxel or doxorubicin) with or without monoclonal antibody showed a significant improvement in response rate and time to progression in antibody treated patients. The combination of antibody with doxorubicin markeadly increased the incidence of cardiotoxicity.

## Bone Disease

Bone is the most common and often the only site of metastatic disease in patients with breast cancer. Patients with bone-only disease may have an indolent course, and the physician must remain alert to treat or prevent common debilitating complications such as hypercalcemia, spinal cord compression, and pathologic fracture of long bones (Sherry 1986). Certain specific considerations apply to treating bony disease.

## Evaluation

Diagnosis is usually made on the basis of bone scan, which is more sensitive, though less specific than bone radiographs (Hortobagyi 1984). Radiographically, bone metastases from breast cancer usually appear lytic, though they may also be osteoblastic or mixed. Lytic lesions will occasionally not be visualized on bone scan, which is a marker of osteoblastic (bone synthetic) activity. However, evaluation of response with bone scan is unsatisfactory. Responding patients will often have no immediate improvement on bone scan, and may even have more intense radiotracer uptake or new areas of uptake in the first 1–6 months of therapy. These "scintigraphic flares" have been reported to occur in 30%–50% of patients experiencing a response to either systemic or hormonal therapy (Vogel 1995; Janicek 1994). Patient symptoms and, tumor markers may aid in response evaluation, although tumor markers may also flare.

## Treatment

Like other sites of metastases, bony disease is frequently palliated by hormonal or chemotherapy. In addition, local or systemic radiation will effectively relieve pain. Strontium-89 and samarium-153 are radioisotopes which can be intravenously administered, and are preferentially taken up at sites of active bone mineral turnover. Strontium is a beta emitter with tissue penetration of 8 mm and a half-life of about 50 days. It has been reported to produce pain improvement in 80% of breast cancer patients, with about 20% becoming pain free. Toxicity is primarily hematologic, and, given the long half-life, treatment with strontium may limit future use of myelosuppressive therapies. Bisphosphonates, which inhibit osteoclast function and can effectively treat hypercalcemia, can also inhibit bone destruction by tumor. A number of trials have reported a decrease in bone pain with bisphosphonate use; in one report 25% of patients with lytic bone disease had sclerosis of their lesions (Theriault 1997, Bloomfield 1998). Two randomized trials of chemotherapy alone versus chemotherapy plus intravenous pamidronate in breast cancer patients with lytic bony disease demonstrated less bony pain and prolonged time to progression in bone in pamidronate-treated patients. Overall survival was not affected (Conte 1996, Hortobagyi 1996).

## References

Aberizk WJ, Silver B, Henderson C, et al (1986) The use of radiotherapy for treatment of isolated locoregional recurrence of breast carcinoma after mastectomy. Cancer 58:1214–1218

Abner AL, Recht A, Eberlein T, et al (1993) Prognosis following salvage mastectomy for recurrence in the breast after conservative surgery and radiation therapy for early-stage breast cancer. J Clin Oncol 11:44–48

Abraham DC, Jones RC, Jones SE, et al (1996) Evaluation of neoadjuvant chemotherapeutic response of locally advanced breast cancer by magnetic resonance imaging. Cancer 78:91–100

Allred DC, Bustamante MA, Daniel CO, et al (1990) Immunocytochemical analysis of estrogen receptors in human breast carcinomas. Arch Surg 125:107–113

American Joint Committee on Cancer Breast (1998) In: Fleming ID, Cooper JS, Henson DE, et al (eds) AJCC Cancer Staging Handbook, Lippincott-Raven, Philadelphia, p 149

American Society of Clinical Oncology (1996) Clinical practice guidelines for the use of tumor markers in breast and colorectal cancer. J Clin Oncol 14:2843–2877

American Society of Clinical Oncology (1998) 1997 Update of recommendations for the use of tumor markers in breast and colorectal cancer. J Clin Oncol 16:793–795

Antman KH, Rowlings PA, Vaughan WP, et al (1997) High-dose chemotherapy with autologous hematopoietic stem-cell support for breast cancer in North America. J Clin Oncol 15:1870–1879

Ayash LJ, Wheeler C, Fairclough D, et al (1995) Prognostic factors for prolonged progression-free survival with high-dose chemotherapy with autologous stem-cell support for advanced breat cancer. J Clin Oncol 13:2043–2049

Ayash LJ, Elias A, Ibrahim J, Schwartz G, et al (1998) High-dose multimodality therapy with autologous stem-cell support for stage IIIB breast carcinoma. J Clin Oncol 16:1000–1007

Baral E, Ogenstad S, Wallgren A (1985) The effect of adjuvant radiotherapy on the time of occurrence and prognosis of local recurrence in primary operable breast cancer. Cancer 56:2779–2782

Bartelink H, Rubens RD, van der Schueren E, et al (1997) Hormonal therapy prolongs survival in irradiated locally advanced breast cancer: a European organization for research and treatment of cancer randomized phase III trial. J Clin Oncol 14:207–215

Baselga J, Tripathy D, Mendelsohn J, et al (1996) Phase II study of weekly intravenous recombinant humanized anti-p185HER2 monoclonal antibody in patients with HER2/neu-overexpressing metastatic breast cancer. J Clin Oncol 14:737–744

Beck TM, Hart NE, Woodard DA, et al (1983) Local or regionally recurrent carcinoma of the breast: results of therapy in 121 patients. J Clin Oncol 1:400–405

Bezwoda WR, Seymour L, Dansey RD (1995) High-dose chemotherapy with hematopoietic rescue as primary treatment for metastatic breast cancer: a randomized trial. J Clin Oncol 13:2483–2489

Bloomfield DJ (1998) Should bisphosphonates be part of the standard therapy of patients with multiple myeloma or bone metastases from other cancers? An evidence-based review. J Clin Oncol 16:1218–1225

Borner M, Bacchi M, Goldhirsch A, et al (1994) First isolated locoregional recurrence following mastectomy for breast cancer: results of a phase III multicenter study comparing systemic treatment with observation after excision and radiation. J Clin Oncol 12:2071–2077

Boyages J, Bilous M, Barraclough B, et al (1988) Fat necrosis of the breast following lumpectomy and radiation therapy for early breast cancer. Radiother Oncol 13:69

Brufman G, Colajori E, Ghilezan N, et al (1997) Doubling epirubicin dose intensity (100 mg/m2 versus 50 mg/m2) in the FEC regimen significantly increases response rates. An international randomised phase III study in metastatic breast cancer. Ann Oncol 8:155–162

Buchanan RB, Blamey RW, Durrant KR, et al (1986) A Randomized comparison of tamoxifen with surgical oophorectomy in premenopausal patients with advanced breast cancer. J Clin Oncol 4:1326–1330

Buzdar AU, Hortobagyi GN (1998) Tamoxifen and toremifene in breast cancer: comparison of safety and efficacy. J Clin Oncol 16:348–353

Buzdar AU, Hortobagyi G (1998) Update on endocrine therapy for breast cancer. Clin Cancer Res 4:527–534

Canney PA, Griffiths T, Latief TN, et al (1987) Clinical significance of tamoxifen withdrawal response. Lancet 1:36

Chan DW, Beveridge RA, Muss H, Fitsche HA, et al (1997) Use of truquant BR radioimmunoassay for early detection of breast cancer recurrence in patients with stage II and stage III disease. J Clin Oncol 15:2322–2328

Coates A, Gebski V, Bishop JF, et al (1987) Improving the quality of life during chemotherapy for advanced breast cancer. N Engl J Med 317:1490–1495

Conte PF, Latreille J, Calabresei MF, et al (1996) Delay in progression of bone metastases in breast cancer patients treated with intravenous pamidronate: results from a multinational randomized controlled trial. J Clin Oncol 14:2552–2559

Derman DP, Browde S, Kessel IL, et al (1989) Adjuvant chemotherapy (CMF) for stage III breast cancer: a randomized trial. Int J Radiat Oncol Biol Phys 17:257–261

Dombernowsky P, Smith I, Falkson G, et al (1998) Letrozole, a new oral aromatase inhibitor for advanced breast cancer: double-blind randomized trial showing a dose effect and improved efficacy and tolerability compared with megestrol acetate. J Clin Oncol 16:453–461

Elledge RM, Green S, Ciocca D, et al (1998) HER-2 expression and response to tamoxifen in estrogen receptor-positive breast cancer: a Southwest Oncology Group Study. Clin Cancer Res 4:7–12

Falkson G, Holcroft C, Gelman RS, et al (1995) Ten-year follow-up study of premenopausal women with metastatic breast cancer: an Eastern cooperative oncology group study 13:1453–1458

Fentiman IS, Lavelle MA, Caplan D, et al (1986) The significance of supraclavicular fossa node recurrence after radical mastectomy. Cancer 57:908

Fentiman IS, Matthews PN, Davison OW, et al (1985) Survival following local skin recurrence after mastectomy. Br J Surg 72:14–16

Fisher B, Anderson S, Fisher ER, et al (1991) Significance of ipsilateral breast tumor recurrence after lumpectomy. Lancet 338:327–331

Fisher B, Redmond C, Fisher ER, et al (1985) Ten-year results of a randomized clinical trial comparing radical mastectomy and total mastectomy with or without radiation. N Engl J Med 312:674–681

Fisher B, Wolmark N, Bauer M, et al (1981) The accuracy of clinical nodal staging and of limited axillary dissection as a determinant of histologic nodal status in carcinoma of the breast. Surg Gyn Obstet 152:765–772

Flamm Honig S (1996) Treatment of metastatic disease. Ch 22 In: Harris JR, Lippman ME, Morrow M, et al (eds) Diseases of the breast. Lippincott-Raven, Philadelphia, p 669

Fourquet A, Campana F, Zafrani B, et al (1989) Prognostic factors of breast recurrence in the conservative management of early breast cancer: a 25-year follow-up. Int J Radiat Oncol Biol Phys 17:719–725

Fowble B, Solin L, Schultz D, et al (1989) Frequency, sites of relapse, and outcome of regional node failures following conservation surgery and radiation for early breast cancer. Int J Radiat Oncol Biol Phys 17:703

Fowble B, Solin L, Schultz D, et al (1991) Breast recurrence following conservative surgery and radiation: patterns of failure, prognosis, and pathologic findings from mastectomy specimens with implications for treatment. Int J Radiat Oncol Biol Phys 19:833

Gage I, Schnitt SJ, Recht A, et al (1998) Skin recurrences after breast-conserving therapy for early-stage breast cancer. J Clin Oncol 16:480–486

Gianni L, Munzone E, Capri G, et al (1995) Paclitaxel by 3-hour infusion in combination with bolus doxorubicin in women with untreated metastatic breast cancer: high antitumor efficacy and cardiac effects in a dose-finding and sequence-finding study. J Clin Oncol 13:2688–2699

Gilliland MD, Barton RM, Copeland EM (1983) The implications of local recurrence of breast cancer as the first site of therapeutic failure. Ann Surg 197:284

Greenberg PAC, Hortobagyi GN, Smith TL, et al (1996) Long-term follow-up of patients with complete remission following combination chemotherapy for metastatic breast cancer. J Clin Oncol 14:2197–2205

Gregory WM, Smith P, Richard MA et al (1993) Chemotherapy of advanced breast cancer: outcome and prognostic factors. Br J Cancer 68:988–995

Haagensen CD (1943) Ann Surg 118:859–870

Haffty BG, Reiss M, Beinfield M, et al (1996) Ipsilateral breast tumor recurrence as a predictor of distant disease: implications for systemic therapy at the time of local relapse. J Clin Oncol 14:52–57

Halverson KJ, Perez CA, Kuske RR, et al (1992) Locoregional recurrence of breast cancer: a retrospective comparison of irradiation alone versus irradiation and systemic therapy. Am J Clin Oncol 15:93–101

Heimann R, Powers C, Halpern HJ, et al (1996) Breast preservation in stage I and II carcinoma of the breast. Cancer 78:1722–1730

Hortobagyi GN, Singletary SE, McNeese MD (1996) Treatment of locally advanced and inflammatory breast cancer. Ch 18 In: Harris JR, Lippman ME, Marrow M, et al (eds) Diseases of the breast. Lippincott-Raven, Philadelphia, p 585–599

Hortobagyi GN, Theriault RL, Porter L, et al (1996) Efficacy of pamidronate in reducing skeletal complications in patients with breast cancer and lytic bone metastases N Engl J Med 335:1785–1837

Jaiyesimi IA, Buzdar AU, Hortobagyi G (1992) Inflammatory breast cancer: a review. J Clin Oncol 10:1014–1024

Janicek M, Hayes DF, Kaplan WD (1994) Healing flare in skeletal metastases from breast cancer. Radiology 192:201–204

Kamby C, Sengelov L (1997) Patterns of dissemination and survival following isolated locoregional recurrence of breast cancer. Breast Cancer Res Treat 45:181–192

Klijn JGM, Beex L, Mauiac L, et al (1996) Addition of LHRH-agonist to tamoxifen improves survival in premenopausal patients with metastatic breast cancer: detailed analysis of EORTC study 10881. Ann Oncol 7:840

Kumar PP, Good RR, Jones EO, et al (1989) Breast carcinoma en cuirasse: pathology and rotational subtotal skin electron beam therapy (SSEBT), a new technique. Radiat Med 7:95–104

Kurtz JM, Amalric R, Brandone H, et al (1989) Local recurrence after breast-conserving surgery and radiotherapy: frequency, time course, and prognosis. Cancer 63:1912–1917

Lamovec J, Bracko M (1991) Metastatic pattern of infiltrating lobular carcinoma of the breast: an autopsy study. J Surg Oncol 48:28–33

Leitzel K, Teramoto Y, Konrad K, et al (1995) Elevated serum c-erbB-2 antigen levels and decreased response to hormone therapy of breast cancer. J Clin Oncol 13:1129–1135

Levine P, Steinhorn S, Ries et al (1985) Inflammatory breast cancer. The experience of the Surveillance Epidemiology and End Result (SEER) Program. J Natl Cancer Inst 74:291–297

Lucas FV, Perez-Mesa C (1978) Inflammatory carcinoma of the breast. Cancer 41:1595–1605

Merajver SD, Weber BL, Cody R, et al (1997) Breast conservation and prolonged chemotherapy for locally advanced breast cancer: the University of Michigan experience. J Clin Oncol 15:2873–2881

Mourali N, Muenz LR, Tabbane F, et al (1980) Epidemiologic features of rapidly progressing breast cancer in Tunisia. Cancer 46:2741–2746

Mouridsen HT (1992) Systemic therapy of advanced breast cancer. Drugs 44:17–28

Mundt AJ, Sibley GS, Williams S, et al (1994) Patterns of failure of complete responders
following high dose chemotherapy and autologous bone marrow transplantation
for metastatic breast cancer: implications for the use of adjuvant radiation therapy.
Int J Radiat Oncol Biol Phys 30:151–160

Muss HB, Case LD, Richards F, et al (1991) Interrupted versus continuous chemotherapy in patients with metastatic breast cancer. N Engl J Med 325:1342–1348

Nolvadex Adjuvant Trial Organisation (1988) Controlled trial of tamoxifen as a single
adjuvant agent in the management of early breast cancer. Br J Cancer 57:608–611

Orel SG, Troupin RH, Patterson EA, et al (1992) Breast cancer recurrence after lumpectomy and irradiation: role of mammography in detection. Radiology
183:201–206

Overgaard M, Hansen PS, Overgaard J, et al (1997) Postoperative radiotherapy in high-
risk premenopausal women with breast cancer who receive adjuvant chemotherapy.
N Engl J Med 337:949–962

Parker SL, Tong T, Bolden S (1997) Cancer Statistics, 1997. CA Cancer J Clin 47:5–27

Pierce LJ, Lippman M, Ben Baruch N, et al (1992) The effects of systemic therapy on
local-regional control in locally advaned breast cancer. Int J Radiat Oncol Biol Phys
23:949–960

Recht A, Hayes DF, Eberlein TJ, et al (1996) Local-regional recurrence after mastectomy or breast-conserving therapy. Ch 21 In Diseases of Breast, ed Harris JR,
Lippman ME, Morrow M, Hellman S. Lippincott-Raven Publishers, Philadelphia pp
649

Recht A, Pierce SM, Abner A, et al (1991) Regional nodal failure after conservative surgery and radiotherapy for early-stage breast carcinoma. J Clin Oncol 9:988–996

Recht A, Schnitt SJ, Connolly JL, et al (1989) Prognosis following local or regional
recurrence after conservative surgery and radiotherapy for early stage breast carcinoma. Int J Radiat Oncol Bio Phys 16:3–9

Rodger A, Jack WJL, Hardman PDJ, et al (1991) Locally advanced breast cancer: report
of phase II study and subsequent phase III trial. Br J Cancer 65:761–765

Rubens RD, Bajetta E, Bonneterre J, et al (1994) Treatment of relapse of breast cancer
after adjuvant systemic therapy – review and guidelines for future research. Eur J
Cancer 30 A:106–111

Saphner T, Tormey DC, Gray R (1996) Annual hazard rates of recurrence for breast
cancer after primary therapy. J Clin Oncol 14:2738–2746

Schaake-Koning C, Hamersma Von der Linden E, Hart G, et al (1985) Adjuvant chemo-
and hormonal therapy in locally advaned breast cancer: a randomized clinical
study. Int J Radiat Oncol Biol Phys 11:1759–1763

Seidman H, Gelb SK, Silverberg E, et al (1987) Survival experience in the breast cancer
detection demonstration project. CA Cancer J Clin 37:258

Sherry MM, Greco FA, Johnson DH, et al (1986) Metastatic breast cancer confined to
the skeletal system. Am J Med 81:381–386

Solin LJ, Fowble BL, Schultz DJ, et al (1990) The detection of local recurrence after definitive irradiation for early stage carcinoma of the breast: an analysis of the results
of breast biopsies performed in previously irradiated breasts. Cancer 65:2497

Swain SM, Whaley FS, Gerber MC, et al (1997) Delayed administration of dexrazoxane
provides cardioprotection for patients with advanced breast cancer treated with
doxorubicin-containing therapy. J Clin Oncol 15:1333–1340

Swain SM, Whaley FS, Gerber MC, et al (1997) Cardioprotection with dexrazoxane for doxorubicin-containing therapy in advanced breast cancer. J Clin Oncol 15:1318–1332

Tannock IF, Boyd NF, DeBoer G, et al (1988) A randomized trial of two dose levels of cyclophosphamide, methotrexate, and fluorouracil chemotherapy for patients with metastatic breast cancer. J Clin Oncol 5:1377–1387

Taylor CW, Green S, Dalton WS, et al (1998) Multicenter randomized clinical trial of goserelin versus surgical ovariectomy in premenopausal patients with receptor-positive metastatic breast cancer: an intergroup study. J Clin Oncol 16:994–999

Tennvall-Nittby L, Tengrup I, Landberg T (1993) The total incidence of loco-regional recurrence in a randomized trial of breast cancer TNM stage II. Acta Oncol 32:614–646

Theriault RL, Hortobagyi GN (1997) Medical treatment of bone metastases. In: Harris JR, Lippman ME (eds) Diseases of the breast updates 1 (3):1–11

Ueno NT, Buzdar AU, Singletary SE, et al (1997) Combined-modality treatment of inflammatory breast carcinoma: twenty years of experience at M.D. Anderson Cancer Center. Cancer Chemother Pharmacol 40:321–329

Valagussa P, Bonadonna G, Veronesi U (1978) Patterns of relapse and survival following radical mastectomy. Cancer 41:1170–1178

Valagussa P, Brambilla C, Zambetti M, et al (1989) In: Recent Results in Cancer Research, Springer-Verlag, Berlin-Heidelberg, p 69–76

Valagussa P, Zambetti M, Bonadonna G, et al (1990) Prognostic factors in locally advanced noninflammatory breast cancer. Long-term results following primary chemotherapy. Breast Cancer Res Treat 15:137–147

Veronesi U, Marubini E, Del Vecchio M, et al (1995) Local recurrences and distant metastases after conservative breast cancer treatments: partly independent events. J Natl Cancer Inst 87:1927

Vogel CL, Azevedo S, Hilsenbeck S, et al (1992) Survival after first recurrence of breast cancer. Cancer 70:129–135

Vogel CL, Schoenfelder J, Shemano I, et al (1995) Worsening bone scan in the evaluation of antitumor response during hormonal therapy of breast cancer. J Clin Oncol 13:1123–1128

Wittliff JL (1984) Steroid-hormone receptors in breast cancer. Cancer 53:630–643

# Tumors of the Head and Neck

# Head and Neck Tumors

R. Stupp

## Epidemiology and Risk Factors

Cancer of the head and neck accounts for approximately 5% of all malignancies with over 40,000 new cases and 12,000 deaths per year in the US [1, 2]. Although the incidence and death rates have been decreasing over the last twenty years, there is a striking increase in females reflecting changing smoking and drinking habits in women. Head and neck cancer is also more common in blacks and Asians.

Squamous cell carcinoma of the head and neck is strongly associated with heavy smoking and drinking with a 15- to 40-fold increase in the relative risk, when both risk factors are present. The varying mortality rates between countries (e.g. oral cancer in France 12.0, Israel 1.5, USA 3.4) can be explained by the different alcohol habits of their populations [3] (Table 1). Over 75% of all oropharyngeal cancers are associated with heavy smoking or drinking, or both. There appears do be a linear dose-risk effect, where duration is more important than intensity [4], suggesting that the development of invasive cancer is a multistep process.

In Asia and the Mediterranean basin undifferentiated nasopharyngeal carcinoma are found endemically with a strong association with

**Table 1.** Mortality of oral cancer (males)

| Country | Deaths/100,000 |
|---------|----------------|
| France | 12.0 |
| Russia | 9.2 |
| Germany | 6.7 |
| USA | 3.4 |
| UK | 3.0 |
| Israel | 1.5 |

Ebstein Barr virus [5]. Nasopharynx cancer in endemic areas are among the most frequent causes of cancer death [6].

Other risk factors for head and neck cancer include vitamin deficiency and malnutrition, poor orodental care and chronic inflammation by malfitting dentures. Occupational exposure to wood dust is associated with an increased risk for adenocarcinoma of the paranasal sinuses [7].

## Pathology and Stage

Over 90% of all head and neck cancers are squamous cell carcinomas, occurring in middle aged and elderly patients. Undifferentiated carcinoma of the nasopharynx type, commonly EBV associated and expressing part of the Ebstein-Barr specific genome need to be distinguished. This subtype is very sensitive to radiation and chemotherapy and can be cured by combined modality treatment. Other histologies are adenocarcinoma, mucoepidermoid carcinoma and adenoid cystic carcinoma of the salivary glands. Lymphoma and Hodgkin's disease, primary melanoma and sarcoma do also arise in the head and neck. Metastatic lung, stomach and pancreas cancer may initially present in the neck.

According to the amount of keratinization, four grades of differentiation can be distinguished, but this carries only little clincially relevant prognostic significance: well, moderately, poorly and undifferentiated carcinoma. New histological staining techniques and flow cytometry allow characterization of nuclear grading and poidy. Lymphatic involvement and extracapsular spread remain the most important prognostic predictors and should always be reported in the pathological reports.

Head and neck cancer stage is best described by the TNM classification [8], defining T-stage according to site, size and local extension (e.g. glottic tumor: $T_1$; limited to vocal cord with intact mobility, $T_2$; Tumor extension to the supra- or subglottis, $T_3$; cord fixation, $T_4$; Cartilage invasion or extension beyond the larynx). The N-stage distinguishes the number, size and localization of the nodes in the neck (Fig. 1). The UICC/AJCC stage grouping separates early stages I + II ($T_1$, $T_2$ tumors, $N_0$), intermediate stage III ($T_3N_1$) and locally advanced stage IV any ($T_4$ or $N_2$, $N_3$). Distant metastases, present in 10%–20% of patients at diagnosis are also included in stage IV.

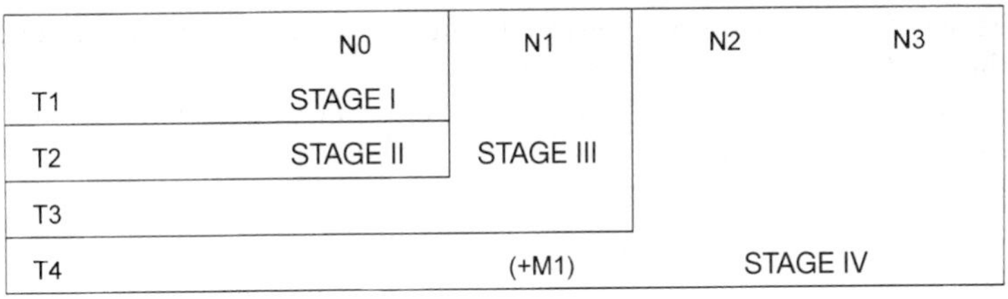

| | N0 | N1 | N2 | N3 |
|---|---|---|---|---|
| T1 | STAGE I | | | |
| T2 | STAGE II | STAGE III | | |
| T3 | | | | |
| T4 | | (+M1) | STAGE IV | |

**Fig. 1.** AJCC and TNM staging. N0, No regional lymph node involvement; N1, one single ipsilateral neck node, 3 cm; N2, multiple neck nodes, >3–6 cm; N2a, metastasis in a single ipsilateral node; N2b, metastases in multiple ipsilateral nodes; N2c, metastases in bilateral, or in a contralateral node; N3, lymph node >6 cm

## Work-up and Staging

Any patient presenting with a persisting lump in the neck needs to be evaluated for a malignant disease. Fine needle aspiration, or better true cut biopsy or an excisional biopsy will reveal a cytological or histological diagnosis. In a young patient the differential diagnosis should exclude an infectious cause like infectious mononucleosis (EBV infection), mumps, measles or cat scratch disease (bordetella henselae). Hodgkin's disease and non-Hodgkin's lymphoma frequently present in the neck as initial site of disease. In patients older than 40 years squamous cell carcinoma are the most frequent cause of a neck mass and the staging procedures should evaluate primary site and extension of disease.

In squamous cell carcinoma of the head and neck, panendoscopy including bronchosopy and esophagoscopy with multiple biopsies and a chest X-ray are mandatory. In 5%–10% of the patients simultaneous second malignancies will be detected [9]. A CT-scan or MRI of the neck is commonly performed to evaluate local tumor extension, invasion in surrounding tissues and bone erosion as well as regional lymph node involvement. Ultrasound of the neck may be even more precise for evaluation of neck nodes. In locally advanced disease a CT-scan of the chest and upper abdomen and a bone scan are recommended to exclude distant metastases.

Laboratory evaluation should include a CBC, liver and renal function tests including calcium and alkaline phosphatase. Tumor markers have no role in the evaluation of head and neck cancer.

Because of the common heavy exposure to nicotine and alcohol in these patients significant comorbidity is frequent. A careful history and physical exam should evaluate for possible cardiac and pulmonary disease.

## Stage-Specific Standard Treatment Options

Over 60% of the patients present at diagnosis with a locally advanced stage. Distant metastases are found in 10% of the patients at diagnosis, another 10% will develop symptomatic metastases during the course of the disease. Autopsy series indicate systemic metastases in up 40% of the patients [10]. Only one third of the patients are diagnosed early and can be cured by surgery and/or radiation. Treatment decision depends on extension and site of the primary tumor, operability and goal of treatment. Historically the role of chemotherapy was limited to palliative treatment in recurrent and metastatic disease. Today chemotherapy is an integral part of a multimodality treatment approach in patients with locally advanced larynx and hypopharynx cancer with organ preservation as primary goal. In inoperable patients chemotherapy may prolong time to progression and survival.

The general concepts of different treatment strategies are outlined in Fig. 2. While early and intermediate stage disease can be cured with surgery and/or radiation alone, the majority of patients presenting with locally advanced disease will require chemotherapy or chemoradiotherapy in addition to surgery. In inoperable patients induction chemotherapy may be indicated, followed by radiation or chemoradiotherapy. Hyperfractionated radiation may be equivalent to chemoradiotherapy for loco-regional control, however more patients will fail with distant metastases. In metastatic disease, radiation and/or surgery should be reserved for patients requiring immediate local palliation. Usually these patients are treated with chemotherapy alone.

## Surgery [11, 12]

Surgical resection as the sole treatment modality will cure up to 90% of patients with stage I squamous cell carcinoma of the head and neck. Results depend on localization of the primary tumor and tumor resec-

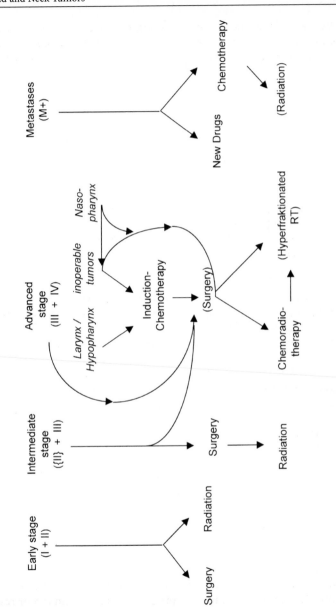

**Fig. 2.** Different treatment strategies. (From [82])

tion margins; in carcinoma of the vocal cords a 1–2 mm margin is sufficient and local recurrences rare. In contrast, tumors of the oropharynx
will frequently show microscopic tumor extension of over 1 cm and
tumor margins of ≥2 cm are required. If resection margins are found to
be positive, reexcission or additional radiotherapy are recommended.

The morbidity and functional impairment by surgery depends not
only on primary tumor size but also on its localization. Small tumors of
the larynx may be resected by a supraglottic laryngectomy, large tumors
(T3) will require a total laryngectomy. Similarly, some early stages of
hypopharynx tumors can be controlled by a partial laryngeophayngec-
tomy, while advanced stages need a complete laryngectomy. Hemi-
laryngectomy and supracricoid partial laryngectomy [13, 14] with improved functional results has been advocated in the last years by skilled surgeons, but whether these procedures do not impair survival remains to be
demonstrated. Recent advances in surgery allow for complex reconstruction with vascularized myocutenous flaps for oral cavity cancers.

Neck Dissection

Elective neck dissection in the clinically N0-neck remains controversial
[15] and should be performed when the result will change the overall
treatment plan (e.g. additional radiotherapy). Exceptions are tumors of
the tongue and pyriform sinus where neck dissection is indicated since
they frequently develop delayed neck metastases. In the clinically involved neck (N1, N2), neck dissection should remove all gross disease and
the uninvolved adjacent lymph nodes according to anatomic localization
and lymphatic drainage. Four principal types of neck dissection are
distinguished [16].

*Radical Neck Dissection.* Resection of all lymph nodes in the neck as well
as internal jugular vein, sternocleidomastoid muscle and spinal accessory nerve. This extensive resection is only rarely performed today.

*Modified radical neck dissection* preserves the spinal accessory nerve
and sternocleidomastoid muscle.

*Functional Neck Dissection.* Removes all the lymph nodes, but preserves
normal tissue and structures with no functional or cosmetic impair-

ment. In skilled hands this can be an alternative to elective radiation to the neck.

*Selective neck dissection* removes a compartment of lymph nodes according to tumor localization, e.g. suprahyoid neck dissection, lateral neck dissection.

Radiotherapy

*Standard Radiation*

Radiation therapy [17] can be an alternative treatment for compliant patients with early stage disease. In patients with advanced disease, radiation is usually given after surgery. Radiation therapy given once daily (180–200 cGy/fraction), five days a week for a total dose of 66–70 Gy to the primary tumor is widely accepted. In patients with larger tumors adjuvant radiation after surgery for 60 Gy with a boost to the tumor bed (66–76 Gy) is indicated [18]. Subclinical neck disease is frequent even in patients with small primary tumors (up to one third of the patients), and elective neck irradiation (50 Gy) is commonly recommended. In patients who have undergone primary neck dissection, adjuvant radiation will be given to patients with multiple positive lymph nodes or extracapsular spread. Although recurrent disease in the previously untreated neck can be salvaged with radiation and/or surgery, primary disease control is preferred. With the exception of well lateralized lesions of the oropharynx bilateral neck irradiation is usually recommended. Macroscopic neck disease should receive 70–76 Gy, and 60 Gy to the uninvolved sites and contralateral side. Subsequent neck dissection for residual disease shows frequently necrotic tissue only, underscoring the effectiveness of radiation for neck disease.

*Hyperfractionated Radiotherapy*

Different radiation schedules and fractionation schemes have been investigated in the last decade [19, 20]. Hyperfractionation (smaller doses per fraction, short treatment intervals, e.g. twice daily) allows for higher total tumor doses with less toxicity to the normal tissue. Treatment accelera-

**Table 2.** Hyperfractionated radiotherapy: randomized trials

| Trial | Treatment | n | Locoregional control | Survival | Remarks |
|---|---|---|---|---|---|
| EORTC 22791, 1992 [21] | RT 35x200 cGy, 1x/d<br>RT 70x115 cGy, 2x/d | 159<br>166 | 5 y: 40%<br>5 y: 59% (p=0.02) | 5 y: 30%<br>5 y: 40% (p=0.08) | |
| EORTC 22851, 1996 [23] | RT 35x200 cGy, 1x/d<br>RT 18 x160 cGy, 3x/d, break 2 wks + RT 45x115 cGy, 2x/d | 511 | Improved (p=0.01) | No difference | Prolonged DFS (p<0.004) |
| RTOG 1987 [24] | RT 33x200 cGy, 1x/d<br>RT 50 x120 cGy, 2x/d | 93<br>94 | 2 y: 29%<br>2 y: 30% (ns) | 2 y: 28%<br>2 y: 32% | CR 62%<br>CR 65% |
| CHART 1997 [25] | RT 36x150 cGy, 3x/dx12d<br>RT 33x200 cGy, 1 x/dx5d/wk | 552<br>356 | No difference | No difference | Increased acute, but decreased late toxicity with CHART |
| Sachchiz 1990 [22] | RT 30x2 Gy<br>RT 64x1.1 Gy<br>RT 30x2 Gy + 5FU qod | 294<br>292<br>306 | Median: 25.2 mo.<br>Median: 51.1 mo.<br>Median: 60.2 mo. | Median: 38 mo.<br>Median: 84 mo.<br>Median: 85 mo. | CR 68%<br>CR 90%<br>CR 96% |

**Table 3.** Induction chemotherapy: landmark trials

| Trial | Treatment | RR | CR | 3-Year survival | Metastases | Remarks |
|---|---|---|---|---|---|---|
| VA; 1991 [26] | PFx3/RT<br>Sx+RT | 54% | 31% | 3y: 53%<br>56% | 11%<br>17% (ns) | Larynx preservation |
| EORTC; 1996 [27] | PFx3/RT<br>Sx+RT | 86% | 54% | 3y: 57%<br>43% | 25%<br>36% (p=0.04) | |
| Paccagnella 1994 [28] | PF/(Sx)/RT<br>(Sx)/RT | 83% | 31% | 3y: 29%<br>20% | 14%<br>38% (p=0.02) | |

P, Cisplatin; F, 5-fluorouracil, RT, radiotherapy; Sx, surgery; VA, Veterans Administration; EORTC, European Organization for Research and Treatment of Cancer.

tion (total dose in a shorter treatment time) increases treatment intensity and acute tissue reaction. A randomized study by the EORTC (Table 2) demonstrated a significantly improved locoregional control with hyperfractionated radiotherapy [21]. The RTOG completed accrual for a randomized trial comparing standard fractionation to hyperfractionation (2x1.2 Gy/d) and split course hyperfractionated, accelerated (2x1.6 Gy/d) radiation. In a Spanish trial reported by Sanchiz in 1990 hyperfractionated radiotherapy was equivalent to chemoradiotherapy with 5-FU and conventional fractionation, but with a significantly better local control and overall survival than standard fractionation radiotherapy alone [22].

## Combined Modality Therapy

### Induction Chemotherapy

Less than 30%–50% of the patients with locally advanced disease will be alive at 5 years. Extensive and possibly mutilating surgery may be required in many patients, other patients may not be operable at all because of tumor stage or other concurrent medical morbidity. Chemotherapy given before surgery and/or radiation, called induction or neoadjuvant chemotherapy has been extensively investigated in the 1980s. Several randomized trials have failed to demonstrate an improved survival after induction chemotherapy (Table 3). The Veterans Affairs Laryngeal Study Group trial tested whether larynx preservation was achievable with induction chemotherapy followed by radiation, reserving surgery for nonresponding patients only [26]. Patients were randomized to induction chemotherapy followed by standard radiation versus surgery and radiotherapy. Of the surviving patients over 60% maintained a functional larynx at 3 years. There was no difference in survival between the two groups. A similar trial was conducted by the European Organization for Research and Treatment of Cancer (EORTC) in larynx and hypopharynx cancer [27]. However, in this trial only patients achieving a complete remission were considered for organ preservation. Again organ preservation could be achieved without detriment in survival. In an Italian trial reported by Paccanella 72% of the patients were considered primarily inoperable [28]. Subgroup analysis of the inoperable patients showed a prolonged survival with induction chemotherapy.

Several conclusions can be drawn from trials with induction chemotherapy: Primary chemotherapy induces high response rates of 50%–80%. A decreased incidence of distant metastases has consistently been shown. Neoadjuvant chemotherapy allows for organ preservation in 60% of advanced larynx and hypopharynx cancer. Induction chemotherapy may prolong survival in patients with inoperable or N2 disease. Outside clinical trials, organ preservation in larynx and hypopharynx cancer remains the sole proven indication for induction chemotherapy.

Chemoradiotherapy,

Simultaneous chemoradiotherapy, rather than sequential chemotherapy followed by radiation has been investigated with promising results over the last years. The rationale for the concomitant use of chemotherapy and radiation has been extensively reviewed [29–34]:
- Locoregional recurrence remains the main cause of failure in advanced head and neck cancer.
- Activity of chemotherapy has been demonstrated by high response rates and decreased distant metastases with induction chemotherapy (spatial cooperation).
- Chemotherapy may act as a radiosensitizer by making tumor cells more sensitive to radiation, and thus eliminating radiation resistant tumor cells.

The goal of concomitant chemo- and radiation therapy must be to administer both modalities at full doses at the usual time intervals. This increase in treatment intensity may by itself improve outcome, however, increased toxicity often requires possibly detrimental treatment interruptions. Three different, but in their principle similar ways of concomitant chemoradiotherapy can be distinguished:
- Standard, uninterrupted radiotherapy with concomitant or intermittent administration of low dose, usually single agent chemotherapy. This approach has a solely radiosensitizing objective.
- Modified radiotherapy schedule with administration of systematically active, commonly combination chemotherapy. This approach may require planned treatment breaks to account for the increased toxicity.
- Alternating chemoradiotherapy; e.g. one week of chemotherapy is followed by two weeks of radiation, again one week of chemotherapy, two weeks of radiation, etc.

**Table 4.** Concepts and selected randomized trials of chemoradiotherapy

| Trial | Treatment | n | Local control | Survival | RR, remarks |
|---|---|---|---|---|---|
| Concomitant, uninterrupted | | | | | |
| Bachaud 1991 [37] | RT 54–74 Gy | 44 | 59% (2 yrs.) | 44% | Resectable pts, postop. RT |
| | P/RT | 39 | 79% (p<0.05) | 75% (p<0.05) | |
| Browman 1994 [35] | Placebo/RT | 87 | N/A | 2 y: 50% | CR 6% |
| | 5-FU/RT | 88 | | 63% | 68% |
| Brizel 1997 [36] | PF wk 1+6/RT bid | 121 | DFS 3 y: 69% | 3y: 51% | Mets: 19% |
| | RT bid | | 31% (p=0.002) | 28% (p=0.06) | 37% (p=0.3) |
| Split course | | | | | |
| Adelstein 1994 [38] | PF, followed by RT (sequential) | 24 | 30 mo.: 39% | 30 mo.: 43% | CR 76%, PR 33% |
| | PF + RT concomitant (split course) | 24 | 60% (p=0.03) | 68% (ns) | |
| Taylor 1994 [39] | PF, followed by RT (sequential) | 107 | 45% (p=0.003) | No sign. difference | Marked differences in RR and toxicity depending on treatment site |
| | PF + RT concomitant qow | 107 | 61% | | |
| Wendt 1998 [40] | RT (70 Gy) bidx2 wks, break 1 wkx3 courses | 140 | 3 y: 17% | 3 y: 24% | |
| | PF + RT bidx2 wks, 1 wk break,x3 courses | 130 | 3 y: 36% (p<0.004) | 3 y: 48% (p<0.003) | Increased toxicity and prolonged breaks with chemoradiotherapy |
| Alternating | | | | | |
| Merlano 1992 [41] | RT | 77 | 3 y: 35% | 23% | CR 22% |
| | PF/RT alternating | 80 | 59% (p<0.01) | 41% (p<0.05) | CR 43% |

Several trials have demonstrated improved locoregional control and survival with concomitant chemoradiotherapy (Table 4). In a placebo controlled, randomized trial with 5-FU given as a 72-h continuous infusion during the first and third week of radiation there was a trend for improved survival (at 2 years: 63% vs. 50%; p=0.07) [35]. In a three arm trial investigators from Spain showed significantly improved survival and local control with either hyperfractionated radiation or standard fractionation with concomitant 5-fluorouracil (250 mg/m2 i.v. bolus qod), compared to standard radiotherapy alone [22]. Brizel et al. added two courses of cisplatin/5-FU chemotherapy (week 1+6) to hyperfractionated radiotherapy (2x125 cGy/d). In a randomized trial with 121 patients with T3/T4 tumors they showed an improved 3 year survival (51% vs. 28%, p=0.06) and a decrease in distant metastases [36].

Split course chemoradiotherapy has been extensively investigated at the University of Chicago. Feasibility of intensive chemoradiotherapy with 5-FU as continuous infusion over 120 h, hydroxyurea p.o. twice daily, and cisplatin on day 1 or paclitaxel as continuous infusion with concurrent standard or accelerated hyperfractionated radiotherapy, treatment given every other week, has been demonstrated [42–45]. Results on local control are encouraging, however, toxicity with these regimens is considerable and requiring attentive supportive care. Investigation of equally effective, but less toxic regimens is warranted. The importance of supportive care and center experience became evident in a randomized trial comparing sequential cisplatin/5-FU with concomitant chemoradiotherapy with cisplatin (60 mg/m2, d1) and 5-FU (800 mg/m2 per day, d1–5 cont. infusion) and once daily radiation [39]. Local control, but not survival was improved with the concomitant treatment. Marked differences in response rates and toxicity were observed depending on treatment site and experience. In a randomized German multicenter trial 270 patients were treated with either hyperfractionated radiotherapy (2x180 cGy/d) for two weeks followed by a one week break, for three courses or the same radiotherapy with concomitant PFL-chemotherapy (cisplatin, infusional 5-FU, leucovorin) during the first 5 days of each treatment block [40]. Prolonged treatment breaks due to toxicity were necessary in the concomitant chemoradiotherapy arm accounting for a longer overall treatment duration, nevertheless both local control (17% vs. 35%) and survival (24% vs. 49%) at 3 years were significantly superior with concomitant therapy [40]. The treatment breaks in the control arm may be considered unnecessary.

The concept of rapidly alternating chemoradiotherapy has been pursued by two European groups [41, 46, 47]. In a randomized trial rapidly alternating chemoradiotherapy with cisplatin and 5-FU was superior to standard radiotherapy only (survival at 3 years: 41% versus 23%, at 5 years: 24% versus 10%, p=0.008) [41, 46]. Rapidly alternating chemoradiotherapy with hyperfractionated accelerated radiation provided encouraging results but toxicity was substantial [47].

The value of chemotherapy in a combined modality approach for treatment of advanced squamous cell carcinoma has also been demonstrated on a recent metaanalysis [48]. This work merits special consideration, because the investigators were able to obtain updated, individual patient data (and not published data as in other metaanalyses) on over 10.000 patients included in 63 randomized trials. Comparing chemotherapy versus no chemotherapy irrespective of administration schedule did not demonstrate an improvement in survival, but a reduced incidence of distant failures. However, when considering only trials with concomitant chemoradiotherapy a significant improvement in local control and survival is suggested.

In conclusion, concomitant chemoradiotherapy for locally advanced head and neck cancer appears to be superior to standard radiotherapy alone and should be considered as standard practice. However, optimal radiation schedule and chemotherapy regimen are not yet defined. The role of hyperfractionation or accelerated radiation remains to be determined. Clearly, treatment regimens with less acute toxicity need to be developed. Integration of new agents, colony stimulating factors and cytoprotective agents may be the way. Patients with advanced head and neck cancer require evaluation by an experienced multidisciplinary team of head and neck surgeons and oncology specialists, enrollment in a clinical trial should be encouraged.

Chemotherapy

For recurrent or metastatic disease chemotherapy is usually the treatment of choice. Many single agents have demonstrated activity against squamous cell carcinoma of the head and neck:

– Methotrexate [49, 50]
– Cisplatin [56, 59]
– Carboplatin [60]

- 5-Fluorouracil [56]
- Ifosfamide [64–66]
- Doxorubicin [57, 58]
- Paclitaxel [51–53]
- Docetaxel [54, 55, 61]
- Vinorelbine [62, 63]

Methotrexate has been considered for many years as the standard treatment. Methotrexate is simple and can be given weekly as an outpatient. Response rates of single agent methotrexate are modest with only 10%–15% of the patients responding [49, 50]. Therefore many other agents and combination regimens have been investigated (Table 5). Response rates of up to 40% with single agent paclitaxel and docetaxel have been reported in selected patients in non-randomized trials [51–55]. The combination of cisplatin and infusional 5-FU is the most widely investigated regimen. Response rates of up to 90% with 40% complete responses has been demonstrated in previously untreated patients. In patients with recurrent disease after surgery and radiation this combination regimen remains the most active treatment and is the treatment of choice in patients who require rapid tumor regression for palliation. In a randomized trial in patients with recurrent disease the combination of cisplatin and 5-FU achieved a response rate of 32%, compared with 17% for single agent cisplatin and 13% for 5-FU [56]. However, there was no survival difference, with a median of 5.7 months.

Biological Response Modifiers

Biological response modifiers have a limited role in the treatment of head and neck cancer [67]. Colony stimulating factors (G-CSF) have been used in clinical trials investigating new and intensive treatment regimens allowing for dose escalation. The modest dose escalation achievable with growth factors will probably not improve outcome of therapy. Interferons have been investigated alone and in conjunction with chemotherapy. Interferon-gamma induced tumor regression in 5 of 13 patients with nasopharynx cancer [68] and 3 of 8 patients with squamous cell carcinoma [69]. The combination of alpha-interferon and cis-retinoic acid failed to show significant responses in two small pilot trials [70, 71]. In vitro, the combination of cisplatin and 5-FU shows synergy with

**Table 5.** Treatment of recurrent or metastatic disease

| Regimen | Dose | Frequency | Response rate | Response duration | Median survival | Reference |
|---|---|---|---|---|---|---|
| Methotrexate | 40–60 mg/m2 | Weekly | 10%–25% | 4.1 mo | 4.2–5.6 mo. | [49, 78] |
| Cisplatin/5-FU | 60–100 mg/m2 600–1000 mg/m2 a | q 3–4 weeks | 32% | 4.2 mo | 5.6–6.4 mo. | [49, 79] |
| Carboplatin/5-FU | 300–400 mg/m2 600–1000 mg/m2 a | q 3–4 weeks | 21% | 5.1 mo | 5.0 mo. | [49] |
| Docetaxel | 100 mg/m2 | q 3–4 weeks | | | | [54, 55, 61, 80] |
| Paclitaxel | 135–175 mg/m2 + G-CSF: 250 mg/m2 | q 3–4 weeks | 31% | 4.4 mo | N/A | [51, 53] |
| Vinorelbine | 20–25 mg/m2 | Weekly | 22% | 5.8 mo | N/A | [81] |

a Daily dose, continuous infusion for 4–5 days.

alpha-interferon. In clinical trials the addition of interferon to this combination regimen resulted in added toxicity (mainly myelosuppression
and mucositis) without evidence of enhanced antitumor activity. A randomized trial with 244 patients failed to demonstrate an improved response rate or survival when alpha-interferon was added to chemotherapy with cisplatin and 5-FU [72].

## Special Entities

### Nasopharynx Cancer

Nasopharynx cancer needs to be considered separately. It causes symptoms only late in the course of the disease and usually presents at an
advanced stage. Nasopharyngeal carcinoma is frequently associated with
EBV and is one of the most frequent cancers in Southeast Asia.
Metastatic disease is frequent. Nasopharynx cancer is exquisitely responsive to both chemotherapy and radiation. Furthermore, as surgical
access is usually difficult, radiotherapy and chemotherapy become the
primary treatment modalities. A recent randomized trial showed the
superiority of concomitant chemoradiotherapy with cisplatin
(100 mg/m2 d1, 22, 43) and once daily RT versus radiation alone. Overall
survival at 3 years was 45% with radiation alone and 83% (p<0.001) with
chemoradiotherapy [73, 74]. A role of neoadjuvant chemotherapy in
nasopharynx cancer is also suggested, although only improvement in
disease free, but not overall survival could be shown in a large, international randomized trial [75].

### Salivary Gland Carcinoma

A tumor found in the minor salivary gland is most likely malignant. In
contrast, up to 85% of the tumors of the parotid gland are found to be
benign. Histology of salivary gland cancer is frequently adenocarcinoma, mucoepidermoid carcinoma adenoid cystic carcinoma. According
to their histological picture and natural history low grade malignancies
can be distinguished from high grade tumors. Low grade tumors like aci-
nic cell carcinoma or mucoepidermoid carcinoma tend to recur locally
and only rarely metastasize. High grade tumors are frequently adenoc-

arcinoma. Adenoid cystic carcinoma may have a slow and long evolution with late recurrences, but more aggressive variants are not infrequent. Surgery is the critical treatment modality for all salivary gland tumors. Despite extensive surgery local recurrence may occur in up to half of the patients. Postoperative radiotherapy is usually recommended for all high grade tumors and for adenoid cystic carcinoma. This allows to reduce the recurrence rate to about 15%–20%. Chemotherapy has a limited role in salivary gland carcinoma and is usually restricted to recurrent unresectable or metastatic disease.

## Current Key Questions

Progress has been made over the last decade in the management of head and neck cancer. Chemotherapy is now an integral part of the multidisciplinary treatment of head and neck cancer. Hyperfractionated radiation and chemotherapy allowed for better loco-regional control, consequently distant failures are becoming a more common problem. Second malignancies are another frequent problem in patients cured of the primary disease. Chemoprevention strategies are currently under investigation.

In a subset of patients organ preservation omitting surgery or limiting surgery to residual neck disease can be achieved with induction chemotherapy or chemoradiotherapy. Better identification of the patients who will benefit from such an approach is warranted. Toxicity of concomitant chemoradiotherapy is increased when compared to each modality alone. Development of treatment regimens of shorter duration and with less toxicity are required. Current treatments are restricted to specialized oncology centers experienced in multimodality treatment approaches and offering regular and intensive supportive care.

Progress in molecular biology and recognition of tumor pathogenesis may lead to more specific treatments and prophylaxis. Identification of the frequent p53 gene mutation and restoration with a viral vector of its function are the first attempts bringing this knowledge into the clinic.

## Investigational Approaches

Whenever possible, patients should be enrolled in clinical trials. An RTOG and Intergroup trial is comparing different organ preservation strategies for larynx cancer: Induction chemotherapy vs. radiotherapy alone and vs. laryngectomy. The EORTC compares induction chemotherapy vs. alternating chemoradiotherapy for organ preservation in advanced hypopharynx cancer. In recurrent disease the main focus is on identifying new and more active treatment regimens. Many of the recently available cytotoxic agents have shown some activity in head and neck cancer. Recent clinical trials are aiming at restoring the lost p53 function in patients with locally accessible disease. Using an adenoviral vector the p53 gene is to be reintroduced into the tumor cell, subsequently inducing apoptosis [76]. Similarly, the onyx-015 virus uses the absence of the p-53 gene as a target for selective replication and thus tumor lysis [77].

## References

1. Vokes EE, Weichselbaum RR, Lippman SM, Hong WK. Medical progress: Head and neck cancer. N Engl J Med (1993);328:184–194
2. Parker S, Tong T, Bolden S, Wingo P. Cancer statistics, 1997. CA, Cancer J Clin (1997);47:5–27
3. Black R, Bray F, Ferlay J, Parkin D. Cancer incidence and mortality in the European Union: Cancer registry data and estimates of national incidence for 1990. Eur J Cancer (1997);33:1075–1107
4. Blot WJ, μlaughlin JK, Winn DM, Austin DF, Greenberg RS, Preston Martin S, Bernstein L, Schoenberg JB, Stemhagen A, Fraumeni JF, Jr. Smoking and drinking in relation to oral and pharyngeal cancer. Cancer Res (1988);48:3282–3287
5. Liebovitz D. Nasopharyngeal carcinoma: The Epstein-Barr virus association. Semin Oncol (1994);21:376–381
6. Fandi A, Altun M, Azli N, Armand JP, Cvitkiovic E. Nasopharyngeal cancer: epidemiology, staging, and treatment. Semin Oncol (1994);21:382–397
7. Vader J, Minder C. Die Sterblichkeit an Krebsen der Nasen- und Nasennebenhöhlen bei Schweizer Schreinern. Schweiz Med Wschr (1987);117:481–486
8. TNM Classification of malignant tumours. (5th ed.) New York: Wiley-Liss, 1997
9. Schwartz LH, Ozsahin M, Zhang GN, Touboul E, De Vataire F, Andolenko P, Lacau Saint Guily J, Laugier A, Schlienger M. Synchronous and metachronous head and neck carcinomas. Cancer (1994);74:1933–1938
10. Zbären P, Lehmann W. Frequency and sites of distant metastases in head and neck squamous cell carcinoma. An analysis of 101 cases at autopsy. Arch Otolaryngol Head Neck Surg (1987);113:762–764
11. Sloan D, Goepfert H. Conventional therapy of head and neck cancer. Hematol Oncol Clin North Am (1991);5:601–625
12. Scher N, Panje WR. New concepts in head and neck surgery. Hematol Oncol Clin North Am (1991);5:627–634
13. Naudo P, Laccourreye O, Weinstein G, Hans S, Laccourreye H, Brasnu D. Functional outcome and prognosis factors after supracricoid partial laryngectomy with cricohyoidopexy. Annals of Otology, Rhinology & Laryngology (1997);106:291–296
14. Naudo P, Laccourreye O, Weinstein G, Jouffre V, Laccourreye H, Brasnu D. Complications and functional outcome after supracricoid partial laryngectomy with

cricohyoidoepiglottopexy. Otolaryngology Head & Neck Surgery (1998);118: 124–129

15. Alvi A, Johnson JT. Extracapsular spread in the clinically negative neck (N0) Implications and outcome. Otolaryngol Head Neck Surg (1996);114:65–70

16. Robbins KT, Medina JE, Wolfe GT, Levine PA, Sessions RB, Pruet CW. Standardizing neck dissection terminology. Official report of the Academy's Committee for Head and Neck Surgery and Oncology [see comments]. Arch Otolaryngol Head Neck Surg (1991);117:601–605

17. Million R, Cassisi N. Management of head and neck cancer. A mulitdisciplinary approach. (Second ed.) J.B. Lippincott, Philadelphia 1994

18. Peters LJ, Goepfert H, Ang KK, Byers RM, Maor MH, Guillamondegui O, Morrison WH, Weber RS, Garden AS, Frankenthaler RA, Oswald MJ, Brown BW. Evaluation of the dose for postoperative radiation therapy of head and neck cancer: First report of a prospective randomized trial. Int J Radiat Oncol Biol Phys (1993);26:3–11

19. Peters LJ, Ang KK, Thames HD, Jr. Accelerated fractionation in the radiation treatment of head and neck cancer. A critical comparison of different strategies. Acta Oncol (1988);27:185–194

20. Dische S. Radiotherapy – new fractionation schemes. Semin Oncol (1994); 21:304–310

21. Horiot JC, Le Fur R, N'Guyen T, Chenal C, Schraub S, Alfonsi S, Gardani G, Van Den Bogaert W, Danczak S, Bolla M, Van Glabbeke M, De Pauw M. Hyperfractionation versus conventional fractionation in oropharyngeal carcinoma: Final analysis of a randomized trial of the EORTC cooperative group of radiotherapy. Radiother Oncol (1992);25:231–241

22. Sanchiz F, Milla A, Torner J, Bonet F, Artola N, Carreno L, Moya LM, Riera D, Ripol S, Cirera L. Single fraction per day versus two fractions per day versus radiochemotherapy in the treatment of head and neck cancer. Int J Radiat Oncol Biol Phys (1990);19:1347–1350

23. Horiot JC, Bontemps P, Begg AC, Le Fur R, Van Den Bogaert W, Bolla M, N'Guyen T, Van Den Weijngaert D, Bernier J, Lusinchi A, Stuschke D, Lopez Torrecilla D, Jancar B, Collette L, Van Glabbeke M, Pierart M. Hyperfractionated and accelerated radiotherapy in head and neck cancer: Results of the EORTC trials and impact on clinical practice. Bull Cancer Radiother (1996);83:314–320

24. Marcial VA, Pajak TF, Chu C et al. Hyperfractionated photon radiation therapy in the treatment of advanced squamous cell carcinoma of the oral cavity, pharynx, larynx, and sinuses, using radiation therapy as the only planned modality: Preliminary report by the Radiation Therapy Oncology Group (RTOG). Int J Radiat Oncol Biol Phys (1987);13:41–47

25. Dische S, Saunders M, Barrett A, Harvey A, Gibson D, Parmar M. A randomised multicentre trial of CHART versus conventional radiotherapy in head and neck cancer. Radiother Oncol (1997);44:123–136

26. The Department of Veterans Affairs Laryngeal Cancer Study Group. Induction chemotherapy plus radiation compared with surgery plus radiation in patients with advanced laryngeal cancer. N Engl J Med (1991);324:1685–1690

27. Lefebvre J, Chevalier D, Luboinski B, Kirkpatrick A, Collette L, T S, for the EORTC Head and Neck Cooperative Group. Larynx preservation in pyriform sinus cancer: preliminary results of a European Organization for Reserach and Treatment of Cancer phase III trial. J Natl Cancer Inst (1996);88:890–899

28. Paccagnella A, Orlando A, Marchiori C, Zorat PL, Cavaniglia G, Sileni VC, Jirillo A, Tomio L, Fila G, Fede A, Endrizzi L, Bari M, Sampognaro E, Balli M, Gava A, Pappagallo GL, Fiorentino MV. Phase III trial of initial chemotherapy in stage III

or IV head and neck cancers: A study by the Gruppo di Studio sui Tumori della Testa e del Collo. J Natl Cancer Inst (1994);86:265–272

29. Vokes EE, Weichselbaum RR. Concomitant chemoradiotherapy: Rationale and clinical experience in patients with solid tumors. J Clin Oncol (1990);8:911–934

30. Vokes E. Interactions of chemotherapy and radiation. Semin Oncol (1993); 20:70–79

31. Dimery IW, Hong WK. Overview of combined modality therapies for head and neck cancer. J Natl Cancer Inst (1993);85:95–111

32. Stupp R, Vokes EE. Progress in treatment of head and neck cancer. Part 2: chemoradiotherapy. Strahlenther Onkol (1995);171:140–148

33. Stupp R, Vokes EE. 5-fluorouracil plus radiation for head and neck cancer. J Infus Chemother (1995);5:55–60

34. Tannock IF. Treatment of cancer with radiation and drugs. J Clin Oncol (1996);Journal-of-Clinical-Oncology. 14:3156–3174

35. Browman GP, Cripps C, Hodson DI, Eapen L, Sathya J, Levine MN. Placebo-controlled randomized trial of infusional fluorouracil during standard radiotherapy in locally advanced head and neck cancer. J Clin Oncol (1994);12:2648–2653

36. Brizel D, Albers M, Fisher S, Scher R, Richtsmeier W, Clough R, George S, Prosnitz L. A phase III trial of hyperfractionated irradiation±concurrent chemotherapy for locally advanced carcinoma of the head and neck: superiority of combined modality treatment. Proc Am Soc Clin Oncol (1997);16:384a (abstract #1368)

37. Bachaud JM, David JM, Boussin G, Daly N. Combined postoperative radiotherapy and weekly cisplatin infusion for locally advanced squamous cell carcinoma of the head and neck: Preliminary report of a randomized trial. Int J Radiat Oncol Biol Phys (1991);20:243–246

38. Adelstein DJ, Saxton JP, Van Kirk MA, Wood BG, Eliachar I, Tucker HM, Lavertu P. Continuous course radiation therapy and concurrent combination chemotherapy for squamous cell head and neck cancer. Am J Clin Oncol (1994);17:369–373

39. Taylor SG, Murthy AK, Vannetzel JM, Colin P, Dray M, Caldarelli DD, Shott S, Vokes E, Showel JL, Hutchinson JC, Witt TR, Griem KL, Hartsell WF, Kies MS, Mittal B, Rebischung JL, Coupez DJ, Desphieux JL, Bobin S, LePajolec C. Randomized comparison of neoadjuvant cisplatin and fluorouracil infusion followed by radiation versus concomitant treatment in advanced head and neck cancer. J Clin Oncol (1994);12:385–395

40. Wendt T, Grabenbauer G, Rödel C, Thiel H, Aydin H, Rohlof R, Wustrow T, Iro H, Popella C, Schallhorn A. Simultaneous radiochemotherapy versus radiotherapy alone in advanced headn and neck cancer: A randomized study. J Clin Oncol (1998);16:1318–1324

41. Merlano M, Vitale V, Rosso R, Benasso M, Corvo R, Cavallari M, Sanguineti G, Bacigalupo A, Badellino F, Margarino G, Brema F, Pastorino G, Marziano C, Grimaldi A, Scasso F, Sperati G, Pallestrini E, Garaventa G, Accomando E et al. Treatment of advanced squamous-cell carcinoma of the head and neck with alternating chemotherapy and radiotherapy. N Engl J Med (1992);327:1115–1121

42. Vokes EE, Panje WR, Schilsky RL, Mick R, Awan AM, Moran WJ, Goldman MD, Tybor AG, Weichselbaum RR. Hydroxyurea, fluorouracil, and concomitant radiotherapy in poor-prognosis head and neck cancer: A phase I-II study. J Clin Oncol (1989);7:761–768

43. Vokes EE, Haraf DJ, Mick R, McEvilly JM, Kozloff M, Stupp R, Wenig B, Moran W, Panje W, Weichselbaum RR. Concomitant chemoradiotherapy for intermediate stage head and neck cancer. Proc Am Soc Clin Oncol (1994);13:282 (abstract #909)

44. Vokes EE, Haraf DJ, Mick R, McEvilly JM, Weichselbaum RR. Intensified concomitant chemoradiotherapy with and without filgrastim for poor-prognosis head and neck cancer. J Clin Oncol (1994);12:2351–2359

45. Brockstein B, Haraf D, Stenson K, Fasanmade A, Stupp R, Glisson B, Lippman S, Ratain M, Sulzen L, Klepsch A, RR W, Vokes E. A phase I study of concomitant chemoradiotherapy with paclitaxel, 5-FU, and hydroxyurea with granuloccyte colony stimulating factor support for patients with poor prognosis cancer of the head and neck. J Clin Oncol (1998);16:735–744

46. Merlano M, Benasso M, Corvo R, Rosso R, Vitale V, Blengio F, Numico G, Margarino G, Bonelli L, Santi L. Five-year update of a randomized trial of alternating radiotherapy and chemotherapy compared with radiotherapy alone in treatment of unresectable squamous cell carcinoma of the head and neck. J Natl Cancer Inst (1996);88:583–589

47. Leyvraz S, Pasche P, Bauer J, Bernasconi S, Monnier P. Rapidly alternating chemotherapy and hyperfractionated radiotherapy in the management of locally advanced head and neck carcinoma: Four-year results of a phase I/II study. J Clin Oncol (1994);12:1876–1885

48. Bourhis J, Pignon J, Designé L, Luboinski B, Guérin S, Domenge C, on behalf of the MACH-NC Collaborative Group. Metaanalysis of chemotherapy in head and neck cancer (MACH-NC): Locoregional treatment vs same treatment + chemotherapy. Proc Am Soc Clin Oncol (1998);17:386a (abstract #1486)

49. Forastiere AA, Metch B, Schuller DE, Ensley JF, Hutchins LF, Triozzi P, Kish JA, McClure E, VonFeldt E, Williamson SK, Von Hoff DD. Randomized comparison of cisplatin plus fluorouracil and carboplatin plus fluorouracil versus methotrexate in advanced squamous-cell carcinoma of the head and neck: A Southwest Oncology Group study. J Clin Oncol (1992);10:1245–1251

50. Schornagel J, Verweij J, De-Mulder P, Cognetti F, Vermorken J, Cappelaere P, Armand J, Wildiers J, De-Graeff A, Clavel M, Sahmoud T, Kirkpatrick A, Lefebvre J. Randomized phase III trial of edatrexate versus methotrexate in patients with metastatic and/or recurrent squamous cell carcinoma of the head and neck: A European Organization for Research and Treatment of Cancer Head and Neck Cancer Cooperative Group study. J Clin Oncol (1995);13:1649–1655

51. Forastiere AA. Paclitaxel (Taxol) for the treatment of head and neck cancer. Semin Oncol (1994);21:49–52

52. Smith RE, Thornton DE, Allen J. A phase II trial of paclitaxel in squamous cell carcinoma of the head and neck with correlative laboratory studies. Semin Oncol (1995);22:41–46

53. Thornton D, Singh K, Putz B, Gams R, Schuller D, Smith R. A Phase II trial of Taxol in squamous cell carcinoma of the head and neck (Meeting abstract). Proc Annu Meet Am Soc Clin Oncol (1994);13:A933

54. Dreyfuss AI, Clark JR, Norris CM, Rossi RM, Lucarini JW, Busse PM, Poulin MD, Thornhill L, Costello R, Posner MR. Docetaxel: An active drug for squamous cell carcinoma of the head and neck. J Clin Oncol (1996);14:1672–1678

55. Couteau C, Chouaki N, Leyvraz S, Oulid-Aissa D, Lebecq A, Domenge C, Groult V, Janot F, de Forni M, Armand J. A phase II study of docetaxel in patients with metastatic squamous cell carcinoma of the head and neck. in press (1998)

56. Jacobs C, Lyman G, Velez Garcia E, Sridhar KS, Knight W, Hochster H, Goodnough LT, Mortimer JE, Einhorn LH, Schacter L, Cherng N, Dalton T, Burroughs J, Rozencweig M. A phase III randomized study comparing cisplatin and fluorouracil as single agents and in combination for advanced squamous cell carcinoma of the head and neck. J Clin Oncol (1992);10:257–263

57. Stewart DJ, Cripps MC, Lamothe A, Laframboise G, Odell P, Gerin Lajoie J. Doxorubicin plus metronidazole in the treatment of recurrent or metastatic squamous cell carcinoma of the head and neck. Am J Clin Oncol (1993);16:113–116

58. Al-Sarraf M. Head and Neck Cancer: Chemotherapy Concepts. Semin Oncol (1988);15:70–85

59. Liverpool Head and Neck Oncology Group. A phase III randomised trial of cisplatinum, methotrexate, cisplatinum + methotrexate and cisplatinum + 5-FU in end stage squamous carcinoma of the head and neck. Br J Cancer (1990);61:311–315

60. Aisner J, Sinibaldi V, Eisenberger M. Carboplatin In the Treatment Of Squamous Cell Head and Neck Cancers. Semin Oncol (1992);19:60–65

61. Catimel G, Verweij J, Mattijssen V, Hanauske A, Piccart M, Wanders J, Franklin H, Le Bail N, Clavel M, Kaye SB. Docetaxel (Taxotere ®): An active drug for the treatment of patients with advanced squamous cell carcinoma of the head and neck. Ann Oncol (1994);5:533–537

62. Canfield V, Saxman S, Kolodziej M, Harrison-Mann B, Loehrer P, Vokes E. Phase II trial of vinorelbine in advanced or recurrent squamous cell carcinoma of the head and neck. Proc Am Soc Clin Oncol (1997);16:387a (abstract #1382)

63. Oliveira J, Geoffrois L, Rolland F, Degardin M, Armand J, Boudillet J, P Tresca P, Lentz M, Vanglabbeke M, Fumoleau P. Activity of Navelbine on lesions within previously irradiated fields in patients with metastatic and/or local recurrent squamous cell carcinoma of the head and neck: an EORTC-ECSG study. Proc Am Soc Clin Oncol (1997);16:406a (abstract #1449)

64. Huber MH, Lippman SM, Benner SE, Shirinian M, Dimery IW, Dunnington JS, Waun Ki H. A phase II study of ifosfamide in recurrent squamous cell carcinoma of the head and neck. Am J Clin Oncol Cancer Clin Trials (1996);19:379–383

65. Cervellino JC, Araujo CE, Pirisi C, Francia A, Cerruti R. Ifosfamide and mesna for the treatment of advanced squamous cell head and neck cancer. A Getlac Study. Oncology (1991);48:89–92

66. Buesa JM, Fernandez R, Esteban E, Estrada E, Baron FJ, Palacio I, Gracia M, Lacave AJ. Phase II trial of ifosfamide in recurrent and metastatic head and neck cancer. Ann Oncol (1991);2:151–152

67. Hamasaki VK, Vokes EE. Interferons and other cytokines in head and neck cancer. Med Oncol (1995);12:23–33

68. Dimery IW, Jacobs C, Tseng AJ, Saks S, Pearson G, Hong WK, Gutterman JU. Recombinant interferon-gamma in the treatment of recurrent nasopharyngeal carcinoma. J Biol Response Mod (1989);8:221–226

69. Richtsmeier WJ, Koch WM, μguire WP, Poole ME, Chang EH. Phase I-II study of advanced head and neck squamous cell carcinoma patients treated with recombinant human interferon gamma. Arch Otolaryngol Head Neck Surg (1990);116:1271–1277

70. Roth AD, Abele R, Alberto P. 13-cis-Retinoic acid plus interferon-alpha: A phase II clinical study in squamous cell carcinoma of the lung and the head and neck. Oncology (1994);51:84–86

71. Cascinu S, Del Ferro E, Ligi M, Graziano F, Castellani, Catalano G. Phase II trial of 13-cis retinoic acid plus interferon-alpha in advanced squamous cell carcinoma of head and neck, refractory to chemotherapy. Ann Oncol (1996); 7:538–539

72. Schrijvers D, Johnson J, Jiminez U, Gore M, Kosmidis P, Szpirglas H, Robbins K, Oliveira J, Lewenson R, Schüller J, Riviere A, Arvay C, Langecker P, Jacob H, Cvitkovic C, Vokes E, for the Head and Neck Interferon Cooperative Group. Phase III trial of modulation of cisplatin/fluorouracil chemotherapy by interferon alfa-2b in patients with recurrent or metastatic head and neck cancer. J Clin Oncol (1998);16:1054–1059

73. Al-Sarraf M, LeBlanc M, Shanker Giri PG, Fu KK, Cooper J, Vuong T, Forastiere AA, Adams G, Sakr WA, Schuller DE, Ensley JF. Chemoradiotherapy versus radiotherapy in patients with advanced nasopharyngeal cancer: Phase III randomized Intergroup study 0099. J Clin Oncol (1998);16:1310–1317

74. Al-Sarraf M, LeBlanc M, Giri PG, Fu K, Cooper J, Vuong T, Forastiere A, Adams G, Sakr W, Schuller D, Ensley J. Chemo-radiotherapy vs radiotherapy in patients with advanced nasopharyngeal cancer. Preliminary results of intergroup (0099) (SWOG 8892, RTOG 8817, ECOG 2388) phase III study: Progress report. Proc Annu Meet Am Soc Clin Oncol (1998);17:385a (abstract #1483)

75. El Gueddari B, on behalf of the International Nasopharynx Study Group. Final results of the VUMCA I randomized trial comparing neoadjuvant chemotherapy (BEC) plus radiotherapy to RT alone in undifferentiated nasopharyngeal carcinoma. Proc Am Soc Clin Oncol (1998);17:385a (abstract #1482)

76. Clayman G, El-Naggar A, Merritt J, Bruso P, Roth J, Lippman S, Hong W, Goepfert H. Adenovirus-mediated p53 gene transfer ina a phase I trial of patients with advanced head and neck squamous carcinoma. Proc Am Soc Clin Oncol (1997);16:383a (abstract #1363)

77. Kirn D, Nemunaitis J, Ganly I, Posner M, Vokes E, Kuhn C, Heise C, Maack C, Kaye S. A phase II trial of intratumoral injection with an E1B-deleted adenovirus, Onyx-015, in patients with recurrent, refractory head and neck cancer. Proc Am Soc Clin Oncol (1998);17:391a (abstract #1509)

78. Eisenberger M, Krasnow S, Ellenberg S, Silva H, Abrams J, Sinibaldi V, Van Echo D, Aisner J. A comparison of carboplatin plus methotrexate versus methotrexate alone in patients with recurrent and metastatic head and neck cancer. J Clin Oncol (1989);7:1341–1345

79. Browman GP, Cronin L. Standard chemotherapy in squamous cell head and neck cancer: What we have learned from randomized trials. Semin Oncol (1994);21: 311–319

80. Ebihara S, Fujii H, Sasaki Y, Inuyama Y. A late phase II study of docetaxel (Taxotere) in patients with head and neck cancer. Proc Am Soc Clin Oncol (1997);16:399a (abstract #1425)

81. Gebbia V, Testa A, Valenza R, Zerillo G, Restivo G, Ingria F, Cannata G, Gebbia N. Weekly vinorelbine in recurrent and/or metastatic squamous cell carcinoma of the head and neck (Meeting abstract). Fourth International Congress on Anti cancer Chemotherapy. February (1993).

82. Stupp R, Vokes E Kopf- und Halstumoren. In: Seeber S, Schütte J, eds. Therapiekonzepte Onkologie. 3rd ed. Berlin & Heidelberg: Springer, 1998,: 436–475

# Carcinoma of the Esophagus

# Carcinoma of the Esophagus

A.M. Mauer, E.E. Vokes

## Epidemiology, Risk Factors

### Incidence

Carcinoma of the esophagus represents a leading cause of cancer relatal mortality worldwide, but accounts for only 2% of adult cancers in the United States [1]. This malignancy displays changing epidemiologic features and tremendous geographic variation. Within the U.S., the incidence of adenocarcinoma of the esophagus and proximal stomach is rising at an annual rate exceeding that any other malignancy [2]. In 1998, 12,300 new cases and 11,900 deaths from cancer of the esophagus are anticipated in the United States [1].

### Race, Sex, Age Distribution, Predisposition

The incidence of esophageal cancer increases with advancing age and the median age of onset is 67 years [3]. In most countries, this disease occurs two to four times more frequently in males than females [3]. Within the United States there are racial differences in incidence and disease histology with squamous cell carcinoma more commonly affecting blacks and adenocarcinoma more commonly affecting whites [3].

### Localization

Marked geographic variation in the incidence and mortality related to esophageal cancer exists. In areas of Iran and China, mortality rates exceed 100 per 100,000 population (U.S. rate <5 per 100,000 per year)

[3]. Substantial regional variation in incidence also occurs; these differences suggest that dietary and environmental factors may influence the development of this malignancy. The esophageal cancer mortality rate remains stable in most countries. While mortality from esophageal cancer is increasing in the United States and parts of western Europe, deaths related to this disease are decreasing in parts of Asia, possibly as a result of dietary modification and other factors such as earlier detection [4].

Risk Factors and Etiology

The etiology of carcinoma of the esophagus is unknown. A number of factors have been implicated in the pathogenesis of squamous cell carcinoma of the esophagus. Excessive ethanol intake and tobacco use increase risk, and appear to act synergistically [5]. A number of case control studies confirmed that dietary factors, independent of alcohol and tobacco use, contribute to esophagus cancer risk [3]. In the areas with the highest incidence of esophageal cancer, the diet is deficient in fruits and vegetables. Nutritional deficiencies of riboflavin, vitamin C, beta-carotene, magnesium, and zinc occur and may contribute to the pathogenesis [6]. Other conditions which predispose for esophageal cancer include: achalasia, caustic or thermal injury, chest radiotherapy, nitrosamine ingestion, and esophageal webs or diverticula [3, 7].

The reasons for the recent emergence of adenocarcinoma of the esophagus in the Western world are not well understood, although obesity and tobacco use have been implicated [8, 9]. The coexistence of Barrett's esophagus, a well-recognized and important risk factor for the development of adenocarcinoma of the esophagus, is not responsible for the increase observed. In Barrett's esophagus, chronic gastroesophageal reflux leads to replacement of the normal squamous epithelium by metaplastic columnar epithelium which may be followed by the development of dysplasia and carcinoma. In individuals with Barrett's esophagus, the annual rate of cancer development is 0.8% [10]. Endoscopic surveillance is mandatory for individuals with Barrett's esophagus, although there is disagreement regarding the optimal frequency [11]. Total esophagectomy is advocated for individuals with severe dysplasia as the frequency of coexisting microscopic adenocarcinoma is high, ranging between 43% and 83%, and the detection of early invasive adenocarcinoma is difficult [12, 13]. A number of potential markers, such as p53 gene deletion and cytogenetic aberrations, are under study to determine their role in the tumor progression of Barrett's esophagus to adenocarcinoma [14, 15].

The development and progression of esophageal cancer probably results from the mutation of multiple genes whose products regulate growth and differentiation. Analyses of molecular events underlying the development of esophageal have yielded several potential suppressor oncogenes (p53, APC, DCC, rb) and proto-oncogenes (cyclin-D, EGFR, HER-2, TGF-alpha) involved in tumorigenesis [16]. As more is understood about the details of carcinogenesis in the malignancy, new therapeutic strategies might be targeted at reversing the various pathways important for malignant development.

## Pathology and Staging

In recent years, adenocarcinoma has replaced squamous cell carcinoma as the predominant disease histology in the United States [3]. Most prior therapy trials included patients with epidermoid esophageal cancer. As more patients with adenocarcinoma of the esophagus accrue to studies and subgroup analyses can be completed, differences in natural history and therapeutic response rates between histologic subtypes may emerge.

The staging and stage grouping of esophageal cancer as proposed the American Joint Commission on Cancer is listed in Tables 1 and 2 [17]. The depth of tumor invasion through the esophageal wall determines the

**Table 1.** TNM classification of esophageal cancer by the AJCC

| | |
|---|---|
| Primary tumor | |
| Tis | Carcinoma in situ |
| T1 | Invades submucosa |
| T2 | Invades muscularis propria |
| T3 | Invades adventitia |
| T4 | Invades adjacent tissues |
| Regional lymph nodes[a] | |
| N0 | No lymph nodes involved |
| N1 | Regional lymph nodes involved |
| Distant metastases | |
| M0 | No distant metastases |
| M1 | Distant metastases evident |

For thoracic esophagus, regional lymph nodes include thoracic nodes only. For abdominal esophagus and gastroesophageal junction, celiac lymph nodes are considered, regional.
[a] For cervical esophagus, regional lymph nodes include cervical and supraclavicular nodes only.

**Table 2.** Esophageal cancer stage grouping

| Stage 0 | Tis N0 M0 |
|---|---|
| Stage I | T1 N0 M0 |
| Stage IIA | T2 N0 M0 |
| Stage IIA | T3 N0 M0 |
| Stage IIB | T1 N1 M0 |
| Stage IIB | T2 N1 M0 |
| Stage III | T3 N1 M0 |
| Stage III | T4 any N M0 |
| Stage IV | Any T any N M1 |

extent of the primary tumor (T). The definition of regional lymph node metastases (N) changes based upon the location of the primary tumor within the esophagus. Lymph node involvement outside of the regional lymph nodes represents M1 metastatic disease. Frequent sites of distant metastasis include the liver, bone, lung, and adrenal gland.

Prognosis

The low overall five year survival rate of <10% and the short median survival of 9 months associated with esophageal carcinoma reflect the poor prognosis [18]. Prognostic factors identified which predict survival include: depth of primary tumor invasion, length of primary tumor, lymph node involvement, and weight loss greater than 10%. The over-expression of several growth factors and growth factor receptors, such as epidermal growth factor and HER-2/neu receptor, has been recently correlated with survival, but none reliably predict clinical course [19, 20]. The poor prognosis of esophageal carcinoma may be attributed to the its early spread into the submucosal lymphatic network and lymph nodes, as well as the absence of a serosal wall to limit local extension. By the time symptoms develop, the disease is often systemic. Autopsy reports confirm that the majority of patients have occult metastases at the time of presentation [21, 22]. In addition, many individuals have poor nutritional status or comorbid conditions related to ethanol and tobacco use which make the delivery of therapy for carcinoma of the esophagus challenging.

## Work-up and Staging

The diagnosis of esophageal cancer generally requires upper gastrointestinal endoscopy and biopsy. Recommended preoperative clinical evaluation includes: chest roentgengram, barium swallow, and computed tomography of the chest and upper abdomen [23]. The CT scan is useful for assessing the liver, lungs, and adrenal glands for metastatic involvement. However, computed tomography does not accurately determine the primary tumor depth of invasion or lymph node metastatic disease. Nuclear magnetic resonance imaging provides the same staging information as CT scan and may better assess the extent of invasion into adjacent structures, but it is not as widely used. As the rate of second malignancy within the aerodigestive tract is high for individuals with squamous cell carcinoma, bronchoscopy should be performed to exclude synchronous lesions. For individuals with cancers involving the cervical esophagus, rigid bronchoscopy is required to exclude tracheoesophageal fistula. Bone scan is indicated only for individuals with clinical findings or laboratory abnormalities suggestive of bone metastases.

A number of other imaging techniques are available for the esophageal cancer staging, but their use is still considered investigational. Endoscopic ultrasonography offers improved resolution of the esophageal wall and may provide a more accurate assessment of tumor wall invasion [24]. This technique allows identification of lymph nodes in greater detail than the CT scan; however, it does not accurately differentiate benign from malignant nodes. Laparoscopy and positive emission tomography may aid detection of systemic tumor dissemination [25, 26]. As the current methods available for staging are limited, these newer techniques may provide more accurate staging and a better determination of appropriate treatment.

## Stage-Specific Standard Treatment Options

Two primary local control modalities, surgery and radiation therapy, exist for the management of esophageal cancer clinically limited to the local regional area, stages I to III. Unfortunately, distant and locoregional treatment failures are common following primary surgical resection or radiotherapy, and these interventions infrequently result in long term survival. The low survival rates achieved with single modality therapy have prompted the investigation of multimodality therapy for locally advanced esophageal cancer.

Surgical Treatment

Surgical resection offers good long term palliation of dysphagia, and may provide cure in patients with carcinoma in situ or stage I carcinoma. However, only 40%–50% of patients have resectable tumors and the prognosis for patients able to undergo surgical resection is poor. Most series report five year survival rates of <10% following primary surgical resection [27]. Contemporary series from centers with experience managing esophageal cancer report acceptable morbidity and mortality rates in the range of 5%–12% [28].

Several technical approaches may be employed for esophageal resection. Surgical resection generally involves a laparotomy to mobilize the gastrointestinal structures and to evaluate for metastases which would preclude a curative resection. The Ivor Lewis esophagectomy technique includes thoracotomy, dissection of regional lymph nodes, and intrathoracic gastroesophageal reanastomosis. Another technique, the transhiatal esophagectomy, utilizes an abdominal approach without thoracotomy for esophageal resection and lymph node resection. With this technique, the gastroesophageal anastomosis is completed through a cervical incision. Other more radical approaches sometimes advocated involve en bloc resection or three-field lymph node dissection. Although the technique of surgical resection remains vigorously debated, none appears to offer a survival benefit [28].

Radiotherapy

External beam radiation as primary therapy for advanced esophageal cancer offers palliation of dysphagia, but relief is short term and long term survival is a dismal 6% at 5 years [29]. Radiotherapy is often extended to poor prognosis patients with technically unresectable tumors or medical conditions which make them unsuitable for surgery. Consequently, comparisons between radiotherapy and surgical series are not meaningful. Two prospective randomized trials comparing surgery and radiotherapy as primary therapy were initiated in the U.S. and Europe, but never completed due to poor accrual [30].

Curative intent radiotherapy studies employ cumulative doses of 6000–7000 cGy in 180–200 cGy fractions. The toxicities commonly encountered include: skin irritation, fatigue, nausea, esophagitis, esophageal stricture, and less commonly, pneumonitis, pericarditis, and myelitis. Curative intent single modality radiation is being used less frequently as recent investigations demonstrate benefit of chemoradiotherapy over radiotherapy alone as definitive therapy.

A number of randomized studies have addressed neoadjuvant and adjuvant radiotherapy. The potential benefits of preoperative radiotherapy may include increased resectability and improved local control. Four randomized studies of preoperative radiotherapy failed to demonstrate an impact on overall survival in patients who received preoperative radiotherapy [31–34]. Two studies reported improved survival with preoperative radiotherapy, but the difference did not reach statistical significance [35, 36,]. Overall, the resectability was not improved in the group that received neoadjuvant therapy. Randomized studies of postoperative radiotherapy demonstrated that adjuvant postoperative therapy may improve locoregional control in node-negative patients; however, it provides no improvement in overall survival [37–39]. Based on these studies, there is no role for neoadjuvant radiotherapy, and the only definite role for adjuvant radiotherapy is in the setting of positive margins.

## Chemotherapy

A number of neoplastic agents have undergone testing for metastatic or recurrent esophageal cancer. In phase II studies, the most active single agents identified include: cisplatin, 5-fluorouracil, bleomycin, mitomycin, methotrexate, vindesine, doxorubicin, mitoguazone, paclitaxel, and vinorelbine [40, 41]. Overall, these single agents yield objective response rates between 15% and 35%, with higher response rates seen in localized disease. The response rates for cisplatin-based combination therapies which range from 30%–60% suggest that cisplatin-based combinations are superior to single agents; however, randomized studies comparing survival outcomes with single agent to combination therapy have not been completed. Cisplatin and fluorouracil is considered a standard combination regimen for treatment of squamous cell carcinoma. Single agent and combination regimens are not as well studied in adenocarcinoma, and there exists no therapy which is considered standard.

Based on the brief duration of response and minimal palliation of symptoms achieved with single agent and combination regimens, chemotherapy alone is not an effective primary therapy for esophageal cancer. Chemotherapy has a role in the multimodality therapy for esophageal cancer.

Combined Modality Therapy

Investigation of multimodality therapy for esophageal cancer has been undertaken to gain better local control and manage the systemic disease. Many phase II studies investigating multimodality therapy employing various combinations of chemotherapy, radiotherapy, and surgery have reported higher response rates than historical controls of surgery alone [42]. Based on the suggested improvement, a number of randomized trials have been completed to determine whether combined modality therapy is truly associated with an improved outcome. A second objective of these studies is the comparison of the toxicity of combined modality therapy against the current standard therapy of surgery.

In theory, preoperative (induction) chemotherapy may downstage local disease, facilitate resection, and eradicate micrometastatic disease. In addition, neoadjuvant chemotherapy allows for assessment of a tumor's sensitivity to the agent. Several phase II or pilot studies investigating various combination chemotherapy regimens in the preoperative setting have demonstrated the feasibility of this approach. Three small, randomized trials comparing preoperative chemotherapy to surgery alone are outlined in Table 3.

One trial conducted by Roth et al. enrolled 39 patients to surgery alone or two cycles of preoperative chemotherapy with cisplatin, bleomycin and vindesine, followed by surgery then six months of postoperative chemotherapy with cisplatin and vindesine [43]. Despite the 47% response rate to preoperative chemotherapy, there was no difference in median survival or resectability for the two treatment groups.

A study reported by Schlag included 46 patients randomized to immediate surgery or preoperative chemotherapy with cisplatin and fluorouracil for two cycles then surgery [44]. The preoperative chemotherapy produced a response rate of 47%, and was associated with considerable toxicity. There was no difference in the surgical resectability or median survival between treatment groups, but the chemotherapy group

**Table 3.** Preoperative chemotherapy randomized trials

| Reference | Histology | Regimen | n | Response rate (%) | Median survival (months) |
|---|---|---|---|---|---|
| Roth et al. [43] | Squam | Surgery | 20 | – | 9 |
| | | Preoperative cisplatin, bleomycin, vindesine x2 cycles then surgery followed by postoperative cisplatin, vindesinex6 months | 19 | 47 | 9 |
| Schlag [44] | Squam | Surgery | 40 | – | 9 |
| | | Preoperative cisplatin, 5-FU x3 cycles, surgery | 29 | 47 | 8 |
| Nygaard et al. [36] | Squam | Surgery | 50 | – | 3-yr 9% |
| | | Preoperative cisplatin, bleomycinx2 cycles, surgery | 56 | NR | 3-yr 3% |
| Kelsen et al. [45] | Squam, adeno | Surgery | 221 | B | 16.1 |
| | | Preoperative cisplatin, 5-FU x3 cycles, surgery, postoperative cisplatin, 5-FU x2 cycles | 202 | NR | 16.8 |

NR, Not reported. Squam, squamous cell. Adeno, adenocarcinoma.

had higher postoperative mortality. Based on the above interim analysis, the study was closed.

Nygaard et al completed a randomized study with four treatment arms: surgery alone; preoperative chemotherapy and surgery; preoperative radiotherapy and surgery; and preoperative chemotherapy plus sequential radiotherapy then surgery [36]. There was no significant difference in the survival for the surgery alone and preoperative chemotherapy groups, with 3-year survival rates of 9% and 3%, respectively.

An interim analysis of Intergroup study 113 (RTOG 89–11), a phase III study comparing neoadjuvant chemotherapy followed by surgery to surgery alone, has been reported by Kelsen et al [45]. The neoadjuvant treatment group received 3 cycles of cisplatin and fluorouracil then surgery. Patients who had stable disease or responding disease following the neoadjuvant therapy, received two additional cycles of chemotherapy postoperatively. This large study enrolled 467 patients with squamous cell or adenocarcinoma histologies. There was no increase in operative morbidity or mortality reported in the group receiving preoperative chemotherapy. At preliminary review, there was no benefit for preoperative chemotherapy in terms of resection rate, relapse free survival, or overall survival.

To date, all completely reported randomized studies have failed to demonstrate a survival benefit for preoperative chemotherapy followed by surgery over surgery alone. Until mature results of the Intergroup trial 113 become available, preoperative chemotherapy should be considered investigational for localized esophageal cancer.

Neoadjuvant Chemoradiation

The theoretical benefits of concomitant chemoradiation have been described by Vokes [46]. Concurrent administration of radiation and a chemotherapeutic agent with radiosensitizing properties may improve local control. Several phase II trials of neoadjuvant chemoradiotherapy have been conducted with conflicting results [42]. Many studies report increased, yet tolerable, toxicity with this combined modality approach. Based on the high rates of pathologic response and the encouraging survival results in these phase II studies, five randomized trials comparing preoperative chemoradiation followed by surgery with surgery alone were undertaken as outlined in Table 4.

**Table 4.** Neoadjuvant chemoradiotherapy randomized trials

| Reference | Histology | Regimen | n | Median survival (months) |
|---|---|---|---|---|
| Bosset et al. [48] | Squam | Surgery | 139 | 18.6 |
| | | Preoperative concurrent cisplatin x2 cycles and XRT 3750 cGy then surgery | 143 | 18.6 |
| Walsh et al. [49] | Adeno | Surgery | 55 | 11 |
| | | Preoperative concurrent cisplatin/5-FU x2 cycles and XRT 4000 cGy then surgery | 58 | 16 (p=0.01)* |
| Urba et al. [50] | Squam 25% Adeno 75% | Surgery | 50 | 3-yr 15% |
| | | Preoperative concurrent cisplatin, 5-FU, vinblastine and XRT 4500 cGy then surgery | 50 | 3-yr 32% (p=0.0402) |
| Le Prise et al. [47] | Squam | Surgery | 45 | 3-yr 13.8% |
| | | Preoperative sequential cisplatin, 5-FU x2 cycles then XRT 2000 cGy followed by surgery | 41 | 3-yr 19% (p=0.10) |
| Nygaard et al. [36] | Squam | Surgery | 50 | 3-yr 9% |
| | | Preoperative sequential cisplatin, bleomycin x2 cycles then XRT 3500 cGy followed by surgery | 53 | 3-yr 17 (p=0.3) |

Squam, squamous cell. Adeno, adenocarcinoma.

Two of the trials investigated sequential chemoradiotherapy followed by surgery versus surgery alone. In the study reported by LePrise et al., the multimodality therapy included a course of chemotherapy with cisplatin and fluorouracil followed by radiotherapy then a second course of cisplatin/5-FU chemotherapy before surgery [47]. The chemotherapy doses and cumulative radiotherapy dose (2,000 cGy) were low. A total of 86 patients were enrolled and there was no difference in 1- or 3-year survival rates.

The other study investigating sequential chemoradiotherapy reported by Nygaard utilized a chemotherapy regimen of cisplatin and bleomycin followed by radiation therapy of 3500 cGy the surgery [36]. There was no difference in the toxicity or survival outcome between the surgery alone and sequential chemoradiotherapy arms.

The trial reported by Bosset et al randomized 297 patients with stage I or II squamous cell carcinoma to surgery alone or preoperative combined therapy [48]. Concurrent chemoradiotherapy was delivered as two one-week courses separated by several weeks: cisplatin of 80 mg/m$^2$ each week and radiotherapy in five daily fractions of 3.7 Gy. This study was criticized for the use of single agent chemotherapy and the low cumulative radiation dose. The chemoradiation group experienced longer disease-free survival and higher frequency of curative resection. However, the postoperative mortality rate was higher with combined modality therapy, and there was no difference in survival between the two groups.

A randomized study by Walsh et al compared surgery alone to multimodality therapy in 113 patients with adenocarcinoma histology [49]. Multimodality therapy included two courses of chemotherapy (fluorouracil 15 mg/m$^2$ daily times five days and cisplatin 75 mg/m$^2$ on day 7) on weeks 1 and 6. Radiotherapy was administered beginning with the first course of chemotherapy for 15 fractions over 3 weeks to a cumulative dose of 4000 cGy. The chemoradiotherapy regimen was reportedly well tolerated. A comparison of the treatment groups revealed a survival advantage for the multimodality group, with 3-year survival rates of 37% for the multimodal group and 7% for the surgery alone group (p=0.01).

Urba and colleagues completed a phase III study of surgery alone versus trimodality therapy [50]. The preoperative chemotherapy included a 21-day continuous infusion of 5-FU combined with cisplatin and vinblastine. The concurrent radiotherapy was administered in 150 cGy fractions twice daily to a total dose of 4500 cGy. For the 100 patients accrued, a significant survival difference favoring the multimodality arm became evident only after several years of follow-up. Three-year survival rates for the surgery alone and multimodality arms were 15% and 32%, respectively (p=0.0402).

A phase III intergroup study is currently in progress to compare trimodality therapy to surgery alone for squamous cell carcinoma or adenocarcinoma of the esophagus. The multimodality therapy consists of cisplatin and fluorouracil with concurrent radiotherapy followed by surgery. This study designed accrue 620 patients will compare survival rates, toxicities and sites of failure for both treatment arms.

Thus to date, two phase III trials comparing concurrent chemoradiation plus surgery versus surgery alone demonstrate a survival benefit from multimodality therapy. Based on these studies, the continued investigation of preoperative concurrent chemoradiotherapy is warranted, but this approach should not be undertaken outside the setting of a clinical trial. For patients with resectable locoregional disease, surgery alone is the standard therapy.

## Combined Chemoradiotherapy as Definitive Therapy

Three randomized studies have compared concurrent chemoradiation to radiation therapy alone as definitive therapy for patients with unresectable esophageal carcinoma. A small randomized study reported from Brazil compared a regimen of concurrent mitomycin and bleomycin with radiation therapy (5,000 cGy) versus radiation therapy (5,000 cGy) alone [49]. There was no significant difference in survival between the groups.

A study conducted by the Eastern Cooperative Oncology Group randomized 119 patients with squamous cell carcinoma to fluorouracil and mitomycin with radiation (4,000 cGy) or radiation alone (4,000 cGy; Table 1) [52]. Individuals were allowed surgical resection after the 4000 cGy of radiation therapy; those who did not have surgery received an additional 2000 cGy of radiotherapy. A preliminary report in abstract form showed a difference in median survival in favor of the combined modality arm, 14.8 months versus 9.1 months (p=0.03). These results are difficult to interpret as some of the patients underwent surgery. An Intergroup study initiated by the RTOG conducted a randomized phase III study (RTOG 85-01) comparing combined chemoradiotherapy and radiotherapy alone in 123 patients with squamous cell carcinoma or

**Table 5.** Chemoradiation vs. radiation as primary therapy randomized trials

| Reference | Histology | Regimen | n | Median survival (months) |
|---|---|---|---|---|
| Sischy et al. [52] | Squam | Radiotherapy (6000 cGy) | 118 | 18.6 |
| | | Concurrent cisplatinx2 cycles and XRT 3750 cGy then surgery | 118 | 18.6 |
| Herskovic et al. [53, 54] | Adeno | Radiotherapy (6400 cGy) | 62 | 14.1 |
| | | Concurrent cisplatin, 5-FU and XRT 5000 cGy | 61 | 9 (p=0.01)* |
| Araujo et al. [51] | Squam | Radiotherapy (5000 cGy) | 31 | 3-yr 15% |
| | | Preoperative concurrent cisplatin, 5-FU, vinblastine and XRT 4500 cGy then surgery | 28 | 3-yr 32% (p=0.0402) |

adenocarcinoma [53, 54]. The chemoradiation arm included two courses of chemotherapy concomitant with radiation therapy to a cumulative dose of 5000 cGy then two additional courses of the same chemotherapy. The chemotherapy regimen consisted of cisplatin 75 mg/m² on day 1 and fluorouracil 1000 mg/m² per day on days 1 through 4 administered every 4 weeks during radiotherapy then every 3 weeks after radiotherapy. The radiation therapy alone arm included 6.4 weeks of therapy to a cumulative dose of 6400 cGy. Systemic toxicity was greater in the multimodality arm with 64% experiencing grade 3 or 4 toxicity, but the local toxicity was similar in both arms. The initial report and an update with all patients followed to 5 years demonstrated a survival advantage for concurrent chemoradiation [54]. At five years, thirty percent in the chemoradiation group were alive compared to no patients in the radiotherapy alone arm. A lower rate of the local failure and decreased incidence of systemic metastases was also evident in the chemoradiation therapy arm. This study provides strong evidence that concurrent chemoradiation is superior to radiotherapy alone for patients with unresectable esophageal cancer, especially squamous cell carcinoma; thus this regimen has been accepted as a standard therapy for those individuals with localized esophageal cancer who require nonsurgical therapy.

Based on the positive results of RTOG 85-01, a phase II study was undertaken to intensify the regimen [55]. The fluorouracil chemotherapy infusion was increased from a four day to a five day infusion of fluorouracil 1000 mg/m² per day on days 1 through 5. The total number of chemotherapy cycles was increased to five and the cumulative radiotherapy dose was modified from 5000 cGy to 6400 cGy. By preliminary report, the incidence of grade 3–4 toxicity was similar to that reported for the RTOG 85-01 trial; however, increased treatment-related mortality noted with this intensified regimen limited its further application.

## Current Questions Regarding Multimodality Therapy

For multimodality therapy, the relative contributions of each modality to survival advantage are not known. The reported failure patterns following treatment with a multimodality approach vary [54, 56]. At present, no consensus exists regarding the need for surgery in patients with localized disease. Many favor surgical resection when possible, as this approach may confer long term survival in the individual with infield residual microscopic disease following chemoradiation. For patients with unresectable disease, chemoradiation appears superior to radiation alone and may be curative.

It remains unclear whether differences in the natural history and responsiveness to therapy occur based on tumor histology. Results of ongoing larger scale trials statistically powered to these detect such differences will be available in the near future.

Palliative Therapy

For metastatic esophageal cancer, the goals of therapy are entirely palliative, specifically, the improvement of pain and the restoration of swallowing function. Local control measures including radiotherapy, brachytherapy, expansile stents, and photodynamic therapy often provide sufficient short term palliation [58-60]. Chemotherapy, if active, may contribute to local control, but its effect upon survival is unknown. Due to the short median survival for metastatic disease, surgical bypass is generally not indicated for palliation of dysphagia.

Current and Future Investigational Approaches

Although significant advances have been made in the management of patients with carcinoma of the esophagus, the disease continues to be associated with an extremely poor prognosis. With a better understanding of the biology of esophageal cancer, targeted strategies for the prevention, diagnosis, and treatment of the disease will be developed. Multimodality therapy has a definite role in this disease, but current treatments are limited by the lack of effective cytotoxic therapy. The investigation of newer agents and approaches may provide enhanced activity while producing less toxicity. The accrual to well designed clinical trials is essential for progress.

## References

1. Landis SH, Murray T, Bolden S, Wingo PA. (1998) Cancer Statistics. CA J Clin. 48:6-29
2. Blot W, Devesa S, Kneller R et al. (1991) Rising incidence of adenocarcinoma of the esophagus and gastric cardia. JAMA 265:1287-1289

3. Blot WJ. Esophageal cancer trends and risk factors. (1994) Semin Oncol 21:403–410
4. Zheng W, Jin F, Devesa SS et al. Declining incidence is greater for esophageal than gastric cancer in Shanghai, People's Republic of China. (1993) Br J Can 68:978–982
5. Blot WJ. Alcohol and Cancer. (1992) Cancer Res 52:2119s-2123 s (suppl)
6. VanRensburg SJ. Epidemiologic and dietary evidence for a specific nutritional predisposition to esophageal cancer. (1981) JNCI 67:243–251
7. Sherrill DJ, Grishkin BA, Golal FS, Zajtchuk R, Graeber GM. (1984) Radiation associated malignancies of the esophagus. Cancer 54:726–728
8. Brown MB, Swanson CA, Gridley G et al. (1995) Adenocarcinoma of the esophagus: role of obesity and diet. J Natl Cancer Inst 87:104–109
9. Chow WH, Finkle WD, µlaughlin J et al. (1995) The relation of gastroesophageal reflux disease and its treatment to adenocarcinomas of the esophagus and gastric cardia. JAMA 274:474–477
10. Spechler SJ. (1992) The frequency of esophageal cancer in patients with Barrett's esophagus. Acta Endoscopica 22:541–544
11. Provenzale D, Kemp JA, Arora S, Wong JB. (1994) A guide for surveillance of patients with Barrett's esophagus. Am J Gastr 89:670–680
12. Heitmiller RF, Redmond M, Hamilton SR. (1996) Barrett's esophagus with high-grade dysplasia, an indication for prophylactic esophagectomy. Annals Surg 224:66–71
13. Edwards MJ, Gable DR, Lentsch AB et al. (1996) The rationale for esophagectomy as the optimal therapy for Barrett's esophagus with high grade dysplasia. Annals Surg 223:585–591
14. Casson AG, Mukhopadhyay T, Clear KR et al. (1991) p53 gene mutations in Barrett's epithelium and esophageal cancer. Cancer Res 51:4495–4499
15. Blount PL, Galipeau PC, Sanchez CA et al. (1994)17p Allelic losses in diploid cells of patients with Barrett's esophagus who develop aneuploidy. Cancer Res 54:2292–2295
16. Rosen N. (1994) The molecular basis for cellular transformation: implications for esophageal carcinogenesis. Semin Oncol 21:416–424
17. American Joint Committee on Cancer. Esophagus. In: Fleming ID, Cooper JS, Henson DE, et al. eds. Manual for staging of cancer, ed 5. Philadelphia: JB Lippincott, 1997:65–69
18. Kosary CL, Ries L, Miller BA et al. (1996) SEER Cancer Statistics Review, 1973–1992. Bethesda, MD, DHHS, NIH Pub No. 96–2789
19. Mukaida H, Toi, Hirai et al. (1991) Clinical significance of the expression of epidermal growth factor and its receptor in esophageal cancer. Cancer 68:142–148
20. Nakamura T, Nekarda H, Hoelscher AH et al. (1994) Prognostic value of DNA ploidy and c-erb-2 overexpression in adenocarcinoma of Barrett's esophagus. Cancer 73:1785–1794
21. Anderson LL, Lad TE. (1982) Autopsy findings in squamous-cell carcinoma of the esophagus. Cancer 50:1587–1590
22. Bosch A, Frias Z, Caldwell WL et al. (1972) Autopsy findings in carcinoma of the esophagus. Acta Radiologica Oncol 18:103–112
23. Koch J, Halvorsen RA. (1994) Staging of esophageal cancer: Computed tomography, magnetic resonance imaging, and endoscopic ultrasound. Semin Roentgenol 29:364–372
24. Lightdale CJ. (1992) Endoscopic ultrasonography in the diagnosis, staging, and follow-up of esophageal and gastric cancer. Endoscopy 24:297–303
25. O'Brien MG, Fitzgerald EF, Lee G, et al (1995) A prospective comparison of laparoscopy and imaging in the staging of esophagogastric cancer before surgery. Am J Gastroenterol 90:2191–2194

26. Leketich JD, Schauer PR, Meltzer CC et al. (1997) Role of positron emission tomography in staging esophageal cancer. Ann Thorac Surg 64:765–769
27. Earlam R, Cunha-Melo. (1980) Oesophageal squamous cell carcinoma: I. A critical review of surgery. Br J Surgery 67:381–390
28. Roth JA, Putnam JB. (1994) Surgery for cancer of the esophagus. Semin Oncol 21:453–461
29. Earlam R, Cunha-Melo JR. (1980) Oesophageal squamous cell carcinoma: II. A critical review of radiotherapy. Br J Surgery 67:457–461
30. Earlam R. (1991) An MRC prospective randomized trial of radiotherapy versus surgery for operable squamous cell carcinoma of the esophagus. Ann R Coll Surg Engl 73:8–12
31. Mei W, Xian-Zhi G, Weibo Y et al. (1989) Randomized clinical trial on the combination of preoperative irradiation and surgery in the treatment of esophageal carcinoma: Report on 206 patients. Int J Radiat Oncol Biol Phys 16:325–327
32. Gignoux M, Roussel A, Paillot B et al. (1987) The value of preoperative radiotherapy in esophageal cancer: Results of a study of the E.O.R.T.C.. World J Surg 11:426–432
33. Launois B, Delarue D, Campion JP et al. (1981) Preoperative radiotherapy for carcinoma of the esophagus. Surg Gynecol Obstet 153:690–692
34. Arnott SJ, Duncan W, Kerr GR et al. (1993) Low dose preoperative radiotherapy for carcinoma of the oesophagus: Results of a randomized clinical trial. Radiother Oncol 24:108–113
35. Huang GJ, Gu XZ, Wang LJ, et al. Combined preoperative irradiation and surgery for esophageal carcinoma, in Delarue NC (ed): International Trends in General Thoracic Surgery. St. Louis, MO, Mosby, 1988, pp 315–318
36. Nygaard K, Hagen S, Hansen HS, et al. (1992) Pre-operative radiotherapy prolongs survival in operable esophageal carcinoma: A randomized, multicenter study of preoperative radiotherapy and chemotherapy. The second Scandinavian trial in esophageal cancer. World J Surg 16:1104–1110
37. Kasai M, Mori S, Watanabe T. (1978) Follow-up results after resection of thoracic esophageal carcinoma. World J Surg 2:543–551
38. Fok M, Sham JST, Choy D et al. (1993) Postoperative radiotherapy for carcinoma of the esophagus: A prospective, randomized controlled trial. Surgery 113:138–147
39. Teniere P, Hay J, Fingerhut A et al. (1991) Postoperative radiation therapy does not increase survival after curative resection for squamous cell carcinoma of the middle and lower esophagus as shown by a multicenter controlled trial. Surg Gynecol Obstet 173:123–130
40. Ajani JA. (1994) Contributions of chemotherapy in the treatment of carcinoma of the esophagus: results and commentary. Semin Oncol 21:474–482
41. Conroy T, Etienne PL, Adenis A et al. (1996) Phase II trial of vinorelbine in metastatic squamous cell esophageal carcinoma. J Clin Oncol 14:164–170
42. Ilson DH, Kelsen DP (1994) Combined modality therapy in the treatment of esophageal cancer. Semin Oncol 21:493–507
43. Roth JA, Pass HU, Flanagan MM et al. (1988) Randomized clinical trial of preoperative and postoperative adjuvant chemotherapy with cisplatin, vindesine, and bleomycin for carcinoma of the esophagus. J Thorac Cardiovasc Surg 96:242–248
44. Schlag PM. (1992) Randomized trial of preoperative chemotherapy for squamous cell cancer of the esophagus. Arch Surg 127:1446–1450
45. Kelsen DP, Ginsberg R, Qian C, Gunderson L et al. (1997) Chemotherapy followed by operation versus operation in the treatment of patients with localized esophageal cancer: a preliminary report of intergroup study 113 (RTOG 89–11) Proc Am Soc Clin Oncol 16:276a (abstract #982)

46. Vokes EE, Weichselbaum RR. (1990) Concomitant chemoradiotherapy: Rationale and clinical experience in patients with solid tumors. J Clin Oncol 8:911–934

47. Le Prise E, Etienne P, Meunier B, et al (1994) A randomized study of chemotherapy, radiation therapy, and surgery versus surgery for localized squamous cell carcinoma of the esophagus. Cancer 73:1779–1784

48. Bosset JF, Gignoux M, Triboulet JP et al. (1997) Chemoradiotherapy followed by surgery compared with surgery alone in squamous-cell cancer of the esophagus. N Engl J Med 337:161-167

49. Walsh T, Noonan N, Hollywood D, et al (1996) A comparison of multimodal therapy and surgery for esophageal adenocarcinoma. N Engl J Med 335:462–467

50. Urba S, Orringer M, Turrisi A et al. (1997) A randomized trial comparing surgery (S) to preoperative concomitant chemoradiation plus surgery in patients (pts) with resectable esophageal cancer (CA): updated analysis. Proc Am Soc Clin Oncol 16:277a (abstract)

51. Araujo CMM, Souhami L, Gil RA, et al (1991) A randomized trial comparing radiation therapy versus concomitant radiation therapy and chemotherapy in carcinoma of the thoracic esophagus. Cancer 67:2258–2261

52. Sischy B, Ryan L, Haller D et al. (1990) Interim report of EST 1282 phase III protocol for the evaluation of combined modalities in the treatment of patients with carcinoma of the esophagus. Proc Am Soc Clin Oncol 9:105 (abstr)

53. Herskovic A, Martz L, Al-Sarraf M et al. (1992) Combined chemotherapy and radiotherapy compared with radiotherapy alone in patients with cancer of the esophagus. N Engl J Med 326:1593–1598

54. Al-Sarraf M, Martz K, Herskovic A et al. (1997) Progress report of combined chemotherapy versus radiotherapy alone in patients with esophageal cancer: an intergroup study. J Clin Oncol 15:277–284

55. Minsky BD, Neuberg D, Kelsen D et al. (1996) Neoadjuvant chemotherapy plus concurrent chemotherapy and high dose radiation for squamous cell carcinoma of the esophagus – A preliminary analysis of the phase II Intergroup trial 0122. J Clin Oncol 14:149–155

56. Gill PG, Denham JW, Jamieson GG et al. (1992) Patterns of treatment failure and prognostic factors associated with the treatment of esophageal carcinoma with chemotherapy and radiotherapy either as sole treatment or followed by surgery. J Clin Oncol 10, 1037–1043

57. Whittington R, Coia LR, Haller DG et al. (1990) Adenocarcinoma of the esophagus and esophago-gastric junction: the effects of single and combined modalities on the survival and patterns of failure following treatment. Int J Radiat Oncol Biol Phys 19:593–603

58. Moni J, Armstrong JG, Minsky BD et al. (1996) High dose rate intraluminal brachytherapy for carcinoma of the esophagus. Dis Esoph 9:123–12

59. Sur RK, Sigh DP, Sharma SC. (1992) Radiation therapy of esophageal cancer: Role of high dose rate brachytherapy. Int J Radiat Oncol Biol Phy 22:1043–1046

60. Heier SK, Rothman KA, Heier LM, Rosenthal WS. (1996) Photodynamic therapy for obstructing esophageal cancer: light dosimetry and randomized comparison with Nd:YAG laser therapy. Gastroenterology 109:63–72

# Lung Cancer

# Non-Small-Cell Lung Cancer

E.E. Vokes

## Epidemiology and Risk Factors

Lung Cancer is the second most common malignancy in and females; its incidence ranks behind only prostate and breast cancer, respectively. However, it is by far the most common cause of death from a malignancy in both genders indicating that it is diagnosed at later stages and less successfully treated than breast and prostate cancer [1, 2]. In 1997, the incidence of lung cancer was 180,000 in the United States and 160,000 patients died of this disease. An estimated 160,000 patients have non-small cell lung cancer (NSCLC) histology. In recent years the death rate from lung cancer has begun to decrease in males reflecting successful smoking intervention programs. In women the death rate continues to rise reflecting the increased incidence of smoking in women. The disease occurs in all races with no known specific racial predisposition. Approximately 40%–50% of patients with NSCLC present with metastatic disease (stage IV, or M1 disease) and an additional 30% with locally or regionally advanced disease confined to the chest (stage IIIA or IIIB). Only a minority of patients present with early stage disease defined as stages I or II (Table 1). The latter is due to the lack of a clinical early warning signs and the absence of successful screening methods in high risk populations.

A variety of risk factors have been described. Of these, tobacco smoking is by far the most important. In fact, until the early 20th century and the introduction of cigarettes to a large proportion of the population, lung cancer was a rare disease. There is evidence of a tobacco dose-cancer risk relation. This risk increases with a higher number of cigarettes smoked and the number of years of smoking. This knowledge emphasizes the need for smoking prevention programs. Potential additional risk factors include asbestos exposure (the latter appears to be synergistic

**Table 1.** Stage grouping (with permission of the AJCC)

| | |
|---|---|
| Primary tumor | |
| TX | Primary tumor cannot be assessed, or tumor proven by the presence of malignant cells in sputum or bronchial washings but not visualized by imaging or bronchoscopy |
| T0 | No evidence of primary tumor |
| Tis | Carcinoma in situ |
| T1 | Tumor 3 cm or less in greatest dimension, surrounded by lung or visceral pleura, without bronchoscopic evidence of invasion more proximal than the lobar bronchusa (i.e., note in the main bronchus) |
| T2 | Tumor with any of the following features of size or extent: More than 3 cm in greatest dimension. Involves main bronchus, 2 cm or more distal to the carina. Invades the visceral pleura |
| T3 | Tumor of any size that directly invades any of the following: chest wall (including superior sulcus tumors), diaphragm, mediastinal pleura, parietal pericardium; or tumor in the main bronchus less than 2 cm distal to the carina, but without involvement of the carina; or associated atelectasis or obstructive pneumonitis of the entire lung |
| T4 | Tumor of any size that invades any of the following: mediastinum, heart, great vessels, trachea, esophagus, vertebral body, carina; or separate tumor nodules in the same lobe; or tumor with a malignant pleural effusionb |
| Regional lymph nodes | |
| NX | Regional lymph nodes cannot be assessed |
| N0 | No regional lymph node metastasis |
| N1 | Metastasis to ipsilateral peribronchial and/or ipsilateral hilar lymph nodes, and intrapulmonary nodes including involvement by direct extension of the primary tumor |
| N2 | Metastasis to ipsilateral mediastinal and/or subcarinal lymph node(s) |
| N3 | Metastasis to contralateral mediastinal, contralateral hilar, ipsilateral or contralateral scalene, or supraclavicular lymph nodes(s) |
| Distant metastasis | |
| MX | Distant metastasis cannot be assessed |
| M0 | No distant metastasis |
| M1 | Distant metastasis presentc |
| Stage grouping | |
| Occult carcinoma | TX N0 M0 |
| Stage 0 | Tis N0 M0 |
| Stage IA | T1 N0 M0 |
| Stage IB | T2 N0 M0 |
| Stage IIA | T1 N1 M0 |
| Stage IIB | T2 N1 M0 |
| | T3 N0 M0 |
| Stage IIIA | T1 N2 M0 |
| | T2 N2 M0 |

|           |              |
|-----------|--------------|
|           | T3 N1 M0     |
|           | T3 N2 M0     |
| Stage IIIB | Any T N3 M0 |
|           | T4 any N M0  |
| Stage IV  | Any T any N M1 |

a The uncommon superficial tumor of any size with its invasive component limited to the bronchial wall, which may extend proximal to the main bronchus, is also classified T1.

b Most pleural effusions associated with lung cancer are due to tumor. However, there are a few patients in whom multiple cytopathologic examinations of pleural fluid are negative for tumor. In these cases, fluid is nonbloody and is not an exudate. When these elements and clinical judgment dictate that the effusion is not related to the tumor, the effusion should be excluded as a staging element and the patient should be staged T1, T2, or T3.

c M1 includes separate tumor nodule(s) in a different lobe (ipsilateral or contralateral).

with tobacco smoking). Exposure to radon is considered to be a potential risk factors as well.

## Pathology

NSCLC is classically divided into three subtypes, including adenocarcinoma, squamous cell carcinoma, and large cell carcinoma [2]. More than one histologic pattern may be observed in a given tumor. When a specific tumor subtype can not be described, tumors are sometimes classified as poorly differentiated NSCLC or as just NSCLC without a further subspecification. An additional infrequent entity is bronchioalvelar carcinoma. Bronchioalvelar carcinoma arises frequently in scars of previous sites of inflammation (e.g., tuberculosis), has a less firm association with smoking, and is frequently multicentric.

## Staging

The most recent staging classification of the UICC is shown in Table 1 [3]. Based on the TNM classification, stage I denotes a small primary lesion with no lymphadenopathy. Stage II includes T2 primaries with hilar lymphadenopathy or T3 primaries with no lymph node involvement. Stage III is divided into stage IIIA and IIIB. Stage IIIA represents technically resectable disease that is confined to one hemithorax while stage IIIB describes regionally advanced disease involving the contralateral mediastinum or supraclavicular lymph nodes; stage IIIB is usually not thought to be resectable. Finally, stage IV is identified by the presence of distant metastases (M1). This includes metastases to the contralateral lung or sites outside of the chest.

The prognosis of NSCLC is closely related to this staging process. Patients with stage I disease can be cured in over 50% of cases particularly if this is pathological stage I disease (i.e., pathologically confirmed after surgery). Patients with stage II disease have a long-term cure rate of approximately 40%. For patients with stage III disease, utilizing combined modality approaches, long term cure rates are between 10% and 25%. Stage IV disease is treated with palliative intent and can not be cured. Median survival time of patients treated with currently available therapies are 8 to 10 months.

## Patient Work-up

Since NSCLC frequently disseminates early, a minimal staging work-up includes a CT scan of the chest and upper abdomen including the liver and adrenal glands [2]. Additional studies should be directed by the presence or absence of clinical symptoms. Many patients will receive a CT scan of the brain and/or a bone scan if specific symptoms suggest possible involvement of these sites. Aggressive work-up of potential bony metastases is indicated since bone involvement is frequent and can lead to local complications including spinal cord compression. There are no specific tumor markers currently available. The identification of specific oncogenes that may indicate a favorable or less favorable prognosis is currently under investigation. In particular, the K-ras oncogene has been postulated to confer a less favorable prognosis; however, these observations still require confirmation in larger studies [2].

## Stage-Specific Therapy: Early Stage Disease (Stage I, Stage II)

Patients with clinical stage I or II disease should be treated with curative intent. Therapy should consist of surgical removal of the tumor and hilar lymph nodes if involved. A mediastinoscopy should be performed to rule out pathological N2 or N3 disease with microscopic involvement of mediastinal lymph nodes. Postoperative radiotherapy has not been demonstrated to increase survival times, although it may increase local and regional control. Nevertheless, at many institutions patients would receive postoperative radiation therapy at least for stage II disease. Whether adjuvant chemotherapy should be administered is also unclear [4]. Until more definitive data from recent and current large randomized trials become available, adjuvant chemotherapy cannot be considered a standard therapy option. Similarly, patients with stage I disease are known to be not only at risk of recurrence of their primary cancer, but also at risk of developing another malignancy if they are cured of their first cancer. It has been postulated that the administration of 13-cis-retinoic acid could prevent the formation of such second malignancies. Therefore, a large randomized trial in which patients received either placebo or three years of 13-cis-retinoic acid was conducted. With over 1000 patients enrolled, this study recently was closed to accrual and an analysis is expected within the next few years.

Patients with poor performance status or compromised pulmonary function that would prohibit the performance of pulmonary resection are frequently treated with single modality radiation therapy. Cure rates following radiation therapy alone are lower than those achieved with surgery. Therefore, patients treated with this "inferior" single agent treatment modality need to be carefully selected in order to avoid withholding a potentially more curative surgical option from the patient.

## Stage III Disease

Stage III disease is clinically divided into stage IIIA (potentially resectable) and stage IIIB (unresectable) disease. Previous staging classification systems included patients with T3No disease in the group of stage IIIA patients. Since these patients have now been recognized to have a distinctly more favorable prognosis more akin to patients with stage II disease, they are now classified as stage IIB [3]. Traditionally, patients with stage III disease received surgery (for resectable disease) followed by postoperative radiotherapy or single modality radiotherapy alone. During the 1980s, the addition of chemotherapy was investigated. Both sequential approaches (induction chemotherapy or adjuvant chemotherapy) and concurrent chemoradiotherapy approaches were explored. In addition, novel radiation therapy schedules, i.e., hyperfractionated or accelerated radiation therapy have been pursued. More definitive data regarding these multimodality therapy approaches are currently available for patients with unresectable disease. Stage IIIA is less common and, with the inclusion of surgery in the overall treatment plan, more complex from a logistical point of view. Combined modality therapy is therefore reviewed largely as currently described for patients with unresectable stage III disease.

## Induction Chemotherapy

Induction chemotherapy is the most thoroughly and successfully studied approach to combined modality therapy of stage IIIB NSCLC to date [4]. Its rationale is based on the early use of systemically active drugs. These are hoped to eradicate potential present microscopic systemic tumor cells. In addition, active chemotherapy agents may be able to reduce the locoregional tumor burden prior to the administration of subsequent locoregional therapy [2]. Early pilot studies indicated the feasibility of induction chemotherapy. Furthermore, response rates were consistently demonstrated to be higher than those previously documented in patients with stage IV disease. Several randomized studies evaluating this approach have been completed. In CALGB study 8433, patients were randomized to receive radiotherapy alone (60 Gy with standard fractionation) or 2 cycles of cisplatin/vinblastine followed by identical radiation therapy [5]. In this study, patients receiving chemotherapy were found to have a significantly longer median survival time (14 vs. 10 months); in addition, chemotherapy treated patients had a higher 5 year survival rate at 17% vs. 7% observed for patients treated with radiotherapy alone. Since this study was closed early to patient accrual (after identification of a statistically significant survival difference) a confirmatory trial was undertaken [6]. Patients again received either radiotherapy alone to 60 Gy vs. 2 cycles of induction chemotherapy with cisplatin and vinblastine followed by radiotherapy to 60 Gy; in this trial, a third arm was added investigating the use of hyperfractionated radiotherapy at 1.2 Gy twice daily to a 69.6 Gy total dose. This trial confirmed a significant survival advantage for induction chemotherapy followed by radiotherapy over radiotherapy alone. Median survival times were 13 months for chemotherapy vs. 11 months for standard radiotherapy. Of interest, with intermediate follow up it appears that hyperfractionated radiation therapy results in a similar long term survival rate as induction chemotherapy. A pattern of failure analysis has been conducted in this trial. It confirms previous observations that the effects of induction chemotherapy are mediated through increased systemic control, confirming the ability of induction chemotherapy to eradicate microscopic systemic disease. Induction chemotherapy has no effect on local and regional control. Since induction chemotherapy has been shown to increase survival in these and other large studies, it can now be considered a possible standard treatment option for patients with regionally advanced unresectable stage III NSCLC.

## Concomitant Chemoradiotherapy

Concomitant chemoradiotherapy aims at the simultaneous administration of systemic therapy while also enhancing the local and regional effects of radiation therapy. For this postulate to transform into clinical reality, it requires the administration of systemically active chemotherapy that can eradicate micrometastatic disease while also enhancing the effects of radiation therapy locoregionally [7]. In clinical practice, most randomized trials have reported on the use of single agent cisplatin with concurrent radiation therapy [2, 8]. Although cisplatin is an active drug in NSCLC, its use as a single agent and at frequently suboptimal doses may compromise its ability to eradicate potential micrometastatic disease. Of four randomized trials comparing radiotherapy alone vs. radiotherapy with cisplatin administered during radiation, three were negative with no clinically or statistically significant difference with regards to survival. A fourth study, however, indicated a benefit for the daily administration of cisplatin [8]. In this study, patients received radiotherapy alone (55 Gy administered over 8 weeks) vs. the same radiotherapy administered with either daily cisplatin at 6 mg/m$^2$ per day or weekly cisplatin at 30 mg/m$^2$ per week; on both treatment arms the total cisplatin dose was 120 mg/m$^2$. Patients receiving radiotherapy with concurrent cisplatin had a statistically significantly superior locoregional control and survival than patients receiving radiotherapy alone. Unfortunately, the trial is difficult to interpret since patients on the "control arm" received a fairly low dose of radiotherapy over a prolonged period of time. Nevertheless, it is of interest that the administration of cisplatin at low doses did not increase systemic control but did increase locoregional control when compared with radiotherapy alone. This finding suggests that concomitant chemoradiotherapy may be of benefit in unresectable NSCLC.

## Hyperfractionated or Accelerated Radiotherapy

The use of more aggressive radiation therapy schedules in stage IIIB NSCLC has also been investigated. The rationale here is that more frequently administered radiotherapy may decrease the proliferation of tumor cells between radiation fractions. This, in turn, may translate into increased locoregional control which in the most optimistic scenario would also decrease the chance of the tumor to disseminate systemically. Hyperfractionated radiotherapy has been investigated in the large Intergroup study mentioned above [6]. Preliminary data suggest no impact on median survival time but a possible increased long term survival rate that may be equivalent to that achieved with induction chemotherapy. Accelerated radiotherapy has been investigated in one large randomized trial. In this British study, patients received either a standard radiotherapy to 60 Gy over 6 weeks or a regimen of continuous hyperfractionated accelerated radiation therapy ("CHART" consisting of three daily fractions of 1.5 Gy each, administered over 12 consecutive days) [9, 10]. In this trial, patients treated with CHART had increased local and regional control and an increased 2 year survival (29% vs 20%); however, this study population differs from that studied in the previously mentioned trials investigating concomitant chemoradiotherapy or induction chemotherapy. A large proportion of patients had earlier stage disease (stages I through IIIA); in addition, approximately 80% of patients had squamous cell NSCLC histology. Since both early stage disease and squamous cell histology are thought to represent a lower risk of micrometastatic dissemination, this trial must be interpreted with some caution. Nevertheless, it is exciting that a more aggressive radiation therapy schedule may improve survival of NSCLC patients and that this effect may be mediated through a mechanism that differs from that involved in mediating the beneficial effects of induction chemotherapy.

## Key Questions and Current Investigations in Stage IIIB Disease

Combined modality therapy has clearly been shown to be of benefit. While induction chemotherapy is currently best supported, there is also available evidence supporting the use of concomitant chemoradiotherapy or intensified radiotherapy schedules. Current efforts are therefore focused on identifying whether induction chemotherapy is truly superior to concomitant chemoradiotherapy (i.e., the optimal schedule of drug administration) or on exploiting the differential mechanisms underline the beneficial effects observed with induction chemotherapy and concomitant chemoradiotherapy. For example, a study in the USA is currently studying induction chemotherapy with two cycles of cisplatin and vinblastine versus the simultaneous administration of this chemotherapy with radiotherapy and a third arm exploring hyperfractionated radiation therapy with concurrent cisplatin and oral etoposide. Japanese investigators have already presented a preliminary analysis of a similar trial investigating the administration of mitomycin, vinblastine, and cisplatin either prior to or during radiation therapy. In their trial, the median survival times with induction chemotherapy were 13 months compared with 16 months for the concurrent administration of this multiagent regimen with radiation therapy [11]. If confirmed, the latter observation would suggest that administration of multiagent systemically active chemotherapy with concurrent radiotherapy may indeed be the most successful combined modality therapy approach to NSCLC.

Other efforts are currently investigating the administration of more than one combined modality approach. For example, one larger randomized trial is comparing induction chemotherapy followed by radiotherapy versus induction chemotherapy followed by accelerated radiotherapy. Similarly, in the Cancer and Leukemia Group B (CALGB) a trial is evaluating the administration of two cycles of chemotherapy followed by two additional chemotherapy cycles administered during radiation therapy. Of note, in this trial several new chemotherapy agents with activity in NSCLC are included in the chemotherapy regimens [12] (see below).

## Stage IIIA Disease

Combined modality investigations in stage IIIA disease have been similar to those outlined above for unresectable disease. However to date, there is no conclusive evidence favoring the addition of chemotherapy when compared with surgery and radiation therapy alone. Nevertheless, two small randomized trials (60 patients each) indicated a marked gain in survival through the use of induction chemotherapy [13, 14]; however, a third even smaller study failed to confirm a survival advantage. Efforts at identifying the optimal approach to resectable stage III NSCLC are therefore continuing. In addition, the value of surgery is being explored. In a large randomized study, patients receive cisplatin, etoposide, and concomitant radiotherapy followed by either surgery or a chemoradiotherapy boost. This study is based on promising phase II data utilizing a combination of cisplatin/etoposide and concomitant radiotherapy prior to surgery [15].


**Stage IV Non-Small Cell Lung Cancer**

Patients with stage IV NSCLC are treated with palliative intent [16, 17]. This includes palliative radiotherapy for painful bony involvement or lesions obstructing parts of the lung leading to post-obstructive pneumonia. It may also involve the selective use of surgical procedures to relieve airway obstructions.

For the large majority of patients, the use of chemotherapy should be considered. Single agents with activity NSCLC (defined as a response rate of approximately 10%–15% or higher) are listed the following:
– Before 1990
  – Cisplatin
  – Carboplatin
  – Etoposide
  – Vinblastine
  – Vindesine
– Since 1990
  – Vinorelbine
  – Paclitaxel
  – Docetaxel
  – Gemcitabine
  – Irinotecan

During the 1980s it was questioned whether chemotherapy resulted in a prolongation of survival when compared with best supportive care. As a result, a large number of such studies was undertaken [18, 19]. While the majority of these studies were too small to allow for independent conclusions, some studies did confirm a survival benefit while virtually all others demonstrated the same statistical trend. Meta-analyses of these trials have been performed and confirm an increase in survival of approximately two months (6 vs. 8 months) [4]. Similarly, cost analyses have indicated that the financial cost of administering chemotherapy for NSCLC cancer is similar to that of other widely accepted interventions in medicine. More recently, quality of life analyses have been added. Although the available literature studying the quality of life in lung cancer is only emerging at this time, there is clear indication that patients receiving chemotherapy also have a higher quality of life when compared with best supportive care alone.

In recent years, several new drugs with single agent activity have been identified (see above) [20]. Several of these drugs have already been compared to a previous standard regimens of the 1980s (usually cisplatin, etoposide, or cisplatin with a vinca-alkaloid such as vinblastine or vindesine). For example, vinorelbine combined with cisplatin has been demonstrated to be superior to vindesine combined with cisplatin (median survival 40 weeks vs. 30 weeks) [21]. This combination has also been shown to be superior to administration of its individual components as single agents [21, 22]. The combination of paclitaxel and cisplatin has also been studied. When compared with cisplatin and etoposide, it results in higher response rates and an increased median survival [23]. Similarly, this regimen was shown to result in a higher response rate (but not increased survival) than cisplatin and VM-26 [24]. Gemcitabine, a novel antimetabolite, has been demonstrated to have encouraging single agent activity. When combined with cisplatin, this regimen has also been shown to be superior to single agent cisplatin [25]. Tirapazamine, a drug with selective toxicity for hypoxic cells, has also been shown to be superior when combined with cisplatin [26]. Therefore, at the present time, four cisplatin-based regimens have been demonstrated to be superior to previous cisplatin-based regimens and can be considered potential standard treatment options. These include the regimens of cisplatin and vinorelbine, cisplatin and paclitaxel, cisplatin and gemcitabine and cisplatin and tirapazamine. Another regimen of interest is the combination of carboplatin and paclitaxel. Phase II studies indicate encouraging activity and good tolerance of this regimen [27]. This regimen is currently undergoing definitive evaluation in large randomized trials.

Docetaxel, another taxane, is also of interest. Docetaxel has been demonstrated to have an approximately 15%–20% response rate in patients who failed previous cisplatin-based chemotherapy [28]. As such, it is the first drug to be studied in this setting with the possibility of patient benefit.

## Key Questions and Current Investigations in Stage IV Disease

While available evidence supports the use of recent chemotherapy regimens in stage IV NSCLC, the current median survival times remain highly unsatisfactory. Therefore, aggressive clinical investigation of additional new agents and treatment principles is necessary. Drugs currently undergoing phase II testing include the topoisomerase I inhibitors, novel thymidylate synthase inhibitors, analogues of cisplatin, and other investigational compounds. In addition, the use of angiogenesis inhibitors and other biologically defined agents are under investigation. With the observed responses to docetaxel given as second line therapy to NSCLC patients, the impact of continued chemotherapy on survival times needs to be investigated.

## References

1. Parker SL et al. Cancer Statistics (1997). CA: Cancer J Clin 47:5–27
2. Ginsberg R, Vokes EE, Raben A. Non-small cell lung cancer (1997). In: DeVita VT Jr, Hellman S, Rosenberg SA, eds. Cancer Principles and Practice of Oncology (5th edn). Philadelphia: Lippincott, 858–911
3. Mountain CF. Revisions in the international system for staging lung cancer (1997). 111:1710–1717
4. Non-Small Cell Lung Cancer Collaborative Group. Chemotherapy in non-small cell lung cancer: a meta-analysis using updated data on individual patients from 52 randomized clinical trials (1995). BMJ 311:899–909
5. Dillman RO et al. Improved survival in stage III non-small cell lung cancer: seven-year follow-up of Cancer and Leukemia Group B (1996). J Natl Cancer Ins 88:1210–1215
6. Komaki R et al. Randomized study of chemotherapy/radiation therapy combinations for favorable patients with locally advanced inoperable non-small cell lung cancer: radiation therapy oncology group (RTOG) 92–04 (1997). Int J Rad Oncol Biol Phys 38 (1):149–155
7. Vokes EE, Weichselbaum RR: Concomitant chemoradiotherapy: Rationale and clinical experience in patients with solid tumors (1990). J Clin Oncol 8:911–934
8. Schaake-Koning et al. Effects of concomitant cisplatin and radiotherapy on inoperable non-small cell lung cancer (1992). N Engl J Med 326:524–530
9. Saunders M et al. Continuous hyperfractionated accelerated radiotherapy (CHART) versus conventional radiotherapy in non-small cell lung cancer: a randomised multicentre trial (1997). Lancet 350:161–165
10. Vokes EE. CHART for non-small cell lung cancer: promises and limitations (1997). Lancet 350:156–157
11. Furuse K et al. A randomized phase III study of concurrent versus sequential thoracic radiotherapy (TRT) in combination with mitomycin (M), vindesine (V), and cisplatin (P) in unresectable stage III non-small cell lung cancer (NSCLC): preliminary analysis (1997). Proc Am Soc Clin Oncol 16:1649a

12. Vokes EE et al. A CALGB randomized phase II study of gemcitabine or paclitaxel or vinorelbine with cisplatin as induction chemotherapy (Inc CT) and concomitant chemotherapy (XRT) in stage IIIB non-small cell lung cancer (NSCLC): feasibility data (CALGB study #9431) (1997). 16:455a

13. Roth JA et al. A randomized trial comparing perioperative chemotherapy and surgery with surgery alone in resectable stage IIIA non-small cell lung cancer (1994). 86 (9):673–680

14. Rosell R et al. A randomized trial comparing preoperative chemotherapy plus surgery with surgery alone in patients with non-small cell lung cancer (1994). 330 (3):153–158

15. Albain KS et al. Concurrent cisplatin/etoposide plus chest radiotherapy followed by surgery for stages IIIA (N2) and IIIB non-small-cell lung cancer: mature results of Southwest Oncology Group Phase II Study 8805 (1995). 13 (8):1880–1892

16. Shepherd FA. Treatment of advanced non-small cell lung cancer. Semin Oncol (1994). 21 (suppl 7):7–18

17. Bunn PA, Kelly K. New chemotherapeutic agents prolong survival and improve quality of life in non-small cell lung cancer: a review of the literature and future directions (1998). 5:1087–1100

18. Rapp E et al. Chemotherapy can prolong survival in patients with advanced non-small cell lung cancer-report of a Canadian multicenter randomized trial (1988). J Clin Oncol 6:633–641

19. Vokes EE, Bitran JD. Non-small cell lung cancer: towards the next plateau (1994) (editorial). Chest 106:659–661

20. Lilenbaum RC, Green MR. Novel chemotherapeutic agents in the treatment of non-small cell lung cancer (1993). J Clin Oncol 11:1391–1402

21. Le Chevalier T et al. Randomized study of vinorelbine and cisplatin versus vindesine and cisplatin versus vinorelbine alone in advanced non-small cell lung cancer: results of a European multicenter trial including 612 patients (1994). J Clin Oncol 12:360–367

22. Wozniak AJ et al. Randomized phase III trial of cisplatin (CDDP) vs CDDP plus navelbine (NVB) in treatment of advanced non-small cell lung cancer (NSCLC): report of a Southwest Oncology Group study (1996). Proc am Soc Clin Oncol 15:374

23. Bonomi P et al. Phase III trial comparing etoposide-cisplatin versus Taxol with cisplatin-G-CSF versus Taxol-cisplatin in advanced non-small cell lung cancer. An Eastern Cooperative Oncology Group trial (1996) Proc Am Soc Clin Oncol 16:382

24. Giaccone G et al. Final results of an EORTC phase III study of paclitaxel versus teniposide, in combination with cisplatin in advanced NSCLC (1997). Proc Am Soc Clin Oncol 16:460a

25. Sandler A et al. Randomized phase III study of cisplatin (P) and vinblastine (V) followed by thoracic radiotherapy with or without hydroxyurea (HX) in previously untreated limited unresectable non-small cell lung cancer (NSCLC): a Hoosier Oncology Group (HOG) Study (1998). Proc Am Soc Clin Oncol 17:454a.

26. von Pawel J, von Roemeling R. Survival benefit from Tirazone (Tirapazamine) and cisplatin in advanced non-small cell lung cancer (NSCLC) patients: final results from the International Phase III Catapult Trial (1998). Proc Am Soc Clin Oncol 17:454a

27. Langer et al. Paclitaxel and carboplatin in combination in the treatment of advanced non-small cell lung cancer: a phase II toxicity, response and survival analysis (1995). J Clin Oncol 13:1360–1370

28. Fosella FV et al. Phase II study of docetaxel for advanced or metastatic platinum-refractory non-small cell lung cancer (1995). J Clin Oncol 13:645–651

# Small-Cell Lung Cancer

F. Cappuzzo, C. Le Pechoux, T. Le Chevalier

## Epidemiology and Risk Factors

Currently lung cancer is the first cause of cancer deaths in the world and is one of the few to exhibit an ever-increasing incidence. In the United States it was estimated that 178,000 new cases of lung cancer would occur in 1997 and approximately 20% of these cases would be of the small-cell histologic sub-type (SCLC) [1]. Of all histologic types of lung cancer, SCLC has the strongest association with cigarette smoking. Only 3% of patients with this cancer have no history of active exposure, and the elimination of cigarette smoking is the most powerful way to drastically reduce the risk of developing this disease in the future [2]. Lung cancer is also associated with other environmental factors, such as arsenic, asbestos, beryllium, chloromethylethers, chromium, hydrocarbons, mustard gas, nickel, and radiation.

## Pathology and Staging

SCLC represents 20% of all lung tumors in autopsy series. As there are major differences in the biological behavior and treatments of SCLC and non-SCLC (NSCLC), SCLC has been classified differently from NSCLC. The Veterans Administration Lung Cancer Study Group (VALCSG) has divided patients with SCLC into two categories: limited-stage disease and extensive-stage disease. Limited-stage disease is when tumor is confined to one hemithorax, with regional lymph node metastases (including hilar, ipsi- and contralateral mediastinal, and/or supraclavicular nodes, and/or malignant pleural effusion). Extensive-stage disease is defined as a tumor with contralateral thoracic and/or extrathoracic involvement. The VALCSG system was recently supplanted by the revised

**Table 1.** TNM staging system

| | |
|---|---|
| Stage 0 | Carcinoma in situ |
| Stage IA | T1 N0 M0 |
| Stage IB | T2 N0 M0 |
| Stage IIA | T1 N1 M0 |
| Stage IIB | T2 N1 M0 |
| | T3 N0 M0 |
| Stage IIIA | T3 N1 M0 |
| | T1-3 N2 M0 |
| Stage IIIB | T1-3 N3 M0 |
| | T4 N0-3 M0 |
| Stage IV | Any T any N M1 |

TNM staging system, in which limited-stage disease is equivalent to stage I-III, and extensive-stage disease is equivalent to stage IV (Table 1) [3].

Primary tumor and regional nodal spread are evaluated by chest-X-ray. Bronchoscopy with bronchial washings and biopsy are essential to confirm the diagnosis and to document the extent of local disease and tumor response during follow-up. Chest CT-scan is mandatory for an appraisal of local and regional disease extension. The most common sites of metastases are the bone, liver, bone marrow and brain. Extra-thoracic disease is therefore assessed by bone scan, brain and abdominal CT-scan, and bone marrow biopsy. Recently, Seto suggested that magnetic resonance imaging (MRI) of bone marrow is useful for staging SCLC and MRI findings represent a prognostic factor in patients with limited disease [4]. SCLC produces high levels of neuron-specific enolase (NSE), carcinoembryonic antigen (CEA), creatinine kinase-BB (CK-BB), and chromogranin A (CGA). NSE and CEA are currently used as serum markers in clinical practice. It is noteworthy that none of these markers has been demonstrated to be capable of replacing conventional staging procedures nor of being useful as a screening test. They do, nonetheless, provide additional information for the prognosis and disease management [5].

## Stage-Specific Standard Treatment Options

Before the introduction of systemic chemotherapy, median survival did not exceed 12–15 weeks for patients with extensive disease and about 6 months for patients with limited-stage, with anecdotal cases surviving more than 5 years. Chemotherapy led to a marked improvement in median survival (12 months for patients with limited disease and 9–10 months for patients with extensive disease) and in 5-year survival (5%–10%) [6]. Treatment of limited and extensive SCLC is different: chemotherapy is the cornerstone of the therapeutic strategy for extensive SCLC, whereas a multimodality approach is mandatory for the management of limited diesease.

## Limited-Stage SCLC

Formerly, there was some controversy about whether surgery should be used and, if so, whether it should be performed before or after chemotherapy and radiotherapy in limited-stage SCLC. Up to the 1980s, surgery was abandoned based on strong evidence that SCLC must be considered as a systemic disease, which can be controlled by chemotherapy and radiotherapy and sometimes cured. More recently, several studies have been performed to clarify the role of surgery particularly in the subset of patients with very-limited disease (stage I and II) and for some selected patients with more advanced stage disease (III). For stage I-II SCLC, several trials have shown that surgery followed by chemotherapy, with or without radiotherapy, yields a 5-year survival rate of 54% [7–11]. These results suggest that it is reasonable to propose surgery followed by chemotherapy for very limited disease. In 1983, the Lung Cancer Study Group initiated a prospective randomized trial to determine whether surgical resection was beneficial in cases of residual disease following response to induction chemotherapy. This study showed no significant differences in terms of median or overall survival in patients who underwent or did not undergo surgery [12]. At the present time, surgery is not recommended in stage III SCLC outside clinical trials. Several randomized trials have been conducted to evaluate the role of radiotherapy combined with chemotherapy in limited-stage SCLC. Many of these trials showed a significant advantage for combined modality treatment, but the results were not always consistent and remained unconvincing. More recently, two meta-analyses, one of which was based on individual data, found a modest but statistically significant improvement in overall survival for combined therapy [13–14]. Pignon et al. demonstrated a decreased relative risk of death of 0.86 (p=0.001) with a 14% reduction in the mortality rate and evidence of a 5% absolute advantage for survival after chemoradiotherapy compared to chemotherapy alone in a total of 2140 patients. This finding represents the only important survival gain for patients with this disease in the last two decades [13]. As a consequence, the standard treatment of limited-stage SCLC became chemotherapy combined with radiotherapy. There are many ways of combining chemotherapy and radiotherapy; they can be administered concurrently, sequentially or alternated, but the optimal combination is yet to be established. Based on promising preliminary observations and supported by theoretical evidence, Arriagada et al. utilized an alternating chemoradiotherapy schedule and highly promising response and survival results were reported with acceptable toxicity [15–16]. Recently, the European Organization for Research and Treatment of Cancer (EORTC) conducted a trial of alternating versus sequential radiochemotherapy in 335 patients with limited-stage SCLC [17]. This trial failed to confirm the superiority of an alternating schedule over a sequential combination, but another clinical trial suggested that an alternating schedule was superior to a concurrent approach [18] and that a concurrent schedule was better than sequential radiochemotherapy [19]. The optimal timing of radiotherapy is also unknown. Three randomized trials have compared early thoracic irradiation versus late thoracic irradiation and only the NCI study (Canada) yielded a statistically significant difference in overall survival in favor of early irradiation (21.2 versus 16 months, p=0.008) [20–22]. Recently, Jeremic conducted a randomized trial in which initial radiotherapy produced better local control and survival than delayed administration (median survival=34 versus 26 months, 5-year survival 30% versus 15%, p=0.052) [23]. The optimal radiotherapy dose and schedule have yet to be established. Conventional fractionation at 2.0 Gy per day is the most frequently used, but in vitro studies suggest that hyperfractionated radiotherapy is a logical approach [24]. Clearly a dose-response relationship exists up to 45–50 Gy, the conventional dose [25], but whether this relationship is sustained beyond 50 Gy is not certain. Arriagada et al. increased the total thoracic dose of 45–65 Gy and found no significant improvement in local control [16]. For the time being, we can only conclude that combined-modality treatment with concurrent or alternating radiotherapy, given early during the chemotherapy course, is the strategy preferred.

## Extensive-Stage SCLC

Chemotherapy is the standard treatment for extensive-stage SCLC.

### Single Agents

Several drugs, such as cyclophosphamide (CTX), doxorubicin (ADM), methotrexate (MTX), etoposide (VP16), vincristine (VCR), ifosfamide (IFO), cisplatin (CDDP), and carboplatin (CBDCA) are considered active in SCLC. Response rates attain 30%–50% in chemotherapy-naive patients. Most of the new agents such as taxanes, vinorelbine, gemcitabine, and topoisomerase inhibitors are equally active.

### Combination Chemotherapy

During the 1970s, the CAV combination (CTX, ADM, VCR) achieved better response and overall survival rates than single agent chemotherapy. This regimen yielded an 80% objective response rate, with complete responses in 40% of patients with limited disease and in 10% of patients with extensive disease; it has become the standard treatment for SCLC [6]. During the 1980s, the activity of the PE (CDDP-VP16) regimen proved irrefutable, and randomized trials suggested that this combination was less toxic than the CAV combination and moreover equally active [26–27] (Table 2). Successive trials demonstrated that alternating CAV and PE regimens yielded a gain in survival in patients with extensive-stage disease but not in those with limited-stage disease [28–29]. Several trials evaluated the role of maintenance chemotherapy and its optimal

**Table 2.** Randomized trials comparing PE versus CAV versus alternating PE with CAV

| Reference | Regimen | $n$ | Complete response (%) | Median survival (months) |
|-----------|---------|-----|----------------------|--------------------------|
| Roth      | CAV     | 140 | 7                    | 8.3                      |
|           | PE      | 140 | 10                   | 8.6                      |
|           | CAV/PE  | 140 | 7                    | 8.1                      |
| Fukuoka   | CAV     | 97  | 16                   | 9.9                      |
|           | PE      | 97  | 14                   | 9.9                      |
|           | CAV/PE  | 92  | 16                   | 11.8                     |

**Table 3.** Combination chemotherapy commonly used in SCLC

| Regimen | Dose, route, day of administration |
|---|---|
| Regimen 1 | |
| CAV | Cycle every three weeks |
| Cyclophosphamide | 1000 mg/m$^2$ IV day 1 |
| Doxorubicin | 45 mg/m$^2$ IV day 1 |
| Vincristine | 2 mg IV day 1 |
| Regimen 2 | |
| PE | Cycle every three weeks |
| Etoposide | 100 mg/m$^2$ IV days 1, 2, 3 |
| Cisplatin | 100 mg/m$^2$ IV day 1 |
| Regimen 3 | |
| Alternating CAV with PE | Cycle of CAV as above alternating, every 3 weeks, with cycle of PE as above |

duration. The most important among them and the recent study conducted by the European Lung Cancer Working Party (ELCWP) showed that maintenance therapy may improve progression-free survival but not overall survival [30]. A consensus panel therefore concluded that four to six cycles of chemotherapy could be recommended without maintenance therapy (Table 3) [31].

## Intensified Regimens and High-Dose Chemotherapy

Randomized studies comparing the efficacy of the CAV or PE regimen at standard doses versus the same regimens with intensified doses demonstrated that the latter induced considerably more toxicity but efficacy was not unequivocally improved [32–33]. In patients relapsing after the PE regimen, no apparent benefit was obtained when the same combination was intensified [34]. Some investigators have attempted high-dose chemotherapy with autologous bone marrow or peripheral stem cell rescue in patients with SCLC. A number of trials have evaluated the effect of high-dose chemotherapy after induction chemotherapy or as initial therapy. After induction therapy, a randomized trial comparing high-dose versus conventional-dose chemotherapy in patients with both limited or extensive-stage SCLC, showed a significant difference in relapse-free survival (28 weeks versus 10 weeks p=0.002) in favor of the high-dose arm but no advantage was gained for overall survival [35].

The main cause of treatment failure is the early emergence of chemoresistant cells. Survival could be improve by increasing initial drug doses. Arriagada et al conducted a retrospective analysis of 52 patients with limited-stage SCLC which evidenced that higher initial doses of CTX and CDDP reduced the frequency of distant metastases and increased the overall survival rate [36]. A larger retrospective study confirmed that a 20% increase in initial CTX and CDDP doses resulted in an increase in overall survival of 20% at 2 years [37]. Based on these results a randomized trial was designed to compare higher initial doses of CTX and CDDP (CTX 1200 mg/m2 and CDDP 100 mg/m2) plus standard doses of ADM and VP16 (40 mg/m2 and 75 mg/m2 for 3 days respectively) versus standard doses of the same drugs (CTX 225 mg/m2 for 4 days and CDDP 80 mg/m2 one day) plus the same standard doses of ADM and VP16 in limited-stage SCLC. This study clearly showed that higher doses of CTX and CDDP during the first cycle of chemotherapy resulted in significantly higher complete response and survival. In this trial the relative risk of death was 0.5 and the absolute survival benefit at two years was 17% [38].

How is it that initial high-dose chemotherapy or trials based on increased dose-intensity have failed to show a clear benefit for survival? Using dose intensity incrementation to describe variations in initial doses is inappropriate; very high doses are often associated with toxicity which may preclude completion of induction therapy and in-so-doing compromise its overall effectiveness. In summary, the PE regimen at standard doses or alternating CAV and PE combinations, must be considered the standard chemotherapy options for patients with SCLC. The delivery of higher initial doses of CDDP and/or CTX prevents the emergence of chemoresistant cells and therefore low initial doses should be avoided in clinical practice. High-dose chemotherapy or dose-intensified regimens are not recommended, at present, outside clinical trials.

## Prophylactic Cranial Irradiation

Prophylactic cranial irradiation (PCI) in patients with SCLC is the subject a long-standing debate in oncology. Several randomized trials conducted in 1970s concluded that PCI reduced the rate of brain metastases but had no impact on overall survival. A retrospective analysis of these studies suggested that PCI might be useful but only for patients in complete remission [39]. During the 1980s, PCI was incriminated in the emergence of side effects such as neuropsycological syndromes and brain abnormalities, and toxicity appeared to be exacerbated when the total radiotherapy dose exceeded 30 Gy, when fractions were above 3 Gy, and when PCI was administered simultaneously or before chemotherapy containing radiosensitising drugs. Routine use of PCI was therefore abandoned and low-dose PCI (<30 Gy) was reserved for complete responders. More recently the results of both the French and the UK/EORTC trials suggested that PCI reduces the incidence of brain metastases without a statistically significant risk of neurological side-effects, but with a debatable impact on survival [40]. The optimal dose and ideal timing of PCI were not clarified in these studies. The ongoing meta-analysis of all randomized studies should better indicate the extent of the benefit for survival. Other unresolved questions await investigation in prospective randomized trials [41–43].

## Treatment of Elderly Patients

Many physicians and patients imagine that SCLC is less tractable in elderly patients due to the presence of concomitant illnesses. In fact, older patients who are able to tolerate standard chemotherapy have an overall survival rate which is not different from that of their younger counterparts. Elderly patients who cannot tolerate standard chemotherapy fare worse for reasons which remain obscure. For several years, oral VP16 was considered ideal for elderly patients with SCLC because it can be administered easily, it is relatively nontoxic and the activity provided by this drug is sustained. Recently, both the trials conducted by The Medical Research Council and the London Lung Cancer Group demonstrated that oral VP16 is less efficient than standard chemotherapy (CAV or alternating CAV and PE regimens) in terms of response (39% versus 61%, p<0.01), median survival (146 days versus 189 days), and 1-year survival (6.5% versus 16.9%) [44–45]. Standard combination chemotherapy should therefore be used as initial therapy for elderly SCLC patients. The PE regimen seems to be particularly appropriate for elderly patients because it is less myelosuppressive than CTX or ADM-based combinations [26].

## Current and Future Investigational Approaches

Recently, the attention of investigators has focused on the development of chemotherapeutic agents with novel mechanisms of action, new biologic therapies, and new agents based on biological principles such as anti-growth factors. During the last few years, several new drugs have been evaluated in SCLC. Ifosfamide, topotecan and CPT-11, paclitaxel, docetaxel, gemcitabine and vinorelbine have demonstrated promising activity (Table 4). Ongoing clinical trials are evaluating the efficacy of these drugs in combination with more established agents. The alleged activity of interferon and interleukin-2, suggested in some in vitro studies, has not been confirmed in randomized clinical trials. The role of interferon as maintenance therapy in SCLC is doubtful, but a recent Finnish trial has suggested that interferon-alpha improves the long-term survival of patients with limited SCLC [46]. Matrix metalloproteinase and angiogenesis inhibitors are very promising agents. Preliminary data from early phase I-II studies suggest that metalloproteinase inhibitors such as batimastat and marimastat are active and well tolerated in SCLC patients [47–48].

Promising activity has also been observed with angiogenesis inhibitors such as analogs of suramin [49], and angiostatin, a potent compound [50]. Several hormones are known to induce the proliferation of SCLC by acting as autocrine growth factors. A new potential therapeutic approach could consist in interfering with autocrine activity using blocking antibodies, peptide hormone antagonists, enzymes hydrolyzing growth factors, peptide/toxin fusion proteins, and inhibitors of signal trasduction. Tumor vaccines are also under investigation, and anticoagulant agents, such as warfarin seem to counteract metastasis, but the potential impact of these drugs on survival when combined with che-

**Table 4.** New agents in SCLC

| Drug | Response rate (%) |
| --- | --- |
| CPT-11 | 33–50 |
| Docetaxel | 25 |
| Paclitaxel | 34–41 |
| Gemcitabine | 27 |
| Topotecan | 21–39 |
| Vinorelbine | 15 |
| Ifosfamide | 49 |

motherapy remains to be established. Correcting tumor genetic abnormalities by gene transfer approaches is possible and may lead to a therapeutic effect, but the ongoing gene therapy trials have not yielded any data indicating activity in SCLC.

Acknowledgements. The authors thank Lorna Saint Ange for her valuable assistance in editing the text.

## References

1. Parker SL, Tong T, Bolden S (1997) Cancer statistics, 1997. CA Cancer J Clin 47:5–27
2. Wynder EL, Graham EA (1950) Tobacco smoking as a possible etiologic factor in bronchogenic carcinoma: A study of six hundred and eighty-four proved cases. JAMA 143:329–346
3. Mountain CF (1997) Revision in the International System for Staging Lung Cancer. Chest 111:1710–1717
4. Seto T, Imamura F, Kuriyama T, et al (1997) Effect on prognosis of bone marrow infiltration detected by magnetic resonance imaging in small cell lung cancer. Eur J Cancer 33:2333–2337
5. Fizazi K, Cojean I, Pignon JP, et al (1998) Normal serum neuron specific enolase (NSE) value after the first cycle of chemotherapy. Cancer 82:1049–1055
6. Bunn PA, Cohen MH, Ihde DC, et al (1977) Advances in small cell bronchogenic carcinoma: a commentary. Cancer Treat Rep 61:333–342
7. Karrer K, Shields TW, Denck H, et al (1986) The importance of surgical and multimodality treatment for small cell bronchial carcinoma. J Thorac Cardiovasc Surg 97:168–176
8. Salzer GM, Muller LC, Huber H, et al (1990) Operation for N2 small cell lung carcinoma. Ann Thorac Surg 49:759–762
9. Ginsberg RJ (1989) Surgery and small cell lung cancer: an overview. Lung Cancer 5:232–236
10. Ohta M, Hara N, Ichinose Y, et al (1986) The role of surgical resection in the management of small cell carcinoma of the lung. Jpn J Clin Oncol 16 (3):289–296
11. Meyer JA, Gullo JJ, Ikins PM, et al (1984) Adverse prognostic effect of N2 disease in treated small cell carcinoma of the lung. J Thorac Cardiovasc Surg 88:495–501
12. Lad T, Piantadosi S, Thomas P, et al (1994) A prospective randomized trial to determine the benefit of surgical resection of residual disease following response of small cell lung cancer to combination chemotherapy. Chest 106 (suppl): 320s-323 s
13. Pignon JP, Arriagada R, Ihde DC, et al (1992) A meta-analysis of thoracic radiotherapy for small-cell lung cancer. N Engl J Med 327:1618–1624
14. Warde P, Payne D (1992) Does thoracic irradiation improve survival and local control in limited-stage small-cell carcinoma of the lung? A meta-analysis. J Clin Oncol 10:890–895
15. Arriagada R, Le Chevalier T, Baldeyrou P, et al (1985) Alternating radiotherapy and chemoherapy schedules in small cell lung cancer limited disease. Int J Radiat Oncol Biol Phys 11:1461–1467
16. Arriagada R, Le Chevalier T, Ruffie P, et al (1990) Alternating radiotherapy and chemotherapy in 173 consecutive patients with limited small cell lung carcinoma. GROP and the French Cancer Centre's Lung Group. Int J radiat Oncol Biol Phys 19:1135–1138

17. Gregor A, Drings P, Burghouts J, et al (1997) Randomized trial of alternating versus sequential radiotherapy/chemotherapy in limited-disease patients with small-cell lung cancer: A European Organization for Research and Treatment of cancer Lung Cancer Cooperative Group Study. J Clin Oncol 15:2840–2849
18. Lebeau B, Chastang C, Urban T, et al (1996) A randomized clinical trial comparing concurrent and alternating thoracic irradiation in limited small cell lung cancer (SCLC). Proc Am Soc Clin Oncol 15:383 (abstract)
19. Takada M, Fukuoka M, Furuse K, et al (1996) Aphase III study of concurrent versus sequential thoracic radiotherapy in combination with cisplatin and etoposide for limited-stage small cell lung cancer: preliminary results of the Japan Clinical Oncology Group. Proc Am Soc Clin Oncol 15:372 (abstract)
20. Murray N, Coy P, Pater JL, et al (1993) Importance of timing for thoracic irradiation in the combined modality treatment of limited-stage small-cell lung cancer. J Clin Oncol 11:336–344
21. Perry MC, Eaton WL, Propert KJ, et al (1987) Chemoyherapy with or without radiation therapy in limited small cell carcinoma of the lung. N Engl J Med 316:912–918
22. Schultz HP, Nielsen OS, Sell A, et al (1988) Timing of chest irradiation with respect to combination chemotherapy in small cell lung cancer, limited disease. Lung Cancer 4 (suppl):153 (abstract)
23. Jeremic B, Shibamoto Y, Acimovic L, et al (1997) Initial versus delayed accelerated hyperfractionated radiation therapy and concurrent chemotherapy in limited small-cell lung cancer: a randomized study. J Clin Oncol 15:893–900
24. Carney DN, Mitchell JB, Kinsella TJ, et al (1983) In vitro radiation and chemotherapy sensitivity of established cell lines of human small cell lung cancer and its cell morphological variants. Cancer Res 43:2806–2811
25. Choi N, Carey R (1989) Importance of radiation dose in achieving improved locoregional tumor control in limited stage small-cell lung carcinoma: an update. Int J Radiat Oncol Biol Phys 17:307–310
26. Fukuoka M, Furese K, Saijo N, et al (1991) Randomized trial of cyclophosphamide, doxorubicin, and vincristine versus cisplatin and etoposide versus alternation of these regimens in small cell lung cancer. J Natl Cancer Inst 83:855–861
27. Roth BJ, Johnson DH, Einhorn LH, et al (1992) Randomized study of cyclophosphamide, doxorubicin and vincristine versus etoposide and cisplatin versus alternation of these two regimens in extensive small cell lung cancer. J Clin Oncol 10:282–291
28. Evans WK, Feld R, Murray N, et al (1987) Superiority of alternating non-cross resistant chemotherapy in extensive small cell lung cancer. A multicenter, randomized clinical trial by the National Cancer Institute of Canada. Ann Intern Med 107:451–458
29. Feld R, Evans WK, Coy P, et al (1987) Canadian multicenter randomized trial comparing sequential and alternating administration of two non-cross-resistant chemotherapy combinations in patients with limited small cell carcinoma of the lung. J Clin Oncol 5:1401–1409
30. Sculier JP, Paesmans M, Bureau G, et al (1996) Randomized trial comparing induction chemotherapy followed by maintenance chemotherapy in small-cell lung cancer. J Clin Oncol 14:2337–2344
31. Bunn PA Jr, Cullen M, Fukuoka M, et al (1989) Chemotherapy in small cell lung cancer: A consensus report. Lung Cancer 5:127–134
32. Ihde DC, Johnson BE, Mulshine JL, et al (1994) Randomized trial of high dose versus standard dose etoposide and cisplatin in extensive stage small cell lung cancer. J Clin Oncol 12:2022–2034
33. Johnson DH, Einhorn LH, Birch R, et al (1987) A randomized comparison of high-dose versus conventional dose cyclophosphamide, doxorubicin, and vincristine

for extensive-stage small cell lung cancer: A phase III trial of the Southeastern Cancer Study Group. J Clin Oncol 5:1731–1738

34. Masuda N, Fukuoka M, Matsui K, et al (1990) Evaluation of high dose etoposide combined with cisplatin for treating relapsed small cell lung cancer. Cancer 65:2635–2640

35. Humblet Y, Symann M, Bosly A, et al (1987) Late intensification chemotherapy with autologous bone marrow transplantation in selected small-cell carcinoma of the lung: A randomized study. J Clin Oncol 5:1864–1873

36. Arriagada R, de Thè H, Le Chevalier T, et al (1989) Limited small cell lung cancer: possible prognostic impact of initial chemotherapy doses. Bull Cancer (Paris) 76:604–615

37. De Vathaire F, Arriagada R, de Thè H, et al (1993) Dose intensity of initial chemotherapy may have an impact on survival in limited small cell lung carcinoma. Lung Cancer 8:301–308

38. Arriagada R, Le Chevalier T, Pignon JP, et al (1993) Initial chemotherapeutic doses and survival in patients with limited small-cell lung cancer. N Engl J Med 329:1848–1852

39. Bumm PA, Kelly K (1995) Prophylactic cranial irradiation for patients with small-cell lung cancer. J Natl Cancer Inst 87:16–17

40. Arriagada R, Le Chevalier T, Borie F, et al (1995) Prophylactic cranial irradiation for patients with small-cell lung cancer in complete remission. J Natl Cancer Inst 87:183–190

41. Le Chevalier T, Arriagada R (1997) Small cell lung cancer and prophylactic cranial irradiation (PCI): Perhaps the question is not who needs PCI but who wants PCI? Eur J Cancer 33:1717–1719

42. Gregor A, Cull A, Stephens RJ, et al (1997) Prophylactic cranial irradiation is indicated following complete response to induction therapy in small cell lung cancer: Results of a multicentre randomised trial. Eur J Cancer 33:1752–1758

43. Wagner H, Kim K, Turrisi A, et al (1996) A randomized phase III study of prophylactic cranial irradiation (PCI) in patients (Pts) with small cell lung cancer (SCLC) achieving a complete response: Final report of an incomplete trial by the Eastern Cooperative Oncology Group and Radiation Therapy Oncology Group (E3589/R92–01). Proc Am Soc Clin Oncol 15:1120 (abstract)

44. Clark PI (1996) Oral etoposide alone is inadequate palliative chemotherapy for small cell lung cancer: A randomized trial. Proc Am Soc Clin Oncol 15:377 (abstract)

45. Harper P, Underhill C, Ruiz de Elvira MC, et al (1996) A randomized study of oral etoposide versus combination chemotherapy in poor prognosis small cell lung cancer. Proc Am Soc Clin Oncol 15:27 (abstract)

46. Mattson K, Niiranen A, Ruotsalainen T, et al (1997) Interferon maintenance therapy for small cell lung cancer: improvement in long-term survival. J Interf Cyt Res 17:103–105

47. Rosemurgy A, Harris J, Langleben A, et al (1996) Marimastat, a novel matrix metalloproteinase inhibitor in patients with advanced carcinoma of the pancreas. Proc Am Soc Clin Oncol 15:207

48. Malfetano J, Teng N, Moore D, et al (1996) Marimastat, a novel matrix metalloproteinase inhibitor in patients with advanced cancer of the ovary: a dose-finding study. Proc Am Soc Clin Oncol 15:283

49. De Cupis A, Ciomei M, Pirani P, et al (1997) Anti-insulin-like growth factor-1 activity of a novel polysulphonated distamycin A derivative in human lung cancer cell lines. Br J Pharmacology 120:537–543

50. O'Reilly MS, Holmgren L, Shing Y, et al (1994) Angiostatin: a novel angiogenesis inhibitor that mediates the suppression of metastases by a Lewis lung carcinoma. Cell 79:315–328

# Mesothelioma

# Mesothelioma

H. L. Kindler, N. J. Vogelzang

## Epidemiology and Risk Factors

Malignant mesothelioma was first associated with asbestos in 1960, when Wagner et al [1] observed an unusually high incidence of the disease in South African asbestos miners. Since that time, the risk of malignant mesothelioma following *asbestos* exposure has been more precisely defined [2–6], and the demographics and natural history of the disease have become more widely known [6–9]. About 2200 cases are diagnosed in the United States each year [7]. Men are more commonly affected, reflecting their greater occupational exposure. The average age of onset is 55 to 60 [10].

For individuals with significant asbestos exposure, there appears to be a relationship between genetic polymorphisms in the metabolic genes GSTM1 and NAT2 and the risk of developing mesothelioma [11]. Several other causes of mesothelioma have been described. Mesothelioma has been reported in patients previously treated with thoracic radiation [12], however a retrospective cohort analysis of over 265,000 patients irradiated for breast cancer or Hodgkin's disease found no increase in the relative risk of mesothelioma [13]. Mesothelioma is the leading cause of cancer death in some Turkish villages, where erionite fibers, which have the same physical characteristics as asbestos, contaminate the soil [14]. Other rarer causes include iatrogenic pneumothorax for treatment of tuberculosis [15], and thorotrast, which induces mesothelioma in a dose-dependent fashion by chronic release of $\alpha$-particles [16].

Mesothelioma can develop when the DNA virus SV-40 is injected into hamsters. Carbone et al observed SV-40-like DNA sequences in 29 of 48 mesothelioma specimens resected at the NIH, and concluded that SV-40 may be a co-carcinogen for human mesothelioma [17]. SV-40 contaminated rhesus monkey kidney cells were used to prepare early polio vaccines; to date there is no evidence that this has resulted in an increased incidence of mesothelioma [17].

## Pathology and Staging

The three histologic subtypes of malignant mesothelioma are epithelial, fibrosarcomatous, and biphasic; the epithelial form predominates. Epithelial mesotheliomas can demonstrate tubular, tubulopapillary, cord-like, or sheetlike patterns. Fibrosarcomatous mesotheliomas are comprised of spindle-shaped or ovoid cells in a variable fibrous stroma. The biphasic, or mixed form contains both epithelial and sarcomatous cell types [15, 18].

A panel of immunohistochemical stains is often required to distinguish the epithelial subtype of mesothelioma from adenocarcinoma. Adenocarcinomas may stain for CEA, mucicarmine, Leu-M1, B72.3, and periodic acid-Schiff with diastase; mesotheliomas should be negative for these stains and may react with vimentin, colloidal iron, or alcian blue. Electron microscopy can differentiate the long, slender, branching microvilli of a mesothelioma from the short, stubby microvilli of an adenocarcinoma [18].

No specific chromosomal abnormalities have been characterized, but aneuploidy and frequent deletions and translocations of chromosomes 1, 2, 3, 4, 5, 7, 9, 11, 17, and 22 have been described. Loss of heterozygosity in the short arm of chromosome 3, and homozygous deletions of p16 have been observed in some samples. The role of p53 is controversial [19].

At least 5 staging systems were in use in 1994 when the International Mesothelioma Interest Group developed a TNM based system for staging malignant mesothelioma (Table 1) [20]. This system incorporates prognostic information derived from prior clinical series, and divides patients with surgically evaluated early disease into separate stages. For example, Boutin et al. [21] observed that patients whose tumors involve only the parietal pleura had a significant survival advantage (32.7 vs. 7 months, p <0.001) over those with visceral pleural involvement. Butchart stage I was therefore divided into Ia and Ib, based on whether the visceral pleura was intact or invaded. Sugarbaker et al. [22] demonstrated that one and two year survival following extrapleural pneumonectomy was significantly better for patients with negative lymph nodes (71% and 46%, respectively) than for those with positive lymph nodes (41% and

0%, respectively), hence all patients with positive bronchopulmonary, hilar, or mediastinal lymph nodes were reclassified into stage III.

The median survival of patients with malignant mesothelioma ranges from 6 to 15 months [23]. Prognostic factors predictive of poor survival vary between series, and include: poor performance status, nonepithelial histology, chest pain, platelet count greater than 400,000/μL, age greater than 75, LDH greater than 500 IU/L, fewer than 6 months since symptom onset, elevated WBC, weight loss, low hemoglobin, and male gender [8, 23, 24]. Smoking status and history of prior asbestos exposure do not appear to influence prognosis [8].

## Workup and Staging

Patients with malignant pleural mesothelioma present with the insidious onset of dyspnea and chest pain; other symptoms include cough, fever, weight loss, and fatigue. Peritoneal mesothelioma may present with abdominal discomfort and increasing abdominal girth from ascites. Symptoms may persist for months prior to diagnosis. The physical exam is often unrevealing except for dullness to percussion or reduced air entry on ascultation.

Chest X-ray usually demonstrates a pleural effusion or diffuse pleural thickening; in advanced disease the mediastinal structures may shift toward the effusion. Pleural plaques or calcifications may be present. Computed tomography of the chest and abdomen can identify subdiaphragmatic extension of the tumor, as well as involvement of the mediastinum and contralateral thorax. Because magnetic resonance imaging can image in multiple planes, it can complement computed tomography for assessment of diaphragmatic, mediastinal and chest wall invasion [25]. Screening computed tomography scans of the brain and nuclear medicine bone scans are not routinely necessary since asymptomatic distant metastatic disease is uncommon [26]. If surgery is planned, pulmonary function tests and echocardiography are essential.

Although most patients with pleural mesothelioma develop a pleural effusion, cytology or pleural biopsy alone are indeterminate in most cases. Thoracoscopic biopsy has a diagnostic sensitivity of 98% [27], and can be used for diagnosis, staging, and palliation if talc pleurodiesis is also performed. Bronchoscopy is used to exclude a primary bronchogenic carcinoma. Laparoscopy can evaluate disease below the diaphragm if peritoneal disease cannot be ruled out before resection [26].

There are no established tumor markers, however CEA is elevated in less than 5% of patients and can be used to exclude a diagnosis of mesothelioma [15]. Staging criteria are provided in Table 1.

**Table 1.** New international staging system for diffuse malignant pleural mesothelioma (from [20])

| | |
|---|---|
| Primary tumor | |
| T1 | T1a Tumor limited to the ipsilateral parietal pleura, including mediastinal and diaphragmatic pleura. No involvement of the visceral pleura |
| | T1b Tumor involving the ipsilateral parietal pleura, including mediastinal and diaphragmatic pleura. Scattered foci of tumor also involving the visceral pleura |
| T2 | Tumor involving each of the ipsilateral pleural surfaces (parietal, mediastinal, diaphragmatic, and visceral pleura) with at least one of the following features: (a) involvement of diaphragmatic muscle, (b) confluent visceral pleural tumor (including the fissures) or extension of tumor from visceral pleura into the underlying pulmonary parenchyma |
| T3 | Describes locally advanced but potentially resectable tumor Tumor involving all of the ipsilateral pleural surfaces (parietal, mediastinal, diaphragmatic, and visceral pleura) with at least one of the following features: (a) involvement of the endothoracic fascia, (b) extension into the mediastinal fat, (c) solitary, completely resectable focus of tumor extending into the soft tissues of the chest wall, (d) nontransmural involvement of the pericardium |
| T4 | Describes locally advanced technically unresectable tumor Tumor involving all of the ipsilateral pleural surfaces (parietal, mediastinal, diaphragmatic, and visceral) with at least one of the following features: (a) diffuse extension or multifocal masses of tumor in the chest wall, with or without associated rib destruction, (b) direct transdiaphragmatic extension of tumor to the peritoneum, (c) direct extension of tumor to the contralateral pleura, (d) direct extension of tumor to one or more mediastinal organs, (e) direct extension of tumor into the spine, (f) tumor extending through to the internal surface of the pericardium with or without a pericardial effusion; or tumor involving the myocardium |
| Lymph nodes | |
| NX | Regional lymph nodes cannot be assessed |
| N0 | No regional lymph node metastases |
| N1 | Metastases in the ipsilateral bronchopulmonary or hilar lymph nodes |
| N2 | Metastases in the subcarinal or the ipsilateral mediastinal lymph nodes, including the ipsilateral internal mammary nodes |
| N3 | Metastases in the contralateral mediastinal, contralateral internal mammary, ipsilateral, or contralateral supraclavicular lymph nodes |

| Metastases | |
|---|---|
| MX | Presence of distant metastases cannot be assessed |
| M0 | No distant metastasis |
| M1 | Distant metastasis present |

| Staging | |
|---|---|
| Stage Ia | T1aN0M0 |
| Stage Ib | T1bN0M0 |
| Stage II | T2N0M0 |
| Stage III | Any T3M0 |
| | Any N1M0 |
| | Any N2M0 |
| Stage IV | Any T4 |
| | Any N3 |
| | Any M1 |

## Treatment

Malignant mesothelioma usually arises from the pleura or peritoneum; less common sites of origin include the pericardium and the tunica vaginalis. Extensive local progression results in death either from respiratory failure or from bowel obstruction and inanition. Therefore treatment of this disease usually includes attempts at local control. Unfortunately, surgical and radiotherapeutic intervention has been fraught with complications, and is only possible in a small percentage of patients. Less than 25% of patients eligible for aggressive surgical intervention will be alive at five years; even fewer will be disease-free [22, 28]. Although there have been a number of recent reports on combined modality therapy with extrapleural pneumonectomy, postoperative radiation and chemotherapy [22, 28, 29], the vast majority of patients with malignant pleural mesothelioma have locally advanced disease, advanced age or other co-morbid medical illnesses, precluding surgical or radiotherapeutic intervention. Therefore, the use of a systemic anticancer agent is the only treatment option for the majority of mesothelioma patients (Fig. 1).

## Surgery

Surgery for malignant mesothelioma can be diagnostic, palliative, or curative in intent. Thoracoscopy with talc pleurodiesis provides equivalent palliation to the more invasive partial pleurectomy, and may be the procedure of choice for recurrent symptomatic effusions. More aggres-

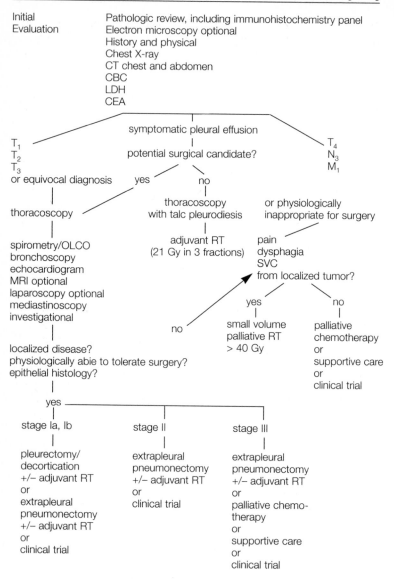

**Fig. 1.** Therapeutic decision tree for malignant mesothelioma

sive surgical approaches, such as *pleurectomy* or *extrapleural pneumonectomy,* cannot be recommended as standard therapy. They may be appropriate, however, for the physiologically fit patient with early-stage disease treated by an experienced surgeon, especially in the context of a clinical trial.

Pleurectomy with decortication involves stripping the pleura from the lung apex to the diaphragm, leaving the lung in place. Operative mortality is low at 1–2%; median survival ranges from 7–21 months [30]. Extrapleural pneumonectomy, the en bloc removal of the parietal and visceral pleura, lung, hemidiaphragm, and pericardium, with subsequent reconstruction of the hemidiaphragm and pericardium, is the only procedure possible when a thick tumor rind obliterates the pleural space. Operative mortality is higher, ranging from 5–31%, major morbidity is up to 25%, and median survival ranges from 4–21 months [30]. There are occasional long-term survivors following extrapleural pneumonectomy, suggesting that this procedure may alter the natural history of the disease in appropriately selected early-stage patients.

It is difficult to assess the impact of surgical resection on survival. There are no randomized trials, and there is significant heterogeneity in patient selection, staging, surgical techniques, and adjuvant therapies. In a prospective, non-randomized trial of the Lung Cancer Study Group, extrapleural pneumonectomy without adjuvant therapy improved disease-free, but not overall survival [31]. Sugarbaker et al. reported on 120 patients treated with extrapleural pneumonectomy followed by chemotherapy and radiation. Two and five year survival in this select group were 45% and 22% respectively; this increased to 65% and 27% for patients with epithelial histology, versus 20% and 0% respectively for all other cell types [32]. In a series of 131 patients who underwent either pleurectomy/decortication for minimal visceral pleural tumor or extrapleural pneumonectomy for more locally advanced disease, Rusch observed superior local control with extrapleural pneumonectomy. Survival was not affected, however, because those patients developed distant metastatic disease with an increased frequency [33].

### Radiotherapy

Radiation therapy for mesothelioma is limited by the large treatment volumes required (the entire hemithorax), the radiation sensitivity of the surrounding organs (heart, lung, esophagus, spinal cord), and technical difficulties in treating the multiple surfaces of the pleura [10]. Radiation doses of 40 Gy or above are required to adequately palliate pain or dysphagia [34, 35]. High-dose hemithorax irradiation can cause a significant radiation fibrosis; the resultant deterioration in pulmonary function is equivalent to a pneumonectomy [36].

Mesothelioma frequently seeds along the tracts of biopsies, chest tubes, thoracoscopy trocars and surgical incisions, producing uncomfortable subcutaneous nodules. This can be prevented with adjuvant radiotherapy. In a small randomized trial, Boutin demonstrated that 21 Gy administered in 3 daily fractions 10 to 15 days after thoracoscopy decreased local recurrence from 40% to 0% [37].

Multimodality approaches commonly include radiation as an adjuvant following surgery, although there have been no randomized trials of its efficacy. Because the lung remains in place after pleurectomy, radiotherapy doses must be lower than when extrapleural pneumonectomy is performed. Brachytherapy to sites of gross residual disease has also been evaluated. Hilaris et al. reported on 41 patients who underwent pleurectomy followed by brachytherapy with $^{125}$I, $^{192}$Ir, or $^{32}$P and 4500 cGY external beam radiotherapy. Median survival was 21 months and 2 year survival was 40% [38].

## Chemotherapy

The chemotherapy of mesothelioma has recently been reviewed [39, 40]. Although some agents appear to have modest activity, response duration is usually less than four months and patients treated with chemotherapy do not appear to have an overall survival advantage compared to untreated patients [41]. Since no phase III studies have been performed in this disease comparing the survival of patients treated with various types of systemic therapy versus supportive care, the survival of "untreated" mesothelioma can only be inferred from retrospective studies. Such studies suggest a median survival of five to six months [8, 9, 23, 39].

The evaluation of chemotherapy regimens has been hampered by the relative rarity of the disease and by the difficulty of uniformly assessing response in the pleura. Response rates greater than 20% have not been consistently demonstrated for any drug, nor has combination therapy proven superior to single-agent treatment [39]. Response rates of 10 to

20% have been reported for cyclophosphamide, cisplatin, carboplatin, ifosfamide, dihydro-5-azacytidine, and mitomycin [39, 40, 42–45] (Tables 2, 3). Inactive drugs include the vinca alkaloids, mitoxantrone, and etoposide [40]. Doxorubicin is generally considered the most active agent; responses rates ranged from 28 to 44% in older trials [39, 40]. In a retrospective review of the ECOG experience with mesothelioma, however, the single agent activity of doxorubicin was only 14% [46].

**Table 2.** Representative "active" single-agent chemotherapy for malignant mesothelioma

| Drug | Dose/Schedule | p | Response rate | Reference |
|------|---------------|---|---------------|-----------|
| Adriamycin | 20 mg/m$^2$/d x 3, q3 wk or 70 mg/m$^2$ q3 wk | 51 | 14% | [46] |
| Carboplatin | 150 mg/m$^2$/d x3 q4 wk | 31 | 16% | [42] |
| Cisplatin | 100 mg/m$^2$ q 3 wk | | | |
| Gemcitabine | 1250 mg/m$^2$ d1, 8, 15 q 28d | 28 | 11% | [57] |
| | 1250 mg/m $^2$ d1, 8, 15 q 28d | 16 | 31% | [58] |
| Ifosfamide | 1.2 or 1.5 g/m$^2$ x qd x 5 q 21d | 17 | 24% | [44] |
| Methotrexate | 3 g/m$^2$ q 10d x 4, then q3 wk leucovorin rescue 15 mg q6 hr 24 hrs after MTX | 60 | 37% | [47] |
| Mitomycin | 10 mg/m$^2$ q4 wk x 3, then q6 wk | 19 | 21% | [45] |
| Onconase | 480 μg/m$^2$ q wk | 25 | 19% | [61] |

**Table 3.** Representative combination chemotherapy regimens for malignant mesothelioma

| Drugs | Dose/Schedule | n | Response | Reference |
|-------|---------------|---|----------|-----------|
| Adriamycin | 60 mg/m$^2$ | 35 | 14% | [70] |
| Cisplatin | 75 mg/m $^2$ q4 wk | | | |
| Mitomycin | 10 mg/m $^2$ q4 wk | 35 | 26% | [70] |
| Cisplatin | 75 mg/m $^2$ q4 wk | | | |
| Adriamycin | 60 mg/m $^2$ q4 wk | 24 | 21% | [71] |
| Mitomycin | 10 mg/m $^2$ q4 wk | | | |
| Cisplatin | 60 mg/m $^2$ q4 wk | | | |
| Gemcitabine | 1000 mg/m $^2$ d1, 8, 15 q4 wk | 21 | 48% | [59] |
| Cisplatin | 1000 mg/m $^2$ q4 wk | | | |

The folic acid antagonists may have the greatest activity in this disease. Solheim et al. observed a 37% response rate and a median survival of 11 months in 60 patients treated with *high-dose methotrexate;* there have been no large confirmatory trials of this report [47]. An increased dose of the methotrexate analogue *trimetrexate* apparently led to an improved median survival in a phase II trial by the CALGB [48]. Belani et al. reported a 25% response rate to edatrexate; toxicity was ameliorated with leucovorin rescue [49, 50]. Preliminary experience with the antifolate MTA *(Multitargeted Antifolate, LY231514)* suggests that it has definite activity against malignant mesothelioma. Partial responses were noted in 5 out of 13 patients in a phase I study when MTA was administered with cisplatin; this combination will be the subject of a large multicenter trial [51].

Many of the newer generation of chemotherapy agents have already been evaluated in mesothelioma. There have been two studies of single-agent paclitaxel: the EORTC observed no responses, although median survival was nine months [52], and the CALGB noted a partial response rate of 13% [53]. Topotecan was inactive in an NCCTG trial [54]. A small Japanese study demonstrated a 20% response rate for irinotecan plus cisplatin [55]; the CALGB is presently evaluating single-agent irinotecan in a phase II trial. It is unclear if the antimetabolite gemcitabine has activity in mesothelioma. In three single-agent trials in a total of 57 patients, gemcitabine demonstrated response rates of 0%, 11%, and 31%, respectively [56–58]. In a recently reported trial of gemcitabine in combination with cisplatin, a response rate of 48% was observed in 21 patients [59]; this data awaits confirmation. Phase I activity has been noted for the combination of oxaliplatin and tomudex; further evaluation of these agents is planned [60]. Other new drugs, including docetaxel and suramin, are being tested in cooperative group studies.

Onconase is a ribonuclease isolated from the eggs of the leopard frog. A response rate of 10% was observed in 21 evaluable patients; median survival was 18.5 months [61]. This compound is presently being compared with doxorubicin in a multicenter phase III trial.

## Intrapleural Therapy

Because local control is so difficult to achieve with surgery and radiotherapy, a variety of approaches to intrapleural therapy of malignant mesothelioma have been evaluated. Intracavitary chemotherapy can produce increased local drug concentrations and prolonged drug exposure with less systemic toxicity [62]. Rusch administered intrapleural cisplatin and mitomycin after pleurectomy to 27 patients, followed by systemic therapy with the same agents; median survival was 17 months, and 2 year survival was 40% [29].

Cytokines have also been delivered intrapleurally. Boutin et al. administered intrapleural recombinant γ-interferon and observed 4 thoracoscopically documented complete responses and one partial response in 9 patients with stage I disease; only one partial response was observed in 10 pts with stage II disease [63]. After 89 patients were accrued, the overall response rate was 20%; it was 45% for patients with stage I disease [64].

Photodynamic therapy combines light with a photosensitizer which has selective uptake in malignant cells. In a phase III randomized trial reported by Pass et al., 63 patients underwent maximal debulking surgery and post-operative cisplatin, interferon $\alpha$-2b, and tamoxifen with or without intraoperative photodynamic therapy with photofrin. No differences were noted in median survival or sites of first recurrence [65]. Second-generation photosensitizers are now under investigation.

Adenovirus vectors carrying the herpes simplex thymidine kinase gene can transfect mesothelioma cells; treatment with gancyclovir kills these cells as well as uninfected neighboring cells. This intrapleural approach has been evaluated in phase I trials; gene transfer has been demonstrated, and phase II trials are ongoing [66, 67].

## Key Questions and Future Investigational Approaches

A large population of asbestos exposed workers and their families are at an increased risk of developing mesothelioma. Screening efforts are hampered by the lack of known predictors for the development of this disease [68]. It is possible that with further follow-up, the patients who received SV-40 contaminated polio vaccines may also develop mesothelioma with an increased frequency [17]. Clearly, as we begin to understand the mechanisms of carcinogenesis mediated by asbestos and SV-40, chemopreventive agents will need to be evaluated.

The mechanisms of drug resistance in malignant mesothelioma are also poorly understood. Ogretmen et al. observed coordinate overexpression of mRNA for the multidrug resistance-associated protein (MRP) and the γ-glutamylcysteine synthetase heavy subunit genes, but not the P-glycoprotein gene, in mesothelioma cell lines; MRP expression correlated with doxorubicin resistance [69]. As we continue to test new drugs, we will need to learn more about the molecular mechanisms which make this tumor so resistant to standard chemotherapeutic agents. New drugs with novel mechanisms of action are also desperately needed.

What is the most appropriate way to assess response in the pleura? In most solid tumors, responses are evaluated in a standard two-dimensional format; reproducibly assessing response in pleural-based disease is more problematic. Bidimensionally measurable disease is uncommon, documenting regression may be inaccurate, measuring multiple levels in a single dimension may not be reproducible, and volumetric computed tomography is still investigational. The lack of a measurement standard makes comparisons between trials difficult. Does response correlate with survival or quality of life? Without randomized trials, this is uncertain.

Locoregional tumor, rather than distant metastatic disease, is the principal source of major morbidity in patients with malignant mesothelioma. Intrapleural drug delivery can achieve increased local drug concentrations; cytotoxicty is limited by tissue penetration of drug. Previous trials administered intrapleural chemotherapy after pleurectomy; insufficient cytoreduction may have hampered adequate drug delivery [29, 62]. One innovative approach currently under evaluation uses intracavitary lavage with hyperthermic cisplatin following maximal debulking by extrapleural pneumonectomy [72]. Other strategies for targeting local disease deserve further study.

Have we made any headway in our management of this disease since 1960, when asbestos was first recognized as the principal cause of mesothelioma? Despite numerous trials of surgery, radiotherapy, and countless chemotherapeutic drugs, it is unclear if any of our interventions have had significant impact on more than a few highly selected patients. Yet we have learned a great deal in the past four decades about staging, prognostic factors, and the molecular biology of malignant mesothelioma. As we deepen our understanding of malignant mesothelioma, we have reason to believe that future trials of novel chemotherapeutic agents and combined modality treatments will help us to finally make progress for patients with this disease.

# References

1. Wagner JC, Slegg CA, Marchand P (1960) Diffuse pleural mesotheliomas and asbestos exposure in Northwestern Cape Province. Br J Ind Med 17: 260-271
2. Selikoff JJ (1987) Cancer Risk of Asbestos Exposure. Origins of Human Cancer. Cold Spring Harbor Laboratory, pp 1765-1784
3. Mossman BT, Gee JBL (1989) Asbestos-related diseases. New Engl J Med 320: 1721-1730
4. Longo WE, Rigler MW, Slade J (1995) Crocidolite Asbestos Fibers in Smoke from Original Kent Cigarettes. Cancer Res 55: 2232-2235
5. Leigh J, Rogers AJ, Ferguson DA, Mulder HB, Ackad M, Thompson R (1991) Lung Asbestos Fiber Content and Mesothelioma Cell Type, Site, and Survival. Cancer 68: 135-141
6. Connelly RR, Spirtas R, Myers MH (1987): Demographic Patterns for Mesothelioma in the United States. J Natl Cancer Inst 78: 1053-1060
7. Antman KH (1993) Natural History and Epidemiology of Malignant Mesothelioma. Chest 103: 373S-376S
8. Antman K, Shemin R, Ryan L, Klegar K, Osteen R, Herman T, Lederman G, Corson J (1988): Malignant Mesothelioma: Prognostic Variables in a Registry of 180 Patients, the Dana-Farber Cancer Institute and Brigham and Women's Hospital Experience Over Two Decades, 1965-1985. J Clin Oncol 6: 147-153
9. Vogelzang NJ, Schultz S, Iannuci AM, Kennedy BJ (1984) Malignant Mesothelioma: The University of Minnesota Experience. Cancer 53: 353-377
10. Rusch VW (1990) Diagnosis and Treatment of Pleural Mesothelioma. Sem Surg Oncol 6: 279-285
11. Hirvonen A, Pelin K, Tammilehto L, Karjalainen A, Mattson K, Linnainmaa K (1995) Inherited GSTM1 and NAT2 Defects as Concurrent Risk Modifiers in Asbestos-related Human Malignant Mesothelioma. Cancer Res 55: 2981-2983
12. Weissmann LB, Corson JM, Neugut AI, Antman KA (1996) Malignant Mesothelioma Following Treatment for Hodgkin's Disease. J Clin Oncol 14: 2098-2100
13. Neugut AI, Ahsan H, Antman K (1997) Incidence of Malignant Pleural Mesothelioma after Thoracic Radiotherapy. Cancer 80: 948-950
14. Baris I, Simonato L, Artvinli M, Pooley F, Saracci R, Skidmore J, Wagner C (1987) Epidemiological and Environmental Evidence of the Health Effects of Exposure to Erionite Fibres: A Four-Year Study in the Cappadocian Region of Turkey. Int J Cancer 39: 10-17
15. Baas P, Schouwink H, Zoetmulder FAN (1998): Malignant pleural mesothelioma. Ann Oncol 9: 139-149
16. Andersson M, Wallin H, Jonsson M, Nielsen LL, Visfeldt J, Vyberg M, Bennett WP, De Benedetti VMG, Travis LB, Storm HH (1995) Lung Carcinoma and Malignant Mesothelioma in Patients Exposed to Thorotrast: Incidence, Histology and p53 Status. Int J Cancer 63: 330-336
17. Carbone M, Pass HI, Rizzo P, Marinetti MR, Di Muzio NI, Mew DJY, Levine AS, Procopio A (1994) Simian virus 40-like DNA sequences in human pleural mesothelioma. Oncogene 9:1781-1790
18. Suzuki Y (1980): Pathology of Human Malignant Mesothelioma. Semin Oncol 8: 268-282
19. Donington JS, Mew DJY, Pass HI (1995) Malignant pleural mesothelioma: newer aspects of carcinogenesis, molecular genetics, and prospects for future therapies. Surg Oncol 4: 175-185

20. International Mesothelioma Interest Group (1995) A Proposed New International TNM Staging System for Malignant Pleural Mesothelioma. Chest 108: 1122-1128

21. Boutin C, Rey F, Gouvernet J, Viallat JR, Astoul Ph, Ledoray V (1993) Thoracoscopy in Pleural Malignant Mesothelioma: A Prospective Study of 188 Consecutive Patients. Part 2: Prognosis and Staging. Cancer 72: 394-404

22. Sugarbaker DJ, Strauss GM, Lynch TJ, Richards W, Mentzer SJ, Lee TH, Corson JM, Antman KH (1993) Node Status Has Prognostic Significance in the Multimodality Therapy of Diffuse, Malignant Mesothelioma. J Clin Oncol 11: 1172-1178

23. Curran D, Sahmoud T, Therasse P, van Meerbeeck J, Postmus P, Giaccone G (1998) Prognostic factors in Patients with Pleural Mesothelioma: The European Organization for Research and Treatment of Cancer Experience. J Clin Oncol 16: 145-152

24. Herndon JE, II., Green MR, Chahinian AP, Corson JM, Suzuki Y, Vogelzang NJ (1998) Factors Predictive of Survival Among 337 Patients with Mesothelioma Treated Between 1984 and 1994 by the Cancer and Leukemia Group B. Chest 113: 723-731

25. Patz EF, Shaffer K, Piwnica-Worms DR, Jochelson M, Sarin M, Sugarbaker DJ, Pugatch RD (1992) Malignant Pleural Mesothelioma: Value of CT and MRI Imaging in Predicting Resectability. Am J Roentgenol 159: 961-966

26. Sugarbaker DJ, Jaklitsch MT, Liptay MJ (1995) Mesothelioma and Radical Multimodality Therapy: Who Benefits? Chest 107: 345S-350S

27. Boutin C, Rey F (1993) Thoracoscopy in Pleural Malignant Mesothelioma: A Prospective Study of 188 Consecutive Patients. Part 1: Diagnosis. Cancer 72: 389-393

28. Sugarbaker DJ, Heher EC, Lee TH, Couper G, Mentzer S, Corson JM, Collins JJ, Jr., Shemin R, Pugatch R, Weissman L, Antman KH (1991) Extrapleural pneumonectomy, chemotherapy, and radiotherapy in the treatment of diffuse malignant pleural mesothelioma. J Thorac Cardiovasc Surg 102: 10-15

29. Rusch V, Saltz L, Venkatraman E, Ginsberg R, McCormack P, Burt M, Markman M, Kelsen D (1994) A Phase II Trial of Pleurectomy/Decortication Followed by Intrapleural and Systemic Chemotherapy for Malignant Pleural Mesothelioma. J Clin Oncol 12: 1156-1163

30. Aisner J (1995) Current Approach to Malignant Mesothelioma of the Pleura. Chest 107: 332S-344S

31. Rusch VW, Piantadosi S, Holmes EC (1991) The role of extrapleural pneumonectomy in malignant pleural mesothelioma. A Lung Cancer Study Group trial. J Thorac Cardiovasc Surg 102: 1-9

32. Sugarbaker DJ, Norberto JJ (1998) Multimodality Management of Malignant Pleural Mesothelioma. Chest 113: 61S-65S

33. Rusch VW, Venkatraman E (1996) The Importance of Surgical Staging in the Treatment of Malignant Pleural Mesothelioma. J Thorac Cardiovasc Surg 111: 815-826

34. Gordon W, Antman KH, Greenberger JS, Weichselbaum RR, Chaffey JT (1982) Radiation Therapy in the Management of Patients with Mesothelioma. Int J Radiation Oncol Biol Phys 8: 19-25

35. Ball DL, Cruickshank DG (1990) The Treatment of Malignant Mesothelioma of the Pleura: Review of a 5-Year Experience, with Special Reference to Radiotherapy. Am J Clin Oncol 13: 4-9

36. Maasilta P (1991) Deterioration in Lung Function Following Hemithorax Irradiation for Pleural Mesothelioma. Int J Radiation Oncol Biol Phys 20: 433-438

37. Boutin C, Rey F, Viallat J-R (1995) Prevention of Malignant Seeding After Invasive Diagnostic Procedures in Patients with Pleural Mesothelioma. Chest 108: 754-758

38. Hilaris BS, Nori D, Kwong E, Kutcher GJ, Martini N (1984) Pleurectomy and Intraoperative Brachytherapy and Postoperative Radiation in the Treatment of Malignant Pleural Mesothelioma. Int J Radiation Oncol Biol Phys 10: 325-331

39. Ong ST, Vogelzang NJ (1996) Chemotherapy in Malignant Pleural Mesothelioma: A Review. J Clin Oncol 14: 1007-1017

40. Ryan CW, Herndon J, Vogelzang NJ (1998) A Review of Chemotherapy Trials for Malignant Mesothelioma. Chest 113: 66S-73S

41. Alberts AS, Falkson G, Goedhals L, Vorobiof DA, Van Der Merwe CA (1988) Malignant Pleural Mesothelioma: A Disease Unaffected by Current Therapeutic Maneuvers. J Clin Oncol 6: 527-535

42. Raghavan D, Gianoutsos P, Bishop J, Lee J, Young I, Corte P, Bye P, McCaughan B (1990) Phase II Trial of Carboplatin in the Management of Malignant Mesothelioma. J Clin Oncol 8: 151-154

43. Zidar BL, Green S, Pierce HI, Roach R,W., Balcerzak SP, Militello L (1988) A phase II evaluation of cisplatin in unresectable diffuse malignant mesothelioma: A Southwest Oncology Group Study. Invest New Drugs 6: 223-226

44. Alberts AS, Falkson G, van Zyl L (1988) Malignant Pleural Mesothelioma: Phase II Pilot Study of Ifosfamide and Mesna. J Nat Canc Inst 80: 698-700

45. Bajorin D, Kelsen D, Mintzer DM (1987): Phase II Trial of Mitomycin in Malignant Mesothelioma. Ca Treat Rep 71: 857-858

46. Lerner HJ, Schoenfeld DA, Martin A, Falkson G, Borden E (1983) Malignant Mesothelioma: The Eastern Cooperative Oncology Group (ECOG) Experience. Cancer 52: 1981-1985

47. Solheim OP, Saeter G, Finnanger AM, Stenwig AE (1992) High-dose Methotrexate in the Treatment of Malignant Mesothelioma of the Pleura. A Phase II Study. Br J Cancer 65: 956-960

48. Vogelzang NJ, Weissman LB, Herndon JE, II., Antman KH, Cooper R, Corson JM, Green MR (1994) Trimetrexate in Malignant Mesothelioma: A Cancer and Leukemia Group B Phase II Study. J Clin Oncol 12: 1436-1442

49. Belani CP, Herndon J, Vogelzang NJ, Green MR (1994) Edatrexate for Malignant Mesothelioma: A Phase II Study of the Cancer and Leukemia Group B, 9131. Proc Am Soc Clin Oncol 13: 329

50. Belani CP, Herndon J, Vogelzang NJ, Green MR (1995) Edatrexate with Oral Leucovorin Rescue for Malignant Mesothelioma: A Phase II Study of the Cancer and Leukemia Group B-CALGB 9131. Proc Am Soc Clin Oncol 14: 352

51. Thoedtmann R, Kemmerich M, Depenbrock H, Blatter J, Ohnmacht U, Hanauske A-R (1998) A Phase I Study of MTA (Multi-Targeted Antifolate, LY231514) Plus Cisplatin in Patients with Advanced Solid Tumors. Proc Am Soc Clin Oncol 17: 254a

52. van Meerbeeck J, Debruyne C, van Zandwijk N, Postmus PE, Pennucci MC, van Breukelen F, Galdermans D, Groen H, Pinson P, van Glabbeke M, van Marck E, Giaccone G (1996) Paclitaxel for malignant pleural mesothelioma: a phase II study of the EORTC Lung Cancer Cooperative Group. Br J Ca 74: 961-963

53. Vogelzang NJ, Herndon J, Clamon GH, Mauer AM, Cooper MR, Green MR (1994) Paclitaxel (Taxol) for Malignant Mesothelioma (MM): A Phase II Study, of the Cancer and Leukemia Group B (CALGB 9234). Proc Am Soc Clin Oncol 13: 405

54. Maksymiuk AW, Jung S-H, Marschke RF, Nair S, Jett JIR (1995) Phase II Trial of Topotecan in Pleural Mesothelioma: A North Central Cancer Treatment Group (NCCTG) Trial. Proc Am Soc Clin Oncol 14: 435

55. Nakano T, Shinjo M, Togawa N, Yamashita H, Tonomura A, Miyake M, Ninomiya K, Higashino K (1997) A Pilot Phase II Study of Irinotecan (CPT-11) in Combination with Cisplatin Administered Intravenously to Patients with Malignant

Mesothelioma. International Mesothelioma Interest Group, Fourth International Conference 50

56. Millard FE, Herndon J, Vogelzang NJ, Green MR (1997) Gemcitabine for Malignant Mesothelioma: A Phase II Study of the Cancer and Leukemia Group B (CALGB 9530). Proc Am Soc Clin Oncol 16: 475a

57. van Meerbeeck JP, Baas P, Debruyne C, Groen HJM, Manegold CH, Ardizzoni A, Gridelli C, Galdermans D, Lenz M-A, Giaccone G (1997) Gemcitabine in malignant pleural mesothelioma: A phase II study. Lung Ca 18: 17

58. Bischoff HG, Manegold C, Knopp M, Blatter J, Drings P (1998) Gemcitabine (Gemzar) May Reduce Tumor Load and Tumor Associated Symptoms in Malignant Pleural Mesothelioma. Proc Am Soc Clin Oncol 17: 464a

59. Byrne MJ, Davidson JA, Musk AW, Dewar J, van Hazel G, Buck M, de Klerk N, Robinson BWS (1998) Cisplatin and Gemcitabine Treatment for Malignant Mesothelioma: A Phase II Study. Proc Am Soc Clin Oncol 17: 464a

60. Fizazi K, Soria JC, Bonnay M, Ruffie P, Ducreux M, LeChevalier T, Couturas O, Poterre M, Armand JP (1998) Phase I/II Dose-Finding and Pharmacokinetic Study of "Tomudex" in Combination with Oxaliplatin in Advanced Solid Tumors. Proc Am Soc Clin Oncol 17: 201a

61. Costanzi J, Darzynkiewicz Z, Chun H, Mittelman A, Partella T, McCachren S, Puccio C, Taub R, Shogen K, Mikulski S (1997) The Use of Onconase for Patients with Advanced Malignant Mesothelioma. International Mesothelioma Interest Group, Fourth International Conference 59

62. Rusch VW, Niedzwiecki D, Tao Y, Menendez-Botet C, Dnistrian A, Kelsen D, Saltz L, Markman M (1992) Intrapleural Cisplatin and Mitomycin for Malignant Mesothelioma Following Pleurectomy: Pharmacokinetic Studies. J Clin Oncol 10: 1001-1006

63. Boutin C, Viallat JR, van Zandwijk N, Douillard JT, Paillard JC, Guerin JC, Mignot P, Migueres J, Varlet F, Jehan A, Delepoulle E, Brandely M (1991) Activity of Intrapleural Recombinant Gamma-Interferon in Malignant Mesothelioma. Cancer 67: 2033-2037

64. Boutin C, Nussbaum E, Monnet I, Bignon J, Vanderschueren R, Guerin JC, Menard O, Mignot P, Dabouis G, Douillard JY (1994): Intrapleural Treatment with Recombinant Gamma-Interferon in Early Stage Malignant Pleural Mesothelioma. Cancer 74: 2460-2467

65. Pass HI, Temeck BK, Kranda K, Thomas G, Russo A, Smith P, Friauf W, Steinberg S (1997) Phase III Randomized Trial of Surgery With or Without Intraoperative Photodynamic Therapy and Postoperative Immunochemotherapy for Malignant Pleural Mesothelioma. Ann Surg Oncol 4: 628-633

66. Treat J, Kaiser L, Recio A, Roberts J, Wilson J, Litsky L, Sterman D, Amin K, Coonrad L, Alston J, Albelda S (1997) Adenoviral-mediated intrapleural HSVtk gene therapy (AdRSVtk) for malignant mesothelioma: a phase I clinical trial. Proc Am Soc Clin Oncol 16: 433a

67. Treat J, Kaiser LR, Sterman DH, Litzky L, Davis A, Wilson JM, Albelda SM (1996) Treatment of Advanced Mesothelioma with the Recombinant Adenovirus H5.010RSVTK: A Phase 1 Trial (BB-IND 6274). Human Gene Therapy 7: 2047-2057

68. Sanden A, Jarvholm B (1991) A Study of Possible Predictors of Mesothelioma in Shipyard Workers Exposed to Asbestos. J Occup Med 33: 770-773

69. Ogretmen B, Bahadori HR, McCauley MD, Boylan A, Green MR, Safa AR (1998) Coordinated Over-Expression of the MRP and $\gamma$-Glutamylcysteine Synthetase Genes, but not MDR-1, Correlates with Doxorubicin Resistance in Human Malignant Mesothelioma Cell Lines. Int J Cancer 75: 757-761

70. Chahinian AP, Antman K, Goutsou M, Corson JM, Suzuki Y, Modeas C, Herndon JE, II., Aisner J, Ellison RR, Leone L, Vogelzang NJ, Green MR (1993) Randomized Phase II Trial of Cisplatin with Mitomycin or Doxorubicin for Malignant Mesothelioma by the Cancer and Leukemia Group B. J Clin Oncol 11: 1559-1565
71. Pennucci MC, Ardizzoni A, Pronzato P, Fioretti M, Lanfranco C, Verna A, Giorgi G, Vigani A, Frola C, Rosso R, for the Italian Lung Cancer Task Force (FONICAP) (1997) Combined Cisplatin, Doxorubicin, and Mitomycin for the Treatment of Advanced Pleural Mesothelioma. Cancer 79: 1897-1902
72. Sugarbaker DJ. Personal communication

# Gastrointestinal Cancers

# Colorectal Cancer

R.L. Schilsky

## Epidemiology, Risk Factors

Incidence

Colorectal cancer is a major public health problem in western countries with the highest incidence rates reported in North America, Australia, New Zealand and western Europe. An estimated 132,000 cases will be diagnosed in the United States in 1998 and approximately 57,000 people will die of the disease [1]. Colorectal cancer is the third most common cancer in men and women and is the third most common cause of cancer death in both sexes. Colon cancer is 2.5 times more common than rectal cancer and, because it has a different natural history than rectal cancer, is usually treated and reported separately from rectal cancer.

Race, Sex, Age Distribution

The incidence rates for colorectal cancer are similar in Caucasians and African-Americans, approximately 61 cases/100,000 for males and 45/100,000 for females, regardless of racial group. During the period 1973–1989, colorectal cancer mortality among whites decreased significantly, by 20% in females and 8.5% in males, whereas mortality increased significantly in blacks, by 22.5% in males and 2.6% in females. The age-adjusted colorectal cancer mortality in the United States for 1988–1992 was highest in black males (28.2/100,000) and exceeded by 33% the mortality in black females (20.4). Corresponding rates in white males (22.9) exceeded by 48% the mortality in white females (15.3) [2].

The age-specific incidence of colorectal cancer rises sharply after age 40, with 90 percent of cancers occurring in individuals age 50 and older. The average age at diagnosis is 60–65 years.

## Localization

Within the large intestine, 69% of cancers occur in the colon and 31% in the rectum. More than half of all colonic cancers occur either in the sigmoid colon (35%) or in the cecum (22%), although, in recent years, right-sided lesions are becoming more common [3].

## Risk Factors, Etiology

Although the specific etiology of colorectal cancer remains unknown, it is likely that the disease results from the accumulation of genetic mutations in the colonic epithelium that ultimately result in the neoplastic phenotype. In some cases, genetic mutations may be inherited as germline mutations, often manifest as familial colon polyp or cancer syndromes. In other cases, somatic mutations in the colon epithelium, perhaps related to environmental or nutritional exposures, ultimately result in the formation of colon cancer. In most cases, adenomatous polyps are believed to be precursor lesions to the development of invasive cancer.

Familial syndromes associated with an increased risk of colorectal cancer are summarized in Table 1. Familial adenomatous polyposis (FAP) is inherited in an autosomal dominant pattern and is characterized by the development of hundreds or thousands of adenomatous polyps throughout the colon and rectum. The average age of onset of polyps is during the 20s and virtually 100% of affected individuals will develop colorectal cancer by age 35–40 if total colectomy is not performed [4]. Germline mutations of the FAP gene located at chromosome 5q22 are detectable in all affected individuals and provide a means of diagnosing the disease prior to the onset of symptoms. Widespread genetic testing may be difficult, however, because each kindred is likely to have a unique FAP mutation.

The hereditary nonpolyposis colorectal cancer syndromes (Lynch syndromes I and II) are characterized by early age of onset of colorectal cancer, autosomal dominant pattern of inheritance, preponderance of

**Table 1.** Familial colon cancer syndromes: familial adenomatous polyposis (FAP) and hereditary non-polyposis colon cancer (HNPCC)

| Feature | Syndrome | |
| | FAP[a] | HNPCC |
| --- | --- | --- |
| Age of onset | 20s | 40s |
| Number of adenomas | >100 | <10 |
| Adenoma distribution | Left or total | Right |
| Cancer distribution | Random | Right |
| Other cancers | Periampullary | Endometrial, ovarian, periampullary, ureteral |
| Germline mutation | APC gene at 5q22 | hMSH2, hMLH1, hPMS1, hPMS2 |

[a] Includes Gardner's syndrome of colon polyps, multiple osteomas, desmoid tumors, neoplasms of thyroid, adrenal, biliary tree, liver.

right sided colon tumors and an excess of synchronous and metachronous colonic and extra-colonic tumors [5]. Endometrial and ovarian cancers have been noted to occur in excess in Lynch syndrome I families while gastric, periampullary and ureteral tumors are increased in frequency in families with Lynch syndrome II. Recently, genetic linkage analysis has demonstrated a high frequency of microsatellite instability in the germline DNA of Lynch syndrome families. Further studies have demonstrated mutations in the human homologues of the bacterial DNA mismatch repair genes (hMSH2, hMLH1, hPMS1, hPMS2) in these families that likely contribute to the development of epithelial tumors [6].

Adenomatous polyps are widely believed to be precursors to the development of most colorectal cancers and the genetic abnormalities that accumulate during the progression from adenoma to carcinoma have now been extensively characterized by Vogelstein and colleagues [7]. This progression typically involves mutations in oncogenes such as FAP, ras and c-myc as well as mutations in tumor suppressor genes such as p53 and DCC [8–10]. The sequence of genetic events thought to occur in the adenoma-carcinoma sequence is depicted in Table 2. There is approximately a 5% probability that carcinoma will be present in an adenoma. Adenomatous polyps less than 1 cm in diameter have a slightly greater than 1% chance of being malignant whereas those greater than 2 cm in diameter contain invasive carcinoma in about 40% of cases.

Patients with inflammatory bowel disease are well known to be at increased risk of developing colorectal cancer. Carcinoma complicating ulcerative colitis is related to the duration of active disease, extent of colitis, duration of symptoms and development of mucosal dysplasia [11]. It

**Table 2.** Postulated genetic changes during colon cancer progression

| Genetic alteration | Normal mucosa | Early adenoma | Late adenoma | Non-invasive carcinoma | Invasive carcinoma | Metastatic carcinoma |
|---|---|---|---|---|---|---|
| APC | WT/mutant | WT/mutant | Loss/mutant | Loss/mutant | Loss/mutant | Loss/mutant |
| K-ras | WT/WT | WT/mutant | WT/mutant | WT/mutant | WT/mutant | WT/mutant |
| p53 | WT/WT | WT/WT | WT/WT | WT/mutant | Loss/mutant | Loss/mutant |
| DCC | WT/WT | WT/WT | WT/WT | WT/WT | Loss/WT | Loss/WT |
| nm23 | WT/WT | WT/WT | WT/WT | WT/WT | WT/WT | Loss/WT |

WT, Wild type

has been estimated that the risk of developing carcinoma in those with total colitis is 10–25 times that of the general population. A similar increase in risk has been estimated for those with Crohn's disease. In patients with this disease, there is an increased risk of small bowel as well as colon carcinomas.

Based on epidemiological studies, as well as studies in animals, a variety of nutritional factors have been implicated in the development of colorectal cancer including diets high in fat or low in fiber as well as deficiency in vitamin D, vitamin E, calcium and selenium [12–15]. While the specific pathobiology resulting in the formation of cancer has not been elucidated for any of these dietary states, these observations have prompted study of various dietary interventions in an attempt to protect against the development of colorectal cancer [16, 17]. Although none have yet produced definitive results, studies examining the importance of calcium, selenium, dietary fiber and folic acid are ongoing.

## Pathology and Staging

Adenocarcinomas account for 90%–95% of all colorectal tumors with the remainder being squamous cell, neuroendocrine or undifferentiated carcinomas. Adenocarcinoma variants that may be associated with a worse prognosis include mucinous and signet ring tumors. In addition to depth of invasion through the bowel wall and extent of regional lymph node involvement, other histopathologic features that may be of prognostic importance are perineural and/or lymphatic invasion, evidence of obstruction or perforation and grade of differentiation [18–20]. The current TNM staging system for colorectal cancer is as follows:

- T1: involves the submucosa but does not invade the muscularis propria
- T2: invades, but does not penetrate, the muscularis propria
- T3: penetrates through the muscularis propria into subserosa, or into nonperitonealized pericolonic or perirectal tissues
- T4: invades other organs or involves the free peritoneal cavity
- N0: no nodal metastases
- N1: one to three pericolic or perirectal nodes involved
- N2: four or more pericolic or perirectal nodes involved
- N3: involvement of any regional node along a named vascular trunk
- M0: no distant metastases
- M1: distant metastases present

The AJCC group staging criteria and corresponding modified Aster-Coller classification are shown in Table 3. The estimated 5-year survival for patients with node negative tumors depends primarily on depth of invasion through the bowel wall but is generally in the range of 70%–85% following surgery only. The survival of patients with regional lymph node metastases depends to a great extent on the number of involved nodes, ranging from 40%–60% for those with 1–3 positive nodes to as low as 25% for those with more than 4 positive nodes follo-wing surgery alone. Patients with rectal cancer are also at high risk of local recurrence in the pelvis. For early stage, node negative tumors, the risk of local recurrence is in the range of 5%–10% but increases to 50% or more if there is transmural penetration of the tumor and involvement of multiple regional nodes.

Recent studies have attempted to identify biological characteristics of the tumor cells that may be of prognostic importance. Factors such as DNA ploidy and S phase fraction, deletion of the DCC gene, overexpres-sion of thymidylate synthase and sucrase-isomaltase and mutation of the Ki-ras and p53 genes have been associated with a worse prognosis in small series of patients, although none have yet been validated as pro-gnostic markers in prospective, large scale clinical trials [21–29]. The impact of such markers may vary based on the pathologic stage of the tumor and the therapy employed.

Preoperative CEA level is the only clinical feature of colorectal cancer that has been consistenly predictive of a poor prognosis.

Table 3. AJCC and modified Aster-Coller staging of colorectal cancer:

|           | AJCC         | Aster-Coller |
|-----------|--------------|--------------|
| Stage I   | T1N0M0       | A            |
|           | T2N0M0       | B1           |
| Stage II  | T3N0M0       | B2           |
|           | T4N0N0       | B3           |
| Stage III | T1-2N1-3M0   | C1           |
|           | T3N1-3M0     | C2           |
|           | T4N1-3M0     | C3           |
| Stage IV  | Tany Nany M1 | D            |

## Work-up and Staging

Evaluation of the Primary Tumor

The presenting symptoms of colorectal cancer, while highly variable and often non-specific, usually include rectal bleeding, change in bowel habits and/or abdominal pain and discomfort. Right sided tumors frequently present with fatigue from the anemia that results from chronic occult blood loss. Left sided tumors are more likely to present with bright red blood per rectum, constipation or diarrhea alternating with constipation, change in stool caliber or left lower quadrant abdominal pain. Tenesmus, rectal bleeding and a sense of incomplete evacuation are symptoms characteristic of rectal cancer. Systemic symptoms such as anorexia and weight loss occur most commonly in the setting of metastatic disease and jaundice or right upper quadrant pain is a frequent harbinger of advanced liver metastases.

The initial evaluation of a patient suspected of having colorectal cancer should include a complete physical examination, including rectal exam with evaluation of the stool for occult blood. Laboratory testing should include a complete blood count with platelet count and white blood cell differential and a chemistry panel that includes renal and liver function tests. A colonoscopy should be performed to exam the entire length of the colon and any detected lesions should be biopsied. Proctocsigmoidoscopy alone is insufficient since even flexible instruments are able to examine only the distal 60 cm of the colon and may miss right sided lesions. A carefully performed air contrast barium enema is a useful diagnostic tool but needs to be followed by colonoscopy if lesions are detected. Therefore, colonoscopy has become established as the preferred diagnostic test for patients suspected of having colorectal cancer. This test also enables detection of multiple, synchronous primary tumors of the bowel.

Once a diagnosis of colorectal cancer has been confirmed by biopsy, additional preoperative evaluation should include measurement of serum CEA level and chest X-ray. The use of pre-operative abdominal CT scans to search for metastatic disease remains controversial for several reasons. First, synchronous metastatic disease is quite uncommon, occurring in less than 5% of patients with a normal physical examination, no significant weight loss, normal liver function tests and a normal preoperative CEA level. Thus, in the majority of patients, abdominal CT scans are likely to be unrevealing and the test is not cost-effective. Further, even if metastatic disease is detected preoperatively, most patients will still require surgical resection of the primary tumor to prevent complications of obstruction, perforation or bleeding. While the detection of metastases preoperatively might impact on the nature of the operation performed, it is not likely to eliminate surgery from the treatment options to be considered. Useful information can occasionally be obtained from preoperative CT scans. Detection of liver metastases might allow the surgeon to plan for metastatectomy during the laparotomy. In addition, since cysts and hemangiomas of the liver are common, baseline CT scans can provide useful information that might be important in clinical decision making at a future time.

At the present time, there is no role for other diagnostic modalities prior to laparotomy. In particular, new scanning techniques that employ radiolabelled monoclonal antibodies have not been demonstrated to be cost-effective in the preoperative evaluation of patients with colorectal cancer.

Work-up for Metastatic Disease

The evaluation of patients suspected of having metastatic disease is based entirely on the clinical signs and symptoms that initiate the workup. The most common sites of metastasis of colorectal cancer are liver, lung and bone. Peritoneal metastases may also occur and local tumor recurrence in the pelvis is a common problem in patients with rectal cancer. Most often, metastases are asymptomatic and may first be detected by palpation of hepatomegaly or abdominal mass on physical exam or by the occurrence of abnormal liver functions tests or a progressively rising CEA level. Symptoms that suggest the presence of metastatic disease include dyspnea with non-productive cough, bone pain, anorexia and weight loss, abdominal pain, jaundice, pelvic pain or urinary frequency. The initial diagnostic test of choice is usually a CT scan of the affected area.

Radio-immunodiagnostic scans such as the Oncoscint scan or the CEAscan can provide useful complementary information, particularly for detection of metastatic deposits in the retroperitoneum, peritoneal cavity or pelvis. Both imaging techniques have superior sensitivity to CT scanning in these areas of the body [30, 31].

## Treatment of Colorectal Cancer

Early Stage Disease

*Colon Cancer*

Surgery is the initial therapy of choice for localized, potentially curable colon cancer. Disease-free and overall survival following surgical resection depend primarily on the pathologic stage of the tumor. Within each pathologic stage, a number of biological characteristics of the tumor, summarized previously, may have prognostic importance as well. Adjuvant chemotherapy has clearly been shown to reduce the risk of recurrence and increase the likelihood of survival of patients with node positive colon cancer. The combination of 5-FU and levamisole administered for one year post-operatively results in a 41% reduction in risk of recurrence and a 33% reduction in risk of death compared with no adjuvant therapy [32]. The recommended doses and schedule of drug administration are shown in Table 4. The combination of 5-FU and leucovorin has also been shown to be acceptable adjuvant therapy for patients with stage III colon cancer [33–36]. INT-0089, a large, multi-center randomized clinical trial, compared 5-FU plus levamisole to 5-FU with high dose leucovorin, 5-FU with low dose leucovorin or the three drug combination of 5-FU, low dose leucovorin and levamisole. With a median follow-up of 5 years, preliminary analysis revealed no significant differences in relapse-free or overall survival for 5-

**Table 4.** Commonly used adjuvant chemotherapy regimens for colon cancer

5-FU/levamisole (duration of therapy: 1 year)
  5-FU 450 mg/m$^2$ daily x5 plus levamisole 50 mg po q 8h x 3 days
  28 days later begin:
  5-FU 450 mg/m$^2$ weekly
  Levamisole 50 mg po q8 hx3 days every 2 weeks

5-FU/leucovorin (high dose) (duration of therapy: 48 weeks)
  Leucovorin 500 mg/m$^2$ weeklyx6
  5-FU 500 mg/m$^2$ weeklyx6
  Two week break, then repeat

5-FU/leucovorin (low dose) (duration of therapy: 6 months)
  Leucovorin 20 mg/m$^2$ daily x5
  5-FU 425 mg/m$^2$ dailyx5
  Repeat every 28 days

FU/high dose leucovorin vs 5-FU/low dose leucovorin; 5-FU/levamisole vs. 5-FU/high dose leucovorin; 5-FU/levamisole vs. 5-FU/low dose leucovorin; or 5-FU/low dose leucovorin vs. 5-FU/low dose leucovorin/levamisole [37]. In each case, 5 year DFS and OS were approximately 60% and 66% respectively.

The three drug combination of 5-FU/low dose leucovorin and levamisole did produce superior survival compared with 5-FU/levamisole. The overall conclusion from the study was that 6 months of chemotherapy with 5-FU/leucovorin should be considered the standard adjuvant regimen for patients with resected high risk colon cancer. A similar trial conducted by the National Surgical Adjuvant Breast and Bowel Project (NSABP CO-4) compared 5-FU/levamisole with 5-FU/high dose leucovorin or 5-FU/high dose leucovorin/levamisole. Preliminary results suggest that 5-FU/high dose leucovorin is superior to 5-FU/levamisole and equivalent to the three drug regimen [38]. A trial conducted by the North Central Cancer Treatment Group has demonstrated that leucovorin does not add to the benefits of 12 months of adjuvant therapy with 5-FU/levamisole but that 6 months of therapy with 5-FU/levamisole is inferior to 6 months of therapy with the three drug combination [39]. Acceptable 5-FU/leucovorin regimens for adjuvant therapy of colon cancer are summarized in Table 3. NSABP CO-5 has addressed whether the addition of interferon alpha to 5-FU/high dose leucovorin provides any additional benefit in the adjuvant setting. The preliminary results of this trial have recently been reported and demonstrate no benefit for the addition of interferon but an increase m toxicity [39a].

Ongoing adjuvant chemotherapy trials are evaluating the role of continuous intravenous infusion of 5-FU in the perioperative or postoperative settings. INT-0136 compares perioperative administration of a seven day infusion of 5-FU followed by conventional 5-FU/levamisole to surgery followed by 5-FU/levamisole while INT-0153 compares 5-FU/low dose leucovorin/levamisole to continuous intravenous infusion of 5-FU plus levamisole in the post-operative setting. In a conceptually similar study, the NSABP is comparing protracted exposure to a fluoropyrimidine, using the orally administered combination of UFT/leucovorin, to standard IV 5-FU/high dose leucovorin. The next generation of adjuvant chemotherapy trials, now being designed, will incorporate the topoisomerase I inhibitor irinotecan (CPT-11) in combination with 5-FU/lecovorin and will compare this 3 drug program to 5-FU/leucovorin alone.

The use of adjuvant chemotherapy for patients with stage II (node negative) colon cancer remains controversial. The intergroup 5-FU/levamisole trial (INT 0035) included a separate randomization for stage II patients to surgery alone or surgery followed by 5-FU/levamisole. With a median follow-up of 7 years, administration of 5-FU/levamisole reduced the risk of recurrence by 31%, a difference that was not statistically significant [40]. Overall survival was virtually identical in the two arms. The NSABP performed a retrospective analysis of outcomes in 1567 stage II patients treated on a series of adjuvant chemotherapy protocols (C01–C04) [41]. The results suggested that stage II patients may benefit from adjuvant therapy to the same extent as stage III patients. While it may be possible to identify stage II patients at particularly high risk of relapse based on biochemical or molecular features of their tumors, prospective trials have not yet shown that the prognosis of such patients can be improved with the use of adjuvant chemotherapy. At the present time, the use of adjuvant chemotherapy for node negative patients should be an individualized decision based on the clinical, pathologic and biologic characteristics of the tumor, the patient's general medical condition and willingness to receive chemotherapy.

An alternative to chemotherapy is the use of immunotherapy in the adjuvant post-operative setting. Active specific immunotherapy with autologous tumor vaccines has been investigated in patients with colon cancer but has yet to demonstrate a significant benefit [42]. More recently, results were reported of a randomized clinical trial comparing administration of the murine monoclonal antibody 17–1A to surgery alone for patients with potentially curable cancer of the colon and rectum. With a median follow-up of 7 years, treated patients had a significant reduction in risk of recurrence (27%) and improvement in survival (30%) with the magnitude of the benefit similar to that originally reported for 5-FU/levamisole [43]. These intriguing results are being pursued in confirmatory trials of antibody versus surgery alone in stage II patients and 5-FU/leucovorin plus or minus antibody in patients with stage III disease.

Perioperative infusion of chemotherapy directly into the portal vein has also been studied as a means of reducing the risk of developing hepatic metastases. Several randomized trials have now been completed and report inconsistent results [44–46]. The largest of these, NSABP CO-2, randomly assigned 1158 patients with Dukes' A, B and C disease to curative resection alone or resection followed by perioperative portal vein infusion of 5-FU at a dose of 600 mg/m$^2$ per day for 7 days. With 7 years of followup, there was a significant improvement in disease-free (68% vs 60%) and overall survival (76% vs 71%) for the treated group, however, there was no reduction in the incidence of hepatic metastases [46]. These results suggested that, while perioperative administration of chemotherapy might be beneficial, the route of administration directly into the portal vein might not be critically important. A recent meta-analysis of ten randomized trials of adjuvant portal vein infusion of chemotherapy suggests a significantly lower mortality for patients treated with portal vein infusion of 5-FU (10%–15% reduction in risk of death compared with surgery alone) [47].

## Rectal Cancer

Local/regional recurrence in the pelvis occurs in 25%–50% of patients with rectal cancer with the magnitude of the risk related to the depth of penetration of the primary tumor and the number of involved regional nodes. Both pre-operative and post-operative pelvic radiation (RT) have been shown to reduce the risk of local failure although most randomized trials have failed to demonstrate a beneficial effect of pelvic RT on survival [48]. Recently, a Swedish multi-center randomized trial demonstrated that preoperative RT given as 25 Gy delivered in five fractions in one week followed by surgery within one week later resulted in a significant reduction in risk of local recurrence as well as a significant improvement in overall survival (58% vs 48% at 5 years) compared with surgery alone [49].

In the United States, combined modality, post-operative adjuvant therapy has been considered the standard based on the results of a series of randomized clinical trials conducted over the past two decades (Table 5). Most studies have employed sequential administration of chemotherapy followed by pelvic RT plus concurrent chemotherapy followed by additional cycles of chemotherapy. Treatment typically begins within six weeks of surgery and is completed over approximately six months. These studies have clearly demonstrated that combined modality therapy results in superior local control and overall survival compared to surgery alone or surgery followed by pelvic RT [50–52]; that chemotherapy with the combination of methyl CCNU and 5-FU is not superior to 5-FU alone [53]; that continuous infusion of 5-FU during pelvic RT

**Table 5.** Rectal cancer: selected completed adjuvant trials

| Series | Accruals | Treatment | Results |
|---|---|---|---|
| GITSG 7175 | 227 | Control<br>MF<br>RT+MF<br>RT | RT + MF results in 59% 5-year survival; 43% in controls ($p<0.01$) |
| NCCTG 79-47-51 | 204 | MF→RT+5FU→MF<br>RT | RT + MF resulted in 63% 7-yr survival; 48% for RT alone ($p=0.04$) |
| NSABP R01 | 555 | Control<br>Pelvic RT<br><br>MOF | MOF resulted in 52% 5-yr survival; 42% in controls (and RT); significantly superior DFS |
| GITSG 7189 | 210 | RT+5FU→5FU<br>RT+MF→MF | 3-yr DFS is 45% for MF and 69% for 5FU |
| NCCTG 86-47-51 | 453 | MF→RT+5FU→MF<br>5FU→RT+5FU→5FU<br>(infusion vs bolus for 5FU) | With 46-mo median follow-up MF was not superior to 5FU; 5FU infusion superior to bolus in time to relapse and survival |
| INT-0114 | 1378 | 5FU→RT+5FU→5FU<br>5FU+LV→RT+5FU+LV→5FU+LV<br>5FU+LEV→RT+5FU→5FU+LEV<br>5FU+LV+LEV→RT+5FU+LV→5FU+LV+LEV | Addition of LEV, LV or LEV + LV to 5-FU results in increased toxicity without increased efficacy |
| NSABP RO2[a] | 750 | MOF<br>MOF→RT+5FU→MOF<br>5FU+LV<br>5FU+LV→RT+5FU→5FU+LV | Not yet reported |

M, Methyl-CCNU; GITSG, Gastrointestinal Tumor Study Group; 5FU, fluorouracil; NCCTG, North Central Cancer Treatment Group; MOF, methyl-CCNU, vincristine, fluorouracil; NSABP, National Surgical Adjuvant Breast and Bowel Project; LEV, levamisole; INT, Intergroup; LV, leucovorin.
[a]Women are not randomized to MOF.

reduces both locoregional and distant failure compared to intermittent bolus administration of 5-FU during RT [54]; and that the addition of levamisole, leucovorin or their combination to 5-FU results in increased systemic toxicity without a clear improvement in local tumor control or overall survival [55]. Thus, at the present time, standard post-operative adjuvant therapy for patients with stages II and III rectal cancer consists of two cycles of systemic administration of 5-FU alone followed by pelvic RT with concomitant administration of continuous intravenous infusion of 5-FU followed by two additional cycles of 5-FU chemotherapy (Table 6).

The ongoing rectal adjuvant trials are summarized in Table 7. INT-0144 compares the standard approach described above to continuous IV infusion of 5-FU given for two months before and after pelvic RT as well as during pelvic irradiation. The third arm is identical to the three drug combination given in INT-0114 in which bolus 5-FU, leucovorin and levamisole are administered prior to and following pelvic RT with concurrent bolus 5-FU plus leucovorin. NSABP R03 addresses the important question of whether combined modality therapy is most effective when administered before or after operation. Of note, an intergroup trial with a similar design was closed prematurely due to poor patient accrual raising some concern as to whether the NSABP study can be successfully completed.

Selected patients with early stage rectal cancer and distal rectal lesions can be managed successfully with local excision of the tumor, thereby preserving normal sphincter function. Tumors amenable to this approach are often small, exophytic, mobile tumors without adverse pathologic features (ie, high grade, blood or lymphatic vessel invasion, perineural invasion, penetration into or through the muscularis propria). T1 tumors generally require no further therapy following excision, however, more deeply invasive tumors or those with adverse pathologic features may have risks of local recurrence or positive regional nodes in the range of 15%–20% and therefore require additional postoperative therapy. A recently completed multi-institutional phase II trial for patients with distal rectal T1/T2 lesions employed transanal excision of the tumor followed by post-operative combined modality therapy for patients with T2 tumors [56]. Preliminary results have demonstrated the feasibility of this approach. After a median followup of 24 months, 4/113 patients had died of cancer and only 2/113 had isolated local recurrences, both of which were successfully treated with surgical resection.

**Table 6.** Adjuvant combined modality regimen for rectal cancer

5-Fluorouracil 500 mg/m$^2$ dailyx5; repeat day 29
Pelvic RT with concurrent 5-FU 250 mg/m$^2$ per day by continuous intravenous infusion during RT
5-Fluorouracil 500 mg/m$^2$ dailyx5; repeat 28 days later

**Table 7.** Ongoing rectal cancer adjuvant randomized trials

| Series | Stage | Target no. | Therapy |
|---|---|---|---|
| NSABP R-03 | Clinically T3 resectable | 900 | 5FU+LV→5FU+LV+RT→S→5FU+LV<br>S→5FU+LV→5FU+LV+RT→5FU+LV |
| INT 0144 | T3-4 and/or N+ | 2400 | Bolus 5FU→RT+PVI 5FU→bolus 5FU<br>PVI 5FU→RT+PVI 5FU→PVI 5FU<br>Bolus 5FU+LV+LEV→RT+5FU+LV→bolus 5FU+LV+LEV |

INT, Intergroup study; 5FU, 5-fluorouracil; LV, leucovorin; RT, radiation therapy; S, surgery; NSABP, National Surgical Adjuvant Breast and Bowel Project; PVI, prolonged venous infusion; LEV, levamisole.

Metastatic Colorectal Cancer

*Surgical Therapy*

Metastases to the liver and lungs account for the great majority of non-nodal metastases from colorectal cancer. Resection of metastases is a reasonable consideration for selected patients and has been associated with long term disease free survival in as many as 25%–40% of patients able to undergo resection. Patients most likely to benefit from resection of hepatic metastases include those with an early stage primary tumor and long disease-free interval (>1 year) from therapy of the primary tumor to the appearance of the metastastic lesions; patients with asymptomatic metastases; patients with no more than 4 liver lesions; and patients in whom a negative 1 cm surgical margin can be obtained at resection [57–60]. The size and location of metastases in the liver do not by themselves impact on prognosis as long as adequate surgical margins can be obtained. Resection of hepatic metastases is contraindicated in patients with extra-hepatic disease. Therefore, all operative candidates should be carefully evaluated with a preoperative CT scan of the chest, abdomen and pelvis, colonoscopy, serum chemistries and CEA determination. Intra-operative biopsy of all suspicious lesions should occur prior to proceeding with definitive hepatic resection and intra-operative ultrasound of the liver should be performed in an attempt to identify small lesions that might have been missed by other radiographic procedures.

Resection of pulmonary metastases can be considered for patients with disease confined to the lungs who have sufficient pulmonary function to be able to tolerate resection. Thus, candidates for resection require extensive pre-operative evaluation before a decision is reached regarding whether surgery is appropriate. Operative mortality averages 1% in contemporary surgical series and 5 year survival ranges from 15%–40% [61].

*Systemic Chemotherapy*

The development of systemic chemotherapy for colorectal cancer has paralleled the development of 5-fluorouracil as an effective antineoplastic agent. Synthesized by Heidelberger et al in 1957 and introduced into clinical trials soon thereafter, 5-FU remains the most widely used chemotherapy drug for colorectal cancer [62]. During the past 40 years, the biochemical pharmacology of the drug has been clearly elucidated and a variety of routes and schedules of administration have been explored in the clinic. Knowledge of the biochemical and clinical pharmacology of the drug has led to the development of rationally designed strategies to enhance its effectiveness and has permitted the design of a new group of orally active agents that may simplify drug administration as well as enhance the efficacy of therapy.

The modulation of 5-FU by leucovorin is perhaps the most successful biochemical modulation strategy to be brought from the laboratory to the clinic. By repleting intracellular stores of reduced folates, the addition of leucovorin results in more sustained inhibition of thymidylate synthase by fluorodeoxyuridylate and increased 5-FU cytotoxicity [63–67]. At least nine prospective randomized clinical trials in patients with metastatic colorectal cancer have demonstrated improved response rates for the use of 5-FU/leucovorin compared with 5-FU alone and two studies have demonstrated an improvement in survival for 5-FU/LV combinations [68–76]. A meta-analysis of nine randomized trials comparing 5-FU/LV to 5-FU alone also concluded that the combination produced superior response rates but could not confirm a survival advantage [77]. Commonly used 5-FU/LV regimens for patients with metastatic disease are the same as those summarized in Table 4 for use in the adjuvant setting. It can be anticipated that such therapy will result in objective tumor regression in 20%–25% of patients with measurable disease and in a median time to disease progression of 6 months. Median survival of patients can be expected to be in the range of 10–12 months. Toxicity varies with schedule of 5-FU administration with the weekly regimen causing more diarrhea and the monthly regimen causing more stomatitis and neutropenia. Other attempts at improving the efficacy of 5-FU chemotherapy by the addition of cisplatin, interferon or N-(phosphonacetyl)-L-aspartate (PALA) have not been demonstrated to be effective in multi-center randomized clinical trials [78]. The administration of methotrexate prior to 5-FU does appear to result in increased response rates compared to 5-FU alone provided that the two drugs are administered 24 h apart [79]. A meta-analysis of several randomized trials examining this strategy has revealed a small survival advantage for the combination [80]. This approach is currently being pursued further with the use of a lipid soluble antifolate, trimetrexate, administered 24 h prior to a 5-FU/LV combination. Phase II studies of this regimen have demonstrated response rates in the range of 35%–50% with acceptable toxicity rates [81, 82]. Thus, this combination is presently being compared to 5-FU/LV in a multi-center, prospective, randomized placebo-controlled clinical trial.

In view of the variety of 5-FU based chemotherapy regimens and schedules developed over the past 20 years, two randomized trials were conducted by the United States cooperative groups in an attempt to define the optimal regimen [83, 84]. The design and results of these studies are shown in Table 8. Neither study was successful in identifying a clearly superior regimen. Indeed both studies demonstrated similar response rates and survival duration for all of the regimens. A consistent observation was that prolonged continuous intravenous infusion of 5-FU was as effective as any other mode of administration of the drug and was associated with substantially less grade 3–4 toxicity. A recent meta-analysis of randomized trials that compared IV bolus to continuous IV infusion of 5-FU has demonstrated a modest survival advantage for infusional therapy (median survival 11.3 vs 12.1 months) [85]. A regimen of LV 200 $mg/m^2$ as a 2 hour infusion followed by bolus 5-FU 400 $mg/m^2$ and 22 hour infusion 5-FU 600 $mg/m^2$ for 2 consecutive days every 2 weeks has been compared to standard 5-FU/LV administered for 5 consecutive

**Table 8.** Randomized trials in metastatic colorectal cancer

| Treatment | Response rate (%) | Median survival (mos) | ≥Grade 4 toxicity (%) |
|---|---|---|---|
| ECOG/CALGB phase III trial | | | |
| 5-FU 24-h infusion, weekly | – | 14.8 | 11 |
| PALA→5-FU 24 h infusion, weekly | – | NR | 11 |
| 5-FU/oral LV weekly | – | 13.2 | 27 |
| 5-FU/IV LV weekly | – | 13.6 | 23 |
| 5-FU/Interferon | – | 15.3 | 21 |
| SWOG phase II trial | | | |
| 5-FU LV push | 29 | 14 | 41 |
| 5-FU/LV (low dose) | 27 | 14 | 40 |
| 5-FU/LV (high dose) | 21 | 13 | 23 |
| 5-FU, CVI | 29 | 15 | 5 |
| 5-FU/lV, CVI | 26 | 14 | 9 |
| 5-FU 24 h infusion, weekly | 25 | 15 | 9 |
| PALA→5-FU 24-h infusion, weekly | 15 | 11 | 9 |

ECOG, Eastern Cooperative Oncology Group; CALGB, Cancer and Leukemia Group B; SWOG, Southwest Oncology Group.  NR = not reported

days each month [86]. The infusional regimen was less toxic and produced superior response rates (32.6 vs 14.4%) and progression-free survival although median survival was not significantly different between the treatments. These observations have led to a resurgence of interest in the use of prolonged exposure to 5-FU as therapy for colorectal cancer and have spawned the development of a number of oral fluoropyrimidines designed to facilitate protracted drug exposure without the need for indwelling catheters and infusion pumps.

5-Fluorouracil itself cannot be administered orally due to rapid metabolism to inactive metabolites by dihydropyrimidine dehydrogenase (DPD) located in the gut wall and liver. In an attempt to circumvent this problem, 5-FU prodrugs that are not substrates for DPD have been designed or 5-FU has been administered in combination with specific DPD inhibitors. Both strategies have been effective in permitting delivery of pharmacologically active concentrations of 5-FU into the systemic circulation. UFT, a combination of uracil and tegafur [87, 88], and capecitabine [89] are both metabolized to 5-FU following oral administration and have shown activity in treatment of metastatic colorectal cancer. Both agents are currently being compared to standard 5-FU/LV regimens in randomized clinical trials. When administered with eniluracil, a specific inactivator of DPD, 5-FU becomes 100% orally bioavailable, and has demonstrated effectiveness in therapy of metastatic colorectal cancer [90]. This regimen is also being compared to standard intravenous therapy with 5-FU/LV. Each of these oral regimens offers both theoretical and practical advantages compared with standard chemotherapy for metastatic colorectal cancer. Whether any will replace standard therapy will be determined by the outcome of the ongoing studies.

There a few therapeutic options for patients whose tumors fail to respond or progress following response to conventional 5-FU based chemotherapy. Irinotecan (CPT-11), a novel topoisomerase 1 inhibitor, has recently been approved for use in this setting. Response rates to CPT-11 range from 15%–20% and the response duration is typically in the range of 4 months [91, 92]. The dosage schedule most commonly used in the United States is 125 mg/m$^2$ weekly for 4 weeks followed by a two week rest period while that most often used in Europe is 350 mg/m$^2$ every three weeks. The regimens seem to be equivalent in both efficacy and toxicity. A recently reported randomized trial has demonstrated that CPT-11, administered on the every three week schedule, results in improved survival compared with best supportive care in patients with 5-FU-refractory colorectal cancer [93]. Toxicities of CPT-11 include diarrhea and neutropenia. Intensive loperamide therapy is necessary to minimize the severity and duration of diarrhea in patients receiving CPT-11.

Patients whose tumors progress following CPT-11 are unlikely to respond to any other conventional chemotherapy treatment and should be considered for participation in clinical trials of novel therapies if they have adequate performance status and organ function. Among the most interesting drugs currently being investigated for treatment of colorectal cancer is oxaliplatin, a novel platinum-containing compound that has produced objective tumor regression in 10% of patients with 5-FU refractory disease and in 27% of previously untreated patients [94]. When administered in combination with infusional 5-FU regimens to patients without prior chemotherapy, response rates as high as 50% have been reported with this drug [95].

## Regional Therapy of Metastatic Disease

The delivery of chemotherapy into the hepatic artery has been facilitated by the development, in recent years, of implantable infusion pumps. The rationale for this approach stems from the fact that the liver is the most common site of metastases from colorectal cancer and that liver metastases derive more than 80% of their blood supply from the hepatic artery. The drug most commonly employed in this setting is fluorodeoxyuridine (FUDR) because of its exceptionally high hepatic extraction. Seven prospective randomized trials comparing systemic fluoropyrimidine therapy with HAI FUDR have now been completed (Table 9) [96–101]. In each study, the response rate to HAI therapy was significantly higher than to systemic treatment yet no study demonstrated a clear survival advantage for HAI, in part because many patients receiving systemic therapy crossed over to HAI treatment at the time of disease progression. A recently reported meta-analysis of these studies has confirmed the significantly higher response rates for HAI therapy and has revealed a survival advantage as well [102].

The toxicity of HAI, once considerable, has been ameliorated with the introduction of new drug combinations and new schedules of drug administration. The most significant toxicity is jaundice secondary to sclerosing cholangitis induced by chemotherapy. Ulceration of the gastric and/or duodenal mucosa has also been reported due, primarily,

**Table 9.** Randomized trials of hepatic artery infusion chemotherapy

| Group | n | Drug | HAI Response rate (%) | Survival (mos) | Drug | Systemic therapy Response rate (%) | Survival (mos) |
|---|---|---|---|---|---|---|---|
| MSKCC | 162 | FUDR | 53 | 17 | FUDR | 21 | 12 |
| NCOG | 143 | FUDR | 42 | 16.8 | FUDR | 10 | 16.1 |
| NCI | 64 | FUDR | 62 | 17 | FUDR | 17 | 12 |
| Consortium | 43 | FUDR | 58 | n.r. | 5-FU | 38 | n.r. |
| City of Hope | 41 | FUDR | 56 | n.r. | 5-FU | 0 | n.r. |
| Mayo Clinic | 69 | FUDR | 48 | 12.6 | 5-FU | 21 | 10.5 |
| France | 163 | FUDR | 43 | 15 | 5-FU | 9 | 11 |

MSKCC, Memorial Sloan Kettering Cancer Center; NCOG, Northern California Oncology Group; NCI, National Cancer Institute.

to inadvertent perfusion of the mucosa of the stomach or duodenum via collateral branches of the hepatic artery. New approaches that appear to reduce the toxicity of HAI therapy include addition of dexamethasone to the infusate, decreasing the duration of the infusion and alternating intraarterial (IA) administration of FUDR with IA 5-FU. Final assessment of the role of HAI chemotherapy in treatment of metastatic colorectal cancer awaits completion of a definitive randomized trial with adequate numbers of patients, prohibition of crossover and inclusion of quality of life as well as economic endpoints in addition to response rate and survival. Such a trial is presently being conducted by the Cancer and Leukemia Group B.

## Summary

As our understanding of the biology of colorectal cancer improves, it will inevitably lead to more effective strategies for prevention, early detection and treatment. The biological characterstics of tumors can already be used to assess prognosis and the likelihood of response to fluoropyrimidine therapy. Current therapeutic strategies, summarized in Table 10 and Figures 1–3, will no doubt soon be modified to incorporate biological markers into the current staging systems and to include new chemotherapeutic agents in the mangement of all stages of colorectal cancer.

**Table 10.** Guidelines for follow-up of patients after completion of primary therapy

| | |
|---|---|
| Physical examination | Every 3 months for 2 years then every 6 months to 5 years |
| CBC and serum chemistries | Same as for physical exam |
| CEA | If elevated at diagnosis or post-colectomy then repeat every 3 months for 2 years, then annually for 5 years |
| Abdominal/pelvic CT | Obtain 4–6 weeks after surgery as baseline, repeat annually for 3 years or sooner if clinically indicated |
| Chest X-ray | Every 6 months for 2 years then annually |
| Colonoscopy | Repeat annually for 2 years; if negative x2 then repeat every 3 years; if polyps detected, repeat annually |

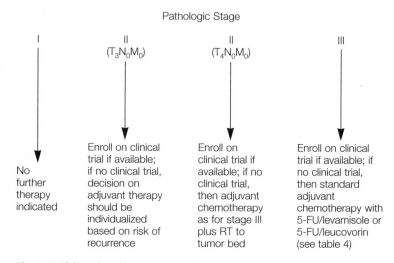

Pathologic Stage

| I | II ($T_3N_0M_0$) | II ($T_4N_0M_0$) | III |
|---|---|---|---|
| No further therapy indicated | Enroll on clinical trial if available; if no clinical trial, decision on adjuvant therapy should be individualized based on risk of recurrence | Enroll on clinical trial if available; if no clinical trial, then adjuvant chemotherapy as for stage III plus RT to tumor bed | Enroll on clinical trial if available; if no clinical trial, then standard adjuvant chemotherapy with 5-FU/levamisole or 5-FU/leucovorin (see table 4) |

**Fig. 1.** Guidelines for adjuvant therapy of colon cancer

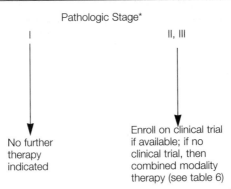

Pathologic Stage*

I                                                    II, III

No further                                          Enroll on clinical trial
therapy                                            if available; if no
indicated                                          clinical trial, then
                                                   combined modality
                                                   therapy (see table 6)

* In patients who receive pre-operative chemotherapy plus radiation, pathologic stage
  cannot be determined reliably. Therefore, such patients should receive post-operative
  chemotherapy for up to four cycles with 5-FU alone or 5-FU/leucovorin.

**Fig. 2.** Guidelines for adjuvant therapy of rectal cancer

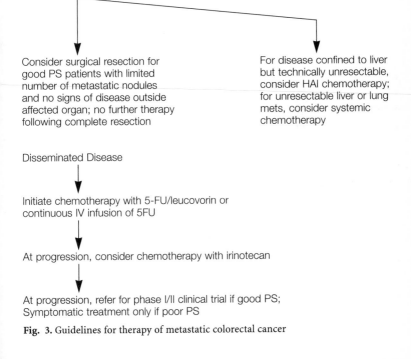

Organ confined (liver or lung)

Consider surgical resection for              For disease confined to liver
good PS patients with limited                but technically unresectable,
number of metastatic nodules                 consider HAI chemotherapy;
and no signs of disease outside              for unresectable liver or lung
affected organ; no further therapy           mets, consider systemic
following complete resection                 chemotherapy

Disseminated Disease

Initiate chemotherapy with 5-FU/leucovorin or
continuous IV infusion of 5FU

At progression, consider chemotherapy with irinotecan

At progression, refer for phase I/II clinical trial if good PS;
Symptomatic treatment only if poor PS

**Fig. 3.** Guidelines for therapy of metastatic colorectal cancer

# References

1. Landis, SH, Murray, T, Bolden, S, Wingo, PA: Cancer Statistics, 1998, CA:A Cancer Journal for Clinicians, 48:6–29, 1998
2. Schottenfeld, D: Epidemiology, *in* Cancer of the Colon, Rectum and Anus, Cohen, AM, Winawer, SJ, Friedman, MA, Gunderson, LL (eds). McGraw-Hill, Inc, New York, 1995, pp:11–24
3. Cohen, AM, Minsky, BD, Schilsky, RL: Cancer of the Colon, *in* Devita, VT, Hellman, S, Rosenberg, SA (eds) Cancer: Principles and Practice of Oncology, Lippincott-Raven, Philadelphia, 5<sup>th</sup> edition, 1997, pp: 1144–1197
4. Rustgi, AK: Hereditary gastrointestinal polyposis and non-polyposis syndromes. N. Engl. J. Med. 331:1694–1702, 1994
5. Lynch, HT, Smyrk, T: Hereditary non-polyposis colorectal cancer (Lynch Syndrome) Cancer 78:1149–1167, 1996
6. Rhyu, MS: Molecular mechanisms underlying hereditary non-polyposis colorectal carcinoma. J. Natl. Cancer Inst. 88:240–251, 1996
7. Fearon, ER, Vogelstein, B: A genetic model for colorectal tumorigenesis. Science 61:759–767, 1990
8. Kinzler, KW, Nilbert, MC, Vogelstein, B, et al. Identification of a gene located at chromosome 5q21 that is mutated in colorectal cancers. Science 251:1366–1369, 1991
9. Baker, SJ, Fearon, ER, Nigro, JM et al. Chromosome 17 deletions and p53 gene mutations in colorectal carcinomas. Science 244:217–221, 1989
10. Fearon, ER, Cho, KR, Nigro, JM et al. Identification of a chromosome 18q gene that is altered in colorectal cancer. Science 247:49–56, 1990
11. Riddell, RH: Inflammatory bowel disease and colorectal cancer, *in* Cohen, AM, Winawer, SJ, Friedman, MA, Gunderson, LL (eds) Cancer of the Colon, Rectum and Anus, McGraw-Hill, Inc. New York, 1995, pp: 105–119
12. Winawer, SJ, Shike, M: Dietary factors in colorectal cancer and their possible effects in earlier stages on hyperproliferation and adenoma formation. J. Natl. Cancer Inst. 84:74–75, 1992
13. Giovannucci, E, Stampfer, MJ, Colditz, G, et al. Relationship of diet to risk of colorectal adenoma in men. J. Natl. Cancer Inst. 84:91–98, 1992
14. Stone, WL, Papas, AM: Tocopherols and the etiology of colon cancer. J. Natl. Cancer Inst. 89:1006–1014, 1997
15. Martinez, ME, Giovannucci, EL, Colditz, GA et al. Calcium, vitatmin D and the occurrence of colorectal cancer among women. J. Natl. Cancer Inst. 88:1375–1382, 1996
16. Alberts, DS, Ritenbaugh, C, Story, JA et al. Randomized, double-blinded, placebo-controlled study of effect of wheat bran fiber and calcium on fecal bile acids in patients with resected adenomatous colon polyps. J. Natl. Cancer Inst. 88:81–92, 1996
17. MacLennan, R, Macrae, F, Bain, C, et al. Randomized trial of intake of fat, fiber and beta carotene to prevent colorectal adenomas. J. Natl. Cancer Inst. 87:1760–1766, 1995
18. Minsky, BD, Mies, C, Rich, TA et al. Lymphatic vessel invasion is an independent prognostic factor for survival in colorectal cancer. Int. J. Radiat. Oncol. 17:311–318, 1989
19. Knudsen, JB, Nilsson, T, Sprechler, M, et al. Venous and nerve invasion as prognostic factors in postoperative survival of patients with resectable cancer of the rectum. Dis Colon and Rectum 26:613–617, 1983

20. Krasna, MJ, Flancbaum, L, Cody, RP et al. Vascular and neural invasion in colorectal carcinoma: incidence and prognostic significance. Cancer 61:1018–1023, 1988

21. Witzig, TE, Loprinzi, CL, Gonchoroff, NJ et al. DNA ploidy and cell kinetic measurements as predictors of recurrence and survival in stages B2 and C colorectal adenocarcinoma. Cancer 68:879–888, 1991

22. Enker, WE, Kimmel, M, Cibas, ES, et al. DNA/RNA content and proliferative fractions of colorectal cancers: a five year prospective study relating flow cytometry to survival. J. Natl. Cancer Inst. 83:701–707, 1991

23. Shibata, D, Reale, MA, Lavin, P et al. The DCC protein and prognosis in colorectal cancer. New Engl. J. Med. 335:1727–1732, 1996

24. Lenz, H-J, Danenberg, KD, Danenberg, P, et al. p53 status and thymidylate synthase expression are associated and predict for recurrence in patients with stage II colon cancer. Proc. Am. Soc. Clin. Oncol. 15:215, 1996

25. Jessup, JM, Lavin, PT, Andrews, CW et al. Sucrase-isomaltase is an independent prognostic marker for colorectal carcinoma. Dis. Colon Rectum 38:1257–1264, 1995

26. Ahnen, DJ, Feigl, P, Quan, G, et al. Ki-ras mutation and p53 overexpression predict the clinical behavior of colorectal cancer: a Southwest Oncology Group study. Cancer Res. 58:1149–1158, 1998

27. Bell, SM, Scott, N, Cross, D, et al. Prognostic value of p53 overexpression and c-Ki-ras gene mutations in colorectal cancer. Gastroenterology 104:57–64, 1993

28. Bosari, S, Viale, G, Bosse, P, et al. Cytoplasmic accumulation of p53 protein: an independent prognostic indicator in colorectal adenocarcinomas. J. Natl. Cancer Inst. 86:681–687, 1994

29. Ogunbiyi, OA, Goodfellow, PJ, Herfarth, K, et al. Confirmation that chromosome 18q allelic loss in colon cancer is a prognostic indicator. J. Clin. Oncol 16:427–433, 1998

30. Patt, YZ, Hogue, A, Podoloff, DA, et al. CEA-Scan, a $^{99}$Tc-labeled Fab fragment of moAb anti-CEA immu-4 for radioimmunodetection of occult metastatic colorectal cancer in patients with rising serum CEA: a multi-institutional study. Proc. Am. Soc. Clin. Oncol. 15:208, 1996

31. Tempero, M, Brand, R, Holdeman, K, Matamoros, A: New imaging techniques in colorectal cancer. Sem. in Oncol. 22:448–471, 1995

32. Moertel, CG, Fleming, TR, MacDonald, JS, et al. 5-FU plus levamisole as effective adjuvant therapy after resection of stage III colon carcinoma: A final report. Ann. Intern. Med. 122:321–326, 1995

33. Wolmark, N, Rockette, H, Fisher B, et al. The benefit of leucovorin-modulated fluorouracil as postoperative adjuvant therapy for primary colon cancer: Results from National Surgical Adjuvant Breast and Bowel Project Protocol C-03. J. Clin. Oncol. 11:1879–1887, 1993

34. International Multicenter Pooled Analysis of Colon Cancer Trials (IMPACT) Investigators. Efficacy of adjuvant fluorouracil and folinic acid in colon cancer. Lancet 345:939–944, 1995

35. Zaniboni, A: Adjuvant chemotherapy in colorectal cancer with high dose leucovorin and fluorouracil: impact on disease-free survival and overall survival. J. Clin. Oncol. 15:2432–2441, 1997

36. O'Connell, MJ, Mailliard, JA, Kahn, MJ, et al. A controlled trial of 5-fluorouracil and low dose leucovorin given for 6 months as postoperative adjuvant therapy for colon cancer. J. Clin. Oncol. 15:246–250, 1997

37. Haller, DG, Catalano, DJ, MacDonald, JS, et al. Fluorouracil (FU), leucovorin (LV) and levamisole (lev) adjuvant therapy for colon cancer: Five year final report of INT-0089. Proc. Am. Soc. Clin. Oncol. 256a, 1998

38. Wolmark, N, Rockette, H, Mamounas, EP, et al. The relative efficacy of 5-FU + leu-covorin (FU-LU), 5-FU and levamisole (FU-Lev), and 5-FU + leucovorin and leva-misole (FU-LV-lev) in patients with Dukes' B and C carcinoma of the colon: First report of NSABP C-04. Proc. Am. Soc. Clin. Oncol. 15:205, 1996

39. O'Connell, MJ, Laurie, JA, Kahn, M, et al. Prospectively randomized trial of post-operative adjuvant chemotherapy in patients with high risk colon cancer. J. Clin. Oncol 16:295–300, 1998

39a. Wolmark N, Bryant, J. Hyams DN, et al. The rektive efficaly of 5-FU + lucovorin and 5-FU-LV + interferon in patents with Dukes' B and C Carcinoma of the color: First report of NSABP C-05. Proc. Am. Soc. Clin. Oncol. 17: 255a, 1998

40. Moertel, CG, Fleming, TR, MacDonald, JS, et al. Intergroup study of fluorouracil plus levamisole as adjuvant therapy for stageII/Dukes' B2 colon cancer. J. Clin. Oncol 13:2936–2943, 1995

41. Mamounas, EP, Rockette, H, Jones J. et al. Comparative efficacy of adjuvant che-motherapy in patients with Dukes' B vs. Dukes' C colon cancer: results from four NSABP adjuvant studies. Proc. Am. Soc. Clin. Oncol. 15:205, 1996

42. Shulman, K, Schilsky, RL: Adjuvant therapy of colon cancer. Sem. in Oncol. 22:600–610, 1995

43. Riethmuller, G, Schneider-Gadicke, E, Schlimok, G, et al. Randomized trial of monoclonal antibody for adjuvant therapy of resected Dukes' C colorectal carci-noma. Lancet 343:1177–1183, 1994

44. Taylor, I, Machint, D, Mulleet, M, et al. A randomized controlled trial of adjuvant portal vein cytotoxic perfusion in colorectal cancer. Br. J. Surg. 72:359–363, 1985

45. Wolmark, N, Rockette, H, Wickerham, DL, et al. Adjuvant therapy of Dukes' A, B, and C adenocarcinoma of the colon with portal vein fluorouracil hepatic infusion: Preliminary results of National Surgical Adjuvant Breast and Bowel Project Protocol C-02. J. Clin. Oncol. 8:1466–1475, 1990

46. Wolmark, N, Rockette, H, Petrelli, N, et al. Long-term results of the efficacy of perioperative portal vein infusion of 5-FU for treatment of colon cancer: NSABP C-02. Proc. Am. Soc. Clin. Oncol 13:194, 1994

47. Liver Infusion Meta-analysis Group: Portal vein chemotherapy for colorectal can-cer: a meta-analysis of 4000 patients in 10 studies. J. Natl. Cancer Inst. 89:497–505, 1997

48. Freedman, GM, Coia, LR: Adjuvant and neoadjuvant treatment of rectal cancer. Sem. in Oncol. 22:611–624, 1995

49. Swedish Rectal Cancer Trial: Improved survival with preoperative radiotherapy in resectable rectal cancer. New Engl. J. Med. 336:980–987, 1997

50. Gastrointestinal Tumor Study Group. Prolongation of the disase-free interval in surgically treated rectal carcinoma. N. Engl. J. Med. 312:1465–1472, 1985

51. Gastrointestinal Tumor Study Group. Survival after postoperative combination treatment of rectal carcinoma. N. Engl. J. Med. 315:1294–1295, 1986

52. Krook, JE, Moertel, CG, Gunderson, LL, et al. Effective surgical adjuvant therapy for high-risk rectal carcinoma. N. Engl. J. Med. 324:709–715, 1991

53. Gastrointestinal Tumor Study Group: Radiation therapy and 5-FU with or without semustine for the treatment of patients with surgical adjuvant adenocarcinoma of the rectum. J. Clin. Oncol. 10:549–557, 1992

54. O'Connell, MJ, Martenson, JA, Wieand, HS, et al. Improving adjuvant therapy for rectal cancer by combining protracted-infusion 5-FU with radiation therapy after curative surgery. N. Engl. J. Med. 331:502–507, 1994

55. Tepper, J, O'Connell, M, Petroni, G, et al. Toxicity in the adjuvant therapy of rectal cancer: a preliminary report of intergroup 0114. Proc. Am. Soc. Clin. Oncol. 15:210, 1996

56. Steele, GD, Herndon, JE, Burgess, AM, et al. Sphincter sparing treatment for distal rectal adenocarcinoma: a phase II intergroup study. Proc. Am. Soc. Clin. Oncol. 16:256a, 1997

57. Dalton, RR, Eisenberg, BL: Surgical management of recurrent liver tumors. Sem. in Oncol. 20:493–505, 1993

58. Hughes, KS, Simon, R, Songhorabodi, S, et al. Resection of the liver for colorectal metastases; a multi-institutional study of indications for resection. Surgery 103:278–288, 1988

59. Doci, R, Gennari, L, Bignami, P, et al. One hundred patients with hepatic metastases from colorectal cancer treated by resection: analysis of prognostic determinants. Br. J. Surg. 78:797–801, 1991

60. Steele, G, Ravikumar, TS: Resection of hepatic metastases from colorectal cancer. Ann. Surg. 210:127–138, 1989

61. McCormack, PM, Burt, ME, Bains, MNS, et al. Lung resection for colorectal metastases: 10 year results. Arch. Surg. 127:1403, 1992

62. Heidelberger, C, Chaudhuari, NK, Danenberg, P, et al. Fluorinated pyrimidines: A new class of tumor inhibitory compounds. Nature 179:663–666, 1957

63. Lockshin, A, Danenberg, PV: Biochemical factors affecting the tightness of 5-fluorodeoxyuridylate binding to human thymidylate synthetase. Biochem. Pharmacol. 30:247–257, 1981

64. Ullman, B, Lee, M, Martin, DW, et al. Cytotoxicity of 5-fluoro-2'-deoxyuridine: requirement for reduced folate cofactors and antagonism by methotrexate. Proc. Natl. Acad. Sci. USA 75:980–983, 1978

65. Evans, RM, Laskin, JD, Hakala, MT: Effects of excess folates and deoxyinosine on the activity and site of action of 5-fluorouracil. Cancer Res. 41:3288–3295, 1981

66. Yin M-B, Zakrzewski, SF, Hakala, MT: Relationship of cellular folate cofactor pools to the activity of 5-fluorouracil. Mol. Pharmacol. 23:190–197, 1983

67. Keyomarsi, K, Moran, RG: Folinic acid augmentation of the effects of fluoropyrimidines on murine and human leukemic cells. Cancer Res. 46:5229–5235, 1986

68. Petrelli, N, Douglass, HO, Herrera, L, et al. The modulation of fluorouracil with leucovorin in metastatic colorectal carcinoma: A prospective randomized phase III trial. J. Clin. Oncol. 7:1419–1426, 1989

69. Valone, FH, Friedman, MA, Wittlinger, PS, et al. Treatment of patients with advanced colorectal carcinomas with fluorouracil alone, high-dose leucovorin plus fluorouracil, or sequential methotrexate, fluorouracil, and leucovorin: A randomized trial of the Northern California Oncology Group. J. Clin. Oncol. 7:1427–1436, 1989

70. Di Costanzo, F, Bartolucci, R, Calabresi, F, et al. Fluorouracil alone vs. high-dose folinic acid and fluorouracil in advanced colorectal cancer: A randomized trial of the Italian Oncology Group for Clinical Research (COIRC). Ann. Oncol. 3:371–376, 1992

71. Labianca, R, Pancera, G, Aitini, E, et al. Folinic acid + 5-fluorouracil (5-FU) versus equidose 5-FU in advanced colorectal cancer: Phase III study of "GISCAD" (Italian group for the Study of Digestive Tract Canacer). Ann. Oncol. 2:673–679, 1991

72. Nobile, MT, Rosso, R, Sertoli, MR, et al. Randomized comparison of weekly bolus 5-fluorouracil with or without leucovorin in metastatic colorectal carcinoma. Eur. J. Cancer 28 A:1823–1827, 1992

73. Erlichman, C, Fine, S, Wong, A, et al. A randomized trial of fluorouracil and folinic acid in patients with metastatic colorectal carcinoma. J. Clin. Oncol. 6:469–475, 1988

74. Doroshow, JH, Multhauf, P, Leong, L, et al. Prospective randomized comparison of fluorouracil versus fluorouracil and high-dose continuous infusion leucovorin calcium for the treatment of advanced measurable colorectal cancer in patients previously unexposed to chemotherapy. J. Clin. Oncol. 8:491–501, 1990

75. Petrelli, N, Herrera, L, Rustum, Y, et al. A prospective randomized trial of 5-flu-
    orouracil versus 5-fluorouracil and high-dose leucovorin versus 5-fluorouracil and
    methotrexate in previously untreated patients with advanced colorectal carci-
    noma. J. Clin. Oncol. 5:1559–1565, 1987
76. Poon, MA, O'Connell, MJ, Wieand, HS, et al. Biochemical modulation of fluoroura-
    cil with leucovorin: Confirmatory evidence of improved therapeutic efficacy in
    advanced colorectal cancer. J. Clin. Oncol. 9:1967–1972, 1991
77. Advanced Colorectal Cancer Meta-Analysis Project (ACCNAP): Modulation of flu-
    orouracil by leucovorin in patients with advanced colorectal cancer: Evidence in
    terms of response rate. J. Clin. Oncol. 10:896–903, 1992
78. Sotos, GA, Allegra, CJ: Biochemical modulation of cancer chemotherapy in
    Schilsky, RL, Milano, GA, Ratain, MJ (eds) Principles of Antineoplastic Drug
    Development and Pharmacology, Marcel Dekker, Inc. New York, 1996, pp 143–187
79. Marsh, JC, Bertino, JR, Katz, KH, et al. The influence of drug interval on the effect
    of methotrexate and fluorouracil in the treatment of advanced colorectal cancer. J.
    Clin. Oncol. 9:371–380, 1991
80. Advanced Colorectal Cancer Meta-analysis Project. Meta-analysis of randomized
    trials testing the biochemical modulation of fluorouracil by methotrexate in meta-
    static colorectal cancer. J. Clin. Oncol. 12:960–969, 1994
81. Blanke, CD, Kasimis, B, Schein, P, et al. Phase II study of trimetrexate, fluorouracil
    and leucovorin for advanced colorectal cancer. J. Clin. Oncol. 15:915–920, 1997
82. Kreuser, ED, Szelenyi, H, Hohenberger, P et al. Trimetrexate, 5-fluorouracil and
    folinic acid: an effective regimen in previously untreated patients with advanced
    colorectal carcinoma. Proc. Am. Soc. Clin. Oncol. 16:294a, 1997
83. O'Dwyer, PJ, Ryan, LM, Valone, FH, et al. Phase III trial of biochemical modulation
    of 5-fluorouracil by IV or oral leucovorin or by interferon in advanced colorectal
    cancer: an ECOG/CALGB phase III trial. Proc. Am. Soc. Clin. Oncol. 15:207, 1996
84. Leichman, CG, Fleming, TR, Muggia, FM, et al. Phase II study of fluorouracil and
    its modulation in advanced colorectal cancer: a Southwest Oncology Group Study.
    J. Clin. Oncol 13:1303–1311, 1995
85. Meta-analysis Group in Cancer. Efficacy of intravenous continious infusion of
    fluorouracil compared with bolus administration in advanced colorectal cancer. J.
    Clin. Oncol. 16: 301–308, 1998
86. deGramont, A, Bosset, J-F, Milan, C, et al. Randomized trial comparing monthly low
    dose leucovorin and fluorouracil bolus with bimonthly high dose leucovorin and
    fluorouracil bolus plus continuous infusion for advanced colorectal cancer: a
    French Intergroup study. J. Clin. Oncol. 15:808–815, 1997
87. Pazdur, R, Lassere, Y, Diaz-Canton, E, et al. Phase I trial of uracil-tegafur (UFT) plus
    oral leucovorin: 28 day schedule. Cancer Investigation 16:145–151, 1998
88. Pazdur, R, Lassere, Y, Rhodes, V, et al. Phase II trial of uracil and tegafur plus oral
    leucovorin; an effective oral regimen in the treatment of metastatic colorectal car-
    cinoma. J. Clin. Oncol. 12:2296–2300, 1994
89. Findlay, M, Van Cutsem, E, Kocha, W, et al. A randomized phase II study of Xeloda in
    patients with advanced colorectal cancer. Proc. Am. Soc. Clin. Oncol. 16:227a, 1997
90. Schilsky, RL, Bukowski, R, Burris, H, et al. A phase II study of a five day regimen of
    oral 5-fluorouracil plus 776C85 with or without leucovorin in patients with meta-
    static colorectal cancer. Proc. Am. Soc. Clin. Oncol 16:271a, 1997
91. Rougier, P, Bugat, R, Douillard, JY, et al. Phase II study of irinotecan in the treat-
    ment of advanced colorectal cancer in chemotherapy-naïve patients and patients
    pretreated with fluorouracil-based chemotherapy. J. Clin. Oncol. 15:251–260, 1997
92. Pitot, HC, Wender, DB, O'Connell, MJ, et al. Phase II trial of irinotecan in patients
    with metastatic colorectal carcinoma. J. Clin. Oncol. 15:2910–2919, 1997

93. Cunningham, D, Pyrhonen, S, James, RD, et al. A phase III multicenter randomized study of CPT-11 versus supportive care alone in patients with 5-FU resistant metastatic colorectal cancer. Proc. Am. Soc. Clin. Oncol. 17:1a, 1998

94. Becouarn, Y, Ychou, M, Duereux, M, et al. Oxaliplatin as first-line chemotherapy in metastatic colorectal cancer patients: preliminary activity/toxicity report. Proc. Am. Soc. Clin. Oncol. 16:229a, 1997

95. Bertheault-Cvitkovic, F, Jami, A, Ithzak, M, et al. Biweekly intensified ambulatory chronomodulated chemotherapy with oxaliplatin, fluorouracil and leucovorin in patients with metastatic colorectal cancer. J. Clin. Oncol. 14:2950–2958, 1996

96. Hohn, DC, Stagg, RJ, Friedman, MA, Hannigan, JF Jr, Raynor, A, Ignoffo, RJ, et al. A randomized trial of continuous intravenous versus hepatic intraarterial floxuridine in patients with colorectal cancer metastatic to the liver: the Northern California Oncology Group trial. J. Clin. Oncol. 7:1646–1654, 1989

97. Kemeny, N, Daly, J, Reichman, B, et al. Intrahepatic or systemic infusion of fluorodeoxyurdine in patents with liver metastases from colorectal carcinoma. A randomized trial. Ann. Intern. Med. 107:459–465, 1987

98. Martin, JK Jr, O'Connell, MJ, Wieand, HS, et al. Intra-arterial floxuridine vs systemic fluorouracil for hepatic metastases from colorectal cancer. A randomized trial. Arch. Surg. 125:1022–1027, 1990

99. Chang, AE, Schneider, PD, Sugarbaker, PH, et al. A prospective randomized trial of regional versus systemic continuous 5-fluorodeoxyuridine chemotherapy in the treatment of colorectal liver metastases. Ann. Surg. 206:685–693, 1987

100. Kemeny, MM, Goldberg, D, Beatty, JD, et al. Results of a prospective randomized trial of continuous regional chemotherapy and hepatic resection as treatment of hepatic metastases from colorectal cancer. Cancer 57:492–498, 1986

101. Rougier, P, Laplanche, A, Huguier, M, et al. Hepatic arterial infusion of floxuridine in patients with liver metastases from colorectal carcinoma: long-term results of a prospective randomized trial. J. Clin. Oncol. 10:1112–1118, 1992

102. Meta-analysis Group in Cancer. Reappraisal of hepatic arterial infusion in the treatment of non resectable liver metastases from colorectal cancer. J. Natl. Cancer Inst. 88:252–258, 1996

# Anal Cancers

B.J. Cummings

## Epidemiology, Risk Factors

### Incidence

The average incidence of anal cancer in the United States between 1973 and 1989 was 0.67 per 100,000 for white women and 0.41 per 100,000 for white men [32]. The incidence is rising in both men and women, for unknown reasons [32].

### Race, Sex, Age Distribution, Predisposition

Anal cancer is thought to be more common in European than in African or Eastern races, although data for the latter groups are incomplete. Cancers of the canal occur more commonly in women, but perianal cancers are found in men and women with equal frequency. The risk increases with age, the median age at diagnosis being about 60 years. There are no known hereditary factors.

### Localization

A distinction should be made between cancers which arise in the anal canal and those in the perianal skin. The risk of lymphatic and/or extrapelvic metastases, and of local recurrence after initial treatment, is greater for anal canal cancers.

The anal canal is 3–4 cm in length and extends from the rectum to the perianal skin [3, 50]. The superior margin of the canal is identified by palpation or radiologically as the upper border of the anal sphincter and puborectalis muscle of the anorectal ring. The distal limit of the canal, or anal verge, is the level at which the walls of the canal come into contact in the resting state at about the lower border of the anal sphincter. Around the anal verge, the normal hair and glandular elements of the perianal skin are lost. The distal canal is lined by squamous epithelium, and the upper canal by squamous and transitional epithelia. Perianal cancers arise from the skin within a 5 cm radius of the anal verge. The term anal margin is used by some authors for the skin immediately adjacent to the anal verge, and by others as a synonym for all of the perianal skin [12]. When it is unclear clinically where a tumor arose, it is usual to classify it as an anal canal cancer.

The major lymphatic pathways from the perianal skin, anal verge and canal below the dentate line drain predominantly to the superficial inguinal nodes. Lymphatics from the canal about and superior to the dentate line flow to the pararectal and internal iliac nodes. There are numerous interconnections between lymphatics from all levels of the canal.

## Risk Factors and Etiology

Benign conditions such as hemorrhoids and fissures do not increase the risk of anal cancer [20]. Cigarette smoking [16], chronic medication-induced immunosuppression [46], and sexually transmitted substances or infections [19] have been implicated as risk factors. Human papilloma virus (especially type 16) is often identified in anal cancers [55], and herpes simplex virus (type 2) and human immunodeficiency virus (HIV) are also thought to have a role greater than simple association [38, 49]. It has been suggested that anoreceptive intercourse is an associated factor in the development of anal cancer rather than HIV infection per se [19].

## Pathology and Staging

The World Health Organization recommends that anal canal cancers be classified as squamous cell carcinomas (synonym cloacogenic carcinomas), and adenocarcinomas, small cell, and undifferentiated cancers [26]. Squamous cell cancers make up about 80% of cancers of the canal, and are subdivided into large cell keratinizing and non-keratinizing types, together making up about two thirds of squamous cancers, and basaloid type. These variants of squamous cell cancer are often grouped as epidermoid cancers, because of their similar natural histories. The AJC/UICC staging classification for anal canal cancers is shown in Table 1 [3, 50].

Cancers of the perianal skin are most commonly squamous cell. Adenocarcinomas and basal cell cancers occur infrequently. The

**Table 1.** Classification and staging of carcinoma of the anal canal (ICD-O C21.1, 2; from [3, 50])

| | |
|---|---|
| **Primary tumor** | |
| TX | Primary tumor cannot be assessed |
| T0 | No evidence of primary tumor |
| Tis | Carcinoma in situ |
| T1 | Tumor ≤2 cm in greatest dimension |
| T2 | Tumor >2 cm but ≤5 cm in greatest dimension |
| T3 | Tumor >5 cm in greatest dimension |
| T4 | Tumor of any size invades adjacent organ(s), e.g., vagina, urethra, bladder (involvement of the sphincter muscle(s) alone is not classified as T4) |
| **Regional lymph nodes** | |
| NX | Regional lymph nodes cannot be assessed |
| N0 | No regional lymph node metastasis |
| N1 | Metastasis in perirectal lymph nodes(s) |
| N2 | Metastasis in unilateral iliac or inguinal lymph node(s) |
| N3 | Metastasis in perirectal and inguinal lymph nodes and/or bilateral internal iliac and/or inguinal lymph nodes |
| **Distant metastases** | |
| MX | Distant metastasis cannot be assessed |
| M0 | No distant metastasis |
| M1 | Distant metastasis |
| **Staging grouping** | |
| Stage 0 | Tis N0 M0 |
| Stage I | T1 N0 M0 |
| Stage II | T2 N0 M0 |
| | T3 N0 M0 |
| Stage IIIA | T4 N1 M0 |
| | T1 N1 M0 |
| | T2 N1 M0 |
| | T3 N1 M0 |
| Stage IIIB | T4 N1 M0 |
| | Any T N2/3 M0 |
| Stage IV | Any T any N M1 |

AJC/UICC staging classification for skin cancers, with which perianal cancers are grouped, is shown in Table 2 [3, 50].

The observed 5-year survival rate for the 1044 cases of anal carcinoma recorded in the U.S. National Cancer Data Base in 1988 was 54% [34]. In those patients, the 5 year survival rates were 58% for epidermoid cancer and 41% for adenocarcinoma. Overall 5-year survival rates of patients with epidermoid anal canal cancers reported from single center studies range from 50% to 70% if the patient has no demonstrable regional node or extrapelvic metastases at presentation. Survival rates fall to about half that range if regional node metastases are found. If systemic metastases occur, the median survival is about 10 months. Cure rates for perianal squamous cell cancer are about 80% or better; death from either uncontrolled loco-regional disease or extrapelvic cancer is uncommon unless

**Table 2.** Classification and staging of perianal carcinoma (trunk including anal margin and perianal skin, ICD-O C44.5; from [3, 50])

| Primary tumor | |
|---|---|
| TX | Primary tumor cannot be assessed |
| T0 | No evidence of primary tumor |
| Tis | Carcinoma in situ |
| T1 | Tumor ≤2 cm in greatest dimension |
| T2 | Tumor >2 cm but ≤5 cm in greatest dimension |
| T3 | Tumor >5 cm in greatest dimension |
| T4 | Tumor invades deep extradermal structures, i.e. cartilage, skeletal muscle or bone |
| **Regional lymph nodes** | |
| NX | Regional lymph nodes cannot be assessed |
| N0 | No regional lymph node metastasis |
| N1 | Metastasis to ipsilateral inguinal lymph nodes |
| **Distant metastases** | |
| MX | Distant metastasis cannot be assessed |
| M0 | No distant metastasis |
| M1 | Distant metastasis |
| **Staging grouping** | |
| Stage 0 | Tis N0 M0 |
| Stage I | T1 N0 M0 |
| Stage II | T2 N0 M0 |
| | T3 N0 M0 |
| Stage III | T4 N0 M0 |
| | Any T N1 M0 |
| Stage IV | Any T any N M1 |

the cancer is poorly differentiated or massive and neglected. The prognosis for adenocarcinomas is fair, but nearer that of adenocarcinomas of the rectum than epidermoid cancers of the anal canal. Small cell carcinomas have a very poor prognosis because of their high proclivity for metastasis.

## Work-up and Staging

The investigations which contribute most to determining the type and extent of anal cancers are shown in Table 3. Many also help assessment of whether a patient is likely to tolerate standard treatment. Limited studies of serum markers have not established any value to their routine use [25].

**Table 3.** Work-up of anal cancers obligatory studies

|  | Anal canal | Perianal |
| --- | --- | --- |
| General |  |  |
| History | X | X |
| Physical Examination | X | X |
| Adjacent organs for direct invasion | X | X |
| Regional lymph nodes | X | X |
| Primary tumor |  |  |
| Biopsy to establish type and grade | X | X |
| Regional nodes |  |  |
| Fine needle aspiration or excision biopsy of enlarged inguinal nodes | X | X |
| Pelvic computerized tomography (also localizes kidneys prior to radiation) | X | X |
| Extrapelvic Metastases |  |  |
| Abdominal computerized tomography (liver and paraaortic nodes) | X | Only if inguinal or pelvic node metastases |
| Chest X-ray | X | X |
| Skeletal imaging | Only if symptoms | Only if symptoms |
| Biochemical/Hematological |  |  |
| Liver and renal chemistry (for staging and for selection of treatment) | X | X |
| Complete blood cell count | X | X |
| HIV antibodies, if risk factors present | X | X |

## Standard Treatment Options

Anal Canal Cancer

Except where specifically indicated, the comments below apply only to epidermoid cancers.

Surgical Treatment

With the success of treatment with combined radiation and chemotherapy, the role of radical surgery for epidermoid cancers has been narrowed greatly. Anorectal excision, usually in the form of abdominoperineal resection with colostomy (APR), is now generally reserved for treatment of cancer residual or recurrent after initial combined modality therapy. However, APR is appropriate initial treatment for those few patients (<5% overall) who are incontinent at presentation due to irreversible destruction of anal sphincter function or fistulae. It is important to establish that a patient is truly incontinent for solid feces, and does not have only a fecal-stained discharge. The risk of local recurrence in large surgical series treated prior to the introduction of combined modality therapy was about 1 in 3 [4, 21, 22], so that adjuvant radiation and chemotherapy in the doses and schedules used for primary treatment are usually recommended after APR, although the value of such adjuvant treatment has not been established. An alternative approach for the incontinent patient is to perform a colostomy prior to standard radiation and chemotherapy. However, it is rarely possible to close the colostomy later in such patients, even if the primary cancer is eradicated.

Radical surgical resection is usually recommended for adenocarcinomas of the anal canal, and is sometimes coupled with adjuvant radiation and chemotherapy as used for rectal adenocarcinomas. Again, the merits of this adjuvant treatment are not known.

Local excision may be considered for superficial squamous cell cancers less than 2 cm in size which arise in the distal canal, since the risk of lymph node metastases from small cancers which have not invaded the sphincter muscles is less than 5% [1, 4]. However, surgery should be avoided if possible when it is anticipated that anal function will be compromised.

Inguinal node metastases may be managed by the same principles. That is, surgery is reserved for the treatment of residual cancer after radiation and chemotherapy. Some authors recommend initial local excision of enlarged inguinal nodes prior to combined modality treatment, and have obtained excellent local control rates [15, 40]. Extensive groin dissections are not necessary: they do not improve outcome and are associated with a high risk of complications such as infection and swelling of the leg.

*Radiotherapy*

Radiation therapy alone also now has a relatively limited role. Some authors recommend radiation for small cancers ≤2 cm in size, in view of the excellent results reported [31, 42]. Most however, prefer combined radiation and chemotherapy [15, 39]. Radiation alone should be considered for patients in whom cytotoxic chemotherapy is contraindicated. The techniques and doses are described elsewhere [13, 40].

*Combined Modality Treatment*

The current standard treatment for epidermoid cancers of the anal canal is radiation therapy with concurrent 5-fluorouracil (5 FU) and mitomycin (MMC). Two multicenter randomized trials have demonstrated the superiority of this combination over the same doses of radiation without concomitant chemotherapy [2, 53] (Table 4). The larger UKCCCR trial included patients with both anal canal and perianal cancers [53].

Radiation doses in both studies consisted of 45 Gy/25 fractions/5 weeks (optionally 20 fractions/4 weeks in the UK study), with further boost radiation 6 weeks later, depending on the extent of tumor regression. If the tumor showed less than a partial response, APR was recommended. The local tumor control and colostomy-free survival rates reported indicate that the primary cancer was eradicated permanently by combined modality treatment in about 60%. Non-randomized studies have examined other radiation doses, ranging from 30 Gy/15 fractions/3 weeks [30, 37] to 50 Gy/20 fractions/4 weeks [15] and 59.4 Gy/33 fractions/6.5 weeks [29]. Primary tumor control rates in these non-randomized studies have typically been in the range of 70% to 90%, likely reflecting differences in the sizes of the cancers treated.

The most effective radiation doses and techniques are not known. Current studies are directed at tailoring dose to the size of the primary

**Table 4.** Randomized comparisons of radiation-5 fluorouracil-mitomycin with radiation alone for anal cancer

| Trial | n | Radiation | 5 FU | MMC | 3-Year colostomy-free survival rate | 3-Year cause-specific survival rate | 3-Year overall survival rate |
|---|---|---|---|---|---|---|---|
| UKCCCR [53] | 577 | 45 Gy/20–25 fns/4–5 wk. Boost of 15–25 Gy at 6 wk if CR or PR; Surgery if NR. | 1000 mg/m² per 24 h IVI d1–4, 29–32 | 12 mg/m² IVB d1 | 61% vs 39%, p<0.0001 (local failure free) | 72% vs 61%, p=0.02 | 65% vs 58%, p=0.25 |
| EORTC [2] | 103 | 45 Gy/25 fns/5 wk; boost of 15–20 Gy at 6 wk if CR or PR; Surgery if NR. | 750 mg/m² per 24 h IVI, d1–5, 29–34 | 15 mg/m² IVB, d1 | 70% vs 45%, p=0.002 | Not reported | 65% vs 63%, p=0.17 |

**Table 5.** Randomized comparison of radiation plus 5-fluorouracil with/without mitomycin (RTOG/ECOG; from [18])

| n | Radiation | 5 FU | MMC | Positive biopsy after first treatment course | 3-Year colostomy-free survival rate | 3-Year overall survival rate |
|---|---|---|---|---|---|---|
| 310 | 45–50.4 Gy/25–28 fns/5–6 wk | 1000 mg/m² per 24 hr IVI, d1–4, 29–32 (max daily dose 2000 mg) | 10 mg/m² IVB, d1 and 29 (max 20 mg per cycle) | 8% vs 14%, p=0.135 | 77% vs 60%, p=0.014 | 82% vs 75%, p=0.31 |
| – | Biopsy 4–6 wk later; if positive 9 Gy/5 fns/1 wk | 1000 mg/m² per 24 h IVI, d1–4 (max daily dose 2000 mg) | No MMC; cisplatin 1000 mg/m² over 4–6 h, d2 | | | |

tumor. In general, there seems little need to exceed about 45 Gy in 5 weeks or an equivalent dose for tumors up to about 4 cm in diameter. More intensive schedules for larger tumors are best examined in formal studies, since the risks of acute and late morbidity at high doses are considerable [10, 29].

The standard cytotoxic drug combination with concomitant radiation is 5 FU and MMC, in the schedules shown in Tables 4 and 5. The Radiation Therapy Oncology Group (RTOG) and the Eastern Cooperative Oncology Group (ECOG) conducted a randomized trial in which patients received radiation together with either 5 FU and MMC or 5 FU alone [18] (Table 5). This trial established the importance of MMC in the schedule used, but it did not address whether the chemotherapy schedules or drugs used were optimal. Non-randomized studies indicate that delivery of a 4-day continuous infusion of 5 FU and a bolus injection of MMC concomitantly with radiation is more effective than giving the drugs in the week prior to radiation [30, 33]. Other schedules investigated include continuous infusion of 5 FU (with or without MMC or Cisplatin) throughout a standard 5 week course of radiation [47], or throughout weekly courses of radiation repeated several times [6]. Although continuous infusions of 5 FU delivered on each day of radiation are attractive by virtue of the theoretical ability of 5 FU to sensitize tumors to radiation [7, 51], the relative merits of different schedules of 5 FU, and of other cytotoxic drugs, remain to be established in formal clinical studies.

Acute toxicity is common with the combination of 5 FU, MMC and radiation, particularly depression of hematologic indices, and acute perineal dermatitis and anoproctitis. Nearly all series have recorded a 1% to 3% risk of acute mortality, generally due to sepsis in neutropenic patients. The severity of the soft tissue reactions associated with medium to high radiation doses with concurrent chemotherapy often prevents a patient completing the scheduled treatment without interruption [10]. It has been suggested, though not proven, that protraction of overall treatment time to accommodate recovery from toxicity may reduce the efficacy of treatment by allowing tumor repopulation [11, 28].

Severe late toxicity affecting the perianal skin and anorectal function is infrequent, particularly following schedules of moderate radiation doses in the range of 40 Gy to 50 Gy, delivered at the rate of 1.8 Gy to 2 Gy per day, with concurrent chemotherapy [10]. However, mild to moderate persistent late morbidity, especially anorectal dysfunction, perianal dermatitis and dyspareunia, is common, after even intermediate dose radiation [14].

The combination of Cisplatin and 5 FU with radiation has been proposed as an alternative to 5 FU and MMC. Pilot studies indicate complete response rates similar to those reported with 5 FU and MMC. The effectiveness of the combination also appears to be less dependent on delivery concurrently with radiation than is the case for 5 FU and MMC [5, 47, 48, 52, 54]. However, there are as yet few reports of long term results of treatment with 5 FU, Cisplatin and radiation. A randomized trial in which these drug combinations would be compared has been discussed by RTOG, but has not yet been opened.

The eradication of cancer from the primary site following treatment may be assessed either clinically or by biopsy. False negative biopsy results are found in 10% to 15% of those who have elective biopsies shortly after complete clinical regression of the cancer [36]. There is no evidence of better outcome following earlier diagnosis of residual cancer by elective biopsy in comparison with deferring biopsy until regrowth is suspected clinically. Unfortunately, the survival rates in both settings are poor, presumably because biologically more aggressive cancers are those most likely to persist and recur [23]. Whichever policy is adopted, patients should be followed at 2–3 month intervals for about 3 years. Most recurrences are found in the first 2 years. Clinical examination of the anal area and adjacent node regions is sufficient, unless the patient has symptoms which warrant other investigations.

The steps in selecting treatment for epidermoid cancers are outlined in Figure 1.

Small cell cancers are rare, and widespread metastases are generally found at diagnosis or shortly after [4]. If the primary tumor is causing symptoms it may be irradiated. Most patients receive a trial of multiple agent chemotherapy, as for small cell cancers elsewhere, but response and survival rates are poor.

## Perianal Cancer

### Surgical Treatment

Wide local excision is an effective and expedient treatment for perianal cancers of all histological types, provided it can be performed without

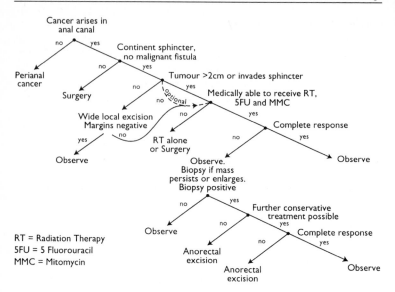

**Fig. 1.** Decision pathway for epidermoid cancer of the anal canal

compromising anorectal function [1, 22]. Where more radical surgery would be required, it is now usual to treat perianal squamous cell cancers according to the same principles as those arising in the anal canal. In these protocols, radical surgery is reserved for the management of residual cancer after initial treatment designed to conserve anal function. Large perianal adenocarcinomas are usually managed by APR and wide perineal excision.

*Radiotherapy*

Several non-randomized studies have shown that radical radiation alone, in doses similar to those used for cutaneous squamous cell cancers elsewhere, is effective [41, 44]. However, the results of the recent UKCCCR randomized trial suggest that combined modality treatment may be preferable (see below). Radiation alone is indicated for basal cell cancers, either as primary therapy or for tumors not amenable to excision with preservation of anorectal function [35].

## Combined Modality Treatment

The UKCCCR randomized trial, in which the combination of radiation with 5 FU and MMC was compared with radiation alone, included cancers which arose in the canal (75% of those entered) and the anal margin (23%) [53]. Although results were not presented separately for anal canal and anal margin (perianal) cancers, this trial demonstrated the superiority of combined modality therapy over radiation alone [53] (Table 4). Accordingly, it may be better to combine 5 FU and MMC with radiation, at least for large, deeply invasive or poorly differentiated perianal squamous cell cancers.

Figure 2 summarizes a decision pathway for perianal epidermoid cancers.

## Biological Response Modifiers

Biological response modifiers have not yet been studied in anal cancer.

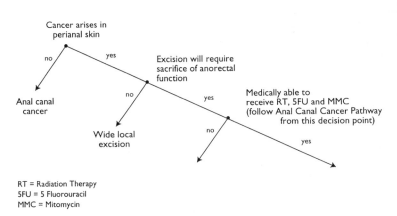

RT = Radiation Therapy
5FU = 5 Fluorouracil
MMC = Mitomycin

**Fig. 2.** Decision pathway for epidermoid cancer of the perianal skin

## Current Key Questions

How Can Survival and Local Control Rates Be Further Improved?

The combination of 5 FU, MMC and radiation leads to cure in from 50% to 70% of those treated [10, 13]. Anorectal function is preserved in about two-thirds overall, and in about 90% of those in whom the primary cancer is eradicated by chemoradiation [10, 13].

Analyses of the sites of failure following combined modality therapy support the direction of current research protocols which are designed primarily to further improve loco-regional control rates. The sites of cancer present at the time of death were reported for the UKCCCR trial [53]. In those treated by radiation combined with 5FU and MMC, extra-pelvic metastases were identified in only 10%, and locoregional failure in 16%. Extrapelvic metastases were twice as common in patients with locoregional failure (17% vs 7%). Because relatively few patients exhibit extrapelvic metastases alone, the value of systemic adjuvant treatment has not been formally studied or established. Those protocols which include more chemotherapy than the one or two courses common in earlier trials should provide further information on the relative importance of improved locoregional control and systemic adjuvant treatment.

What Changes Occur in the Biology of Anal Cancers that Make Extrapelvic Metastases Difficult To Control?

The single most effective agent against extrapelvic metastases is Cisplatin, either alone or in combination with 5 FU [17]. However, complete responses are rare, and the duration of both complete and partial responses brief. Unpublished data from Princess Margaret Hospital show that irradiation of the whole or part of an organ harboring metastases, with concurrent 5 FU and MMC or 5 FU and Cisplatin, rarely produces complete response, even in tumors of small volume which would be expected to be readily eradicated were they at the primary site. Histological and molecular features examined have failed so far to identify patients at risk of metastases or to suggest new strategies for treatment [9].

## How Should Patients with HIV Infection/AIDS Who Develop Anal Cancer Be Managed?

Opinions vary on the most effective, and best tolerated, treatment for these patients [24, 43]. Patients infected with HIV but who do not have AIDS usually exhibit normal tolerance to radiation and chemotherapy. Those with AIDS may develop severe mucositis and dermatitis at unexpectedly low radiation doses. Many of the antiviral medications in use currently may cause marrow depression, and patients are often reluctant to accept cytotoxic chemotherapy which could lower blood counts further. While some authors electively modify the doses of cytotoxic drugs, or omit them entirely, others prefer standard schedules and alter treatment according to the acute reactions produced in each patient. All series are small, but local tumor control rates appear to be similar, stage for stage, to those in patients who do not have HIV infection. Survival is usually determined by the course of AIDS.

## Is Combined Modality Treatment Effective Against Anal Adenocarcinoma?

There are anecdotal reports of cure and preservation of anorectal function in patients with adenocarcinoma of the anal canal or perianal area treated with radiation, 5 FU and MMC in the schedules used for epidermoid cancer. For example, unpublished data from the Princess Margaret Hospital show local control for 2 years or longer in 5 of 11 patients. However, the standard treatment is surgery, and combined modality treatment should at present be considered investigational.

### Current and Future Investigational Approaches

Current standard treatments are summarized in Table 6. Efforts to intensify treatment by additional chemotherapy offer promise, since early results suggest that this strategy may produce less late normal tissue damage than increasing the dose of radiation. A French Cooperative Anal Cancer Group described complete regression at 2 months after treatment in 28 of 29 patients who received 2 courses of induction 5 FU and Cisplatin, followed by a further 2 courses given concurrently with radia-

**Table 6.** Summary of usual first treatment by site and histology

|                                                              | Treatment                                                                                       |
| ------------------------------------------------------------ | ----------------------------------------------------------------------------------------------- |
| Anal canal                                                   |                                                                                                 |
| Squamous cell (cloacogenic):                                 |                                                                                                 |
| keratinizing, non-keratinizing, basaloid                     | Radiation, 5 FU and MMC                                                                          |
| Undifferentiated                                             | Radiation and chemotherapy<br>(5 FU and MMC or 5 FU and cisplatin)                              |
| Adenocarcinoma                                               | Surgery                                                                                          |
| Small cell                                                   | Chemotherapy±radiation                                                                           |
| Perianal                                                     |                                                                                                 |
| Squamous cell                                                | Local excision, or radiation, or radiation +<br>5 FU and MMC according to size, location        |
| Basal cell                                                   | Surgery or radiation                                                                            |
| Adenocarcinoma                                               | Surgery                                                                                          |

tion [45]. Cancer and Leukemia Group B is conducting a Phase II study in which patients receive 2 courses of 5 FU and Cisplatin prior to 2 courses of 5 FU and MMC given concurrently with radiation [8]. Other investigators are studying the scheduling of drugs in relation to radiation in efforts to separate further the effects on cancer and normal tissues [51]. There is some evidence that radiation technique affects the severity of side-effects, perhaps independently of dose, so that this too is the subject of investigation [10, 13].

Greater understanding of the cellular and molecular biology of anal cancer offers the prospect of new treatment approaches, such as the use of hypoxic cell radiation sensitizers or biological response modifiers. Identification of drugs which protect normal tissues in the pelvis from the effects of radiation will facilitate manipulation of radiation doses and techniques.

The relative effectiveness of the current standard for epidermoid cancers of radiation, 5 FU and MMC is such that alterations in treatment must now be carried out with care and circumspection, so that the gains already made in improved locoregional control rates and colostomy-free survival rates are not lost.

## References

1. Al-Jurf AS, Turnbull RB, Fazio VW (1979) Local treatment of squamous cell carcinoma of the anus. Surg Gynecol Obstet 148:576–8

2. Bartelink H, Roelofsen F, Eschwege F, et al (1997) Concomitant radiotherapy and chemotherapy is superior to radiotherapy alone in the treatment of locally advanced anal cancer: results of a Phase III randomized trial of the European Organisation for Research and Treatment of Cancer Radiotherapy and Gastrointestinal Cooperative Groups. J Clin Oncol 15:2040–9

3. Beahrs OH, Henson DE, Hutter RVP, et al. eds (1998) American Joint Committee on Cancer. Manual for staging of cancer, 3rd edn, Lippincott, Philadelphia

4. Boman BM, Moertel CG, O'Connell M, et al (1984) Carcinoma of the anal canal: a clinical and pathological study of 188 cases. Cancer 54:114–6

5. Brunet R, Becouarn Y, Pigneux J, et al (1991) Cisplatine (P) et flurouracile (FU) en chimiotherapie neoadjuvante des carcinomes epidermoides du canal anal. Lyon Chir 87:77–8

6. Byfield JE, Barone RM, Sharp TR, et al (1985) Conservative management without alkylating agents of squamous cell anal cancer using cyclical 5-FU alone and X-ray therapy. Cancer Treat Rep 67:709–12

7. Byfield JE, Calabro-Jones P, Klisak I, et al (1982) Pharmacologic requirements for obtaining sensitization of human tumor cells in vitro to combined 5-fluorouracil or ftorafur and X-rays. Int J Radiat Oncol Biol Phys 8:1923–33

8. Cancer and Leukemia Group B. CALGB 9281 (1992) A phase II trial of induction chemotherapy followed by radiation therapy plus concurrent chemotherapy for poor prognosis, locally advanced, previously untreated carcinomas of the anal canal. CALGB 1992

9. Cummings BJ (1995) Anal canal carcinoma. In: Hermanek P, Gospodarowicz MK, Henson DE, et al (eds) Prognostic factors in cancer. Springer-Verlag, Berlin, pp 80–7

10. Cummings BJ (1995) Anal cancer: Treatment with and without chemotherapy. In: Cohen AM, Winawer SJ (eds) Cancer of the colon, rectum and anus. McGraw-Hill Inc, New York, pp 1025–42

11. Cummings BJ (1996) Anal cancer: to split or not to split (editorial). Cancer J Sci Am 2:194–6

12. Cummings BJ (1996) The anal margin. Oncology 10:1853–4

13. Cummings BJ (1997) Anal canal. In: Perez CA, Brady LW (eds) Principles and practice of radiation oncology. 3rd edn. Lippincott-Raven Publishers, Philadelphia, pp 1511–24

14. Cummings BJ (1998) Preservation of structure and function in epidermoid cancer of the anal canal. In: Rosenthal CJ, Rotman M (eds) Chemotherapy infusion – radiation therapy interaction: its biology and significance for organ salvage and prevention of second primary neoplasms. Elsevier Scientific Publishing Co, Amsterdam, pp 167–78

15. Cummings BJ, Keane TJ, O'Sullivan B, et al (1991) Epidermoid anal cancer: treatment by radiation alone or by radiation and 5-fluorouracil with and without mitomycin C. Int J Radiat Oncol Biol Phys 21:1115–25

16. Daling JR, Weiss NS, Hislop TG, et al (1987) Sexual practices, sexually transmitted diseases, and the incidence of anal cancer. N Engl J Med 317:973–7

17. Flam MS (1995) Chemotherapy of persistent, recurrent, or metastatic cancer. In: Cohen AM, Winawer SJ (eds) Cancer of the colon, rectum and anus. MGraw-Hill Inc, New York, pp 1051–60

18. Flam M, John M, Pajak TF, et al (1996) The role of mitomycin C in combination with 5-fluorouracil and radiotherapy, and of salvage chemoradiation in the definitive nonsurgical treatment of epidermoid carcinoma of the anal canal: Results of a phase III randomized Intergroup study. J Clin Oncol 14:2527–39

19. Frisch M, Glimelius B, van den Brule A, et al (1997) Sexually transmitted infection as a cause of anal cancer. N Engl J Med 337:1350–8
20. Frisch M. Olsen JH, Bautz A, et al (1994) Benign anal lesions and the risk of anal cancer. N Engl J Med 331:300–2
21. Golden GT, Horsley JS III (1976) Surgical management of epidermoid carcinoma of the anus. Am J Surg 131:275–80
22. Greenall MJ, Quan SHQ, Decosse JJ (1985) Epidermoid cancer of the anus. Br J Surg 72 (suppl):S97–S103
23. Herrera L, Luna P, Garcia C (1995) Surgical therapy of recurrent epidermoid carcinoma of the anal canal. In: Cohen AM, Winawer SJ (eds) Cancer of the colon, rectum and anus. McGraw-Hill Inc, New York, pp 1043–50
24. Höcht S, Wiegel T, Kroesen AJ, et al (1997) Low acute toxicity of radiotherapy and radiochemotherapy in patients with cancer of the anal canal and HIV-infection. Acta Oncologica 36:799–802
25. Indinnimeo M, Reale MG, Cicchini C, et al (1997) CEA, TPA, CA 19–9, SCC and CYFRA at diagnosis and in the follow-up of anal canal tumors. Int Surg 82:275–9
26. Jass JR, Sobin LH, eds (1989) Histological typing of intestinal tumours, 2nd edn. Springer-Verlag, Berlin
27. John M, Flam M, Berkey B, et al (1998) Five year results and analyses of a Phase III randomized RTOG/ECOG chemoradiation protocol for anal cancer (abstract). Proc ASCO 17:258a
28. John M, Pajak T, Flam M, et al (1996) Dose acceleration in chemoradiation for anal cancer: preliminary results of RTOG 9208. Cancer J Sci Am 2:205–11
29. John M, Pajak T, Kreig R, et al (1997) Dose escalation without split-course chemoradiation for anal cancer: results of a phase II RTOG study. (abstract) Int J Radiat Oncol Biol Phys 39: Suppl:203
30. Leichman L, Nigro N, Vaitkevicius VK, et al (1985) Cancer of the anal canal: model for preoperative adjuvant combined modality therapy. Am J Med 78:211–5
31. Martenson JA, Gunderson LL (1993) Radiation therapy without chemotherapy in the management of cancer of the anal canal. Cancer 71:1736–40
32. Melbye M, Rabkin CS, Frisch M, et al (1994) Changing patterns of anal cancer incidence in the United States, 1940–1989. Am J Epidemiol 139:772–80
33. Michaelson RA, Magill GB, Quan SHQ, et al (1983) Preoperative chemotherapy and radiation therapy in the management of anal epidermoid carcinoma. Cancer 51:390–5
34. Myerson RJ, Karnell LH, Menck HR (1997) The National Cancer Data Base report on carcinoma of the anus. Cancer 80:805–15
35. Nielsen OV, Jensen SL (1981) Basal cell carcinoma of the anus – a clinical study of 34 cases. Br J Surg 68:856–7
36. Nigro ND (1984) An evaluation of combined therapy for squamous cell cancer of the anal canal. Dis Colon Rectum 27:763–6
37. Nigro ND, Vaitkevicius VK, Considine B (1974) Combined therapy for cancer of the anal canal: a preliminary report. Dis Colon Rectum 17:354–6
38. Noffsinger A, Witte D, Fenoglio-Preiser CM (1992) The relationship of human papillomaviruses to anorectal neoplasia. Cancer 70:1276–87
39. Northover J, Meadows H, Ryan C, et al (1997) Combined radiotherapy and chemotherapy for anal cancer. Lancet 349:205–6
40. Papillon J (1982) Rectal and anal cancers: conservative treatment by irradiation – an alternative to radical surgery. Springer Verlag, New York, pp 107–85
41. Papillon J, Chassard JL (1992) Respective roles of radiotherapy and surgery in the management of epidermoid carcinoma of the anal margin. Series of 57 patients. Dis Colon Rectum 35:422–9

42. Papillon J, Montbarbon JF (1987) Epidermoid carcinoma of the anal canal: a series of 276 cases. Dis Colon Rectum 30:324–33
43. Peddada AV, Smith DE, Rao AR, et al (1997) Chemotherapy and low-dose radiotherapy in the treatment of HIV-infected patients with carcinoma of the anal canal. Int J Radiat Oncol Biol Phys 37:1101–5
44. Peiffert D, Bey P, Pernot M, et al (1997) Conservative treatment by irradiation of epidermoid carcinomas of the anal margin. Int J Radiat Oncol Biol Phys 39:57–66
45. Peiffert D, Seitz JF, Rougier P, et al (1997) Preliminary results of a phase II study of high-dose radiation therapy and neoadjuvant plus concomitant 5-fluorouracil with CDDP chemotherapy for patients with anal canal cancer: a French cooperative study. Ann Oncol 8:575–81
46. Penn I (1986) Cancer is a complication of severe immunosuppression. Surg Gynecol Obstet 162:603–10
47. Rich TA, Ajani JA, Morrison WH, et al (1993) Chemoradiation therapy for anal cancer: Radiation plus continuous infusion of 5-fluorouracil with or without cisplatin. Radiother Oncol 27:209–15
48. Roca E, Pennella E, Milano C, et al (1993) Efficacy of cisplatin (DDP) with fluorouracil (5-FU) and alternating radiotherapy (RT) as first line treatment in anal cancer (ACC): long term results (abstract). Proc ASCO 12:206
49. Scurry J, Wells M (1992) Viruses in anogenital cancer. Path Cell Biol 1:138–45
50. Sobin LH, Wittekind C (eds), (1997) Union Internationale Contre le Cancer. TNM classification of malignant tumours, 5th edn. Springer-Verlag, Berlin
51. Steel GG (1988) The search for therapeutic gain in the combination of radiotherapy and chemotherapy. Radiother Oncol 11:31–5
52. Svensson C, Kaigas M, Goldman S (1992) Induction chemotherapy with carboplatin and 5-fluorouracil in combination with radiotherapy in loco-regionally advanced epidermoid carcinoma of the anus – preliminary results. Int J Colorectal Dis 7:122–4
53. UKCCCR Anal Canal Cancer Trial Working Party (1996) Epidermoid anal cancer: results from the UKCCCR randomized trial of radiotherapy alone versus radiotherapy, 5-fluorouracil and mitomycin. Lancet 348:1049–54
54. Wagner JP, Mahe MA, Romestaing P, et al (1994) Radiation therapy in the conservative treatment of carcinoma of the anal canal. Int J Radiat Oncol Biol Phys 29:17–23
55. Williams GR, Lu QL, Love SB, et al (1996) Properties of HPV-positive and HPV-negative anal carcinomas. J Pathol 180:378–82

# Gastric Cancer

J.S. Macdonald

## Epidemiology, Risk Factors

Some 22,400 new cases of gastric carcinoma occurred in the United States in 1997. There were 14,000 deaths resulting from this disease [1]. Gastric cancer has fallen significantly in incidence over most of this century in the United States with rates decreasing from roughly 32/100,000 in 1930 to approximately 3.5/100,000 in the 1970s [2]. Although no adequate explanation for this change has been provided the decrease in gastric cancer has occurred in the "endemic" or intestinal form of disease usually associated with pre-existing intestinal metaplasia. There has been a relative increase in adenocarcinomas occurring in the proximal stomach and distal esophagus over the last 15 years. These tumors do not occur on the background of intestinal metaplasia but may be associated with Barrett's epithelium (gastric metaplasia of the distal esophagus) developing from chronic gastroesophageal reflux disease (GERD). These tumors occur most commonly in middle-aged Caucasian males and they are of particular concern because they may have a worse prognosis stage for stage than more distally located tumors [3].

There is a large international variation in gastric cancer incidence and death rates. High incidence countries include Costa Rica (death rate 54.7/100,000 for men) and Japan (death rate 34.9/100,000 for men) [2]. In most countries the incidence and death rates for men are 2 times those of women. In high incidence countries intestinal form of gastric cancer developing upon the background of intestinal metaplasia of the stomach is more common than the diffuse form.

## Risk Factors

Gastric cancer is environmentally caused in most cases and studies of migrant populations strongly support environmental causation of stomach cancer. For example, migrant populations from Japan to the US develop a lower incidence rate of stomach cancer approaching the US rate within a generation. These populations also experience an increase in colon cancer incidence rates as US diet and lifestyle are adopted. A number of case control epidemiologic studies have examined various associations in the development of gastric cancer. The unifying hypothesis in many of these studies is that N-nitrosamine compounds act as carcinogens or co-carcinogens for gastric cancer. Positive associations with cancer in multiple studies have been diets rich in cured and smoked meats, salted fish, and bacon. Diets high in fruit, raw vegetables, fiber-rich bread, and increased amounts of vitamin C appear to provide some protection from stomach cancer [4]. The mechanism by which protection is afforded is unknown and possibly related to the antioxidant properties of vitamin C leading to inhibition of N-nitrosamine formation.

Convincing evidence of a strong positive association of gastric cancer incidence with tobacco smoking and alcohol intake has not been documented for the intestinal form but is clearly correlated for proximal stomach and cardioesophageal junction lesions. As noted previously, these latter tumors are associated with a history of GERD, obesity, along with alcohol and cigarette use.

In the endemic (intestinal) form of gastric cancer, lower socioeconomic class and lack of education correlate positively with cancer incidence. It is likely that these socioeconomic and educational factors are not independent variables but rather are characteristic of groups in societies consuming diets conducive to the development of stomach cancer. Occupational exposures also have been associated with stomach cancer. Increased incidence has been shown in workers in coal, nickel, and asbestos mining, and in individuals who process timber and rubber [5]. Previous surgery for benign ulcer disease and infection with the bacteria *Helicobacter pylori* an organism associated with chronic gastritis, have been shown to be risk factors for subsequent development of the intestinal form of gastric cancer [6].

## Pathology and Staging

95% of all malignant tumors of the stomach are adenocarcinomas [7]. The histopathologic differentiation may vary from well- to poorly differentiated. The well- and moderately well-differentiated tumors tend to be associated with intestinal metaplasia of the stomach, more distal presentations and occurrence in high incidence countries. The poorly differentiated proximal lesions are more commonly seen in association with distal esophageal cancers and proximal gastric cancers. As described previously, these tumors are increasing in incidence in the US. Rare tumors [8] of the stomach include adenoacanthoma, squamous cell carcinoma, carcinoid tumors, and leiomyosarcoma (gastrointestinal stromal tumors). Lymphoma [9] occurs in the gastrointestinal tract and the stomach is the most common site for gastrointestinal lymphomas. The most common form of aggressive lymphomas are the large non-cleaved B-cell neoplasms. Maltoma (mucosa-associated lymphatic tissue) neoplasms [10] are low grade neoplastic processes associated with H. pylori colonization. These neoplastic B-cell proliferations appear to initially develop as polyclonal proliferations which may be successfully treated with antibiotic therapy directed at eradication of H. *pylori* before the maltoma has evolved to a monoclonal truly malignant neoplasm [11].

The TNM staging [12] for adenocarcinoma of the stomach is indicated below.

## Staging

Staging according to the AJCC's TNM system is listed in Table 1.

## Prognosis

Survival after gastric resection with curative intent for gastric cancer can be summarized as follows. In patients with early gastric cancer (T1N0 lesions rarely seen in the US) 5-year post resection survival can be expected to be at least 90%. With T2-T3N0 lesions survival is approximately 50%. When lymph nodes are involved (typically Stages IIIA, IIIB, IV M0) survival drops to 20% or below after gastric resection [2, 13].

**Table 1.** TNM classification

| Primary tumor | |
|---|---|
| Tx | Minimum requirements to assess primary tumor cannot be met |
| T0 | No evidence of primary tumor |
| Tis | Tumor limited to mucosa without penetration into the lamina propria |
| T1 | Tumor invades lamina propria or submucosa |
| T2 | Tumor invades muscularis propria or subserosa |
| T3 | Tumor penetrates serosa without invasion of adjacent organs |
| T4 | Tumor penetrates through serosa and involves adjacent organs |

| Lymph node involvement | |
|---|---|
| Nx | Regional nodes cannot be assessed |
| N0 | No regional lymph node metastasis |
| N1 | Metastases in perigastric lymph nodes within 3 cm of the edge of primary tumor |
| N2 | Metastases in perigastric lymph nodes >3 cm from the edge of the primary tumor, or in lymph nodes along the left gastric, common hepatic, splenic, or celiac arteries |

| Distant metastases | |
|---|---|
| Mx | Presence of distant metastases cannot be assessed |
| M0 | No known distant metastases |
| M1 | Distant metastases present |

| Stage | |
|---|---|
| Stage 0 | Tis, N0, M0 |
| Stage IA | T1, N0, M0 |
| Stage IB | T1, N1, M0 |
| | T2, N0, M0 |
| Stage II | T1, N2, M0 |
| | T2, N1, M0 |
| | T3, N0, M0 |
| Stage IIIA | T2, N2, M0 |
| | T3, N1, M0 |
| | T4, N0, M0 |
| Stage IIIB | T3, N2, M0 |
| | T4, N0, M0 |
| Stage IV | T4, N2, M0 |
| | Any T, any N, M1 |

## Work-up and Staging

The symptoms of gastric cancer are frequently vague and non-specific. They include such complaints as epigastric discomfort, nausea, vomiting, fatigue, and weight loss. Other symptoms may include dysphagia, with proximal lesions, anorexia, regurgitation, early satiety and belching.

Patients may present with gastric outlet obstruction as well as partial bowel obstruction, depending on the location of the tumor within the stomach and the extent of its regional progression. Dysphagia and symptoms of esophageal partial obstruction will become increasingly common because of the increase in incidence of cardioesophageal junction tumors. It is not uncommon for gastric cancer to be discovered in patients undergoing evaluation for iron-deficiency, anemia, and/or positive stool occult blood tests. It should be noted, however, that patients with gastric cancer rarely present with significant bleeding. In the setting of acute upper intestinal bleeding, gastrointestinal stromal tumors (leiomyosarcomas) or benign ulcers are more common diagnoses than adenocarcinoma.

In the US, patients with gastric cancer unfortunately usually present at a stage when their neoplasms are not curable by gastric resection, although they may be palliated by such a procedure. Physical signs [7] of dissemination of gastric cancer include palpable lymph node metastases in the supraclavicular area (Virchow's node) or the left axilla (Irish's node). Periumbilical nodules (Sister Joseph's nodes) represent peritoneal dissemination of tumor. Hepatomegaly or ascites may be present and epigastric mass or pelvic masses due to Krukenburg tumor (ovarian drop metastasis) or pelvic peritoneal dissemination (Blumer's shelf) may be palpated on pelvic and/or rectal examination.

The work-up for patients suspected of gastric carcinoma is first oriented towards making a tissue diagnosis. The primary diagnostic procedure is fiberoptic upper endoscopy. A tumor of the stomach may usually be directly visualized and multiple biopsies may be obtained [7]. The double contrast barium upper gastrointestinal series may be helpful in providing anatomic definitions of a gastric lesion (mucosal based mass, malignant appearing ulcer, or peristaltic abnormality). Some gastric tumors may not present with a mass lesion, but rather extensively infiltrate the submucosa and muscularis of the stomach. These lesions result in a rigid stomach on upper gastrointestinal series. There is also a decrease or absence of peristalsis through the areas of tumor infiltration that may be seen both with endoscopy and on upper Barium gastrointestinal series. In patients suspected of having infiltrating submucosal tumor blind endoscopic biopsies of the stomach may be helpful in establishing diagnosis.

Endoscopic ultrasound [14] may be a useful tool in defining tumor penetration of the gastric wall (T stage), and has been shown to be superior to CT scanning for this purpose. However, this technique is less accurate for detecting the presence of metastatic disease in perigastric lymph nodes. The accuracy rate for detecting lymph node metastases is approximately 70%–80%. Although initial T-staging of tumors is accurate with endoscopic ultrasound, the technique loses sensitivity when used after chemotherapy and particularly after irradiation. CT scanning and conventional ultrasound examinations provide additional information for staging prior to laparotomy and assist in decision making regarding curative vs. palliative resections. CT scanning [2], however, is an imperfect staging tool having an accuracy of between 30%–72% and understaging appears to be more of a problem than overstaging. There are no reliable serum tumor markers for gastric cancer. Both CEA and CA19–9 have been noted to be elevated in some patients with disseminated disease.

### Stage-Specific Treatment Options

Surgical Resection

The curative therapy for gastric cancer is surgical resection [15]. Surgical resection of a primary gastric cancer is appropriate palliative therapy even when cure is not possible. Because of the unreliability of non-surgical staging, most patients should be offered surgical exploration unless there is clear evidence of widely disseminated disease or the patient is a poor surgical candidate for medical reasons. Resection, even if done only for palliation, often offers an effective and safe means of decreasing pain and bleeding, and preventing obstruction. Palliative resection, as long as total gastrectomy is not required, may result in improvement of overall quality of life.

For patients with disease potentially resectable for cure (Stages 0-IV M0) the surgical aim should be to perform tumor resection entailing at least a partial gastrectomy with an en bloc lymphatic dissection. For at least 20 years [15, 16] there has been an international debate regarding the most appropriate surgical procedures to use in cases of potentially curative stomach cancer. The main point at issue is whether extensive lymph node dissection improves survival. If the surgeon dissects in en bloc fashion, the tumor plus the N1 nodes (lymph nodes within 3 cm of the primary tumor) and the N2 nodes (lymph nodes greater than 3 cm from the tumor) a D2 resection has been performed. Currently it is unclear whether this improves survival compared to gastrectomy and nodal resection limited to the N1 nodes (D1 resection).

The development of extended nodal dissection (D2 resections) occurred in Japan. Japanese surgeons [16] for a number of years have reported superior results with this plan of surgical resection for patients with gastric cancer. Small Phase III comparisons of D1 and D2 resections have been completed in South Africa [17] and Hong Kong [18]. These studies were underpowered (less than 30 patients per arm) and showed no survival benefit for D2 resection. At present, a larger Phase III study [19] with 996 cases is testing D2 vs. D1 resection. This is a study being carried out in the Netherlands and partial results were reported upon by Bunt et al [20]. in 1995. In this initial publication the Dutch investigators addressed the effects of lymph node resection upon staging. Pathologists were asked to review pathology on patients who had D2 dissections. Pathologic staging was first performed by assessing the N1 nodes, and then subsequently examining the N2 nodes.

The object of bunt et al's study was to apply a pathologic stage to patients looking first at the cases as if a D1 dissection had been performed and then by looking at the complete nodal resection specimen to determine what the final stage would be after the D2 dissection. These workers demonstrated (Table 2) that the reports of improved survival with D2 dissection may actually be due to improved surgical staging resulting from the more complete nodal dissection. For example, Bunt and colleagues showed that the overall survival of all patients was not significantly improved by D2 dissections but stage-specific survival appeared to be improved in D2 patients since the D2 surgical staging assured more accurate staging than if only the N1 nodes had been evaluated. From 60% to 75% of cases (Table 2) had their stages changed (typically Stage II to IIIA, or IIIA to IIIB) by examination of the N2 nodes.

**Table 2.** Stage migration: R1 vs. R2 staging (from [20])

| n | R1 TNM stage | R2 TNM stage | | | | % Stage migration |
|---|---|---|---|---|---|---|
| | | II | IIIa | IIIb | IV | |
| 48 | II | 30 | 18 | – | – | 60 |
| 49 | IIIa | – | 19 | 29 | 1 | 61 |
| 24 | IIIb | – | – | 6 | 18 | 75 |

Although the impact of D2 resection upon staging is impressive, before a definitive conclusion can be drawn about the value of extended lymphadenopathy, the complete outcome results of the Netherlands trial need to be made available. Initial results [19] reported at the American Society of Clinical Oncology in 1997 failed to show significant differences in favor of more extensive lymphadenectomies, but these results must be considered to be preliminary.

## Radiotherapy

External beam radiotherapy has only a palliative role in locally unresectable gastric cancers. There is no evidence that survival can be improved significantly by such approaches in these patients. There is, however, interesting evidence provided by the Gastrointestinal Tumor Study Group (GITSG) in the 1980s [21] that combined modality chemotherapy plus radiation is superior to radiation alone in patients with small volumes of residual gastric cancer. GITSG investigators demonstrated that approximately 20% of a small number of patients with small volume residual cancer receiving radiation plus fluorinated pyrimidine were long-term disease-free survivors, i.e. cured, of their cancer. Essentially no patients receiving radiation alone were long-term survivors. The concept of combined modality radiation plus chemotherapy (Fig. 1) is being tested as adjuvant therapy in the National Intergroup Adjuvant Study (INT 0116). Radiotherapy also may have other roles in the management of gastric cancer such as being a component of combined modality neoadjuvant programs which typically are administered before gastric resection.

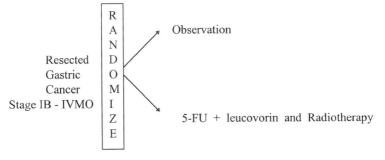

**Fig. 1.** Schema of INT 0116

## Chemotherapy, Combined Modality Therapy

The use of chemotherapy in gastric cancer falls into three major categories: (a) adjuvant chemotherapy used after gastric resection as a strategy to curatively treat microscopic residual disease and prevent relapse; (b) chemotherapy as a palliative strategy for patients with established incurable metastatic disease; (c) chemotherapy used preoperatively either alone or in combination with radiation as neoadjuvant therapy.

First, in regard to adjuvant chemotherapy, it is important to understand that this approach has been studied for a number of years both in the US and abroad. The studies performed in the US have generally not shown benefit for post-operative adjuvant chemotherapy alone. A study [22] of 193 cases performed by the Southwest Oncology Group and published in 1995 showed no benefit for FAM (5-FU, Adriamycin, mitomycin-C) chemotherapy in a controlled randomized study vs. surgery alone. Also, it should be noted that a meta analysis [23] of Phase III adjuvant chemotherapy trials published in 1993 demonstrated no significant benefit in survival for patients treated with adjuvant chemotherapy.

Although the weight of data reported with currently available chemotherapy regimens suggests there is no rate of adjuvant chemotherapy alone in patients with resected stomach cancer, there may be a rationale to use chemotherapy plus radiation. One attractive strategy for adjuvant therapy is to build upon the GITSG data [21] with known local residual disease. The GITSG data demonstrated that combined radiation plus fluorinated pyrimidine may be of value in such patients. For the first time in the US a national intergroup gastric cancer adjuvant study is being performed. This study is the Southwest Oncology Group Study 9008 (Intergroup 0116) (Fig. 1). This study randomizes patients with resected Stage IB through Stage IVMo adenocarcinoma of the stomach to surgery alone or surgery followed by combined 5-FU, leucovorin and radiation therapy. INT 0116 has compeled accrual closed on the July of 1998. The analysis of this study will require approximately 2 more years. This large, well-powered, prospectively randomized study will define whether or not this regimen of combined modality chemoradiation is a valuable adjuvant strategy after gastric resection.

Another area that is of significant interest in gastric cancer therapy is the use of neoadjuvant approaches. With this strategy chemotherapy alone or combined radiation chemotherapy is used preoperatively in patients with gastric cancer. The aim of this approach is to reduce the primary tumor size and stage and increase the ease, safety, and efficacy of surgical resection. Another obvious goal of this approach is based upon the assumption that early systemic therapy as part of a neoadjuvant approach will treat microscopic metastatic disease and help prevent systemic relapse.

Neoadjuvant therapy has not been tested in gastric cancer in controlled or randomized studies. However, the results of Phase II studies have been published. Clinical investigators at Memorial Sloan-Kettering Cancer Center in New York [24] and the University of Southern California [25] have reported results of this therapeutic approach. Both of these groups have used systemic preoperative chemotherapy along with a post resection intraperitoneal chemotherapy strategy designed to prophylax the peritoneal cavity from relapse. Intraperitoneal chemotherapy is a rational approach since the peritoneal cavity is a common site of recurrence after gastric cancer resection.

An example of aggressive neoadjuvant therapy is the 1997 study reported by Cookes et al. from the University of Southern California [25]. In this study 59 patients received combined modality therapy consisting of continuous infusion 5-FU with weekly leucovorin and cisplatinum, followed by surgical resection of the primary gastric tumor. Postoperatively resected cases received 2 cycles of intraperitoneal 5-fluoro-2'-deoxyuridine (FUDR) and cisplatinum. This study demonstrated that 56 of 59 patients (95%) receiving a neoadjuvant therapy were able to undergo surgical exploration. Forty cases (71%) underwent resections with curative intent. Only 9 of 40 patients who had curative resections developed recurrent carcinoma. The median time in the follow-up now exceeds 45 months. Since the relapse rate demonstrated in well-designed perspective studies after gastric cancer resection is in the range of 60%–70%, the 23% relapse rate in the USC study with median follow-up of almost 4 years is an impressive Phase II result. What must be done in the future is to subject neoadjuvant therapeutic approaches such as that described by Cookes et al. evaluation by prospectively randomized clinical trials. A neoadjuvant approach will be one of the strategies tested in the next national Intergroup early gastric cancer study.

Chemotherapy for metastatic gastric cancer has been an interesting area of investigation for medical oncologists. The regimens with considerable activity reported recently in the literature are summarized in

Table 3. EAP-type regimens encompassing etoposide, Adriamycin, cis-platinum as pioneered by Preusser and colleagues [26] in Germany led to a new era in combination chemotherapy in which response rates in excess of 30% could be expected along with some complete tumor regressions. The EAP regimen is not used in the late 1990s as widely as previously because of its significant toxicity [27]. However, there are other regimens that are widely used and are major regimens of interest. Strategies of chemotherapy being frequently used include Methotrexate-directed 5-FU [29], infusional 5-FU [25], with and without other agents and Etoposide-based regimens [28].

**Table 3.** Current regimens for metastatic adenocarcinoma of the stomach

| Drug combinations | Dose (mg/m$^2$) per schedule | Response rate |
|---|---|---|
| FAMTX [29, 30, 32] | | |
|   Methotrexate | 1,500 d1, h0 | 30%–70% overall, 12% CR |
|   Leucovorin | 15 po q6 x 8, starting h 24 | |
|   Fluorouracil | 1,500 d1, h1 | |
|   Doxorubicin | 30 d15 | |
| ELF [28] | | |
|   Leucovorin | 300 d1–3 | 48% overall, 12% CR |
|   Etoposide | 120 d1–3 | |
|   Fluorouracil | 500 d1–3 | |
| EAP [26, 27] | | |
|   Etoposide | 120 d4–6 | 20%–70% overall, 15% CR |
|   Doxorubicin | 20 d1, 7 | |
|   Cisplatin | 40 d2, 8 | |
| ECF [34–36] | | |
|   Epirubicin | 50 d1 | 37%–45% overall, 17% CR |
|   Cisplatin | 60 d1 | |
|   5-FU | 200 qd by CI | |
| PELF [37] | | |
|   Cisplatin | 40 weekly x 8 | 37%–45% overall, 17% CR |
|   Fluorouracil | 500 weekly x 8 | |
|   Epirubicin | 35 weekly x 8 | |
|   Leucovorin | 250 weekly x 8 | |
|   G-CSF | 5 µg/kg qd except for the day of chemotherapy | |
|   Glutathione | 1.5 g/m$^2$ with cisplatin | |
| FLC [25] (Repeat every 28 days) | | |
|   5-FU | 200 qd by CI x 21 | 52% overall |
|   Leucovorin | 20 weekly x 3 | |
|   Cisplatin | 100 iv d1 | |

h, Hour; d, day; CI, continuous infusion; CR, complete response.

A fairly standard regimen widely used in the 1990s is the FAMTX program (see Table 3). FAMTX uses moderately high doses of methotrexate followed by 5-FU on day 1. A single dose of Adriamycin is given on day 14. The FAMTX regimen has been reported to have response rates as high as 60% [29] and as many as 12% of metastatic disease patients demonstrated complete regression of tumor. However, a large Phase II multiinstitution study performed by the European Organization for Research and Treatment of Cancer (EORTC) evaluated the FAMTX regimen [30] and found an overall response rate of 33% with 15% complete responses. This regimen does contain high-dose methotrexate and therefore careful attention must be paid to hydration, alkalinization of the urine, and plasma methotrexate levels. methotrexate level monitoring is essential to ensure adequate Leucovorin rescue and to avoid potentially life-threatening toxicity. Another issue with the high-dose Methotrexate in FAMTX is that many patients with gastric cancer late in their diseases will have ascites and high-doses of Methotrexate must be used with caution in patients with ascites, since the possibility of sequestration of Methotrexate in the ascitic fluid can lead to prolonged toxicity.

FAMTX has been tested in Phase III fashion in at least 3 studies. A randomized comparison of FAMTX to EAP was reported by Kelsen and colleagues [31]. This study was terminated before full accrual goals were reached because an interim analysis demonstrated increased toxicity in the EAP arm. The response rates were 33% for FAMTX and 20% for EAP. Complete response was seen in the FAMTX arm but not in the EAP arm. In Europe [32], FAMTX was compared to the FAM chemotherapy regimen in a Phase III study. There were 103 patients randomized to the FAM arm and 105 to the FAMTX arm. The response rate for FAMTX was 41% vs. 9% response for FAM. This was a significant difference and the median survival differences between FAMTX patients (10.5 months) and FAM cases (7.2 months) for FAM were also significant. Five patients on FAMTX had complete tumor responses. There were no complete responses on the FAM regimen.

Etoposide has also been an agent of interest for inclusion in combination chemotherapy of gastric cancer. The same German investigators who reported the EAP regimen also reported results of another regimen in which 5-FU and leucovorin were combined with etoposide [28]. This regimen was designated ELF and is described in Table 3. The ELF regimen was originally tested in patients with advanced gastric cancer who were not considered good candidates for EAP because of the toxicity potential of this regimen. A total of 51 patients were treated. The response rate initially was in excess of 50% with a 12% complete response rate. Phase III [33] results with ELF have yet not been reported but the European Organization for Research and Treatment of Cancer carried out such a study and its results will be important in defining the true activity of ELF. The ELF regimen is well-tolerated with the grade III and IV toxicities being diarrhea and leucopenia. ELF is generally thought not to have the same level of activity as first line gastric cancer regimens but is a well-tolerated acceptable alternative treatment option for patients with advanced gastric cancer who may not be candidates for the most aggressive therapy.

There has been significant interest in prolonged infusion of 5-FU as part of combination chemotherapy treatment for a gastric cancer. As noted previously in this publication, Cookes and colleagues [25] have used continuous infusion 5-FU as a major component of a neoadjuvant program (Table 2). Cunningam and colleagues [34] reported interesting results with a combination designated ECF. The ECF regimen is described in Table 3. Of note, the ECF uses protracted infusion of 5-FU at a rate of 200 mg/m2 per day with intermittent Epirubicin and Cisplatinum. Epirubicin is an anthracycline analogue that is available in Western Europe but is not available in the United States. Caccia et al [35]. reported an ECF trial involving 52 patients. The overall response rate was 37% and there were 17% complete responses. ECF has also been tested in Phase III trials. A recently published randomized trial [36] compared ECF to FAMTX in patients with advanced gastroesophageal junction adenocarcinoma. In this study, 274 patients with adenocarcinoma or undifferentiated cancer were randomized between FAMTX and ECF. The FAMTX regimen caused significant hematologic toxicity and was inferior in regard to response rate when compared to ECF. The overall response rate for ECF was 45% vs. 21% for FAMTX (p=0.002). The median survival for ECF was 8.9 months vs. 5.7 months for FAMTX (p=0.0009). The one-year survival for ECF was 36% vs. a one-year survival of 21% for FAMTX. Webb and colleagues [36] also assessed global quality of life in their study. The quality of life with ECF was superior at 24 weeks. This advantage in quality of life, however, did not persist as patients were followed further in the study.

Another study recently reported was of the regimen PELF (Table 3). This Phase II study [37] reported impressive results in patients with advanced gastric cancer. This cooperative multi-institution study from

Italy was an intensive weekly chemotherapy program entailing the use of 5-FU, cisplatin, epirubicin, leucovorin, glutathione, G-CSF. This regimen has been given the eponym of PELF and is an intensive weekly regimen as noted on Table 3. The regimen requires the use of G-CSF on the days the patients are not receiving weekly chemotherapy. Glutathione is given in an attempt to ameliorate platinum toxicity. The 6S-stereoisomer of Leucovorin is administered with the 5-FU.

The results of PELF in 105 patients with either locally advanced or metastatic gastric cancer were striking. After 1 8-week cycle of therapy, the overall response rate was 65/105 or 62%. Eighteen patients had complete responses and 47 patients had partial responses. The median duration of survival for all patients was 11 months. The 1-year survival was 42% and for 2-year survival was 5%.

The Phase II experience with PELF certainly demonstrates that this aggressive intensive regimen is active in gastric cancer and should be tested in a Phase III fashion. The toxicity was surprisingly mild and was characterized by Grade III or IV anemia, neutropenia, thrombocytopenia, and mucositis in 38% of patients. There were no treatment-related deaths. One should be cautious in that the aggressive use of these drugs, which requires colony stimulating factor support, would represent a very expensive chemotherapeutic approach in gastric cancer.

## Key Questions for Gastric Cancer

- Understanding the causes of the increase in incidence of cardioesophageal junction adenocarcinomas. Are there newly present environmental risk factors associated with this disease? Are there molecular genetic differences between proximal and distal tumors?
- Will eradication of gastric H. pylori infection decrease subsequent risk of gastric cancer?
- What is the "best" surgical procedure for patients with resectable gastric carcinoma? Does extended lymph node dissection (D2 dissection) result in improved overall survival in patients with localized gastric carcinoma? Is morbidity/mortality acceptable for such procedures?
- Can less radical surgical resections, including D1 dissections, result in improved survival if combined with either preoperative or postoperative neoadjuvant or adjuvant therapy?

- What are the most appropriate adjuvant and neoadjuvant approaches? Will postoperative chemoradiation therapy result in improved survival in patients with resected gastric carcinoma? Do neoadjuvant approaches with or without intraperitoneal therapy improve resectability and improve overall survival?
- What are the most appropriate advanced disease therapies? What is the best way to interface current drugs in the treatment of metastatic gastric cancer? What is the optimal way to use infusional fluorinated pyrimidines? What are roles for newer drugs, including the new oral fluorinated pyrimidine compounds (UFT, S1, capecitabine, etc.) taxanes, topoisomerase-1 inhibitors, gemcitabine, and combinations of these new agents?

**Acknowledgements.** The author appreciates the excellent technical assistance of Mr. John Bazos in preparing this manuscript.

### References

1. Parker SL, Tong L, Bolden S, Wingo PA (1997) Cancer Statistics. Ca Cancer J Clin 47:5–27
2. Gunderson LL, Donohue JH, Burch PA (1995) Stomach. In: Abeloff MD, Armitage JO, Lichter AS, Niederhuber JE (eds) Clinical Oncology. Churchill Livingstone, New York, pp 1209–1241
3. Graham DY, Schwartz JT, Cain GD, Gyorkey F (1982) Prospective evaluation of biopsy number in the diagnosis of esophageal and gastric carcinoma. Gastroenterology 82:228
4. Boeing H (1991) Epidemiological research in stomach cancer: Progress over the last ten years. J Cancer Res Clin Oncol 117:133–143
5. Wu-Williams AH, Yu MC, Mack TM (1990) Life-style, workplace, and stomach cancer by subsite in young men of Los Angeles county. Cancer Res 50:2569–2576
6. Parsonnet J, Friedman GD, Vandersteen, DP, et al (1991) Helicobacter pylori infection and the risk of gastric carcinoma. N Engl J Med 325:1127–1131
7. Macdonald JS, Hill MC, Roberts IM (1992) Gastric cancer: Epidemiology, pathology, detection and staging. In: Ahlgren JD, Macdonald JS (eds) Gastrointestinal Oncology. J.B. Lippincott, Philadelphia, pp 151–158
8. Ganesan TS, Slavin M (1988) Rare Gastric Tumours. In: Williams GJ, Krikorian JG, Green MR, Raghavan D (eds) Textbook of uncommon cancers. John Wiley & Sons, New York, pp 461–469
9. Perren TJ, Blackledge G (1986) Gastrointestinal lymphomas. In: Fielding JWL, Priestman TJ (eds) Gastrointestinal oncology. Lea & Febiger, Philadelphia, p 237
10. Isaacson P, Spencer J (1987) Malignant lymphoma of mucosa-associated lymphoid tissue. Histopathol 11:445
11. Wotherspoon A, Doglioni C, Diss T, Pan L, Moschini A, de Boni M (1993) Regression of primary low-grade B-cell gastric lymphoma of mucosa-associated lymphoid tissue type after eradication of Helicobacter pylori. Lancet 342:575

12. Beahrs OH, Hansen DE, Hutter RVP, Kennedy BJ (1992) Stomach. In: Manual for staging of cancer, 4th Ed. JB Lippincott, Philadelphia
13. Noguchi Y, Imada T, Matsumoto A, et al (1989) Radical surgery for gastric cancer. A review of the Japanese experience. Cancer 64:2053
14. Botet JF, Lightdale CJ, Zauber AG et al. (1991) Preoperative staging of gastric cancer: Comparison of endoscopic US and dynamic CT. Radiology 181:426
15. Wanebo HJ, Koness RJ (1992) Pancreatic Cancer: Surgical approach. In: Ahlgren JD, Macdonald JS (eds) Gastrointestinal oncology. JB Lippincott, Philadelphia, pp 209–214
16. Kodama Y, Sugimachi K, Soejima K et al. (1981) Evaluation of extensive lymph node dissection for carcinoma of the stomach. World J Surg 5:241–248
17. Dent DM, Madden MV, Price SK (1988) Randomized comparison of R1 and R2 gastrectomy for gastric carcinoma. Br J Surg 75:110
18. Robertson CS, Chung SCS, Woods SDS et al. (1994) A prospective randomized trial comparing R1 subtotal gastrectomy for antral cancer. Ann Surg 220:176
19. van de Velde for the Dutch Gastric Cancer Group Leiden University Hospital (1997) Lymph node dissection in gastric cancer: 5-year results of a randomized trial of D1 and D2 dissection in 996 Dutch patients (Abstract #987). Proc Amer Soc Clin Oncol 16:278a
20. Bunt AMG, Hermans J, Smit VTHBM, van de Velde CJH, Fleuren GJ, Bruijn JA (1995) Surgical/pathologic-stage migration confounds comparisons of gastric cancer survival rates between Japan and western countries. J Clin Oncol 13 (1):19–25
21. Gastrointestinal Tumor Study Group (1982) A comparison of combination chemotherapy and combined modality therapy for locally advanced gastric carcinoma. Cancer 49:1771–1777
22. Macdonald JS, Fleming TR, Peterson RF, Berenberg JL, McClure S, Chapman RA, Eyre HJ, Solanki D, Cruz AB, Gagliano R, Estes NC, Tangen CM and Rivkin S (1995) Adjuvant chemotherapy with 5-FU, adriamycin, and mitomycin-C (FAM) versus surgery alone for patients with locally advanced gastric adenocarcinoma: A Southwest Oncology Group Study. Ann Surg Oncol 2 (6):488–494
23. Hermans J, Bonenkamp JJ, Boon MC et al. (1993) Adjuvant therapy after curative resection for gastric cancer: Meta-analysis of randomized trials. J Clin Oncol 11:1441
24. Atiq OT, Kelsen DP, Shiu MH, Saltz L, Tong W, Niedzwiecki D et al. (1993) Phase II trial of postoperative adjuvant intraperitoneal cisplatin and fluorouracil and systemic fluorouracil chemotherapy in patients with resected gastric cancer. J Clin Oncol 11:425–433
25. Crookes P, Leichman CG, Leichman L, Tan M, Laine L, Stain S, Baranda J, Casagrande Y, Groshen S, Silberman H (1997) Systemic chemotherapy for gastric carcinoma followed by postoperative intraperitoneal therapy. Cancer 79 (9):1767–1775
26. Preusser P, Wilke H, Achterrath W et al. (1989) Phase II study with the combination etoposide, doxorubicin and cisplatin in advanced measurable gastric cancer. J Clin Oncol 7:1310–1317
27. Lerner A, Gonin R, Steele GD et al. (1992) Etoposide, doxorubicin and cisplatin chemotherapy for advanced gastric adenocarcinoma: Results of a phase II trial. J Clin Oncol 10:536–540
28. Wilke H, Preusser P, Fink U, et al (1990) High dose folinic acid/etoposide/5-flurorouracil in advanced gastric cancer – a phase II study in elderly patients or patients with cardiac risk. Invest New Drugs 8:65–70
29. Klein H, Wickramanayake P, Farrokh G (1986) 5-FU, adriamycin and methotrexate – a combination protocol (FAMTX) for treatment of metastasized stomach cancer. Proc Am Soc Clin Oncol 5:84

30. Wils J, Beliberg H, Blijham G, et al (1986) An EORTC gastrointestinal evaluation of the combination of sequential methotrexate, and 5-fluorouracil combined with adriamycin, in advanced measurable gastric cancer. J Clin Oncol 4:1799

31. Kelsen D, Atiq OT, Saltz L et al. (1992) FAMTX versus etoposide, doxorubicin, and cisplatin: A random assignment trial in gastric cancer. J Clin Oncol 10:541–548

32. Wils JA, Klein HO, Wagener DJT et al. (1991) Sequential high-dose methotrexate and fluorouracil combined with doxorubicin: a step ahead in the treatment of advanced gastric cancer: a trial of the European Organization for Research and Treatment of Cancer Gastrointestinal Tract Cooperative Group. J Clin Oncol 9:827

33. Wils JA, Wagener DJT, Coombes RC et al. (1995) Phase III trial of fluorouracil, methotrexate and epirubicin (FEMTX) versus FEMTX plus cisplatin (FEMTX-P) in advanced gastric cancer. Abstracts of the Second International Conference on Biology, Prevention and Treatment of GI Malignancy. Koln, Germany p 74

34. Cunningham D, Cahn A, Menzies-Gow N (1990) Cisplatin, epirubicin and 5-fluorouracil (CEF) has significant activity in advanced gastric cancer. Proc Am Soc Clin Oncol 9:123

35. Caccia G, Alasino C, Fein L (1990) 5-Fluorouracil + epirubicin + cisplatin in patients with advanced gastric cancer. Proc Am Soc Clin Oncol 9:123

36. Webb A, Cunningham D, Scarffe JH, Harper P, Norman A, Jaffe J, Hughes M, Mansi J, Findlay M, Hill A, Oates J, Nicolson M, Hickish T, O'Brien M, Iveson T, Watson M, Underhill C, Wardley A and Meehan M (1997) Randomized trial comparing epirubicin, cisplatin and fluorouracil versus fluorouracil, doxorubicin, and methotrexate in advanced esophagogastric cancer. J Clin Oncol 15 (1):261–267

37. Cascinu S, Labianca R, Allesandroni P et al. (1997) Intensive weekly chemotherapyfor advanced gastric cancer using fluorouracil, cisplatin, epi-doxorubicin, 6S-leucovorin, glutathione, and filgrastim: A report from the Italian Group for the Study of Digestive Tract Cancer. J Clin Oncol 15 (11):3313–3319

# Hepatobiliary Cancer

# Hepatobiliary Cancer, Pancreatic Cancer, and Neuroendocrine Cancers of the GI Tract

S. Mani

## Hepatocellular Carcinoma

### Epidemiology, Risk Factors

*Incidence*

Hepatoma (hepatocellular carcinoma, HCC) is one of the most common malignancies in the world. Worldwide the annual incidence is nearly 1 million and it causes an estimated 1,250,000 deaths every year. There is striking geographic variation – the highest rates are found in China, Southeast Asia, and Africa (>20/100,000 males per year); the lowest rates in the United Kingdom, North America, and Latin America [1–3].

*Race*

The incidence of hepatomas is higher in Asians and blacks which correlate with the geographical differences in incidence rates [1, 2].

*Sex*

Hepatomas are more commonly found in males with a male to female ratio of 6:1 in Asia, 3:1 worldwide and 2:1 in the United States [1, 2].

*Age Distribution*

The incidence rate is age proportional. In high risk areas, there is a tendency towards an increased incidence in the younger age group. Notably, the mean age at diagnosis in Asia is 53 years which is a decade earlier than in the United States (62 years).

## Predisposition

Hepatomas generally always occur in the context of chronic underlying liver disease. Although well defined familial syndromes have not been described for adult onset liver cancer, there are some well known risk factors associated with this disease.

## Localization

Hepatomas are usually multicentric on presentation and diffusely involve liver parenchyma; however, in most patients there is a dominant mass which determines resectability. Only 5%–30% of patients present with localized disease to the liver that is amenable to curative resection; the majority of patients have locally advanced disease and a fewer number present with metastases to regional lymph nodes, malignant ascites, bone, lung and brain.

## Risk Factors, Etiology

Hepatitis B and to a lesser extent hepatitis C chronic carriage is most strongly associated with the development of hepatomas. Other risk factors in the context of cirrhosis and development of hepatomas include aflatoxin exposure, alcoholic liver disease, autoimmune chronic active hepatitis, genetic hemochromatosis, and hereditary tyrosinemia. Other liver inflammatory conditions like alpha-1 antitrypsin deficiency are only moderately associated with hepatomas, while conditions like primary biliary cirrhosis is weakly associated with hepatomas [4].

## Pathology and Staging

Hepatomas are typically described as nodular, diffuse and massive; >90% are massive or diffuse while the nodular variety is multifocal.

Several histologic types have been documented ranging from trabecular to pseudoglandular and clear cell. Fibrollamellar is a distinctive variant with large eosinophilic cells arranged in thin or thick trabeculae that are separated by fibrous strands with lamellar stranding. This variant typically occurs in young adults, arising in noncirrhotic liver. The serum alpha-fetoprotein (AFP) is usually normal but levels of serum B12-binding globulin and neurotensin are usually increased [5]. The staging of hepatomas is based on primary tumor size, nodal involvement and distant metastatic spread based on the TNM classification as shown in Table 1. In summary, this staging is based on number and size of lesions as well as involvement of the portal system.

Work-up and Staging

The clinical scenario dictates the work-up of hepatic neoplasms. For patients with known cirrhosis, in high risk populations, screening for hepatomas with repetitive ultrasounds of the liver and serum AFP twice a year has been recommended. For patients who are older than 35 years and HbsAg-positive or with a family history of HCC should be screened by AFP and aminotransferase levels once a year [6, 7]. For patients with hepatomegaly and/or history of predisposing factors to liver cancer or cirrhosis with progressive weight loss and/or ascites, we recommend either ultrasonography or lipiodal scan with computed tomograms (CT), CT portography, or a dedicated liver CT study. In some institutions where magnetic resonance image (MRI) is readily available, T1 and T2 weighted MRI may be preferred. We recommend simultaneous screening serum alpha-fetoprotein, hepatitis B (Ag and antibody) and C antibody, liver function tests, serum albumin and a coagulation screen with prothrombin time and partial thromboplastin time. A needle biopsy (usually a core) is the preferred method for obtaining biopsies. Additional evaluation includes chest CT scan and a bone scan (especially if a curative intervention is entertained or if serum alkaline phosphatase is elevated in the absence of extrahepatic ductal obstruction).

**Table 1.** Staging for hepatoma

| | |
|---|---|
| **Primary tumor** | |
| TX | Primary tumor cannot be assessed |
| T0 | No evidence of primary tumor |
| T1 | Solitary tumor 2 cm or less in greatest dimension without vascular invasion |
| T2 | Solitary tumor 2 cm or less in greatest dimension with vascular invasion, or multiple tumors limited to one lobe, none more then 2 cm in greatest dimension without vascular invasion, or a solitary tumor more than 2 cm in greatest dimension without vascular invasion |
| T3 | Solitary tumor more than 2 cm in greatest dimension with vascular invasion, or multiple tumors limited to one lobe, none more than 2 cm in greatest dimension, with vascular invasion, or multiple tumors limited to one lobe, any more than 2 cm in greatest dimension, with or without vascular invasion |
| T4 | Multiple tumors in more than one lobe or tumor(s) involve(s) a major branch of the portal or hepatic vein(s) or invasion of adjacent organs other than the gallbladder or perforation of the visceral peritoneum |
| **Regional lymph nodes** | |
| NX | Regional lymph nodes cannot be assessed |
| N0 | No regional lymph node metastasis |
| N1 | Regional lymph node metastasis |
| **Distant metastasis** | |
| MX | Distant metastasis cannot be assessed |
| M0 | No distant metastasis |
| M1 | Distant metastasis |
| **Stage grouping** | |
| Stage I | T1 N0 M0 |
| Stage II | T2 N0 M0 |
| Stage IIIA | T3 N0 M0 |
| Stage IIIB | T1 N1 M0 |
| | T2 N1 M0 |
| | T3 N1 M0 |
| Stage IVA | T4 Any N M0 |
| Stage IVB | Any T any N M1 |

## Treatment

*Curative (Stages I, II, and Selected III)*

Surgical resection remains the only curative modality for HCC. Patients with stage I and II disease are virtually always cured with surgical resection; however these stages of presentation especially in an unscreened population are uncommon. Operative mortality is a function of the degree of "normal" functioning liver remaining after surgery and can range between 5% and 30% [8]. With complete resections, the one year survival rates range between 70%–80% with 5-year survival rates ranging between 30%–46%. At present, there is no established role for adjuvant chemotherapy or radiotherapy and patients should be referred for protocol based treatments. Cryosurgery as an alternative to resection is ideal for patients with cirrhosis who have poor hepatic reserve and/or multifocal tumor involvement. There does not seem to be a clear improvement in survival with cryosurgery and its use should still be in a research setting [9].

Liver transplantation is curative especially in very early stage disease. The indications for transplantation are dependant on the age and risks of the individual concerned – the best results are obtained with stage I or II disease, those with incidental tumors, epithelioid hemangioendothelioma or fibrolamellar histology. The overall world-wide experience suggests that all patients with resectable tumors are potential transplant candidates with 2-month post-operative mortalities ranging between 5%–32%. Tumor recurrence rates vary between 11% and 69% and overall 3-year survival rates between 20%–75%. 5-year survival is not uncommon which may also vary depending on the histology between 17% and 57% [10].

Transarterial embolization (TACE) consists of intra-arterial infusion of an anti-cancer agent in the feeding artery of the tumor followed by embolization. The embolization material consists of very small particles such as gelatin sponge, polyvinyl alcohol, collagen, lipiodol or gelfoam. The most common anti-cancer agents used include but are not limited to doxorubicin, epirubicin, mitomycin C and cisplatin. The material together undergoes degradation and reabsorption in to the circulation within 48–72 h. The response rates (>50% reduction in size of the embolized lesion) may be noted in 15%–75% of cases while reductions in alpha-fetoprotein levels observed in 23%–100% of cases [11, 12]. This procedure may be used while patients await transplantation or for those with unresectable disease and must be performed in centers experienced in TACE (Fig. 2).

An alternative to resection is percutaneous ethanol injection (PEI; Figs. 1, 2). Larger experience from European and Japanese patients suggest that PEI may be safely administered to patients with <3 lesions none

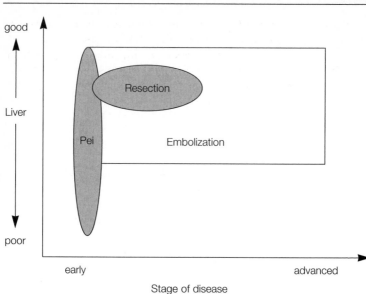

**Fig. 1.** Resection vs. PEI

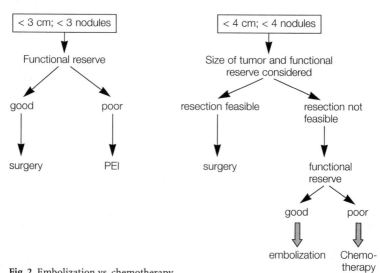

**Fig. 2.** Embolization vs. chemotherapy

of which are >3 cm in size or for patients with poor functional hepatic reserve or for those who are inoperable but have accessible tumor for needle injections. For patients with good functional reserve, surgical resection remains the treatment of choice [13, 14]. Patients eligible for TACE or PEI should, however, always be referred to specialized centers for protocol based management especially protocols combining chemotherapy with these approaches.

## Palliative

Unresectable disease may be approached with TACE or PEI depending on the availability of protocols. It is now routine practice that other modalities be considered in the treatment of advanced disease.

## Chemotherapy

This remains an option for most patients with HCC; however, there is no effective palliative therapy available. Doxorubicin yields a response rate around 20% with most responses being partial and no obvious survival benefit. Other approaches of intra-hepatic infusion of chemotherapy such as floxuridine (FUDR), mitomycin, and interferon have yielded response rates of nearly 50% but these are not durable. Other more novel chemotherapies have yielded more modest response rates of less than 10% [15, 16, 17]. Patients who are candidates for chemotherapy should be referred for protocol based therapy as there is no current standard for chemotherapy in this disease.

## Radiation Therapy

External beam radiotherapy, although investigational, has a role in palliation in this disease, especially for patients with inordinate liver pain/discomfort. Radiation hepatitis and fibrosis are likely complications with whole liver radiation especially at doses >30 Gy. This effect may be lessened with conformal radiotherapy. Patients who have a large dominant mass and are not eligible for chemotherapy protocols or who have inordinate discomfort from the liver mass may should be referred for investigation radiotherapy options. Some emerging investigational options include 131-I polyclonal antiferritin antibody therapy (48% remission rate), 90-Y antiferritin isotope therapy and other monoclonal preparations against ferritin [18].

## Biliary Tract Cancers

Epidemiology, Risk Factors

*Incidence*

Cancer of the biliary tract is uncommon with 8000 cases reported annually. Two-third of cases arise in the gallbladder, with one-third arising from the bile duct or peri-ampullary region.

*Race, Sex, Age, Distribution, Predisposition*

**Gallbladder Cancer.** The median age at diagnosis is 73 years. Women are more commonly affected than men with a ratio of 2.7:1. The incidence is greater in southwestern Native Americans, Mexicans, Hispanics, and Alaskans and in these populations is estimated to be 5–6 times that of the general population.

**Bile Duct Cancer.** The median age at presentation is 70 years. Extrahepatic bile duct tumors occur primarily in older individuals. Men are equally affected as women [19, 20].

*Risk Factors, Etiology*

The risk factors for gallbladder cancer are not precisely known but these cancers tend to arise more frequently in porcelain gallbladders and in patients with chronic cholecystitis. Other factors that may contribute to carcinogenesis include nitrosamines and inflammatory processes like ulcerative colitis [19].

## Pathology and Staging

Morphologically, most gallbladder and bile duct tumors are adenocarcinomas; <20% are squamous or mixed call tumors. In bile duct tumors, the papillary and nodular types occur more frequently in the distal duct while the sclerosing variety is more common in the proximal bile duct. Papillary lesions have the best prognosis. The clinical staging for these tumors are described in the TNM classification in Tables 1 and 2.

## Work-up and Staging

The work-up of a suspected gallbladder cancer starts with a right upper quadrant ultrasound, especially in patients with a normal bilirubin level but elevated alkaline phosphatase or other liver function abnormalities. This may be supplemented with a CT scan which can aide in defining gallbladder wall thickness. In most cases, however, an endoscopic retrograde cholangiopancreatography demonstrates a filling defect in the gallbladder or common duct. Further, staging usually requires a chest-X-ray after a biopsy or cytology diagnosis is confirmed. Other tests including bone scan or MRIs are not indicated except in situations of clinical suspicion for bone metastases.

## Treatment

### Curative (Stages I and II)

For early-stage gallbladder carcinoma, mucosa or muscularis tumor invasion requires only a cholecystectomy alone. If there is extension in to or through the serosa, the resection should include segments IV and V of the gallbladder bed and porta hepatis lymph node dissection. For early stage bile duct tumors, distal lesions are more amenable to resection than proximal lesions. For proximal bile duct lesions, local excision will suffice. Hepatic resection is indicated for tumors invading the quadrate lobe or intrahepatic ductal or vascular involvement. Stent placements are not routinely indicated in the pre-operative setting for biliary decompression. The goal of surgical intervention is to obtain a complete resection with clear margins. For mid-ductal lesions, duct skeletonization may

**Table 2.** Staging for gallbladder cancer

| | |
|---|---|
| Primary tumor | |
| TX | Primary tumor cannot be assessed |
| T0 | No evidence of primary tumor |
| Tis | Carcinoma in situ |
| T1 | Tumor invades lamina propria or muscle layer |
| T1a | Tumor invades lamina propria |
| T1b | Tumor invades muscle layer |
| T2 | Tumor invades perimuscular connective tissue; no extension beyond serosa or into liver |
| T3 | Tumor perforates the serosa (visceral peritoneum) or directly invades one adjacent organ, or both (extension 2 cm or less into liver) |
| T4 | Tumor extends more than 2 cm into liver, and/or into two or more adjacent organs (stomach, duodenum, colon, pancreas, omentum, extrahepatic bile ducts, any involvement of liver) |
| Regional lymph nodes | |
| NX | Regional lymph nodes cannot be assessed |
| N0 | No regional lymph node metastasis |
| N1 | Metastasis in cystic duct, pericholedochal, and/or hilar lymph nodes (i.e., in the hepatoduodenal ligament) |
| N2 | Metastasis in erperipancreatic (head only), periduodenal, periportal, celiac, and/or superior mesenteric lymph nodes. |
| Distant metastasis | |
| MX | Distant metastasis cannot be asssessed |
| M0 | No distant metastasis |
| M1 | Distant metastasis |
| Stage grouping | |
| Stage 0 | Tis N0 M0 |
| Stage I | T1 N0 M0 |
| Stage II | T2 N0 M0 |
| Stage IIIA | T1 N0 M0 |
| | T2 N1 M0 |
| | T3 N1 M0 |
| | T3 N1 M0 |
| Stage IVA | T4 N0 M0 |
| | T4 N1 M0 |
| Stage IVB | Any T any N M1 |

be sufficient for tumor removal. For more distal lesions, the surgery of choice is pancreaticoduodenectomy. The resulting biliary-enteric reconstruction is a jejunal loop after pancreaticoduodenectomy or a Roux-en-Y anastomosis for more proximal lesions. Overall, for gallbladder resections, the 5-year survival rate is 10%–30% with locoregional recurrences seen in about 80% of patients [21].

Outside of a protocol setting, there is no established role for adjuvant chemoradiation for gallbladder or bile duct tumors. In most instances, however, patients are referred for 5-FU-based chemotherapy in conjunction with radiation to the biliary bed and may be appropriate for patients who are not protocol candidates and who have transmural tumor involvement and/or regional lymph node metastases.

## Palliative (Unresectable Stage III and IV Disease)

Palliative treatments for gallbladder or bile duct tumors depends on the symptom being palliated. For symptomatic cholestasis, percutaneous or endoscopic stents (wall or expandable) should be placed. For symptoms of tumor growth such as cachexia or pain, chemotherapy and/or radiotherapy are most appropriate. For locally advanced disease, both modalities are useful in tumor control although randomized prospective studies have not been conducted comparing chemoradiotherapy to chemotherapy alone in this setting. For patients without major symptoms or those with metastatic disease, chemotherapy in the investigational setting should be the standard approach. This is because there are no standard chemotherapy agents for this disease. 5-FU based chemotherapy yields response rates in the order of 10%–15% although higher response (>30%) rates have been demonstrated with prolonged infusion 5-FU with interferon. However, these responses are not durable and have a negligible impact on survival. Newer agents with a potential for use in the disease include the oral 5-FU analogs like oral 5-FU and eniluracil, capecitabine, UFT and S-1. These drugs may be combined with the more traditional drugs like gemcitabine, cisplatin or adriamycin to augment single agent response rates and such trials are underway [22, 23, 24].

## Pancreatic Cancer

### Epidemiology, Risk Factors

#### Incidence

Cancer of the exocrine pancreas continues to be a devastating health issue with approximately 28,000 new cases and 27,000 deaths due to disease per year. The incidence rates are identical to mortality rates. With current modes of treatment less than 4% of patients with adenocarcinoma of the pancreas will be alive 5 years after diagnosis. The world-wide incidence of pancreatic cancer is approximately 185,000 new cases per year (1985) with a death/incidence ratio of 0.99. The disease is predominantly seen in developed countries and parallels the distribution of colorectal cancer.

*Race*

The incidence in the Hispanic and African-American population is higher (by approximately 30%–40%) than other populations. Another US subpopulation with high incidence (16.4/100,000) is Koreans in Los Angeles, CA.

*Sex*

The ratio of males to females affected differs according to age, with a 2:1 ratio in patients younger than 40 years and 1:1 in those over 80. There is a slight male predominance (10.1/100,000 person-years among males compared with 7.5/100,000 among females) in both whites and non-whites.

*Age Distribution*

The incidence of pancreatic cancer increases with age with most cases presenting between ages 65 and 79 years.

*Predisposition*

There is a relative excess of pancreatic cancer among first-degree relatives of cases, and anecdotal reports of familial aggregations. Furthermore, there are familial associations of pancreatic and extrapancreatic cancers including breast and ovarian cancer. Other genetic disorders that predispose to pancreatic cancer include hereditary pancreatitis (autoso-

mal dominant, AD), multiple endocrine neoplasia type I (AD), glucagonoma syndrome (? AD), hereditary nonpolyposis colorectal cancer,
Lynch II variant (AD), Gardner's syndrome (AD), a subset of familial atypical mole melanoma (FAMMM) syndrome kindreds, Von Hipple-
Lindau syndrome, and in association with insulin dependant diabetes
mellitus and exocrine insufficiency [25–28].

## Localization

The majority of cancers of the pancreas (~95%) arise within exocrine
portions of the gland usually from the proximal portions including the
head, neck and uncinate process. Only 20% arise from the body and
5%–10% from the tail of the pancreas. At presentation, however, 85% of
patients have clinically evident metastases or micrometastases.
Approximately, 20% are organ confined, 40% locally advanced (inoperable) and 40% with visceral metastases. The most common sites of metastases are liver (>90%), peritoneum, regional lymph nodes (pancreatico-
duodenal, inferior pancreatic head and subpyloric nodes) and lung [29].

## Risk Factors, Etiology

There appears to be a relationship between pancreatic cancer and environmental carcinogens; however, this relationship is inconsistent for
many carcinogens with the exception of cigarette smoking.

Cigarette smoke has been most strongly linked to pancreatic cancer
based on published case-control studies and autopsy studies linking
cigarette exposure to ductal hyperplasia. Also, there is an increased risk
of pancreatic cancer as a second malignancy in patients with a first-ciga-
rette related malignancy (head and neck, lung, and bladder cancer). A VA
hospital study showed almost twice incidence rate of carcinoma of the
pancreas in cigarette smokers as for nonsmokers. The risk increases with
increase in pack-years which levels off 10–15 years after cessation of
smoking.

Dietary carcinogens have also been linked to pancreatic cancer.
Laboratory animals (e.g. Syrian golden hamsters) develop pancreatic
cancer after administration of 2, 2'-dihydroxy-di-N-propylnitrosamine
and the incidence of such cancers increase with dietary fat and protein

intake. A significant association between dietary fat and cancer has been shown in two studies; however, other studies in different populations have not corroborated influence of dietary meat on cancer incidence. Alcohol use and pancreatic cancer have been linked through some retrospective studies such that chronic pancreatitis has shown to be a major risk factor for pancreatic cancer. Reviews on this subject conclude that there is insufficient evidence for a causal relationship and since then few studies have clarified the role of alcohol consumption and pancreatic cancer. A similar conclusion has been reached with collating studies showing a higher relative risk of cancer among subjects exposed to coffee or tea [30–36].

Pathology and Staging

Adenocarcinoma arising from ductal epithelium of the exocrine glands within the pancreas accounts for 95% of the pathology. Most of these ductal carcinomas are mucin-producing and usually associated with a dense desmoplastic reaction. Other uncommon pathology includes acinar cell carcinoma and cystadenocarcinomas. The most important aspect of pancreatic carcinoma is that it is microscopically multicentric and in many cases perineural invasion portends a poor prognosis. Pancreatitis is an attendant feature surrounding the carcinoma in most cases. Staging of pancreatic carcinoma is based on local primary tumor size, nodal involvement and distant metastatic spread based on the TNM classification as shown in Table 3. For purposes of prognostication, tumor size, lymph node metastases and histology (degree of differentiation) are important determinant of survival such that small lymph node negative well-differentiated tumors that are completely resected have the best survival rates.

Work-up and Staging

The minimum but cost-effective work-up of pancreatic cancer depends on the clinical presentation. Most patients present with jaundice (elevated conjugated bilirubin) and directed work-up with either a liver ultrasound or Computerized Tomography (CT) scan (a spiral scan with contrast is advocated) is warranted. If a mass is documented with no evidence of metastatic disease, the location of the mass further dictates work-up. If the mass is in the head of the pancreas and the patient has symptoms of cholestasis, cholangitis or fever, we advocate an endoscopic stent placement. Most patients, however, have endoscopic stent placement if there is documented bile duct obstruction whether or not they have symptoms at the time of placement. This is especially relevant to patients in whom you contemplate further treatment of their disease. If the mass is present in the body of the pancreas, we advocate either an endoscopic ultrasound and/or laparoscopic biopsy. In most cases, howe-

**Table 3.** Staging system for pancreatic tumors

| | |
|---|---|
| Primary tumor | |
| TX | Primary tumor cannot be assessed |
| T0 | No evidence of primary tumor |
| Tis | In situ carcinoma |
| T1 | Tumor limited to the pancreas 2 cm or less in greatest dimension |
| T2 | Tumor limited to the pancreas more than 2 cm in greatest dimension |
| T3 | Tumor extends directly into any of the following: duodenum, bile duct, peripancreatic tissues |
| T4 | Tumor extends directly into any of the following: stomach, spleen, colon, adjacent large vessels |
| | |
| Regional lymph nodes | |
| NX | Regional lymph nodes cannot be assessed |
| N0 | No regional lymph node metastasis |
| N1 | Regional lymph node metastasis |
| PN1a | Metastasis in a single regional lymph node |
| PN1b | Metastasis in multiple regional lymph nodes |
| | |
| Distant metastasis | |
| MX | Distant metastasis cannot be assessed |
| M0 | No distant metastasis |
| M1 | Distant metastasis |
| | |
| Stage grouping | |
| Stage 0 | Tis N0 M0 |
| Stage I | T1 N0 M0 |
| | T2 N0 M0 |
| Stage II | T3 N0 M0 |
| Stage III | T1 N0 M0 |
| | T2 N1 M0 |
| | T3 N1 M0 |
| | T3 N1 M0 |
| Stage IVA | T4 any N M0 |
| | T4 N1 M0 |
| Stage IVB | Any T any N M1 |

ver, patients require a laparotomy due to inconclusive pathology or inadequete biopsy material. Masses documented in the tail of the pancreas are rarely curable and also rarely present with jaundice; however, if one is documented by routine ultrasound or CT, we advocate a spiral CT scan to determine resectability.

In patients in whom a mass in the head or body of the pancreas is found on routine ultrasound or abdominal CT scan without evidence of metastatic disease, we advocate a dedicated spiral CT scan with contrast to determine criteria for resectability. Patients presenting with or without jaundice should all be evaluated with a good chest film (both posterior-anterior and lateral views). For those patients with a histologic diagnosis of pancreatic cancer, a serum marker CA19–9 does not add to the diagnosis (especially for stages I and II); however, serial CA19–9 levels have been found to correlate with survival of pancreatic cancer in both surgical and chemotherapy series. This antigen, a sialylated Lewis A blood group member, is nonspecific but highly sensitive (67.6%–92% dependent on cut-off levels) and its levels may be useful in differentiating pancreatic adenocarcinoma from inflammatory conditions of the pancreas. The higher the cut-off level of CA19–9, the higher the specificity of the test in detecting pancreatic cancer. For those patients without histologic diagnosis who are not surgical candidates or for whom the disease is metastatic, CA19–9 is nonspecific and usually does not aide in the diagnosis of pancreatic cancer. The use of this marker for diagnosis, especially in this situation is problematic and there is no consensus. Bone scans, head and/or pelvic CT scans, bone marrow examination, or other MRI and/or nuclear scans have no role in the routine work-up of patients with pancreatic cancer.

The American Joint Committee on Cancer (AJCC) has developed staging criteria for adenocarcinoma of the pancreas; however, this criteria has not been widely adopted by many centers with surgical expertise in pancreatic cancer management (Table 3) [37, 38]. We encourage use of these criteria so that clinical trial results from different centers are comparable and hence, interpretable.

Treatment

*Curative (Stages I, II and III)*

Determination of resectability is the first step in the management of patients with pancreatic cancer. Pancreaticoduodenectomy or Whipple resection is the standard operation for cancer of the head of the pancreas. There is no accepted universal standard criteria for resection; however, collating our experience with those of others, certain guidelines are useful in the assessment of resectability. Clearly high-resolution (helical or spiral) CT scans are paramount in establishing preoperative staging of resectability with the following conditions being met: a) no extrapancreatic disease b) no direct extension to (or invasion of) the celiac and superior mesenteric artery c) unobstructed superior mesenteric-portal vein confluence. Additional criteria, usually indicating borderline resectability is dependent on the scan resolution and patient factors, as indicated in Table 4 [38]. At present using such and similar criteria for operability, mortality rates in most experienced centers are low (<5%); however, despite the most optimal conditions, the median survival of resected patients is 12–18 months with 90% dying of recurrent disease in the first 2 years after resection [39, 40].

*Adjuvant*

The initial basis for radiation therapy (RT) in combination with chemotherapy for pancreatic cancer came from the Mayo Clinic and Duke University. In the Mayo report, patients with locally unresectable gastrointestinal cancer were randomized to receive RT (35–40 Gy) plus placebo, or RT plus 5-FU. The median survival of 64 patients with adenocarcinoma of the pancreas who received radiation and placebo was 6.3 months compared with 10.4 months for patients who received 5-FU plus RT (p<0.05) [41, 42]. The Duke report showed 69% of patients radiated using a double split course of RT survived 6 months and 34% 1 year survival rate [43]. These statistics were far better than historical data from Mayo on the natural history of untreated pancreatic cancer with 26% and 8%, 6 month and 1 year survival, respectively [41, 42, 43]. The early Mayo and Duke studies set the stage for future randomized studies by the Gastrointestinal Tumor Study Group (GITSG) between the years 1973

**Table 4.** Criteria defining resectability status

| | Head | Body | Tail |
|---|---|---|---|
| Resectable | No distant metastases | No distant metastases | No distant metastases |
| | Clear fat plane around celiac and superior mesenteric arteries | Clear fat plane around celiac and superior mesenteric arteries | Clear fat plane around celiac and Patent SMV/PV |
| | Patent SMV/PV | Patent SMV/PV | superior mesenteric arteries |
| Borderline resectable | Severe unilateral SMV/portal impingment | Severe unilateral SMV/portal impingment | Adrenal, colon, or kidney invasion |
| | Tumor abutment on SMA | Tumor abutment on SMA | |
| | GEDA encasement up to origin at hepatic artery | GEDA encasement up to origin at hepatic artery | |
| | Colon invasion | Colon invasion | |
| Unresectable | Distant metastases | Distant metastases | Distant metastases |
| | SMA, celiac encasement | SMA, celiac hepatic encasement | SMA, celiac encasement |
| | SMV/portal occlusion | SMV/portal occlusion | Rib, vertebral invasion |
| | Aortic, IVC invasion or encasement | Aortic invasion | |
| | Invasion of SMV below | | |
| | Transverse mesocolon | | |

and 1985 for resectable (one study) and unresectable disease (four studies) [44].

GITSG protocol G9173 compared no adjuvant therapy with 40 Gy plus 5-FU following apparently curative resection. RT was given as single split course and 5-FU was given on the first and last 3 days of the radiation course and subsequently continued on a weekly basis at a dose of 500 mg/m². Treatment was continued for 2 years unless recurrence was demonstrated. The median survival was 20 months for the treated group. This compared with only 11 months for surgery-only patients (p=0.03). The analysis was, however, conducted on 43 patients who were randomized over 8 years and 3 months. Subsequent to initial analysis, 32 patients were registered in 28 months and treated according to protocol specifications with combined modality therapy. The overall survival in this group mirrored the randomized group [45, 46]. Since no successor trial has been conducted, this protocol is the only randomized study showing survival benefit from adjuvant therapy. A similar study has been conducted by the European Organization for Research and Treatment of Cancer (EORTC) and the results will soon be available. Subsequent to the report of the GITSG study, NCI reported on the efficacy of adjuvant intraoperative RT (20 Gy) which resulted in a disease-free interval of 20 months in 16 patients compared with 12 months for the 16 patients who did not receive adjuvant radiation [47]. Another study from the University of Pennsylvania utilized a 96-hour 5-FU infusion given during weeks 1 and 5 of radiation (45–48.6 Gy) and they reported a 59% 2-year and 47% 3-year survival in patients who had undergone a complete resection [48]. Despite these results, we have not yet established a standard practice in the adjuvant treatment of pancreatic cancer. Hence even for patients with resected cancer, investigational options especially combined modality approaches should be pursued.

*Locally Advanced Disease*

In the first GITSG study 9273, the protocol was a three arm comparison as illustrated in Table 5. In the first phase of the trial with nearly equal patients in each arm during interim analysis, the results showed a significant survival advantage for the combined modality arms over the radiotherapy alone arm. The final analysis showed a modest survival advantage (not significant) for patients receiving 60 Gy plus 5-FU over those

**Table 5.** G1 9273: initial GITSG protocol for locally unresectable disease

Radiotherapy alone (60 Gy)[a] vs
Radiotherapy (60 Gy) plus 5-FU[a,b] vs
Radiotherapy (40 Gy) plus 5-FU[a,b]

Treatment given with parallel opposed anterior posterior fields (AP/PA) (maximum volume 400 cm[2]). During final 20-Gy treatment given to tumor and pancreas only
[a] Radiotherapy given as 20 Gyx3 double split course (single split for 40 Gy plus 5-FU arm) in daily fractions of 2 Gy with 2 weeks of between courses as in Duke University Series.
[b] 5-Fluorouracil, 5-given in 500 mg/m[2] bolus days 1 through 3 of each of the three courses followed by weekly maintenance indefinitely.

receiving 40 Gy plus5-FU (Fig. 3) [49]. The successor protocol tested 60 Gy plus 5-FU versus 40 Gy plus doxorubicin. There were no significant differences in survival; however, toxicity was significantly increased in the RT plus doxorubicin arm [50]. In a single arm pilot study (n=18 evaluable patients) using hyperfractionated RT with SMF chemotherapy, the median survival was only 35 weeks with 39% 1-year survival rate [51].

The ECOG randomized patients to receive SMF alone or SMF plus 40 Gy. The median survival was identical in both groups; however, the incidence of severe toxicities were doubled in the SMF plus RT arm when compared with the SMF alone arm [52]. The non-GITSG trial experience also document the efficacy of chemoradiation but still the overall survival does not exceed 50 weeks. In one study the 2-year survival was 46.7% and other studies employing prophylactic liver irradiation suggests that the frequency of failure in the liver may decrease but not affect the over-

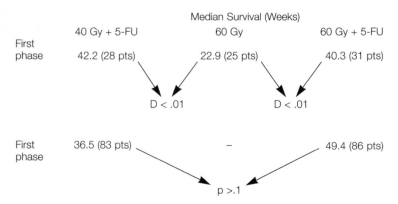

**Fig. 3.** GI-9273 results: treatment of locally unresectable disease

all survival [53, 54]. Despite the use of 5-FU based therapy in conjunction with radiation, patients should be encouraged to participate in chemoradiotherapy protocols assessing novel radiosensitizer therapy or radiation delivery.

**Surgical Palliation.** Biliary decompression is an important aspect in the overall management of patients with pancreatic cancer. In situations where there is cholestasis from extrahepatic obstruction without attendant fever, or symptoms of cholangitis, one may consider elective placement of a biliary drain or internal stent. When there is attendant fever or other related symptoms, expandable metal stents (preferable) or conventional polyethylene prostheses should be placed immediately. The issue as to whether surgical bypass is better or worse than nonsurgical drainage becomes important when dealing with patients with good performance status and localized disease who are otherwise unresectable. The principal advantage of nonoperative stents is avoidance of a major surgical proceedure, expense and attendant mortality rate (15%–40%). However, the disadvantages include higher infection and occlusion rate requiring frequent (sometimes every 2–3 months) stent changes. Bornman et al studied stent placement versus surgical bypass in a prospective randomized study but was unable to show clear superiority of one approach over the other. Thirty day mortality rates were similar; however, the jaundice recurrence rate was higher in the endoprosthesis group [55]. Despite higher initial costs for surgery, the effect of cost savings with endoprosthesis is lost over time as patients require repeated placements for obstruction and cholangitis. Nonetheless, results from nonoperative stents continue to improve as more superior prostheses (e.g. expandable wall metal stents) are developed. In fact, in a prospective randomized trial, metal stents showed less tendency to obstruct and was more durable. Finally, the option of either surgery or nonsurgical decompression should take into account the patient's status and wishes and will also depend on expertise from center to center [56].

*Metastatic Disease: Chemotherapy*

5-Fluorouracil (5-FU) based chemotherapy has been used extensively in the past with little success yielding response rates of 0%–28% (95%CI

0%–43%) [57]. Combination chemotherapy with 5-FU with leucovorin or interferon or PALA have also produced disappointingly low rates of tumor response [58, 59]. Most of these studies were published between 1965 and 1991 with a majority of newer regimens published in the 1980s. During this period there has been a tremendous flux in our understanding and interpretation of CT scans and associated imaging modalities and hence, there is tremendous interobserver variability in measurement of tumor size. Furthermore, given the high degree of fibrosis within pancreatic lesions, tumor cells may respond to chemotherapy without apparent change in tumor size or vice-versa. The collating of different small studies done over time is not without error since the dosages of any one or more drugs varied from study to study and in selected studies some patients had received previous chemotherapy.

Therefore a more reasonable approach to assessing the impact of chemotherapy in pancreatic cancer would be through randomised trials that have accrued quickly and published survival rates in each arm. No randomized trial has demonstrated that 5-FU based combination therapy is superior to single agent 5-FU [60]. In the 1980s a combination chemotherapy regimen "Mallinson regimen" was developed. Forty patients with advanced pancreatic cancer were randomly assigned to either symptomatic supportive care only or chemotherapy with an induction course of 5-FU, cyclophosphamide, methotrexate, and vincristine, followed by maintenance treatment with 5-FU plus mitomycin C. Median survival in the control arm was 9 weeks in comparison with 44-week median survival in the treatment group. In a follow-up comparison study the "Mallinson regimen" was studied versus FAP and 5-FU alone and there was no difference in overall survival between the arms [61, 62]. Further support of the efficacy of single agent 5-FU come from published randomized trials comparing 5-FU plus streptozotocin, FAM, or 5-FU plus leucovorin combination therapy versus single agent 5-FU [63, 64]. These studies underscore the need for randomized trials of new agents for pancreatic cancer.

Until recently 5-FU was considered standard chemotherapy for pancreatic cancer. In 1996, the US Food and Drug Administration approved Gemzar (gemcitabine HCL) for patients with locally advanced or metastatic adenocarcinoma of the pancreas. Based on phase I studies, a dose of 1000 mg/m2 once per weekx7 weeks followed by a 1 week rest then weeklyx3 repeated every 4 weeks given as a 30 minute infusion, was selected as a dosage regimen in the Phase III Gemzar pancreas pivotal trial [65, 66]. The rationale for such a trial was based on earlier pilot trials with gemcitabine in which some patients experienced objective improvement in analgesic requirements and performance status even without tumor response. The pivotal phase III trial randomized 126 patients with advanced symptomatic pancreas cancer after completing a lead-in period for symptom control to receive either gemcitabine or 5-FU (600 mg/m2 weekly). The median survival duration for the gemcitabine versus 5-FU arm was 5.65 versus 4.41 months (Fig. 4; p=0.0025).

The clinical benefit (an objective measure of pain, performance score, weight changes) response rate in the gemcitabine arm was 23.8% versus 4.8% in the 5-FU arm (p=0.0022) [67]. The main aspects of the trial were that the patients were moderately symptomatic at trial entry and the objective response rate was only 5.4% for patients treated with gemcitabine. Although the treatment is effective, it is likely to be mos useful to those patients with moderate symptoms. For asymptomatic patients or patients with slow growing tumors, clinical trials investigating newer drugs should be offered and they should be encouraged to participate.

## Neuroendocrine Tumors of the Gastrointestinal Tract

### Carcinoid Tumors

*Epidemiology, Risk Factors*

#### Incidence
In the US, fewer than 2000 cases are diagnosed yearly. Neuroendocrine tumors constitute approximately 2% of all malignant gastrointestinal cancers. Carcinoid tumors (approximately 650 cases per 100,000 autopsies) are more common than pancreatic islet-cell carcinomas. Of the latter, gastrinomas (0.4 cases per million individuals) and insulinomas (0.9 cases per million individuals) are most common [68].

#### Race
Typically a disease of Western Hemisphere – the actual incidence varies in certain racial groups and clear predilection is not discernable. For carcinoid tumors, for example, the annual incidence in Ireland is 13 cases per million; in Scandinavia 7 per million population while the US SEER data indicates an annual rate of 2.8 per million population [68, 69, 77, 78]

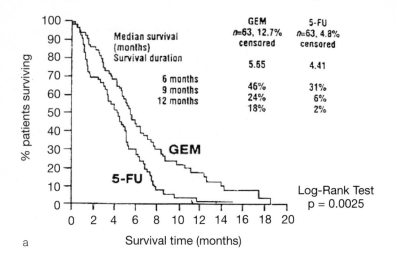

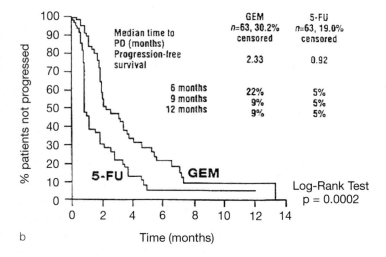

**Fig. 4a,b.** 5-FU versus Gemcitabine: Randomized trial in pancreatic cancer

## Sex
Males and females are equally affected.

## Age Distribution
Young adults are most frequently affected especially in the third and fourth decades of life.

## Predisposition
These tumors may occur as part of the multiple endocrine neoplasia (MEN) syndromes, particularly MEN I (Wermer's syndrome). This disorder is characterized as a familial autosomal disorder involving tumors of the pituitary gland, parathyroids and pancreatic islet cells. More recently, the genetic locus predisposing to this disorder has been linked to the muscle phosphorylase locus on chromosome 11q13 [69, 70].

## Localization
Carcinoids most commonly originate in the gastrointestinal tract; however there has been a recent trend for an increase in the percentage of carcinoids arising from the bronchus and a relative decrease in the number arising from the jejunoileum and rectum. The small bowel (jejunoileum) is the most common site for carcinoids that metastasize to the liver. They are also most hormonally active in that these patients present with the carcinoid syndrome. Based on an institutional study, the majority of carcinoids arise from the appendix [45%], small intestines [30%] and rectum [15%] [68, 69].

## Risk Factors and Etiology
Risk factors involved in the pathogenesis of these tumors are unknown. The tumors originate from amine precursor uptake and decarboxylation (APUD) cells and therefore, they contain high levels of carboxyl groups and nonspecific esterase. In addition, they share several genetic and biochemical markers in common with other APUD tumor derivatives like small cell carcinoma, medullary carcinoma of the thyroid gland, neuroblastoma, and Merkel-cell tumor of the skin [71, 72]. Furthermore, various growth factors have been implicated in its pathogenesis including aberrant expression of TGF-beta that may directly influence matrix formation and fibrosis seen with carcinoids [73]. In endocrine pancreatic tumors, CD44 expression correlates with the tumor's ability to metastasize to the regional lymph nodes [74].

## Pathology and Staging

A variety of carcinoid tumor patterns have been characterized histologically – insular, glandular, mixed and undifferentiated. Pancreatic islet cells have similar histology. Carcinoids, however, may have extensive necrosis associated with it and in cases of midgut tumors also present with extensive stromal fibrosis. Further diagnostic tests are usually performed on the pathology specimen including histochemical, electron microscopic and immunohistochemical analysis. Silver staining (limited to well differentiated cells) is the classic stain for revealing the presence of well differentiated neuroendocrine cells; however, in most centers these tests have been replaced by staining for secretory granule contents including chromogranin A and synaptophysin. In addition, staining for cytoplasmic constituents like neuron-specific (nonspecific esterase) enolase also aids in the diagnosis. In cases of doubt, electron microscopy reveals dense core granules for cells of neuroendocrine origin [68–72].

## Work-up and Staging

Once there is a clinical suspicion for carcinoid tumor (nearly 1/3 present with symptoms), the work-up and staging are simple. Seventy-five percent of patients with the carcinoid syndrome present with attacks of flushing and watery diarrhea. Tumors of bronchial origin tend to produce long-lasting flush associated with hypotension, facial edema, lacrimation, and sweating. Gastric carcinoids are associated with a red geographic flush of the head and neck while ileal carcinoid flush is typically violaceous. Other associated phenomenon of relevance is asthma (15%) and pellagroid rash due to depletion of tryptophan for synthesis of niacin (5%), arthralgias (<5%), encephalopathy and endomyocardial fibrosis (35%) leading to tricuspid regurgitation and right heart failure [68, 75–83].

The work-up includes measurement of urinary 5-HIAA (Fig. 5) and at baseline a CT scan of the abdomen and/or pelvis. More than 90% of patients with carcinoid syndrome have liver metastases. In cases of suspected bronchial carcinoid, a chest CT scan and preferably bronchoscopy (with biopsy) should be performed. For localized ileal carcinoids, a dedicated small bowel X-ray study is advocated. Angiography, octreotide scans (OctreoScan), and 131-metaiodobenzylguanidine scans have limi-

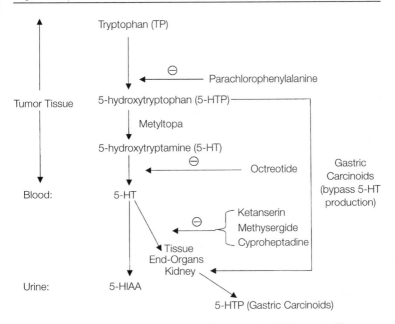

**Fig. 5.** Synthesis, secretion, and metabolism of serotonin (5-HT) in carcinoid tumors

ted diagnostic potential except is rare situations outside the scope of this chapter. A urinary 5-HIAA >150micromol/24 h, is diagnostic of carcinoid syndrome and directly correlates with disease extent and prognosis. It is very important to obtain urinary 5-HIAA levels when avoiding certain food substances prior to tests like bananas as they may interfere with the assay false high or low values [83]. In the rare patient with foregut carcinoid, 5-hydroxytryptophan is not measured in the 5-HIAA assay, so one should measure urinary or platelet serotonin for diagnosis [68, 80].

The classic TNM staging system is not useful in providing prognostic or therapeutic information, instead curability is dependant on complete removal of the primary lesion in the absence of liver metastases. After complete resection, 20-year survivors may be seen which may approach 20%. In the presence of liver metastases, longer survival have been reported with aggressive embolization and surgical extirpation; however, it is not certain that long-term cure may be achieved as median survival varies between 3–8 years [81–89].

*Treatment*

Curative

**Appendiceal Carcinoids.** For tumors <1 cm, local excision is sufficient. For tumors between 1 and 2 cm, the risk for subsequent metastases is 50% and the need for further management depends on the patients age and co-morbidities; however for tumors >2 cm a standard cancer-type right hemicolectomy should be performed [68, 76–78].

**Rectal Carcinoids.** For tumors <1 cm, metastasis is rare and local fulguration is adequate. Tumors <2 cm almost always metastasize and should be treated with a standard cancer-type procedure appropriate for its location within the rectum [68, 76–78].

**Small Intestinal Carcinoids.** All primaries when located should be resected, especially in those without liver metastases. In addition, despite metastases, obstructing primaries should be resected for symptom control. The resection should typically include a wedge lymphadenectomy [68, 76–78].

Palliative

**Carcinoid Syndrome.** The carcinoid syndrome characterized by paroxysmal flushing, watery diarrhea, abdominal cramping, facial telangiectasia, pellagra-like lesions of skin and oral mucosa, endomyocardial fibrosis and or asthma/wheezing. Several treatment options exist and these have been tabulated in Table 6. Perhaps the two most effective modalities to treat or control the syndrome is the use of the somatostatin analogue SMS 201–995 and/or hepatic arterial embolization. Hepatic arterial embolization involves cannulating the hepatic artery and applying embolic material with or without selected chemotherapy. Several uncontrolled studies have shown that embolization produces marked symptomatic response in 75% or more of patients, with a reduction of flushing and diarrhea and lowering of urinary 5-HIAA excretion [83, 87]. SMS 201-995 or octreotide has a half-life of 100 min (unlike native somatostatin which has a half-life of only a few minutes) and may be safely given three times a day. In 62 patients treated with this analogue at doses between 200 and 1500 microgm/day for more than one month and for as long as 18 months, >90% of patients exhibited improvement in flushing or diarrhea [88, 89]. The urine 5-HIAA decreased while on treatment in

**Table 6.** Symptomatic therapy for carcinoid syndrome[a]

| Drug | Dosage | Flush reduced | Diarrhea reduced | Comments |
|------|--------|---------------|------------------|----------|
| α-Adrenergic antagonist | 10–30 mg daily | Yes | No | Causes severe drowsiness in some patients phenoxybenzamine hydrochloride |
| Chlorpromazine | 10–25 mg every 8 h | Yes (foregut) | No | Anticholinergic, weak antihistamine and anti-serotonin; may have antikinin actions |
| methyldopa | 4–6 g daily | Occasionally | No | Partial blocker of tryptophan decarboxylase; also α-adrenergic antagonist |
| Parachlorophenylalanine | 0.5–1.0 g every 6 h | Occasionally | Yes | Blocks aromatic amino acid hydroxylase; causes depression, eosinophilia in 50%, necessitating stopping use of drug |
| cyproheptadine | 4–8 mg every 6 h | No | Yes | Also has histamine H$_1$ antagonist activity |
| Ketanserin | 40–160 mg daily | Occasionally | Yes | 5HT$_2$ antagonist, histamine H$_1$, α-adrenergic, and dopamine antagonist activity |
| Methysergide | 3–8 mg daily | No | Yes | Anticholinergic H$_1$ antagonist, and vasospastic actions; causes retroperitoneal fibrosis |
| diphenhydramine hydrochloride plus cimetidine | 50 mg and 300 mg every 6 h | Yes (gastric) | – | Uniquely effective in gastric carcinoids |
| Others | | | | |
| Prednisolone | 10–20 mg daily | Yes (foregut) | No | |
| Tamoxifen | 40 mg daily | Occasionally | Occasionally | Antiestrogen; rrely antitumor effects |
| Leukocyte interferon | 6x10$^6$ U i.m. daily | Yes | Yes | Antitumor effects in minority |
| Somatostain analogue SMS 201–995 | 150 g every 8 h | Yes | Yes | Useful in long-term and in crisis; no rebound reported; some antitumor effect |

[a]The effect of drugs on symptoms is only a general guide. Responses vary from patient to patient.

the majority of patients but none of the patients had normalized values. In patients who have increased symptoms while on the lower doses of octreotide can benefit from higher doses.

Side-effects are mild and include transient diarrhea, abdominal pain, steatorrhea, and possible gallstone formation. Another option for patients refractory to SMS 201–995 includes treatment with leukocyte alpha interferon. In one study, of 30 patients treated, 70% had improvement in flushing symptoms; 35% noted improvement in diarrheal frequency; and 42% had lowering of urinary 5-HIAA excretion. However, there was significant side-effects including flu-like symptoms, fatigue and myelosuppression [90]. In another study, of 27 patients treated with doses of alpha interferon between 6 and 24x106 U/m2 three times per week, 20% experienced objective tumor response and 39% had a biochemical response. In another study, patients were given a combination of octreotide plus alpha interferon. Biochemical responses (4 of 22 had a complete response) were observed in 77% of patients. The median response duration was 15 months [91]. In these situations, however, it is advisable to refer patients who are refractory to SMS 201–995 or an equivalent somatostatin analogue to a tertiary care center for the option of protocol based management.

*Metastatic Carcinoid Disease*

Chemotherapy may be palliative in patients with refractory carcinoid syndrome or in whom the urinary 5-HIAA excretion is >150 mg/24 h and/or those who have dominant symptomatic metastases or who have lost weight on account of tumor metabolism. Carcinoids are in general resistant to most chemotherapies. The two most active agents include fluorouracil and doxorubicin. Single agent response rates vary between 10%–25% and response durations are invariable less that 4–6 months. Doxorubicin-based combination therapy produce higher response rates (~30%); however, response durations are still less than 6 months [92–94]. Anaplastic variants may respond to combination etoposide and cisplatin [95]. If chemotherapy is an anticipated modality for the patient, referral at this stage to a tertiary care center is appropriate and encouraged so that these patients may be offered novel approaches towards palliating their tumor burden.

Gastrinomas

*Epidemiology, Risk Factors*

Incidence
In the US, 1 in 2000 peptic ulcers present as a Zollinger-Ellison syndrome.

Sex
The ZES is more common in males (60%).

Age Distribution
The mean age at diagnosis is 45–50 years almost a decade later than those with carcinoid disease.

Predisposition
These tumors may occur as part of the multiple endocrine neoplasia (MEN) syndromes, particularly MEN I (Wermer's syndrome). Approximately, 20% of ZES cases occur as part of MEN I. Patients with duodenal ulcer and hypercalcemia should be suspected of having multiple gastrinomas in the setting of an MEN I syndrome. The most common associated tumor is parathyroid adenoma.

Localization
Most gastrinomas are located in the gastrinoma triangle, defined by the junction of the second and third portions of the duodenum and the junction of the neck and body of the pancreas. 50% of patients have multiple tumors, especially those with MEN I syndrome. 60% of gastrinomas are malignant; 50% have established metastases at diagnosis [96–99].

Risk Factors, Etiology
Risk factors involved in the pathogenesis of these tumors are unknown. The tumors originate from amine precursor uptake and decarboxylation (APUD) cells and therefore, they contain high levels of carboxyl groups and nonspecific esterase. In addition, they share several genetic and biochemical markers in common with other APUD tumor derivatives like small cell carcinoma, medullary carcinoma of the thyroid gland, neuroblastoma, and Merkel-cell tumor of the skin.

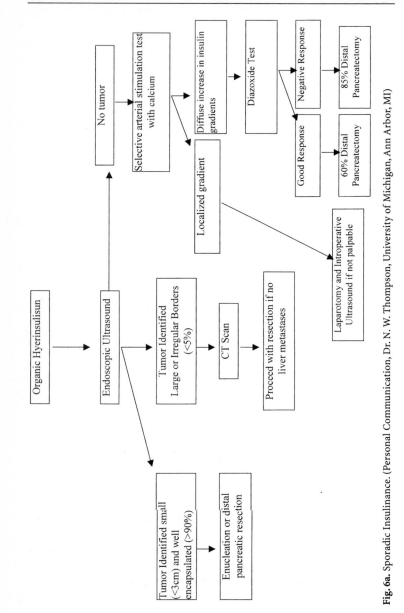

**Fig. 6a.** Sporadic Insulinance. (Personal Communication, Dr. N. W. Thompson, University of Michigan, Ann Arbor, MI)

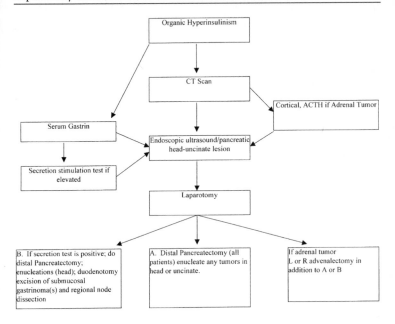

**Fig. 6b.** MEN I Hyperinsulinism. (Personal Communication, Dr. N. W. Thompson, University of Michigan, Ann Arbor, MI)

## Pathology and Clinical Diagnosis

Pathology is helpful in identifying neuroendocrine origin of these tumors; however, the diagnosis of gastrinomas are clinical. The presence of a neuroendocrine tumor in a patient with gastrin hypersecretion, hyperacidity, peptic ulceration, abdominal pain and diarrhea (ZE syndrome) is diagnostic of a gastrinoma. Alternatively, an elevated concentration of gastrin in the blood sample of a fasting patient and increased basal gastric acid secretion (>15 mEq/hr in the absence of prior peptic ulcer surgery or appropriate medications) is highly suggestive of a gastrinoma. In eqiuvocal situations, a gastrin-provocative test (secretin test) is required to differentiate gastrinomas from these other causes.

## Work-up and Staging

Once there is a clinical suspicion for gastrinoma, localization of the tumor is important. Most gastrinomas are indolent and metastases uncommon. Median survival ranges between 3 and 6 years; however, in patients with completely resected disease, 5- and 10-year survival rates are 70% and 100% [100–102]. Therefore, localization of gastrinomas by imaging techniques is imperative to achieve curability for some patients.

The work-up includes measurement of serum gastrin and basal gastric-acid secretion levels in fasting patients, CT scan of the abdomen (chest X-ray to include evaluation for pulmonary metastases), and selective arteriography (this test needs to be individualized) which could be combined with selective sampling of vessels draining the pancreas and duodenum for gastrin levels pre- and post secretin stimulation.

The classic TNM staging system is not useful in providing prognostic or therapeutic information, instead curability is dependant on complete removal of the primary lesion in the absence of liver metastases. In the presence of liver metastases, longer survival have been reported with aggressive embolization and surgical extirpation; however, it is not certain that cure may be achieved.

## Treatment

### Curative

Surgical excision is the treatment of choice for gastrinomas; however, this is only possible in 20% of patients with sporadic tumors. For patients with MEN-1 syndrome, there is an increased likelihood of occult early metastases making them less likely to benefit from surgery. However, since these patients are young and could potentially be spared of metastatic disease, explorative surgery with debulking may be a preferred option. Enucleation of pancreatic lesions are the treatment of choice; however, with duodenal tumors, pancreaticoduodenectomy may be necessary. The role for post-operative adjuvant therapy has not been demonstrated although for patients with positive nodes and/or margins post-operative radiation given concurrently with 5-FU based chemotherapy may be considered. Palliative therapy for metastatic disease will be discussed at the end of this chapter for all islet cell carcinomas.

Insulinomas

*Epidemiology, Risk Factors*

Incidence
Insulinomas are the most common islet cell tumors with an incidence of 0.8–0.9 cases per million population each year.

Sex
In most reported series, 60% of patients are women

Age
The peak incidence is between ages 20–75 years; the average age of presentation is 44–46 years.

Predisposition
These tumors may occur as part of the MEN syndrome with sporadic LOH on chromosome 11 [103–105] (see section on gastrinomas).

Localization
Most sporadic tumors are benign (90%), solitary and small and usually confined within the pancreas (100%). Patients are typically overweight and may suffer form psychiatric disturbances with episodic symptoms of hypoglycemia (confusion, altered conciousness, visual disturbances, weakness, sweating, tremulousness, sezures) due to insulin secretion. Usually when symptoms are unclear, a provocative test with 48-hour fast and repeated glucose monitoring should be performed in the hospital. At nadir glucose levels, insulin and C-peptide should be assayed (both will be inappropriately high for patients with insulinomas). CT, arteriography and ultrasounds fail to detect 40% of insulinomas (see Fig. 6). Although these are the initial recommended studies, a negative study for a patient suspected to harbour an islet cell tumor, additional studies increase the diagnostic yield. These studies include octreotide scans and portal venous sampling for hormones. A laparotomy should be performed if these studies are non-diagnostic and intra-operative ultrasonography should be performed to localize the tumor [106–108].

## Work-up and Staging

Once the diagnosis is established, the tumor is either amenable to surgical resection or only amenable to single or multimodalitiy palliation. The TNM staging does not apply to these tumors.

## Treatment

Curative
As described for gastrinomas, surgery is curative for localized insulinomas.

## Other Tumors

Glucagonomas, Somatostatinoma, VIPomas, Pancreatic Polypeptideoma

A detailed analysis of these tumors is outside the scope of this chapter and more detailed reviews are available [109–112]. The treatment of hormonal syndromes for each of these tumors is still the use of long acting somatostatin analogs at doses used to treat carcinoid syndrome.

## Management of Advanced Islet Cell Carcinoma

The treatment of hormonal excess syndromes have been discussed in the section dealing with carcinoid syndrome. The use of palliative therapy for advanced islet cell tumors is useful in controlling refractory symptoms and tumor growth and in some instances leads to prolonged survival. Islet cell carcinomas in contrast to carcinoids are more sensitive to chemotherapy and active chemotherapeutic drugs include streptozotocin, chlorozotocin, doxorubicin, fluorouracil, and dacarbazine [113–118]. The earliest report of streptozotocin activity in islet cell tumors showed a 50% objective tumor regression rate and a median duration of response >12 months. The side-effects included kidney failure, nausea/vomiting, and myelosuppression. The first randomized trial compared 5-FU plus streptozotocin versus streptozotocin alone. In this study, the complete remission rate was 12% in the streptozotocin alone arm versus

33% in the combined drug arm and patient survival was significantly prolonged in patients receiveing both drugs [118]. The follow-up study was a three arm multi-instiututional trial comparing chlorozotocin alone, streptozotocin plus 5-FU, and streptozotocin plus doxorubicin. The combination of streptozotocin plus doxorubicin was superior to streptozotocin plus fluorouracil (objective response rate 69% versus 45%, p=0.05) but the time to tumor progression was significantly longer for patients receiving streptozotocin plus doxorubicin (20 versus 6.9 months, p=0.001) and the median survival was prolonged by a median of 9.6 months (2.2 versus 1.4 years, p=0.004) [117]. Despite these advances and an established standard of treatment for islet cell tumors, patients must be encouraged to enroll in trials investigating novel drugs for this disease. The long term remission rates for progressive metastatic islet cell tumors is still poor as less than 5%–10% outlive 5 years.

## References

1. International Union Against Cancer: Workshop on Biology of Human Cancer. Rep. 17: Hepatocellular carcinoma. Geneva, 1982
2. Bosch FX, Munoz N. Hepatocellular carcinoma in the world: epidemiological questions. In Tabor E, DiBisceglie AM, Purcell RH (eds): Etiology, Pathology, and Treatment of Hepatocellular Carcinoma. Portfolio, The Woodlands, Texas, 1991
3. Parker SL, Tong T, Baden S, Wingo PA, Cancer statistics, 1996. CA 1996, 46:5
4. Tabor E, DiBisceglie AM, Purcell RH (eds). Etiology, pathology, and treatment of hepatocellular carcinoma in North America. Adv Appl Biotechnol Ser 1991, 13
5. Craig JR, Peters RL, Edmondson HA, Omata M. Fibrolamellar carcinoma of the liver: a tumor of adolescents and young adults with distinctive clinicopathologic features. Cancer 1980, 46:372–379
6. McMahon BJ, London T. Workshop on screening for hepatocellular carcinoma. J Natl Cancer Inst 1991, 83:916–919
7. Colombo M. Early diagnosis of hepatocellular carcinoma in Italy. A summary of a consensus development conference held in Milan, 16 November 1990 by the Italian Association for the Study of the Liver (AISF). J Hepatol 1992, 14:401–403
8. Adson MA. Primary hepatocellular cancers: Western experience in Blumgart LH (eds): Surgery of the Liver and Biliary Tract, p. 1155. New York, Churchill-Livingstone
9. Zhou XD, Tang ZY, Yu YQ et al. Clinical evaluation of cryosurgery in the treatment of primary liver cancer. Cancer 61:1889–92, 1988
10. Mazzaferro V, Regalia E, Doci R et al. Liver transplantation for the treatment of small hepatocellular carcinomas in patients with cirrhosis. N Engl J Med 1996, 14:728–29
11. Venook AP. Treatment of hepatocellular carcinoma: too many options? J Clin Oncol 1994, 12:1323–1334
12. Venook AP, Stagg RJ, Lewis BJ et al. Chemoembolization for hepatocellular carcinoma. J Clin Oncol 1990, 8:1108–1114

13. Livraghi T, Bolondi L, Buscarini L et al. No treatment, resection and ethanol injection in hepatocellular carcinoma: a retrospective analysis of survival in 391 patients with cirrhosis. J Hepatol 1995; 22:522–26

14. Okuda K, Takayasu K, Okada S. Treatment selection. In Liver Cancer Okuda K, Tabor E (eds) p 435–39, Churchill Livingstone. 1997

15. Lewis BJ, Friedman MA. Current status of chemotherapy for hepatoma, in Ogawa M (ed): Chemotherapy of Hepatic Tumors, p63–74, Princeton NJ, Excerpta Medica, 1998

16. Atiq OT, Kemeny N, Niedzweicki D et al. Treatment of unresectable primary liver cancer with intrahepatic floxuridine and mitomycin C through an implanted pump. Cancer 69:920–924, 1992

17. Okada S. Chemotherapy for hepatocellular carcinoma. In Liver Cancer Okuda K, Tabor E (eds) p 441–47, Churchill Livingstone. 1997

18. Order SE, Pajak T et al. A randomized prospective trial comparing full dose chemotherapy to 131-I antiferritin: An RTOG study. Int J Radiat Oncol Biol Phys 20:953–63, 1991

19. Vaittinen E. Carcinoma of the gallbladder: A study of 390 cases diagnosed in Finland 1953–1967. Ann Chir Gynaecol 168 (suppl): 1–18, 1970

20. Krain L. Gallbladder and extrahepatic bile duct carcinoma: Analysis of 1808 cases. Geriatrics 27:1111–17, 1972

21. Bosset JF et al. Primary carcinoma of the gallbladder: Adjuvant postoperative external irradiation. Cancer 64:1843–47, 1990

22. Altaee MY, Johnson PJ, Farrant JM et al. Etiologic and clinical characteristics of peripheral and hilar cholangiocarcinoma. Cancer 1991; 68:2051–55

23. Schoenthaler R, Philips TL, Castro J et al. Carcinoma of the extrahepatic bile ducts: the University of California at San Francisco experience. Ann Surg 1994, 219:267

24. Harvey JH, Smith FP, Sehien PS. 5-fluorouracil, mitomycin and doxorubicin (FAM) in carcinoma of the biliary tract. J Clin Oncol 1984, 2:1245

25. Aoki K, Owawa H. Cancer of the pancreas, international mortality trends. Wold Health Stat Q 31:2–27, 1978

26. Boyle P, Hsieh CC, Maisonneuve P et al. Epidemiology of pancreas cancer. Int J Pancreatol 5:327–346, 1989

27. Mack TM. Pancreas in Schottenfeld D, Fraumeni JF (eds): Cancer Epidemiology and Prevention, London, England, Saunders, 1982, pp 638–677

28. Lunch HT, Smyrk T, Kern SE et al. Familial pancreatic cancer: a review. Sem Oncol 23:2, 251–275

29. Warshaw AL, Fernandez-del Castillo C. Pancreatic carcinoma. New Engl J Med 1992, 326:455

30. Durbec JP, Chevillotte C, Bidart JM et al. Diet, alcohol, tobacco, and risk of cancer of the pancreas: A case-control study. Br J Cancer 43:463–470, 1983

31. Norell SE, Ahlbom A, Erwald R et al. Diet and pancreatic cancer: A case-control study. Am J Epidemiol 124, 894–902, 1986

32. Howe GR, Ghadirian P, Bueno de Mesquita HB et al. A collaborative case-control study of nutrient intake and pancreatic cancer within the SEARCH programme. Int J. Cancer 51:365–372, 1992

33. Ghadirian P, Simard A, Baillargeon J. Tobacco, alcohol, and coffee and cancer of the pancreas. Cancer 67:2664–2670, 1991

34. Doll, Peto R. Mortality in relation to smoking: Twenty years observation on male British doctors. Br Med J 2:1525–1536, 1976

35. Kahn HA. The Dorn study of smoking and mortality among US Veterans: Report on eight and one-half years of observation. Natl Cancer Inst Monograph 19:1–125, 1966

36. Lossing EH, Best EWR, µgregor JT et al. A Canadian study of smoking and health. Ottawa, Canada, Department of National Health and Welfare, 1986
37. AJCC Cancer Staging Manual, Fifth Edition, American Joint Committee on Cancer, American Cancer Society, Lippincott-Raven, 1997
38. NCCN Practice Guidelines for Pancreatic Cancer. NCCN Oncology Practice Guidelines, Oncology 11 (11 A):41–55, 1997
39. Crist DW, Sitzmann JV, Cameron JL. Improved hospital morbidity, mortality, and survival after the Whipple procedure. Ann Surg 206:358–365, 1987
40. Yeo CJ, Cameron JL, Lillemoe KD et al. Pancreaticoduodenectomy for adenocarcinoma of the pancreas. J Clin Oncol 15:928–937, 1997
41. Moertel CG, Reitemeier RJ. Advanced Gastrointestinal Cancer – Clinical Management and Chemotherapy. New York, NY, Hoeber, Medical Division, Harper and Row, 1969, p7
42. Moertel CG, Childs DS, Reitemeier RJ et al. Combined 5 fluorouracil and supervoltage radiation therapy of locally unresectable gastrointestinal cancer. Lancet 2:865–867, 1969
43. Haslam JB, Cavanaugh PJ, Stroup SL. Radiation therapy in the treatment of irresectable adenocarcinoma of the pancreas. Cancer 32:1341–1345, 1973
44. Thomas PRM. Radiotherapy for carcinoma of the pancreas. Sem Oncol 23 (2):213–219, 1996
45. Gastrointenstional Tumor Study Group: Pancreatic cancer. Adjuvant combined radiation and chemotherapy following curative resection. Arch Surg 120:899–903, 1985
46. Gastrointestinal Tumor Study Group: Effective surgicaladjuvant therapy for pancreatic cancer. Cancer 59:2006–2110, 1987
47. Sindelar WF, Kinsella TJ. Randomized trial of intraoperative therapy in resected carcinoma of pancreas. Int J Rad Oncol Biol Phys 12:148, 1986 (abstr) (suppl 1)
48. Whittington R, Bryer MP, Haller DG et al. Adjuvant therapy of resected adenocarcino of the pancreas. Int J Rad Oncol Biol Phys 21:1137–1143, 1991
49. Gastrointestinal Tumor Study Group. Therapy of locally unresectable pancreatic carcinoma: A randomized comparison of high dose (6000 rads) radiation alone, moderate radiation (4000 rads) plus 5-fluorouracil and high dose radiation plus 5-fluorouracil. Cancer 58:1705–1710, 1981
50. Gastrointestinal Tumor Study Group: Radiation therapy combined with Adriamycin or 5-fluorouracil for the treatment of locally unresectable pancreatic carcinoma. Cancer 56:2563–2568, 1985
51. Seydel HG, Stabllein DM, Leichman LP et al. Hyperfractionated radiation and chemotherapy for unresectable localized adenocarcinoma of the pancreas. The Gastrointestinal Tumor Study Group Experience. Cancer 65:1478–1482, 1990
52. Gastrointestinal Tumor Study Group: Treatment of locally unresectable carcinoma of the pancreas: Comparison of combined modality therapy (chemotherapy plus radiotherapy) to chemotherapy alone. J Natl Cancer Inst 80:751–755, 1988
53. Treurniet-Donker AD, Van Mierlo MJM, Van Putten WLJ: Localized unresectable pancreatic cancer. Int J Rad Oncol Biol Phys 18:59–62, 1990
54. Komaki R, Wadler S, Peters T et al. High-dose local irradiation plus prophylactic hepatic irradiation and chemotherapy for imoperable adenocarcinoma of the pancreas. Cancer 69:2807–2812, 1992
55. Bornman PC, Harris-Jones EP, Tobias R et al. Prospective controlled trial of transhepatic biliary endoprothesis versus bypass surgery for incurable carcinoma of head of pancreas. Lancet 1:69–71, 1986
56. µgrath PC, Sloan DA, Kenady DE. Surgical management of pancreatic carcinoma. Sem Oncol 23:200–212, 196 1

57. Schnall SF, Macdonald JS. Chemotherapy of adenocarcinoma of the pancreas. Sem Oncol 23 (2):220–228, 1996
58. Morrell LM, Bach A, Richman SP et al. A phase II multi-institutional trial of low-dose N-(phosphonacetyl)-L-asparate and high-dose 5-fluorouracil as a short-term infusion in the treatment of adenocarcinoma of the pancreas. Cancer 67:363–366, 1991
59. Ardalan B, Sridhar KS, Benedetto P et al. A phase I, II study of high-dose 5-flu-orouracil and high-dose leucovorin with low-dose phosphonacetyl-L-aspartic acid in patients with advanced malignancies. Cancer 68:1242–1246, 1991
60. Schultz RM. Future directions for the treatment of human pancreatic carcinoma. Expert Opin Invest Drug 1995 Dec; 4:1273–9
61. Mallinson CN, Rake MO, Cocking JB et al. Chemotherapy in pancreatic cancer: Results of a controlled prospective, and randomised, multicentre trial. Br Med J 281:1589–1591, 1980
62. Cullinan S, Moertel CG, Wieand HS et al. A phase III trial on the therapy of advanced pancreatic carcinoma. Cancer 65:2207–2212, 1990
63. The Gastrointestinal Tumor Study Group: Phase II studies of drug combinations in advanced pancreatic carcinoma: Fluorouracil plus doxorubicin plus mitomycin-C and two regimens of streptozotocin plus mitomycin-C plus fluorouracil. J Clin Oncol 4:1794–1798, 1986
64. Oster MW, Gray R, Panasci L et al. Chemotherapy for advanced pancreatic cancer. Cancer 57:29–33, 1986
65. Casper ES, Green MR, Kelsen DP et al. Phase II trial of gemcitabine (2, 2'-difluoro-deoxycytidine) in patients with adenocarcinoma of the pancreas. Invest New Drugs 12:29–34, 1994
66. Rothenberg ML, Burris III HA, Andersen JS et al. Gemcitabine: Effective palliative therapy for pancreas cancer patient failing 5-FU. Proc Am Soc Clin Oncol 14:198, 1995
67. Burris HA III, Moore Malcolm J, Andersen J et al. Improvements in survival and clinical benefit with gemcitabine as first-line therapy for patients with advanced pancreas cancer: A randomized trial. J Clin Oncol 15 (6):2403–2413, 1997
68. Moertel CG. An odyssey in the land of small tumors. J Clin Oncol 5:1503–1522, 1987
69. Buchanan KD, Johnston CF, O'Hare MMT: Neuroendocrine tumors. Am J Med 81:14, 1986
70. Larsson C, Shogseid B, Oberg K et al. MEN-1 gene maps to chromosome 11 and is lost in insuloma. Nature 332:85–87, 1988
71. Pearse AGE: The diffuse neuroendocrine system and the APUD concept: Related endocrine peptides in brain, intestine, pituitary, placenta and anuran cutaneous glands. Med Biol 55:115–125, 1977
72. Wilander E. Diagnostic pathology of gastrointestinal pancreatic neuroendocrine tumors. Acta Oncol 288:363–369, 1989
73. Waltenberger J, Lundin L, Obergk et al. Involvement of transforming growth factor-beta in the formation of fibrotic lesions in carcinoid heart disease. AM J Pathol 142:71–78, 1993
74. Chaudhry A, Gobl A, Eriksson B et al. Different splice variance of CD44 are expressed in gastrinomas but not in other subtypes or endocrine pancretic tumors. Cancer Res 54:981–986, 1994
75. Wynick D, Williams SJ, Bloom SR. Symptomatic secondary hormone syndromes in patients with established malignant pancreatic endocrine tumors. N Engl J Med 319:605–607, 1988

76. Thompson GB, van heerden JA, Martin JK et al. Carcinoid tumors of the gastrointestinal tract: Presentation, management, and prognosis. Surgery 98:1054, 1985
77. Wtson RGP, Johnston CF et al. The frequency of gastrointestinal endocrine tumors in a well-defined population. Northern Ireland 1970–1985. Q J Med 72:647, 1989
78. Norheim I, Oberg K, Theodorsson-Norheim E et al. Malignant carcinoid tumors. Ann Surg 206:115, 1987
79. Weiss NS, Yang CP. Incidence of histologic types of cancer of the small intestine. J Natl Cancer Inst 78:653, 1987
80. Jensen R, Norton JA. Cancer of the endocrine system, in De Vita VT, Hellman S, rosenberg SA (eds): Cancer Principles and Practice of Oncology, pp 1705–1719. Philadelphia, JB Lippincott, 1997
81. Moertel CG. Treatment of carcinoid tumors and the malignant carcinoid syndrome. J Clin Oncol 1:727–740, 1983
82. Oberg K. Treatment of neuroendocrine tumors. Cancer Treat Rev 20:331–355, 1994
83. Maton PN. The Carcinoid Syndrome. JAMA 260 (11):1602–1605, 1988
84. Norheim I, Oberg K, Theordorsson-Norheim E et al. Malignant carcinoid tumors. Ann Surg 206:115–126, 1987
85. Davis Z, Moertell CG, Mellrath DC. The malignant carcinoid syndrome. Surg Gyn Obstet 137:637–644, 1973
86. Maartensson H, Norbin A, Bengmarks S et al. Embolization of the liver in the management of metastatic carcinoid tumors. J Surg Oncol 27:152–158, 1984
87. Mitty HA, Warner RRP, Newman LH. Control of carcinoid syndrome with hepatic artery embolization. Radiology 155:623–626, 1982
88. Kvols LK, Moertel CG, O'Connell MJ et al. Treatment of malignant carcinoid syndrome: Evaluation of a long-acting somatostatin analogue. N Engl J Med 315:663–666, 1986
89. Proceedings of Somatostatin, 85. Scand J Gastroenerol 21 (suppl 119), 1986
90. Oberg K, Norheim I, Lind E. Treatment of malignant carcinoid tumors with human leukocyte interferon: Long-term results. Cancer Treat Rep 70:1297–1304, 1986
91. Legha SS, Valdivieso M, Nelson RS et al. Chemotherapy for metastatic carcinoid tumors: Experience with 32 patients and a review of the literature. Cancer Treat Rep 61:1699–1703, 1977
92. Stolinsky DC, Sadoff L, Braunwald J et al. Streptozotocin in the treatment of cancer: Phase II study. 30–61–67, 2972
93. Kissinger A, Foley FJ, Lemon JH. Use of DTIC (dacabazine) in the malignant carcinoid tumors. Cancer Treat Rep 61:101–102, 1977
94. Ajani JA, Kegha SS, Karlin DA et al. Combination chemotherapy of metastatic carcinoid tumors with 5-FU, adriamycin, and cytoxan (FAX) and 5-FU, adriamycin, mitomycin-C, and methyl CCNU (FAMMe) (abstract). Proc Am Soc Clin Oncol 2:124, 1983
95. Moertel CG, Kvols LK, O'Connell MJ et al. Treatment of neuroendocrine carcinomas with combined etoposide and cisplatin. Evidence of major therapeutic activity in the anaplastic variants of these neoplasms. Cancer 68:227–232, 1991
96. Schimke RN. Multiple endocrine neoplasia: how many syndromes? Am J Med Genet 37:375–383, 1990
97. Jensen RT, Gardner JD. Zollinger-Ellison syndrome: Clinical presentation, pathology, diagnosis and treatment, in Dannenberg A Zakim D (eds): Peptic Ulcer and Other Acid-Related Diseases, p. 117. New York, Academic Research Association, 1991
98. Townsend CM, Lewis BG, Gourley WK et al. Gastrinoma. Curr Prob Cancer 7:1–33, 1982
99. Townsend CM, Thompson JC. Gastrinoma. Sem Surg Oncol 691–697, 1990

100. Malagelada JR, Edis AJ, Adson MA et al. Medical and surgical options in the management of patients with gastrinoma. Gastroenterology 84:1524–1532, 1983
101. Norton JA, Doppman JL, Jensen RT. Curative resection in Zollinger-Ellison syndrome: Results of a 10 year prospective study. Ann Surg 215:218, 1992
102. Ellison EC, Carey LC, Sparks J et al. Early surgical treatment gastrinoma. Am J Med 82:17, 1987
103. Larson C, Skogseid B, Oberg K et al. Multiple endocrine neoplasia type 1 gene maps to chromosome 11 and is lost in insulinoma. Nature 332:85–87, 1988
104. Bale AE. Allelic loss on chromosome 11 in hereditary and sporadic tumors related to familial multiple endocrine neoplasia type 1. Cancer Res 51:1154–1157, 1991
105. Jensen RT, Norton JA. Endocrine tumors of the pancreas. In: Yamada T, Alpers BH, Owyang C et al. Eds. Textbook of gastroenterology. Philadelphia: JB lippincott, 1995:2131
106. Rosch T, Lighdale CJ, Botit JF et al. Localization of pancreatic endocrine tumors by endoscopic ultrasonography. N Engl J Med 326:1721–1726, 1992
107. Doppmann J. Pancreatic endocrine tumors – the search goes on (editorial). New Engl J Med 326:1770–1772, 1992
108. Pasieka JL, McLeod MK, Thompson NW et al. Surgical approach to insulinomas: assessing the need for preoperative localization. Arch Surg 127:442–447, 1992
109. Stacpoole PW. The glucagonoma syndrome: Clinical features, diagnosis, and treatment. Endocrin Rev 2:347, 1981
110. Vinik AI, Strodel WE, Eckhauser FE et al. Somatostatinom Pomas, neurotensinomas. Semin Oncol 14:263–281, 1987
111. Verner JV, Morrison AB. Islet cell tumor and a syndrome refractory watery diarrhea and hypokalemia. Am J Med 25:375, 1958
112. Adrian TE, Uttenthal LO, Williams SJ et al. Secretion pancreatic polppeptide in patients with pancreatic endocrine tumors. N Engl J Medi 315:287–291, 1986
113. Ajani JA, Kavanagh J, Patt Y et al. Roferon and doxorubicin combinations active against advanced islet cell or carcinoid tumors. Proc Am Assoc Cancer Res 30:293, 1989
114. Haller I, Schutt A, Sayal Y et al. Chemotherapy for metastatic carcinoid tumors: An ECOG phase II-III trial (abstract). Proc Am Soc Clin Oncol 9:395, 1990
115. Hahn RG, Cnaan A, Kissinger A et al. A phase II study of DTIC in the treatment of non0resectable islet cell carcinoma: An ECOG treatment protocol (abstract) Proc Am Soc Clin Oncol 9:417, 1990
116. Broder LE, Carter SK. Pancreatic islet cell tumors with streptozotocin. Ann Intern Med 79:108, 1973
117. Moertel CG, Lefkopoulos M, Lipsitz S et al. Streptozocin, doxorubicin, streptozocin-fluorouracil or chlorozotocin in the treatment of advanced islet cell carcinoma. N Engl J Med 326:519–523, 1992
118. Moertel CG, Hahnley JA, Johnsson LA. Streptozocin alone compared with streptozocin plus fluorouracil in the treatment of advanced islet cell carcinoma. N Engl J Med 303:1189, 1980

# Genitourinary Malignancies

# Prostate Cancer

N.J. Vogelzang, C.W. Ryan

## Introduction

Prostate cancer is the most common cancer in American men. Though prostate cancer does affect younger men, it is mostly a disease of the elderly, with a median age at diagnosis of 66 years [1]. Although the 1996 estimated number of new cases of prostate cancer was over 340,000 [2] in 1998 it is estimated that only 174,000 new cases of prostate cancer will be diagnosed in the United States [3] (Table 1). Nonetheless, with nearly 42,000 deaths attributable to the disease, prostate cancer is the second leading cause of cancer death in men. At autopsy, over two thirds of men over 80 have asymptomatic or latent prostate cancer [4]. Older age remains the greatest risk factor for the development of prostate carcinoma with a 70 year old male having an approximately one in eight risk compared to a 50 year old with a one in 100 risk.

The cause of prostate cancer is unknown, though racial, genetic, and dietary factors have been implicated [1]. Approximately 9% of prostate

**Table 1.** Epidemiology of prostate cancer

---

Incidence
  Incidence rapidly rose from 1982 to 1992 with the widespread use of PSA screening and the spring-loaded and ultrasound directed biopsy "gun."
  Incidence was 128,000 new cases in 1982, 341,000 in 1991, but is now predicted to be only 175,000 cases in 1997 in the U.S.A.

Race, age distribution, and predisposition
  African-Americans have the highest "racial" rate in the world.
  Scandinavian countries have the highest "national" rates in the world.
  African rates are poorly defined due to lower life expectancies, but Senegal and Nigeria have the very high "national" rates.
  Carribean islanders of African descent also have very high rates.
  The rate of autopsy detected or true "latent" prostate cancer is identical worldwide. Clinical prostate cancer rates very widely possibly due to detection bias.

---

cancers can be attributed to inherited mutations in prostate cancer susceptibility genes [5]. A major susceptibility locus for prostate cancer has been mapped to chromosome 1q and has been designated HPC1 (hereditary prostate cancer 1) [6]. No research has yet linked aging to mutations of this gene. Recent evidence suggests that a CAG repeat polymorphism in the androgen receptor gene confers risk for prostate cancer, with fewer repeats in the germline associated with an increased likelihood of developing the disease [7].

The increasing (and now decreasing) incidence of prostate cancer can be attributed to wide-spread screening using prostate-specific antigen (PSA). Increasing use of the assay in the late 1980s, coupled with the ease of transrectal prostate biopsies using spring-loaded devices and transrectal ultrasonography caused an explosion in prostate cancer detection peaking in 1991–1993. Increasing public awareness of the disease has also contributed to this rapid growth.

Risk factors for prostrate cancer are:
– African-American race
– One or more first-degree relatives (grandfather, father, son or brother) with the disease
– A PSA level above the age-specific reference range for the respective race (Table 2)
– Age >60

The American Cancer Society recommends annual digital rectal examination (DRE) in combination with PSA testing for prostate cancer scre-

**Table 2.** Age and race as risk factors for prostate cancer: PSA level (95% CI) above the age-specific reference range for Caucasians and African-Americans (from [12])

| Age (years) | Serum PSA concentration (ng/ml) |
|---|---|
| Caucasians | |
| 40–49 | 0.0–2.5 |
| 50–59 | 0.0–3.5 |
| 60–69 | 0.0–4.5 |
| 70–79 | 0.0–6.5 |
| African-Americans | |
| 40–49 | 0.0–2.7 |
| 50–59 | 0.0–4.4 |
| 60–69 | 0.0–6.7 |
| >70 | 0.0–7.7 |

ening beginning at age 50, or at a younger age for African Americans or those with a family history [8]. Retrospective analysis has suggested that biannual PSA testing may be an acceptable screening interval when the initial PSA level is less than 2.0 ng/ml [9]. Families with an altered HPC1 gene exhibit more advanced stage and younger age at diagnosis, thus supporting initiation of annual screening at age 40 in susceptible families [10].

The use of the PSA assay as a screening tool has been the center of much controversy. PSA is a serine protease of the kallikrein family [11] that is found only in prostatic tissue. Increases in prostatic volume, prostatic infarctions, ejaculation and other nonspecific factors lead to PSA elevation as men age, even in the absence of malignancy. The low specificity of the PSA test can lead to unnecessary work-ups for men with false-positive results. Conversely, 20% of prostate cancers are diagnosed in men with low PSAs (< 4 ng/ml). The normal range that is in common use, regardless of age, is 0–4.0 ng/ml. Some investigators have recommended the institution of age-specific reference ranges, with higher levels of PSA accepted as normal for older patients (Table 2) [12, 13].

The use of PSA density (amount of PSA per unit volume of prostate gland, as determined by transrectal ultrasound) and PSA velocity (prostate cancer causes a more rapid increase in PSA over time) have been investigated as methods to increase screening specificity but neither refinement has proven useful [14, 15]. PSA complexed with alpha-1-antichymotrypsin bound-PSA is the form preferentially elevated in prostate carcinoma, and the combined measurements of free (non-bound) PSA with total PSA may increase the positive predictive value of the test [16]. Before employing the PSA assay to screen a patient for prostate cancer, discussion with the patient should be undertaken to explain the nature of the test and the implications and consequences of the potential results. Some investigators have concluded that PSA screening may be highly cost-effective, costing less than $5,000 per year of life saved, which compares well to the cost of other cancer-screening practices, such as the $50,000 per year of life saved with mammography [17].

PSA is most commonly used to measure response to therapy. PSA values should drop to undetectable levels after radical prostatectomy for localized disease [18]. Detectable and rising PSA levels after surgery (so-called biochemical failure) may indicate residual local disease or distant metastases. Increasing PSA levels after treatment of metastatic disease is usually the earliest sign of relapse. Likewise, a decreasing PSA during treatment of metastatic disease can be used as a response marker and may be indicative of improved survival [19]. Acid phosphatase level is another serum marker that was formerly most useful for detecting extra-capsular disease in untreated patients, and is helpful in determining which patients may benefit from surgery.

Prostate cancer usually causes few clinical symptoms in its early sta-ges. As prostate cancer progresses, symptoms of urinary obstruction may occur, including hesitancy, weakness of stream, postvoid dribbling, incomplete voiding, nocturia and occasionally hematospermia. Pain

**Table 3.** Prostate cancer staging (from [21])

| | | |
|---|---|---|
| **Primary tumor** | | |
| T0 | No evidence or primary tumor | |
| T1 | Clinically inapparent tumor not palpable nor visible by imaging | |
| | T1a | Incidental tumor in ≤5% of resected tissue |
| | T1b | Incidental tumor in >5% of resected tissue |
| | T1c | Found at time of TRUS* biopsy, prompted by elevated PSA |
| T2 | Organ confined | |
| | T2a | Tumor involves one lobe |
| | T2b | Tumor involves both lobes |
| T3 | Tumor extends through the prostate capsule | |
| | T3a | Extracapsular extension, unilateral or bilateral |
| | T3b | Tumor invades seminal vesicles |
| T4 | Tumor invades bladder neck, external sphincter, rectum, levator muscles and/or pelvic wall | |
| **Lymph nodes** | | |
| N0 | No regional nodes | |
| N1 | Regional node metastasis | |
| **Distant metastasis** | | |
| M0 | No distant metastasis | |
| M1a | Non-regional node metastasis | |
| M1b | Bone metastasis | |
| M1c | Other metastasis | |
| **Staging** | | |
| Stage I | T1a N0 M0, Gleason Score 2–4 | |
| Stage II | T1a N0 M0, Gleason Score ≥5 | |
| | T1b,T1c | |
| | T2 N0 M0 | |
| Stage III | T3 N0 M0 | |
| Stage IV | T4 N0 M0 | |
| | Any T N1 M0 | |
| | Any T any N M1 | |

* TRUS, Transrectal ultrasound.

from bony metastases occurs in late stage disease. Anemia or pancyto-penia may result from bone marrow replacement in very advanced disease.

Staging of prostate cancer was formerly described by the older Whitmore-Jewett classification system, but since 1998 the tumor, node, and metastases (TNM) system has been in widespread clinical use (Table 3) [20, 21]. A typical staging work-up includes measurement of PSA and serum acid phosphatase, chest X-ray, and bone scan (if the PSA is >10 ng/ml). Although, there is a high rate of inaccurate clinical staging, as extracapsular or lymph node spread is often difficult to assess clinically and may not be detected until the time of surgery, PSA levels are increasingly being used as a surrogate staging tool. PSA levels over 20 ng/ml are virtually synonymous with poor-risk disease (Table 4).

The most common histologic grading system in use is the Gleason system. A score of two through 10 is applied, based on the primary and secondary growth patterns of the tumor. The higher the grade, the more undifferentiated the tumor and the less discrete the glandular architecture. Higher grade is associated with a higher rate of local tumor spread and metastasis [22].

Kattan et al. have published a useful nomogram for calculating the probability of disease recurrence following radical prostatectomy based on pre-operative clinical findings and biopsy results (Fig. 1) [23]. The

Table 4. Studies for complete staging and diagnosis of prostate cancer

Obligatory studies
A. A complete history and physical examination including diagram of clinical T stage of primary tumor.
B. Baseline PSA within one to two weeks of definitive local therapy.
C. A histologic diagnosis of cancer must be available before proceeding with definitive local therapy (either surgery or radiotherapy).
D. Bone scan/pelvic CT if PSA >10 ng/ml.

Systemic tumor dissemination
A. None if PSA < 10 ng/ml, clinical T stage is T1C or T2a and Gleason score <7. Laboratory/radiographs as required pre-op.
B. If PSA >10 ng/ml, Gleason score >7 or clinical T stage >T2a, perform bone scan, other radiographs (CT scan of abdomen/pelvis, chest radiographs) and serum chemistry screen. Serum prostatic acid phospatase, if elevated, is still useful to predict for nodal/systemic disease.
C. PSA levels >20 ng/ml are predictive of 70%–80% PSA failure rate at four to five years of follow-up. Such levels are also strongly predictive for seminal vesical invasion, extra-capsular disease and positive lymph nodes.

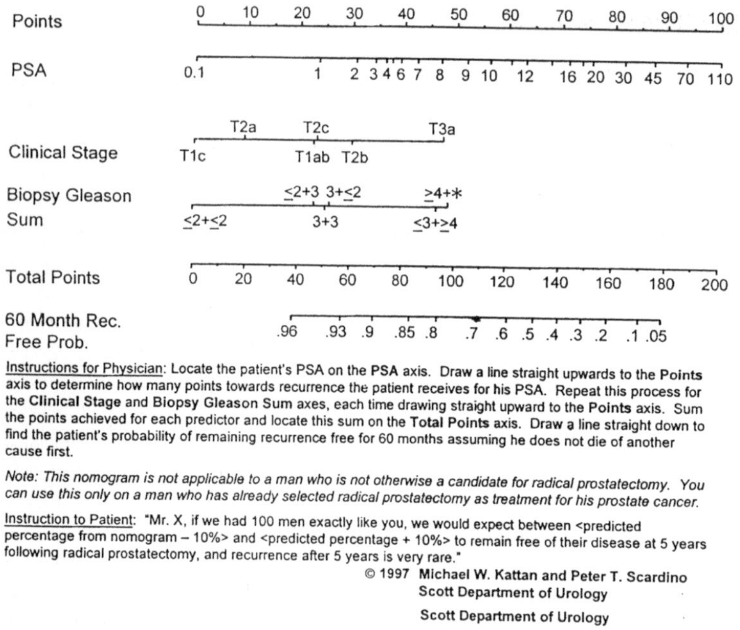

**Fig. 1.** Preoperative nomogram for prostate cancer recurrence. (From [23]) Reprinted from Ref. [23] with permission by Peter T. Scardino, M.D. and Michael W. Kattan, Ph.D.

Copyright 1997, Peter T. Scardino, M.D. and Michael W. Kattan, Ph.D. Patent pending. Nomogram to be used as reference material only and cannot be used for any commercial purposes.

Cancer and Leukemia Group B is developing a set of standardized criteria that can be used prospectively to define poor risk patients using pre-operative PSA values and pathological features of the surgical specimen. Such criteria will be used to prospectively test adjuvant therapy strategies (Table 5).

**Table 5.** Proposed criteria for classifying patients with a high (>50%) risk of PSA failure within 2 years of radical prostatectomy

| |
|---|
| Positive seminal vesicles |
| Gleason 6 and PSA >18 ng/ml |
| Gleason 7 and PSA >14 ng/ml |
| Gleason 8–10 and any PSA |

## Localized Prostate Cancer

Stage I prostate cancer (T1a) is found at the time of transurethral resection of the prostate (TURP) for obstructive symptoms and is defined as a normal gland on DRE with 5% or less of tissue containing well-differentiated adenocarcinoma (Gleason sum less than 5) from the TURP specimen. Stage I prostate cancer is often treated with observation alone, as disease progression is found to occur in only 2% of patients [24]. Such conservative therapy has been challenged, as longer follow-up has shown disease progression in 16% of men followed for at least eight years after diagnosis [25]. Lowe and Listrom found that the probability of disease progression increases with age, and recommend further treatment for patients with a life expectancy of at least five years and have Gleason 4 or greater disease [26]. Though T1a disease is unlikely to progress to clinical significance in the life span of many elderly men, annual PSA and DRE remain necessary.

Among incidentally discovered prostate cancers, Stage II disease includes T1a tumors with a Gleason score of 5 or greater and T1b disease (greater than 5% of tissue containing adenocarcinoma). Radical prostatectomy or radiation therapy is offered, especially to men under 65, as median time to disease progression is four to five years and death from untreated cancer will occur in 50% of untreated patients within 10–15 years [27]. Survival can improve to 70%–90% at 10–15 years with such treatment [28]. Thus, it is important to distinguish these more aggressive cancers from Stage I disease.

Stage T1c was added to the TNM staging system in 1992, and is defined as carcinoma found on needle biopsy performed solely for an elevated PSA with no palpable tumor. These carcinomas have a tendency to be of higher grade and have higher tumor volumes than T1a tumors and clinically behave like T1b tumors. A 93% disease-free survival at eight years has been reported in T1c patients treated with radical prostatectomy [29]. With mass PSA screening there appears to have been a progressive decline in median PSA values at diagnosis of T1c disease since 1992 [30].

Among clinically detectable tumors, stage T2a disease is defined as a palpable nodule localized to one lobe of the gland with a normal serum acid phosphatase. Radical prostatectomy or radiotherapy have nearly the same efficacy with a 50%–60% survival at 10 years, though some evidence indicates a higher recurrence rate with radiotherapy [31]. Interestingly, Alexander et al., noted that older patients with clinical stage T2 disease had a higher pathological stage and grade at radical prostatectomy, possibly due to masking of prostatic induration by benign glandular hypertrophy [32]. Stage T2b disease is defined as a palpable nodule involving both lobes of the gland. The lateral sulcus is not obliterated. Pathologic distinction between T2a and T2b disease is difficult since the pathologic specimen commonly shows diffuse malignancy throughout the gland. Molecular micro-dissection studies have demonstrated multi focal carcinoma within the majority of glands.

The management of clinically localized prostate cancer is challenging. Without PSA substaging, nearly half of patients thought to have organ-confined disease are found to have cancer spread beyond the prostate at the time of radical prostatectomy [33]. With PSA-driven substaging there is an increasing risk of non-organ confined disease with each incremental increase in the PSA above 4.0 ng/ml. For example, with PSA levels over 10 ng/ml, about 50% of patients have non-organ-confined disease. The use of PSA testing combined with clinical stage and Gleason score can help predict the likelihood of lymph node spread, and thus stratify those patients who are more likely to achieve cure from radical prostatectomy [34].

The efficacy of radical prostatectomy versus external beam radiotherapy in the management of localized prostate cancer has been a controversial topic for many years. The only randomized trial to date indicated an advantage for radical prostatectomy, but the study was small and not controlled for pre-treatment PSA values [31]. During the last five years, the concept of PSA or biochemical failure as a surrogate endpoint for survival has been used to compare radiation with surgery. Biochemical failure is defined as detectable levels of PSA (usually >0.2 ng/ml) after radical prostatectomy or a rising PSA on two to three consecutive occasions following a radiotherapy-induced nadir (usually < 1.0 ng/ml). Pretreatment PSA and Gleason score are used to stratify patients and "level the playing field" when comparing surgery to radiotherapy. Although some series suggest that radical prostatectomy offers improved biochemical relapse free survival compared to radiation therapy, [35] that position is highly controversial. For example, Lattanzi et al., estimate that a PSA of less than 8.0 ng/ml is the level at which the majority of patients can obtain long-term biochemical relapse free control with radiation [36]. A study of surgically staged cases of node negative, localized prostate cancer revealed that although biochemical "cure" was less commonly achieved with radiation therapy than with surgery, cause specific survival at 10 years still exceeded 80% [37]. In summary, we believe that radiotherapy or surgery for prostate cancer, as they are for breast cancer, are equivalent modalities when stratified by pre-treatment PSA and Gleason scores.

Elderly men are often given the option of watchful waiting in the case of clinically localized disease and several studies have shown that this is a reasonable approach. The Veterans Administration Cooperative Urological Research Group (VACURG) was unable to show a survival benefit in patients with localized disease undergoing radical prostatectomy compared to observation alone, but this study lacked statistical power [38]. The study did conclude that localized prostate cancer in patients greater than 70 years of age with a low Gleason score (less than 7) is unlikely to decrease that patient's life expectancy if no initial treatment is instituted. A non-randomized observational study by Albertsen et al., suggested that observation alone may be appropriate in older men who have low-volume, low-grade disease [39]. The study retrospectively examined men aged 65–75 years who were treated with observation or hormonal therapy alone. Men with low grade (Gleason 2–4) cancer showed no loss of life expectancy in comparison to the general population, while men with moderate grade (Gleason 5–7) disease showed up to a four to five year loss of life expectancy, and those with high grade (Gleason 8–10) showed up to six to eight years of loss of life expectancy. In 1993, the Prostate Patient Outcomes Research Team (PORT) published a decision analysis for management of clinically localized prostate cancer that showed little benefit to curative intent therapy in elderly men [40]. The group modeled radiation therapy, radical prostatectomy, and watchful waiting, with the benefit of treatment being a decrease in death or disability from metastatic disease. They determined that there was less than six month improvement in quality-adjusted survival for men between 70 and 75 years who received radiotherapy or radical prostatectomy, and that in men older than 75 years, no benefit from these therapies were seen in comparison to watchful waiting. The methodology of the PORT analysis was criticized by those favoring surgical or radiation treatment, and a repeat decision analysis with updated data suggested benefit for aggressive therapy in men with moderately or poorly differentiated cancers up to age 75 [41, 42]. A prospective trial, the Prostate Cancer Intervention Versus Observation Trial (PIVOT) started in 1994 to compare the effectiveness of radical prostatectomy versus observation in localized prostate cancer and has accrued over 400 out of planned 2100 men [43]. Hopefully, the results of such a study will help to better define appropriate treatment of localized prostate cancer.

The decision between conservative versus aggressive management is an important one, as poorer quality of life has been reported in men undergoing radical prostatectomy or radiation therapy, including significantly worse sexual, urinary, and bowel function [44]. An analysis of radical prostatectomies performed on Medicare patients reported a 1.4% mortality rate for men aged 75–79, and a 4.6% mortality rate in those over 79 years [45]. Besides the risk of perioperative mortality, other long-term complications from surgery include impotence, incontinence, and urethral stricture. A survey of Medicare patients 65 years and older who had undergone radical prostatectomy reported that over 30% of men needed to use pads or clamps for wetness and 60% had absence of partial or full erections [46]. The impairment of post-operative sexual function has been shown to be related to the age of the patient, with older patients faring worse [47, 48]. Several types of treatment are available for post-operative or post-radiation sexual dysfunction, including vacuum devices, pharmacologic injection therapy, and implantation of penile protheses [49].

The complications of radiotherapy include acute toxicity such as diarrhea, cystitis, and fatigue, and late toxicity, including proctitis, urinary incontinence, impotence, and urethral stricture [50]. The incidence of urinary or rectosigmoid sequelae has been reported to be 3% for severe and 7%–10% for moderate complications [51]. Despite these risks, definitive radiation therapy is generally well tolerated if comorbid conditions are absent.

Despite the adverse effects associated with curative-intent therapy, a study of a veteran population indicated that a majority of older patients were willing to accept both impotence and incontinence if there was a chance of at least a 10% five year survival advantage with treatment [52]. Frank discussions need to be undertaken between the physician and patient explaining the risks and benefits of the various treatment options. Other investigational therapies for localized prostate cancer include brachytherapy and cryosurgery [53]. These methods have the potential to be reasonable, well-tolerated alternatives for patients, but a detailed discussion of them is beyond the scope of this chapter.

## Locally Invasive Disease

Stage III and locally invasive Stage IV disease is defined as extension of cancer beyond the capsule of the gland, or involving the seminal vesicles, pelvic side wall, bladder, or rectum. Serum acid phosphatase level is elevated and PSA (not used in formal staging) is often above 20 ng/ml. Surgery, radiation therapy, and hormone therapy may be used singly but most patients receive radiation therapy, which helps to control local symptoms, plus hormonal therapy prior to and during radiation to decrease the amount of tissue to be irradiated and increase symptom-free survival [54, 55]. Though previous studies have not shown a survival advantage, a recent study comparing external radiation alone versus radiation plus hormone ablation with goserelin (a gonadotropin-releasing hormone agonist) showed that combination therapy resulted in an improved five year overall survival of 79% compared to 62% in patients treated with radiation alone [56]. The use of hormonal therapy alone is attractive for some patients and may be a viable choice in men with significant co-morbidity. A currently open international trial is attempting to compare hormonal therapy alone to hormonal therapy plus radiotherapy. Based upon the Pilepich et al., and Bolla et al., data, we currently recommend radiation therapy plus hormonal therapy for one to three years for treatment of stage T3/T4 disease in those men not entering a clinical trial.

## Metastatic Disease

Before the advent of the TNM staging system, metastatic disease was referred to as Stage D and had been divided into Stage D0, defined as an elevated acid phosphatase level without evidence of metastatic disease (probably indicating micrometastatic disease), Stage D1 defined as metastatic disease localized to the pelvic nodes only, and Stage D2 defined as bony metastases. Some clinical trials refer to Stage D3 as hormone-refractory metastatic disease but D3 is not an accepted staging term. Twenty-five to 30% of newly diagnosed prostate cancers in older men are metastatic at the time of diagnosis, but this figure is dropping with the use of PSA screening [57].

The management of node-positive (N1) cancer is controversial. Most patients will eventually die of their disease while a minority survive long periods apparently free of further metastases. Five year survival rates vary from 61%–97%, partly as a function of the number and size of positive nodes [58]. Some advocate aggressive therapy with radical prostatectomy or radiotherapy to control local, symptomatic spread of the disease. External beam radiation as single modality treatment has shown mixed results, with some evidence suggesting a delay in disease progression, but no long-term survival benefit [59, 60]. There is some evidence that radical prostatectomy may show improved local control in comparison to expectant management [58]. There is also evidence that adjuvant hormonal therapy may improve outcome following radical prostatectomy, especially in patients with diploid tumors [61]. Hormonal ablation as sole therapy is frequently used in node-positive disease, but whether treatment should be initiated early or late in the course of metastatic prostate cancer long been debated [62]. Recent data from a British Medical Research Council Phase III trial in over 900 men has suggested an advantage to early initiation of hormonal therapy. A decrease in metastatic complications and cancer-related deaths was seen in those patients who received hormonal treatment immediately at the time of diagnosis of locally advanced or asymptomatic metastatic prostate cancer as compared to those who began treatment when clinical progression occurred [63]. We therefore recommend radiotherapy combined with hormonal therapy for up to three years in patients with advanced local disease (T3/T4) or positive nodes.

Hormone ablation has been the mainstay for distant metastatic disease since Huggins and Hodges documented the palliative effects of castration in 1941 [64]. Options for primary androgen withdrawal include orchiectomy or injection of luteinizing-hormone-releasing hormone (LHRH) agonists. Orchiectomy remains the standard modality by which all other forms of hormonal therapy are measured. Though effective, this procedure can be psychologically detrimental and, like all forms of hormonal therapy, will cause decreased potency and hot flashes. Orchiectomy has the advantage of immediate hormonal control, relatively low cost, and elimination of issues of patient compliance. Despite these advantages, the majority of men choose an LHRH agonist when given a choice between orchiectomy and the LHRH agonist [65]. LHRH agonists have become the most popular form of hormonal therapy, though these expensive agents have similar side effects and are less convenient than orchiectomy. The two analogs in common use in the United States are leuprolide and goserelin, which initially were administered as monthly injections, and now are available as three monthly or four monthly depots. LHRH agonists have been shown to be equally efficacious as orchiectomy [66]. LHRH agonists rapidly bind to all luteinizing hormone (LH) receptors causing an initial surge in LH production followed by down regulation of LH production. The initial LH release and a resultant rise in testosterone will cause a flare of disease activity when treatment is first begun. Because of this, patients with severe vertebral metastases or acute urethral obstruction should not be given LHRH agonists without the co-administration of an antiandrogen during the first few weeks of treatment [67]. Diethylstilbesterol, in spite of being a cheap and non-surgical alternative to surgical castration [64] is associated with excessive cardiovascular complications and has been withdrawn from the market.

Androgen blockade can also be accomplished by administration of antiandrogen agents which competitively block binding of dihydrotestosterone to the androgen receptor. Examples include flutamide, bicalutamide, and nilutamide. These drugs do not have the progestational side effects of the steroidal anti-androgens cyproterone acetate and megesterol acetate nor are they as effective as medical or surgical castration [68]. The antiandrogens have hepatotoxic effects, and monitoring of liver function during the first three to four months is necessary. Past enthusiasm for so-called "total androgen blockade" using a combination of an antiandrogen with orchiectomy or LHRH agonist has been lessened by results of a meta-analysis showing only minor effects [69] and a recent 1300 patient randomized trial comparing orchiectomy to orchiectomy plus flutamide in which the flutamide arm was not superior and was more toxic [70, 71]. The extra cost of such oral treatment may be a drawback in older patients. Flutamide costs $200 to $300 per month and is not covered by Medicare, but is covered by the Veterans Administration [72].

Nearly all patients will eventually progress after initial hormone therapy, with a median time to PSA progression of 15–18 months and clinical progression of 24–36 months. These so called hormone-refractory cancers (HRPC) are particularly difficult to manage. Withdrawal of antiandrogens should be the initial intervention in the management of HRPC, as 15%–25% of patients demonstrate an objective and/or PSA response with this maneuver [73]. Whether anti-androgens should be added after failure of medical or surgical castration is unknown but is widely done [74]. Administration of low-dose glucocorticoids is also an accepted practice that improves pain and can induce both pain and PSA response [75, 76]. Recent evidence indicates that mutations in the androgen-receptor (AR) gene may be a factor in the development of hormone resistance and that responses to withdrawal of antiandrogen therapy may be related to stimulation of the mutated AR by antiandrogens [77].

Cytotoxic chemotherapy plays a major role in the palliation of HRPC [78]. Chemotherapy is surprisingly well tolerated even in elderly patients, although the common occurrence of bone marrow involvement may curtail the use of chemotherapy. A phase III trial of cyclophosphamide versus 5-fluorouracil versus standard treatment demonstrated a survival advantage to chemotherapy [79]. Numerous phase II studies have been performed in patients with hormone refractory prostate cancer, and the following drugs have demonstrated activity; mitoxantrone, [80] doxorubicin, oral cyclophosphamide, and estramustine. The combination of estramustine and vinblastine has shown reproducible activity, with approximately one-third of patients obtaining PSA reduction of greater than 50% [81]. Estramustine in combination with either etoposide, docetaxel, paclitaxel or vinorelbine is as an active regimen [78, 82, 83]. Because of its favorable toxicity profile, mitoxantrone has been investigated as a potential agent for elderly patients and has shown beneficial effects on disease-related symptoms [80]. Two randomized phase III trials have compared mitoxantrone plus a glucocorticoid to a glucocorticoid alone in HRPC [84, 85]. Both trials showed an advantage for mitoxantrone in terms of pain control, improved quality of life, time to tumor progression, and decline in PSA. There was no survival advantage for mitoxantrone in either trial, perhaps due to the widespread use of other drugs as second-line therapy. Additional studies with mitoxantrone are ongoing, including dose-intensive regimens [86]. More effective and less toxic agents need to be developed, but currently chemotherapy should be offered to all patients with HRPC.

The management of bony pain in patients with metastatic disease is an important component of care. The use of narcotic analgesics or nonsteroidal anti-inflammatory agents must be carefully administered, given their propensity to cause side effects in older patients. External beam radiation is an effective modality in controlling individual sites of painful metastasis [87]. Suramin, a drug with unique mechanisms of action benefits 20%–35% of patients with bone pain from HRPC although response rates were confounded (in early trials) by simultaneous withdrawal of flutamide and the activity of coadministered corticosteroids [88, 89]. Radiopharmaceuticals such as strontium-89 and samarium-153 are also effective in pain control of skeletal disease [90, 91]. Some degree of myelosuppression can be expected with both external beam therapy and radiolabeled compounds, which may exacerbate preexisting anemia from marrow infiltration or chronic disease. Administration of bisphsophonates may also be helpful in controlling symptoms from diffuse bony metastases and in treating or preventing osteoporosis which regularly accompanies androgen deprivation therapy [92]. Spinal cord compression and pathologic fractures are two feared complications of bone metastases for which the clinician must retain a high index of suspicion.

**Acknowledgements.** Adapted from "Genitourinary Cancer in the Elderly," in *Cancer in the Elderly,* eds CP Hunter, KA Johnson, HB Muss. Marcel Dekker, New York, 1998, (in press).

# References

1. Oesterling J, Fuks Z, Lee CT, Scher HI. Cancer of the prostate. In: DeVita VT, Jr., Hellman S, Rosenberg SA. Cancer: principles and practice of oncology. Philadelphia: Lippincott-Raven, 1997:1322–1386
2. Parker SL, Tong T, Bolden S, Wingo PA. Cancer Statistics, 1997. CA Cancer J Clin 1997; 47:5–27
3. Wingo PA, Landis S, Ries LAG. An adjustment to the 1997 estimate for new prostate cancer cases. CA Cancer J Clin 1997; 47:239–242
4. Franks LM, Durh MB. Latency and progression in tumors: the natural history of prostate cancer. Lancet 1956; 17:1036–1037
5. Carter BS, Beaty TH, Steinberg GD, Childs B, Walsh PC. Mendelian inheritance of familial prostate cancer. Proc Natl Acad Sci USA 1992; 89:3367–3371
6. Smith JR, Freije D, Carpten JD et al. A genome-wide search reveals a major susceptibility locus for prostate cancer on chromosome 1. Science 1996; 274: 1371–1373
7. Giovannucci E, Stampfer MJ, Krithivas K et al. The CAG repeat within the androgen receptor gene and its relationship to prostate cancer. Proc Natl Acad Sci USA 1997; 94:3320–3323
8. Mettlin C, Jones G, Averette H, Gusberg SB, Murphy GP. Defining and updating the American Cancer Society guidelines for the cancer related check up: prostate and endometrial cancer. CA Cancer J Clin 1993; 43:42–46
9. Carter HB, Epstein JI, Chan DW, Fozard JL, Pearson JD. Recommended prostate-specific antigen testing intervals for the detection of curable prostate cancer. JAMA 1997; 277:1456–1460
10. Gronberg H, Isaacs SD, Smith JR, Carpten JD, Bova GS, Freije D, Xu J, Meyers DA, Collins FS, Trent JM, Walsh PC, Isaacs WB. Characteristics of prostate cancer in families potentially linked to the hereditary prostate cancer (HPC1) locus. JAMA 1997; 278:1251–1255
11. Watt KWK, Lee PJ, M'Timkulu T, Chan WP, Loor R. Human prostate-specific antigen: structural and functional similarity with serine protease. Proc Natl Acad Sci USA 1986; 83:3166–3170
12. Oesterling JE, Jacobsen SJ, Chute CG, Guess HA, Girman CJ, Panser LA, Lieber MM. Serum prostate-specific antigen in a community-based population of healthy men. JAMA 1993; 270:860–864

13. Deantoni EP, Crawford ED, Oesterling JE et al. Age- and race-specific reference ranges for prostate-specific antigen from a large community-based study. Urology 1996; 48:234–239

14. Hostetler RM, Mandel IG, Marshburn J. Prostate cancer screening. Med Clin N America 1996; 80:83–98

15. Carter HB, Pearson JD, Metter EJ, Brant LJ, Chan DW, Andres R, Fozard JL, Walsh PC. Longitudinal evaluation of prostate-specific antigen levels in men with and without prostate disease. JAMA 1992; 267:2215–2220

16. Woodrum DL, Brawer MK, Partin AW, Catalona WJ, Southwick PC. Interpretation of free prostate specific antigen clinical research for detection of prostate cancer. J Urol 1998; 159:5–12

17. Benoit RM, Naslund MJ. The economics of prostate cancer screening. Oncology 1997; 11:1533–1543

18. Stamey TA, Yang N, Hay AR, McNeal JE, Freiha FS, Redwine E. Prostate-specific antigen as a serum marker for adenocarcinoma of the prostate. N Engl J Med 1987; 317:909–916

19. Kelly WK, Scher HI, Mazumdar M, Vlamis V, Schwartz M, Fossa SD. Prostate-specific antigen as a measure of disease outcome in hormone-refractory prostatic cancer. J Clin Oncol 1993; 11:607–615

20. Whitmore WF Jr. Natural history and staging of prostate cancer. Urol Clin N Amer 1984; 11:205–220

21. American Joint Committee on Cancer: Prostate, in Fleming ID, Cooper JS, Henson DE et al. (eds): Manual for staging of cancer, 5th ed. Philadelphia: Lippincott, 1997:219–222

22. Gleason DF. Histologic grading of prostate cancer: a perspective. Hum Pathol 1992; 23:273–279

23. Kattan MW, Eastham JA, Stapleton AMF, Wheeler TM, Scardino PT. A preoperative nomogram for disease recurrence following radical prostatectomy for prostate cancer. J Natl Cancer Inst 1998, 90:766–771

24. Cantrell BB, DeKlerk DP, Eggleston JC, Boitnott JK, Walsh PC. Pathological factors that influence prognosis in stage A prostatic cancer: the influence of extent versus grade. J Urol 1981; 125:516–520

25. Epstein JI, Paull G, Eggleston JC, Walsh PC. Prognosis of untreated stage A1 prostatic carcinoma: a study of 94 cases with extended follow up. J Urol 1986; 136:837–839

26. Lowe BA, Listrom MB. Incidental carcinoma of the prostate: an analysis of the predictors of progression. J Urol 1988; 140:1340–1344

27. Brockstein BE, Vogelzang NJ. Chemotherapy of genitourinary cancers. In: The chemotherapy source book. Baltimore: Williams and Wilkins, 1996:1215–1251

28. Elder JS, Gibbons RP, Correa RJ Jr., Brannen GE. Efficacy of radical prostatectomy for stage A2 carcinoma of the prostate. Cancer 1985; 56:2151–2154

29. Epstein JI, Walsh PC, Carmichael M, Brendler CB. Pathologic and clinical findings to predict tumor extent of nonpalpable (stage T1c) prostate cancer. JAMA 1994; 271:368–374

30. Carter HB, Sauvageot J, Walsh PC, Epstein JI. Prospective evaluation of men with stage T1c adenocarcinoma of the prostate. J Urol 1997; 157:2206–2209

31. Paulson DF, Lin GH, Hinshaw W, Stephani S, and the Uro-Oncology Research Group. Radical surgery versus radiotherapy for adenocarcinoma of the prostate. J Urol 1982; 128:502–504

32. Alexander RB, Maguire MG, Epstein JI, Walsh PC. Pathological stage is higher in older men with clinical stage B1 adenocarcinoma of the prostate. J Urol 1989; 141:880–882

33. Garnick MB, Fair WR. Prostate cancer: emerging concepts. Part I. Ann Intern Med 1996; 125:119–125

34. Partin AW, Kattan MW, Subong ENP, Walsh PC, Wojno KJ, Oesterling JE, Scardino PT, Pearson JD. Combination of prostate-specific antigen, clinical stage, and Gleason score to predict pathological stage of localized prostate cancer. JAMA 1997; 277:1445–1451

35. Kupelian P, Katcher J, Levin H et al. External beam radiotherapy versus radical prostatectomy for clinical stage T1–2 prostate cancer: therapeutic implications of stratification by pretreatment PSA levels and biopsy Gleason scores. Cancer J Sci Am 1997; 3:78–87

36. Lattanzi JP, Hanlon AL, Hanks GE. Early stage prostate cancer treated with radiation therapy: stratifying an intermediate risk group. Int J Radiation Oncology Biol Phys 1997; 38:569–573

37. Powell CR, Huisman TK, Riffenburgh RH et al. Outcome for surgically staged localized prostate cancer treated with external beam radiation therapy. J Urol 1997; 157:1754–1759

38. Graversen PH, Nielsen KT, Gasser TC, Corle DK, Madsen PO. Radical prostatectomy versus expectant primary treatment in stages I and II prostate cancer: a fifteen year follow-up. Urology 1990; 36:493–498

39. Albertsen PC, Fryback DG, Storer BE, Kolon TF, Fine J. Long-term survival among men with conservatively treated localized prostate cancer. JAMA 1995; 274:626–631

40. Fleming C, Wasson JH, Albertsen PC, Barry MJ, Wennberg JE. A decision analysis of alternative treatment strategies for clinically localized prostate cancer. JAMA 1993; 269:2650–2658

41. Beck JR, Kattan MW, Miles BJ. A critique of the decision analysis for clinically localized prostate cancer. J Urol 1994; 152:1894–1899

42. Kattan MW, Cowen ME, Miles BJ et al. Modeling the impact of comorbidity on the decision to treat clinically localized prostate cancer. Med Decis Making 1996; 16:460

43. Wilt TJ, Brawer MK. The prostate cancer intervention versus observation trial: a randomized trial comparing radical prostatectomy versus expectant management for the treatment of clinically localized prostate cancer. J Urol 1994; 152:1910–1914

44. Litwin MS, Leake B, Hays RD, Fink A, Ganz PA, Leake B, Leach GE, Brook RH. Quality-of-life outcomes in men treated for localized prostate cancer. JAMA 1995; 273:129–135

45. Lu-Yao GL, McLerran D, Wasson J, Wennberg JE, for the Prostate Patient Outcomes Research Team. An assessment of radical prostatectomy. JAMA 1993; 269:2633–2636

46. Fowler FJ, Barry MJ, Lu-Yao G, Roman A, Wasson J, Wennberg JE. Patient-reported complications and follow-up treatment after radical prostatectomy. The national Medicare experience: 1988–1990* (updated June 1993). Urology 1993; 42:622–629

47. Quinlan DM, Epstein JI, Carter BS, Walsh PC. Sexual function following radical prostatectomy: influence of preservation of neurovascular bundles. J Urol 1993; 145:998–1002

48. Walsh PC. Retropubic prostatectomy for benign and malignant diseases. In: Marshall FF ed. Operative Urology. Philadelphia: WB Sauanders, 1991; 264–289

49. NIH Consensus Development Panel on Impotence. JAMA 1993; 270:83–90

50. Dreicer R, Cooper CS, Williams RD. Management of prostate and bladder cancer in the elderly. Urol Clin N America 1996; 23:87–97

51. Perez CA, Hanks GE, Leibel SA, Zietman AL, Fuks Z, Lee WR. Localized carcinoma of the prostate (stages T1B, T1 C, T2, and T3) review of management with external beam radiation therapy. Cancer 1993; 72:3156–3173

52. Mazur DJ, Merz JF. Older patients' willingness to trade off urologic adverse outcomes for a better chance at five-year survival in the clinical setting of prostate cancer. J Am Geriatr Soc 1995; 43:979–984

53. Garnick MB, Fair WR. Prostate cancer: emerging concepts. Part II. Ann Int Med 1996; 125:205–212

54. Forman JD, Kumar R, Haas G, Montie J, Porter AT, Mesina CF. Neoadjuvant hormonal downsizing of localized carcinoma of the prostate: effects on the volume of normal tissue irradiation. Cancer Invest 1995; 13:8–15

55. Pilepich MV, Krall JM, Al-Sarraf M, John MJ, Doggett RL, Sause WT, Lawton CA, Abrams RA, Rotman M, Rubin P. Androgen deprivation with radiation therapy compared with radiation therapy alone for locally advanced prostate carcinoma: a randomized comparative trial of the Radiation Therapy Oncology Group. Urology 1995; 45:616–623

56. Bolla M, Gonzalez D, Warde P, Dubois JB, Mirimanoff RO, Storme G, Bernier J, Kuten A, Sternberg C, Gil T, Collette L, Pierart M. Improved survival in patients with locally advanced prostate cancer treated with radiotherapy and goserelin. N Engl J Med 1997; 337:295–300

57. Stephenson RA, Smart CR, Mineau GP, James BC, Janerich DT, Dibble RL. The fall in incidence of prostate cancer: on the down side of a prostate specific antigen induced peak in incidence-data from the Utah Cancer Registry. Cancer 1995; 77:1342–1348

58. Kongrad A, Lai H, Lai S. Survival after radical prostatectomy. JAMA 1997; 278 (1):44–46

59. Smith JA, Haynes TH, Middleton RG. Impact of external irradiation on local symptoms and survival free of disease in patients with pelvic lymph node metastasis from adenocarcinoma of the prostate. J Urol 1984; 131:705–707

60. Paulson DF, Cline WA, Koefoot RB et al. Extended field radiation therapy versus delayed hormonal therapy in node positive prostatic adenocarcinoma. J Urol 1982; 172:935

61. Myers RP, Larson-Keller JJ, Bergstralh EJ, Zincke H, Oesterling JE, Leiber MM. Hormonal treatment at the time of radical retropubic prostatectomy for stage D1 prostate cancer: results of long-term follow up. J Urol 1992; 147:910–915

62. Frose GS, Messing EM. Optimal management of stage D1 prostate cancer. In: Dawson NA, Vogelzang NJ, eds. Prostate Cancer. New York: Wiley-Liss, 1994: 197–213

63. The medical research council prostate cancer working party investigators group. Immediate versus deferred treatment for advanced prostatic cancer: initial results of the medical research council trial. Br J Urol 1997; 79:235–246

64. Huggins C, Hodges CV. Studies on prostatic cancer I: the effect of castration, estrogen and androgen injections on serum phosphatase in metastatic carcinoma of the prostate. Cancer Res 1941; 1:293–297

65. Cassileth BR, Soloway MS, Vogelzang NJ, Schellhammer PS, Seidmon EJ, Hait HI, Kennealey GT. Patient's choice of treatment in stage D prostate cancer. Urology 1989; 33 (Suppl 5):57–62

66. Vogelzang NJ, Chodak G, Soloway MS, Block NL, Schellhammer PH, Smith JA, Caplan RJ, Kennealey GT of the Zoladex Prostate Study Group. Goserelin versus orchiectomy in the treatment of advanced prostate cancer: Final results of a randomized trial. Urology 1995; 46:220–226

67. Thrasher B, Crawford ED. Combined androgen blockade. In: Vogelzang NJ, Scardino PT, Shipley WU, Coffey D, eds. Comprehensive textbook of genitourinary oncology. Baltimore: Williams & Wilkins, 1995:875–884

68. Kolvenbag GJCM, Furr BJA. Bicalutamide ("Casodex") development: from theory to therapy (Review). Can J Scien Am 1997; 3:192–203

69. Prostate Cancer Trialist's Collaborative Group. Maximum androgen blockade in advanced prostate cancer: an overview of 22 randomized trials with 3283 deaths in 5710 patients. Lancet 1995; 346:265–269

70. Eisenberger M, Crawford ED, μleod D, Loehrer P, Wilding G, Blumenstein B. A comparison of bilateral orchiectomy (orch) with or without flutamide in stage D2 prostate cancer (PC) (NCI INT-0105 SWOG/ECOG). Proc Am Soc Clin Oncol 1997, 16 (suppl):2a

71. Monipour CM, Savage M, Lovato L, Troxel A et al. Quality of life (QOL) endpoints in advanced stage prostate cancer: a randomized, double blind study comparing flutamide to placebo in orchiectomized stage D2 prostate patients (pts). Proc Am Soc Clin Oncol 1997, 16 (suppl):53a

72. Matchar DB, McCrory DC, Bennett C. Treatment considerations for persons with metastatic prostate cancer: survival versus out-of-pocket costs. Urology 1997; 49:218–224

73. Scher HI, Kelly WK. Flutamide withdrawal syndrome: its impact on clinical trials in hormone-refractory prostate cancer. J Clin Oncol 1993; 11:1566–1572

74. Small EJ, Vogelzang NJ. Second line hormonal therapy for advanced prostate cancer: a shifting paradigm. J Clin Oncol 1997; 15:382–388

75. Tannock I, Gospodarowicz M, Meakin W, Panzarella T, Stewart L, Rider W. Treatment of metastatic prostate cancer with low-dose prednisone: evaluation of pain and quality of life as pragmatic indices of response. J Clin Oncol 1989; 7:590–597

76. Storlie JA, Buckner JC, Wiseman GA, Burch PA, Hartmann LC, Richardson RL. Prostate specific antigen levels and clinical response to low dose dexamethasone for hormone-refractory metastatic prostate carcinoma. Cancer 1995; 76:96–100

77. Taplin ME, Bubley GJ, Shuster TD, Frantz ME, Spooner AE, Ogata GK, Keir HN, Balk, SP. Mutation of the androgen-receptor gene in metastatic androgen-independent prostate cancer. N Engl J Med 1995; 332:1393–1398

78. Vogelzang NJ, Crawford ED, Zietman A. Current clinical trial design issues in hormone-refractory prostate cancer: Report of a consensus panel. Cancer 1998; 82:2093–2101

79. Scott WW, Gibbons RP, Johnson PE, Prout GR, Schmidt JD, Saroff J, Murphy GD. The continued evaluation of the effects of chemotherapy in patients with advanced carcinoma of the prostate. J Urol 1976; 116:211–213

80. Moore MJ, Osoba D, Murphy K, Tannock IF, Armitage A, Findlay B, Coppin C, Neville A, Venner P, Wilson J. Use of palliative end points to evaluate the effects of mitoxantrone and low-dose prednisone in patients with hormonally resistant prostate cancer. J Clin Oncol 1994; 12:689–694

81. Seidman AD, Scher HI, Petrylak D, Dershaw DD, Curley T. Estramustine and vinblastine: use of prostate specific antigen as a clinical trial end point in hormone refractory prostatic cancer. J Urol 1992; 147:931–934

82. Hudes GR, Nathan F, Khater C, Haas N, Cornfield M, Giantonio B, Greenberg R, Gomella L, Litwin S, Ross E, Roethke S, McAleer C. Phase II trial of 96-hour paclitaxel plus oral estramustine phosphate in metastatic hormone-refractory prostate cancer. J Clin Oncol 1997; 15:3156–3163

83. Pienta KJ, Redman BG, Bandekar RG, Bandekar R, Strawderman M, Cease K, Esper PS, Naik H, Smith DC. A phase II trial of oral estramustine and oral etoposide in hormone refractory prostate cancer. Urology 1997; 50:401–407

84. Tannock IF, Osoba D, Stockler MR, Ernst DS, Neville AJ, Moore MJ, Armitage GR, Wilson JJ, Venner PM, Coppin CM, Murphy KC. Chemotherapy with mitoxantrone plus prednisone or prednisone alone for symptomatic hormone-resistant prostate cancer: a Canadian randomized trial with palliative endpoints. J Clin Oncol 1996; 14:1756–1764

85. Kantoff PW, Conaway M, Winer E, Picus J, Vogelzang NJ. Hydrocortisone (HC) with or without mitoxantrone (M) in patients (pts) with hormone refractory prostate cancer (HRPC): preliminary results from a prospective randomized Cancer and Leukemia Group B study (9182) comparing chemotherapy to best supportive care (abstr). J Clin Oncol 1996; 14:1748

86. Levine EG, Halabi S, Hars V, Rago R, Vogelzang NJ. Preliminary results of CALGB 9680: a phase II trial of high dose mitoxantrone/GM-CSF and low dose steroids in hormone-refractory prostate cancer (HRPC). Proc Am Soc Clin Oncol 1998, 17 (suppl):336a

87. Benson RC, Hasan JM, Jones AG, Schlise S. External beam radiotherapy for palliation of pain from metastatic carcinoma of the prostate. J Urol 1981; 127:69–71

88. Kobayaski K, Vokes EE, Vogelzang NJ, Janisch L, Soliven B, Ratain MJ. A phase I study of suramin (NSC 34936) given by intermittent infusion without adaptive control in patients with advanced cancer. J Clin Oncol 1995; 13:2196–2207

89. Rosen PJ, Mendoza EF, Landaw EM, Mondino B, Graves MC, McBride JH, Turcillo P, deKernion J, Belldegrun A. Suramin in hormone-refractory metastatic prostate cancer: A drug with limited efficacy. J Clin Oncol 1996; 14:1626–1636

90. Porter AT, McEwan AJB, Powe JE, Reid R, μgowan DG, Lukka H, Sathyanarayana JR, Takemchuk VN, Thomas GM, Erlich LE. Results of a randomized phase III trial to evaluate the efficacy of strontium-89 adjuvant to local field external beam irradiation in the management of endocrine resistant prostate cancer. Int J Rad Onc Biol Phys 1993; 25:805–813

91. Serafini AN, Houston SJ, Resche I, Quick DP et al. Palliation of pain associated with metastatic bone cancer using Samarium-153 Lexidronam: a double-blind placebo-controlled clinical trial. J Clin Oncol 1998, 16:1574–1581

92. Purohit OP, Anthony C, Radstone CR, Owen J, Coleman RE. High dose intravenous pamidronate for metastatic bone pain. Br J Cancer 1994; 70:554–558

# Testicular Cancer

J.A. McCaffrey, R.J. Motzer

## Introduction

Testicular germ cell tumors (GCT) serve as a model of a curable cancer. Patient management requires the coordinated efforts of the pathologist, surgeon, and medical oncologist. Modern-day combined-modality therapy cures 70% to 80% of such patients, in contrast to the pre-cisplatin era when most patients with advanced disease died from the disease.

## Epidemiology and Etiology

Most malignant testicular tumors are of germ cell origin. Despite their rarity (1% of all cancers in men), GCT constitute the most common solid tumor malignancy in males between the ages of 15 and 35 (average incidence in this group is 9.0 cases per 100,000 population), [1] and there is evidence that the incidence of this disease in young males is rising [2]. The annual incidence of GCT in the United States is 2.1 cases per 100,000 males (all ages), with 6000 new cases diagnosed each year [3, 4]. In the United States, testicular cancer occurs more commonly in Caucasian men than in other races, [5, 6] and geographic differences exist, with Denmark having one of the highest incidences (6.3/100,000 males) [2].

Although the cause of testicular cancer is not known, several hypotheses have been formulated. Young, postpubertal males with a history of abnormal testicular development or descent have a higher than normal incidence, with cryptorchidism [undescended testis] increasing the risk of testicular cancer 10- to 40-fold [7]. Testicular feminization syndromes increase the risk of cancer in the gonads by 40-fold, [8] whereas Klinefelter's syndrome and hypogonadism are associated with mediastinal rather than with testicular primary sites [9]. Trauma, torsion of the testis, [10] testicular atrophy from mumps orchitis, [11] a familial HLA predisposition, [12, 13] industrial exposure, and exposure to radiation have also been postulated as possible causes of testis cancer, but none are considered definitive.

## Pathology and Staging

Germ cell tumors may be either nonseminomas or seminomas. These may be distinguished histologically and clinically. Nonseminomas are heterogeneous and display a variety of clinical behaviors characterized by early dissemination, usually to the retroperitoneum and lungs, and produce elevated serum levels of either alpha-fetoprotein (AFP) or human chorionic gonadotropin (HCG). Nonseminomas consist of embryonal carcinoma, mature and immature teratoma, choriocarcinoma, and endodermal sinus (yolk sac) tumor, each element appearing alone or in combination with others (mixed GCT). Nonseminomatous GCT may also be associated with seminomatous components, and such tumors are managed for the more aggressive nonseminomatous component. Pure choriocarcinoma is extremely rare, accounting for fewer than one percent of all testicular GCT, [14] and is known for its extraordinarily aggressive metastatic behavior.

Seminoma is the most common histology, representing 40% to 45% of all testicular GCT [15]. Unlike patients with nonseminomas who present at a median age of 25, seminoma affects an older population, with a median age of 35 years. Most patients present with early stage disease, although approximately 15% of patients have nodal metastases [16]. There is a low tendency to metastasize, and this is predominantly via the lymphatic system and rarely hematogenously. When the disease does metastasize beyond the retroperitoneal lymph nodes, metastatic sites include lung and, occasionally, bone. Seminomas are exquisitely radiosensitive and generally have an excellent prognosis [17].

The diagnosis, prognosis, and determination of response to therapy in GCT has been facilitated by the use of serum tumor markers HCG and AFP. The HCG, AFP, or both markers are abnormally elevated in approximately 60% to 70% of patients with advanced GCT [18]. HCG may be elevated in patients with either nonseminomatous GCT or seminoma, but AFP is only elevated in patients with nonseminomatous histologies. Thus, finding an elevated AFP in a patient with a "pure seminoma" indicates that an occult or unrecognized nonseminomatous component is present, and the patient should be treated accordingly. The serum tumor markers are useful in predicting both prognosis and response to surgery and chemotherapy. The serum half-life decline for HCG is about 30 h and that of AFP is five to seven days. The presence of residual disease after surgery or an inadequate response to chemotherapy may be evidenced by failure of AFP and/or HCG to decline by half-life following initiation of therapy [19]. Lactate dehydrogenase (LDH) may be elevated in 50% to 80% of patients with testicular cancer, including some in whom HCG and AFP levels are normal [20]. In patients with advanced disease, the degree of elevation of serum LDH is of prognostic significance [21].

The use of diverse eligibility criteria for allocation to clinical trials (Table 1) and their implications resulted in the formation of the International Germ Cell Tumor Collaborative Group. This group analyzed data from GCT trials in Europe, North America, and Australia to determine independent prognostic factors for use in one classification system [21–27]. This study, performed in over 5000 GCT patients, found that the pre-treatment levels of the LDH, HCG, AFP and the site of the primary tumor, i.e., mediastinal versus testis or retroperitoneal, and the presence of non-pulmonary visceral metastases were independent factors for survival [28–30]. The inclusion of such a large number of patients identified pre-treatment AFP levels as an additional independent factor for survival. Good, intermediate and poor prognosis groups of patients were developed based on their response to chemotherapy (Table 2). This consensus provided uniform eligibility criteria that could be used for all clinical trials in patients with advanced GCT. The allocation of all mediastinal NSGCT to the poor risk category and seminoma patients to only good and intermediate risk subsets support the diverse outcome associated with each of these prognostic factors when modelled by linear regression.

The findings of the International Germ Cell Tumor Consensus Group have been utilized to develop the new testicular cancer staging system for the American Joint Committee on Cancer (AJCC) and the Union Internationale contre le Cancre (UICC). AJCC/UICC staging for GCT is unique in that, for the first time, a serum tumor marker category (S) is used to supplement the prognostic stages defined by anatomy alone, i.e., the new TNMS modification now replaces the older TNM system (Table 3).

**Table 1.** Selected criteria used to assign poor prognosis in clinical trials

Indiana University "advanced disease" [85]
  Category 7: advanced pulmonary metastases
  Mediastinal mass >50% of intrathoracic diameter; or primary mediastinal NSGCT
  >10 pulmonary metastases per lung field
  Pulmonary metastases with largest. >3 cm (±non-palpable retroperitoneal disease)
  Category 8: palpable abdominal mass plus pulmonary metastases
  Category 9: hepatic, osseous, or central nervous system metastases
MSKCC "poor-risk disease" [21]
  All patients with NSGCT of extragonadal origin
  Testicular NSGCT with probability of CR <0.5 calculated by: probability CR=exp
  h/(1 + exp h) where h=8.514–1.973 log (LDH + 1) – 0.530 log (HCG + 1) – 1.111
  TOTMET, and TOTMET=0, 1, or 2 depending on whether there are 0, 1, or 2 or
  more sites of metastases
National Cancer Institute: "poor-prognosis testicular cancer" [87]
  Advanced abdominal disease
  Palpable abdominal disease (>10 cm); or obstructive uropathy; or hepatic involve-
  ment
  Central nervous system involvement
  Advanced lung disease
  Pulmonary or mediastinal mass >5 cm; or 5 metastases per lung field; or pleural
  effusion
  Stage III disease with AFP >2000 ng/ml, or HCG >10,000 mIU/ml
Medical Research Council: second classification of poor prognosis [142]
  Lung metastases (any size) >20 in number
  Brain, liver or bone metastasis
  HCG >10,000 IU/1 or AFP >1000/kU/1
  Mediastinal mass >5 cm
Institut Gustave-Roussy Model [143]
  Testis NSGCT with probability CR <70% where probability CR=exp (h)/(1+exp
  (h)) where h=1.90–0.033 (the square root of AFP) – 0.021 (the square root HCG)
  + 0.033 (HCG)

exp, Exponential; AFP, serum a-fetoprotein; HCG, serum human chorionic gonadotropin; LDH,
serum lactate dehydrogenase level; NSGCT, nonseminomatous germ cell tumor; CR, complete
response.

## Work-up and Staging

The most typical presentation of testicular cancer is a painless swelling
or nodule in one testis, noted incidentally by the patient. This may follow
an episode of trauma to the testis which preceded the swelling and draws
attention to the preexisting tumor. Patients may present with painful
testicular enlargement because of bleeding or infarction in the tumor or
with symptoms of acute epididymitis. Testicular cancer can also present
as back pain secondary to retroperitoneal metastases, which can mimic
the more common, nonspecific musculoskeletal pain [31]. A small pro-

**Table 2.** International Germ Cell Cancer Collaborative Group (IGCCCG) consensus prognostic classification [30]

| Risk | Seminoma | NSGCT |
|------|----------|-------|
| Good | Any marker<br>NPVM absent<br>Any primary site | AFP<1000 ng/ml<br>HCG <5000mIu/ml<br>LDH <1.5xupper limit of normal<br>NPVM absent<br>Primary gonadal or retroperitoneal site |
| Intermediate | Any marker<br>NPVM present<br>Any primary site | AFP 1000–10,000 ng/ml<br>HCG 5000–50,000mIu/ml<br>LDH 1.5–10xupper limit of normal<br>NPVM absent<br>Primary gonadal or retroperitoneal site |
| Poor | Not applicable | AFP >10,000 ng/ml<br>HCG >50,000 mIu/ml<br>LDH >10xupper limit of normal<br>NPVM present<br>Mediastinal primary site |

NSGCT, non-seminomatous germ cell tumor; NPVM, non-pulmonary visceral metastases (e.g., bone, brain, liver); AFP, alpha-fetoprotein; HCG, human chorionic gonadotropin; LDH, lactate dehydrogenase.

**Table 3.** New TNM staging of testis tumors (AJCC)

Primary tumor

| | |
|------|------|
| pTX | Primary tumor cannot be assessed (if no radical orchiectomy has been performed, TX is used) |
| pT0 | No evidence of primary tumor |
| pTis | Intratubular germ cell neoplasia |
| pT1 | Tumor limited to the testis and epididymis and no vascular-lymphatic invasion; tumor may invade into tunica albuginea but not tunica vaginalis |
| pT2 | Tumor limited to the testis and epididymis with vascular-lymphatic invasion or tumor extending through the tunica albuginea with involvement of tunica vaginalis |
| pT3 | Tumor invades the spermatic cord with or without vascular-lymphatic invasion |
| pT4 | Tumor invades the scrotum with or without vascular-lymphatic invasion |

Regional lymph nodes:
clinical involvement

| | |
|------|------|
| NX | Regional lymph nodes cannot be assessed |
| N0 | No regional lymph node metastasis |
| N1 | Lymph node mass 2 cm or less in greatest dimension; or multiple lymph nodes, none more than 2 cm in greatest dimension |

**Table 3.** Continued

| N2 | Lymph node mass more than 2 cm but not more than 5 cm in greatest dimension; or multiple lymph nodes, any one mass more than 2 cm but not more than 5 cm in greatest dimension |
|----|----|
| N3 | Lymph node mass more than 5 cm in greatest dimension |

**Pathologic involvement**

| pN0 | No evidence of tumor in lymph nodes |
|----|----|
| pN1 | Lymph node mass 2 cm or less in greatest dimension and 5 nodes or less positive; none more than 2 cm in greatest dimension |
| pN2 | Lymph node mass more than 2 cm but not more than 5 cm in greatest dimension; more than 5 nodes positive, none more than 5 cm in greatest dimension |
| N3 | Lymph node mass more than 5 cm in greatest dimension |

**Distant metastases**

| M0 | No evidence of distant metastases |
|----|----|
| M1 | Nonregional nodal or pulmonary metastases |
| M2 | Nonpulmonary visceral metastases |

**Serum tumor markers**

| S1 | LDH <1.5xnormal |
|----|----|
| | HCG <5,000 (mIU/ml) |
| | AFP <1,000 (ng/ml) |
| S2 | LDH 1.5–10xnormal |
| | HCG 5,000–50,000 (mIU/ml) |
| | AFP 1,000–10,000 (ng/ml) |
| S3 | LDH >10xnormal |
| | HCG >50,000 (mIU/ml) |
| | AFP >10,000 (ng/ml) |

**Stage grouping**

| | | | | |
|----|----|----|----|----|
| Stage IA | T1 | N0 | M0 | S0 |
| Stage IB | T2 | N0 | M0 | S0 |
| | T3 | N0 | M0 | S0 |
| | T4 | N0 | M0 | S0 |
| Stage IS | Any T | N0 | M0 | Any S |
| Stage IIA | Any T | N1 | M0 | S0 |
| | Any T | N1 | M0 | S1 |
| Stage IIB | Any T | N2 | M0 | S0 |
| | Any T | N2 | M0 | S1 |
| Stage IIC | Any T | N3 | M0 | S0 |
| | Any T | N3 | M0 | S1 |
| Stage IIIA | Any T | Any N | M1 | S0 |
| | Any T | Any N | M1 | S1 |
| Stage IIIB | Any T | Any N | M0 | S2 |
| | Any T | Any N | M1 | S2 |
| Stage IIIC | Any T | Any N | M0 | S3 |
| | Any T | Any N | M1 | S3 |
| | Any T | Any N | M2 | Any S |

portion of patients have gynecomastia as their sole presenting sign as a consequence of an abnormally elevated serum human chorionic gonadotropin level (HCG), and may have associated infertility. Germ cell tumor may arise in extragonadal sites including the mediastinum or, rarely, the pineal gland.

When a patient is found to have a testicular mass on physical examination, a complete work-up for a germ cell neoplasm is necessary. Ultrasonography of the testis demonstrates whether a mass is intratesticular or extratesticular, and may detect an occult neoplastic process in the controlateral testis. Radical inguinal orchiectomy is the indicated surgical procedure. If a malignant tumor is confirmed, the cord and its tunica should be dissected up to the retroperitoneal tissue proximal to the internal ring. A transscrotal biopsy or orchiectomy is not the correct procedure, as this can facilitate tumor metastases to inguinal and scrotal lymph nodes and alter the normal lymphatic drainage of the testis, resulting in a high recurrence rate [32]. Treatment is determined by tumor histology (seminoma vs. nonseminoma) on pathologic evaluation of the specimen and by clinical staging.

A cytogenetic abnormality which is highly specific to GCT has been identified. Most GCT express an isochromosome of the short arm of chromosome 12 [i (12p)] [33, 34]. This isochromosome has been found in seminomas, nonseminomas, and mature teratomas of gonadal and extragonadal primary tumors and in established germ-cell tumor cell lines, and has been shown to aid in the diagnosis of midline tumors of uncertain histogenesis [35].

Clinical staging work-up includes a complete physical examination, chest radiograph (a chest CT scan is required if mediastinal or hilar disease is suspected), CT scan of the abdomen and pelvis and serum tumor marker levels of HCG, AFP, and LDH. Bilateral pedal lymphangiography has been replaced as a diagnostic test by CT scan, although it may be used as an adjunct to CT in evaluating low-stage seminoma where radiation therapy is considered in clinical management. Assignment of patients with advanced disease to good- or poor-risk categories can then be made and treatment selected accordingly.

## Treatment

Early Stage Disease

*Nonseminoma*

Clinical Stage I
In patients with nonseminomatous histologies, it is important to differentiate clinical staging from pathologic staging. Clinical stage is determined by results of all radiographic procedures, blood tests, and physical exam. In contrast, pathologic stage is defined by a surgical procedure, i.e., an inguinal orchiectomy and/or a retroperitoneal lymph node dissection (RPLND). After an orchiectomy is performed for nonseminomatous GCT (NSGCT), if there is no radiographic or biochemical evidence of metastatic disease (clinical stage I), two options of further therapy exist. One is a nerve-sparing RPLND and the second is close observation. The rationale for doing a RPLND is that approximately 20% of clinical stage I patients with normal radiographic studies will have lymph nodes involved by malignancy (pathologic stage II) [36]. The full and bilateral template RPLND involves a more extensive dissection of retroperitoneal nodes, which results in retrograde ejaculation due to damage of the sympathetic ganglia and hypogastric plexus and hence infertility in the vast majority of patients [37, 38]. Therefore, a nerve-sparing RPLND should be performed when RPLND is chosen as a treatment option for clinical stage I GCT, since ejaculatory function is preserved in as many as 90% of patients. In this regard, an adequate dissection is essential.

Observation alone for clinical stage I nonseminomatous GCT patients is an alternative approach to RPLND, and results in a similar survival rate [39–46]. Observation is an option since a minority of patients have GCT at RPLND, and nearly all patients who relapse following surveillance will be cured with systemic chemotherapy. The following criteria must be met for clinical stage I patients to be candidates for observation alone:
– Tumor is confined to the testis (T1)
– Nonseminoma histology
– Absence of vascular or lymphatic invasion in the primary tumor
– Negative staging work-up [normal CT scan of abdomen, chest radiograph, ipsilateral lymphangiogram may be indicated in some patients]
– Normal serum tumor markers or appropriate decline by half-life
– Compliance with close follow-up.

Patients who do not meet the above criteria, e.g., non-compliant, having vascular or lymphatic invasion in the tumor or a more advanced T stage, undergo RPLND [39].

The surveillance schedule should include monthly chest radiographs, AFP, HCG, LDH, and physical exam in the first year and alternating months during the second and third year. CT scans of the abdomen should be done every three months for the first year, and every four months in the second year.

The surveillance study conducted at MSKCC accrued 105 patients [47]. When last reviewed, 78 (74%) of patients have been continuously free of disease for 4.1–16.8 years following orchiectomy, with a median duration of 11.6 years. The median time to relapse in 27 patients (26%) was five months (range 2–24 months). The relapse rate was higher in patients with the presence of vascular or lymphatic invasion in the primary tumor: 60% of 20 patients with vascular or lymphatic invasion relapsed compared with 17% without vascular or lymphatic invasion. It was concluded from this study that surveillance following orchiectomy appears to be a reasonable option in carefully selected patients with clinical stage I (T1) NSGCT of the testis without evidence of vascular invasion in the primary tumor, and those who are reliable for close follow-up. A similar surveillance trial was conducted by the Medical Research Council in 396 patients [41]. The two-year actuarial relapse-free rate was 75% (95% confidence interval, 71% to 79%), and this decreased to only 73% five years after orchiectomy. A multivariate analysis showed venous invasion to be the most important individual variable, giving a high-risk group with a relapse-free rate of 65%. This study confirmed the effectiveness of surveillance as a policy for stage I NSGCT of the testis with a five-year survival rate of 98%. A consensus of studies including the Memorial Sloan-Kettering Cancer Center (MSKCC) study has shown an overall relapse proportion of 30% with observation alone [40–46].

The modified nerve-sparing technique was developed to permit preservation of ejaculatory function as knowledge was gained about the distribution of nodal metastases and about the neuroanatomy of the retroperitoneal sympathetic chain [36]. Investigation of the patterns of nodal spread in 104 patients with pathological stage II NSGCT revealed that the interaortocaval zone just below the left renal vein was the most common site of metastasis in patients with right-sided testicular tumors, followed by the precaval and preaortic nodes [48]. When the primary tumor was in the left testis, the most common areas of spread were the true para-aortic, preaortic, and interaortocaval zones [48]. Surgical modifications were developed which usually preserved ejaculatory function when nerves were prospectively identified [49]. It has been shown that a successful RPLND could be performed with maintenance of normal ejaculatory function in the majority of patients by avoiding injury to the hypogastric plexus (i.e., by limiting dissection of the contralateral side superior to the inferior mesenteric artery) [50]. In a recent series, modified nerve-sparing RPLND preserved ejaculation in 94% patients undergoing such a resection [51]. Patients undergoing this procedure have survivals comparable to those undergoing the classic RPLND.

Pathologic Stage II

In cases with vascular invasion in the primary tumor or if clinical staging suggests low-volume retroperitoneal disease, a RPLND is indicated to resect disease, provide prognostic information, and direct further therapy [52].

Prior to the introduction of cisplatin-based chemotherapy, patients with completely resected stage N2–3 disease were offered either no adjuvant chemotherapy (i.e., therapy given to patients after surgery without clinically detectable disease but at a high risk of recurrence), minimally effective [non-cisplatin-based] chemotherapy, or post-operative radiation therapy [53–59]. The relapse rate for such patients ranged from 20% to 70%, with an average of 50% to 60% shown in most series [57]. It is now evident that two cycles of cisplatin-based chemotherapy almost invariably results in a cure. Only two cycles of adjuvant chemotherapy are recommended, since treatment with four cycles has yielded greater toxicity with an equal survival proportion [60].

It has been shown that the relapse proportion for patients with N1 and N2a disease is only 15%, and hence observation only is indicated [55, 61–63]. An alternative option to cisplatin adjuvant therapy in compliant patients with stage II N2b and N3 disease is close observation with a full three or four cycles of chemotherapy given to patients who relapse. One randomized trial has shown that close surveillance of patients with stage II disease, with chemotherapy reserved for those patients who relapsed (three or four cycles of chemotherapy with or without adjunctive surgery), had a survival rate equivalent to that obtained with the routine use of two cycles of adjuvant chemotherapy. However, it must be noted that only 5% of patients in this trial had extranodal disease, and 51% had N1 and N2a disease [64]. Furthermore, the cisplatin regimens have been modified since the cisplatin, vinblastine, and bleomycin-containing regimens of the 1970s, which resulted in substantial toxicity. Adjuvant programs used today are two cycles of cisplatin and etoposide with or without bleomycin. These are effective and well tolerated.

## Seminoma

Stage I Disease
Inguinal orchiectomy followed by infradiaphragmatic radiation therapy is the standard treatment for stage I seminoma, and cures more than 95% of such patients [65]. Adjuvant radiotherapy to the retroperitoneal lymph nodes, which are involved in approximately 15% of cases, is given to prevent relapse. A dose of 2500 cGy is given over a three-week period of time, and prophylactic mediastinal radiotherapy is not necessary since this is not the site of most recurrences. In general, infradiaphragmatic radiation therapy is well tolerated, and the most frequent long-term sequela are dyspepsia or peptic ulcer disease, reported in about 5% of patients [66]. Usually, there is no associated permanent azoospermia or oligospermia after infradiaphragmatic radiation therapy.

Since observation was shown to be an option for patients with Stage I nonseminoma and because of the high success rate with cisplatin-containing chemotherapy in the setting of advanced disease, surveillance alone has been studied in Stage I seminoma. A surveillance program has been conducted in 113 patients with a median follow-up period of 33 months [67]. The probability of recurrence at one year was 6.2%, at two years 12.1%, and at three years, 14.9% [68]. The majority of relapses occurred in the retroperitoneal region, although occasionally patients demonstrated intrathoracic disease. A second surveillance trial followed 81 stage I seminoma patients for three to 43 months (median 19 months) [69]. Results showed that three patients had relapsed at three, five, and 18 months after orchiectomy with non-bulky retroperitoneal disease. This study has since been extended to 119 patients, and the number of relapses has risen to seven (6%). A third surveillance study followed 274 patients for a median of 30 months and demonstrated similar results: 43 (15.7%) patients relapsed, and the median time to relapse was 12 months (2.5–38.5 months) [70]. In view of the low morbidity associated with infradiaphragmatic radiation therapy, it is the approach for men with clinical stage I seminoma preferred over the surveillance approach.

Non-bulky Stage II

Patients with seminoma having non-bulky retroperitoneal disease (Stage IIA, B; <5 cm in diameter) are treated with radiation therapy to the retroperitoneal lymph nodes with an additional 500–1000 cGy delivered to areas of known nodal disease (i.e., total 3000–3500 cGy). Prophylactic mediastinal and supraclavicular radiation are not necessary for patients with non-bulky Stage II seminoma [65]. This was demonstrated in a trial conducted at the Princess Margaret Hospital, in which 444 patients with seminoma were treated (Stages I, II, and III). Prophylactic mediastinal irradiation was not used for patients with Stage II disease, and none of 40 Stage II patients without palpable abdominal disease recurred in the non-irradiated mediastinum. A greater than 90% survival rate may be achieved in patients with stage II seminoma with infradiaphragmatic radiation therapy alone. Earlier reviews reported a survival rate of 69%, but this included patients with bulky stage II disease who had higher failure rates [71]. A marked difference in relapse-free survival has been documented in patients with stage IIA and IIB (with retroperitoneal masses <5 cm diameter) disease compared with those having bulky stage IIC disease, with the relapse-free survival of the former resembling that of stage I patients [17].

Advanced Disease

*Nonseminoma*

Patients with more advanced stage II and stage III GCT are treated with cisplatin plus etoposide-based combination chemotherapy with surgical resection of all residual disease, and complete remissions (CR defined as complete disappearance of all clinical evidence of tumor for one month) are achieved in 70% to 80% of patients. Unfortunately, 20% to 30% of patients do not achieve a CR, and an additional 4% to 10% of patients relapse after CR and require salvage therapy. Pretreatment characteristics define patients likely to achieve CR, and treatment is directed according to good- or poor-risk category.

Prognostic Factors

Until recently, no universally accepted criteria existed for identifying good- and poor-risk GCT patients. A number of centers in the USA, notably Indiana University (IU) and MSKCC, and in Europe recently defined good- and poor-risk patients using various pretreatment prognostic factors (Table 1) [72]. Previously, no universally accepted risk classification existed. At MSKCC, a mathematical equation was derived via a multivariate analysis based on pretreatment serum levels of HCG and LDH and number of metastatic sites of disease [21]. From this equation, the probability of CR was calculated for each patient. Those with a probability of CR >0.50 were considered "good risk", whereas those having a probability of CR <0.50 were considered "poor risk" [73]. At IU, patients ranged from minimal through advanced disease based on similar criteria. The lack of consensus and the difficulty in comparing clinical trial results based on these differences led to the establishment of the International Germ Cell Cancer Collaborative Group (IGCCCG), which yielded a consensus and, ultimately, a new staging system for the disease. The good- and poor-risk criteria are shown in Table 2, and the new staging system in Table 3.

## Good-Risk Trials
### Optimizing Good-Risk Therapy

Standard cisplatin-containing regimens with or without bleomycin are shown in Table 4. Given an anticipated cure rate greater than 90% in patients identified as good-risk, attempts to reduce toxicity focused on the elimination of bleomycin, reducing the number of cycles of therapy (Table 5) and substituting carboplatin for cisplatin (Table 6).

**Table 4.** Treatment scheme

| Regimen | Agents | Schedule |
|---|---|---|
| Good risk | | |
| EP | Etoposide 100 mg/m$^2$ d1–5 (USA) Cisplatin 20 mg/m$^2$ d1–5 | Repeat every 3 weeks, 4 cycles |
| BEP | Bleomycin 30 mg d1, 8, 15 Etoposide 100 mg/m$^2$ d1–5 Cisplatin 20 mg/m$^2$ d1–5 | Repeat every 3 weeks, 3 cycles |
| Poor risk | | |
| BEP | Bleomycin 30 mg d1, 8, 15 Etoposide 100 mg/m$^2$ d1–5 Cisplatin 20 mg/m$^2$ d1–5 | Repeat every 3 weeks, 4 cycles |

**Table 5.** Randomized trials of bleomycin in good-risk GCT

| Regimen (cycles) | | Accrual | CR (%) | Durable CR (%) | Conclusion |
|---|---|---|---|---|---|
| 1 | $BE_{500}P$ (4) [74] | 96 | 97 | 92 | Equivalent |
|   | $BE_{500}P$ (3) | 88 | 98 | 92 | |
| 2 | VAB-6 (3) [75] | 82 | 96 | 85 | Equivalent |
|   | $E_{500}P$ (4) | 82 | 93 | 82 | |
| 3 | $PVB^a$ [144] | 110 | 87 | – | PV inferior |
|   | $PV^a$ | 108 | 82 | – | |
| 4 | $BE_{500}P$ (3) [145] | 86 | 95 | 86 | $E_{500}P$ (3) inferior |
|   | $E_{500}P$ (3) | 78 | 90 | 70 | |
| 5 | $BE_{360}P$ (4) [78] | 211 | 95 | 93 | $E_{360}P$ (4) inferior |
|   | $E_{360}P$ (4) | 208 | 87 | 90 | |

$BE_{500}P$, bleomycin, etoposide (500 mg/m$^2$), cisplatin; $E_{500}P$, etoposide (500 mg/m$^2$), cisplatin; VAB-6, cyclophosphamide, vinblastine, bleomycin, dactinomycin and cisplatin; $BE_{360}P$, bleomycin, etoposide (360 mg/m$^2$), cisplatin; $E_{360}P$, etoposide (360 mg/m$^2$), cisplatin; PVB, cisplatin, vinblastine, bleomycin; PV: cisplatin, vinblastine.
[a] Two cycles beyond best response

**Table 6.** Randomized trials of carboplatin in good-risk GCT

| Regimen (cycles) | | CR (%) | Durable CR (%) | Conclusion |
|---|---|---|---|---|
| 1 | EP (4) [83] | 90 | 87 | EC inferior |
|   | EC (4) | 88 | 76 | |
| 2 | CEB (4) [84] | 87 | $77^a$ | CEB inferior |
|   | BEP (4) | 94 | $91^a$ | |

EP, Etoposide, cisplatin; EC, etoposide, carboplatin; CEB, carboplatin, etoposide, bleomycin; BEP, bleomycin, etoposide, cisplatin.

[a] Failure-free at 1 year.

## The Role of Bleomycin and Number of Cycles

Using the IU classification system, duration of therapy was examined in 184 good-risk patients in a randomized trial of BE500P (bleomycin, etoposide 500 mg/m2, cisplatin) for either four cycles (12 weeks) or three cycles (9 weeks) [74]. Any clinically evident pulmonary toxicity resulted in the discontinuation of bleomycin. Of the patients randomized to receive three cycles, 86/88 (98%) achieved disease-free status, compared with 93/96 (97%) who received four cycles., Overall disease-free survival was identical (92% for both arms) with minimal follow-up of 12 months. Although toxicity was comparable per course, the shorter duration arm was associated with less overall toxicity. As a result, three cycles of

BE500P is preferable to four cycles due to equivalent efficacy with reduced toxicity and cost.

At MSKCC, etoposide and cisplatin (E500P) were compared in a randomized trial to the five-drug, bleomycin-containing regimen VAB-6 in 164 patients deemed good-risk by MSKCC criteria [75]. Disease-free status was observed in 79/82 (96%) patients receiving VAB-6, and in 76/82 (93%) receiving E500P. Relapse from CR (11% and 12%, respectively) was virtually identical, and no late relapses were observed for E500P patients, with a median follow-up five years in a subsequent analysis. Higher nadir platelet and leucocyte counts, no pulmonary toxicity and less emesis, stomatitis and magnesium wasting were observed in patients receiving E500P. The standard chemotherapy regimen offered to patients with good-risk germ cell cancer seen at MSKCC became four cycles of etoposide and cisplatin, based on these data.

The Eastern Cooperative Oncology Group (ECOG) randomized good-risk (IU criteria) patients to three cycles of either E500P or BE500P, extending the observation in an earlier trial that established the equivalence of three cycles of BE500P over four cycles of BE500P [76]. Disease-free status was achieved in 82/86 (95%) patients assigned to BE500P, and in 78/86 (90%) patients randomized to E500P. Pulmonary toxicity was not reported in either arm. Significant myelosuppression occurred in 57% of patients treated with the bleomycin-containing arm, and in 45% of E500P patients. However, an interim analysis revealed an increased number of adverse events (relapse, persistent or progressive cancer and death) for the two-drug arm, resulting in early termination of the study. Only 60/86 (70%) E500P patients were continuously disease-free compared to 74/86 (86%) BE500P patients. E500P for three cycles was deemed inferior therapy.

The European Organization on Research and Treatment of Cancer (EORTC) randomized over 450 patients to receive four cycles of cisplatin and etoposide (EP) or the combination with bleomycin (BEP) [77, 78]. Good-prognosis patients had serum AFP and HCG levels less than 1000 IU/l and 10,000 IU/l, respectively, with lung and lymph-nodal metastases measuring less than 2 cm and 5 cm respectively [79, 80]. The regimen utilized etoposide in a dose and schedule which differs from the U.S. regimens, resulting in a lower total dose (360 mg/m2 over three days as compared to 500 mg/m2 over five days). Dose attenuations of both cisplatin and etoposide were mandated for leucocytosis and thrombocytopenia. The three-drug regimen of BE360P was significantly superior (p=0.0075) to E360P in inducing complete response to chemotherapy with or without post-chemotherapy surgery, with 189/200 (95%) BE360P patients and 169/195 (87%) E360P patients achieving CR. There was no difference in time to progression or overall survival, at a median follow-up of over seven years. Greater toxicity, including two deaths from pulmonary toxicity, was documented on the bleomycin-containing regimen, and Raynaud's phenomenon was observed only on the BE360P arm. The investigators conclude that four cycles of "European" EP (E360P) are inferior to four cycles of "European" BEP (BE360P).

These data confirm that bleomycin may be omitted in good-risk therapy provided that four cycles are administered and American doses are used (E500P). Three cycles of BE500P are considered to be the therapeutic equivalent of four cycles of E500P. The effect of etoposide dose on European results compared to US trials has been examined using the new IGCCCG criteria. When controlled for prognostic factors, the regimens appear to be therapeutically equivalent. Until prospective comparison determines therapeutic equivalence between the different doses, U.S. investigators continue to advise using etoposide 500 mg/m² [81].

*The Substitution of Cisplatin for Carboplatin*

With the activity of carboplatin observed in a pilot study of chemotherapy-naïve patients, and a toxicity profile superior to cisplatin, a further reduction in toxicity was sought through the replacement of cisplatin by carboplatin. Studies varied in the dose of carboplatin, either using the Calvert formula [82 [(defined area under the curve) or a fixed dose per square meter. Two randomized trials have evaluated the comparison of carboplatin with cisplatin. In a multi-institutional trial through a collaboration of MSKCC and the Southwestern Oncology Group (SWOG), 270 good-risk patients (MSKCC criteria) were randomized to four cycles of etoposide with either carboplatin ([E500C] using body surface area to determine dose) or cisplatin (E500P) [83]. While CR proportions were similar with 121/134 (90%) E500P patients and 115/131 (88%) E500C patients achieving disease-free status, patients receiving E500C experienced an inferior event-free (incomplete response or relapse [13% E500P versus 24% E500C; p=0.02]) and relapse-free (p=0.005) survival after a median follow-up of 22 months.

In a confirmatory randomized trial conducted by MRC/EORTC, similar results were observed. The regimen used bleomycin on day one only (B1) [84]. Four cycles of either B1E360P or CE360B were administered to

598 patients using the Calvert formula to calculate carboplatin dose. Among 268 patients who received B1E360P, 253 (94%) achieved disease-free status compared with 227/260 (87%) CE360B patients. Disease-free survival at one year was 91% and 77%, respectively, confirming the superiority of cisplatin over carboplatin. There were ten deaths on the B1E360P arm compared to 27 on the CE360B arm (p=0.003). These data confirm that conventional-dose carboplatin is inferior to cisplatin in good-risk disease.

Poor-Risk Trials
*Clinical Trials in Poor-Risk Germ Cell Tumors*
In a randomized trial in unselected patients with germ cell tumors performed at Indiana University, cisplatin, vinblastine, and bleomycin was compared with cisplatin, etoposide and bleomycin (BEP) [85]. In the poor-prognosis sub-group (Indiana University criteria), 37 patients were randomized to PVB and 35 to BEP. Sixty-three percent of those patients receiving BEP achieved disease-free status compared with only 38% of patients receiving PVB. The etoposide arm was also associated with less toxicity. As a result of this trial, despite the limitations of sub-group analysis, four cycles of BEP became the "standard" therapy for patients with poor-prognosis GCT.

A number of studies have been performed attempting to improve upon the results with standard BEP, focusing on increased dose intensity (especially of cisplatin), the use of alternate or additional cytotoxic agents, and strategies of alternating or sequencing chemotherapy regimens.

*Randomized Trials*
Pre-clinical models and clinical trials suggest a dose-response relationship for cisplatin [86]. Double-dose cisplatin (200 mg/m2 per cycle) with vinblastine, etoposide and bleomycin was compared to standard-dose PVB (100 mg/m2 per cycle of cisplatin) at the National Cancer Institute [87]. In a small group of patients, there was a higher response rate with the more aggressive therapy, and relapses were less frequent. The results are summarized in Table 7. A number of factors, including the addition of etoposide and the value of an increased dose intensity of cisplatin, may account for the apparent superiority of the more aggressive regimen, but this remains uncertain. The higher-dose regimen was associated with increased toxicity.

**Table 7.** Results of randomized trials in patients with poor-risk germ cell tumors

| Study | Treatment arm | n | Complete response rate (%) | Durable response Rate (%) | Benefit over control arm |
|---|---|---|---|---|---|
| Williams et al [85] | PVB | 37 | 38 | NS | Yes[a] |
|  | PEB | 35 | 63 | NS |  |
| Ozols et al [87] | PVB | 18 | 67 | 39 | Yes |
|  | P (200)VBE | 34 | 88 | 74 |  |
| Nichols et al [88] | PEB | 77 | 73 | 61 | No |
|  | P (200)EB | 76 | 68 | 63 |  |
| Wozniak et al [146] | PVB | 52 | 73 | NS | No[a] |
|  | PEV | 62 | 65 | NS |  |
| DeWit et al [90] | PEB | 118 | 64 | NS | No |
|  | PEB/PVB | 116 | 67 | NS |  |
| Nichols et al [147] | PEB | 141 | 60 | 57 | No |
|  | VIP | 145 | 63 | 56 |  |
| Kaye et al [91] | BEP | 190 | 57 | 60 | No |
|  | BOP/VIP-B | 190 | 54 | 53[b] |  |
| Droz et al [148] | P (200)VBE | 49 | 61 | 59 | No |
|  | P (200)VBE +ABMT | 53 | 41 | 37 |  |

P, cisplatin 100 mg/m$^2$; P (200), cisplatin 200 mg/m$^2$; V, vinblastine; B, bleomycin; E, etoposide; I, ifosfamide; O, vincristine; NS, not stated; EORTC, European Organization for the Research and Treatment of Cancer; NCI, National Cancer Institute; MRC, Medical Research Council; SWOG, South-West Oncology Group; IGR, Institut Gustave-Roussy.

[a]Description of "poor-prognosis" group as a subset analysis of a larger trial
[b]Failure-free at 1 year.

The importance of cisplatin dose intensity was more directly assessed in a clinical trial performed by the South-eastern Cancer Study Group in patients with advanced germ cell cancer (Indiana University criteria). In this study, patients were randomized to receive standard BEP or the same treatment but with double dose cisplatin [88]. One hundred fifty-nine patients entered the study, of which 153 were evaluable for toxicity and response. There was no significant difference between the two groups in relation to response or disease-free survival (Table 7). The high dose arm was again associated with significantly greater toxicity including ototoxicity, neurotoxicity, and myelosuppression. The conclusion of the trial was that increasing the dose of cisplatin above 100 mg/m2 per cycle offered no advantage.

Ifosfamide is one of the few drugs that has shown activity in relapsed GCT. Its inclusion in the VIP regimen of cisplatin, etoposide and ifosfamide demonstrated significant activity in the salvage setting [89]. VIP was compared to BEP in a subsequent study performed by the Eastern Cooperative Oncology Group (ECOG) [147]. The aim of the study was to assess whether ifosfamide, when substituted for bleomycin, was more active in combination therapy. Three hundred and four advanced-stage patients (Indiana University) were randomized between 1987 and 1992. There was no advantage for the ifosfamide-containing arm (Table 7), the VIP arm was more toxic, and therefore PEB was recommended as standard therapy.

The EORTC Genitourinary Tract Cancer Cooperative Group compared four cycles of PEB to four alternating cycles of PEB plus PVB [90]. There was no advantage to the alternating regimen (Table 7). Investigators of the MRC and EORTC developed a novel regimen termed BOP/VIP-B, comprising initial intensive therapy with cisplatin, bleomycin and vincristine followed sequentially by three cycles of a modified VIP-B regimen (etoposide, ifosfamide, cisplatin and bleomycin). Initial results in a large Phase II study were encouraging. However, results of a randomized comparison to a PEB regimen have failed to demonstrate any benefit, but a higher degree of toxicity was seen with BOP/VIP-B (Table 7) [91].

*High-Dose Chemotherapy with Hemopoietic Stem Cell Support*
Reinfusion of autologous hemopoietic stem cells has enabled the administration of much higher doses of myelosuppressive chemotherapy. This technique has been investigated in the last two decades and continues to develop. Recent advances include the use of harvested, mobilized progenitor cells from the peripheral circulation [92]. Technological improvements and increased physician expertise have reduced the morbidity and mortality from this approach. Initial use in patients with GCT has been in the salvage setting where a proportion of patients refractory to conventional chemotherapy achieve prolonged survival [93, 94]. Success in the salvage setting has led to investigation in the initial therapy of patients with a poor prognosis where less toxicity is expected and greater potential for benefit exists.

High-dose, carboplatin-containing chemotherapy investigated as initial treatment for patients with a poor prognosis has generally incorporated carboplatin, etoposide and cyclophosphamide or ifosfamide [95–98]. Two cycles of conventional chemotherapy were used in the treatment of patients at MSKCC. Those with a slower than expected serum tumor marker decline received two cycles of high-dose carboplatin, etoposide, with or without cyclophosphamide. Two sequential studies have demonstrated feasibility, improved survival compared to historical controls, and the fact that more intensive therapy can be given as initial rather than as salvage treatment [96]. A phase III trial is ongoing to assess the role of high-dose therapy further as initial treatment. Patients with intermediate- or poor-risk features (IGCCC criteria) are randomized to receive either four cycles of PEB or two cycles of PEB, plus two cycles of high-dose carboplatin, etoposide, and cyclophosphamide followed by peripheral blood progenitor cell support.

*Seminoma*

Based on the high cure rate achieved with cisplatin-containing chemotherapy and the relative minimal toxicity associated with recently developed regimens, chemotherapy is the treatment of choice for patients with Stage IIC (RP adenopathy >5 cm) and Stage III (distant metastases) disease. In an MSKCC study, 130 of 140 patients (93%) with advanced seminoma treated with platinum-based chemotherapy achieved a favorable response (defined as a CR or PR with negative tumor markers) [99]. The four-cycle regimen of cisplatin plus etoposide was found to be highly effective therapy for seminoma, with less toxicity than that reported with a five-drug regimen that included vinblastine and bleomycin [75]. Of 389 evaluable patients treated, 336 (86%) demonstrated CR to the various chemotherapy regimens, with 315 (81%) achieving durable CR.

While all patients with seminoma are considered "good risk" certain pretreatment patient characteristics which were studied did have prognostic significance. Elevated pretreatment serum HCG and LDH levels were adverse prognostic factors, while an extragonadal primary tumor site was not associated with an adverse prognosis [99]. Prior radiation therapy was associated with an inferior treatment outcome and more severe hematologic toxicity.

Postchemotherapy Surgery

Resection of metastases after chemotherapy is an integral part of therapy. Indications differ according to seminoma and nonseminoma histology.

## Nonseminoma

Following induction chemotherapy, patients are restaged with tumor marker assays and radiographic evaluation of all previous sites of disease. Patients found to have residual radiographic abnormalities and normal tumor marker values require surgical removal of all sites of remaining disease. Possible findings at resection include viable GCT, mature teratoma, and necrotic tissue. One other rarer possibility is malignant transformation of teratoma to a tumor morphology other than GCT, such as an adenocarcinoma or sarcoma [100]. The incidence of necrotic debris, teratoma, or viable GCT is variable, and, in general, necrotic debris and/or fibrosis tissue comprise about 40%, teratoma another 40%, and viable non-teratomatous GCT in the remaining 20% of resection specimens [36]. Surgery defines response, renders a patient free of viable tumor, and dictates further management. Patients with necrotic tissue and those with mature teratoma require no further chemotherapy, but patients with completely excised viable tumor are routinely treated with two more cycles of chemotherapy. Although such adjuvant chemotherapy improves relapse-free survival over that of historical controls, the relapse-free survival is substantially less than that observed in patients with necrotic debris or fibrosis [80, 101–105]. In patients with viable tumor which is not completely resected, salvage chemotherapy is given.

## Seminoma

Controversy exists regarding surgery in seminoma patients with residual radiographic abnormalities [106–110]. The size of residual disease on postchemotherapy radiographic studies has been the usual indicator of whether or not viable seminoma is present [102–110], but some studies have found no correlation between size of residual mass and persistence of tumor. At MSKCC, 104 advanced seminoma patients were studied retrospectively to determine if size of residual mass could predict persistence of viable disease. Seventy-four of 104 (71%) patients with normal biochemical markers and a complete or partial radiographic response after cisplatin-based chemotherapy had a residual mass less than 3 cm. Only two of these 74 patients (3%) had GCT histology at surgery or had subsequent relapse at the assessed site. In contrast, among 30 patients

(29%) who had a mass 3 cm or greater, eight (27%) had persistent semi-noma or teratoma found at surgery. Therefore, patients who have a CR to chemotherapy or have a residual mass <3 cm in size are observed; however justification for resection exists when a residual mass is >3 cm in diameter. If the tumor is unresectable, multiple biopsies of the mass should be performed, and if viable tumor is found, subsequent treatment with salvage chemotherapy is indicated [111].

*Salvage Therapy*

For the 20% to 30% of patients who fail to achieve a durable CR with initial chemotherapy, salvage chemotherapy is required [112]. Effective salvage therapies include conventional-dose regimens with cisplatin, ifosfamide plus either etoposide or vinblastine, or high-dose chemotherapy and autologous bone marrow transplantation (AuBMT).

Conventional-Dose Regimens
Conventional-dose salvage chemotherapy for patients with GCT has been in evolution for the past decade [113]. Etoposide was shown to be an active single agent after failure of standard chemotherapy [114–116]. The combination of cisplatin plus etoposide was the first salvage regimen to achieve durable CR in patients failing cisplatin plus vinblastine-based therapy [117, 118]. Ifosfamide had antitumor activity both as a single agent as well as in combination with cisplatin plus etoposide or vinblastine [119, 120]. Ifosfamide plus cisplatin plus either etoposide (VIP) or vinblastine (VeIP) achieves CR in about 15% of patients as third-line therapy [121–123]. Using the combination of ifosfamide, cisplatin, and vinblastine as first-line salvage therapy in 124 patients, CR was achieved in 56 patients (45%), with 37 patients (30%) currently disease-free [124].

Dose-Intensive Therapy
Curative third-line therapy for patients who relapse or achieve an incomplete response to ifosfamide-based salvage chemotherapy is observed with high-dose chemotherapy consisting of carboplatin and etoposide with or without an oxazophosphorine (ifosfamide or cyclophospha-mide) followed by AuBMT. High-dose therapy results in long-term disease-free survival in 10% to 20% of patients with cisplatin-refractory disease [113, 133].

However, the morbidity and mortality of high-dose chemotherapy and AuBMT in heavily pretreated patients may be formidable, largely due to cumulative hematologic and renal toxicity [113, 125–127]. Early intervention as directed by prognostic factors is preferable, since high-dose chemotherapy is better tolerated by less heavily pretreated patients [125]. Additionally, the use of hematopoietic growth factors such as granulocyte-colony stimulating factor (G-CSF) has reduced hematologic toxicity. The use of high-dose chemotherapy with AuBMT as first- or second-line therapy in relapsed patients is being studied, with the goal of increasing the durable CR rate while minimizing toxicity [134].

Prognostic Factors For Salvage Therapy
The minority of patients achieving durable CR with cisplatin-based salvage therapy and the cumulative toxicity of therapy has prompted the investigation of prognostic factors. Identification of prognostic variables will direct early use of dose-intensive chemotherapy regimens or new investigational agents [112]. Best prior response and extent of disease have been reported to be significant prognostic factors in patients treated with salvage chemotherapy [112, 117, 118, 122]. Studies at MSKCC have demonstrated that a significantly higher response rate for salvage therapy is observed in patients who have had a prior CR to cisplatin chemotherapy compared with those without a previous CR. Patients with a prior incomplete response had a particularly poor prognosis (p=0.00007); only four of 52 (9%) patients were alive (median follow-up, 37 months) compared with 15 of 42 (36%) patients with a prior best response of a CR (median follow-up, 35 months) [112]. In addition, an extragonadal primary site (i.e., mediastinal, retroperitoneal) was found to adversely affect prognosis; none of 14 patients with an extragonadal primary tumor were alive at 60 months after salvage therapy, compared with 14 of 80 (18%) patients with testis primary site, p=0.00001). Other investigators have similarly found that an extragonadal primary site is an adverse prognostic factor for salvage therapy [135–137].

Salvage Surgery
In general, adjunctive surgery is only attempted in patients who have achieved normal serum tumor markers [138]. Patients with rising or persistently elevated markers after four cycles of chemotherapy are considered to have achieved an incomplete response and are treated with salvage chemotherapy. Recently, a highly select group of patients have been

rendered disease-free by resection despite elevated serum tumor markers (AFP, HCG). Thirty-eight of 48 patients (79%) were rendered grossly free of disease, and 29 (60%) obtained a serologic remission. Ten patients (21%) remain continuously disease-free with no postoperative treatment, with a median follow-up of 46 months (range 31–89) [139]. At MSKCC, 15 patients underwent surgical resection of a solitary site of residual disease despite elevated serum tumor markers. These patients had received initial or salvage chemotherapy and were refractory to cisplatin-based treatment. Seven patients remain free of disease; four of 10 patients with a retroperitoneal mass relapsed versus four of five patients with visceral (bone, mediastinum, lung) disease. All five patients with an elevated HCG relapsed versus four of 10 with an elevated AFP. Although the number of patients was small, it appeared that patients with a retroperitoneal mass as the solitary site and/or an elevated AFP are more likely to benefit [140].

New Agents in Cisplatin-Refractory Patients
Further improvement in the cure rate of patients with cisplatin-resistant tumors depends on the identification of new active agents. Recent investigation has shown a 24% major response rate with paclitaxel (Taxol) [141]. As a result, paclitaxel is being studied in combination with other active agents in patients with cisplatin-resistant GCT.

## Conclusions

With the progress made over the past two decades, testicular cancer has become the model of a curable malignancy. Overall, the survival approaches 94%. The identification of prognostic factors for CR has reduced toxicity in good-risk patients. Prognostic factors for salvage therapy have been delineated which enable dose-intensive therapy to be administered earlier potentially increasing the chance for cure. Future investigation will focus on the development of new active agents, defining the role of high dose therapy plus AuBMT in first-line therapy, and tumor biology studies.

**Acknowledgment.** The authors wish to thank Carol Pearce for her review of the manuscript.

# References

1. Miller BA (ed), et al. Cancer Statistics Review: 1973–1989, National Cancer Institute. NIH Publication No. 92–2789, p. XXIV.4, 1992
2. Brown LM, Pottern LM, Hoover RN, et al. Testicular cancer in the United States: Trends in incidence and mortality. Int J Epidemiol 15:164–170, 1986
3. Mostofi FK: Testicular tumors: Epidemiologic, etiologic and pathologic features. Cancer 32:1186–1201, 1973
4. Boring C, Squires T, Tong T: Epidemiology of cancer, 1991. CA Cancer J Clin 41:19–36, 1991
5. Schottenfeld D, Warshauer ME, Sherlock S, et al. The epidemiology of testicular cancer in young adults. Am J Epidemiol 112:232–246, 1980
6. Henderson BE, Ross RK, Pike MC, et al. Epidemiology of testis cancer. In Skinner DG (ed): Urological Cancer, pp 237–250. New York, Grune & Stratton, 1983
7. Karagas MR, Weiss NS, Strader CH, et al. Elevated intrascrotal temperature and the incidence of testicular cancer in noncryptorchid men. Am J Epidemiol 129: 1104–1109, 1989
8. Federman KK: Abnormal Sexual Development: A Genetic and Endocrine Approach to Differential Diagnosis. Philadelphia, WB Saunders Co., 1967
9. Sogge MR, McDonald SD, Cofold PB: The malignant potential of the dysgenetic germ cell in Klinefelter's syndrome. Am J Med 66:515, 1979
10. Chilvers CED: Torsion of the testis: A new risk factor for testicular cancer. Br J Cancer 35:105, 1987
11. Kaufman JJ: Testicular atrophy following mumps-a cause of testis tumour? Br J Urol 35:67, 1963
12. Tollerud DJ: Familial testicular cancer and urogenital developmental anomalies. Cancer 55:1849, 1985
13. Lynch HT: Familial embryonal carcinoma in a cancer-prone kindred. Am J Med 78:891, 1985
14. Ro JY, Dexeus FH, El-Naggar A, et al. Testicular germ cell tumors: clinically relevant pathologic findings. Pathol Annu 26 (Part 2):59–87, 1991
15. Ulbright TM, Roth LM: Recent developments in the pathology of germ cell tumors. Semin Diagn Pathol 4:304–319, 1987
16. Mason MD, Featherstone J, Olliff J, et al. Inguinal iliac lymph node involvement in germ cell tumours of the testis: Implications of radiological investigation and for therapy. Clin Oncol 3:147–150, 1991
17. Ellerbroek NA: Testicular seminoma: A study of 103 cases treated at UCLA. Am J Clin Oncol 11:93, 1988
18. Bajorin DF, Bosl GJ: The use of serum tumor markers in the prognosis and treatment of germ cell tumors. Principles and Practice of Oncology Updates 6 (1):1–11, 1992
19. Toner GJ, Geller NL, Tan C, et al. Serum tumor marker half-life during chemotherapy allows early prediction of complete response and survival in nonseminomatous germ cell tumors. Cancer Res 50:5904–5910, 1990
20. Von Eyben FE, Blaabjerg O, Petersen PH, et al. Serum lactic dehydrogenase 1 as a marker of testicular germ cell tumors. J Urol 140:986–990, 1988
21. Bosl GJ, Geller NL, Cirrincione C, et al. Multivariate analysis of prognostic variables in patients with metastatic testicular cancer. Cancer Res 48:3403–3407, 1983
22. Einhorn LH. Treatment of testicular cancer: a new and improved model. J Clin Oncol 8:1777–1781, 1990
23. Birch R, Williams S, Cone A et al. Prognostic factors for favorable outcome in disseminated germ cell tumors. J Clin Oncol 4:400–407, 1986

24. Einhorn LH. Testicular cancer as a model for a curable neoplasm: The Richard and Hinda Rosenthal Foundation Award Lecture. Cancer Res 41:3275–3280, 1981

25. Stoter G, Sylvester R, Sleijfer DT et al. Multivariate analysis of prognostic factors in patients with disseminated non-seminomatous testicular cancer: results from a European Organization for Research on Treatment of Cancer Multi-institutional Phase III Study. Cancer Res 47:2714–2718, 1987

26. Prognostic factors in advanced non-seminomatous germ-cell testicular tumours: results of a multi-centre study. Report from the Medical Research Council Working Party on Testicular Tumours. Lancet 1:8–11, 1985

27. Levi JA, Thomson D, Sandeman T et al. A prospective study of cisplatin-based combination chemotherapy in advanced germ cell malignancy: role of maintenance and long-term follow-up. J Clin Oncol 6:1154–1160, 1988

28. Stoter G, Sylvester R, for the EORTC Genito-Urinary Tract Cancer Cooperative Group. Prognostic Factors in disseminated non-seminomatous testicular cancer. Proc Am Soc Clin Oncol 13:230, 1994

29. Bajorin DF, Mazumdar M, Motzer RJ et al. Model comparisons predicting germ cell tumor (GCT) response to chemotherapy (Abstract). Proc ASCO 13:232, 1994

30. International Germ Cell Cancer Cooperative Group: International Germ ell Consensus Classification: A prognostic factor-based staging system for metastatic germ cell cancers. J Clin Oncol 15:594–603, 1997

31. Cantwell BMJ: Back pain-a presentation of metastatic testicular germ cell tumours. Lancet 1:262, 1987

32. Pizzocaro G: Transscrotal surgery and prognosis in resected stage I and II nonseminomatous germ cell tumors of testis. Presented in San Francisco at the Annual Meeting of the Societe Internationale d'Urologie, Sept. 5–10, 1982

33. Atkin NB, Baker MC: Specific chromosome change i (12p) in testicular tumors. Lancet 2:1349, 1982

34. Bosl GJ, Dmitrovsky E, Reuter VE, et al. Isochromosome 12: Clinically useful marker for male germ cell tumors. J Natl Cancer Inst 81:1874–1878, 1989

35. Motzer RJ, Rodriquez E, Reuter VE, et al. Genetic analysis as an aid in diagnosis for patients with midline carcinomas of uncertain histologies. J Natl Cancer Instit 83:341–346, 1991

36. Bajorin DF, Herr H, Motzer RJ, et al. Current perspectives on the role of adjunctive surgery in combined modality treatment for patients with germ cell tumors. Sem Oncol 19:148–158, 1992

37. Nijman JM, Schraffordt Koops H, Oldhoff J, et al. Sexual function after surgery and combination chemotherapy in men with disseminated nonseminomatous testicular cancer. J Surg Oncol 38:182–186, 1988

38. Nijman JM, Schraffordt Koops H, Kremer J, et al. Gonadal function after surgery and chemotherapy in men with Stage II and III nonseminomatous testicular tumors. J Clin Oncol 5:651–656, 1987

39. Sogani PC, Whitmore WF, Herr HW, et al. Orchiectomy alone in the treatment of clinical stage I nonseminomatous germ cell tumor of the testis. J Clin Oncol 2:267–270, 1984

40. Sogani PC, Fair WR: Surveillance alone in the treatment of clinical stage I nonseminomatous germ cell tumor of the testis (NSGCT). Semin Urol 6:53–56, 1988

41. Read G, Stenning SP, Cullen MH, et al. Medical Research Council prospective study of surveillance for stage I testicular teratoma. J Clin Oncol 10:1762–1768, 1992

42. Gelderman WA, Koops HS, Sleifer DT, et al. Orchiectomy alone in stage I nonseminomatous testicular germ cell tumors. Cancer 59:578–580, 1987

43. Jewett MAS, Herman JG, Sturgeon JFJ, et al. Expectant therapy for clinical stage A nonseminomatous germ cell testicular cancer? Maybe. World J Urol 2:57–58, 1984

44. Pizzocaro G, Zanoni F, Milania A, et al. Orchiectomy alone in clinical stage I non-seminomatous testis cancer: A critical appraisal. J Clin Oncol 4:35–40, 1986

45. Rorth M, von-der-Masse H, Nielsen ES, et al. Orchiectomy alone versus orchiectomy plus radiotherapy in stage I nonseminomatous testicular cancer: A randomized study by the Danish Testicular Carcinoma Study Group. Int J Androl 10:255–262, 1987

46. Swanson D, Johnson D, von Eschenbach A, et al. Five years experience with orchiectomy (surveillance) for clinical stage I nonseminomatous germ cell testicular tumors. J Urol 137:211 A, 1987 (abstr)

47. Sogani PC, Perrotti M, Herr HW, et al. Clinical stage I testis cancer: longterm outcome of patient surveillance. J Urol 159:855–858, 1998

48. Donohue JP, Zachary JM, Maynard BR: Distribution of nodal metastases in nonseminomatous testis cancer. J Urol 128:315–320, 1982

49. Donohue JP, Foster RS, Rowland RG, et al. Nerve-sparing retroperitoneal lymphadenectomy with preservation of ejaculation. J Urol 144:287–291, 1990

50. Narayan P, Lange PH, Fraley EE: Ejaculation and fertility after retroperitoneal lymph node dissection for testicular cancer. J Urol 127:685–688, 1982

51. Richie JP: Clinical stage I testicular cancer: The role of modified retroperitoneal lymphadenectomy. J Urol 144:1160–1163, 1990

52. Motzer RJ, Bosl GJ: Role of adjuvant chemotherapy in patients with stage II nonseminomatous germ cell tumors. Urol Clin N Amer 20:111–116, 1993

53. Bredael JJ, Vurgin D, Whitmore WF: Selected experience with surgery and combination chemotherapy in the treatment of nonseminomatous testis tumors. J Urol 129:985–988, 1983

54. Jacobs EM, Muggia FM: Testicular cancer: Risk factors and the role of adjuvant chemotherapy. Cancer 45:1782–1790, 1980

55. Javadpour N: Predictors of recurrence in stage II nonseminomatous testicular cancer after lymphadenectomy: Implications for adjuvant chemotherapy. J Urol 134:629, 1984

56. Skinner DG: Nonseminomatous testis tumors: A plan of management based on 96 patients to improve survival in all stages by combined therapeutic modalities. J Urol 115:65–69, 1976

57. Vogelzang NJ, Fraley EE, Lange PH, et al. Stage II nonseminomatous testicular cancer: A 10-year experience. J Clin Oncol 1:171–178, 1983

58. Vugrin D, Whitmore W, Cvitkovic E, et al. Adjuvant combination of vinblastine, actinomycin D, bleomycin and chlorambucil following retroperitoneal lymph node dissection for stage II testis tumor. Cancer 47:840–844, 1981

59. Walsh RC, Kaufman JJ, Coulson WF, et al. Retroperitoneal lymphadenectomy for testicular tumors. JAMA 2:309–312, 1971

60. Weissbach L, Hartlapp JH: Adjuvant chemotherapy of metastatic stage II nonseminomatous testis tumor. J Urol 146:1295–1298, 1991

61. Johnson DE, Bracken RB, Blight EM: Prognosis for pathologic stage I nonseminomatous germ cell tumors of the testis managed by retroperitoneal lymphadenectomy. J Urol 116:63–65, 1976

62. Vugrin D, Whitmore W, Cvitkovic E, et al. Adjuvant combination of vinblastine, actinomycin D, bleomycin and chlorambucil following retroperitoneal lymph node dissection for stage II testis tumor. Cancer 47:840–844, 1981

63. Richie JP, Kantoff PW: Is adjuvant chemotherapy necessary for patients with stage B1 testicular cancer? J Clin Oncol 9:1393–1396, 1991

64. Williams SD, Stablein DM, Einhorn LH: Immediate adjuvant chemotherapy versus observation with treatment at relapse in pathological stage II testicular cancer. N Engl J Med 317:1433–1438, 1987

65. Thomas GM, Rider WD, Dembo AF, et al. Seminoma of the testis: Results of treatment and patterns of failure after radiation therapy. Rad Oncol Biol Phys 8:165–174, 1982

66. Hamilton C, Horwich A, Easton D, et al. Radiotherapy for stage I seminoma testis: Results of treatment and complications. Radiother Oncol 6:115–120, 1986

67. Duchesne GM, Horwich A, Dearnaley DP, et al. Orchiectomy alone for stage I seminoma of the testis. Cancer 65:1115–1118, 1990

68. Horwich A, Dearnaley DP: Treatment of seminoma. Semin Oncol 19:171–180, 1992

69. Thomas GM, Sturgeon JF, Alison R, et al. A study of post-orchiectomy surveillance in stage I testicular seminoma. J Urol 142:313–316, 1989

70. Horwich A: Surveillance for stage I seminoma of the testis. In Horwich A (ed): Testicular Cancer: Investigation and Management. Baltimore, Williams & Wilkins, Chapter 7, pp 109–116, 1991

71. Smith RB: Testicular seminoma. In Skinner DJ (ed): Genitourinary Cancer. Philadelphia, WB Saunders Co., p. 460, 1978

72. Droz JP, Kramar A, Rey A: Prognostic factors in metastatic disease. Sem Onc 19:181–189, 1992

73. Israel A, Bosl GJ, Golbey RB, et al. The results of chemotherapy for extragonadal germ cell tumors in the Cisplatin era: The Memorial Sloan-Kettering Cancer Center experience (1975–1982). J Clin Oncol 3:1073–1078, 1985

74. Einhorn LH, Williams SD, Loehrer PJ et al. Evaluation of optimal duration of chemotherapy in favorable-prognosis disseminated germ cell tumors: a Southeastern Cancer Study Group protocol. J Clin Oncol 7:387–391, 1989

75. Bosl GJ, Geller NL, Bajorin D et al. A randomized trial of etoposide + cisplatin versus vinblastine + bleomycin + cisplatin + cyclophosphamide + dactinomycin in patients with good-prognosis germ cell tumors. J Clin Oncol 6:1231–1238, 1988

76. Osterlind K, Andersen PK. Prognostic factors in small cell lung cancer: multivariate model based on 778 patients treated with chemotherapy with or without radiation. Cancer Res 46:4189–4194, 1986

77. Stoter G, Kaye S, Jones W, et al. Cisplatin (P) and VP16 (E) + bleomycin (B), (BEP) vs. (EP) in good risk patients with disseminated non-seminomatous testicular cancer: a randomized EORTC GU Group study. Onkologie 14S4:17–22, 1991

78. deWit R, Stoter G, Kaye SB, et al. Importance of bleomycin in combination chemotherapy for good-prognosis testicular non-seminoma: a randomized study of the European Organization for Research and Treatment of Cancer Genitourinary tract Cancer Cooperative Group. J Clin Oncol 15:1837–1843, 1997

79. Peckham MJ, Barrett A, Liew KH et al. The treatment of metastatic germ-cell testicular tumours with bleomycin, etoposide and cis-platin (BEP). Br J Cancer 47:613–619, 1983

80. Dearnaley DP, Horwich A, AHern R et al. Combination chemotherapy with bleomycin, etoposide and cisplatin (BEP) for metastatic testicular teratoma: long-term follow-up. Eur J Cancer 27:684–691, 1991

81. Bajorin DF, Bosl GJ: Bleomycin in germ cell tumor therapy: not all regimens are created equal. J Clin Oncol 15:1717–1719, 1997

82. Calvert AH, Newell DR, Gumbrell LA et al. Carboplatin dosage: prospective evaluation of a simple formula based on renal function. [Abstract] J Clin Oncol 7:1748–1756, 1989

83. Bajorin DF, Sarosdy MF, Pfister DG et al. Randomized trial of etoposide and cisplatin versus etoposide and carboplatin in patients with good-risk germ cell tumors: A multi-institutional study. J Clin Oncol 11:598–606, 1993

84. Horwich A, Sleiifer DT, Fossa SD, et al. Randomized trial of bleomycin, etoposide and cisplatin compared with bleomycin, etoposide and carboplatin in good-pro-

gnosis metastatic non-seminomatous germ cell cancer: A multi-institutional Medical Research Council/European Organization for Research and Treatment of Cancer trial. J Clin Oncol 15:1844–1852, 1997

85. Williams SD, Birch R, Einhorn LH, et al. Treatment of disseminated germ-cell tumors with cisplatin, bleomycin, and either vinblastine or etoposide. N Engl J Med 316:1435–1440, 1987

86. Samson MK, Rivkin SE, Jones SE, et al. Dose-response and dose-survival advantage for high versus low-dose cisplatin combined with vinblastine and bleomycin in disseminated testicular cancer. A Southwest Oncology Group study. Cancer 53:1029–1035, 1984

87. Ozols RF, Ihde DC, Linehan WM, et al. A randomized trial of standard chemotherapy versus a high-dose chemotherapy regimen in the treatment of poor prognosis nonseminomatous germ-cell tumors. J Clin Oncol 6:1031–1040, 1988

88. Nichols CR, Williams SD, Loehrer PJ, et al. Randomized study of cisplatin dose intensity in poor-risk germ cell tumors: a Southeastern Cancer Study Group and Southwest Oncology Group protocol. J Clin Oncol 9:1163–1172, 1991

89. Loehrer PJ, Sr., Lauer R, Roth BJ, et al. Salvage therapy in recurrent germ cell cancer: ifosfamide and cisplatin plus either vinblastine or etoposide. Ann Int Med 109:540–546, 1988

90. de Wit R, Stoter G, Sleijfer DT, et al. Four cycles of BEP versus an alternating regime of PVB and BEP in patients with poor-prognosis metastatic testicular non-seminoma; a randomised study of the EORTC Genitourinary Tract Cancer Cooperative Group. Br J Cancer 71:1311–1314, 1995

91. Kaye SB, Mead GM, Fossa S, et al. Intensive induction-sequential chemotherapy with BOP/VIP-B compared with treatment with BEP/EP for poor-prognosis metastatic nonseminomatous germ cell tumor: a randomized Medical Resaerch Council/European Organization for Research and Treatment of Cancer study. Clin Oncol 16:692–701, 1998

92. Kaye SB, Mead GM, Fossa S, et al. An MRC/EORTC randomised trial in poor prognosis metastatic teratoma, comparing BEP with BOP-VIP. Proc Am Soc Clin Oncol 14:246, 1995 (Abstr)

93. Motzer RJ, Mazumdar M, Bosl GJ, et al. High-dose carboplatin, etoposide, and cyclophosphamide for patients with refractory germ cell tumors: treatment results and prognostic factors for survival and toxicity. J Clin Oncol 14:1098–1105, 1996

94. Broun ER, Nichols CR, Turns M, et al. Early salvage therapy for germ cell cancer using high dose chemotherapy with autologous bone marrow support. Cancer 73:1716–1720, 1994

95. Motzer RJ, Mazumdar M, Gulati SC, et al. Phase II trial of high-dose carboplatin and etoposide with autologous bone marrow transplantation in first-line therapy for patients with poor-risk germ cell tumors. J Natl Cancer Inst 85:1828–1835, 1993

96. Motzer RJ, Mazumdar M, Bajorin DF, et al. High-dose carboplatin, etoposide and cyclophosphamide with autologous bone marrow transplantation in first-line therapy for patients with poor-risk germ cell tumors. J Clin Oncol 15:2546–2552, 1997

97. Droz JP, Pico JL, Ghosn M, et al. A phase II trial of early intensive chemotherapy with autologous bone marrow transplantation in the treatment of poor prognosis non seminomatous germ cell tumors. Bull Cancer 79:497–507, 1992

98. Barnett MJ, Coppin CM, Murray N, et al. High-dose chemotherapy and autologous bone marrow transplantation for patients with poor prognosis nonseminomatous germ cell tumours. Br J Cancer 68:594–598, 1993

99. Mencel PJ, Motzer RJ, Mazumdar M, et al. Advanced Seminoma: Treatment results, survival, and prognostic factors in 142 patients. J Clin Oncol 12:120–126, 1994

100. Ahmed T, Bosl GJ, Hajdu SI: Teratoma with malignant transformation in germ cell tumors in men. Cancer 56:860–863, 1985

101. Geller NL, Bosl GJ, Chan EY: Prognostic factors for relapse after complete response in patients with metastatic germ cell tumors. Cancer 63:440–445, 1989

102. Fossa SD, Aass N, Ous S, et al. Histology of tumor residuals following chemotherapy in patients with advanced non-seminomatous testicular cancer. J Urol 142:1239–1242, 1989

103. Tait D, Peckham MJ, Hendry WF, et al. Post-chemotherapy surgery in advanced non-seminomatous germ cell testicular tumors: The significance of histology with particular reference to differentiated (mature) teratoma. Br J Cancer 50:601–609, 1984

104. Jansen RHL, Sylvester R, Sleyfer DT, et al. Long term follow-up of non-seminomatous testicular cancer patients with mature teratoma or carcinoma at post-chemotherapy surgery. Eur J Cancer 27:695–689, 1991

105. Fox EP, Weathers TD, Williams SD, et al. Outcome analysis for patients with persistent nonteratomatous germ cell tumor in postchemotherapy retroperitoneal lymph node dissections. J Clin Oncol 11:1294–1299, 1993

106. Schultz SM, Einhorn LH, Conces DJJ, et al. Management of postchemotherapy residual mass in patients with advanced seminoma: Indiana University experience. J Clin Oncol 7:1497–1503, 1989

107. Motzer RJ, Bosl GJ, Heelan RT, et al. Residual mass: An indication for further therapy in patients with advanced seminoma following systemic chemotherapy. J Clin Oncol 5:1064–1070, 1987

108. Babaian JR, Zagars GK: Testicular seminoma: The M.D. Anderson experience. An analysis of pathological and patient characteristics, and treatment recommendations. J Urol 139:311–314, 1988

109. Peckham MJ, Horwich A, Hendry WF: Advanced seminoma: Treatment with cisplatin-based combination chemotherapy or carboplatin. Br J Urol 52:7–13, 1985

110. Fossa SD, Kullmann G, Lien HH, et al. Chemotherapy of advanced seminoma: Clinical significance of radiological findings before and after treatment. Br J Urol 64:530–534, 1989

111. Puc HS, Heelan R, Mazumdar M, et al. Management of residual mass in advanced seminoma: results and recommendations from the Memorial Sloan-Kettering Cancer Center. J Clin Oncol 14:454–460, 1996

112. Motzer RJ, Geller NL, Tan C-Y, et al. Salvage chemotherapy for patients with germ cell tumor: The Memorial Sloan-Kettering Cancer Center experience (1979–1989). Cancer 67:1305–1310, 1991

113. Motzer RJ, Bosl GJ: High-dose chemotherapy for resistant germ cell tumors: Recent advances and future directions. J Natl Cancer Inst 84:1703–1709, 1992

114. Vogelzang NJ, Raghaven D, Kennedy BJ: VP-16–213 (etoposide): The mandrake root from Issyk-Kul. Am J Med 72:136–144, 1982

115. Cavalli F, Klepp O, Renard J, et al. A phase II study of oral VP-16–213 in nonseminomatous testicular cancer. Eur J Cancer 17:245–249, 1981

116. Fitzharris Em, Kaye SB, Saverymuttu S, et al. VP-16–213 as a single agent in advanced testicular tumors. Eur J Cancer 16:1193–1197, 1980

117. Bosl GJ, Yagoda A, Golbey RB, et al. Role of etoposide-based chemotherapy with refractory or relapsed germ cell tumors. Am J Med 78:423–438, 1985

118. Hainsworth JD, Williams SD, Einhorn LH, et al. Successful treatment of resistant germinal neoplasms with VP-16 and cisplatin: Results of a Southeastern Cancer Study Group Trial. J Clin Oncol 3:666–671, 1985

119. Bremer K, Niederle N, Krischke W, et al. Etoposide and etoposide-ifosfamide therapy for refractory testicular tumors. Cancer Treat Rev 9:79–84, 1982

120. Wheeler BM, Lowhrer PJ, Williams SD, et al. Ifosfamide in refractory male germ cell tumors. J Clin Oncol 4:28–34, 1986

121. Motzer RJ, Cooper K, Geller NL, et al. The role of ifosfamide plus cisplatin-based chemotherapy as salvage therapy for patients with refractory germ cell tumors. Cancer 66:2476–2481, 1990

122. Loehrer PJ Sr, Lauer R, Rother BJ, et al. Salvage therapy in recurrent germ cell cancer: Ifosfamide and cisplatin plus either vinblastine or etoposide. Ann Intern Med 109:540–546, 1988

123. Ghosn M, Droz JP, Theodore C, et al. Salvage chemotherapy in refractory germ cell tumors with etoposide (VP-16) plus ifosfamide plus high-dose cisplatin. Cancer 62:24–27, 1988

124. Einhorn LH, Weathers T, Loehrer P, et al. Second line chemotherapy with vinblastine, ifosfamide, and cisplatin after initial chemotherapy with cisplatin, VP-16 and bleomycin (PVP16B) in disseminated germ cell tumors (GCT): long term follow-up. Proc Amer Soc Clin Oncol 11:196, 1992 (abstr 599)

125. Motzer RJ, Gulati SC, Tong WP, et al. Phase I trial with pharmacokinetic analyses of high-dose carboplatin, etoposide, and cyclophosphamide with autologous bone marrow transplantation in patients with refractory germ cell tumors. Cancer Res 53:3730–3735, 1993

126. Nichols C, Tricot G, Williams S, et al. Dose-intensive chemotherapy in refractory germ cell cancer-a phase I/II trial of high-dose carboplatin and etoposide with autologous bone marrow transplantation. J Clin Oncol 7:932–939, 1989

127. Nichols CR, Andersen J, Lazarus HM, et al. High-dose carboplatin and etoposide with autologous bone marrow transplantation in refractory germ cell cancer: An Eastern Cooperative Oncology Group protocol. J Clin Oncol 10:558–563, 1992

128. Rosti G, Albertazzi L, Salvioni R, et al. High dose chemotherapy with carboplatin, VP 16 + ifosfamide in germ cell tumors: The Italian Experience. Bone Marrow Transplant 7 (suppl 2):94, 1991

129. Broun ER, Nichols CR, Tricot G, et al. High dose carboplatin/VP-16 plus ifosfamide with autologous bone marrow support in the treatment of refractory germ cell tumors. Bone Marrow Transplant 7:53–56, 1991

130. Linkesch W, Krainer M, Wagner A: Phase I/II trial of ultrahigh dose carboplatin, etoposide, cyclophosphamide with ABMT in refractory or relapsed germ cell tumors. Proc Amer Soc Clin Oncol 11:196, 1992, (abstr 600)

131. Lotz JP, Machover D, Malassagne B, et al. Phase I-II study of two consecutive courses of high-dose epipodophyllotoxin, ifosfamide, and carboplatin with autologous bone marrow transplantation for treatment of adult patients with solid tumors. J Clin Oncol 9:1860–1870, 1991

132. Siegert W, Beyer J, Weisbach V, et al. Treatment of relapsed or refractory germ cell tumors with high dose chemotherapy and autologous stem cell rescue. Onkologie 14 (suppl 4):30, 1991.

133. Broun ER, Nichols CR, Kneebone P, et al. Long-term outcome of patients with relapsed and refractory germ cell tumors treated with high-dose chemotherapy and autologous bone marrow rescue. Ann Intern Med 69:550–556, 1992

134. Motzer RJ, Gulati SC, Crown JP, et al. High-dose chemotherapy and autologous bone marrow rescue for patients with refractory germ cell tumors: Early intervention is better tolerated. Cancer 69:550–556, 1992

135. Logothetis CJ, Samuels ML, Selig DE, et al. Chemotherapy of extragonadal germ cell tumors. J Clin Oncol 8:316–325, 1985

136. Nichols CR, Saxman S, Williams SD, et al. Primary mediastinal nonseminomatous germ cell tumors-a modern single institution experience. Cancer 65:1641–1646, 1990

137. Hainsworth JD, Greco A: Extragonadal germ cell tumors and unrecognized germ cell tumors. Sem in Oncol 19:119–127, 1992

138. Brenner J, Vugrin D, Whitmore W: Cytoreductive surgery for advanced nonseminomatous germ cell tumors of the testis. Urology 19:571–575, 1982

139. Murphy B, Breeden E, Donohue J, et al. Surgical salvage of chemorefractory germ cell tumors. J Clin Oncol 11:324–329, 1993

140. Wood DP, Herr HW, Motzer RJ, et al. Surgical resection of solitary metastases after chemotherapy in patients with non-seminomatous germ cell tumors and elevated serum tumor markers. Cancer 70:2354–2357, 1992

141. Hutter HS, Motzer RJ, Schwartz L: Phase II trial of taxol in cisplatin-resistant germ cell tumor patients. Proc Am Soc Clin Oncol 13:232 (abstr #712), 1994

142. Mead GM, Stenning SP, Parkinson MC, et al. The Second Medical Research Council study of prognostic factors in nonseminomatous germ cell tumors. Medical Research Council Testicular Tumour Working Party. J Clin Oncol 10:85–94, 1992

143. Droz JP, Kramar A, Ghosn M, et al. Prognostic factors in advanced nonseminomatous testicular cancer. A multivariate logistic regression analysis. Cancer 62:564–568, 1988

144. Levi JA, Raghavan D, Harvey V et al. The importance of bleomycin in combination chemotherapy for good-prognosis germ cell carcinoma. J Clin Oncol 11:1300–1305, 1993

145. Loehrer P, Elson P, Johnson DH, et al. A randomized trial of cisplatin plus etoposide with or without bleomycin in favorable prognosis disseminated germ cell tumors. (Abstr 540) Proc Am Soc Clin Oncol 10:169, 1991

146. Wozniak AJ, Samson MK, Shah NT, et al. A randomized trial of cisplatin, vinblastine, and bleomycin versus vinblastine, cisplatin, and etoposide in the treatment of advanced germ cell tumors of the testis: a Southwest Oncology Group study. J Clin Oncol 9:70–76, 1991

147. Nichols CR, Loehrer PJ, Einhorn LH, et al. Phase III study of cisplatin, etoposide and bleomycin or etoposide, ifosfamide and cisplatin in advanced stage germ cell tumors: an intergroup trial. Proc Am Soc Clin Oncol 14:239, 1995 (Abstr)

148. Droz JP, Pico JL, Biron P, et al. No evidence of a benefit of early intensified chemotherapy with autologous bone marrow transplantation in first line treatment of poor risk non seminomatous germ cell tumors: preliminary results of a randomized trial. Proc Am Soc Clin Oncol 11:197, 1992 (Abstr)

# Renal Cancer

N.J. Vogelzang, C.W. Ryan

## Epidemiology and Risk Factors

In 1997 it was estimated that 28,800 new cases of renal cell carcinoma (RCC) occurred in the United States, and that 11,300 people died of the disease. Fifty percent of all patients diagnosed with the disease survive beyond 10 years and thus, over 14,000 long-term survivors of the disease are added to the U.S.A. population each year. The population of RCC survivors is difficult to estimate but probably totals over 200,000 patients. These patients have a risk of developing a cancer in the remaining kidney but the risk has been poorly quantified. The major risk factors beyond male gender and age over 60 include cigarette smoking, obesity, hypertension, and a variety of occupational exposures [1, 2]. Patients with chronic renal failure on or off dialysis have a greater than 30 fold excess risk of RCC [3].

Most cases of kidney cancer are random occurrences, but there are several inherited forms. The short arm of chromosome three (3p) is frequently mutated in both sporadic and familial cases of the disease. Familial clear cell kidney cancer is associated with a germline translocation t(3,8) (p14.2;q24.1) and is inherited in an autosominal dominant pattern [4]. Von Hippel-Lindau (VHL) disease is an autosomal dominant syndrome that leads to development of tumors in multiple organs, including angiomas of the central nervous system and retina, hundreds of renal cysts (all of malignant potential), and pheochromocytomas. VHL families with renal cell carcinoma do not have an increased risk of pheochromocytoma. The VHL gene has been mapped to 3p25–26 and is a tumor suppressor gene [5]. Hereditary papillary renal carcinoma is also an autosomal dominant disorder but it involves chromosome 9 [6] rather than the short arm of chromosome 3. The hereditary forms of RCC tend to occur at younger ages, while kidney cancer in older patients is more likely to represent a sporadic occurrence.

RCC has classically been referred to as the "internist's tumor," owing to its variety of systemic signs and symptoms [7]. Though the most frequent manifestations are hematuria, abdominal pain, and palpable mass, these three findings occur together as the "classic triad" in less than 10% of patients [8]. Non-specific symptoms are the usual way by which RCC presents. Such symptoms include anemia, fatigue, weight loss, fever, and night sweats. In men, a varicocele occasionally results from chronic obstruction of the gonadal vein by RCC tumor thrombus in the renal vein at its junction with the renal vein. Rare, but fascinating paraneoplastic syndromes have been associated with RCC, including erythrocytosis, hypercalcemia, amyloidosis, and nonmetastatic hepatic dysfunction (Stauffer's syndrome). Often, renal carcinomas are found incidentally during imaging studies performed for unrelated reasons. Patients with incidental tumors ("incidentalomas") have a better prognosis, as these carcinomas tend to be smaller and more confined than symptomatic cancers [9].

## Pathology and Staging

The most common histological form of RCC is clear cell carcinoma, which comprises 85% of kidney cancers. "Granular cell" RCC and the "sarcomatoid" variant of RCC, which carries a particularly poor prognosis are subsets of clear cell carcinoma. Clear cell carcinomas all arise from proximal renal tubule cells. Oncocytoma and papillary RCC are unusual histological subtypes which tend to have less aggressive clinical courses, the former with nearly 100% survival. Tumors rarely arise from the collecting ducts of the kidney and are called Duct of Bellini carcinomas. Transitional cell carcinomas can arise from the renal pelvis and are radiographically very similar to RCC.

Intravenous pyelography is often the first imaging study ordered by the clinician, prompted by hematuria, physical findings or a suspicion of a kidney stone. This procedure may detect renal masses but lacks sensitivity or specificity. Ultrasonography and CT are the main imaging modalities which should be used to detect and define renal masses. Non-malignant lesions such as cysts and angiomyolipomas have distinguishing characteristics on ultrasound and CT that often eliminate the need for biopsy. For patients with a strong family history of renal carcinoma, it may be warranted to perform screening ultrasounds beginning at age

35–40. If renal cysts are detected they should be imaged every two to five years to monitor for change. Dialysis patients with intact kidneys should be imaged annually and consideration given to prophylactic nephrectomies. Suspicious mass lesions may be sampled with impunity via percutaneous cyst puncture or needle aspiration biopsy under ultrasound or CT guidance.

CT is the most accurate method for preoperative staging, but is limited in its ability to detect minimally enlarged lymph nodes [10]. MRI is superior to CT for evaluating vena caval involvement, and is comparable to inferior venacavography [11]. Renal arteriography is sometimes used in operative planning or to infarct large tumors prior to nephrectomy. Evaluation for metastatic disease should include blood chemistries, a bone scan, and a chest radiograph. Given the speed and sensitivity of

**Table 1.** Stage grouping in RCC

| | |
|---|---|
| **Primary tumor** | |
| T1 | Tumor 7.0 cm or less in greatest dimension limited to the kidney |
| T2 | Tumor more than 7.0 cm in greatest dimension limited to the kidney |
| T3 | Tumor extends into major veins or invades the adrenal gland or perinephric tissues but not beyond Gerota's fascia |
| T3a | Tumor invades the adrenal gland or perinephric tissues but not beyond Gerota's fascia |
| T3b | Tumor grossly extends into the renal vein(s) or vena cava below the diaphragm |
| T3c | Tumor grossly extends into the vena cava above the diaphragm |
| T4 | Tumor invades beyond Gerota's fascia |
| **Regional lymph nodes**[a] | |
| NX | Regional lymph nodes cannot be assessed |
| N0 | No regional lymph node metastasis |
| N1 | Metastasis in a single lymph node |
| N2 | Metastasis in more than one regional lymph node |
| **Stage grouping** | |
| Stage I | T1 N0 M0 |
| Stage II | T2 N0 M0 |
| Stage III | T1 N1 M0 |
| | T2 N1 M0 |
| | T3 N0/N1 M0 |
| Stage IV | T4 N0,N1 M0 |
| | Any T N2 M0 |
| | Any T any N M1 |

[a]Laterality does not affect the N classification.

chest CT imaging, most oncologists recommend this in addition to a chest X-ray.

RCC is staged by either the older Robson [12] or the 1998 revision of the TNM system (Table 1) [13]. Stage is the most important predictor of survival. Stage I patients have a 75% survival at five years, while stage II patients have a 60%–70% survival. Stage IIIA has a 40%–50% five year survival rate, while survival for stage IIIB (node or renal vein involvement) drops to less than 20% at five years. Those patients with stage IV (metastatic) disease have a median survival of less than one year although 2%–3% survive beyond five years [14].

## Work-up and Staging

Table 2 lists the obligatory studies for complete diagnosis and staging.

## Stage Specific Standard Treatment Options

Surgical Treatment (Early Stages)

Surgery is the mainstay of treatment for localized RCC, as this is the only curative therapy available. In 1969, Robson et al. established radical nephrectomy as the gold standard with a reported survival of greater than 60% in stage I and II disease [12]. Radical nephrectomy involves ligation of

**Table 2.** Obligatory studies for a complete diagnostic work-up of RCC

Primary tumor
  Renal function – serum creatinine
  Diagnostic CT scan of chest and abdomen
  MRI of vena cava is selected cases
  No need for pre-nephrectomy histologic diagnosis in the absence of metastatic
    disease
Systemic tumor dissemination
  Complete history and physical examination
  Serum chemistry tests to include liver, bone and renal function plus calcium level
  Abdominal CT to rule out liver or retroperitoneal nodes
  Bone scan
  CT or MRI of the brain in patients with any suspicious history or physical exami-
    nation findings
Tumor Markers
  None currently available although serum calcium can be useful

the renal vessels and en bloc removal of Gerota's fascia and its contents. The adrenal gland is occasionally spared. Removal of tumor thrombus from the inferior vena cava or vena caval resection is required if the tumor extends into this vessel. A tumor thrombus extending into the chest may require cardiopulmonary bypass with hypothermic circulatory arrest. Regional lymphadenectomy is advocated by some because of a few reports of improved survival in patients with nodal metastases alone [15]. Postoperative radiation may be considered in patients with evidence of deep invasion of Gerota's fascia, adjacent organs, or regional lymph nodes. [16, 17] There is no evidence that adjuvant immunotherapy is beneficial in the management of localized RCC [18]. Four randomized controlled trials have been reported. [19–22] Three of them compared control to interferon, or a vaccine, while one compared ex vivo activated lymphocyte therapy (ALT) plus high dose cimetidine to high dose cimetidine alone. Only the ALT trial showed a statistical advantage for treatment in overall survival.

Nephron-sparing surgery (partial nephrectomy) is indicated if there is anatomical or functional absence of the ipsilateral kidney, or in cases of bilateral RCC, which occurs in less than 2% of patients [23]. Relative indications include impaired kidney function from conditions such as calculus disease, renal artery stenosis, hypertension, or diabetes [24]. Nephron-sparing surgery caries an increased risk of local tumor recurrence, but has been shown to be efficacious in properly selected patients with low-stage RCC. Because of similar overall survival as patients undergoing radical nephrectomy, nephron-sparing surgery is being more commonly performed in patients with small tumors and a normal (or near-normal) contralateral kidney [24].

Radiotherapy (Early Stages)

Radiotherapy is not used in early stage disease because of lack of radiation sensitivity and the risk of damage to adjacent tissues, including radiation nephritis.

Chemotherapy (Advanced Stages)

Thirty percent of patients with RCC present with metastatic disease [14]. The most common site of metastasis is the lung, followed by soft tissues, bone, liver, and central nervous system. Median survival of untreated patients is less than one year, and patient age does not seem to affect prognosis [18].

Unfortunately, metastatic RCC is one of the most chemoresistant cancers. No single agent has yet emerged as a standard therapy for RCC. Vinblastine, 5-FU, and floxuridine (FUDR) have been studied the most, but only 5-FU and its metabolite FUDR have demonstrated a 10%–12% activity rate [25]. A recent trial with vinblastine induced no responses in over 60 patients [26]. RCC cells and tumor lines along with normal proximal renal tubule cells have been shown to highly express mRNA for the multidrug resistance gene MDR1 and its product, P-glycoprotein [27]. This may partially explain the tumor's high-level resistance to cytotoxic chemotherapy. In spite of this "drug resistant" phenotype, a clinical trial of 5FU with or without a biochemical modulator, such as leucovorin, hydroxyurea, or gemcitabine, may be indicated in high performance status patients who wish to try systemic therapy after failure of immunotherapy.

## Biological Response Modifiers, Cytokines, Hormone Therapy (Advanced Stage)

Hormonal therapy for RCC has been investigated in the past because of the discovery that RCC expresses progestin, androgen and estrogen receptors. Success with therapy such as megesterol acetate, flutamide, and or estrogen has been seen but in less than 10% of patients [25].

Because of cases of prolonged disease stabilization and spontaneous regression, RCC has been implicated as being susceptible to host immune responses. Thus, the introduction of biologic response modifier therapy in the 1978–82 period with interferons gave new hope to treatment of disseminated RCC [28]. Interferon (IFN) alpha was initially reported to have a 25%–30% response rate, but after many additional trials, the true response rate is probably only 10% [29]. Of some interest was a phase III trial comparing vinblastine alone to vinblastine plus IFN alpha [30]. That trial showed a significant improvement in median survival for the IFN plus vinblastine group (15 months) compared to vinblastine alone (eight months). Another recent trial from England compared oral medroxyprogesterone acetate to IFN alpha therapy and showed a statistically significant survival advantage to IFN [31]. A trial of gamma IFN compared to placebo [32] showed no survival advantage to gamma IFN. Although IFN is not FDA approved for treatment of RCC, it is widely used as a palliative single agent. Motzer et al. have suggested that adding 13-cis-retinoic acid (CRA) to IFN (based upon preclinical synergy data) improves the response rate to nearly 25%–30% [33]. A phase III trial comparing IFN to IFN plus CRA has been completed, but not yet reported.

Interleukin-2 (IL-2) (T cell growth factor) was approved by the FDA in 1992 for treatment of metastatic RCC based on reports of complete and durable tumor responses. Initial studies performed at the National Cancer Institute using high-dose IL-2 and infusions of autologous lymphokine-activated killer (LAK) cells showed response rates of greater than 30%, though subsequent studies have yielded overall response rates of 15%–20% but with about 2%–5% long-term survivors. [34, 35] Additional studies have indicated that LAK cells are not a necessary component of treatment [36]. No clear benefit has been seen with the addition of IFN-alpha to high-dose intravenous IL-2 therapy, [37] although low-dose subcutaneous IFN may be synergistic or additive when added to low-dose subcutaneous IL-2. [38–40]

High-dose IL-2 is usually administered as a dose of 720,000 IU/kg intravenous bolus every eight hours, up to 14 doses per cycle or until toxicity develops. Toxicity is mainly related to increased vascular permeability with septic shock-like hemodynamics frequently encountered [41]. Capillary leak often leads to pulmonary edema and dysfunction that can be similar to that of the adult respiratory distress syndrome. Cardiac toxicity can be life-threatening, including myocardial ischemia, infarction, and arrhythmias. Oliguria and renal failure can occur and are thought to be pre-renal in origin. Mental status changes range from confusion to obtundation and may continue to progress for several days after IL-2 is discontinued. Thrombocytopenia and anemia are among the hematologic effects of therapy. Obviously, the use of high-dose IL-2 is restricted to healthy, relatively young patients. Normal cardiac, pulmonary, and renal function are prerequisite to treatment, and evaluation of potential candidates should include cardiac stress-testing for patients older than 50 years.

Low-dose IL-2 has been advocated by some as alternative to high-dose IL-2. In animal models prolonged low-dose IL-2 can cause excellent tumor regression. While side effects are not as severe as with high-dose therapy, fatigue, fluid-retention, azotemia, and anemia are still common.

A randomized trial of high-vs. low-dose IL-2 has shown no differences in survival between the two groups [42]. Outpatient-based IL-2 therapy using subcutaneous injections with or without IFN-alpha has been investigated in a large number of phase I and II studies [38]. Response rates seem comparable to high-dose therapy, but randomized trials are still under way. We recommend low-dose IFN and IL-2 to virtually all patients, regardless of age. IL-2 is administered subcutaneously at a dose of one half of 22mu vial- 11mu (fixed dose not adjusted to body surface area) for four consecutive days per week with IFN-alpha at 9-10mu on the first and fourth days of each four day cycle. Four consecutive weeks of therapy are given followed by a two week rest period. This therapy is continued as long as the tumor is stable or responding and in the absence of severe toxicity [43].

## Current Key Questions

The role of surgery in metastatic RCC has been reevaluated with renewed interest since the advent of successful immunotherapy. Evidence suggests that decreasing tumor burden with surgery may improve immunoreactivity against the malignancy by the host and thus intial IL-2 trials routinely required a nephrectomy prior to immunotherapy. However, up-front nephrectomy can result in a high postoperative morbidity and renal dysfunction rate which often prevents administration of subsequent immunotherapy, except in a well selected population [44]. Because we have never observed a complete response (CR) in the primary in spite of CRs in metastatic disease. [43, 45], we advocate a delayed nephrectomy in patients who demonstrate excellent response in the systemic disease to immunotherapy. Surgical excision of residual metastatic lesions after an initial response to nephrectomy and/or immunotherapy [46, 47] is the standard of care. Resection of metastatic lesions which threaten the quality of life such as metastases to the brain, spinal cord, bone or other organs is also standard of care for RCC patients. Such approaches are particularly warranted for patients with grade I-II clear cell carcinomas which display an indolent natural history.

## Current and Future Investigational Approaches

Because of a lack of well-tolerated, effective therapy, treatment of metastatic RCC must be carefully chosen. Withholding treatment until disease progression is evident may be prudent in some cases. Unlike other metastatic genitourinary cancers, systemic therapy cannot not be relied upon to palliate symptoms. Analgesia, surgery, and radiotherapy should be employed as needed to manage complications. Discovery of renal cancer specific tumor antigens, manipulation of the immune system to recognize such antigens, gene therapy trials with the VHL gene and clinical trials with new novel agents are just some of the research areas desperately needed in this field.

**Acknowledgements.** Adapted from "Genitourinary Cancer in the Elderly", in *Cancer in the Elderly*, eds CP Hunter, KA Johnson, HB Muss. Marcel Dekker, New York, 1998 (in press).

## References

1. Coughlin SS, Neaton JD, Randall B, Sengupta A. Predictors of mortality from kidney cancer in 332,547 men screened for the multiple risk factor intervention trial. Cancer 1997; 79:2171–2177
2. Mandel JS, McLaughlin JK, Schlehofer B et al. International renal-cell cancer study. IV. Occupation. Int J Cancer1995; 61:601–605
3. Ishikawa I, Kovacs G. High incidence of papillary renal cell tumours in patients on chronic haemodialysis. Histopathology 1993; 22 (2):135–139
4. LaForgia S, Lasota J, Latif F, Boghosian-Sell L, Kastury K, Ohta M, Druck T, Atchison L, Cannizzaro LA, Barnea G. Detailed genetic and physical map of the 3p chromosome region surrounding the familial renal cell carcinoma chromosome translocation, t(3,8) (p14.2;q24.1). Cancer Res 1993; 53:3118–3124
5. Linehan WM, Lerman MI, Zbar B. Identification of the von Hippel-Lindau gene: its role in renal carcinoma. JAMA 1995; 273:564–570
6. Zbar B, Tory K, Merino M, Schmidt L, Glenn G, Choyke P, Walther MM, Lermann M, Linehan WM. Hereditary papillary renal cell carcinoma. J Urol 1994; 151: 561–566
7. Kiely JM. Hypernephroma-the internist's tumor. Med Clin North Am 1966; 50:1067–1083
8. Ritchie AWS, Chisholm GD. The natural history of renal carcinoma. Semin Oncol 1983; 10:390–400
9. Tsukamoto T, Kumamoto Y, Yamazaki K, Miyao N, Takahashi A, Masumori N, Satoh M. Clinical analysis of incidentally found renal cell carcinomas. Eur Urol 1991; 19:109–113
10. Johnson CD, Dunnick NR, Cohan RH, Illescas FI. Renal adenocarcinoma: CT staging of 100 tumors. Am J Roentgenol 1987; 148:59–63

11. Horan JJ, Robertson CN, Choyke PL, Frank JA, Miller DL, Pass HI, Linehan WM. The detection of renal carcinoma extension into the renal vein and inferior vena cava: a prospective comparison of venacavography and magnetic resonance imaging. J Urol 1989; 142:943–948

12. Robson CJ, Churchill BM, Anderson W. The results of radical nephrectomy for renal cell carcinoma. J Urol 1969; 101:297–301

13. Guinan P, Sobin LH, Algaba F, Badellino F, Kameyama S, MacLennan G, Novick A: TNM staging of renal cell carcinoma, workgroup 3. Cancer, 1997; 80 (5):992–993

14. Guinan PD, Vogelzang NJ, Fremgen AM, Chmiel JS, Sylvester JL, Sener SF, Imperato JP. Renal cell carcinoma: tumor size, stage and survival. J Urol 1995; 153:901–903

15. Guiliani L, Giberti L, Martorana G, Rovida S. Radical extensive surgery for renal cell carcinoma: long-term results and prognostic factors. J Urol 1990; 143:468–474

16. Linehan WM, Shipley WU, Parkinson DR. Cancer of the kidney and ureter. In: DeVita VT Jr., Hellman S, Rosenberg SA. Cancer: principles and practice of oncology. Philadelphia: Lippincott-Raven, 1997:1271–1300

17. Kjaer M, Frederiksen PL, Engelholm SA. Postoperative radiotherapy in stage II and III renal adenocarcinoma. A randomized trial by the Copenhagen Renal Cancer Study Group. Int J Radiation Oncology Biol Phys 1987; 13:665–672

18. Motzer RJ, Bander NH, Nanus DM. Renal cell carcinoma. New England J Med, 1996; 355:865–875

19. Galligioni E, Quaia M, Merlo A, Carbone A, Spada A, Favaro D et al. Adjuvant immunotherapy treatment of renal carcinoma patients with autologous tumor cells and bacillus Calmett-Guerin: Five-year results of a prospective randomized study. Cancer 1996; 77:2560–2566

20. Trump DL, Elson P, Propert K, Pontes J, Crawford E, Wilding P et al. Randomized, controlled trial of adjuvant therapy with lymphoblastoid interferon in resected, high-risk renal cell carcinoma. Proc Amer Soc Clin Oncol (abstract), 1996; 15:648

21. Pizzocaro G, Piva L, Costa A, Silvestrini R. Adjuvant interferon to radical nephrectomy in Robson's stages II and III renal cell cancer, a multicenter randomized study with some biological evaluations. Proc Amer Soc Clin Oncol (abstract) 1997; 16:1132

22. Sawczuk IS, Graham SD, Miesowicz F. Randomized, controlled trial of adjuvant therapy with ex vivo activated T cells (ALT) in T1–3a,b,c or T4 N+,M0 renal cell carcinoma. Proc Amer Soc Clin Oncol (abstract) 1997; 16:326a

23. Nelson JF, Marshall FF. Surgical treatment of locally advanced renal cell carcinoma. In: Vogelzang NJ, Scardino PT, Shipley WU, Coffey DS (eds), Comprehensive Textbook of Genitourinary Oncology. Williams & Wilkins, 1996; 218–236

24. Novick AC. Current surgical approaches, nephron-sparing surgery, and the role of surgery in the integrated immunologic approach to renal-cell carcinoma. Sem Oncology 1995; 22:29–33

25. Motzer RJ, Vogelzang NJ. Chemotherapy for renal cell carcinoma. In: Raghavan D, Scher HI, Leibel SA, Lange PH (eds), Principles and Practice of Genitourinary Oncology. Lippincott-Raven Publishers, Philadelphia. 1997; 85:885–896

26. Samuels BL, Hollis DR, Rosner GL, Trump DL, Shapiro CL, Vogelzang NJ, Schilsky RL. Modulation of vinblastine resistance in metastatic renal cell carcinoma with cyclosporine A or tamoxifen: A CALGB study. Clin Cancer Res 1997; 3:1977–1984

27. Chapman AE, Goldstein LJ. Multiple drug resistance: biologic basis and clinical significance in renal-cell carcinoma. Sem Oncology 1995; 22:17–28

28. Quesada JR, Swanson DA, Trindade A, Gutterman JU. Renal cell carcinoma: Anti-tumor effects of leukocyte interferon. Cancer Res 1983; 43:940–947

29. Minasian LM, Motzer RJ, Gluck L, Mazumdar M, Vlamis V, Krown SE. Interferon alfa-2a in advanced renal cell carcinoma: Treatment results and survival in 159 patients with long-term follow-up. J Clin Oncol 1993; 11:1368–1375

30. Pyrhonen S, Salminen E, Lehtonen T, Nurmi M, Tammela T, Juusela H et al. Recombinent interferon alfa 2a with vinblastine vs. vinblastine alone in advanced real cell carcinoma. Proc Amer Soc Clin Oncol 1996; 15:614 (abstr)
31. Ritchie AWS, Griffiths G, Cook P, Oliver RTD, Hancock B, Parmar MKB. Alpha interferon improves survival in patients with metastatic renal carcinoma – preliminary results of an MRC randomised controlled trial. Proc Amer Soc Clin Oncol 1998; 17:310 (abstr.)
32. Gleave ME, Elhilali M, Fradet Y, Davis I, Venner P, Saad F, Klotz LH, Moore MJ, Paton V, Bajamonde A. Interferon gamma-1b compared with placebo in metastatic renal-cell carcinoma. New Engl J Med 1998; 338:1265–1271
33. Motzer RJ, Schwartz L, Law TM, Murphy BA, Hoffman AD, Albino AP, Vlamis V, Nanus DM. Interferon alfa-2a and 13-cis-retinoic acid in renal cell carcinoma: Antitumor activity in a phase II trial and intereactions in vitro. J Clin Oncol 1995; 13 (8) 1950–1957
34. Rosenberg SA, Lotze MT, Muul JM, Chang AE, Avis FP, Leitman S, Linehan WM, Robertson CN, Rubin JT. A progress report on the treatment of 157 patients with advanced cancer using lymphokine-activated killer cells and interleukin-2 or high-dose interleukin-2 alone. N Engl J Med 1987; 316:889–897
35. Rosenberg SA, Yang JC, Topalian SC, Schwartzentruber DJ, Weber JS, Parkinson DR, Seipp CA, Einhorn JH, White DE. Treatment of 283 consecutive patients with metastatic melanoma or renal cell cancer using high-dose bolus interleukin-2. JAMA 1994; 271:907–913
36. Law TM, Motzer RJ, Mazumdar M, Sell KW, Walther PJ, O'Connell M, Khan A, Vlamis V, Vogelzang NJ, Bajorin DF. Phase III randomized trial of interleukin-2 with or without lymphokine-activated killer cells in the treatment of patients with advanced renal cell carcinoma. Cancer 1995; 76:824–832
37. Atkins MB, Sparano J, Fisher RI, Sunderland M, Margolin K, Ernest ML, Sznol M, Atkins MB, Dutcher JP, Micetich KC, Weiss GR. Randomized phase II trial of high-dose interleukin-2 either alone or in combination with interferon alpha-2b in advanced renal cell carcinoma. J Clin Oncol 1993; 11:661–670
38. Stadler WM, Vogelzang NJ. Low-dose interleukin-2 in the treatment of metastatic renal-cell carcinoma. Sem Oncol 1995; 22:67–73
39. Bukowski RM. Natural history and therapy of metastatic renal cell carcinoma. Cancer 1997; 80:1198–1220
40. Negrier S, Escudier B, Lasset C, Douillard J-Y, Savary J, Chevreau C, Ravaud A, Mercatello A, Peny J, Mousseau M, Philip T, Turz T. Recombinant human interleukin-2, recombinant human interferon alfa-2a, or both in metastatic renal-cell carcinoma. New Engl J Med 1998; 338:1272–1278
41. Siegel JP, Puri RK. Interleukin-2 toxicity. J Clin Oncol 1991; 9:694–704
42. Yang JC, Topalian SL, Parkinson D, Schwartzentruber DJ, Weber JS, Ettinghausen SE et al. Randomized comparison of high-dose and low-dose intravenous interleukin-2 for therapy of metastatic renal cell carcinoma: An interim report. J Clin Oncol 1994; 12 (8):1572–1576
43. Stadler WM, Kuzel T, Dumas M, Vogelzang NJ. A multi-center phase II trial of interleukin-2, interferon-alpha, and 13-cis-retinoic acid in patients with metastatic renal cell carcinoma. J Clin Oncol 1998; 16 (5):1820–1825
44. Levy DA, Swanson DA, Slaton JW, Ellerhorst J, Dinney CPN. timely delivery of biological therapy after cytoreductive nephrectomy in carefully selected patients with metastatic renal cell carcinoma. J Urol, 159:1168–1173, 1998
45. Vogelzang NJ, Lipton A, Figlin RA. Subcutaneous interleukin-2 plus interferon alfa-2a in metastatic renal cancer: An outpatient multicenter trial. J Clin Oncol 1993; 11 (9):1809–16

46. Fleischmann JD, Kim B. Interleukin-2 immunotherapy followed by resection of residual renal cell carcinoma. J Urol 1991; 145:938–941
47. Sella A, Swanson DA, Ro JY, Putman JB Jr., Amato RJ, Markowtiz AB, Logothetis CJ. Surgery following response to interferon-alpha-based therapy for residual renal cell carcinoma. J Urol 1993; 149:19–22

# Genitourinary Malignancies:
# Bladder, Penis, and Urethral Cancers

W. Stadler

## Bladder Cancer

### Epidemiology, Risk Factors

Approximately 54,400 Americans will be diagnosed with bladder cancer in 1998 [1]. The vast majority of these patients will be suffer from superficial disease and thus only 12,500 deaths are expected. Despite an 11.6% increase in the incidence of bladder cancer from 1973 to 1994, the death rate declined by 22.4%, likely reflecting improvements in the diagnosis, management, and monitoring of patients with superficial disease [2]. These opposite trends in incidence and mortality lead to an estimated 582,000 individuals in the United States alive in 1997 who have or who have had a diagnosis of bladder cancer [2]. Incidence increases with age; the median age at diagnosis is 71 and it is unusual for patients younger than 40 to develop bladder cancer. The male to female incidence ratio remains approximately 3:1 in all racial groups despite changes in female occupational exposures and increases in tobacco abuse in women [2].

In the Western hemisphere, the most important epidemiologic risk factor, by far, is tobacco use. The relative risk of developing bladder cancer for a smoker is 2–10 and there is a definite dose response [3, 4]. Quitting leads to a 30%–60% reduction in risk over the first 2–4 years, but the relative risk does not ever appear to return to unity. Smokers of "black," or unfiltered cigarretes have an especially high risk [5]. The exact risk level with cigar smoking and "smokeless" tobacco has not been quantified.

Occupational risk for bladder cancer has been known since the seminal work of Rehn who in 1895 demonstrated an unusual incidence of this disease in German aniline dye workers [6]. Since then a large number of industries, most prominently dye and rubber manufacturing, have been associated with bladder cancer. The common etiologic agent in all these is exposure to arylamines, especially 4-aminobiphenyl, 2-napthylamine, and benzidine [7]. Figure 1 demonstrates the biochemical activation of an arylamine such that carcinogenic DNA adducts are formed. Figure 1 also provides an explanation for the observation that patients with certain polymorphisms in the N-acetyltransferase enzyme (NAT) that lead to slower metabolism rates are at a increased risk for the development of occupationally associated bladder cancer [8]. Arylamines are present in tobacco smoke, but it is doubtful that this is the sole carcinogenic agent.

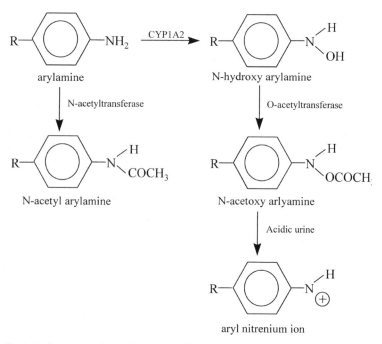

**Fig. 1.** Arylamines can be undergo metabolism via two principle routes, N-hydroxylation or N-acetylation. In the latter pathway subsequent glucuronidation leads to excretion of innocuous metabolites. The N-hydroxy metabolite also undergoes subsequent acetylation, however, the resultant compound is unstable in the acidic urinary enviroment leading to formation of the reactive aryl nitrenium ion which can readily form promutagenic DNA adducts

Chronic bladder infections are a risk factor for bladder cancer, but in these cases the histology is usually squamous cell [9]. Worldwide the most important infection is Schistosomiasis haematobium, which is the leading etiologic agent for bladder cancer in many Middle Eastern and African nations. Pelvic irradiation is also an important risk factor, although the lag time between exposure and disease development may be as long as 15–20 years [10, 11]. Finally, exposure to cyclophosphamide either with chronic low doses administered for immunologic disorders, or with high doses administered in the oncologic setting, can lead to development of bladder cancer [12, 13].

## Cancer Pathology and Staging

In the Western world the most common histologic subtype of bladder cancer, comprising about 90% of cases, is transitional cell cancer, with or without squamous or adenomatous differentiation [14]. Pure squamous cell cancers tend to arise in the setting of chronic infection, pure adenocarcinomas are rare and often arise from urachal remnants. These latter two histologic subtypes tend to present at more advanced stages and have a worse prognosis than pure transitional cell cancer. Table 1 depicts staging information and Table 2 depicts estimates of stage specific survival following appropriate therapy. Importantly, the most recent AJCC staging system classifies all muscle invasive disease as T2, unlike the previous version that classified invasion into the outer half of the muscle layer as T3a [15].

It should also be noted that clinical staging, as determined by cystoscopic biopsy, underestimates pathologic stage, as determined by cystectomy, in up to 30% of cases [22]. Although pathologic stage is the single most important prognostic factor, nuclear grade does add independent information [23]. More recently a number of molecular markers, including p53 and pRb mutations, overexpression of epidermal growth factor receptor and E-Cadherin, and increased neovascularization have all been found to provide some independent prognostic information [24–28]. The greatest number of studies relate to p53, but even in this case there remains some controversy as to the best techniques for detection and the ultimate role in determining therapy.

**Table 1.** Bladder cancer staging (from [15])

| Primary tumor | |
|---|---|
| Ta | Noninvasive papillary carcinoma |
| Tis | Carcinoma in situ |
| T2 | Primary tumor invades muscle |
|    T2a | Primary tumor invades superficial muscle (inner half) |
|    T2b | Primary tumor invades deep muscle (outer half) |
| T3 | Primary tumor invades perivesical tissue |
|    T3a | Microscopic perivesical tissue invasion |
|    T3b | Macroscopic perivesical tissue invasion |
| T4 | Primary tumor invades adjacent organs or structures |
|    T4a | Primary tumor invades prostate, uterus, or vagina |
|    T4b | Primary tumor invades pelvic or abdominal wall |
| | |
| Regional lymph nodes[a] | |
| N1 | Metastasis in single node, 2 cm or less |
| N2 | Metastasis in single node 2—5 cm, or metastasis multiple nodes 5 cm or less |
| N3 | Metastasis in any node greater than 5 cm |
| | |
| Stage grouping | |
| Stage 0a | Ta N0 M0 |
| Stage 0is | Tis N0 M0 |
| Stage I | T1 N0 M0 |
| Stage II | T2 N0 M0 |
| Stage III | T3 N0 M0 |
| | T4a N0 M0 |
| Stage IV | T4b N0 M0 |
| | Any T any N M0/M1 |

[a] Hypogastric, obturator, iliac, perivesical, sacral.

**Table 2.** Survival by stage

| Stage | 5-year survival | References |
|---|---|---|
| 0a | 85%—95% | 2, 16 |
| 0is | 80%—90% | 2, 16, 17 |
| I | 70%—90% | 2, 16, 17 |
| II | 50%—80% | 18, 19, 20, 24 |
| III | 20%—50% | 19, 20, 24 |
| IV | 0%—30% | 2, 21, 54 |

## Work-up and Staging

The single most important staging procedure is an adequate cystoscopic biopsy (Fig. 2). The biopsy sample must contain muscle tissue to deter-

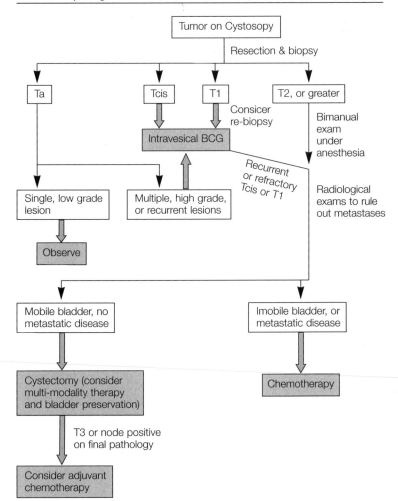

**Fig. 2.** Simplified flow diagram for work-up and therapy of a patient with bladder cancer. Shaded boxes, therapeutic manuevers. Not depicted as part of the work-up is an intravenous pyelogram which is usually required to rule out upper tract disease. See text for details

mine the degree of invasion. If no muscle is seen a repeat biopsy should be performed. Due to the problem of understaging, and the different therapeutic approaches, consideration for re-biopsy should also be given for any diagnosis of T1 disease. Carcinoma in situ (Tcis) has important therapeutic and prognostic implications, but may be difficult to diagnose due to fixation or cautery artifacts. Referral for a second pathologic interpretation at a reference center may be indicated whenever there is any doubt. Patients with suspected muscle invasive disease should have a bimanual examination under anesthesia during the biopsy. A fixed bladder is a poor prognostic indicator and many of these patients will be found to be unresectable during surgical exploration [29]. In experienced hands, a bimanual examination is more sensitive and more accurate than a CT scan. Patients with muscle invasive disease should undergo at least an abdominal/pelvic CT scan and a CXR to rule out metastatic disease. A chest CT scan is more sensitive for detection of lung disease and should be considered in patients with deeply invasive local cancer. An intravenous pyelogram is helpful to rule out upper tract disease. Bone scans are helpful in patients with bony pain, but may lead to excessive false positives in patients who are otherwise free of metastatic disease.

## Therapy

### *Superficial Disease*

Superficial bladder cancer (Ta, Tcis, and T1 disease) can be treated with local therapy only. Single, low grade, Ta lesions can be treated with simple cystoscopic resection or fulguration. Although patients need to be monitored for disease recurrence, the probability of progression to muscle invasive disease is vanishingly small [30, 31]. Patients with frequent recurrences of Ta disease or with higher grade Ta disease can be treated with a course of intravesical BCG. Such an approach will decrease the risk for subsequent recurrence, although it is unclear whether the small risk of subsequent progression to muscle invasive disease is affected significantly [32]. Tcis is a high risk disease that in the abscence of therapy almost invariably progresses to muscle invasive disease. Intravesical BCG therapy is curative in approximately three fourths of Tcis patients [33]. Some reports suggest that a maintenence schedule of BCG for up to 3 years further decreases the risk of recurrence and progression [34]. For patients failing BCG therapy the standard of care in most countries is cystectomy, but a number of investigational agents are being pursued. As previously discussed, clinical T1 disease is often understaged and additional biopsies often reveal muscle invasive disease. If T1 disease is confirmed, then a trial of intravesical BCG therapy is reasonable, especially for grade 2 disease, but the response rate is lower than in patients with Tcis [35]. A low threshold for moving on to more definitive cystectomy thus needs to be maintained.

*Muscle Invasive Disease*

Surgical Therapy
Standard of care in most countries is radical cystectomy. A number of options for redirecting the urinary stream are available. Details are beyond the scope of this chapter, but the most common is to fashion a internal reservoir from intestinal tissue which then empties through an abdominal wall urostomy into a collection bag. Many surgeons are capable of creating continent stomas that need to be catherized at a regular interval. There is thus no need for a urine collection bag and cystectomy thus becomes a more palatable option for the patient. In many specialized centers a functioning neobladder can be connected to the native urethra in which the external urethral sphincter is spared thus maintaining normal anatomic voiding. Patients need to void via a Valsalva manuever and neobladder capacity is less then that of a native bladder, but daytime continence rates are in excess of 90% and patient satisfaction with such neobladders is high [36]. Because of the shorter continence mechanism in women, the vast majority of neobladders have been constructed in men, but many referral institutions are currently performing them in women as well.

Radiotherapy
In the United States and many Western countries, radiotherapy is considered inferior to cystectomy for control of muscle invasive disease. It should be pointed out, however, that because of clinical understaging and patient selection, a necessary bias against radiotherapy exists in most non-randomized, retrospective comparative studies. Furthermore radiotherapy is considered the standard of care in some European countries and comparative studies from Europe, at least one of which was a

prospective randomized trial, suggest that there is little to no difference in survival between patients treated with radical cystectomy and those treated with radiotherapy [37]. This likely reflects the fact that approximately one half of patients with muscle invasive disease will die of metastatic disease, and very few of these patients suffer local recurrence, irrespective of the modality used to treat the primary tumor. Thus, in most cases better therapy for micrometastatic disease is a more important issue than better local therapy.

## Combined Modality, Organ Sparing

Due to patient dissatisfication with urostomy bags, the effectiveness of radiotherapy in localized disease, and the observation that chemotherapy for metastatic disease leads to complete disappearance of local disease in approximately 30% of individuals, a number of investigators have explored a multi-modality approach to muscle invasive bladder cancer with the goals being curative therapy and preservation of a functioning native bladder. Most protocols require aggressive cystoscopic resection of all visible tumor, several cycles of induction chemotherapy, followed by a course of combination chemotherapy and radiotherapy. At specialized centers this approach leads to survival equivalent to matched cystectomy patients with 60%–70% of survivors maintaining their native bladder [38, 39]. It should be noted that a properly performed organ sparing approach requires several months of aggressive chemo-radiotherapy and may thus not be appropriate for patients who are unable to tolerate a cystectomy due to co-morbid conditions. In addition, patients who present with hydronephrosis do not fare will with this approach [40]. Furthermore, in patients who experience a complete response to combined modality therapy, the native bladder remains at high risk for recurrent disease, including recurrent muscle invasive disease [38, 39]. In one of the larger multi-institutional series to date, patients were treated with induction cisplatin, methotrexate, and vinblastine (CMV), followed by RT with concomittant cisplatin. At a median followup of 3.8 years only 26% of the original 91 patients were alive with an intact bladder and continuously free of all disease [39]. It is likely that the better results reported by single institutions reflects patient selection [41].

## Adjuvant and Neoadjuvant Therapy

Because the most common mode of failure for patients with muscle invasive disease is development of metastatic disease, a number of trials have

**Table 3.** Selected Multi-Institutional Neoadjuvant Trials

| Chemotherapy | Local therapy | n | Results | Reference |
|---|---|---|---|---|
| MVAC | Cystectomy | (298) | Pending | |
| CMV | RT or cystectomy | 975 | ND | 43 |
| CMV | cisplatin/RT | 126 | ND | 44 |
| Cisplatin | RT | 255 | ND | 45 |
| MVEC | Cystectomy | 240 | ND | 46 |
| AC/RT | RT/cystectomy | 311 | 15% survival advantage in T3/T4 | 47 |

MVAC, Methotrexate, vinblastine, Adriamycin, cisplatin; CMV, cisplatin, methotrexate, vinblastine; MVEC, methotrexate, vinblastine, epirubicin, cisplatin; RT, radiotherapy; cyst., cystectomy; AC, Adriamycin, cisplatin.

investigated the use of neoadjuvant or adjuvant chemotherapy in conjunction with definitive local therapy. Table 3 depicts the largest randomized, multi-institutional, trials of neoadjuvant chemotherapy. Unfortunately the largest trial to date, an EORTC trial involving almost 1000 patients has been published in abstract form only. Nonetheless, in the absence of new data from this study or the soon to be completed US study, neoadjuvant therapy with standard MVAC or CMV chemotherapy does not appear to affect survival.

Table 4 depicts randomized, adjuvant trials that included a no therapy control group. No trial is adequately powered to detect even a 20% difference in survival between the treated and untreated groups [42]. Furthermore, each trial has a number of methodologic problems that have been discussed in the literature [42]. The cumulative data suggests that adjuvant therapy increases the time to disease recurrence, but it

**Table 4.** Randomized adjuvant trials

| Regimen | n | Results | Reference |
|---|---|---|---|
| CISCA | 91 | Benefit in RFS, survival benefit not statistically significant | 48 |
| CDDP | 77 | No survival benefit | 49 |
| MVAC/MVEC | 49 | Benefit in RFS, survival not reported | 50 |
| CM | 83 | No benefit | 51 |
| CMV | 49 | Benefit in RFS, no survival benefit | 52 |

CISCA, Cyclophosphamide, cisplatin, adriamycin; CDDP, cisplatin, MVAC/MVEC, methotrexate, vinblastine, adriamycin (epirubicin), cisplatin; CM, cisplatin, methotrexate; CMV, cisplatin, methotrexate, vinblastine.

remains unclear whether survival is affected. Participation in ongoing adjuvant chemotherapy trials is encouraged.

*Metastatic Disease*

Metastatic bladder cancer is a chemoresponsive disease and tumor shrinkage can be observed with a large number of single agents [53]. Although cisplatin has traditionally been considered the single most active agent, the response rate in a randomized MVAC versus cisplatin trial was only 12% [54]. This reflects, in part, more rigorous modern response evaluations as well as patient selection in smaller phase II trials from referral institutions. This latter problem also plagues more recent phase II trials that report very encouraging data from treatment with single agent paclitaxel or gemcitabine [55, 56]. Nonetheless, the number of complete responses and responses in sites traditionally resistant to chemotherapy, such as liver, lead to the conclusion that these two agents are an important addition to our therapeutic armanterium. One additional important, often overlooked, class of agents with impressive single agent activity is the antifolates [53]. Whether second and third generation antifolates such as piritrexim have an advantage over methotrexate remains to be determined.

Despite encouraging data from trials of novel single agent therapy in metastatic bladder cancer, the standard of care remains combination chemotherapy. The standard combination regimen is MVAC (methotrexate, vinblastine, Adriamycin, and cisplatin). MVAC has been proven to be superior to both single agent cisplatin as well as to a combination of cyclophosphamide, cisplatin, and adriamycin (CISCA). [54, 57] A combination of CMV (cisplatin, methotrexate, and vinblastine), which uses a higher dose of cisplatin than MVAC, has also been used extensively. Although no randomized data exists, most investigators believe that CMV and MVAC are equivalent in efficacy.

Long term results with MVAC are, however, disappointing. In the randomized multi-institutional trial of MVAC versus cisplatin, the complete response rate to MVAC was 13%, median survival was only 12.5 months, and only 5/133 were continuously free of disease after 6 years of followup [58]. Toxicity was also not insignificant with grade 3 or 4 neutropenia in 24% (with fever in 10%), grade 3–4 mucositis in 17%, and grade 3 or 4 renal insuffiency in 7% of treated patients [58]. Dose escalation or substitution of various analogs for the individual components of MVAC has not lead to significant improvements in survival either (see reference 40 for review). Thus, the development of better combination chemotherapy regimens for metastatic bladder cancer remains a priority.

Finally, it should be noted that pure squamous or adenocarcinomas respond poorly to standard MVAC therapy. Data from centers with a high rate of schistosomiasis associated squamous cell cancer suggests that a combination of vincristine, etoposide, ifosfamide, and a doxorubicin analog leads to an overall response rate of 46% [60].

Current Key Questions

Some of the important clinical questions in bladder cancer therapy are:
– What is the role of maintenence BCG?
– Are there options besides radiotherapy or radical cystectomy for patients with Tcis who fail BCG therapy?
– What are the relative merits of cystectomy with continent urinary diversion versus combined modality therapy and attempted organ preservation?
– Does adjuvant chemotherapy prolong survival?
– Is there a more effective and less toxic combination chemotherapy regimen than MVAC?
– Can molecular markers be used to guide therapy?

Current and Future Investigational Approaches

Ongoing and planned clinical trials are attempting to answer the above questions. Newer intravesical agents are being investigated for refractory superficial disease. A number of surgeons continue to improve on their techniques for construction of a neobladder and several trials are examining novel approaches to combined modality therapy and organ preservation. Unfortunately, due to provider and patient biases, it is unlikely that a trial of cystectomy with neobladder versus combined modality therapy and organ preservation will ever be initiated in the United States. Several large north American and international groups are performing trials of MVAC versus novel combinations for metastatic disease as well as for adjuvant therapy of high risk disease. Although an adjuvant trial with observation as one arm is scientifically valid, it may be difficult to complete accrual in a timely fashion in the United States. Many of these trials are incorporating molecular markers to prospectively evaluate their role and determine whether they can be used to guide therapy.

## Penile and Urethral Cancer

Penile and urethral cancers are both rare cancers in the United States together comprising less than 1% of all genitourinary cancers. Because a number of specific treatment issues for the various stages of each disease must be entertained, and because these cancers often require a multimodality approach, referral to a institution with special expertise in genitourinary cancer is recommended. More detailed discussions with appropriate references are available in textbooks of genitourinary oncology (e.g. [61]).

In general, penile cancer is most common in uncircumcised males with poor hygiene. Some association with human papilloma virus infection has also been reported. Superficial disease can be treated with laser fulguration or Moh's microsurgery, but invasive disease must be treated with partial or complete penectomy or radiotherapy. The most common metastatic site is femoral lymph nodes, but these are notoriously difficult to evaluate clinically, because they are often swollen due to associated inflammation in the primary tumor. Treatment of lymph node positive disease is especially controversial. Surgery and radiotherapy can both be curative, but can also lead to debilitating lymphedema. Chemotherapy does play a role in treatment of locally advanced as well as metastatic disease with 5FU, cisplatin, methotrexate, and bleomycin all being active agents. Clinical studies, however, include too few patients to confidently compare their relative merits or to determine the most active combination regimen.

Etiologies for urethral cancer are more difficult to determine. The disease is also very heterogenous. Proximal disease is often transitional cell histology and can safely be approached like a bladder cancer. More distal disease is often squamous cell cancer and it may be reasonable to approach it like invasive penile cancer, but few studies have been performed. Adenocarcinomas of the urethra are not uncommon and tend to have a very poor prognosis with standard surgical or radiotherapy approaches. Novel combined modality therapy with surgical debulking, and concomittant chemo-radiotherapy have been successful in small series and case reports.

# References

1. Landis SH, Murray T, Bolden S, Wingo PA. Cancer statistics, 1998. CA 48:6–29, 1998
2. Ries, LAG, Kosary CL, Hankey BF, Miller BA, Harras AA, Edwards BK (eds). SEER cancer statistics review, 1973–1994. National Cancer Institute, NIH Pub. No. 97-2789, Bethesda, MD, 1997
3. Hartge P, Silveman D, Hoover R et al. Changing cigarette habits and bladder cancer risk: a case-control study. J Natl Cancer Inst 78:1119–1125, 1987
4. Engeland A, Andersen A, Haldorsen T, Tretli S. Smoking habits and risk of cancers other than lung cancer: 28 years' follow-up of 26,000 Norwegian men and women. Cancer Causes Control 1996 Sep;7 (5):497–506
5. Vineis P. Black (air-cured) and blond (flue-cured) tobacco and cancer risk. I: Bladder cancer. Eur J Cancer 1991, 27 (11):1491–1493
6. Rehn L. Blasengeschw?lste bei Buchsin-Arbeitern. Arch Klin Chir 50:588–600, 1895
7. Swaminathan S, Reznikoff C. Biochemical and molecular carcinogenesis. In: Comprehensive Textbook of Genitourinary Oncology, Vogelzang NJ, Scardino PT, Shipley WU, Coffey DS eds. Williams & Wilkins, 1996, pp 305–313
8. Yu MC, Skipper PL, Taghizadeh K, Tannenbaum SR, Chan KK, Henderson BE, Ross RK. Acetylator phenotype, aminobiphenyl-hemoglobin adduct levels, and bladder cancer risk in white, black, and Asian men in Los Angeles, California. J Natl Cancer Inst 1994 May 4, 86 (9):712–716
9. Kantor AF, Hartge P, Hoover RN, Narayana A, Sulivan JW, Fraumeni JF Jr. Urinary tract infection and risk of bladder cancer. Am J Epidemiol 119:510–515, 1984
10. Maier U, Ehrenbock PM, Hofbauer J. Urological complications and malignancies after curative radiotherapy for gynecological carcinomas: A retrospective analysis of 10,709 patients. J Urol 158:814–817, 1997
11. Neugut AI, Ahsan H, Robinson E, Ennis RD. Bladder carcinoma and other second malignancies after radiotherapy for prostate carcinoma. Cancer 79:1600–1604, 1997
12. Travis LB, Curtis RE, Glimelius B et al. Bladder and kidney cancer followign cyclophosphamide therapy for non-hodgkins lymphoma J Natl Cancer Inst 87:524–530, 1995
13. Talar-Williams C, Hijazi YM, Walther MM, Linehan WM, Hallahan CW, Lubensky I, Kerr GS, Hoffman GS, Fauci AS, Sneller MC. Cyclophosphamide-induced cystitis and bladder cancer in patients with Wegener granulomatosis. Ann Intern Med 1996 Mar 1, 124 (5):477–484
14. Tumors Of The Kidney, Bladder, And Related Urinary Structures. AFIP Electronic Fascicle v2.0, 1997
15. AJCC staging manual, Fleming ID, Cooper JS, Henson DE, Hutter RV, Kennedy BJ, Murphy GP, O'Sullivan B, Sobin LH, Yarbro J. eds. Lippencott-Raven, 1997
16. Koch MO, Smith JA. Natural history and surgical management of superficial bladder cancer. In: Comprehensive Textbook of Genitourinary Oncology, Vogelzang NJ, Scardino PT, Shipley WU, Coffey DS eds. Williams & Wilkins, 1996, 405–415
17. Cookson MS, Herr HW, Zhang A-F, Soloway S, Sogani PC, Fair WR. The treated natural history of high risk superficial bladder cancer: 15-year outcome. J Urol 158:62–67, 1997

18. Wishnow KI, Levinson AK, Johnson DE et al. Stage B (P2/3 A/N0) transitional cell carcinoma of bladder highly curable by radical cystectomy. Urology 39:12–16, 1992
19. Schoenberg MP, Walsh PC, Breazeale DR, Marshall FF, Mostwin JL, Brendler CB. Local recurrence and survival folowing nerve sparing radical cystoprostatectomy for bladder cancer: 10pyear followup. J Urol 155:490–494, 1996
20. Pagano F, Bassi P, Galetti TP et al. Results of contemporary radical cystectomy for invasive bladder cancer: a clinicopathological study with an emphasis on the inadequacy of the tumor, nodes, and metastases classification. J Urol 145:45–50, 1991
21. Lerner SP, Skinner DG, Lieskovsky G et al. The rationale for en bloc pelvic lymph node dissection for bladder cancer patients with nodal metastases: Long term results. J Urol 149:758–765, 1993
22. Herr HW, Scher HI. Surgery of invasive bladder cancer: Is pathologic staging necessary? [Review]. Semin Oncol 17:590–597, 1990
23. Carbin BE, Ekman P, Gustafson H et al. Grading of human urothelial carcinoma based on nuclear atypia and mitotic frequency II. Prognostic importance. J Urol 145:972–975, 1991
24. Esrig D, Elmajian D, Groshen S et al. Accumulation of nuclear p53 and tumor progression in bladder cancer. N Engl J Med 331:1259–1264, 1994
25. Cordon-Cardo C, Wartinger D, Petrylak D, Dalbagni G, Gair WR, Fuks Z, Reuter VE. Alterec expression of the retinoblastoma gene product: Prognostic indicator in bladder cancer. J Natl Cancer Inst 84:1251–1256, 1992
26. Mellon K, Wright C, Kelly P, Wilson Horne CH, Neal DE. Long term outcome related to epidermal growth factor receptor status in bladder cancer. J Urol 153:919–925, 1995
27. Shimazui T, Schalken JA, Giroldi LA, Jansen CF, Akaza H, Koiso K, Debruyne FM, Bringuier PP. Prognostic value of cadherin-associated molecules (alpha-, beta-, and gamma-catenins and p120cas) in bladder tumors. Cancer Res 1996 Sep 15, 56 (18):4154–4158
28. Bochner BH, Cote RJ, Weidner N, Groshen S, Chen SC, Skinner DG, Nichols PW. Angiogenesis in bladder cancer: relationship between microvessel density and tumor prognosis. J Natl Cancer Inst 1995 Nov 1, 87 (21):1603–1612
29. Fossa SD, Ous S, Berner A. Clinical significance of the "palpable mass" in patients with muscle-infiltrating bladder cancer undergoind cystectoy after pre-operative radiotherapy. Br J Urol 67:54–60, 1991
30. Lutzeyer W, Rubben H, Dahm H. Prognostic parameters in superficial bladder cancer: an analysis of 315 cases. J. Urol 127:250–254, 1982
31. Raghavan D, Shipley WU, Garnick MB et al. Biology and management of bladder cancer. N Eng J Med 322:1129–1138, 1990
32. Krege S, Giani G, Meyer R, Otto T, Rubben H et al. A randomized trial of adjuvant therapy in superficial bladder cancer: Transurethral resection only versus transurethral resection plus mitomycin C versus transurethral resection plus bacillus Calmette-Guerin. J Urol 156:962–966, 1996
33. Lamm DL. Long-term results of intravesical therapy for superfical bladder cancer. Urol Clin North Am 19:573–580, 1992
34. Witjes JA, Fransen MPH, van der Meijden APM et al. Use of maintenance intravesical bacillus Calmette-Guerin (BCG) with or without intradermal BCG in patients with recurrent superficial bladder cancer. Urol Int 51:67–72, 1993
35. Zhang GK, Uke ET, Sharer WC, Borkon WD, Bernstein SM. Reassessment of conservative management for stage T1N0M0 transitional cell carcinomal of the bladder. J Urol 155:1907–1909, 1996
36. Bales GT, Kim H, Steinberg G. Surgical therapy for locally advanced bladder cancer. Sem Oncol 23:605–613, 1996

37. Bloom HJ, Hendry WF, Wallace DM, Skeet RG. Treatment of T3 bladder cancer: Controlled trial of pre-operative radiotherapy and radical cystectomy versus radical radiotherapy. Br J Urol 54:136–151, 1982

38. Douglas RM, Kaufman DS, Zietman AL, Althausen AF, Heney NM, Shipley WU. Conservative surgery, patient selection, and chemoradiation as organ-preserving treatment for muscle-invading bladder cancer. Sem Oncol 23:614–620, 1996

39. Tester W, Caplan R, Heaney J, Venner P, Whittington R, Byhardt R, True L, Shipley W. Neoadjuvant combined modality program with selective oran preservation for invasive bladder cancer: results of radiation therapy oncology group phase II trial 8802. J Clin Oncol 14:119–126, 1996

40. Kaufman DS, Shipley WU, Griffen PP, Heney NM, Althausen AF, Efird JT. Selective bladder preservation by combination treatment of invasive bladder cancer. N Engl J Med 329:1377–1382, 1993

41. Kachnic LA, Kaufman DS, Heney NM, Althausen AF, Griffen PP, Zietman AL, Shipley WU. Bladder preservation by combined modality therapy for invasive bladder cancer. J Clin Oncol 15:1022–1029, 1997

42. Sternberg CN. Neoadjuvant and adjuvant chemotherapy in locally advanced bladder cancer. Sem Oncol 23:621–632, 1996

43. Hall RR, for the MRC Advanced Bladder Cancer Working Party, EORTC GU Group. Neo-adjuvant CMV chemotherapy and cystectomy or radiotherapy in muscle invasive bladder cancer. First analysis of MRC/EORTC intercontinental trial. Proc Amer Soc Clin Oncol 15:612, 1996 (abst)

44. Shipley WU, Winter KA, Lee R, Kaufman DS et al. Initial results of RTOG 89-03: A phase III trial of neoadjuvant chemotherapy in patietns with invasive bladder cancer treated with selective bladder preservation by combined radiation therapy and chemotherapy. Int J Rad Onc Biol Physics 39 (Supplement 2) 155, 1997

45. Wallace DM, Raghavan D, Kelly KA et al. Neo-adjuvant (pre-emptive cisplatin therapy in invasive transitional cell carcinoma of the bladder. Br J Urol 67:608–615, 1991

46. Pellegrini A, for GISTV. Neoadjuvant treatment for locally advanced bladder cancer: A randomized prospective clinical trial. Proc Fourth In Symp Adv Urol Oncol 29 A:S229, 1993

47. Malmstrom PU, Rintala E, Wahlqvist R et al. Five year follow up of a prospective trial of radical cystectomy and neoadjuvant chemotherapy. Nordic cystectomy trial I. J Urol 1996 Jun;155 (6):1903–1906

48. Skinner DG, Daniels JR, Russell CA et al. The role of adjuvant chemotherapy following cystectomy for invasive bladder cancer: A prospective comparraive trial. J Urol 145:459–467, 1991

49. Studer UE, Bacchi M, Biedermann C et al. Adjuvant cisplatin chemotherapy following cystectomy for bladder cancer: Results of a prospective randomized trial. J Urol 152:81–84, 1992

50. Stoeckle M, Meyenburg W, Wellek S, Voges G, Gertenbach U, Thueroff JW, Huber C, Hohenfellner R. Advanced bladder cancer (Stages pT3b, pT4a, pN1, and pN2) Improved survival after radical cystectomy and 3 cycles of chemotherapy. Results of a controlled prospective study. J Url 148:302–307, 1992

51. Bono AV, Benvenuti C, Reali L, Pozzi E, Gibba A, Cosciani-Cunico S, Comuzzi U, Anselmo G. Adjuvant chemotherapy in advanced bladder cancer. Italian Uro-Oncologic Cooperative Group. Prog Clin Biol Res 1989, 303:533–540

52. Freiha F, Reese J, Torti FM. A randomized trial of radical cystectomy versus radical cystectomy plus cisplatin, vinbastine, and methotrexate chemotherapy for muscle invasive bladder cancer. J Urol 155:495–500, 1996

53. Fagbemi SO, Stadler WM. New chemotherapy regimens for advanced bladder cancer. Semin Urol Oncol 16:23–29, 1998

54. Loehrer, P., Einhorn, L.H., Elson, P.J., Crawford, E.D., Kuebler, P., Tannock, I., Raghavan, D., Stuart-Harris, R., Sarosdy, M.F., Lowe, B.A., Blumenstein, B., and Trump, D. (1992). A randomized comparison of cisplatin alone or in combination with methotrexate, vinblastine and doxorubicin in patients with metastatic urothelial carcinoma: A cooperative group study. J. Clin. Oncol., 10, 1066–73

55. Roth, B.J., Dreicer, R., Einhorn, L. H., Neuberg, D., Johnson, D.H., Smith, J.L., Hudes, G.R., Schultz, S.M., and Loehrer, P.J. (1994). Significant activity of paclitaxel in advanced transitional-cell carcinoma of the urothelium: A phase II trial of the Eastern Cooperative Oncology Group. J. Clin. Oncol., 12, 2264–70

56. Stadler WM, Kuzel T, Roth B, Raghavan D, Dorr FA. A phase II study of single agent gemcitabine in previously untreated patients with metastatic urothelial cancer. J Clin Oncol. 15:3394–3398, 1997

57. Logothetis CJ, Dexeus FH, Finn L, Sella A, Amato RJ, Ayala AG, Kilbourn RG. A prospective randomized trial comparing MVAC and CISCA chemotherapy for patietns with metastatic urothelial tumors. J Clin Oncol 8:1050–1055, 1990

58. Saxman SB, Propert KJ, Einhorn LH, Crawford ED, Tannock I, Raghavan D, Loehrer PJ, Trump D. Long-term follow-up of a phase III intergroup study of cisplatin alone or in combination with methotrexate, vinblastine, and doxorubicin in patients with metastatic urothelial carcinoma: A cooperative group study. J Clin Oncol. 15:2564–2569, 1997

59. Fagbemi SO, Stadler WM. New chemotherapy regimens for advanced bladder cancer. Semin Urol Oncol 16:23–29, 1998

60. Khaled HM, Gad el-Mawla N, el-Said A, Hamza MR, Gaafar R, el-Attar I, Abu Rabia A, Magrath I. Combination chemotherapy for advanced bilharzial bladder carcinoma. Ann Oncol 1996 Sep;7 (7):751–754

61. Vogelzang NJ, Scardino PT, Shipley WU, Coffey DS eds, Comprehensive Textbook of Genitourinary Oncology, Williams & Wilkins, 1996

# Gynecologig Cancers

# Endometrial Cancer

S.E. Waggoner

## Epidemiology, Risk Factors

Endometrial carcinoma is the most common gynecologic malignancy in North America, with an estimated 36,000 new cases in the United States in 1997 [1]. Approximately 6300 deaths will occur from uterine cancer this year, reflecting its relatively favorable prognosis when compared to ovarian and cervical cancer. Endometrial cancer is primarily a disease of postmenopausal women, with the incidence rising rapidly after menopause and peaking between the ages of 55–65 years. Cases do occasionally develop in women of reproductive age, though account for only about 5% of cases. The incidence of uterine cancer among White women is about twice that of African-American women, possibly reflecting the greater prevalence of hormone replacement therapy among White women. African American women are, however, nearly twice as likely to die from this disease. The age-adjusted mortality rate of endometrial cancer for African American women is 6.0 (per 100,000) versus 3.3 in White women [2]. Five-year survival rate for African American women averages 55% and is substantially less than the 86% survival rate in White women. Black women present more often with tumors of unfavorable histology, higher grade, and possibly more advanced disease.

It is generally believed that most cases of endometrial adenocarcinoma develop from prexisting endometrial hyperplasia, and typically reflect the effect of unopposed estrogen stimulation (either endogenous or iatrogenic). The risk and rate of progression to cancer is not well defined, though hyperplasia with atypical glandular histology is considered to carry a much higher risk of progression to cancer in comparison to simple or complex hyperplasia without cytologic atypia. It is now clear that some cases of endometrial adenocarcinoma develop in the absence of hyperplasia, and are often characterized by poorer grade and histologic subtype, and carry a worse prognosis than the more typical estrogen related carcinomas.

Numerous factors have been identified which are associated with either an increase, or decrease in the risk of developing endometrial adenocarcinoma. Unopposed estrogen stimulation is a strong risk factor, increasing the risk 4–8 times over non-estrogen users. Risk increases with both duration and amount of estrogen exposure, and histologic evidence of endometrial hyperplasia may develop within a few months of unopposed estrogen use. Progestin therapy, either alone or in conjunction with estrogen therapy reduces the risk of endometrial cancer and presently all postmenopausal women with an intact uterus placed on hormone therapy should receive some form of combination estrogen-progestin therapy. Oral contraceptive use also decreases the relative risk of endometrial cancer to about 0.5, with the protective effect beginning about 1 year after starting therapy and lasting for up to 15 years after completion of therapy.

Endogenous long-term estrogen stimulation from feminizing ovarian tumors or polycystic ovarian syndrome also increases the risk of endometrial cancer, though the absolute number of cases due to these diseases is quite small. Obesity, nulliparity, and late menopause also subject the endometrium to relatively high, or prolonged estrogen stimulation and are well established risk factors. The relative risk increases 3 fold for women 20–50 pounds overweight, and 10 times for those greater than 50 pounds overweight. Late menopause (>52 years) and nulliparity increase the relative risk from 2–3 times. Diabetes and hypertension are associated with an increase risk but are commonly present in women with other risk factors including obesity and the biologic explanation underlying the adverse risk associated with these conditions has not been identified.

Tamoxifen use in women with breast cancer increases the relative risk of endometrial cancer 6–7 fold, with the risk being most pronounced after two years of use [3]. Both well differentiated and high grade tumors have been described. Tamoxifen, as a result of its estrogen agonist effect on the uterus, commonly gives rise to an abnormally thickened endometrium. Uterine bleeding is relatively uncommon, though if this occurs, histologic assessment of the uterus to exclude malignancy is required.

**Pathology**

Histologic Types

Approximately 90% of uterine malignancies arise from the endometrium. Several histologic subtypes are recognized, with endometrioid adenocarcinoma comprising about 80% of cases. Primary uterine sarcomas (including mixed carcinosarcomas) are rare and account for approximately 10% of uterine malignancies.

The types of endometrial adenocarcinomas are:
– Typical endometrioid adenocarcinoma
– Adenosquamous carcinoma
– Clear cell carcinoma
– Serous carcinoma
– Secretory carcinoma
– Mucinous carcinoma
– Squamous carcinoma
– Mixed cell types

Endometrial carcinomas are graded depending upon the degree of glandular differentiation and atypical nuclear features (G1, well differentiated; G2, moderately differentiated; G3, poorly differentiated). Grade 1 tumors demonstrate well preserved, though crowded glandular architecture in at least 95% of the tumor. In grade 3 tumors, less than 50% of the tumor retains glandular differentiation, with most areas being solid, without glandular lumens or stroma. The presence of significant nuclear atypia is also considered in tumor grading, and if present will increase the grade in tumors with G1 or G2 glandular architecture. Squamous differentiation is seen in approximately 30% of endometrial tumors and usually consists of benign squamous elements of no prognostic significance (adenoacanthoma). If the squamous component resembles squamous cell carcinoma (adenosquamous carcinoma), the prognosis is generally worse than pure endometrioid tumors. When correcting for coexistent glandular differentiation (typically poor) and myometrial invasion, an independent adverse impact of the malignant squamous component has not been proven.

Clear cell carcinomas of the endometrium resemble clear cell adenocarcinomas of the ovary and cervix. In comparison to typical endometrioid tumors, clear cell adenocarcinoma generally occurs at a later age, is less often associated with hormone use, and carries a much worse prognosis, due to its propensity for early hematogenous and lymphatic dissemination.

Serous carcinomas, which account for approximately 5%–10% of endometrial cancers, are highly aggressive and, like clear cell adenocarcinomas, carry a worse prognosis [4]. Histologically these tumors resemble ovarian papillary serous carcinoma and like ovarian cancer, intraperitoneal metastasis is common, even with tumors grossly confined to the uterus. Several cases of metastatic serous carcinoma have been reported in patients without any apparent myometrial invasion and for these reasons all patients are considered at high risk for recurrence. Adjuvent therapy is typically offered following surgery, though the efficacy of this approach has not been proven.

Secretory adenocarcinomas are extremely rare, and have typically been reported in premenopausal women, often in the presence of progestational influence. Surgery is usually curative, as these tumors tend to be of low grade with little myometrial invasion. Mucinous and primary squamous tumors are also quite rare, with mucinous tumors having a relatively good prognosis and squamous cell carcinomas a less favorable prognosis. Removal of the uterus and adnexa is necessary to exclude the presence of an occult primary cervical or ovarian tumor, and adjuvent therapy should be individualized.

## Signs and Symptoms

An effective screening system for endometrial cancer has not been established. The most common presenting symptom is postmenopausal vaginal bleeding. In the absence of bleeding, endometrial cancer occasionally presents with abdominal pain associated with an obstructed, blood filled uterus, or rarely abnormal endometrial cells on routine Pap screening. An abnormally thickened endometrial stripe, as assessed by ultrasound or MRI, may also suggest the presence of endometrial cancer or hyperplasia, though neither test is likely to be clinically useful in asymptomatic patients.

Diagnosis is established through endometrial biopsy, usually obtained as a minor office procedure. With small tissue samples it is occasionally difficult to distinguish complex hyperplasia from adenocarcinoma. In select cases it may be necessary to perform a dilation and curettage under anesthesia to obtain additional tissue for analysis.

**Table 1.** FIGO classification of endometrial carcinoma

| | | |
|---|---|---|
| Stage | Ia G123 | Tumor limited to endometrium |
| | Ib G123 | Invasion of less than half of the myometrium |
| | Ic G123 | Invasin of more than half of the myometrium |
| | IIa G123 | Endocervical glandular involvement only |
| | IIb G123 | Cervical stromal invasion |
| | IIIa G123 | Tumor invades serosa and/or adnexae and or positive peritoneal cytology |
| | IIIb G123 | Vaginal metastases |
| | IIIc G123 | Metastases to pelvic and/or para-aortic lymph nodes |
| | IVa G123 | Tumor invasion of bladder and/or bowel mucosa |
| | IVb | Distant metastases, including intraabdominal and/or inguinal lymph node |

Histopathology: Degree of differentiation
Cases of carcinoma of the corpus should be grouped according to the degree of differentiation of the adenocarcinoma as follows:
G1 = 5% or less of a nonsquamous or nonmorular solid growth patter
G2 = 6% to 50% of a nonsquamous or nonmorular solid growth pattern
G3 = more than 50% of a nonsquamous or nonmorular solid growth pattern

## Staging and Prognostic Factors

The International Federation of Gynecology and Obstetrics (FIGO) introduced a surgical staging classification system for endometrial carcinoma in 1988 (Table 1). Prior to this time a clinical staging system was utilized, and remains relevant for patients treated only with radiation therapy. With surgical staging, a particular emphasis is placed on the degree of myometrial invasion, which is prognostically important, and not reliably determined with clinical assessment.

The natural history and prognosis of endometrial carcinoma is influenced by a variety of factors [5]. Clinically relevant risk factors include patient age, race, tumor stage and medical co-morbidities. Younger women (<55 years) have a better prognosis than older women, with tumor grade and stage tending to increase with advancing age. Tumor stage is the most well recognized prognostic factor for endometrial adenocarcinoma. Overall, 5-year survival is about 75%, which is due primarily to the early stage of presentation in the majority of cases (Table 2).

Pathologic risk factors are generally grouped into uterine and extrauterine prognostic factors. Uterine factors include histologic cell type, tumor grade, depth of myometrial invasion, tumor size, capillary or lymphatic vessel involvement, and extension to the cervix. Extrauterine fac-

**Table 2.** Carcinoma of the corpus uteri 1987–1989; 5-year survival in collected series of patients; distribution by stage (n=13,040; from [12])

| Stage | 5-Year survival | Proportion of cases |
|-------|-----------------|---------------------|
| I     | 86%             | 72%                 |
| II    | 66%             | 14%                 |
| III   | 44%             | 9%                  |
| IV    | 16%             | 5%                  |

Includes both surgically and clinically staged patients.

tors include adnexal metastasis, intraperitoneal involvement, lymph node metastasis, and positive peritoneal cytology. Risk of extrauterine disease is most strongly related to depth of uterine invasion, followed by tumor grade [6]. The risk of lymph node involvement is <1% for patients whose tumor is confined to the endometrium. With invasion confined to the inner half of the myometrium, the risk of nodal involvement is increased to about 5%, and less if the tumor is grade 1 or 2. If the outer half of the myometrium is involved, the risk of pelvic or para-aortic lymph node involvement is increased to about 25%.

The clinical relevance of molecular markers including estrogen or progesterone receptor status, DNA ploidy, pre-treatment CA 125 level, and tumor p53 mutation status have not been clearly established and are usually not considered in primary treatment decisions.


Preoperative Evaluation

Once endometrial adenocarcinoma has been established through endo-metrial biopsy, a pelvic examination is performed to determine if there is clinically apparent penetration of the tumor beyond the uterus. In >75% of patients there will be no clinical evidence of extrauterine disease, and further indicated studies would normally include only a chest X-ray and routine blood tests. The clinical benefit of more extensive preoperative testing including CT scans, MRI, IVP or barium enema in patients without symptoms of extrauterine pathology is not proven, though occasionally provides useful information in the subset of patients with poor prognostic tumors (serous, clear cell, or poorly differentiated histology). Patients with abnormal liver function tests or symptoms suggesting metastatic disease should undergo confirmatory studies, which can help guide decisions regarding the risks versus benefits of surgery.

## Preoperative Radiotherapy

In the past, it was quite common to administer preoperative radiation therapy to the majority of patients prior to hysterectomy. It was felt that radiation therapy could eradicate occult extrauterine disease confined to the pelvis more efficiently and perhaps more safely if the uterus remained in place during radiation. With this approach, most patients with clinical stage 1 tumors received intracavitary brachytherapy followed shortly thereafter by surgery. This approach led to a proportion of individuals receiving radiation therapy for tumors at very low risk for metastasis. More recently, the emphasis has been on surgical staging, followed occasionally by postoperative adjuvent irradiation after assessment of intraoperative and pathologic findings.

## Surgical Staging

Surgery is performed through an incision adequate to evaluate the upper abdominal structures and to remove para-aortic lymph nodes, if necessary. Peritoneal washing are collected for cytology and the abdomen and pelvis are carefully assessed for any obvious evidence of extrauterine disease. Suspicious lymph nodes should be resected, or biopsied if unresectable. An extrafascial, total hysterectomy and bilateral salpingo-oophorectomy is then performed. In the absence of obvious metastatic disease, the uterus is opened off the field to determine the extent of tumor and to help guide whether to perform selective lymph node sampling in the absence of suspicious nodes. Relative depth of myometrial invasion (none, inner half, outer half), and the presence or absence of cervical involvement can be determined grossly in almost all cases. If necessary, a frozen section analysis can be performed. Indications for selective pelvic and para-aortic lymph node sampling include:
- Invasion into the outer half of the myometrium
- Presence of tumor involving the cervix
- Clinically apparent adnexal metastasis
- Serous, clear cell, squamous or poorly differentiated histology

Para-aortic lymph nodes are removed from below the level of the inferior mesenteric artery; on the right side over the vena cava, and on the left side along the lateral aspect of the aorta. If pelvic lymph nodes are sampled, nodes from the distal common iliac artery, external iliac artery and vein, hypogastric artery, and above the obturator nerve are removed.

Postoperative Therapy

Patients with confirmed extra-uterine endometrial cancer are at high risk for recurrence and death and are appropriate candidates for adjuvent therapy with radiation therapy, chemotherapy, hormone therapy, or a combination of these modalities. The role of adjuvent therapy for women with tumors apparently confined to the uterus is less clear. Most of these patients are at low risk for recurrence and do quite well without additional treatment. Mathematical models are being devised to identify stage I and II patients at increased risk of recurrence (generally considered as a 5-year survival of 80% or less) in an effort to help clinicians and patients with decisions regarding the potential efficacy of adjuvent therapy [6].

The GOG has recently analyzed results of a large, randomized study of surgery versus surgery plus adjuvent pelvic radiation therapy in intermediate risk endometrial adenocarcinoma. All 392 evaluable patients were surgically staged and had stage IB, IC, or II (occult) tumors. Risk factors (depth of invasion and grade) did not differ significantly between the two treatment arms. Grade 3 tumors and outer third myometrial invasion each comprised about 18% of cases. The 2-year recurrence free interval in the surgery plus radiation group was 96% and for the surgery only group, 87%. As some surgery only patients were treated and probably cured with radiation therapy following identification of a localized pelvic recurrence, the differences in 2-year survival between the two groups were less appreciable; 95% with surgery alone versus 97% for surgery plus radiation therapy [7]. The best treatment for patients with myometrial invasion who have not undergone complete surgical staging cannot be answered from this study. Similarly, as only a relatively small proportion of tumors in the GOG study were grade 3 or deeply invasive, some clinicians will continue to recommend that all patients with localized tumors demonstrating high risk cell types (serous, clear cell and grade 3 endometrioid) and especially in conjunction with one or more additional high risk factors (myometrial invasion >50%, vascular space involvement or cervical involvement) should be considered as candidates for adjuvent therapy with either postoperative pelvic radiation (4500–5000 cGy) or chemotherapy.

Vaginal ovoid brachytherapy following surgery is a reasonable approach in patients felt to be at low risk for lymph node metastasis. Following surgery alone, approximately 10% of patients will develop a vaginal recurrence. This risk may be substantially reduced by treatment with intracavitary radiation. Both high-dose rate (HDR) and low-dose rate (LDR) techniques are acceptable. Vaginal cuff brachytherapy is not generally administered in conjunction with external-beam radiation therapy.

Stage II Disease

Cervical involvement with endometrial carcinoma is an adverse prognostic variable, and treatment decisions should be made on an individual basis. Important factors include depth of cervical involvement (whether confined to the endocervical glands or extending to the cervical stroma), occult involvement identified after surgery versus preoperative clinically apparent disease, and the presence or absence of other recognized risk factors (cell type, nodal involvement, and myometrial invasion). It is probably sufficient to treat patients with occult endocervical glandular involvement with surgery alone, or with vaginal cuff brachytherapy. If the cervix is grossly involved with cancer (previously considered as clinical stage II) preoperative pelvic irradiation is given, followed by extrafascial hysterectomy, though primary radical hysterectomy, as utilized for cervical cancer, has also been used with success. The optimal management of patients with smaller tumors penetrating into the cervical stroma (stage II B) has not been identified. Most of these patients will be cured with surgery, though overall, the risk of lymph node involvement and vaginal cuff recurrence is higher than for patients with cancer confined to the uterine fundus. Typically, these tumors are treated with either whole pelvic radiotherapy or vaginal brachytherapy. Given the risk of death associated with distant relapse in stage IIB patients, adjuvent chemotherapy has also been used on occasion, though the small numbers of patients treated in this manner do not permit any conclusions regarding the efficacy of this approach.

Stage III and IV Disease

Extension of endometrial cancer beyond the uterus is correlated with a high risk of relapse and death. Tumor free survival at 3 years for stage III/IV disease averages about 30%, but ranges from near 80% to under 5% depending upon various clinical and pathologic features. For example, uterine serosal involvement, adnexal involvement or positive peritoneal washings (stage IIIa) is associated with survival rates ranging from 50%–80%. With uterine serosal or adnexal involvement postoperative pelvic irradiation is typically administered to 4500–5000 cGy though the efficacy of this approach in comparison to surgery alone or more extensive whole abdominal radiotherapy has not been tested in randomized trials. Management of patients with positive peritoneal cytology is even more unclear. In the absence of significant concurrent intrauterine high risk factors, the impact of malignant peritoneal cytology is uncertain, and many patients are followed without adjuvent therapy. Patients with concurrent high risk pathologic features have typically received adjuvent therapy, often consisting of pelvic or whole abdominal irradiation, chemotherapy, or occasionally intraperitoneal radioactive colloidal P-32.

Extension to pelvic or para-aortic nodes is associated with 3 year relapse free-survival rates of approximately 30%. Standard treatment recommendations include irradiation to the pelvis in the case of isolated pelvic nodal metastasis, though many radiation oncologists will utilize extended-field irradiation to encompass the para-aortic regions in patients with common iliac nodal disease. Para-aortic involvement is treated with extended-field irradiation, though cure is unlikely, primarily due to the development of upper abdominal or distant relapse.

Clinically apparent extension of endometrial adenocarcinoma into the vagina or parametria usually precludes a primary surgical approach. Treatment in these rare cases should be individualized, with most patients receiving definitive radiation therapy. Some patients will experience enough regression of tumor with either radiation or neoadjuvent chemotherapy that a hysterectomy may later be accomplished. Though most of these patients will subsequently develop extrapelvic recurrence, it is generally felt that quality of life is frequently improved with removal of the primary tumor.

Whole abdominal irradiation has been utilized as an adjunctive treatment for patients with stage III and optimally resected (<2 cm) stage IV disease. Some centers have reported favorable results utilizing this approach, with 5 year relapse-free survivals over 50% [9]. The GOG, in a phase II study completed in 1992, prospectively evaluated whole abdominal radiotherapy. Although data analysis is incomplete, toxicity was acceptable, though 3-year survival was only about 33%. Presently the GOG is conducting a phase III trial comparing whole abdominal radiotherapy to chemotherapy with combination doxorubicin-cisplatin in patients with optimally resected, advanced endometrial adenocarcinoma.

## Treatment of Incompletely Resected and Recurrent Disease

The best therapy for endometrial cancer following surgical staging and maximal cytoreduction is not known, and all patients with recurrent or metastatic disease should be encouraged to participate in clinical trials. Patients with locoregional recurrence following surgery can occasionally be cured with radiation therapy, provided this was not administered previously. Small vaginal cuff recurrences are most successfully treated, with therapy usually consisting of external-beam irradiation and the use of vaginal brachytherapy. Patients with isolated central recurrence following standard surgery and radiation therapy may be considered for pelvic exenteration, though there are no large published series describing the efficacy of this approach. Nevertheless, long-term survivors have been reported, and pelvic exenteration remains the only reasonable chance of cure in this rare subset of patients.

Endocrine therapy with progestins, tamoxifen, or both has been tried, with response rates averaging 15%–20%. Duration of response is only about 4 months and median survival less than a year. Occasionally complete responses are noted, typically in patients with well differentiated tumors and late recurrence. Both oral and parenteral regimens have been tried and appear equivalent. Most clinicians begin with 80–320 mg of megestrol acetate daily. Tamoxifen has been shown to increase progestin-receptor expression in previously untreated endometrial cancer though the clinical significance of this observation is unknown. The GOG has completed a phase II trial of daily tamoxifen in combination with alternating weeks of medroxyprogesterone to examine this issue, though no conclusions have yet been reported.

Systemic chemotherapy has been disappointing when given to patients with endometrial carcinoma. Results of a phase III GOG study reported in 1993 noted a 45% response rate, including 22% complete responses, for the combination of cisplatin and doxorubicin (cisplatin 50 mg/m2; doxorubicin 60 mg/m²) in advanced or recurrent endometrial carcinoma [10] with measurable disease. This was significantly superior to the 27% response rate in the doxorubicin alone arm. There was no clinically relevant difference in survival, as shown by the less than 10% progression free survival at two years.

Recently the GOG completed a phase II study of single-agent paclitaxel (24-hour continuous infusion, 250 mg/m², with G-CSF support) in patients with advanced endometrial carcinoma who had not received prior chemotherapy. An overall response rate of 36% with 14% complete response was observed [11]. Given the activity of taxol in endometrial carcinoma, the GOG is presently conducting a randomized, phase III study of doxorubicin plus cisplatin versus doxorubicin plus 24-hour paclitaxel (with G-CSF) in patients with advanced or recurrent endometrial carcinoma.

### References

1. Landis SH, Murray T, Bolden S, Wingo PA: Cancer statistics, 1998. CA Cancer J Clin:48:6–29, 1998
2. Miller BA, Ries LAG, Hankey BF, Kosary CL, Harras A, Devesa SS, Edwards BK (eds): SEER cancer statistics review: 1973–1990. Bethesda, MD: National Cancer Institute; MH Publication 93:2789, 1993
3. Rayter, Sheperd J, Gazrt JC: Tamoxifen and endometrial lesions. Lancet 343:1124, 1993
4. Sutton GP, Brill L: Malignant papillary lesions of the endometrium. Gynecol Oncol 27:294–304, 1987
5. Kosary CL: FIGO stage, histology, histologic grade, age, and race as prognostic factors in determining survival for cancers of the female gynecologic system: an analysis of 1973–1987 SEER cases of cancers of the endometrium, cervix, ovary, vulva and vagina. Sem Surg Oncol 10:31–46, 1994
6. Morrow CP, Bundy BN, Kurman RJ, et al. Relationship between surgical-pathological risk factors and outcome in clinical stage I and II carcinoma of the endometrium: A Gynecologic Oncology Group study. Gynecol Oncol 40:55–65, 1991
7. Roberts JA, Brunetto VL, Keys HM, Zaino R, Spirtos NM, Bloss JD, Pearlman A, Maiman M, Bell J. A phase III randomized study of surgery vs surgery plus adjunctive radiation therapy in intermediate-risk endometrial adenocarcinoma (GOG No. 99). Gynecol Oncol 68:134 1998 (abstract)
8. Zaino RJ, Kurman RJ, Diana KL, et al. Pathologic models to predict outcome for women with endometrial adenocarcinoma: the importance of the distinction between surgical stage and clinical stage: A Gynecologic Oncology Group study. Cancer 77:1115–1121, 1996
9. Martinez A, Schray M, Podratz K, et al. Postoperative whole abdominopelvic irradiation for patients with high risk endometrial carcinoma. Int J Radiat Oncol Biol Phys 17:371–377, 1989

10. Thigpen T, Blessing J, Homesley H et al. Phase III trial of doxorubicin±cisplatin in advanced or recurrent endometrial carcinoma: A Gynecologic Oncology Group study. Proc Am Soc Clin Oncol 12:261, 1993

11. Ball HG, Blessing JA, Lentz SS, et al. A phase II trial of taxol in advanced and recurrent adenocarcinoma of the endometrium: A Gynecologic Oncology Group study. Gynecol Oncol 62:278–281, 1996

12. Pettersson F, Creaseman WT, Shepherd JH, et al. Annual report on the results of treatment in gynecologic cancer: vol. 22, Stockholm, 1995, International Federation of Gynecology and Obstetrics

# Ovarian Cancer

M. Markman

## Epidemiology, Risk Factors [1]

**Incidence.** Ovarian cancer is the leading cause of death from female gynecologic malignancies in the United States, exceeding the death rate from cancers of the endometrium and cervix combined. There are approximately 27,000 new cases of ovarian cancer in the United States each year, and 15,000 deaths. It has been estimated that a woman has a lifetime risk of developing ovarian cancer of approximately 1 in 70 [2].

**Age Distribution.** Ovarian cancer develops most commonly in women beyond the age of 50, with an increasing incidence during the next two decades of life.

**Location.** While ovarian cancer begins in either one or both ovaries, <15%–20% of individuals developing this cancer will be found to have disease confined to the ovaries at the time of diagnosis. Overall, approximately 70% of women will be discovered to have stage III or IV disease at initial presentation.

**Risk Factors/Etiology.** A family history of ovarian cancer appears to be the most important risk factor for the development of this malignancy [2]. With one family member known to have ovarian cancer, the lifetime risk for ovarian cancer for another women in the family increases to approximately 5% (compared to a risk for the general population of 1.5%). This risk increases to 7% for two family members known to have the malignancy. However, in families with a true hereditary component (<5% of patients with the malignancy), with multiple cases of ovarian cancer or breast cancer within the family (strongly suggesting a direct mendelian inheritance pattern), the lifetime risk for development of this cancer can reach 50%. Mutations in BRCA-1 have been demonstrated to be associated with the development of ovarian cancer in approximately 80% of families with a history suggestive of hereditary ovarian cancer [3]. The presence of a specific BRCA-1 abnormality in an individual from a family with a strong history of ovarian cancer has been shown to predict a lifetime risk for the disease (or primary peritoneal carcinoma) as high as 80%.

A second risk factor for the development of ovarian cancer is parity, with a decreasing risk of the malignancy with increasing number of children. This observation supports the "incessant ovulation hypothesis" for the etiology of ovarian cancer. As ovulation requires subsequent proliferation of the epithelial surface to repair damage, the opportunity for the development of cancer in this setting should be reduced with fewer lifetime ovulatory cycles [4].

## Pathology and Staging

**Pathology.** Approximately 90% of ovarian cancers originate from the epithelium, with the large majority being adenocarcinomas. Invasive epithelial cancers are divided into histologic subtypes, including serious, mucinous, endometrioid, clear cell and undifferentiated.

Epithelial ovarian cancer of low malignant potential ("borderline tumor") are ovarian cancers which demonstrate atypia of cellular elements, but lack the invasive features of carcinomas. Even when found at an advanced stage, this group of ovarian cancers can be associated with prolonged survival, in the absence of systemic chemotherapy.

Other less common ovarian cancers include germ cell and sex cord stromal tumors, and ovarian sarcomas. Germ cell tumors of the ovary are quite similar in treatment strategies and outcome to their male counterparts (dysgerminomas (female) and seminomas (male); non-dysgerminomas and non-seminomas). Sex cord stromal tumors and ovarian sarcomas are rare cancers with poorly defined treatment strategies beyond surgical resection.

**Table 1.** FIGO ovarian cancer staging system and survival

| Stage | Status of tumor | Incidence | 5-Year survival |
|-------|-----------------|-----------|-----------------|
| I | Confined to ovaries | 10%–20% | 70%–85% |
| II | Confined to pelvis | 5%–10% | 40%–55% |
| III | Peritoneum or nodes | 60%–70% | 20%–35% |
| IV | Distant metastases | 10%–15% | 5% |

**Staging.** The major staging system for ovarian cancer is that of the International Federation of Gynecology and Obstetrics (FIGO) (Table 1). In this system a laparotomy is required to adequately assess the status of the tumor.

**Prognostic Factors.** Tumor grade is an important prognostic factor in ovarian cancer, and can significantly influence management decisions. For example, the long-term survival of women with grade 1, stage I epithelial ovarian cancer is >90%, without the administration of chemotherapy. In contrast, survival of patients with grade 3, stage I ovarian cancer patients is significantly lower, even with the delivery of cisplatin-based combination chemotherapy. In addition, tumor grade will influence the risk of relapse following the attainment of a surgically documented complete response to chemotherapy. Patients with stage III or IV, grade 3 tumors who achieve this clinical state experience a 50% risk of ultimate relapse, while the risk of developing recurrent disease is less in similar patients with lower grade tumors. Unfortunately, 60%–70% of all patients with advanced ovarian cancer will have high grade (grade 3) cancers.

There is little evidence in epithelial ovarian cancer that histologic subclass has important prognostic significance independent of stage and tumor grade. A potential exception to this are advanced clear cell and mucinous tumors of the ovary which appear to have a particularly poor prognosis.

Factors which negatively influence prognosis in early stage ovarian cancer, in addition to high tumor grade, include the presence of tumor excrescences on the surface of the ovary, dense adhesions between the ovary and other organs or pelvic side wall, and rupture of the ovarian capsule. In patients with advanced disease, response to chemotherapy and ultimate survival is strongly influenced by the amount of residual cancer remaining within the peritoneal cavity at the initiation of cytotoxic chemotherapy. The Gynecologic Oncology Group (GOG) has defined "optimal" stage III ovarian cancer as stage III disease whose largest residual mass is < 1 cm in maximum diameter. Patients whose largest diameter residual mass is >1 cm are considered to have "suboptimal" disease.

Other prognostic factors which have been suggested to be of clinical utility in ovarian cancer include DNA ploidy, p53 mutations, Her 2-neu overexpression, and a variety of drug resistance markers (e.g., MDR phenotype). However, none of these factors have been demonstrated to provide additional clinically relevant information beyond that currently defined through knowledge of surgically defined stage and tumor grade.

## Work-up and Staging

The appropriate pre-operative work-up for patients with suspected ovarian cancer includes the following: CBC, serum chemistries, clotting studies, chest radiograph, EKG, and serum CA-125. If there remains a question regarding the etiology of symptoms (e.g., abdominal pain, bloating) or signs suggestive of ovarian cancer (e.g., pelvic or abdominal mass, ascites), additional tests might include a pelvic ultrasound or CT scan of the abdominal and pelvis, stool test for occult blood, serum CEA, and upper or lower gastrointestinal radiographic studies or endoscopy. Tests which are clearly not indicated in the evaluation of women with suspected ovarian cancer include liver/spleen and bone scans, lymphangiograms or CT scans of the chest or brain.

The serum level of CA-125 is not a useful test for the diagnosis of ovarian cancer as it is elevated in a number of malignancies involving the peritoneal cavity, and is frequently abnormal in several benign conditions which may mimic malignancy (e.g., pelvic inflammatory disease, alcoholic hepatitis or cirrhosis, endometriosis) [5, 6]. In addition, only 50% of patients with early stage ovarian cancer will have an elevated value, and even in the presence of far advanced disease approximately 10%–20% of patients will have normal serum levels. The serum level of CA-125 is of clinical utility in following the course of therapy in patients with known ovarian cancer [7].

## Stage Specific Standard Treatment Options

**Surgical Treatment (Early Stage).** As previously mentioned, surgery plays a major role in management of women with early stage (Stage I and II) ovarian cancer. In a small subset of women with ovarian cancer (Stage I, grade 1) surgical resection of the tumor will be definitive treatment. While there remains some disagreement regarding the need for chemotherapy in patients with Stage I, grade 2 cancers, all other individuals will be treated with chemotherapy in addition to surgical resection [8].

**Radiotherapy (Early Stages).** As standard therapy for ovarian cancer includes surgical staging and aggressive tumor debulking, there is no role for radiation as a substitute for surgical resection. The role of radiotherapy as a substitute for chemotherapy in early stage disease remains highly controversial. There have been no recent studies directly comparing whole abdominal radiotherapy (required in ovarian cancer due to the pattern of spread of the malignancy) to modern chemotherapy (a platinum agent and paclitaxel). In view of the concern for the toxicity of whole abdominal radiation in individuals who have recently undergone an exploratory laparotomy, the absence of a systemic effect of local radiation, and the limited ability to deliver tumoricidal doses of radiation to the upper abdomen (toxicity to normal organs), radiation has been relegated in most centers to a palliative modality in recurrent ovarian cancer.

**Combined Modality Therapy.** The standard initial treatment program for advanced ovarian cancer is surgery followed by combination platinum plus paclitaxel chemotherapy (Table 2) [9, 10]. Based on the results of a large randomized controlled trial it would be appropriate to deliver cisplatin by the intraperitoneal route in women with optimal residual ovarian cancer, in combination with systemic paclitaxel [11]. There is currently no evidence that adding a third or fourth drug to the two drug platinum/paclitaxel combination results in a superior clinical outcome [12]. Several randomized trials have examined the issue of dose intensity for platinum in ovarian cancer [13, 14]. Based on the results of these studies, there is no evidence to suggest a more dose intensive platinum regimen than employed in standard clinical practice results in a superior outcome (progression-free or overall survival).

**Second-Line Chemotherapy.** Despite the high response rate (70%–80%) to initial chemotherapy in advanced ovarian cancer, the majority of women with this malignancy will ultimately relapse and will be candidates for a second-line chemotherapy strategy [2]. Options in this clini-

**Table 2.** Front-line chemotherapy regimens in advanced ovarian cancer

1. Cisplatin (75 mg/m$^2$) plus paclitaxel (135 mg/m$^2$
   delivered over 24 h)
2. Carboplatin (AUC 6–7) plus paclitaxel (175 mg/m$^2$
   delivered over 3 h)

cal setting include the administration of the same therapy previously employed, single agent cisplatin, carboplatin, or paclitaxel, or a new agent. In general, patients who have tolerated the initial regimen, have evidence of a response to the program, and have experienced a treatment-free interval of at least 4–6 months, are appropriate candidates to receive the same drug(s) previously employed [15]. In contrast, with a shorter treatment-free interval, or when there has been no response to initial therapy, alternative drugs or experimental trials should be considered. Antineoplastic drugs with evidence of activity (>10%–15% response rate, generally of short duration) in platinum-resistant ovarian cancer in phase 3 (topotecan only) or phase 2 clinical trials include: topotecan [16], oral etoposide (20 day regimen) [17], liposomal doxorubicin [18], gemcitabine [19], vinorelbine [20], ifosfamide [21], and altretamine [22]. The choice of therapy in this clinical setting should include consideration of the toxicity of the available drugs, the individual's prior experience with side effects of chemotherapy, and performance status.

**High Dose Chemotherapy.** A number of investigators have examined several high dose chemotherapy programs in the management of ovarian cancer, as a component of initial chemotherapy, at the time of relapse or the finding of persistent disease following front-line treatment, or as a consolidation strategy [23]. While high response rates have been reported in phase 1 and 2 clinical trials of high dose chemotherapy, and prolonged survival suggested, all such trials have involved a highly select group of women with this malignancy. A recently activated NCI-sponsored randomized trial will examine the role of high dose chemotherapy, versus continuation of a more standard dose carboplatin/paclitaxel regimen, in women with ovarian cancer who have attained a clinically or surgically defined response to platinum-paclitaxel combination chemotherapy.

**Biological Response Modifiers/Cytokines/Hormone Therapy.** There is currently no evidence of a role for biological response modifiers or cytokines in the management of ovarian cancer. An ongoing Intergroup randomized trial is examining the role of intraperitoneal alpha-interferon as consolidation therapy of patients with ovarian cancer who achieve a surgically defined complete response, but have a >50% risk for ultimate relapse.

Tamoxifen has been demonstrated to be an active agent in platinum-refractory ovarian cancer (10%–15% objective response rate) [24]. This is a reasonable drug to consider as one option in individuals with platinum-refractory disease in view of its favorable toxicity profile compared to alternative antineoplastic agents in this clinical setting.

**Current Key Questions.** Several important issues in the management of ovarian cancer remain unresolved, including: (a) the role of intraperitoneal chemotherapy as initial, second-line, and consolidation therapy; (b) the role of high dose chemotherapy regimens; (c) the role of interval surgical tumor debulking in individuals who have persistent tumor masses despite a response to chemotherapy; (d) the role in initial therapy of the multiple agents which have been demonstrated to have activity in platinum-refractory disease; (f) the importance of a variety of biological factors in prognosis and determining management (e.g., Her 2-neu, p-53); (g) the clinical utility of "neoadjuvant chemotherapy" employed prior to an attempt at maximum surgical tumor removal in patients with large volume intraperitoneal cancer [25]; and (h) the role of biological (e.g, monoclonal antibodies, vaccines), anti-angiogenesis and anti-metastatic agents in patient management.

**Current and Future Investigational Approaches.** Current trials in ovarian cancer have focused on defining optimal chemotherapy as initial treatment of ovarian cancer. Investigative efforts in the second-line setting have attempted to define the level of activity of "new drugs" in individuals with platinum and paclitaxel refractory disease. Future studies will need to examine the clinical utility of adding of a third or fourth drug to platinum and paclitaxel as initial therapy of ovarian cancer, and explore the benefits of novel strategies (e.g. biological therapies, drug resistance reversal agents).

### References

1. Parazzini F, Franceschi S, La Vechia C, et al (1991) The epidemiology of ovarian cancer. Gynecol Oncol 43:9–23
2. Cannistra SA (1993) Cancer of the ovary. N Engl J Med 329:1550–1558
3. Stratton JF, Gayther SA, Russell P, et al (1997) Contribution of BRCA1 mutations to ovarian cancer. N Engl J Med 336:1125–1130
4. Schildkraut JM, Bastos E, Berchuck A (1997) Relationship between lifetime ovulatory cycles and overexpression of mutant p53 in epithelial ovarian cancer. J Natl Ca Inst 89:932–938

5. Carlson KJ, Skates SJ, Singer DE (1994) Screening for ovarian cancer. Ann Intern Med 121:124–132
6. Schapira MM, Matchar DB, Young MJ (1993) The effectiveness of ovarian cancer screening. A decision analysis model. Ann Intern Med 118:38–843
7. Rustin GJS, Nelstrop AE, McClean P, et al (1996) Defining response of ovarian carcinoma to initial chemotherapy according to serum CA 125. J Clin Oncol 14:1545–1551
8. Munoz KA, Harlan LC, Trimble EL (1997) Patterns of care for women with ovarian cancer in the United States. J Clin Oncol 15:3408–3415
9. μguire WP, Hoskins WJ, Brady MF, Kucera PR, Partridge EE, Look KY, Clarke-Pearson DL, Davidson M (1996) Cyclophosphamide and cisplatin compared with paclitaxel and cisplatin in patients with stage III and stage IV ovarian cancer. N Engl J Med 334:1–6.
10. Stuart G, James K, Cassidy J, Kaye S, Hoctin Boes G, Timmers P, Roy JA, Pecorelli S (1997) Is cisplatin-paclitaxel (P-T) the standard in first-line treatment of advanced ovarian cancer (Ov Ca)? The EORTC-GCCG, NOCOVA, NCI-C and Scottish intergroup experience. Proc ASCO 16:352a
11. Alberts DS, Liu PY, Hannigan EV, O'Toole R, Williams SD, Young JA, Franklin EW, Clarke-Pearson DL, Malviya VK, DuBeshter B, Adelson MD, Hoskins WJ (1996) Intraperitoneal cisplatin plus intravenous cyclophosphamide versus intravenous cisplatin plus intravenous cyclophosphamide for stage III ovarian cancer. N Engl J Med 335:1950–1955
12. Omura GA, Bundy BN, Berek JS, et al (1989) Randomized trial of cyclophosphamide plus cisplatin with or without doxorubicin in ovarian carcinoma: a Gynecologic Oncology Group study. J Clin Oncol 7:457–465
13. μguire WP, Hoskins WJ, Brady MF, et al (1995) Assessment of dose-intensive therapy in suboptimally debulked ovarian cancer: a Gynecologic Oncology Group study. J Clin Oncol 13:1589–1599
14. Gore ME, Mainwaring PN, Macfarlane V, et al (1996) A randomized study of high-versus standard-dose carboplatin in patients with advanced epithelial ovarian cancer. Proc ASCO 15:284a
15. Markman M, Rothman R, Hakes T, Reichman B, Hoskins W, Rubin S, Jones W, Almadrones L, Lewis JL Jr (1991) Second-line platinum therapy in patients with ovarian cancer previously treated with cisplatin. J Clin Oncol 9:389–393
16. ten Bokkel Huinink W, Gore M, Carmichael J, Gordon A, Malfetano J, Hudson I, Broom C, Scarabelli C, Davidson N, Spanczynski M, Bolis G, Malmstrom H, Coleman R, Fields SC, Heron J-F (1997) Topotecan versus paclitaxel for the treatment of recurrent epithelial ovarian cancer. J Clin Oncol 15:2183–2193
17. Hoskins PJ, Swenerton KD (1994) Oral etoposide is active against platinum-resistant epithelial ovarian cancer. J Clin Oncol 12:60–63
18. Muggia FM, Hainsworth JD, Jeffers S, Miller P, Groshen S, Tan M, Romon L, Uziel B, Muderspach L, Garcia A, Burnett A, Greco FA, Morrow CP, Paradiso LJ, Liang L-J (1997) Phase II study of liposomal doxorubicin in refractory ovarian cancer: Antitumor activity and toxicity modification by liposomal encapsulation. J Clin Oncol 15:987–983
19. Lund B, Hansen OP, Theilade K, et al (1994) Phase II study of gemcitabine (2', 2'-difluorodeoxycytidine) in previously treated ovarian cancer patients. J Natl Cancer Inst 86:1530–1533
20. Burger RA, Burman S, White R, et al (1996) Phase II trial of navelbine in advanced epithelial ovarian cancer. Proc ASCO 15:286a
21. Markman M, Hakes T, Reichman B, et al (1991) Ifosfamide and mesna in previously treated advanced epithelial ovarian cancer: activity in platinum-resistant disease. J Clin Oncol 10:243–248

22. Vergote I, Himmelmann A, Frankendal B, et al (1992) Hexamethylmelamine as second-line therapy in platinum-resistant ovarian cancer. Gynecol Oncol 47:282–286
23. Stiff PJ, Bayer R, Kerger C, Potkul RK, Malhotra D, Peace DJ, Smith D, Fisher SG (1997) High-dose chemotherapy with autologous transplantation for persistent/relapsed ovarian cancer: A multivariate analysis of survival for 100 consecutively treated patients. J Clin Oncol 15:1309–1317
24. Markman M, Iseminger KA, Hatch KD, et al (1996) Tamoxifen in platinum-refractory ovarian cancer: a Gynecologic Oncology Group ancillary report. Gynecol Oncol 62:4–6
25. Surwit E, Childers J, Atlas I, Nour M, Hatch K, Hallum A, Alberts D (1996) Neoadjuvant chemotherapy for advanced ovarian cancer. Int J Gynecol Cancer 6:356–361

# Cervical, Vulvar, and Vaginal Cancer

S.E. Waggoner

## Cervical Cancer

Epidemiology, Risk Factors

Cervical cancer remains the world's most common gynecologic malignancy and in many developing countries is the leading cause of cancer death. In North America, the incidence of cervical cancer has significantly diminished over the last 50 years, primarily as a result of Pap smear screening. In 1998, it is estimated that about 14,000 American women will develop cervical cancer and 5000 women will die of the disease [1]. The median age at diagnosis is 47 years, with nearly half of all patients diagnosed below the age of 35 years. Older women (age >65 years) account for only about 10% of total cases, yet contribute to over 40% of the deaths from cervical cancer. The mortality rate for cervical cancer is about 25% higher for African American women in comparison to non-Hispanic White women, in spite of a similar reported frequency of Pap smear screening. African American women tend to be diagnosed with cervical cancer at later stage than White women, for unclear reasons.

Cervical cancer generally develops from a premalignant dysplastic lesion arising at the squamocolumnar junction. Cervical dysplasia, in turn, most often develops following infection with human papillomavirus (HPV) [2]. Sexual activity is the most common means of acquiring HPV, though most infections are self limiting and never result in any significant cervical lesion. Many different HPV types have been identified in the female anogenital tract, and several (i.e. types 16, 18, 31, 33, and 35) are strongly associated with cervical cancer. HPV probably exerts its oncogenic effect through interaction and disruption of normal p53 directed apoptosis.

Additional epidemiologic studies have indicated that early (<16 years) age of onset of sexual activity, increased total number of sexual partners (>4), and prior history of genital warts are adverse risk factors. Whether these observations simply reflect a greater risk of exposure to HPV or altered host factors is uncertain.

Cigarette smoking is a significant, independent risk factor for cervical carcinoma. Tobacco specific carcinogens have been identified in the cervical mucus of smokers and women exposed to second hand smoke. Cigarette smoking may also impair the effectiveness of treatment for locally advanced cervical cancer, possibly as a result of radiation resistant tumor hypoxia or diminished immune function.

Other causes of immune dysfunction including HIV infection, use of immunosuppressive medication, and chronic renal failure are associated with a higher risk of preinvasive and invasive cervical cancer. In contrast to immunocompetent individuals, HPV infection in women with immune dysfunction is generally chronic, and treatment of cervical dysplasia and cancer is less effective.

*Signs and Symptoms*

The most common sign of cervical cancer is abnormal vaginal bleeding, typically intermenstrual or postcoital. Less common presenting symptoms include pain, renal failure, or urinary incontinence due to vesicovaginal fistula. Many cases of early, occult, cervical cancer are diagnosed in asymptomatic women as a result of Pap smear screening. It is quite uncommon for an asymptomatic women to present with a clinically apparent cervical malignancy at the time of routine examination.

*Screening*

The exfoliative cervical cytology smear, or Pap smear, is a reliable, cost-effective, well accepted, and proven means of reducing the morbidity and mortality of cervical cancer in at risk populations. It is recommended that screening be initiated at the age of 18 years or the onset of sexual activity, and repeated annually until there have been three consecutive, normal results. In women without significant risk factors for cervical dysplasia, subsequent Pap smears can then be performed at less frequent intervals, though screening intervals longer than every three years should be avoided, as this will increase the likelihood of a precancerous lesion progressing to cancer. All patients with previously identified risk factors, including prior cervical dysplasia, smoking, immune dysfunction, or poor compliance with follow-up should be screened at annual intervals.

## Diagnosis

Though the Pap smear, clinical examination or colposcopy may suggest the presence of an invasive cervical lesion, the diagnosis of cervical cancer is confirmed only after a tissue biopsy. This may include a small punch biopsy from a gross lesion, or a conization specimen if the lesion appears small or possibly microinvasive. It is imperative that the biopsy be of sufficient depth to demonstrate invasion into the underlying stroma, otherwise distinguishing invasive cervical cancer from carcinoma in situ may be impossible.

## Pathology

Approximately 80% of primary cervical carcinomas arise from squamous epithelium. Nearly all squamous cell cancers of the uterine cervix develop from pre-existing squamous dysplasia, the detection of which is the primary goal of Pap smear screening. Adenocarcinoma of the cervix accounts for about 20% of invasive cervical cancers, and some evidence suggests that this proportion may be increasing. The development of cervical adenocarcimoma is not as well understood as that of squamous cancer. Adenocarcinoma in situ is probably the most common precursor lesion, and is detected much less efficiently by Pap smear screening than squamous lesions. As most adenocarcinomas develop within the endocervical canal, it is not uncommon for symptomatic patients to present with large, bulky lesions, and overall, the survival rate for patients with cervical adenocarcinoma is poorer in comparison to squamous lesions. When stage at diagnosis and tumor size are accounted for, the prognosis of squamous cell carcinoma and adenocarcinoma appear similar, and treatment decisions are typically made without regard to cell type.

## Staging and Prognosis

Presently, cervical cancer is staged clinically, and stage assigned primarily on the size of the tumor in the cervix or its extension into the pelvis (Table 1). Recent modifications in the International Federation of Obstetrics and Gynecology (FIGO) staging system have clarified the description of microinvasive cervical cancer (stage IA1 and IA2) and subdivide stage IB into IB1 (tumor <=4 cm) and IB2 (tumor >4 cm). In North America, approximately 60% of patients are diagnosed at stage I, 25% stage II, 10% stage III, and 5% stage IV.

**Table 1.** FIGO staging for carcinoma of the cervix uteri

| | |
|---|---|
| Stage 0 | Carcinoma in situ, intraepithelial carcinoma. |
| Stage I | The carcinoma is strictly confined to the cervix (extension to the corpus should be disregarded). |
| Stage IA | Invasive cancer identified only microscopically. All gross lesions even with superficial invasion are Stage IB cancers. Invasion is limited to measured stromal invasion with maximum depth of 5.0 mm and no wider than 7.0 mm. |
| Stage IA1 | Measured invasion of stroma no greater than 3.0 min in depth and no wider than 7.0 mm. |
| Stage IA2 | Measured invasion of stroma greater than 3.0 mm and no greater than 5.0 mm in depth and no wider than 7.0 mm. |
| Stage IB | Clinical lesions confined to the cervix or preclinical lesions greater than IA. |
| Stage IB1 | Clinical lesions no greater than 4.0 cm in size. |
| Stage IB2 | Clinical lesions greater than 4.0 cm in size. |
| Stage II | The carcinoma extends beyond the cervix but has not extended to the pelvic wall. The carcinoma involves the vagina butt not as far as the lower third. |
| Stage IIA | No obvious parametrial involvement |
| Stage IIB | Obvious parametrial involvement |
| Stage III | The carcinoma has extended to the pelvic wall. On rectal there is no cancerfree space between the tumor and the pelvic wall. The tumor involves the lower third of the vagina. All cases with a hydronephrosis or nonfunctioning kidney are included unless they are known to be due to other causes. |
| Stage IIIA | No extension to the pelvic wall. |
| Stage IIIB | Extension to the pelvic wall and/or hydronephrosis or nonfunctioning kidney. |
| Stage IV | The carcinoma has extended beyond the true pelvis or has clinically involved the mucosa of the bladder or rectum. A bullous edema as such does not permit a case to be allotted to Stage IV. |
| Stage IVA | Spread of the growth to adjacent organs. |
| Stage IVB | Spread to distant organs. |

For smaller lesions (stage IA and IBI), stage is assigned following pelvic examination. Additional evaluation typically includes a chest X-ray and routine blood tests. For larger tumors, patients are staged following pelvic examination (often under anesthesia), and chest X-ray, cystoscopy or proctoscopy, if performed. For advanced tumors the ureters are assessed, traditionally by IVP, though CT scan or MRI have been found to provide better assessment of the extent of pelvic disease and lymph node metastasis. If there is evidence of large pelvic and/or para-aortic nodal metastasis, the adenopathy should be assessed through fine-needle aspiration. If positive, treatment should be individualized, as patients with large lymph node metastasis have a poor survival rate with either surgery or radiation therapy.

Clinical staging is widely applicable and permits comparison of treatment modalities from around the world. It is not without its limitations, however, primarily with regard to detection of occult lymph node metastasis. Surgical staging, which includes retroperitoneal assessment of pelvic and para-aortic lymph nodes in patients with locally advanced tumors, has a theoretical advantage in that patients found to have microscopic nodal disease can be treated with extended-field radiation therapy, often with concurrent chemotherapy, with the aim of increasing long-term survival. In practice, surgical staging of advanced cervical tumors will result in benefit to only a small number of individuals, as most will either have no nodal metastasis, or have unresectable or advanced nodal lesions that are incurable with present treatment modalities. The Gynecologic Oncology Group has studied the pros and cons of surgical staging of cervical cancer quite carefully and presently leaves this as an option for patients with locally advanced tumors being considered for prospective, randomized clinical trials [3].

## Prognostic Factors

Clinical stage is the most important prognostic factor. Five-year survival approaches 100% for patients with stage IA tumors, and averages 75%–85% for stage IB1 and smaller IIA lesions. Survival for more locally advanced tumors (stages IB2 to IV) is quite variable, and is influenced significantly by the bulk of disease, which may vary considerably within a given stage. Overall, 5-year disease free survival approximates 60% for stage IB2, 50% for stage IIB, 30% for stage III and 5% for stage IV [4].

Other important prognostic factors include histology, patient age, and medical co-morbidities. For HIV-seropositive patients with diminished CD4+ counts, prognosis is particularly poor, even for those with apparent early stage disease [5].

For patients treated with radical hysterectomy and lymphadenectomy, adverse risk factors include increasing tumor size and depth of tumor invasion, lymph-vascular vessel involvement [6], positive vaginal or parametrial margins, and lymph node metastasis.


Treatment

*Stage IA*

A cervical conization specimen is required to permit diagnosis of microinvasive squamous cell cervical cancer. The invasive lesion and any coexistent cervical dysplasia must appear to have been removed completely after careful pathologic assessment of the conization margins. Lesions invading no more than 3 mm (stage IA1) and in which there is no evidence of lymphatic or vascular space invasion may be treated by extrafascial hysterectomy. For patients desiring preservation of the uterus, the conization itself is probably sufficient treatment, though long term experience with this approach is not as extensive as with hysterectomy. For lesions invading deeper than 3 mm (stage IA2), or if lymph-vascular space involvement is identified, the risk of lymph node metastasis is of sufficient concern that treatment should entail radical hysterectomy and lymphadenectomy or radiation therapy. As there is no accepted definition of microinvasive adenocarcinoma of the cervix, these lesions should also be treated with radical hysterectomy or radiation therapy.


*Stage IB*

Several different treatment modalities are currently utilized in the management of stage IB cervical cancer, which is not surprising given that the volume of tumor in a large IB cancer may be several hundred fold greater in comparison to an early IB lesion. Smaller tumors ($<=4$ cm) can be treated effectively with either radical hysterectomy and lymphadenectomy or with radiation therapy. Advantages of radical hysterectomy over radiation therapy include a shorter duration of treatment, preservation of ovarian function in younger patients, and no concern of future recurrence in the uterus or cervix. In addition, the information obtained at laparotomy, such as lymph node status or the presence of gross disease beyond the cervix provides the opportunity for selective adjunctive therapy.

Primary radiation therapy usually includes a combination of external irradiation and intracavitary brachytherapy. Whole pelvic irradiation, typically 4000–5000 cGy, is administered over 4–5 weeks, and is used primarily to treat the parametria and lateral pelvic walls. External irradiation usually precedes brachytherapy, as the former will lead to reduction in central tumor bulk and permit a more effective dose of irradiation from the intracavitary device. Either low-dose-rate (LDR) or high-dose-rate (HDR) brachytherapy may be used, with equivalent results. LDR therapy (50–60 cGy/hr) necessitates placement of the implant device under anesthesia and a 2–3 day hospitalization. HDR therapy (200–300 cGy/min) is performed on an outpatient basis, with typically 3–5 insertions placed at weekly intervals. The advantage of radiation therapy over surgery is its applicability to nearly all patients regardless of weight, age, and medical condition. Long term complications involving the gastrointestinal urinary tract are uncommon, though if occur, are more difficult to manage than complications arising after surgery.

Stage IB2, or bulky, barrel-shaped cervical tumors pose a unique challenge to the clinician. It has been recognized for some time that the survival rate for these larger tumors is substantially worse than for smaller primary tumors. Lymph node metastasis in the larger tumors is more common, and the size of the tumor often extends beyond the curative isodose curve of radiation. Both central and distant failures are more common in comparison to stage IB1 lesions. For this reason, many centers choose to treat these patients with a combination of preoperative whole pelvic radiation therapy and brachytherapy, followed by an extrafascial hysterectomy and para-aortic lymph node sampling. Though a randomized GOG study confirmed that the rate of central recurrence is less with adjuvent hysterectomy, this study was not able to identify a survival advantage of radiation followed by extrafascial hysterectomy versus radiation therapy alone [7]. In Europe, it is common to administer preoperative brachytherapy followed by radical hysterectomy and lymphadenectomy for larger stage I tumors. This approach is not widely utilized in the United States, though European data suggests this management gives excellent control of central disease and acceptable morbidity.

More recently, the GOG has been exploring the role of chemotherapy in the management of stage IB2 cervical cancer. In a recently analyzed randomized phase III study involving 374 patients, weekly cisplatin chemotherapy (40 mg/m2, maximum dose 70 mg/wk) during irradiation was found to improve survival and reduce relapse for patients with bulky cervical cancer treated with irradiation and adjuvent hysterectomy. The risk of relapse and death was reduced to about half that seen in the control arm not receiving chemotherapy. Two year survival and recurrence free interval was 89% and 81%, respectively, in the chemotherapy arm vs 79% and 69% respectively, in the control arm [8]. The GOG has also recently completed a randomized trial evaluating the role of adjunctive radiation therapy following radical hysterectomy and pelvic lymphadenectomy in the management of stage IB cervical cancers with selected risk factors including large tumor size, deep cervical stromal invasion, or lymph-vascular space involvement. For the 277 patients studied, the risk of recurrence was reduced 44% in the group receiving adjuvent radiotherapy (5,100 cGy/30 fractions). Patients receiving radiation therapy had a two year recurrence free rate of 88% vs 79% in the group treated with radical hysterectomy alone. Severe urologic and gastrointestinal toxicity were more common in the group treated with adjuvent radiation, and survival analysis awaits further follow-up [9]. Patients discovered to have lymph node metastasis or involvement of parametrial or vaginal margins with cancer following radical hysterectomy and lymphadenectomy are at particularly high risk of recurrence. Most of these patients are offered postoperative pelvic radiation therapy, thought the benefit of this approach has not been proven in a sufficiently large randomized trial. The GOG has completed a randomized comparison of 5-fluorouracil and cisplatin used as an adjunct to radiation therapy vs radiation therapy alone in patients with positive pelvic nodes, positive parametrial or surgical margins following radical hysterectomy for stage IA2, IB, and IIA cervical carcinoma. The results of this study are pending, yet may help to determine the role, if any, of adjuvent chemotherapy in these high risk individuals.

## Stage IIA

The optimal treatment of most stage IIA cervical cancers is definitive radiation therapy. Rarely, there is a sufficiently small amount of extension of cancer into the vaginal fornix that the cancer can be treated effectively with radical hysterectomy, pelvic and para-aortic lymphadenectomy and upper vaginectomy.

## Stages IIB, III, and IVA

Once cervical cancer has extended beyond the confines of the cervix, cure with surgery is unlikely. These patients should be treated with definitive radiation therapy, including both external beam therapy and brachytherapy. Treatment should be individualized based upon the volume of tumor and degree of extension, if any, into the vagina. Extended field radiation therapy encompassing the para-aortic nodes may be used unless surgical staging has previously shown this region to be free of tumor. Using modern radiation therapy techniques, control of central disease with radiation therapy alone is quite good, and averages 80% for stage II disease and 50% for stage III disease.

Many advanced stage patients dying from disease do so with evidence of distant disease, with or without recurrence centrally. In an effort to improve upon both local and distant recurrence, cooperative groups including the GOG and RTOG have studied the influence of concomitant chemoradiation in advanced cervical cancer. A recently completed randomized phase III GOG study compared standard radiation therapy plus hydroxyurea versus hydroxyurea, 5-FU infusion and bolus cisplatin versus weekly cisplatin in advanced, para-aortic node negative patients. 487 eligible patients were studied, and both platinum containing regimens demonstrated improved progression free intervals when compared to hydroxyurea, reducing the risk of progression by over 40%. The proportion of patients recurrence free at two years was nearly 70% for the two platinum containing regimens and 50% for the hydroxyurea regimen. Bone marrow and gastrointestinal toxicity was significantly increased with the 5-FU containing regimen in comparison to weekly cisplatin or hydroxyurea. The impact of chemoradiation on survival from this study awaits further analysis [10]. Currently the GOG is comparing standard radiation plus concurrent weekly cisplatin vs protracted venous infusion

5-FU (225 mg/m2 per day over 5 weeks) in patients with locally advanced tumors.

## Stage IVB, Recurrent or Metastatic Disease

Nearly all patients with stage I-II disease and most patients with stage III disease will experience complete disappearance of pelvic disease following surgery or radiation therapy. Ninety percent of recurrences will be identified within 3 years of initial diagnosis and less than 5% of these patients will be alive 5 years later. The rare, potentially curable patient with recurrent disease would include those with isolated pulmonary metastasis or isolated central recurrence. Solitary lung metastasis, though unusual, can be treated with resection and nearly 25% of these patients will survive at least 5 years. Isolated pelvic recurrence following radical hysterectomy may be treated with radiation therapy, provided radiation was not administered previously. Generally, only small recurrences under 2–3 cm would be considered as potentially curable in this situation, with about 40% of patients alive at 5 years. Patients with central pelvic recurrence following radiation therapy may occasionally be cured with surgery. This normally entails a pelvic exenteration including, in addition to removal of the uterus and cervix, a cystectomy and resection of most of the rectum and vagina. Select patients may be managed with a less extensive procedure and recent advances in reconstructive procedures have led to an improvement in the quality of life for many patients requiring urinary diversion. Nevertheless, only about a third of patients with negative pelvic and para-aortic lymph nodes and free surgical margins treated with pelvic exenteration are alive 5 years later. Radiation therapy is an effective modality for palliation of metastatic disease to distant sites including lymph nodes, bones, lungs or the brain. Most lesions respond to about 3000 cGy given in 10 fractions.

## Chemotherapy

Chemotherapy for advanced or recurrent disease has been and continues to be considered as a palliative procedure. Most cervical carcinomas are refractory to chemotherapy, and only a small proportion of patients experience sufficient tumor regression that quality of life is improved.

Multiple chemotherapy agents have been evaluated, alone or in combination [11, 12]. Response rate in multicenter phase II trials averages 10% to 40%, with complete responses seen only rarely and for short duration. Cisplatin is presently considered the most active agent against cervical carcinoma, and is presently being compared to the combination of cisplatin and paclitaxel in a randomized, phase III GOG study. Factors which appear to influence the effectiveness of chemotherapy in cervical cancer include whether the recurrence is within a previously irradiated field, and perhaps, patient age, with older patients responding more frequently than younger patients [13].

## Vulvar Cancer

Epidemiolgy, Risk Factors

Vulvar carcinoma is the fourth most common gynecologic cancer, yet is quite rare, accounting for about 4% of tumors of the female genital tract. Less than 1000 cases are diagnosed annually in the United States, with most occurring in women over the age of 60 years. While the incidence of pre-invasive vulvar dysplasia appears to be increasing, particularly in younger women, the incidence of invasive tumors has remained stable for several years.

A specific cause for vulvar cancer has not been identified. Identified risk factors, aside from increasing age, include smoking, a history of genital warts or vulvar intraepithelial neoplasia, and increasing number of lifetime sexual partners [14]. Benign vulvar lesions, including lichen sclerosis and squamous cell hyperplasia, are associated with an increased risk of cancer, approaching 5% in individuals followed over many years. Human papillomavirus DNA can be found in approximately 50% of squamous tumors, and is more common in tumors developing in younger women or smokers. HPV containing tumors tend to be multifocal and are commonly associated with preexisting vulvar dysplasia. Tumors lacking HPV DNA are more commonly found in older women, are typically solitary, and frequently lack evidence of a prior pre-invasive lesion. Some evidence suggests that the presence of HPV DNA in vulvar carcinomas may influence biologic behavior [15], but further study of this issue is necessary.

**Table 2.** FIGO staging for carcinoma of the vulva

| | |
|---|---|
| Stage 0 | TIS: Carcinoma in situ; intraepithelial carcinoma. |
| Stage I | T1 N0 M0: Tumor confined to the vulva and/or perineum – 2 cm or less in greatest dimension, nodes are negative. |
| Stage IA | Stromal invasion no greater than 1.0 mm.[a] |
| Stage IB | Stromal invasion greater than 1.0 mm.[a] |
| Stage II | T2 N0 M0: Tumor confined to the vulva and/or perineum – more than 2 cm in greatest dimension, nodes are negative. |
| Stage III | T3 N0 M0, T3 N1 M0: Tumor of any size with (1) Adjacent spread to the lower urethra and/or the vagina, or the anus, and/or, T1 N1 M0, T2 N1 M0: (2) Unilateral regional lymph node metastasis. |
| Stage IVA | T1 N2 M0, T2 N2 M0, T3 N2 M0, T4 any N M0: Tumor invades any of the following: Upper urethra, bladder mucosa, rectal mucosa, pelvic bone, and/or bilateral regional node metastasis. |
| Stage IVB | Any T, Any N, M1: Any distant metastasis including pelvic lymph nodes. |

Rules for clinical staging
(similar to those for carcinoma of the cervix):
TNM classification of carcinoma of the vulva (FIGO)

*Primary tumor*

| | |
|---|---|
| Tis | Preinvasive carcinoma (carcinoma in situ) |
| T1 | Tumor confined to the vulva and/or perineum – < 2 cm in greatest dimension |
| T2 | Tumor confined to the vulva and/or perineum – > 2 cm in greatest dimension |
| T3 | Tumor of any size with adjacent spread to the urethra and/or vagina and/or to the anus |
| T4 | Tumor of any size infiltrating the bladder mucosa and/or the rectal mucosa, including the upper part of the urethral mucosa and/or fixed to the bone. |

*Regional lymph nodes*

| | |
|---|---|
| N0 | No lymph node metastasis |
| N1 | Unilateral regional lymph node metastasis |
| N2 | Bilateral regional lymph node metastasis |

*Distant metastasis*

| | |
|---|---|
| M0 | No clinical metastasis |
| M1 | Distant metastasis (including pelvic lymph node metastasis) |

[a]The depth of invasion is defined as the measurement oft he tumor from the epithelial-stromal junction of the adjacent most superficial dermal papilla to the deepest point of invasion.

## Signs and Symptoms

Grossly, vulvar carcinoma appears as a lump or polypoid mass, often present for many months. Patients typically relate a long history of vulvar pruritis or discomfort. Delays in the diagnosis of vulvar cancer are not uncommon because of patient embarrassment or the hesitancy of physicians to evaluate or biopsy vulvar lesions.

## Diagnosis

Though often obvious on clinical examination, the diagnosis of vulvar cancer requires a tissue biopsy, and is easily obtainable in the office under local anesthesia. It is important to include the full thickness of the epithelium and it is advantageous to include a slim margin or border of normal appearing skin. In the rare situation where the diagnosis remains in doubt following biopsy, the lesion should be excised with a sufficient margin in the event that malignancy is confirmed.

## Pathology

About 90% of vulvar cancers are squamous, with subtypes described as basaloid, warty, or typical on the basis of hematoxylin and eosin (H&E) staining. Other cell types include melanoma, bartholins gland adenocarcinoma, and primary vulvar sarcoma, with each accounting for less than 5% of invasive vulvar tumors. Vulvar Paget's disease, basal cell carcinoma, and veruccus cell carcinoma are typically considered as locally invasive lesions, with little risk of metastatic dissemination. Nevertheless, these lesions may become quite extensive and cause considerable morbidity and occasional death. Tumors metastatic to the vulva are exceedingly rare.

## Staging and Prognosis

FIGO has adopted a modified tumor-node-metastasis (TNM) staging system for vulvar carcinoma (Table 2). With this system, lymph node involvement is assessed surgically prior to assigning stage. Most patients are stage I or II when diagnosed, and overall, the 5-year survival rate for vulvar cancer is approximately 60%. Survival is influenced primarily by the presence or absence of lymph node involvement. Approximately 90% of patients with no evidence of tumor in resected lymph nodes are cured, as compared to about 40% if lymph nodes are involved [16, 17]. The number of involved regional lymph nodes is also important, with survival rates dropping from nearly 90% if a single, small node is involved, to 80% with two nodes involved, to under 20% if three or more nodes are involved with tumor. Other factors shown to correlate with survival or risk of recurrence include lesion size, cell type, tumor grade, and whether or not lymph-vascular space involvement is present [18].

## Treatment

Treatment of vulvar cancer should be individualized. Radical vulvectomy and bilateral inguinofemoral lymph node dissection is curative in a substantial number of patients with local disease or limited metastasis to the inguinal lymph nodes. Despite good results with this approach, dissatisfaction with this procedure has been common, primarily as a result of the associated serious morbidity including wound separation in approximately 50% of patients, lymphedema, voiding difficulties, and gross disfigurement of the vulva. Thus, it is now common to perform more conservative procedures with T1, T2 lesions, with the primary aim to excise all malignant tissue and a 1–2 cm margin of surrounding skin. Depending upon the size and location of the lesion, this approach may result in preservation of the majority of vulvar epithelium and improved cosmetic results. For T1 tumors invading less than 1 mm, the risk of nodal involvement is about 1% and the risk of local recurrence quite low. These lesions may be safely treated with wide local excision without lymph node dissection.

Invasion beyond 1 mm indicates an increasing risk of lymph node involvement, approaching 15% with 5 mm of invasion. With lateralized cancers under 2 cm in diameter and with more than 1 mm invasion, ipsilateral lymphadenectomy and locally radical excision of the primary tumor is acceptable. Whether the extent of nodal dissection can be limited to the superficial inguinal lymph nodes, or should also include the deep femoral lymph nodes is unsettled [19]. Lesions involving the clitoris or posterior perineum may metastasize to either groin, and in this case bilateral groin dissection is indicated.

If inguinal lymph nodes are free of tumor and the primary lesion has been resected with adequate margins, then no further therapy is necessary. If inguinal nodes are involved, then the pelvic nodes are considered at risk for metastatic disease, and post-operative radiation to the groin and pelvis is given. While the addition of inguinopelvic irradiation improves survival over surgery alone in patients with >1 positive inguinal node [20], many such patients will relapse in the groin, pelvis, or distant sites. Some investigators have argued that radiation sensitizing chemotherapy, typically ciplatin with or without 5-FU, may be more beneficial than radiation alone. The GOG recently attempted to examine this question however an insufficient number of patients could be accrued and the study was terminated.

Larger vulvar tumors, particularly those involving the rectum or urethra, pose unique challenges. Traditionally, many of the women with these extensive lesions required fecal or urinary diversion prior to radical vulvectomy. A more recent approach has been to administer preoperative irradiation, or irradiation with chemotherapy to reduce the size of the primary tumor and spare the anogenital region or urethra, which leads to an improvement in quality of life [21, 22]. The most commonly utilized chemotherapy agents have been 5-FU, cisplatin, and mitomycin-C. The GOG has completed a study investigating the use of chemoradiation therapy for locally advanced disease. The results await final analysis, however the approach is feasible, though toxicity is not uncommon. Whether these combined modalities for the treatment of locally advanced vulvar cancer will have a favorable impact on survival has not yet been conclusively determined.

Recurrent vulvar cancer carries a poor prognosis. Occasional long-term remissions or cures can be achieved with local resection, and irradiation is sometimes given to patients not previously irradiated. Effective chemotherapy for recurrent or disseminated squamous cell vulvar cancer has not yet been identified.

## Vaginal Cancer

Primary vaginal cancer is one of the rarest gynecologic malignancies, accounting for less than 2% of tumors of the female genital tract. As with vulvar cancer, most cases are diagnosed in older women, with the peak incidence in the sixth decade of life. Squamous is the predominant cell type, and accounts for over 90% of cases. Vaginal melanoma and adenocarcinoma together comprise about 10% of primary tumors. Vaginal cancer is defined as a primary malignancy arising in the vagina and not involving the cervix superiorly or the vulva inferiorly. Risk factors include prior treatment for cervical neoplasia, prior pelvic irradiation, and, in younger women with clear cell adenocarcinoma, in utero diethylstilbestrol (DES) exposure. Patients typically present with symptoms of abnormal vaginal discharge or bleeding. Women with advanced tumors

**Table 3.** FIGO staging for carcinoma of the vagina

| | |
|---|---|
| Stage 0 | Carcinoma in situ, intraepithelial carcinoma. |
| Stage I | The carcinoma is limited to the vaginal wall. |
| Stage II | The carcinoma has involved the subvaginal tissue but has not extended on to the pelvic wall. |
| Stage III | The carcinoma has extended on to the pelvic wall. |
| Stage IV | The carcinoma has extended beyond the true pelvis or has clinically involved the mucosa of the bladder or rectum. Bullous edema as such does not permit a case to be allotted to Stage IV. |
| Stage IVA | Spread to adjacent organs and/or direct extension beyond the true pelvis. |
| Stage IVB | Spread to distant organs. |

can present with pain, urinary complaints, or constipation, depending upon the location of the neoplasm. With inspection and palpation, the tumor can appearas either an ulcerated, indurated, or fungating mass. Occasionally a malignancy will protrude from the vaginal introitus, though this is unusual as most cases arise in the upper third of the vagina.

Diagnosis is made after analysis of direct biopsy of the tumor mass. Once diagnosed, vaginal cancer is staged clinically according to FIGO criteria (Table 3). Evaluation for the presence of metastatic disease is similar to that previously discussed for cervical cancer. Prognosis depends primarily on the volume of disease present at diagnosis, and stage for stage, is generally less than that reported for cervical and vulvar cancer. Overall, 5-year survival rates average 40%–50%, with no significant change over the last two decades [23, 24]. The survival rate for women with stage I disease averages 75%; stage II 50%; stage III 25%; and stage IV under 5%.

Tumors arising in the upper third of the vagina can spread via lymphatics to the paracervical lymph nodes and drain to the obturator, hypogastric, and external iliac nodes. Tumors arising in the lower vagina, in addition to being capable of draining to the pelvic nodes, can spread via lymphatics to the inguinal nodes shared by the vulva. Depending upon the location and stage of the tumor, radiation, surgery, or both may be utilized, though most patients are treated primarily with radiatherapy. For smaller tumors (generally <1 cm) in the upper vagina, surgery is usually successful and includes radical hysterectomy, partial vaginectomy, and pelvic lymphadenectomy. Smaller tumors are also treated effectively with radiation therapy. If the tumor is less than 0.5 cm thick, brachytherapy delivered via a vaginal cylinder will control over 90% of tumors [25]. For larger or thicker lesions, external beam radiation therapy is usually given first and followed by a subsequent implant [26]. Stage III and IV tumors seldom permit an implant, and are frequently treated with external beam therapy alone, or occasionally with interstitial needles.

A variety of adjuvent chemotherapy regimens have been employed with radiation therapy in the treatment of squamous cell carcinoma of the vagina. The rarity of the tumor and the diversity of agents used does not permit any meaningful conclusions on the efficacy of combined chemoradiation therapy.

## References

1. Landis SH, Murray T, Bolden S, Wingo PA: Cancer statistics, 1998. CA Cancer J Clin 48:6–29, 1998
2. Schiffman MH, Bauer HM, Hoover RN, et al. Epidemiologic evidence showing that human papillomavirus infection causes most cervical intraepithelial neoplasia. J Natl Cancer Inst 85:958–964, 1993
3. National Institutes of Health Consensus Statement on Cervical Cancer. J Natl Cancer Inst, monograph 21, 1996
4. Jones WB, Shingleton HM, Russel AH, et al. Patterns of care for invasive cervical cancer: results of a national survey of 1984 and 1990. Cancer 76:1934–1947, 1995
5. Maiman M, Fruchter RG, Guy L, et al. Human immunodeficiency virus infection and invasive cervical carcinoma. Cancer 71:402–406, 1993
6. Delgado G, Bundy B, Zaino R, et al. Prospective surgical-pathological study of disease-free interval in patients with stage IB squamous cell carcinoma of the cervix: A Gynecologic Oncology Group study. Gynecol Oncol 38:352–357, 1990
7. Treatment of patients with sub-optimal ("bulky") stage IB carcinoma of the cervix: A randomized comparison of radiation therapy versus radiation therapy plus adjuvant extrafascial hysterectomy (GOG #71, RTOG #84–22). Keys HM, Hornback N, Okagaki T, Stehman FB. American Radium Society 1997 (abstract)
8. Keys HM, Bundy BN, Stehman FB, Muderspach LI, Chafe WE, Suggs CL, Walker JL, Gersell D. Weekly cisplatin chemotherapy during irradiation improves survival and reduces relapses for patients with bulky stage Ib cervical cancer treated with irradiation and adjuvent hysterectomy: Results of a randomized GOG trial. Gynecol Oncol 68:100 1998 (abstract)
9. Sedlis A, Bundy BN, Rotman M, Lentz S, Muderspach LI, Zaino R. Treatment of selected patients with stage IB carcinoma of the cervix after radical hysterectomy and pelvic lymphadenectomy: Pelvic radiation therapy (Rt) versus no further therapy (NFT) (A GOG study). Gynecol Oncol 68:105 1998 (abstract)
10. Rose PG, Bundy B, Thigpen T, Deppe G, Maiman M, Clarke-Pearson D. Significant preliminary results of a phase III randomized study of concomitant chemoradiation with hydroxyurea vs hydroxyurea, 5-FU infusion, and bolus cisplatin (HFC) vs weekly cisplatin in advanced cervical cancer, a GOG study. Gynecol Oncol 68:104 1998 (abstract)
11. Lopez A, Kudelka AP, Edwards CL, et al. Carcinoma of the uterine cervix, in Pazdur R (ed): Medical Oncolgy: A Comprehensive Review, 2nd ed. Huntington, NY, PRR, 1996

12. Park RC, Thigpen JT: Chemotherapy in advanced and recurrent cervical cancer. Cancer 71:1446–1450, 1993

13. Brader KR, Morris M, Levenback C, et al. Chemotherapy for cervical carcinoma: factors determining response and implications for clinical trial design. J Clin Oncol 16:1879–1884, 1998

14. Briton LA, Nasca PC, Mallin K, et al. Case-control study of cancer of the vulva. Obstet Gynecol 75:859, 1990

15. Hording U, Junge J, Daugaard S, Lundvall F, Poulsen H, Bock JE: Vulvar squamous cell carcinoma and papillomaviruses: Indications for two different etiologies. Gynecol Oncol 52:241–246, 1994

16. Homesley HD, Bundy BN, Sedlis A, et al. Assessment of current International Federation of Gynecology and Obstetrics staging of vulvar carcinoma relative to prognostic factors for survival (a Gynecologic Oncology Group study). Amer J Obstet Gynecol 164:997–1003, 1991

17. Hacker NF, Berek JS, Lagasse LD, et al. Management of regional lymph nodes and their prognostic influence in vulvar carcinoma. Obstet Gynecol 61:408–412, 1983

18. Creasman WT, Phillips JL, Menck HR: The National Cancer Data Base report on early stage invasive vulvar carcinoma. Cancer 80:505–513, 1997

19. Stehman FB, Bundy BN, Dvoretsky PM, Creasman WT: Early stage I carcinoma of the vulva treated with superficial inguinal lymphadenectomy and modified excision hemivulvectomy: A prospective study of the Gynecologic Oncology Group. Obstet Gynecol 79:490–497, 1992

20. Homesley HD, Bundy BN, Sedlis A, Adcoc L: Radiation therapy versus node resection for carcinoma of the vulva with positive groin nodes. Obstet Gynecol 68:733–740, 1986

21. Boronow RC, Hickman BT, Reagan MT, Smith RA, Steadham RE: Combined therapy as an alternative to exenteration for locally advanced vulvovaginal cancer. Am J Clin Oncol 10:171–181, 1987

22. Landoni F, Maneo A, Zanetta G, et al. Concurrent preoperative chemotherapy with 5-fluorouracil and mitomycin C and radiotherapy (FUMIR) followed by limited surgery in locally advanced and recurrent vulvar carcinoma. Gynecol Oncol 61:321–327, 1996

23. Perez CA, Camel HM, Galakatos AE, et al. Definitive irradiation in carcinoma of the vagina: Long-term evaluation of results. Int J Radiat Oncol Biol Phys 15:1283–1290, 1988

24. Dixit S, Singhal S, Baboo HA: Squamous cell carcinoma of the vagina: a review of 70 cases. Gynecol Oncol 48:80–87, 1993

25. Nanavati PJ, Fanning J, Hilgers RD, Hallstrom J, Crawford D: High-dose-rate brachytherapy in primary stage I and II vaginal cancer. Gynecol Oncol 51:67–71, 1993

26. Urbanski K, Kojs Z, Reinfuss M, Fabisiak W: Primary invasive vaginal carcinoma treated with radiotherapy: Analysis of prognostic factors. Gynecol Oncol 60:16–21, 1996

# Brain Tumors

# Primary and Metastatic Brain Tumors

M.K. Nicholas

## Epidemiology, Risk Factors

Incidence

The estimated annual incidence of newly diagnosed CNS tumors in the United States (U.S.) exceeds 100,000 [1]. Primary tumors comprise the minority of cases with approximately 17,000 newly diagnosed cases per year. Annual age-adjusted incidence rates for primary CNS tumors in the U.S. range from 5.0 to 14.1 per 100,000 population [2]. CNS metastases comprise the remainder of the cases. The average annual incidence rate for CNS metastases in the U.S. is estimated to be 8.4 per 100,000 population [3]. Incidence rates for both primary and metastatic CNS tumors vary widely across series. Autopsy-based studies include asymptomatic and previously undiagnosed tumors, increasing overall incidence and altering distribution by tumor type when compared to clinical series.

## Race, Sex, Age, Distribution, Predisposition

Primary Tumors

Taken altogether, primary tumors are encountered more frequently among Caucasians than Blacks, Asians, or Latinos. This trend holds for studies performed in diverse geographic locations. For example, primary CNS tumors are encountered among Israelis of European descent more often than they are among those of either Asian or African heritage [4]. Particular subsets of CNS tumors may be encountered more frequently in Blacks: meningiomas in adults and craniopharyngiomas in children.

Again, considering all primary CNS tumors collectively, males are affected more often than females: gender ratio=1.4 [5]. However, considerable variation exists between tumor types. For example, the male to female gender ratio for gliomas is 1.5 while that for meningiomas is 0.6 [6].

Age is an important factor in primary CNS tumor susceptibility. They account for approximately 20% of childhood cancers but only 1.4% of adult cancers. The distribution of tumor types differs considerably between these groups, as well. Among adults, an overall increase in primary CNS tumor incidence occurs with age. This is particularly true for high grade astrocytomas and meningioma. The incidence of low grade glioma and oligodendroglioma decreases after middle age [7] .

Primary CNS tumors may be found anywhere within the CNS spaces but histology often dictates tumor location. Thus, ependymomas and choroid plexus tumors are more often encountered within the ventricular system while the commoner astroglial tumors are more evenly distributed throughout the neuraxis. Particular astroglial variants such as optic and brainstem gliomas derive their names by the location from which they arise. Primary CNS tumors rarely metastasize outside the CNS. Extra-CNS metatstases are most common in medulloblastoma [8]. Howwever, case reports of abdominal seeding after ventriculo-peritoneal shunting are reported for most primary tumor types.

Extensive analytic epidemiology has sought to determine environmental, lifestyle, and genetic risks associated with primary CNS tumors. Environmental factors including exposure to various chemicals or ionizing and electromagnetic radiation may play some role in both glioma and meningioma formation [9]. However, data are at times conflicting and methodologic differences between studies make comparisons of them difficult. Lifestyle factors including diet, social class, and smoking history are less convincing than environmental studies in relating particular activities to primary CNS tumor susceptibility.

Genetic factors undoubtedly influence primary brain tumor susceptibility. Persons with neurofibromatosis types 1 and 2 are at increased risk for a variety of primary CNS tumors, as are persons with tuberous sclerosis, Turcot syndrome, the Li-Fraumeni syndrome, and others. These are outlined in Table 1.

**Table 1.** Genetic syndromes associated with primary CNS tumors

| Syndrome | Genetic abnormality | Associated tumor |
|---|---|---|
| Neurofibromatosis type 1 glioma | Neurofibromin | Optic-hypothalamic |
| | | Astrocytoma |
| | | Neurofibroma |
| Neurofibromatosis type 2 | Merlin | Acoustic schwannoma |
| | | Meningioma |
| | | Glioma |
| | | Neurilemoma |
| Li-Fraumeni syndrome | p53 | Glioma |
| Turcot syndrome | APC, hMLH1, hPMS2 | PNET |
| | | Glioblastoma |
| Tuberous sclerosis | a | Giant cell astrocytoma |
| Malignant melanoma | CDKN2 | Glioma |
| | | Astrocytoma |

a, Gene(s) unknown or hypothesized; APC, adenoma polyposis coli; hMLH1 and hPMS2, DNA mismatch repair genes; CDKN2, inhibitor of cyclin-dependent kinase.

## Metastases

The race and sex distribution of CNS metastases parallels that of the primary tumor in question. Thus, although CNS metastases from bronchogenic carcinoma are more commonly encountered in men than in women, a similar gender difference is seen in the prevalence of the primary diagnosis [3].

Age is an important factor in determining susceptibility to CNS metastasis. Furthermore, age determines the type of CNS metastasis one is most likely to encounter. In children, intraparenchymal metastases are most commonly seen with sarcomas and germ cell tumors [10]. Leptomeningeal metastatses in children are most often of hematopoietic origin. Epidural compression in children is most often the consequence of sarcoma, neuroblastoma, or lymphoma. In adults, on the other hand, intraparenchymal metatstases occur most often in the setting of lung, breast, gastrointestinal, skin (melanoma), and genitourinary cancers [3]. Although hematologic malignancies account for a considerable percentage of leptomeningeal metastases in adults, other tumors, especially small cell lung cancer, show a predilection for leptomeningeal dissemination. Epidural compression in adults occurs most often in the setting of systemic lymphoma, renal cell cancer, multiple myeloma, melanoma, prostate cancer, and sarcoma.

Over two thirds of intra-parenchymal brain metatstases are found in the cerebral hemispheres. Most of the remainder are found in the cerebellum, although a small percentage may be found in the brainstem [11]. Leptomeningeal disease may overlie an intraparenchymal metastasis or present as disseminated disease. The skull base is a common site for symptomatic leptomeningeal metatstases.

There are no known risk factors for CNS metastasis. Their etiology involves a complex process that includes tumor cells breaking free of the primary site followed by their spread to and subsequent growth within the CNS. Each of these steps is complex and details are beyond the scope of this manuscript. Interested readers are referred to a recent review [12]. It bears mention that most intraparenchymal tumors are distributed hematogenously in relative proportion to the blood flow to various CNS regions. Many tumors arising in the pelvis, however, tend to metastasize to the cerebellum although the posterior fossa only receives 15% of the cerebral blood supply.

## Pathology

The pathologic grading of primary CNS tumors is complex and evolving. For many tumor types, more than one grading system exists, often with little agreement between them. Thus, the same glial tumor may be of relatively higher or lower grade depending upon the classification system used. This has led to considerable confusion in the clinical literature and likely contributes substantially to differences in treatment outcomes sometimes observed when comparing studies. Members of the international neuropathology community, under the auspices of the World Health Organization (WHO) have gone to considerable length to standardize the criteria for classifying and grading primary CNS tumors. The WHO criteria were most recently updated in 1993 [13]. The major histologic categories by which tumors are classified are shown below:

- Neuroepithelial Tumors
  - Astrocytic tumors
  - Oligodendroglial tumors
  - Ependymal tumors
  - Mixed gliomas
  - Choroid plexus tumors

- - Neuroepithelial tumors of uncertain origin
- - Neuronal and mixed neuronal-glial tumors
- - Pineal parenchymal tumors
- - Embryonal tumors
- Tumors of Cranial and Spinal Nerves
  - - Schwannoma
  - - Neurofibroma
  - - Malignant peripheral nerve sheath tumors
- Tumors of the Meninges
  - - Meningothelial cell tumors
  - - Mesenchymal non-menigothelial tumors
  - - Primary melanocytic tumors
- Lymphomas and Hematopoietic Neoplasms
- Germ Cell Tumors
- Cysts and Tumor-like Lesions
- Sellar Region Tumors
- Local Extension from Regional Tumors
- Metastatic Tumors
- Unclassified Tumors

Many subcategories exist, especially within the neuroepithelial, meningeal, and cranial/spinal nerve categories. In general, tumors are ranked within categories or subcategories according to their relative degree of anaplasia with the lowest grade tumors ranked first. For example, among the astrocytic tumors, fibrillary, protplasmic and gemistocytic variants are listed before anaplastic astrocytoma and glioblastoma multiforme. Astroglial tumors with distinct histologic features, such as pilocytic astrocytoma are grouped seprately.

Attempts to link important molecular parameters and prognosis to classic histology are frequently made. The many molecular abnormalities present in primary CNS tumors are beyond the scope of this chapter but are well described in recent reviews [14]. A summary of molecular changes thought to be of importance in glial tumors and meningiomas are outlined in Table 2.

The prognosis for patients with primary and metastatic CNS tumors varies widely. For example, among the astrocytic tumors surgical cure is a distinct possibility for pilocytic astrocytomas while fewer than 5% of patients with glioblastoma are alive 5 years following the diagnosis, despite extensive treatment [15]. Representative survival times for the

**Table 2.** Molecular changes commonly encountered in some primary CNS tumors

| Tumor | Molecular abnormalities |
|---|---|
| Astrocytoma | p53 mutation, 17p loss, 22q loss, PDGF and PDGFR overexpression |
| Anaplastic astrocytoma | As above plus: RB mutation and 13q loss, 9p loss, 19q loss |
| Glioblastoma | As above plus: loss of 10 p+q, EGFR amplification |
| Oligodendroglioma | 19q and 1p loss |
| Oligoastrocytoma | 19q and 1p loss |
| Meningioma | Loss of 22 p+q, Progesterone receptor overexpression |

p, Chromosomal short arm; q, chromosomal long arm; PDGF, platelet-derived growth factor; PDGFR, platelet-derived growth factor receptor; RB, retinoblastoma gene; EGFR, epidermal growth factor receptor.

**Table 3.** Five-year survivial rates for many tumors discussed in this chapter (from [15])

| Tumor | Five-year survival (%) |
|---|---|
| Astrocytoma | 43 |
| Oligodendroglioma | 47 |
| Glioblastoma | 4 |
| Ependymoma | 59 |
| Other glioma | 30 |
| Medullobalstoma | 41 |
| Malignant meningioma | 50 |

commoner tumor types encountered in the CNS are listed in Table 3. There is considerable variation in survival times for each tumor considered. The values chosen are representative of 5-year survival rates in patients receiving the therapies outlined in this chapter.

## Work-up and Staging

Tumors of the CNS come to diagnosis as a consequence of innumerable symptoms and signs. In general, tumor location dictates symptoms, but non-specific symptoms such as headache, fatique, and mild cognitive impairment are common. Seizures, too, often bring CNS tumors to clinical attention. These are commoner with supratentorial lesions than with their infratentorial counterparts. Whether or not a patient presents with discreet signs or symptoms referable to a specific brain region, other causes of their disabilities including infection, stroke, demyelinating disease, and side effects of prior cancer treatment must be considered in the differential diagnosis.

## Primary Tumors

As a rule, primary CNS tumors rarely metastasize outside the CNS. Thus, systemic staging is rarely, if ever, necessary at the initial diagnosis of a primary CNS tumor. Furthermore, the commonest tumors (astrocytoma and oligdendroglioma) usually present as focal intra-CNS masses. Suspected tumors are usually diagnosed via neuroimaging. Brain or spine imaging with magnetic resonance imaging (MRI) scan is the most common technique employed today, although computed tomography (CT) scans are also used. Tumors of the pineal region, those involving the ventricular system, or those suggestive of medulloblastoma or primitive neuroectodermal tumors (PNET) are more likely to present with intra-CNS dissemnination and craniospinal imaging is warranted. Otherwise, unless symptoms warrant, imaging of the entire neuraxis is seldom necessary at presentation. Functional neuroimaging techniques such as positron electron emission tomography (PET) and magnetic resonance spectroscopy (MRS) can aid in guiding differential diagnosis.

Histologic diagnosis is essential in most CNS tumors. Because prognosis and treatment vary substantially according to tumor type, tissue diagnosis can be essential to management. A few notable exceptions exist. For example, lesions of the optic chiasm and tract with a radiologic appearance consistent with optic glioma are sometimes treated without biopsy, as are presumed brainstem gliomas in infants [16]. Occasionally, tumors with imaging features suggesting meningioma are also not biopsied. Finally, intrinisic spinal cord masses are sometimes not biopsied if their location precludes doing so.

Sampling of the cerebrospinal fluid (CSF) is essential in cases of PNET/medulloblastomas and pineoblastoma as well as primary CNS lymphoma. Rarely is CSF sampling of benefit in staging or treating astroglial or oligodendroglial tumors. Some advocate CSF sampling in the staging of ependymomas of high grade, but CSF dissemination is rare at initial presentation [17]. Cytologic examination for characteristic malignant cells remains the hallmark feature of any CSF analysis. Abnormalities of CSF protein (high) or glucose (low) are suggestive but not diagnostic of CSF involvement. With the exception of germ cell tumors, biochemical markers have not been very useful in the staging or management of primary CNS tumors [18]. In cases of known or suspected germ cell tumors, both beta-hcg and alpha-fetoprotein should be followed. If these proteins are elevated, a fall in their levels correlates with treatment response while an increase may herald disease progression before any other evidence for recurrent disease.

In pateints with primary CNS lymphoma (PCNSL) a detailed opthalomologic examination is recommended. The eyes may be involved in as many as 15% of patients at presentation and the treatment plan differs for this subset [19]. Patients with PCNSL and the acquired immune deficiency syndrome should undergo evaluation for systemic lymphoma.

An outline of the evaluation of a patient with suspected primary CNS tumor is provided in Figure 1.

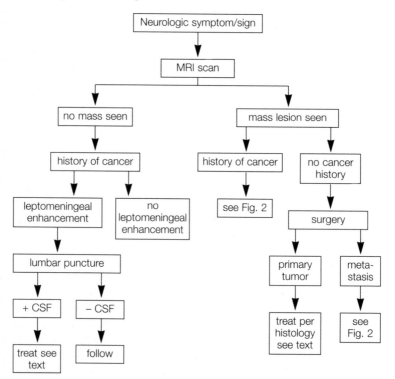

**Fig. 1.** Diagnostic approach to the patient with a suspected primary CNS tumor

## Metastatic Tumors

In contrast to primary CNS tumors, patients with known or suspected metastatic disease must undergo systemic staging. If, at biopsy, a newly diagnosed brain mass reveals metastatic disease in a patient not known to have systemic cancer, a comprehensive work-up is in order. This can, at times, be guided by the histologic diagnosis. At other times, a primary site is unclear and an exhaustive search for a primary source is necessary. More often than not, the patient with brain metastasis from a tumor other than lung cancer has systemic metastases, as well [20]. Knowledge of the extent of systemic disease is essential to appropriate treatment and may impact the modality chosen for treatment of the brain metasasis.

Many CNS masses suggesting tumor on neuroimaging in a patient with known cancer are either biopsied or resected. This is especially true of single or solitary accessible lesions. Exceptions might be made in the case of classic-appearing CNS masses in patients with known systemic cancer with a propensity to metastasize to the CNS where surgery plays no role in treatment. Of note, in a well controlled series studying the effect of surgery and irradiation on outcome in CNS metastases, >10% of presumed metastatic disease was found to represent either a second malignancy or an infection at biopsy [21]. Side effects of prior treatment (both radiation and chemotherapy) can also mimic metastatic masss CNS lesions. Finally, although rarely encountered, both stroke and demyelinating disease can also be confused with CNS tumor.

CSF sampling is important in metastatic disease. In some cases, leptomeningeal metastases exist in isolation from intraparenchymal spread, in others they are coincident. In patients with intraparenchymal lesions the need to assess CSF is guided by either imaging suggesting leptomeningeal disease or clinical features suggesting the diagnosis. As with primary tumors, cytologic confirmation of malignant cells is the cornerstone of diagnosis. Elevated CSF pressure, elevated protein, and depressed glucose can aid in the diagnosis if infection is excluded. Up to three separate lumbar punctures may be necessary to rule out leptomeningeal disease [22]. At times, treatment based on clinical suspicion alone may be warranted. Again, in patients with metastatic germ cell tumors, following CSF beta-hcg and alpha-fetoprotein levels can be of value. Other biochemical markers such as B2-microglobulin, lactate dehydrogenase isoenzymes, and carcinoembryonic antigen are sometimes followed but there is little concensus as to their value [23]. As sensitive tumor markers for specific cancers are developed, their role in assessing CSF dissemination will warrant testing.

An outline of the evaluation of a patient with known or suspected CNS metastasis is provided in Figure 2.

## Standard Treatment Options

Given the varieties of tumor types and because treatment varies considerably by histology, we will concentrate on those tumors arising most often in adults with mention of general principles of treatment for other tumor types. Those tumor types considered in detail below are:
- Low-grade infiltrative glial tumors
  - Astrocytoma
  - Oligodendroglioma
  - Oligoastrocytoma
- Anaplastic glial tumors
  - Anaplastic astrocytoma
  - Anaplastic oligodendroglioma
  - Anaplastic oligoastrocytoma
  - Glioblastoma multiforme
- Ependymoma
- PNET/medulloblastoma
- Primary CNS lymphoma
- Meningioma
- Intraparenchymal metastases
- Spinal (epidural) metastatses
- Leptomeningeal metastases

Treatment of all CNS tumors is directed both at effective anti-tumor therapy and at symptom control. Tumor-directed therapies themselves can have an adverse impact upon symptoms and the medications commonly used to control symptoms have potential negative impact on a patient's neurologic status. Most patients with CNS tumors will use coritcosteroids to relieve swelling-associated symptoms at some time during the course of their illness. Anticonvulsants are also commonly used. In addition to their side effects, the interactions of these drugs with chemotherapies must be considered. Analgesia and narcotics are less often

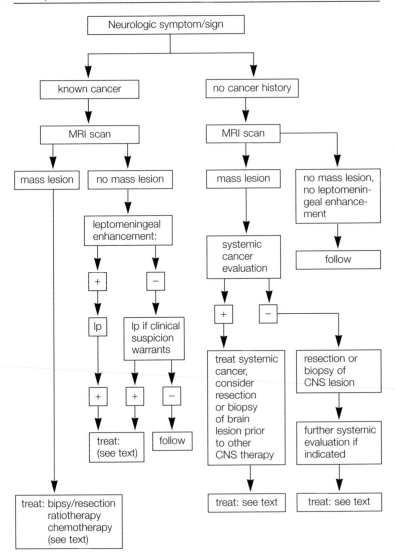

**Fig. 2.** Diagnostic approach to the patient with suspected CNS metastsis

used in brain tumor patients, except as adjuncts in the treatment of headache. A notable exception would be the patient with pain secondary to epidural spinal cord compression. Finally, the role of physical and occupational therapists, speech pathologists, and behavioral medicine specialists cannot be overlooked in the overall approach to the care of these patients.

Multimodality treatment is the rule for most CNS tumors. Treatment algorithms for each tumor type discussed below are provided throughout the text.

Surgical Treatment

*Primary Tumors*

Surgery is, with few exceptions, always recommended for purposes of diagnosis. Tumors of the optic pathway and brainstem, often encountered in children, are not always biopsied (16). Spinal masses may not always be biopsied. Recent advances in surgical techniques such as image-guided stereotaxy and multidisciplinary teams who assist in brain mapping have increased the possiblities for performing larger resections with higher degrees of safety. With the exception of well-circumscribed pilocytic astrocytomas and meningiomas, surgery is not considered potentially curative. However, in some instances, surgery alone may constitute initial therapy (see below).

Low-Grade Infiltrative Glial Tumors
(Astrocytoma, Oligodendroglioma, Oligoastrocytoma)
This diverse group of tumors comprises approximately 25% of all glial neoplams (see Fig. 3). The low grade astrocytoma is commoner in children, but oligodendroglioma and oligoastrocytoma occur more frequently in young adults. Although somewhat controversial, most neuro-oncologists recommend the maximal surgical resection that is safe in the initial management of low grade glial tumors [24]. Although these tumors may be relatively "benign" compared to their higher grade counterparts, most patients succumb to the disease. Five and ten year survival rates of 50% and 20%, respectively, are characteristic, despite treatment [24]. Children characteristically survive longer than do adults. Patients with complete or near complete resections are often observed

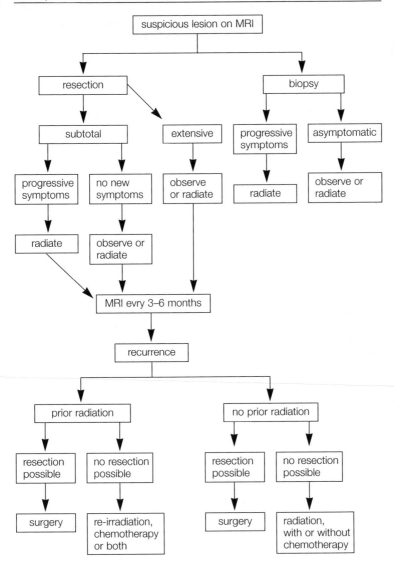

**Fig. 3.** Treatment approach to the patient with a low-grade infiltrative glial tumor

with surveillance MRI scans every 3–6 months and with any new symptoms. Symptomatic patients with subtotal resection are sometimes treated adjuvantly with radiotherapy, (see below). Asymptomatic patients with subtotal resections are more likely to be observed with surveillance MRI scans every 3–6 months [24]. Patients with recurrent disease following initial surgery should always be considered for further debulking procedures. This may be important in reducing disease burden and in assessing progression of the tumor to a higher grade of malignancy. These recommendations derive from retrospective studies often spanning many years. Several series suggest improved survival in patients who undergo extensive resection [24, 25]. The importance of adequate tissue sampling if biopsy alone is performed cannot be overstated, given the heterogeneity of these tumors.

Anaplastic Glial Tumors (Astrocytoma, Oligodendroglioma, Oligoastrocytoma, and Glioblastoma Multiforme) (See Fig. 4)
Anaplastic glial tumors are the commonest primary brain tumors. The highest grade tumor, glioblastoma multiforme, comprises half of these cases and its incidence increases with advancing age. The goals of surgery in these higher grade lesions include: diagnosis, symptom improvement by relief of mass effect, and lower requirements for steroid use. Maximal safe resections are recommended. However, as these lesions are highly infiltrative surgery alone is rarely, if ever, curative. Additional treatment is always recommended after surgery and these considerations should play a role in the surgical approach. The extent of surgical resection has been shown to lengthen survival in patient subsets, both at the time of initial diagnosis and at the time of tumor recurrence [26].

Ependymoma (Low Grade and Anaplastic)
Commoner in children than in adults, ependymomas can occur anywhere along the neuraxis (see Fig. 5). Supratentorial tumors are commoner in adults while infratentorial tumors are seen more often in children. They comprise 6–12% of primary tumors in children and less than 5% in adults. Surgery plays a central role in the management of these tumors, regardless of their grade. Patients with completely resected tumors do far better than their counterparts with subtotal resections (17, 27). Surgery should always be considered in the management of patients with recurrent disease, especially for relief of symptoms. As with most

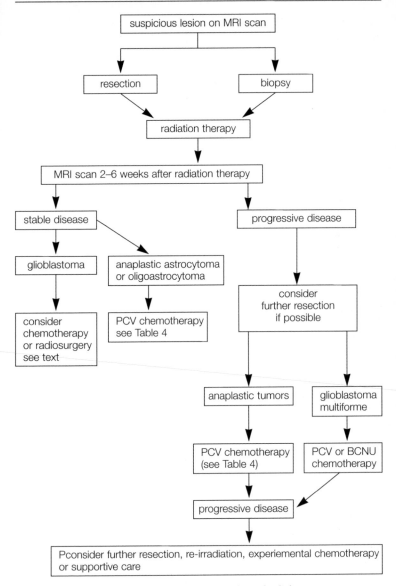

**Fig. 4.** Treatment approach to the patient with a high-grade glial tumor

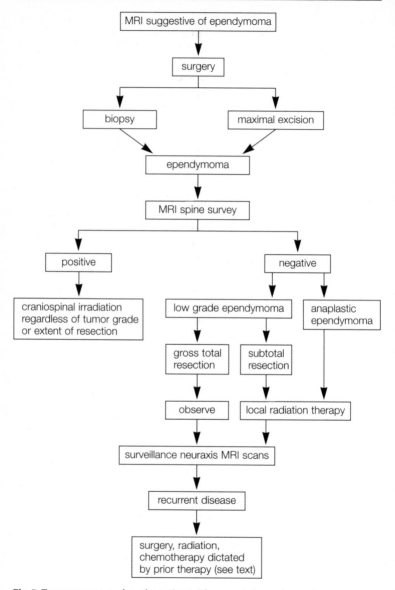

**Fig. 5.** Treatment approach to the patient with suspected ependymoma

primary CNS tumors, age at diagnosis is an important prognostic factor. However, relapse-free survival is also important because recurrent tumors are seldom successfully treated. Despite best available treatment, the 5 year actuarial survival for patients with ependymoma remains approximately 45% [28].

## PNET/Medulloblastoma

These tumors, more common in children, are also encountered in young adults (see Fig. 6). While they comprise approximately 8% of all primary CNS tumors, they represent over 20% of primary pediatric CNS tumors [29]. For purposes of this discussion, medulloblastoma will be considered PNET of the posterior fossa. These tumors have a propensity for subarachnoid spread and surgery alone is not curative. However, patients with gross totally resected tumors, both by the impression of the surgeon and a post-operative MRI scan, fare better than do those with biopsy alone or with limited resection. Patients with minimal residual disease after an extensive resection have outcomes similar to those with more extensive resections. Thus, second operations to attempt complete removal of these tumors are not warranted. Resection of PNET/medulloblastoma at the time of tumor recurrence should be aimed at palliation of symptoms.

## Primary CNS Lymphoma (PCNSL)

This rare tumor comprising approximately 1% of all primary brain tumors is encountered in patients with compromised immune function and, with increasing frequency, among the immunocompetent elderly (see Fig. 7). The only role for surgery in the management of PCNSL is for purposes of diagnosis (19).

## Meningioma

Meningiomas are common tumors of the arachnoid lining, affecting approximately 2 per 100,000 U.S. population [30] (see Fig. 8). Usually histologically benign, these tumors can display anaplastic (malignant) features. Surgery plays an important role in meningioma therapy. Complete resection can result in cure. However, the location of many of these tumors precludes a total resection. In these instances, adjuvant therapy, prinicpally radiation, plays a role (see below).

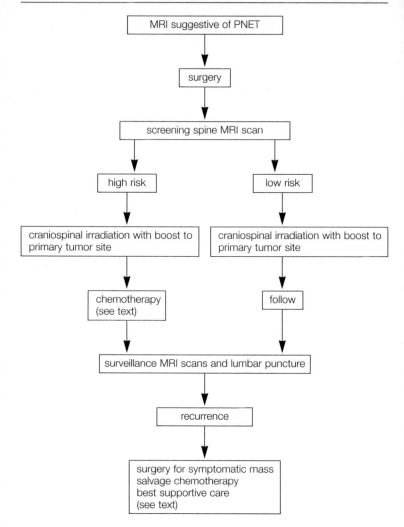

**Fig. 6.** Treatment approach to the patient with suspected PNET/medulloblastoma

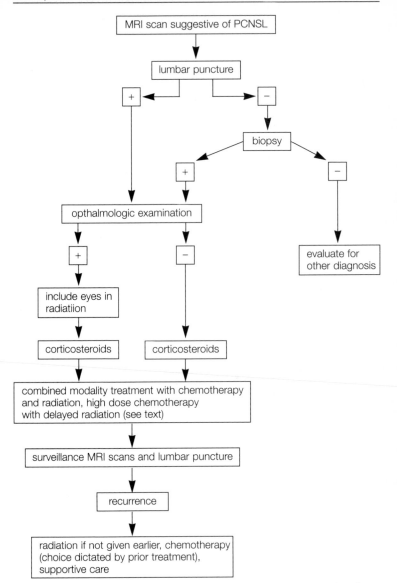

**Fig. 7.** Treatment approach to the patient with suspected primary CNS lymphoma (PCNSL)

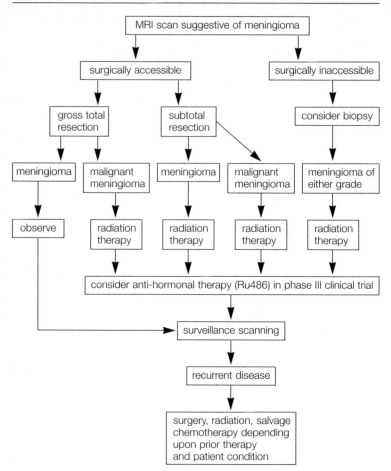

**Fig. 8.** Treatment approach to the patient with suspected meningioma

*Metastases*

**Intraparenchymal Metastases.** Intraparenchymal CNS metastases occur in 20–40% of cancer patients (see Fig. 2). These lesions may be solitary (the only known active tumor in the body), single (the only known active tumor in the CNS), or multiple. Surgery plays a variable role in the management of intraparenchymal CNS metastases depending upon the extent of the systemic disease, the number and surgical accessibility of the metastases, and the radiation and/or chemosensitivity of the original tumor. Strong consideration should be given to the removal of one or two surgically accessible but radioresistant lesions in patients with either controlled systemic disease or limited systemic disease with reasonable treatment options. Patients' with radiation-sensitive tumors (such as small cell lung cancer) should receive radiation, not surgery. If such patients fail to respond to radiation and are symptomatic from tumor mass, then surgery in such cases is appropriate.

**Spinal (Epidural) Metastases.** Metastases to the vertebral bodies and paravertebral spaces is common in systemic cancer. Spinal cord compression may occur as a consequence and is a common cause of substantial cancer-related morbidity, including pain, paraplegia, bowel and bladder dysfunction. The differential diagnosis of epidural spinal cord compression includes similarly located abcesses, hematomas, and herniated disks, as well as leptomeningeal disease and intraparenchymal tumor. Treatment of epidural spinal cord compression is often emergent. Surgery may be employed. Patients usually receive either laminectomy or vertebral body resection. There is considerable controversy as to whether patients undergoing surgical decompression do better than (or even as well as) those receiving radiation only [31]. Typical of such debates, comparison between studies is often difficult and patients in surgical series have often failed other treatments, including radiotherapy. Several indications for surgery include the presence of tumor from an unknown primary site, progression during or after radiotherapy, rapid progression of symptoms, and in the treatment of radioresistant tumors (such as renal cell carcinoma). Spinal instability is a common complication of surgery for relief of epidural spinal cord compression.

**Leptomeningeal Metastases.** There is no role for surgery in the treatment of leptomeningeal metastases excepting the important placement of CSF-systemic shunts for intrathecal therapy and cytologic monitoring (see below).

## Radiotherapy

Radiotherapy plays a central role in the management of most CNS tumors, if not in intitial management, then at the time of recurrence. Improvements in delivery systems have allowed radiotherapists to significantly alter the radiobiology of their treatments. In additional to conventionally administered external beam radiation, options include conformal treatment plans, stereotactic radiosurgery, braychytherapy, proton beam therapy, photodynamic therapy, and even boron neutron capture therapy (see Chapter 2). Re-irradiation is commonly administered in neuro-ocology.

### *Primary Tumors*

Low Grade Infiltrative Glial Tumors
(Astrocytoma, Oligodendroglioma, Oligoastrocytoma)
Considerable debate exists regarding both the timing and dosing of radiotherapy for the low grade infiltrating glial tumors (see Fig. 3). For patients with stable symptoms after surgery some favor adjuvant radiotherapy while others favor deferring radiation until the appearance of radiographic evidence for tumor progression. Small prospective and retrospective studies have been mixed, with some showing a survival advantage to post-operative radiotherapy and others not [32, 33]. A large randomized trial comparing adjuvant radiotherapy to delayed radiotherapy is now underway under the auspices of the Eurpean Orgainzation for Research and Treatment of Cancer (EORTC).

Most investigators do not hesitate to irradiate those patients with low grade infiltrating glial tumors who's symptoms are progressive. In addition, elderly patients with residual disease usually progress quickly without radiation. The conventional dose administered is usually approximately 54 Gy in 30 fractions of 180 cGy each. This dose is based upon the observations of Shaw et al where patients receiving less than 53 Gy had a poorer 5 year survival than those receiving $\geq$ 54 Gy [24].

Patients with recurrent or progressive disease are routinely irradiated with doses ranging from 54–60 Gy. In addition, patients with progressive low grade tumors who had previous external beam radiotherapy may receive stereotactic radiotherapy or focal re-irradiation.

Anaplastic Glial Tumors (Anaplastic Astrocytoma, Anaplastic Oligo-dendroglioma, Oligoastrocytoma, and Glioblastoma Multiforme)

Radiotherapy has been a central component of the initial treatment of high grade glial tumors for the last 25 years [34] (see Fig. 4). Doses of approximately 60 Gy in 33 fractions of 180 cGy each are routinely delivered. There have been many attempts to improve the effectiveness of radiotherapy with altered dose and fractionation schemes. To date, none has proved superior to conventional treatment. However, as stated above, changes in radiation technology such has highly conformal treatment fields may allows to improved survival and/or fewer side effects of treatment. This remains to be tested. Whether or not the addition of a focal stereotactic radiosurgery boost to conventional radiation treatment improves outcome is the subject of an ongoing Radiation Therapy Oncology Group (RTOG) trial, (RTOG 93–05).

Patients with recurrent high grade tumors are often subjected to re-irradiation, especially if they had a response to radiation initially. Several options exist, including brachytherapy, stereotactic radiosurgery, and stereotactic radiotherapy. None has yet been proven superior to the other and tumor location and size as well as treating physician preference often dictate which modality will be used.

Ependymoma (Low Grade and Anaplastic)

Radiotherapy plays a significant role in the initial management of patients with ependymoma (see Fig. 5). Excepting patients with gross totally resected low grade ependymomas and no evidence for dissemination, all patients with ependymoma should receive postoperative radiotherapy [35]. The entire craniospinal axis is irradiated whenever there is MRI evidence for disseminated disease, regardless of enpendymoma grade. Typical doses are 36 Gy to the craniospinal axis with a boost to 50–55 Gy to residual tumor.

Treatment of residual disease in the absence of dissemination depends to some extent upon tumor grade. Subtotally resected low grade tumors should receive local irradiation to a dose of approximately 54 Gy. There is some controversy as to whether patients with subtotally resected anaplastic ependymomas should receive local or craniospinal irradiation. Those who argue in favor of local radiation point out that neither local control rate nor spinal metastasis is prevented by the craniospinal approach (17). Whether or not altered fractionation schemes and/or the addition of stereotactic radiosurgery boosts will improve outcome remain unanswered questions.

PNET/Medulloblastoma)
Radiotherapy is central in the management of PNET/medulloblastoma
[29, 37] (see Fig. 6). Because this is a disease often affecting young children and because radiation has more toxicity in this age group, many
attempts have been made to reduce both the extent and dose of radiation
without success. Craniospinal radiation is recommended for all patients
after surgery because patterns of failure often include dissemination of
disease throughout the craniospinal axis and because attempts at controlling local disease with focal radiotherapy have failed to prevent
disease disemination. The usual dose is 36 Gy to the craniospinal axis
with a boost to the tumor bed to 54 Gy. Hyperfractionated radiation
schemes have been reported from single institutions but are not routinely employed at this time [37].

Primary CNS Lymphoma (PCNSL)
Radiation therapy is central to the management of PCNSL (see Fig. 7).
Complete radiographic responses are seen following the administration
of 40 to 50 Gy conventional whole brain radiation [38]. These responses
are short-lived and PCNSL is usually treated with both radiotherapy and
chemotherapy (see below). If the eyes are involved, 36 Gy is administered
to the posterior 2/3 of the globe as part of initial therapy (19).

Meningioma
Radiotherapy is commonly used in the treatment of meningioma (see
Fig. 8). Tumors that are incompletely resected or surgically inaccessible
are routinely irradiated. This has doubled both time to tumor recurrence
and long-term survival [39]. Patients with progressive disease may be re-
irradiated with further external beam treatment, stereotactic radiosurgery, or brachytherapy [40, 41].

*Metastases*

The role for radiotherapy in patients with brain metastases varies widely
depending upon the clinical circumstances (see Fig. 2) [42]. Patients with
very radiosensitive tumors (small cell lung cancer) should receive whole
brain radiation therapy at the time of diagnosis. Surgery for such patients should be withheld unless large accessible lesions are causing marked acute impairment. 30 Gy, administered in 10 fractions, constitutes

standard therapy. Patients with progressive systemic disease poor systemic treatment options and brain metastases of any number should receive whole brain radiation. Survival has not been improved by the addition of surgery to radiotherapy in such patients when surgically accessible lesions are removed [43]. Patients with recurrent tumors may receive additional external beam radiotherapy or focal treatment such as stereotactic radiosurgery.

## Chemotherapy/Combined Modality Therapy

Treatment for most brain tumors consists of combined modality therapies.

### *Primary Tumors*

Low Grade Infiltrative Glial Tumors
(Astrocytoma, Oligodendroglioma, Oligoastrocytoma)
Chemotherapy has no role in the initial management of low grade glial tumors (see Fig. 3). There are reports suggesting a benefit to the use of adjuvant treatment with several chemotherapy regimens, but these are either non-randomized prospective or retrospective series [44, 45]. Chemotherapy is often used in the treatment of recurrent low grade tumors. However, the histologic grade of such tumors is often of higher grade at the time of recurrence. The same agents used in the treatment of higher grade glial tumors are then employed (see below).

Anaplastic Glial Tumors (Anaplastic Astrocytoma, Anaplastic Oligodendroglioma and Oligoastrocytoma, and Glioblastoma)
Patients with anaplastic tumors of all three types listed above are now routinely treated with chemotherapy following surgery and radiotherapy. In the case of anaplastic oligodendroglioma, chemotherapy is sometimes given after surgery but prior to radiotherapy [46] (see Fig. 4). The most commonly employed drug combination in this context is procarbazine, CCNU, and vincristine (PCV). PCV chemotherapy is also routinely used following radiotherapy in the treatment of anaplastic astrocytoma [47]. PCV chemotherapy is usually given for a total of 6–8 cycles, each separated by 6 weeks. The treatment algorithm is given in

**Table 4.** PCV chemotherapy regimen

| Drug | Administration |
| --- | --- |
| CCNU | 110 mg/m$^2$ p.o. day 1 |
| Procarbazine | 60 mg/m$^2$/day p.o. days 8—21 |
| Vincristine | 1.4 mg/m$^2$ i.v. days 8 and 29 (2 mg maximum dose) |

Table 4. Patients with glioblastoma multiforme are often treated with single agent BCNU. This can be given in single doses of 210 mg/m2 every six weeks, usually for 6 cycles. Some investigators give the first few cycles of BCNU during radiotherapy and continue for a total of six cycles after radiation's completion.

Several drugs are used at the time of relapse in patients with high grade glial tumors. These include BCNU-impregnated wafers (Gliadel) in patients eligible for surgery, intravenous carboplatin, and high dose oral tamoxifen. Gliadel wafers are used to line post-operative surgical cavities and are not intended for the treatment of bulky residual disease. One of the advantages of this approach is minimal systemic side effects of chemotherapy. One of the disadvantages is post-operative cerebral edema often requiring high and prolonged steroid doses [48]. Carboplatin is infused at a dose of 300–400 mg/m2 in patients with normal renal function and given every 3–4 weeks. This is repeated up to twelve times in responding patients [49]. Tamoxifen is given in daily divided doses beginning at 120 mg/day. The dose may be increased to 240 mg/day as tolerated. Cerebellar dysfunction is the usual dose-limiting side effect [50]. Gliadel has been tested in a randomized prospective phase III trial [z]. Carboplatin and tamoxifen have been evaluated in a number of phase II trials [49, 50].

Ependymoma
Chemotherapy does not play a role in the treatment of ependymoma (see Fig. 5). Patients with recurrent disease who have received maximal radiotherapy are sometimes treated palliatively with PCV or platinum-based regimens.

PNET/Medulloblastoma
Chemotherapy plays a role in poor risk patients with PNET/medulloblastoma [29] (see Fig. 6). The factors contributing to poor risk include pri-

mary tumors outside the posterior fossa, residual tumor >1.5 cm2, and subarachnoid metastases at the time of diagnosis. Patients treated with either CCNU, cisplatin, and vincristine or cisplatin and etoposide experience improved disease-free and overall survival when compared to their counterparts receiving surgery and radiotherapy only [51]. Because medulloblastoma is so common in the very young, trials are ongoing to find improved chemotheraeutic regimens that might allows to delayed and/or reduced dose craniospinal radiotherapy.

Patients with recurrent disease are often treated palliatively with either nitrosoureas or platinum, the choice determined by prior treatment. Survival after relapse is poor.

## Primary CNS Lymphoma (PCNSL)

Chemotherapy is routinely used in the treatment of PCNSL (see Fig. 7). Some investigators choose to provide chemotherapy before and after radiotherapy. Others elect to treat patients with high dose chemotherapy and to eliminate or defer radiation. Standard protocols for systemic lymphoma are not any more effective than radiotherapy alone and should not be used.

Methotrexate may be given intravenously at high doses (up to 3.5 $g/m^2$) with or without post-chemotherapy irradiation. This latter approach is favored by some for the treatment of elderly and otherwise debilitated patients who tolerate the radiotherapy poorly [52]. A combination of intravenous methotrexate (1–3.5 g/m2) and intrathecal methotrexate (12 g/dose) followed by cranial irradiation (40 Gy whole brain with 14 Gy boost to bulky disease) and then high dose cytosine arabinoside (3 g/m2) was developed at Memorial Sloan Kettering Cancer Center and variations on this scheme are often used [53]. A RTOG-sponsored phase II trial of this strategy has recently closed. Results are pending. Median survivals of >40 months are reported for most protocols that include chemotherapy and radiation, contrasting favorably with those observed following radiotherapy alone (12 months) (19).

Survial rates similar to those reported above have been reported with post-radiation PCV chemotherapy in a small group of patients [54]. Hydroxyurea was given during radiation treatment to this group.

## Meningioma

Chemotherapy is rarely used in the treatment of meningioma. There are no currently accepted protocols (see Fig. 8). However, patients with progressive disease and no further surgery or radiation options sometimes receive palliative chemotherapy. Favorable responses have been reported in a very small study (four patients) using hydroxyurea [55]. This observation has prompted several phase II trials, all ongoing.

*Metastases*

Chemotherapy plays a variable role in the treatment of CNS metastases (see Fig. 2).

**Intraparenchymal Metastases.** Chemotherapy can be considered for patients with metastatic germ cell, breast, or small cell lung cancer, as well as for patients with metastatic hematologic malignancies. The choice of chemotherapy depends upon the extent of systemic disease, prior treatment history, and histology. In general, many drugs with activity against the tumor in question penetrate the blood brain barrier poorly with resultant unsatisfactory results.

**Spinal (Epidural) Metastases.** Chemotherapy for epidural metastases could be considered for the same tumor histologies listed above, but surgery and radiotherapy play a much more significant role in patient management.

**Leptomeningeal Metastases.** Chemotherapy is often administered in the context of leptomeningeal metastases. Given the complex anatomy and physiology of the subarachnoid space, chemotherapy is often administered via Ommaya resevoir. There are a limited number of agents that can be safely administered into the subarachnoid space, including methotrexate, cytosine arabinoside, and thiotepa. Methotrexate is usually given at 12 mg/dose twice a week for 5 doses and then every 1–4 weeks depending upon the clinical response [56]. Leucovorin rescue is given on the day of treatment and for three days thereafter. Cytosine arabinoside is given at a dose of 50 mg twice per week. Some investigators alternate methotrexate and cytosine arabinoside dosing. Thiotepa is used less frequently than either of the above two drugs as it is rapidly cleared from the CSF. The dose is 10 mg twice per week.

Biological Response Modifiers/Cytokines/Hormone Therapy

Many phase I and II clinical trials are either underway or have been completed that involve biologic response modifiers, cytokines and or hormone therapy, either alone or in combination with conventional therapies. To date, all such treatments remain experimental and none has become standard of care for either newly diagnosed or recurrent CNS disease. Many trials utilizing these agents in the treatment of systemic cancers exclude pateints with known brain metastases from participation.

Tamoxifen, mentioned above as a palliative (salvage) therapy for recurrent high grade glioma, is thought to mediate its antiproliferative effects in brain tumors through protein kinase C inhibition, not hormone antagonism [50].

The progesterone antagonist, Ru486, is presently being tested in a randomized double blind phase III study as therapy for meningioma following surgery and conventional radiotherapy. The trial was still open for enrollment at the time of this publication.

**Current Key Questions and Future Investigational Approaches**

The CNS is a challenging environment for anti-cancer therapies. Many drugs penetrate the blood-brain barrier poorly. Attempts to increase the intra-CNS concentrations of drugs have often resulted in either unacceptable systemic toxicities, CNS toxicity, or both. Strategies have included hyperosmolar and biochemical opening of the blood brain barrier [57], and high dose systemic chemotherapies with or without bone marrow transplant [58].

Intra-arterial chemotherapy with hyperosmolar opening of the blood brain barrier is still utilized at specialized institutions equipped to do so. It is unlikely that this strategy will achieve wide use due to its highly technical nature.

Biochemical modulation of the blood brain barrier is under investigation in an international randomized phase III trial. In this trial, patients with newly diagnosed glioblastoma multiforme are randomized to receive: post-operative pre-irradiation chemotherapy with carboplatin plus either placebo or RMP-7, a bradykinin analogue that transiently opens the blood brain barrier [59]. These patients will receive post-chemotherapy radiation and will be compared to a cohort who receive post-operative radiotherapy with or without adjuvant chemotherapy.

Interstitial chemotherapy may be able to overcome the problem of drug delivery by bypassing the blood brain barrier. BCNU-impregnated (Gliadel) wafers, mentioned above, use this strategy. Other agents are under investigation. This strategy will require the use of agents not dependent upon systemic metabolism for their effect and will require close attention to potential CNS toxicity.

The blood brain barrier contains very high levels of the multidrug resistance gene, p-glycoprotein [60]. Strategies aimed at selectively depleting blood brain barrier pgp activity are underway.

Overcoming drug resistance is as important in the treatment of CNS tumors as it is in any cancer. The commonest primary CNS tumors often have high levels of the enzyme O6-alkylguanine-DNA-alkyltransferase. This renders cells relatively resistant to the most effective drugs currently available in the treatment of primary CNS tumors [61]. Phase I trials utilizing O6-benzylguanine, an inhibitor of this enzyme, are underway in the treatment of high grade glioma.

Therapies directed at abnormalities specific to paritcular CNS tumors are underway. An example is SU-101, an inhibitor of tyrosine kinase [62]. Tyrosine kinases are often over-expressed in high grade glial neoplasms and their selective inhibition may result in tumor shrinkage. Another example is the use of the progesterone antagonist, Ru486, in the treatment of residual meningioma [63].

Radiation therapy remains the most effective means of controlling the growth of most CNS tumors, both primary and metastatic. Many attempts have been made to increase the effectiveness of radiation with altered dose and fractionation schemes as well as with radiation sensitizers. To date, no radiation sensitizers have been found to be convincingly superior to radiation alone. Hydroxyurea is sometimes used, based upon the results of a phase II trial using hydroyurea as a radiation sensitizer in patients with high grade astrocytoma [64].

Gadolinium-Texaphyrin is a radiation sensitizer that appears to exert its effects independent of cell cycle parameters and tumor cell oxygenation state [65]. The agent is currently in phase III testing in the treatment of brain metastases and in phase I testing as a radiation sensitizer in the treatment of glial tumors.

Gene therapies are currently under investigation in the treatment of primary CNS tumors. Using the so-called "suicide gene" approach, mouse fibroblasts producing the herpes simplex thymidine kinase gene have been injected into high grade glial tumors followed by treatment with the antiviral drug, gancyclovir [66]. A phase III trial using this approach is underway and new strategies using both attenuated herpes viruses and adenoviral vectors are in development.

The examples of innovative approaches to brain tumor treatment mentioned above are meant to be representative rather than all inclusive. There are currently more than one hundred phase I, II and III clinical trials available to persons with CNS tumors. A comprehensive list of such trials is unavailable from any single source. However, information on many trials can be obtained via the internet at: http://cancernet. nci.nih.gov/. Additional information may be obtained from the American Brain Tumor Association, 2720 River Road, Des Plaines, IL 60018. http://www.abta.org.

### References

1. Boring CC, Squires TS, Tong T (1993) Cancer Statistics. CA Cancer Clin J 43:7–26
2. Black PM (1990) Brain tumors: part 1. N Engl J Med 324:1555–1564
3. Walker AE, Robins M, Weinfeld FD (1985) Epidemiology of brain tumors: the National Survey of Intracranial Neoplasms. Neurology 24:981–985
4. Bahemuke M (1988) Worldwide incidence of primary nervous system neoplasms: geographical, racial and sex differences, 1960–1977. Brain 111:737–755
5. Velema JP, Walker AM (1987) The age curve of nervous system tumor incidence in adults: common shape but changing levels by sex, race, and geographic location. Int J Epidemiol 16:177–183
6. Doll R, Peto R. (1981) The causes of cancer: quantitative estimates of avoidable risk of cancer in the United States today. J Natl Cancer Inst 66:1291–1308
7. Helseth A, Mork SJ (1989) Neoplasms of the central nervous system in Norway: III. Epidemiological characteristics of intracranial gliomas according to histology. APMIS 97:547–555
8. Packer RJ, Finlay JL (1988) Medulloblastoma: presentation, diagnosis, and management. Oncology 17:35–49
9. Bohnen NI et al (1997) Descriptive and Analytic Epidemiology of Brain Tumors, In: Black PMcl, Loeffler JS (eds) Cancer of the Nervous System. Blackwell Science, Cambridge, MA, pp 3–24
10. Vanucci RC, Baten M (1974) Cerebral metastatic disease in childhood. Neurology 24:981–985
11. Delattre JY et al (1988) Distribution of brain metastases. Arch Neurol 45:741–744
12. Posner JB (1995) Pathophysiology of metastasis to the nervous system, In: Posner JB. Neurologic Complications of Cancer. FA Davis Co., Philadelphia, pp15–22
13. Kleihues P et al. (1993) Histologic Typing of Tumours of the Central Nervous System, Springer-Verlag, Berlin, pp 1–112
14. Louis DN, Gusella JF (1995) A tiger behind many doors: multiple genetic pathways to malignant glioma. Trends Genet 11:412–415

15. Giles GG et al (1993) Incidence and survival from cancers in Victoria 1970–1979 and 1980–1989. Anti-Cancer Council of Victoria, Melbourne
16. Alshail E et al (1997) Optic chiasmatic-hypothalamic glioma. Brain Pathol 7:799–806
17. Vanuytsel LJ et al (1992) Intracranial ependymoma: long-term results of a policy of surgery and radiotherapy. Int J Radiat Oncol Biol Phys 23:313–319
18. Wasserstrom WR et al (1981) Cerebrospinal fluid biochemical markers in central nervous system tumors: a review. Ann Clin Lab SCI 11:239–246
19. Freilich RJ, DeAngelis LM (1995) Primary central nervous system lymphoma. Neurol Clin N Am 13:901–914
20. Cairncross JG et al (1985) Radiation therapy for brain metastases. Ann Neurol 7:570–572
21. Patchell Ra et al (1990) A randomized trial of surgery in single metastases to the brain. N Engl J Med 322:494–500
22. Wasserstrom WR et al (1982) Diagnosis and treatment of leptomeningeal metastases from solid tumors: experience with 90 patients. Cancer 49:759–772
23. Rogers L et al (1987) Cerebrospinal fluid tumor markers as an aid to the diagnosis of meningeal metastasis. Proc Am Soc Clin Oncol 6:8
24. Shaw EG et al (1989) Radiation therapy in the management of low-grade supratentorial astrocytomas. J neurosurg 70:853–861
25. Phillipon JH et al (1993) Supratentorial low grade astrocytomas in adults. Neurosurgery 32:554–559
26. Curran WJ et al (1993) Recursive partitioning analysis of prognostic factors in three Radiation Therapy Oncology Group malignant glioma trials. J Natl Cancer Inst 85:704–710
27. Shaw EG et al (1987) Postoperative radiotherapy of intracranial ependymoma in pediatric and adult patients. Int J Radiat Oncol Biol Phys 13:1457–1462
28. Miller RW et al (1994) Histology of cancer incidence and prognosis: SEER population-based data, 1973–1987. Cancer 75:395–405
29. Rorke LB et al (1997) Primitive neuroectodermal tumors of the central nervous system. Brain Pathol 7:765–784
30. Cushing H (1922) The meningiomas (dural endotheliomas): their source, and favored seats of origin. Brain 45:282–306
31. Gilbert RW et al (1978) Epidural spinal cord compression from metastatic tumor: diagnosis and treatment. Ann Neurol 3:40–51
32. Lindegaard KF et al (1987) Statistical analysis of clincopathological features, radiotherapy, and survival in 170 cases of oligodendroglioma. J neurosurg 67:224–230
33. Shaw EG et al (1994) Mixed oligoastrocytomas: a survival and prognostic factor analysis. Neurosurgery 34:577–582
34. Walker MD et al (1978) Evaluation of BCNU and/or radiotherapy in the treatment of anaplastic gliomas. J Neurosurg 49:333–343
35. Rousseau P et al (1994) Treatment of intracranial ependymomas of children: review of a 15 year experience. Int J Radiat Oncol Biol Phys 22:281–286
36. Deutsch M et al (1996) Results of prospective randomized trial comparing standard dose neuraxis irradiation (3,600 cGy/20) with reduced neuraxis irradiation (2,340 cGy/13) in patients with low stage medulloblastoma: a combine Children's Cancer Group-Pediatric Oncology Group Study. Pediat neurosurg 24:167–177
37. Landverg TG et al (1980) Improvements in the radiotherapy of medulloblastoma 1946–1975. Cancer 45:670–678
38. Nelson DF et al (1992) Can high dose, large volume radiation therapy improve survival? Report on a prospective trial by the Radiation Therapy Oncology Group (RTOG): RTOG 8315. Int J Radiat Oncol Biol Phys 23:9–18

39. Barbaro NM et al (1987) Radiation therapy in the treatment of partially resected menigiomas. Neurosurgery 20:525–528
40. Engenhart R et al (1990) Stereotactic single high dose radiation therapy of benign intracranial meningiomas. Int J Radiat Oncol Biol Phys 19:1021–1026
41. Gutin PH et al (1987) Brachytherpay of recurrent tumors of the skull base and spine with iodine-125 sources. Neurosurgery 20:938–945
42. Coia LR (1992) The role of radiation therapy in the treatment of brain metastases. Int J Radiat Oncol Biol Phys 23:22–29
43. Noordijk EM et al (1994) The choice of treatment of single brain metastasis should be based extracranial tumor activity and age. Int J Radiat Oncol Biol Phys 29:711–717
44. Eyre Hj et al (1993) A randomized trial of radiotherapy versus radiotherapy plus CCNU for incompletely resected low-grade gliomas: Southwest Oncology Group study. J Neurosurg 78:909–914
45. Packer RJ et al (1993) Carboplatin and vincristine for recurrent and newly diagnosed low-grade gliomas of childhood. J Clin Oncol 11:850–856
46. Cairncross G et al (1994) Chemotherapy for anaplastic oligodendroglioma. J Clin Oncol 12:2013–2021
47. Levin VA et al (1995) Radiation therapy and romodeoxyuridine chemotherapy followed by procarbazine, lomustine, and vincristine for the treatment of anaplastic gliomas. Int J Radiat Oncol Biol Phys 32:75–82
48. Brem H et al (1995) Placebo-controlled trial of safety and efficacy of intraoperative controlled delivery by biodegradable polymers of chemotherapy for recurrent gliomas. Lancet 345:1008–1012
49. Yung WKA et al (1991) Intravenous carboplatin for recurrent malignant glioma: a phase II study. J Clin Oncol 9:860–864
50. Vertosik FT et al (1992) The treatment of intracranial malignant gliomas using orally administered tamoxifen therapy: preliminary resluts in a series of failed patients. Neurosurgery 30:897–902
51. Evans AE et al (1990) The treatment of medulloblastoma. Results of a prospective randomized trial of radiation therapy with and without CCNU, vincristine, and prednisone. J Neurosurg 72:572–582
52. Freilich RJ et al (1996) Chemotherapy without radiation therapy as initial treatment for primary CNS lymphoma in older patients. Neurology 46:435–439
53. DeAngelis LM et al (1990) Primary CNS lymphoma: combined treatmetn with chemotherapy and radiotherapy. Neurology 40:80–86
54. Chamberlain MC, Levin VA (1992) Primary central nervous system lymphoma: a role for adjuvant chemotherapy J Neurooncol 14:271–275
55. Schrrell et al (1997) Hydroxyurea for the treatment of unresectable and recurrent meningiomas. II. Decrease in the size of meningiomas in patients treated with hydroxyurea. J Neurosurg 86:845–852
56. Sullivan MP et al (1977) Combination intrathecal therapy for meningeal leukemia: two versus three drugs. Blood 50:471–479
57. Shapiro WR et al (1992) A randomized comparison of intra-artierial versus intravenous BCNU, with or without intravenous 5-fluoouracil, for newly diagnosed patients with malignant glioma. J Neurosurg 76:772–781
58. Nomura K et al (1984) Intensive chemotherapy with autologous bone marrow rescue in the treatment of recurrent malignant gliomas. Neurosurg Rev 7:13–22
59. Chang et al (1995) A pilot study of RMP-7 and carboplatin in patients with recurrent malignant glioma. Proc Am Soc Clin Oncol 14:152
60. Schinkel Ah (1998) Pharmacological insights from p-glycoprotein knockout mice. Int J Clin Pharm Ther 36:9–13

61. Pegg AE (1990) Mammalian O6-alkylguanine-DNA alkyltransferase: regulation and importance in response to alkylating carcinogenic and therapeutic agents. Cancer Res 50:6119–6129
62. Levitzki A, Gazit A (1995) Tyrosine kinase inhibitors: an approach to drug development. Science 267:1787–1788
63. Serfatz D (1995) Ru-486: current and potential indications. Great expectations and strong resistance. Presse Medicale 24:775–778
64. Kornblith PL, Walker M (1988) Chemotherapy for malignant gliomas. J Neurosurg 68:1–17
65. Rosenthal DI et al (1997) Phase I single dose trial of the radiation sensitizer gadolinium-texaphyrin (Gd-Tex) confirms tumor selectivity. Proc Am Soc Clin Oncol 16:480a
66. Culver KW et al (1995) Gene therapy for brain tumors In: Chang PL (ed) Somatic Gene Therapy, CRC Press, Boca Raton pp243–262

# Sarcomas

# Soft-Tissue Sarcomas

B. E. Brockstein, T. D. Peabody, M. A. Simon

## Epidemiology and Risk Factors

Soft-tissue sarcomas affect over 6,000 patients in the United States each year [1]. They are a heterogeneous group of neoplasms located in the upper and lower extremities in two-thirds of the cases but are also diagnosed in the retroperitoneum and trunk, head and neck, and soft-tissues of the gastrointestinal and genitourinary tract. Rarely, they occur in other viscera. While soft-tissue sarcomas are three times as common as their counterparts affecting bone, they are rare in comparison to benign soft-tissue tumors including hemangiomas, lipomas, and benign nerve sheath tumors. The most common anatomical location for a soft-tissue sarcoma is the thigh. Tumors presenting in this location are often large, and intramuscular, and symptoms may be of long duration. However, some soft-tissue sarcomas will be small (less than 5 cm) and up to 30% of extremity sarcomas may be located in subcutaneous tissues [2]. Soft-tissue sarcomas present with highly variable symptoms and physical findings. Similarly their behavior is unpredictable and certain aspects of treatment remain controversial.

The most common histological subtypes of soft-tissue sarcomas of the extremities are presented in Table 1. The relative incidence of these histologies varies by anatomic location. In the extremities, malignant fibrous histiocytoma (MFH) is the most common soft-tissue sarcoma. However, in the retroperitoneum, liposarcoma is more commonly seen and leiomyosarcoma is most common in the uterus. Special note should be made that desmoid tumors, Kaposi's sarcoma, and dermatofibrosarcoma protuberans are not included in most soft-tissue sarcoma series.

Soft-tissue sarcomas do not have any racial predilection and affect men and women equally. They are most commonly diagnosed in patients in the fifth decade of life however these soft-tissue sarcoma occur

**Table 1.** Most common histological subtypes of soft-tissue sarcomas of the extremities

| | |
|---|---|
| Malignant fibrous histiocytoma | 35% |
| Liposarcoma | 20% |
| Synovial Sarcoma | 10% |
| Neurosarcoma | 10% |
| Fibrosarcoma | |
| Leiomyosarcoma | |
| Angiosarcoma | |
| Rhabdomyosarcoma | together, 25% total |
| Epithelioid Sarcoma | |
| Malignant Hemangiopericytoma | |
| Alveolar Soft Parts Sarcoma | |

throughout life. When considering treatment and prognosis, it is useful to separate rhabdomyosarcoma, the most common pediatric soft-tissue sarcoma, from adult soft-tissue sarcoma. Similar to bone sarcomas, little is known about the etiology of these tumors. In a very few cases, heritable conditions such as Li Fraumeni syndrome or Von Recklingausen's neurofibromatosis (NF) may be associated with the development of a soft-tissue sarcoma [3, 4]. While possible, it is rare for a soft-tissue sarcoma to dedifferentiate from a pre-existing benign soft-tissue neoplasm. Multifocal angiosarcoma or lymphgiosarcoma may be seen in edematous upper extremities of women treated with lymph node dissection or radiation for breast carcinoma (Stewart-Treeves syndrome).

## Pathology and Staging

It is important to note that pathologic interpretations and definitions regarding soft-tissue sarcomas are constantly changing. For example, malignant fibrous histiocytoma, the most common soft-tissue sarcoma of the extremities, was formerly classified as fibrosarcoma or rhabdomyosarcoma in many cases. In the future, it may come under the more general term spindle cell sarcoma. Likewise, gastrointestinal stromal tumors (GIST) were formerly classified as leiomyosarcoma. Fortunately, for most extremity sarcomas it does not appear that histology is related in any way to patient prognosis.

The most important prognostic variables are tumor grade, tumor size, the presence or absence of metastases, and possibly tumor depth. Tumor grade is defined as an estimation of a particular tumor's likelihood to metastasize based on histological measures of cell differentiation and growth. This is based on tumor cellularity, nuclear atypia, mitotic activity, and necrosis [5, 6]. Unfortunately, even among expert pathologists, there is a great deal of difficulty in obtaining agreement on histologic grading of soft-tissue sarcomas [2, 7, 8].

The American Joint Commitee on Cancer (AJCC) Staging System is the most commonly used staging system and was revised in the latest edition published in 1997 [9]. This is a "TNM" system which includes tumor grade. The staging system is outlined in Table 2. There are four histological grades numbered 1–4. Well differentiated (G1) and moderately differentiated (G2) tumors are considered low-grade, while poorly differentiated (G3) and undifferentiated (G4) tumors are considered high-grade. The variable T refers to tumor size and depth. Size is defined as less than or equal to 5 cm (T1) or greater than 5 cm (T2). Depth is defined as superficial (a) or deep (b). Superficial lesions do not involve the superficial fascia covering the muscle. Deep lesions are deep to or invade the superficial investing fascia of the muscle and also include all intraperitoneal visceral lesions or lesions with major vessel invasion, intrathoracic lesions, and the majority of head and neck tumors. Adult soft-tissue sarcomas rarely metastasize to lymph nodes [10], although patients with synovial sarcoma and rhabdomyosarcoma are at a higher risk of metastases to lymph nodes than are patients with other histological types of sarcoma. When they do occur, they are associated with a very poor prognosis. Their survival is similar to or worse than those patients with the more commonly noted pulmonary metastases. Any metastases place the patient in stage 4 disease as defined by this system.

Critics of this staging system point to the fact that the AJCC System is based largely on single institution studies which demonstrate that size, grade, and depth are independent prognostic factors. In fact, it is quite possible that the effect of prognostic variables on survival is time dependent. High tumor grade has been noted to be associated with early metastatic disease whereas the negative effect of large size on survival may not be seen for several years [11]. In addition, other studies have demonstrated that tumor depth is not as important a prognostic factor as grade or the presence or absence of metastases [2]. It is clear that not all prognostic variables should be weighted equally.

The use of 5 cm as a dimension of importance in determining prognosis by this Committee should be considered arbitrary. Certainly pati-

**Table 2.** American Joint Committee on Cancer staging protocol for sarcomas of soft-tissue (from [9])

| Staging | | | | |
|---|---|---|---|---|
| Stage IA | G 1–2 | T1a–1b | N0 | M0 |
| Stage IB | G1–2 | T2a | N0 | M0 |
| Stage IIA | G1–2 | T2b | N0 | M0 |
| Stage IIB | G3–4 | T1a–1b | N0 | M0 |
| Stage IIC | G3–4 | T2a | N0 | M0 |
| Stage III | G3–4 | T2b | N0 | M0 |
| Stage IN | Any G | Any T | N0 or 1 | M1 |

Stage characteristics
Stage IA    Low-grade, small, superficial or deep
Stage IB    Low-grade, large, superficial
Stage IIA   Low-grade, large deep
Stage IIB   High-grade, small, superficial or deep
Stage IIIC  High-grade, large, superficial
Stage III   High-grade, large, deep
Stage IV    Any metastases

Primary tumor
T1 Tumor 5 cm or less in greatest dimension
T2 Tumor more than 5 cm in greatest dimension

Distant metastases
MO    No distant metastases
M1    Distant metastases

Histologic grade
G1      Well differentiated
G2      Moderately well differentiated
G3–4    Poorly differentiated; undifferentiated

Depth
a    Superficial: lesion does not involve
     Involve superficial fascia
b    Deep: lesion is deep to or invades the superficial fascia
(Includes all intraperitoneal visceral lesions or lesions with major vessel invasion or
intrathoracic, head, or neck location)

ents with very small tumors, many of which are subcutaneous, have an excellent prognosis. No study, however, has shown that 5 cm is a critical measure in distinguishing low, intermediate, and high-risk patient populations. Size is likely a continuous variable and it may be that tumor volume or weight may be more predictive of patient outcome.

Additionally, this system is based on studies including a number of non-extremity lesions affecting the retroperitoneum, thorax, and head and neck. It is likely that extremity lesions should be considered separately, because as a group they are resectable with wide margins and have a better prognosis than do sarcomas of other anatomic locations of the same stage.

Finally, this system has not been subjected to multi-institutional tests of validity. Its value in estimating an individual's prognosis is not clear. What is apparent from the staging , however, is that the population of patients with large, high-grade and deep tumors are at high risk of metastatic disease. Small low-grade tumors are associated with survival of greater than 90% at five years. In contrast, patients with large high-grade tumors have a long term survival of approximately 50%. These latter patients are those to which innovative adjuvant therapy should be directed [11]. Patients with stage IV disease have a long term survival of approximately 5%.

Certain cytogenetic abnormalities have been noted in soft-tissue sarcomas. A brief list of consistent chromosomal translocations in soft-tissue locations is included in Table 3. Approximately 25–30% of soft-tissue sarcomas are associated with overexpression of p53 [12] and 10–25% with mutation of the p53 gene [13], and this appears to correlate with poor prognosis. In contrast, bcl-2, expressed in approximately 50% of soft-tissue sarcomas, appears to correlate to a good prognosis [14]. It is likely that further advances in our understanding of the underlying genetic and biologic mechanisms responsible for the development of these sarcomas will lead to a more accurate staging system, one based not on crude estimates of tumor size and histologic grade, but on a more fundamental molecular basis.

**Table 3.** Chromosomal translocations in sarcomas

| Diagnosis | Translocation |
| --- | --- |
| Clear cell sarcoma | t(12;22)(q13;q12) |
| Ewing's/PNET | t(11;22)(q24;q12) |
| Extraskeletal myxoid chondrosarcoma | T(9;22)(q31;q12) |
| Myxoid liposarcoma | t(12;16)(q13;p11) |
| Alveolar rhabdomyosarcoma | T(2;13)(q35;q14) |
| Synovial cell sarcoma | T(x;18)(p11;q11) |

## Work-up and Staging

A general systematic evaluation of a patient with a soft-tissue mass is outlined in Figure 1. A mass greater than 5 cm in dimension or located deep to the fascia must be considered malignant until proven otherwise either by biopsy or by magnetic resonance imaging. A large number of patients with soft-tissue sarcomas, especially those in a subcutaneous location, will be referred following marginal excision performed outside

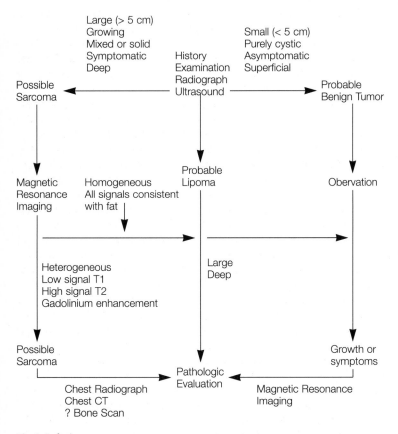

**Fig. 1.** Soft-tissue mass

the operating room under local anesthesia for a presumed benign neoplasm. In these cases, the diagnosis will be known and the patient evaluation will include staging for metastatic disease and imaging for residual disease or local contamination. Because of the risk of local recurrence due to contamination or inadequate resection, a re-excision is frequently necessary, and therefore all soft tissue masses suspected of being a sarcoma should be resected by an orthopedic or surgical oncologist.

The best imaging test for evaluating soft-tissue masses is magnetic resonance imaging. It will demonstrate tumor depth, size, and the relationship of the tumor to the surrounding neurovascular structures. In addition, magnetic resonance imaging may be diagnostic as is the case for most deep and superficial lipomas. Positron emission tomography scanning and thallium scanning are considered investigational tools at this time but they may be of value in evaluating a patient for local disease and non-pulmonary metastases, to measure response to therapy, or to detect tumor recurrence. Computed tomography of the chest is more sensitive than chest x-ray and is an important part of staging the individual known to have a soft-tissue sarcoma. The most common route of metastatic spread for extremity tumors is a hematogenous one to the lungs. For visceral and retroperitoneal sarcomas, the liver should be imaged due to its higher risk of metastases. As stated earlier, metastases to lymph nodes are unusual in soft-tissue sarcomas. However, certain soft-tissue sarcomas such as synovial sarcomas, epithelioid sarcomas, and rhabdomyosarcoma may metastasize to lymph nodes. In these cases, gallium scanning or PET scanning may be effective in detecting non-pulmonary metastases.

The biopsy is ideally performed following all other imaging tests, as the quality of the images may be degraded by postoperative changes, hematoma, or inflammation that results from any intervention. As stated, large or deep tumors are more likely to be malignant and should be referred to a musculoskeletal oncologist prior to biopsy. The biopsy may be an open procedure involving incision or excision of the tumor mass or a closed procedure using fine needles (25 gauge) or Trephines. The decision to proceed with any form of biopsy depends on the experience and availability of qualified pathologists for the interpretation of the results. In addition, the amount of diagnostic tissue needed for electron microscopy or other special tests may impact upon a particular type of biopsy. Because almost all patients with soft-tissue sarcomas are candidates for limb salvage procedures, it is important not to perform the biopsy in such a way that wide resection of the tumor is made more difficult or even impossible. Biopsy placement is critical and should be performed through small longitudinal incisions. Care must be taken not to contaminate other anatomic compartments or surrounding neurovascular structures in the performance of a biopsy. The person performing the biopsy must be aware of the standard approaches made during the performance of limb salvage procedures so that the biopsy tract may be excised at the time of definitive surgery. The biopsy is a technically simple procedure but must be performed by an experienced physician who should be the individual ultimately responsible for the operative management of the patient. Poorly placed biopsies or biopsy complications may lead to the need for an amputation [15].

Histologic evaluation of the biopsy specimen is essential in determining stage and treatment alternatives. While preoperative radiation therapy may be given to tumors of any grade in an effort to make limb salvage possible, chemotherapy is generally reserved for high-grade lesions. Grade is a histological measure that may be more difficult to determine based solely on fine needle aspiration. Trephine or open biopsy will usually reveal the tissue architecture necessary to make such a determination. Additional histochemical stains may allow the pathologist to arrive at a precise histologic diagnosis. However, as stated, histology is generally not as important as grade in determining a patient's prognosis.

## Stage Specific Standard Treatment Options

Surgical Treatment

Operative resection of soft-tissue sarcomas remains the mainstay of treatment at this time. Adjuvant local therapy in the form of radiation therapy (addressed later) may decrease the prevalence of local relapse but, to date, has not been of demonstrated benefit in prolonging survival in these patients. Surgical resection may be defined as (a) intralesional, (b) marginal, (c) wide, or (d) radical [16]. Similar to bone sarcomas, soft-tissue sarcomas tend to grow in a centrifugal manner compressing surrounding soft tissues into a reactive zone or *pseudocapsule*. This pseudocapsule contains compressed fibrous tissue, peritumoral vascular structures, inflammatory cells, and small foci of tumor cells. For this reason, surgical resection in the plane between the neoplasm and the reactive zone in the form of debulking is most commonly performed as a palliative procedure associated with a high incidence of local recurrence. In contrast, marginal resections performed in the plane of this reactive zone may be associated with an acceptable rate of local recurrence if an effective adjuvant is administered. This is commonly in the form of pre or postoperatively administered external beam radiation therapy and/or brachytherapy.

The preferred and most commonly performed surgical treatment of a soft-tissue sarcoma, which may be curative in many instances, is a wide resection. This involves removing the sarcoma in continuity with surrounding normal soft tissues outside of the reactive zone. Obviously it is technically feasible in certain anatomic locations such as the lateral thigh. In other locations such as with a very large tumor immediately adjacent to neurovascular structures or bone, a marginal resection is all that is possible. In these instances, adjuvant radiation therapy is generally administered to decrease the chance of local recurrence. In cases where a presumed benign mass is excised and later is proved to be a sarcoma, a wide re-excision of the biopsy tract and all tumor contaminated tissue is recommended. In a large proportion, the re-excised tissue will show evidence of residual tumor [2, 17].

Radical resections involving removal of the entire anatomic compartment from which the tumor originated are uncommonly performed today for soft-tissue sarcomas. For example, a radical resection for a tumor originating in the anterior compartment of the thigh would involve resection of the entire anterior compartment from anterior iliac crest to tibial tubercle. With conventional imaging and the ability of the surgeon to preoperatively precisely identify the location and extent of the tumor, this is rarely necessary. From an oncological, or survival, standpoint, it does not matter whether surgery is performed in the form of limb sparing resections or amputations. Most patients (80–90%), however, are given the option of limb salvage surgery. Operative treatment must be individualized and the patient educated as to the oncological and functional implications of the various alternative procedures.

Radiation Therapy

Historically, because of the high local recurrence rates following even radical resections of soft-tissue sarcomas and the belief that these tumors were in fact radioresistent, amputation was recommended for patients with soft-tissue sarcomas of the extremities [18]. However, the combination of operative resection and high-dose radiation therapy has been shown in multiple studies to be effective in local control of soft-tissue sarcomas. The theory is that while radiation is not lethal for large bulky tumors, it is effective in destroying microscopic disease at the periphery of the tumor in many cases. For tumors located in the extremities, the combination of radiation therapy and operative resection allows the limb to be salvaged in most instances [19–21]. Unfortunately, demonstrable improvement in survival has not been shown.

Radiation therapy may be administered preoperatively, intraoperatively, or postoperatively. It may be administered in the form of teletherapy or external beam therapy (orthovoltage or supervoltage) or brachytherapy (interstitial or intercavitary) [22]. Currently, many centers treat large soft-tissue sarcomas with preoperative external beam radiation therapy. In theory and practice, radiation given prior to surgery has several advantages. First, the tumor may diminish in size improving the quality and quantity of operative margins, especially about bone and neurovascular structures. Second, a "rind" formed by a thickened and edematous fibrous tissue is found to surround the tumor after radiation, making contamination through inadvertent tumor spillage less likely. Third, if contamination does occur, the tumor cells may be non-viable as a result of the preoperative radiation. Fourth, radiation may be lethal to the microscopic satellite tumor cells located at the periphery of the tumor making recurrence less likely. Last, radiation therapy is most effective in the well oxygenated and vascularized tissue found pre-operatively.

Despite these theoretical advantages, preoperative radiation appears to only have an advantage over postoperative radiation in tumors greater than 15 cm. Tepper & Suit [23] noted no overall difference in local control between pre and postoperative radiation therapy for tumors less than 15 cm. However, in tumors greater than 15 cm, local control was obtained in 78% of the patients treated preoperatively compared to 61% postoperatively. It should be noted in this study, however, that there is some selection bias as tumors of higher stage tended to be treated preoperatively which may underestimate the effect of preoperative treatment.

Preoperative radiation is administered to a dose of 5000 cGy in 200 cGy fractions. Operative resection is performed two to four weeks following completion of radiotherapy. If margins are negative at the time of surgery no additional therapy is recommended. In cases where tumor contamination occurs or positive margins are evident, an addition 1500 cGy radiation boost is given in the form of brachytherapy, intraoperative electron therapy, or postoperative external beam therapy [24].

The disadvantage of preoperative radiation therapy is primarily related to wound healing complications, especially following resection of thigh sarcomas. At times, a musculocutaneous flap should be performed to encourage wound healing. In addition, a potential disadvantage is the relatively large area being treated which often results in significant limb edema, fibrosis, and joint stiffness.

Preoperative radiation therapy has been used in combination with chemotherapy for large high-grade sarcomas. Intraarterial and intravenous therapy is used with no clear differences noted [25]. More recently, Eilber et al. [26] reported promising early results with a regimen using intravenous ifosfamide for two doses followed by preoperative external beam radiation therapy given in 350 cGy fractions to a dose of approximately 2800 cGy. Doxorubicin and cisplatin are administered following the radiation therapy and surgical resection is performed three weeks after the completion of pre-operative chemotherapy. The three cycles of pre-operative chemotherapy are repeated post-operatively.

Brachytherapy refers to the role of ionizing radiation therapy through local implantation of radioisotopes. A high-dose of radiation is supplied to the local area most at risk for local relapse sparing much of the surrounding tissue. It may be given in addition to or in place of external beam radiation therapy. In addition to limiting the tissue volume being treated, in theory, the tissues at the time of tumor resection remain well oxygenated, thus improving the effect of radiation.

Brachytherapy is performed by placing multiple thin plastic canulaes across the surgical field following tumor resection. These tubes are subsequently loaded with a radioisotope, most commonly iridium[192]. These loaded catheters remain in place in the wound for a length of time depending on the total dose to be delivered; 4200 to 4500 cGy over four to six days when brachytherapy is administered alone, or a shorter duration of treatment is given when brachytherapy is combined with external beam radiation therapy.

Pisters et al. [27] demonstrated in a randomized trial that adjuvant brachytherapy improved local control after complete resections of soft-tissue sarcomas. This improvement, however, was limited to patients with high-grade histology. No effect on survival was noted in a similar fashion to all radiation therapy studies. Brachytherapy may have certain advantages in that the treatment course is abbreviated compared to external beam radiation. Disadvantages, however, are that inpatient hospitalization is required and that brachytherapy is associated with a high incidence of wound healing complications. The true value of brachytherapy may lay in treating patients when positive margins are obtained, tumor contamination occurs, or when there is gross tumor residual.

Postoperative radiation therapy is usually administered in doses of 6400 cGy in 200 cGy fractions. A shrinking field technique is used following wound healing [23]. The operative wound drain sites and areas of potential contamination are included in the radiation field. A strip of soft-tissue of the circumference of the extremity should be spared in order to minimize lymphedema, swelling, fibrosis, and joint stiffness.

Yang et al. at the National Cancer Institute published long term follow-up of a randomized trial of 141 patients who received limb sparing surgery followed by adjuvant XRT or no adjuvant XRT [28]. All 91 high grade patients received concurrent chemotherapy, while the 50 low grade patients received no chemotherapy. Ten year follow-up showed only 1 local recurrence in irradiated patients versus 17 patients receiving no radiation (78% local-recurrence free survival in high grade, no radiation group and 63% in low grade no radiation group). Again, no effect on overall survival was seen. A functional and quality of life analysis showed a negative effect of radiation on limb range of motion, limb strength and edema but no difference measured by a global quality of life scale. It should be noted that in this study, chemotherapy with doxorubicin and cyclophosphamide was given concomitant with RT which may have increased both the local control and the toxicity.

Similarly electron beam radiation therapy has been noted to have some effect in soft-tissue sarcomas [29]. Again, the advantage is the ability to deliver a high dose of radiation therapy to a limited area, especially in cases where wide resection is not possible. Doses from 750 cGy to 2000 cGy may be administered through the use of Lucite cylinders. Peripheral neuropathy is the most common adverse effect noted and appears to be a dose limiting adverse effect.

Proton therapy has been used with success in certain anatomic locations. Protons are heavy particles for which penetration is finite and which allow high doses of radiation to be delivered to small volumes of tissues. Protons are particularly important in the treatment of paraspinal and skull based tumors [30]. Neutron beam therapy is another alternative treatment modality. It is most commonly used at this time for patients with non-resectable advanced malignancies [31]. This form of high energy therapy is associated with local tumor control in many cases, however, is associated with a higher incidence of side-effects as compared to proton or photon therapy.

Finally, radiation therapy may be used palliatively in the treatment of patients with advanced non-resectable tumors. It may be effective in slowing local tumor progression and alleviating pain, and may occasionally allow permanent local control.

Not all patients with soft-tissue sarcomas require radiation therapy [32]. Those with small tumors located in anatomic locations that allow wide resections with a large amount of surrounding normal tissue are at low likelihood of recurrence and likely will not require radiation therapy. In addition, subcutaneous sarcomas, for the same reasons, generally do not require additional radiation therapy. For all other patients, an individual decision should be made based on the likelihood of local recurrence and the risk of acute and chronic toxicity.

## Chemotherapy/Combined Modality Therapy

Due to the rarity of soft-tissue sarcomas, issues relating to chemotherapy are frequently generalized to all soft-tissue sarcomas as a whole, despite the existence of differences in clinical behavior amongst some of the numerous subtypes. This section will deal with general chemotherapy issues related to adult soft-tissue sarcomas. Specific subtypes in situations for which the general rules do not apply will be discussed separately.

### Single Agent Chemotherapy

Despite the rarity of soft-tissue sarcomas, most old and new chemotherapy drugs have undergone clinical trials as single agents for the therapy of advanced soft-tissue sarcoma. Only a few drugs have shown consistent activity. Doxorubicin [32–35] and ifosfamide [36–42] are the two most active agents, with single agent activity ranging from 15 to 30% for doxorubicin and 15–40% for ifosfamide, depending on the dose, setting and study. Both doxorubicin [33, 43] and ifosfamide [39, 40] appear to demonstrate a steep dose response relationship. Dacarbazine (DTIC) has consistently produced a response rate of 15 to 20% [44]. Less active drugs, to which 10–15% of patients respond, include cyclophosphamide, methotrexate, cisplatin, and carboplatin. Most of the newly approved drugs of the 1990's, including paclitaxel [45,46], docetaxel [47], topotecan [48] and oral etoposide [49] have undergone clinical trials with response rates of less than 10% in mostly pretreated patients. Gemcitabine [50], edatrexate [51] and navelbine [52] have shown some initial promising responses. Suprisingly, initial trials of Doxil, a liposomal form of doxorubicin, have been disappointing [53].

Thus, in general, if a single agent is to be used for *palliation* of an advanced soft-tissue sarcoma, doxorubicin at a dose of 60 to 90 mg/m$^2$ every three weeks should be used. Infusions of 48 to 96 hours are commonly utilized to minimize cardiac toxicity [54]. Ifosfamide, which is probably more active in short infusions (1 to 4 hours) than as a continuous infusion, is equally acceptable [36, 40]. A total dose of 8 to 14 g/m$^2$ as a daily short infusion divided over 4 to 5 days is commonly used. At these doses, ifosfamide is nearly equally effective in untreated patients as in those who have previously received doxorubicin. Even in patients refractory to low dose ifosfamide, a response rate of up to 30% is seen with higher dose ifosfamide [41]. Ifosfamide and cyclophosphamide have been compared in a randomized trial by the European Organization for the Research and Treatment of Cancer (EORTC) [42]. Amongst a group of 135 patients, ifosfamide had a response rate of (18%) versus (8%) for cyclophosphamide (p = .13). A current EORTC trial is comparing (3 regimens of) ifosfamide or doxorubicin as first line therapy with an accrual goal of 780 patients.

*Combination Chemotherapy*

Numerous chemotherapy combinations have been utilized to treat soft-tissue sarcomas. The four regimens most commonly utilized include:
- CyVADIC. This regimen of cyclophosphamide, vincristine, doxorubicin and dacarbazine utilizes two suboptimally active agents, thereby compromising on the doses of the two most active agents. Although one study [35] showed an equivalent 28% response rate between CyVADIC and AI (doxorubicin and ifosfamide), the doses of doxorubi-

cin and ifosfamide in the AI regimen were on the low end of the dose response curve and less than those used by most sarcoma groups. CyVADIC is not commonly used currently.

- AD. This regimen of doxorubicin and dacarbazine, which is commonly given as a continuous infusion but can be given IV bolus, has been compared in randomized trials to doxorubicin alone as well as the MAID regimen (see below). It yields higher response rates than doxorubicin alone [34, 55] but a lower response rate than the MAID regimen [56]. In these randomized studies, despite the differences in response rates, median survival was not improved in the more aggressive regimens.

- MAID. This regimen of mesna, ifosfamide, doxorubicin, and DTIC become a "standard" in the late 1980's. MAID combines the three most active drugs against soft-tissue sarcoma and has shown response rates in phase II and phase III trials of 30 to 55% [56, 57]. A cooperative group randomized trial of the CALGB and SWOG randomized 340 patients to MAID vs AD. The response rate for the MAID group was 32% versus 17% for the AD group. The median survival however, was better for the AD group (p = 0.04, not significant in multivariate analysis) and toxicity was significantly higher in the MAID group [56].

- AI. Because doxorubicin and ifosfamide are the two most active agents and both demonstrate a steep dose response curve, many sarcoma centers now utilize combinations of doxorubicin and ifosfamide, in various doses, as standard first line treatment for soft-tissue sarcoma. When given at doses of doxorubicin, 60 to 90 mg/m$^2$ with ifosfamide 5 to 10 g/m$^2$ over three to five days, response rates in numerous phase II studies range from 35 to 65% [58–59]. At these higher doses, however, toxicity is profound.

Thus for therapy of metastatic or locally advanced soft-tissue sarcoma in a physiologically healthy individual who is willing to undergo a higher rate of toxicity for a greater chance of response, the combination of adriamycin and ifosfamide may be optimal. The additional benefit of DTIC is probably small. An acceptable alternative is the sequential use of doxorubicin (with or without DTIC), followed by ifosfamide for patients who are either non-responsive to or who progress after an initial response to doxorubicin. The total response rate to these sequential maneuvers is approximately equal to that of the combination. Since no survival benefit has been demonstrated for the combination regimen, the less toxic sequential regimen may be used when initial response rate is not critical.

## Curative Uses of Chemotherapy

With rare exceptions, chemotherapy is not by itself curative in the therapy of soft-tissue sarcoma. Chemotherapy however, may play in integral role in the multimodality curative therapy of large high grade soft-tissue sarcomas.

## Adjuvant Chemotherapy

It became clear in the 1970's that adjuvant chemotherapy reduced the risk of recurrence and death in diseases such as breast cancer and osteosarcoma. Soft-tissue sarcomas, for which relapse and death, as in breast cancer and osteosarcoma are generally attributable to distant metastases, were thus put to the same test. Numerous randomized trials have addressed the possible benefit of adjuvant (post-operative) chemotherapy towards decreasing the risk of recurrence and death in patients with soft-tissue sarcomas. Approximately 15 studies, all or most underpowered to detect small differences between the treatment and non-treatment groups, have been published [60]. Eligibility has been fairly heterogenous as some studies have included patients with extremity sarcomas only and some with retroperitoneal and other sarcomas. Some studies have included only patients with large, high grade (stage IIIB) sarcomas while others have had broader eligibility requirements. Nearly half of these trials have utilized doxorubicin as a single agent and others used combinations generally considered less than optimal today. Only one trial, currently completed but not fully published [61], has utilized the doxorubicin and ifosfamide regimen, and no completed trial used the MAID regimen.

No single trial has clearly demonstrated a statistically significant benefit in overall survival for the adjuvant therapy group. Nonetheless, most of these trials have shown a trend towards benefit in disease free or overall survival or both for the group receiving adjuvant chemotherapy. In an attempt to quantitatively analyze the data from these trials, the Sarcoma Meta-analysis Collaboration retrieved individual patient data from all 14 appropriately randomized trials of adjuvant chemotherapy for soft-tissue sarcoma. These trials involved 1568 patients with 9.4 years median follow -up. The trials spanned the years 1973–1990 and included 54% females, 58% extremity tumors, and mostly high grade tumors. Almost half the patients received doxorubicin alone (versus no treatment), the other half received doxorubicin in addition to cyclophosphamide, dactinomycin, vincristine, methotrexate or dacarbazine (versus no treatment). From the available data the following conclusions were drawn:

- Local relapse free survival, distant relapse free, and overall recurrence free interval were all significantly improved with chemotherapy at 10 years. The absolute benefit was 6%, 10% and 10% (p = 0.016, 0.0003, 0.0001) respectively.
- Overall survival trended toward improval but the difference was not statistically significantly (4% at 10 years, $P = 0.12$).
- Certain subgroups appeared to have a larger survival benefit than others, including 31–60 year old individuals, men, patients with extremity tumors and patients with 5–10 cm tumors.

A single randomized trial by the National Research Council of Italy has been completed comparing 5 cycles of epirubicin 60 mg/m$^2$ x 2 days and ifosfamide 1800 mg/m$^2$ x 5 days with GCSF, versus no chemotherapy [61]. This trial was closed early when a statistically significant difference emerged between the two groups. The most recent report of this trial which randomized 104 patients, 86 de novo and 18 relapsed, had 24 month median follow up. At that time there were 9 deaths in the chemotherapy arm versus 18 in the control arm ($P = 0.005$).

Other recent attempts at randomized trials of chemotherapy for soft-tissue sarcoma have been met with poor accrual, probably due to the bias of many specialists based on the existing data. One trial by the U.S. National Cancer Institute and one by the EORTC, both comparing doxorubicin and ifosfamide vs no adjuvant, are ongoing.

In general, when faced with a patient with a high risk (IIIB) soft-tissue sarcoma, one can counsel a patient about the potential benefits based on the results of the meta-analysis. The clinician should be aware, however, that more aggressive chemotherapy regimens, such as the one used in the Italian study, may actually provide for a more meaningful benefit with chemotherapy, though at greater risk of side effects, than demonstrated in the meta-analysis. In the experience of the authors, the majority of young patients and about half of patients 60 and older will choose adjuvant chemotherapy when carefully counseled.


## Neoadjuvant Chemotherapy

Pre-operative, or neoadjuvant chemotherapy, may provide the same benefits as adjuvant, post-operative chemotherapy in reducing the risk of relapse and death by treating subclinical metastases. Additionally, neoadjuvant chemotherapy may be additive or synergistic to pre-operative radiotherapy in converting unresectable or difficult to resect tumors to resectable tumors by tumor shrinkage. Neoadjuvant chemotherapy is a standard for pediatric rhabdomyosarcoma, osteosarcoma and Ewing's sarcoma. Its use in adult soft-tissue sarcoma remains more investigational.

When utilized with pre-operative radiotherapy, pre-operative chemotherapy provides the potential benefits outlined above, as well as a theoretical "in vivo assay" of the effectiveness of chemotherapy for its potential use post-operatively. While a very strong correlation exists between pathological response to chemotherapy and survival in osteosarcoma, this relationship is less well demonstrated for soft-tissue sarcoma [62]. When utilized in conjunction with radiotherapy, the true benefit of the pre-operative chemotherapy (versus that of the RT) is difficult to evaluate in terms of tumor response. Chemotherapy in this setting, however, is justifiable in order to attempt to convert some of the 20% of patients who are felt to require amputations to candidates for limb salvage, to reduce the 10–20% risk of local relapse in stage IIIB patients, and to treat micrometastases at their earliest.

Perhaps the longest experience with pre-operative chemotherapy is from five consecutive studies at UCLA, beginning in 1974, all of which utilized pre-operative chemotherapy and preoperative radiotherapy [25]. In the first three trials comprising a total of 229 stage IIIB patients, intra-arterial doxorubicin (30 mg/m$^2$/day x 3 days constant arterial infusion) was followed by large fraction RT. A total RT dose of 3500 cGy led to local complications, 1750 cGy led to a 20% rate of local recurrences, and 2800 cGy led to less complications and only 14% local recurrences. In the third trial, intravenous administration of doxorubicin was found to be equally effective to intra-arterial administration. A fourth trial added cisplatin preoperatively with little improvement. The most encouraging results come from the fifth and most recent trial, begun in 1990. Sixty-one patients received two cycles of high dose ifosfamide followed by 2800 cGy in 8 fractions and then a cycle of doxorubicin and cisplatin. Surgery then followed after which the preoperative chemotherapy was repeated. In the first 61 patients (with short follow up), the complete response rate was 34% (7.4% in previous 4 trials) and local recurrence rate only 2%. The overall survival rate was 85%. Encouraging was the similar complete response rate in an additional 52 patients with retroperitoneal, head and neck and chest/flank tumors, groups which typically have a poorer prognosis.

MD Anderson has reported 2 series of patients treated with pre-operative chemotherapy and, in some, pre-operative radiotherapy [62, 63]. The response rate in the first 46 patients treated from 1979 to 1985 with doxorubicin based chemotherapy was 40% [63]. When using modern response criteria, the response rate was 24%. A second series of 76 patients treated between 1986 and 1990 with doxorubicin based chemotherapy (with DTIC in 65) had a response rate of 27%. They concluded, in the second series, that objective response does not predict for various survival parameters, and that radiographic response to pre-operative chemotherapy should not be used to facilitate clinical decision making regarding post-operative chemotherapy. It is notable that response rates in these primary tumors appear to be less than or equal to response rates in distant sites of disease. Of note, ifosfamide was not used in these studies.

## Palliative Chemotherapy

While chemotherapy in the neoadjuvant or adjuvant setting may play a role in the multi-modality curative therapy of soft-tissue sarcomas, chemotherapy alone for metastatic soft-tissue sarcoma, with the exception of alveolar and embryonal rhabdomyosarcoma, is rarely curative. A small percentage of patients with metastatic disease may achieve a cure with pulmonary metastesectomy, with or without chemotherapy. As described in previous sections, response rates to single agent chemotherapy is in the range of 15 to 35%, and to combination chemotherapy 20 to 50%. As with other metastatic cancers, some of those patients who respond to chemotherapy may achieve meaningful palliation. However, since chemotherapy in this setting does not significantly prolong survival, the timing of the initiation of chemotherapy and the aggressiveness of chemotherapy must be carefully chosen. All of the issues regarding risk and benefit must be thoroughly discussed with the patient.

All of the issues discussed under "single agent chemotherapy" and "combination chemotherapy" apply in the palliative situation. Doxorubicin and ifosfamide are the mainstay of palliative chemotherapy, either alone or in combination. For patients who respond poorly to doxorubicin and ifosfamide containing regimens, the probability of a response to further chemotherapy is very low. A possible exception is that high dose ifosfamide may lead to responses in patients who have been previously treated with low dose ifosfamide [41]. These patients failing first line therapy, as well as patients who have yet to be treated with chemotherapy, should be considered as candidates for clinical trials of new drugs or newer treatment approaches.

## Pulmonary Metastesectomy

Soft-tissue sarcomas (and bone sarcomas) are unique in that pulmonary metastases may be resected for cure in a subset of patients. Numerous studies have a shown a long term survival rate of 15 to 40% for appropriately selected patients who undergo pulmonary metastesectomy [64–66]. Prognostic factors for long term survival vary between studies but include: 1) small number of nodules (1 to up to 10 in some series), 2) disease free interval of over a year (although some patients who present with metastases may be suitable candidates); 3) in all cases, no other sites of distant metastasis. Long term survival curves of large series of stage IV patients generally show a "tail" of about 5%. These 5% are generally represented by these select patients undergoing curative pulmonary metastesectomy. Chemotherapy may play a role in select patients who undergo pulmonary metastesectomy. For those patients who have not had prior chemotherapy, adjuvant chemotherapy may decrease the risk of recurrence and death, as extrapolated from the meta-analysis of primary adjuvant chemotherapy. Patients who have had prior adjuvant chemotherapy within a year or two of the development of metastases are unlikely to benefit from further chemotherapy. Patients for whom several years have elapsed since their past chemotherapy or have undergone less aggressive chemotherapy may benefit from re-treatment with aggressive adjuvant chemotherapy. The timing of chemotherapy in this situation remains controversial. Many oncologists will choose to give chemotherapy prior to surgery as an "in vivo" assay of its effectiveness, thereby sparing non-responding patients the side effects of a full regimen of adjuvant chemotherapy.

## High Dose Chemotherapy

Although doxorubicin and ifosfamide have steep dose response relationships, high dose chemotherapy requiring stem cell support has no established role in the therapy of adult soft-tissue sarcomas. Several investigators have conducted small phase I or II trials in these patients [67, 68]. These studies are difficult to interpret in light of their small numbers and patient selection. High dose chemotherapy with stem cell support for adult soft-tissue sarcomas should still be considered experimental. One possible exception is young adults with rhabdomyosarcoma. Although 20 to 30% of patients with metastatic rhabdomyosarcoma will achieve long term remission or cure with non-transplant dose chemotherapy, many investigators have attempted to improve this outcome with high dose chemotherapy and stem cell support. In these studies the long term remission rate appears to be slightly higher than with standard chemotherapy, although this may be the result of patient selection [69]. Therefore more data is needed before conclusively commenting on the role of high dose chemotherapy for rhabdomyosarcoma.

## Special Subtypes

Although the rarity of each of the various tumor types makes comparative differences of response rates within any given trial difficult, data accumulated from multiple trials suggest certain patterns of unique responsiveness and refractoriness.

Perhaps the least responsive of all sarcomas are the gastrointestinal leiomyosarcomas, many of which have been reclassified as gastrointestinal stromal tumors (GIST). These tumors have a response rate to standard sarcoma chemotherapy that is consistently much lower than other soft-tissue sarcomas. Patients with this disease requiring chemotherapy should be considered candidates for clinical trials as first line therapy. Neurofibrosarcomas occurs in 10 to 15% of all neurofibromatosis patients and these sarcomas likewise appear to be less responsive to chemotherapy than other soft-tissue sarcomas.

Synovial sarcomas may be uniquely sensitive to higher doses of Ifosfamide. In two separate studies, the overall response rates in regimens containing high dose Ifosfamide has been near 100% [70, 71].

Desmoid tumors represent benign proliferations of collagen and fibroblast-like cells and occur predominantly in the pelvic and shoulder girdles, and in the abdomen in association with familial adenomatous polyposis (FAP). Although benign, they are locally aggressive and can cause significant morbidity and mortality. These tumors have been reported to respond to nonsteroidal anti-inflammatory drugs [72] and certain hormonal manipulations. Tamoxifin and its analogue Toremefine may cause marked regression of these tumors [73]. In addition, two small studies of combination chemotherapy have shown intriguingly high response rates. Weiss et al. have reported a response rate of 75% in a group of 8 patients with desmoid tumors treated with weekly methotrexate and vinblastine [74]. Patel et al. have published a series of 12 patients receiving doxorubicin and dacarbazine for advanced desmoids. They reported 6 responses in 9 evaluable patients treated with doxorubicin and dacarbazine [75]. Despite the reports of activity with systemic therapy, local control measures of surgery and radiotherapy should be used first whenever feasible.

Aveolar and embryonal rhabdomyosarcomas are the most common soft-tissue tumors in children. Approximately 300 to 400 cases occur per year in this country. A minority of these cases occur in young adults. The treatment principles for these adult patients are borrowed from the experience in children. Prior to the age of effective chemotherapy this disease was lethal in over 80% of all patients despite aggressive locoregional therapy. In the age of modern chemotherapy, 60 to 70% of all patients with rhabdomyosarcoma will be cured [76]. This includes 20 to 30% of patients with metastatic rhabdomyosarcoma. [76]. Although an exact standard does not exist for adults, our group and others have had good experience treating young adults with the regimens based on the Intergroup Rhabdomyosarcoma Study (IRS)-III and IRS-IV. All patients with this disease, pediatric or adult, should be treated at an Institution with a multimodality sarcoma treatment team.

*Conclusions: Chemotherapy*

Chemotherapy has an increasing role in the therapy of soft-tissue sarcomas. Doxorubicin and ifosfamide, both with notable dose response relationships, are the most active drugs in soft-tissue sarcomas. The use of chemotherapy may play a role in the multidisciplinary curative therapy of localized soft-tissue sarcoma. For metastatic soft-tissue sarcoma its role is primarily for palliation. For rhabdomyosarcoma, chemotherapy for all stages of the disease is nearly essential for cure.

Biologic Response Modifier Cytokine Hormone Therapy

Many studies of biological response modifiers and other "immunotherapies" have included patients with soft-tissue sarcomas [77]. Unfortunately, to date, these therapies have met with little success in sarcoma patients. Likewise, with rare exceptions of "benign" but disseminated smooth muscle neoplasms [78], and desmoid tumors [73], hormonal therapy has little role in the treatment of soft-tissue sarcomas.

One arena in which biologic therapy appears to be effective is isolated limb perfusion. Eggermont et al. treated 186 patients who were otherwise candidates only for amputation or function altering procedures, with tumor necrosis factor (TNF) and melphalan. They reported an 82% histologic response (29% complete and 53% partial response) and a 2 year limb salvage rate of 82% [79]. TNF appears to improve outcome over melphalan alone although a controlled comparison has not been performed [80].

**Key Questions**

Several key questions remain regarding soft-tissue sarcomas:
a) Further definition of etiology or risk factors may help improve prevention or early detection and help to target therapeutic strategies.
b) Risk stratification for prognosis or response to chemotherapy and radiation will help separate patients who will benefit from treatment and spare toxicities to those who will not.
c) Can neoadjuvant chemotherapy improve local control and can other measures such as isolated limb perfusion improve upon local control or avoid amputation.

d) Identification of new drugs, including existing but poorly tested drugs, with activity in soft-tissue sarcoma.

e) Can aggressive doxorubicin and ifosfamide regimens improve survival in metastatic disease.

f) Can aggressive ifosfamide and doxorubicin containing regimens improve outcome in the adjuvant setting over that seen with less than aggressive regimens in the meta-analysis.

g) Identification of chemotherapy regimens for the difficult to treat subsets, including GIST and neurofibrosarcoma of NF.

h) Identification of the etiology and appropriate therapy for the "benign" desmoid tumor.

### References

1. Landis SH, Murray T, Bolden S, Wingo PA (1998) Cancer Statistics. In: Murphy G (ed) CA: A Cancer Journal for Clinicians, p 10

2. Peabody TD, Monson D, Montag AJ, Schell MJ, Finn HA, Simon MA (1994) A Comparison of the prognosis for deep and subcutaneous sarcomas of the extremities. J Bone Joint Surg 76A: 1167–1173.

3. Li FP, Froumeni JF (1969) Soft-tissue sarcomas, breast cancer, and other neoplasms: a familial syndrome? Ann Intern Med 71: 747–750

4. Sorensen SA, Mulvihill JJ, Nielsen A (1986) Long-term follow-up of Von Recklinghausen Neurofibromatosis. Survival and Malignant Neoplasms. N Engl J Med 314: 1010–1015.

5. Costa J, Wesley RA, Glatstein E, Rosenberg SA (1984) The grading of soft-tissue sarcomas. Cancer 53: 530

6. Broders AC (1975) The grading of carcinoma. Minn Med 8: 726

7. Alevgard TA, Bern NO (1989) Histopathology peer review of high-grade soft-tissue sarcoma: The Scandinavian Sarcoma Group experience. J Clin Oncol 7: 1845–1857

8. Scholz RB, Kabisch H, Weber B (1992) Studies of the RB 1 gene and the p53 gene in human osteosarcomas. Pediatr Hematol Oncol 9: 125–137

9. American Joint Committee on Cancer: Soft Tissues (1997) In: Beahrs OH, Myers MH (eds) Manual for Staging of Cancer, 5th ed. JB Lippincott, Philadelphia, pp 149–156

10. Mazeron J, Suit HD (1987) Lymph nodes as sites of metastases from sarcomas of soft tissue. Cancer 60: 1800

11. Pisters PWT, Leung DHY, Woodruff J, Shi W, Brennan MF (??) Analysis of prognostic factors in 1041 patients with localized soft-tissue sarcomas of the extremities. J Clin Oncol 14: 1679–1689

12. Drobnjak M, Latres E, Pollack D et al (1994) Prognostic implications of P53 nuclear overexpression and high proliferation index of Ki-67 in adult soft tissue sarcomas. J Natl Cancer Inst 86: 549–554

13. Taubert H, Meye A, Wurl P (1996) Prognosis is correlated with P53 mutation type for soft tissue sarcoma patients. Cancer Res 56: 4134-4136

14. Nakanishi H, Ohsawa M, Naka N et al (1997) Immunohistochemical detection of bcl-2 and P53 proteins and apoptosis in soft tissue sarcoma: their correlations with prognosis oncology 54: 238–244

15. Mankin HJ, Mankin CJ, Simon MA (1997) The Hazards of Biopsy, Revisited. J Bone Joint Surg 78A: 659

16. Enneking WF, Spanier SS, Goodman MA (1980) A system for the surgical staging of musculoskeletal sarcoma. Clin Orthop 153: 106–120

17. Grivano AE, Eilber FR (1985) The rationale for planned reoperation after unplanned total excision of soft-tissue sarcoma. J Clin Oncol 3: 1344–1348

18. Boden L, Booherr (1958) The principles and technique of resection of soft parts for sarcoma. Surgery 44: 963–977

19. Suit HD, Proppe KH, Mankin HJ, Wood WC (1981) Preoperative radiation therapy for sarcomas of soft tissue. Cancer 47: 2269–2274

20. Eilber FE, Morton DC, Eckardt J, Grant T, Weisenburger T (1984) Limb salvage for skeletal and soft-tissue sarcomas. Multidisciplinary preoperative therapy. Cancer: 2579–2584

21. Lindberg RD, Martin RG, Romadahl MM, Barkley HT (1981) Conservative surgery and postoperative radiotherapy in 300 adults with soft tissue sarcomas Cancer 47: 2391

22. Hellman S (1997) Principles of Cancer Management and Radiation Therapy. In: Devita VT, Hellman S, Roseberg SA (eds) Cancer: Principles and Practice of Oncology, 5th ed. Lippincott-Raven, Philadelphia, p 307

23. Tepper J, Suit H (1985) Radiation therapy of soft-tissue sarcomas. Cancer 55: 2273–2277

24. O'Connor MI, Gunderson LL, Edmonson JH (1998) Multimodality management of malignant soft-tissue tumors. In: Simon MA, Springfield DS (eds) Surgery for Bone and Soft-Tissue Tumors. Lippincott-Raven, Philadelphia, pp 567–576

25. Eilber F, Eckardt J et al (1995) Preoperative therapy for soft-tissue sarcoma. Hem/Onc Clin N Amer 9: 817–823

26. Eilber F, Eckhard J, Rosen G, Forscher C, Selch M, Fu Y-S (1994) Improved complete response rate with neoadjuvant high dose Ifosfamide, adriamycin, platinum, and radiation for high grade extremity soft-tissue sarcomas. Proc Am Soc of Clin Oncol 13: 473

27. Pisters P, Harrison L, Leung D, Woodruff J, Casper E, Brennan M (1996) Long term results of prospective randomized trial of adjuvant brachytherapy in soft-tissue sarcoma. J Clin Oncol 14: 859–868

28. Yang JC, Chang AE, Baker AR et al (1998) Randomized prospective study of the benefit of adjuvant radiation therapy in the treatment of soft tissue sarcomas of the extremity. J Clin Oncol 16: 197–203

29. Gunderson L, Shipley W, Suit H, Epp E, Nardi G, Wood W, Cohen A, Nelson J, Bettit G, Biggs P, Russell A, Rockett A, Clark D (1982) Intraoperative irradiation: A pilot study combining external beam photons with boost dose intraoperative electron. Cancer 49: 2257–2266

30. Suit H, Urie M (1992) Proton beams in radiation therapy. J Natl Cancer Instit 84: 155–163

31. Reimers M, Castro J, Lindstadt D, Collier J, Henderson S, Hannigan J, Phillips T (1986) Heavy charge particle therapy of bone and soft-tissue sarcoma. Am J Clin Oncol 9: 488–493

32. Gustafson P, Rooser B, Willen H, Akennan M, Herrlin K, Alvegard T (1991) Limb sparing surgery without radiotherapy based on anatomic location of soft-tissue sarcoma. J Clin Oncol 9: 1757–1765

33. Benjamin R, Wiernik P, Bachur N (1975) Adriamycin, a new effective agent in the therapy of disseminated sarcomas. Med Pediart Oncol 1: 63–67

34. Borden EC, Amato D et al (1987) Randomized comparison of Adriamcyin regimens for treatment of metastatic soft-tissue sarcomas. J Clin Oncol 5: 840–850

35. Santoro A, Tursz T et al (1995) Doxorubicin versus CYVADIC versus doxorubicin plus ifosfamide in first line treatment of advanced soft-tissue sarcoma. A randomized study of the European Organization for Research and Treatment of Cancer Soft-tissue and Bone Sarcoma Group. J Clin Oncol 13: 1537–1545

36. Antman KH, Ryan L et al (1989) Responses to ifosfamide and mesna: 124 previously treated patients with metastatic or unresectable sarcoma. J Clin Oncol 7: 126–131

37. Tursz T (1996) High-dose ifosfamide in the treatment of advanced soft-tissue sarcomas. Semin Oncol 23: 34–39

38. Elias AD, Eder JP et al (1990) High-dose ifosfamide with mesna uroprotection: A phase I study. J Clin Oncol 18: 95–103

39. Benjamin RS, Legha SS et al (1993) Single-agent ifosfamide in sarcomas of soft-tissue and bone: the MD Anderson experience. Cancer Chemother Pharmacol 31: S174–S179

40. Patel SR, Vadhan RS et al (1997) High-dose ifosfamide in bone and soft-tissue sarcomas: result of phase II and pilot studies dose-response and schedule dependence. J Clin Oncol 15: 2378–2384

41. Le-Cesne A, Antoine E et al (1995) High-dose ifosfamide: circumvention of resistance to standard-dose ifosfamide in advanced soft-tissue sarcomas. J Clin Oncol 13: 1600–1608

42. Bramwell V, Mouridsen H et al (1987) Cyclophosphamide vs ifosfamide: Final report of a randomized phase II trial in adult soft-tissue sarcoma. Eur J Cancer Clin Oncol 23: 311–321

43. Schoenfeld D, Rosenbaum C et al (1982) A comparison of Adriamycin versus vincristine and Adriamycin, and cyclophosphamide or advanced sarcoma. Cancer 50: 2757–2762

44. Gottlieg JE, Benjamin RS et al (1976) Role of DTIC (NSC 45388) in the chemotherapy of sarcomas. Cancer Treat Rep 60: 19–203

45. Patel S, Linke K et al (1997) Phase II study of paclitaxel in patients with soft-tissue sarcoma. Sarcoma 1: 95–97

46. Balcerzak SP, Benedetti J et al (1995) A phase II trial of paclitaxel in patients with advanced soft-tissue sarcomas. Cancer 76: 2248–2252

47. Verweij J, Judson D et al (1997) Randomized study comparing docetaxel (Taxotere) (T) to doxorubicin (D) in previously untreated soft-tissue sarcomas (STS). Proc ASCO 16 (abstr 1788)

48. Bramwell VH, Eisenhauer EA et al (1995) Phase II study of topotecan (NSC 6096099) in patients with recurrent or metastatic soft-tissue sarcoma. Ann Oncol 6: 847–849

49. Keizer HJ, Crowther D et al (1997) EORTC Group phase II study of oral etoposide for pretreated soft-tissue sarcoma. Sarcoma: 99–101

50. Späth-Schwalbe E, Koschuth R et al (1998) Gemcitabine (GEM) in pretreated patients with advanced soft-tissue sarcomas (STS). Preliminary results from a phase II trial. Proc ASCO 17 (abstr 1976)

51. Casper ES, Christman KL et al (1993) Edatrexate in patients with soft soft-tissue sarcoma. Activity in malignant fibrous histiocytoma. Cancer 72: 766–770

52. Fidias P, Demetri G, Harman PC (1998) Navelbine shows activity in previously treated sarcoma patients: Phase II results from MGH/Dana Farber Partner's Cancer Care Study. Proc ASCO 17 (abstr 1977)

53. Elson P, Chidiac T et al (1998) Phase II trial of Doxil in advanced soft-tissue sarcomas (STS). Proc ASCO 17 (abstr 1979)

54. Casper ES, Gaynor JJ et al (1991) Prospective randomized trial of adjuvant chemotherapy with bolus versus continuous infusion of doxorubicin in patients with high-grade extremity soft-tissue sarcoma and an analysis of prognostic factors. Cancer 68: 1221–1229

55. Omura GA, Major FJ et al (1985) Randomized clinical trials of adjuvant Adriamycin in uterine sarcomas: A Gynecologic Oncology Group study. J Clin Oncol 552: 626–632

56. Antman K, Crowley J et al (1993) An intergroup phase III randomized study of doxorubicin and dacarbazine with or without ifosfamide and mesna in advanced soft-tissue and bone sarcoma. J Clin Oncol 11: 1276–1285

57. Elias A, Ryan L et al (1989) Response to Mesna, Doxorubicin, Ifosfamide, and Dacarbazine in 108 patients with metastatic or unresectable sarcoma and no prior chemotherapy. J Clin Oncol 7: 1208–1216

58. Steward WP, Verweij J et al (1993) Granulocyte-macrophage colony stimulating factor allows safe escalation of dose-intensity of chemotherapy in metastatic adult soft-tissue sarcomas: a study of the European Organization for Research and Treatment of Cancer Soft-tissue and Bone Sarcoma Group. J Clin Oncol 11: 1–2

59. Patel SR, Vadhan RS et al (1997) Dose intensive therapy does improve response rates – updated results of studies of Adriamycin (A) and ifosfamide with growth factors in patients (pts) with untreated soft-tissue sarcomas (STS). Proc ASCO 16 (abstr 1794)

60. Sarcoma Meta-analysis Collaboration (1997) Adjuvant chemotherapy for localized resectable soft-tissue sarcoma of adults: meta-analysis of individual data. Lancet 350: 1647–1654

61. Picci P, Frustaci S et al (1997) Localized high grade soft-tissue sarcomas of the extremities in adults: Preliminary results of the Italian Cooperative Study. Sarcoma 1: 194

62. Pisters WT, Patel SR et al (1997) Preoperative chemotherapy for stage IIIB extremity soft-tissue sarcoma: long-term results from a single institution. J Clin Oncol 15: 3481–3487

63. Pezzi CM, Pollock RE et al (1990) Preoperative chemotherapy for soft-tissue sarcomas of the extremities. Arm Surg 211: 476–481

64. Masters GA, Golomb HM (1995) Management of pulmonary metastases. Lancet 68: 346 (8967)

65. Vogt-Moykopf I, Butzebruck H et al (1987) Results of surgical treatment of pulmonary metastases. Eur J Cardiotho Surg 2: 224–232

66. Schirren J, Krysa S et al (1995) Results of surgical treatment of pulmonary metastases from soft-tissue sarcomas. In: Bamberg M, Hoffman W, Hossfeld DK (eds) Soft-tissue Sarcomas in Adults. Berlin, Germany, Springer-Verlag, p 130

67. Bonhour D, Biron P et al (1996) High dose chemotherapy (HDCT) with autologous hematopoietic stem cell support for advanced soft-tissue sarcoma (ASTS) of adults. Connective Tissue Oncology Society Annual Meeting, Toronto, Canada (abstr)

68. Dumontet C, Biron P et al (1992) High dose chemotherapy with ABMT in soft-tissue sarcomas. A report of 22 eases. Bone Marrow Transplant 10: 405–408

69. Boulad F, Kernan NA et al (1998) High dose induction chemoradiotherapy followed by autologous bone marrow transplantation as consolidation therapy in rhabdomyosarcoma, extraosseous Ewing's sarcoma, and undifferentiated sarcoma. J Clin Oncol 16: 1697–1706

70. Rosen G, Forscher C et al (1994) Uniform response of metastases to high dose ifosfamide. Cancer 73: 250
71. Edmonson JK et al (1993) Randomized comparison of doxorubicin alone versus ifosfamide plus doxorubicin or mitomycin, doxorubicin, and cisplatin against advanced soft-tissue sarcomas. J Clin Oncol 11: 1269–1275
72. Tsukada K, Church JM et al (1992) Noncytotoxic drug therapy for intra-abdominal desmoid tumor in patients with familial adenomatous polyposis. Dis Colon Rectum 35: 29–33
73. Brooks MD, Ebbs SR et al (1992) Desmoid tumors treated with triphenylethylenes. Eur J Cancer 28A: 1014–1018
74. Weiss AJ, Lackman RD. (1989) Low-dose chemotherapy of desmoid tumors. Cancer 64: 1192–1194
75. Patel SR, Evans HL et al (1993) Combination chemotherapy in adult desmoid tumors. Cancer 72: 3244–3247
76. Crist W, Gehan EA et al (1995) The third intergroup rhabdomyosarcoma study. J Clin Oncol 13: 610–630
77. Brennan MF, Casper ES, Harrison LB (1997) Soft Tissue Sarcoma. In: Devita VT Jr, Hellman S, Rosenberg SA (eds) Cancer Principles and Practice of Oncology. Lippincott-Raven, Philadelphia, PA 1738–1788
78. Taylor JR, Ryu J et al (1990) Lymphangioleiomyomatosis. New Engl J Med 323: 1254–1260
79. Eggermont AM, Schraffordt-Koops H et al (1996) Isolated limb perfusion with tumor necrosis factor and melphalan for limb salvage in 186 patients with locally advanced soft-tissue extremity sarcomas. The cumulative multicenter European experience. Ann Surg 224: 756–765
80. Eggermont AMM, Schraffordt-Koops H et al (1996) Isolated limb perfusion with high dose tumor necrosis factor-AAA in combination with interferon-GGG and melphalan for nonresectable extremity soft-tissue sarcomas: A multicenter trial. J Clin Oncol 14: 2653–2665

# Bone Sarcomas

T. D. Peabody, B. E. Brockstein

## Epidemiology and Risk Factors

Sarcomas of bone are a relatively uncommon and heterogeneous group of malignant tumors with an incidence of approximately 2,000 per year in the United States [1]. Protean manifestations and their rarity often present diagnostic and therapeutic challenges to the physicians caring for these patients. Often, the disease and treatment compromise limb function resulting in disability. More importantly though, most patients with high-grade sarcomas of bone develop metastatic disease and without effective systemic and local therapy will not survive. Recent advances in medical oncology and limb salvage operative techniques have had significant positive effects on the lives of these patients.

The most common histologic diagnoses for bone sarcomas are listed in Table 1. After multiple myeloma, primary high-grade intramedullary sarcoma is the most common biopsy analyzed primary malignancy of bone [2]. Osteosarcomas are twice as common as chondrosarcomas and three times as common as Ewing's sarcoma of bone [3]. The quoted incidence of 1 to 3 cases per million population has not changed significantly with time [4]. Conventional high-grade osteosarcoma is most commonly diagnosed in patients between 15 and 25 years and is most often located in the distal femur, proximal tibia, proximal humerus, proximal femur, and pelvis with over one-half of the tumors involving the metaphyseal bone about the knee (Fig. 1). In osteosarcoma, there has been no demonstrated racial preference, but men are slightly more commonly affected than women.

In the vast majority of cases, the etiology of osteosarcoma is unknown. In some cases, however, osteosarcomas have been associated with dedifferentiation of underlying non-neoplastic bone disease such as Paget's disease of bone, a history of radiation exposure, or in conjunction with certain heritable conditions such as Fraumeni syndrome

**Table 1.** Most common histologic diagnoses in bone sarcomas

Osteosarcoma
    Conventional (high-grade intramedullary)
    Parosteal (low-grade surface)
    Telangiectatic
    Low-grade Central
    Periosteal (high-grade surface)

Chondrosarcoma
    Primary
    Secondary
    Dedifferentiated
    Mesenchymal
    Clear cell

Ewing's Sarcoma, primitive neuroectodermal tumors

Chordoma

Malignant Fibrous Histiocytoma

Fibrosarcoma

Hemangioendothelial Sarcomas

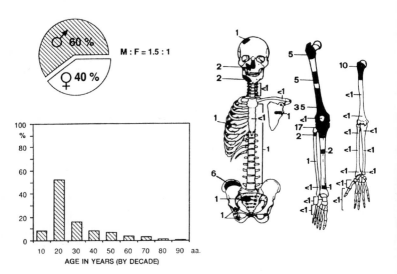

**Fig. 1.** Osteosarcoma, 2525 cases [6]

(germline p53 mutation) or retinoblastoma [5]. Most osteosarcomas are solitary lesions, however, on occasion polyostotic disease is noted.

Chondrosarcomas, in contrast, are most frequently found in older individuals with a peak incidence in the sixth decade of life [6]. These tumors are frequently found in the axial skeleton, that is the pelvis, proximal femur, ribs, spine, and proximal humerus (Fig. 2). There again, is a slight male predominance. There is no racial preference. Chondrosarcomas may be primary, that is without an antecedent bone lesion or secondary. Secondary chondrosarcomas arise from pre-existing benign cartilage lesions such as osteochondromas. Dedifferentiated sarcomas are high-grade lesions, which appear to arise from malignant degeneration of an underlying low grade or benign bone neoplasm. This kind of malignant degeneration of an underlying bone neoplasm is most commonly seen in the autosomal dominant syndrome known as multiple hereditary exostoses or in patients with multiple enchondromas, known by the eponym Ollier's disease.

Ewing's sarcoma and primitive neuroectodermal tumor are unusual bone sarcomas seen most commonly in the second decade of life affecting both males and females equally (Fig. 3). The most common locations

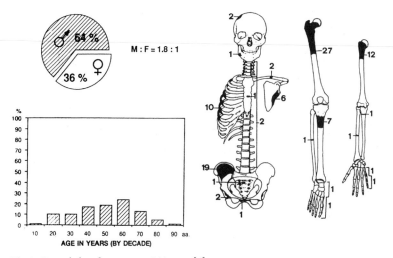

**Fig. 2.** Central chondrosarcome, 746 cases [6]

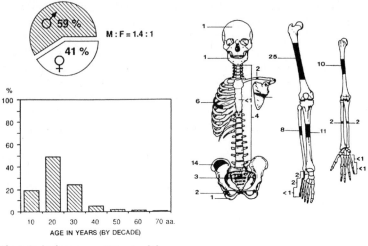

**Fig. 3.** Ewing's sarcoma, 871 cases [6]

are the pelvic girdle and lower extremities and unlike other bone sarcomas is commonly seen in flat bones (ribs, pelvis, scapula) and in the diaphyseal segments of long bones. In addition, PNET tumors are common in the soft tissues. Like other bone sarcomas, there are few known risk factors and the etiology is unclear. However, for Ewing's sarcoma, a characteristic gene translocation has been identified that results in a fusion gene and protein product. The fusion gene EWS-FLI is unique to these tumors and its sequence is determined by two different genes on separate chromosomes juxtaposed by a translocation event t(11;22) (q24:q11.2–12) [7]. The messenger RNA associated with these proteins has been used diagnostically.

## Pathology and Staging Systems

Staging systems have been developed for malignant bone tumors in an attempt to predict prognosis and evaluate the effect of therapeutic intervention by stratifying similar tumors according to various prognostic factors. Unfortunately for bone sarcomas, there is no universally accepted staging system. The reasons are the low incidence of these tumors, their heterogeneous nature, their unpredictable behavior, and disagreement as to the relative importance of various prognostic factors. In addition, unlike staging systems for carcinomas, tumor grade is an important prognostic variable for musculoskeletal malignancies and must be included in any staging system. Therefore a TNM system must also include tumor grade in order to be useful in the treatment of patients with bone sarcomas. Tumor grade should be considered a histologic estimate of a tumor's potential to metastasize based on tumor cellularity, nuclear atypia, mitotic activity, and necrosis.

The American Joint Committee on Cancer Staging Systems for Bone Tumors is presented in Table 2 [8]. Unfortunately, as all staging systems for bone and soft tissue sarcomas, this system has not been validated in multicenter studies. This staging system was first proposed in 1983 and at that time the Committee emphasized that it's task force on bone

**Table 2.** American joint committee, staging protocol for sarcomas of bone (from [8])[a]

| Stage IA   | G1–G2       | T1    | N0    | M0 |
|------------|-------------|-------|-------|----|
| Stage IB   | G1–G2       | T2    | N0    | M0 |
| Stage IIA  | G3–G4       | T1 N0 | M0    |    |
| Stage IIB  | G3–G4       | N0    | M0    |    |
| Stage III  | Not defined |       |       |    |
| Stage IVA  | Any G       | Any T | N1    | M0 |
| Stage IVB  | Any G       | Any T | Any N | M1 |

Primary tumor
T1  Tumor confined within the cortex
T2  Tumor extending beyond the cortex
Note: Juxtacortical (parosteal) sarcomas should be considered separately

Regional lymph nodes
N0  No regional lymph node metastases
N1  Regional lymph node metastases

Distant metastases
M0  No distant metastases
M1  Distant metastases

Histologic grade
G1  Well differentiated
G2  Moderately differentiated
G3  Poorly differentiated
G4  Undifferentiated

[a]Note: Ewing's sarcoma and malignant lymphoma are defined as G4

tumors was still considering the problem of staging, and that further recommendations would be made in the future. This system, however, remains essentially unchanged in the latest edition of the Committee's manual for staging of cancer. In this system, the TNM designation with the addition of grade is used, with T referring to histologic grade and extent of tumor, N to nodal metastases, and M to distant metastases. There are four progressive tumor grades designated 1–4. Grades 1 and 2 define low and intermediate histologic grade and grades 3 and 4 refer to poorly or undifferentiated tumors. A tumor confined by the cortex is considered T1 and one extending beyond the cortex is T2. In this system, stage 3 is undefined, and stage 4 refers to the presence of metastases. Stage 4 is further modified as A (the unusual nodal metastases) or B (the more common pulmonary metastases).

When one carefully considers the staging system, it is apparent that only two histologic grades are utilized. Prognosis in bone sarcomas is most closely related to tumor grade, while tumor extent and location are more important from an operative perspective. Patients with widely resected low-grade sarcomas have a favorable prognosis with surgical resection only. On the other hand, high-grade osteosarcomas were known to have a mortality of 85% prior to modern chemotherapy. With current chemotherapy and surgical intervention, survival now exceeds 60%. It is obvious that tumor grade is the single most important variable determining a patient's prognosis.

## Work-up and Staging: Patient Evaluation and Staging

Imaging studies are essential in the staging of a patient with a bone sarcoma. These examinations allow a determination of anatomical extent and characteristics of the tumor. As a result of this evaluation, information is obtained which may alter the differential diagnosis leading to better clinical, radiographical, and pathological correlation. Certain imaging tests such as bone scintigraphy, magnetic resonance imaging (MRI), or radiography will be degraded by the performance of the biopsy, especially open biopsy, making radiographic interpretation and treatment more difficult. In addition, a more accessible site for biopsy or the best approach may be based on the information gained from staging studies. For these reasons, histological evaluation in the form of a biopsy is the final step of the patient evaluation.

For bone sarcomas, the radiograph provides important information regarding the intraosseous extent of the lesion, internal characteristics such as ossification or calcification, the clarity of the margin between the lesion and the host bone and the presence or absence of fracture. Cortical destruction and periosteal new bone formation are associated with invasive neoplasms.

Computed tomography allows the surgeon to assess the character of bone tumors. Although not as accurate as MRI in determining soft tissue and marrow extent, computed tomography is superior in evaluating cortical erosion, fracture, and internal characteristics such as ossification and calcification.

Computed tomography also reveals associated soft tissue masses and the adjacent important anatomical structures, especially in the pelvis. Computed tomography of the lungs is an essential part of the staging in an individual with a suspected high-grade musculoskeletal malignancy. The lung is the most common site of metastatic disease in these patients and computed tomography is a more sensitive method for determining metastatic disease than is conventional chest radiography.

The best imaging test for evaluating a soft tissue mass, soft tissue extent of a bone tumor or bone marrow extent is MRI. For bone sarcomas, MRI will demonstrate extraosseous and intraosseous extent, joint involvement, and will detect skip metastases defined as neoplastic foci located at a distance from but usually in the same anatomic compartment as the principle tumor mass.

Scintigraphy of bone tumors is sensitive but non-specific. Bone scanning cannot differentiate benign from malignant lesions nor can it accurately determine tumor extent. The value of technetium bone scanning in evaluating patients with bone tumors is the detection of polyostotic bone disease or bone metastases, the second most common site of distant disease in bone sarcomas.

Positron emission tomography scanning and thallium scanning are considered investigational tools at this time. They may be of value in determining local disease, non-pulmonary metastases, response to therapy, or tumor recurrence. How these tests will compliment computed tomography and magnetic resonance imaging is yet to be determined.

In summary, imaging tests as part of the staging process are an essential part of the evaluation of a patient with a bone tumor. These tests allow the clinician to arrive at a differential diagnosis prior to biopsy. If these studies, in addition to clinical information, suggest a primary malignant bone tumor, the patient should be referred without additional tests or biopsy to the multidisciplinary treatment team who will ultimately be responsible for the treatment of the patient.

A biopsy may be an open procedure involving incision or excision of the tumor mass or a closed procedure using needles or trephines. The decision to proceed with any form of biopsy depends on the experience and availability of a qualified pathologist for interpretation of the results. It is essential that the person performing the biopsy and the pathologist discuss the differential diagnosis and findings prior to biopsy. In addition, the pathologist needs to inform the treating physician if tissue is required for additional studies, such as cytogenetic analysis or electron microscopy. Because almost all patients with malignant neoplasms are candidates for limb salvage procedures, it is important not to perform a biopsy in such a way that surgery is made more difficult or impossible. Biopsy placement is critical. The biopsy tract must be excised en bloc with the tumor, most often through a longitudinal incision. No additional contamination of other compartments or neurovascular structures by manipulation or hematoma should occur. Preferentially a soft tissue mass, rather than bone, should be biopsied to minimize the potential for pathologic fracture. Frozen section should be performed to confirm the operative diagnosis prior to any definitive operative treatment. The biopsy is a technically simple procedure but should be done by a thoughtful, knowledgeable, and experienced physician. A poorly placed biopsy incision, poor biopsy, or the complications of biopsy will make it difficult to salvage an extremity and, in some cases, may affect the patients survival [9].

Pathologic evaluation of the biopsy specimen in cases of bone sarcomas will estimate tumor grade based on cellularity, nuclear atypia, mitotic activity, and necrosis. The presence of tumor osteoid should be carefully evaluated and is essential for the diagnosis of osteosarcoma. Except in cases of Ewing's sarcoma, immunohistochemistry has not been of benefit in the diagnosis and treatment of these patients. As stated earlier, Ewing's sarcoma, has a characteristic translocation and the product of this translocation the, "Ewing's specific antigen" or MIC-2 antigen may be exploited for diagnostic benefit. Unfortunately, in bone sarcomas, serologic or urologic testing has not been proven to be useful in diagnosis or treatment. Serum measurements of alkaline phosphatase and sedimentation rate have been known to be elevated in patients with bone sarcomas, but these changes are not specific and studies disagree on the significance of these laboratory values.

## Stage Specific Treatment Options

Operative treatment remains the primary therapy for low-grade sarcomas and all chondrosarcomas and is performed in conjunction with adjuvant chemotherapy for high-grade sarcomas. Operative treatment may be defined as intralesional, marginal, wide, or radical [10]. Radiotherapy is rarely used in primary bone sarcomas and usually only utilized for palliation or after an incomplete resection in the axial skeleton. An exception to this is cases of Ewing's sarcomas in non-expendable bones. For Ewing's sarcoma of the acetabulum, spine, or where amputation would be necessary, radiation therapy is considered as an equal alternative to operative resection.

Bone sarcomas are known to grow centrifugally although their final shape is influenced by local anatomy and the host response. Beginning in the bone of origin, with time, they will invade the cortex and erupt into the surrounding soft tissues. They typically will compress surrounding soft tissues resulting in a reactive zone or *pseudocapsule* containing fibrous tissue, supporting vascular structures, inflammatory cells, and microscopic satellites of tumor.

Intralesional surgery or a resection performed within this pseudocapsule in the form of a curettage or contaminated excision is associated with an extremely high likelihood of local relapse. While this may or may not be associated with development of metastatic disease in low-grade tumors, local recurrence is certainly associated with a high incidence of distant metastases and death in osteosarcoma and Ewing's sarcoma. Intralesional resections are indicated in operations with palliative, not curative, intent.

Marginal resections are those performed in the plane of the reactive zone and in many instances may be performed with an acceptably low risk of local recurrence as long as an effective adjuvant has been administered. Most commonly this is in the form of chemotherapy given preoperatively and postoperatively.

The preferred operative treatment for bone sarcoma is a wide resection or removal of the tumor in continuity with a circumferential cuff of normal tissue, that most commonly being bone, synovium, and muscle.

The precise quantity as a measurable dimension or quality (fascia versus fat) necessary to prevent local relapse is not known.

A radical resection is defined as removal of the entire bone of origin and is rarely performed. It may be indicated in instances where the tumor is associated with a "skip metastases", defined as tumor located within the bone of origin but at some distance from the primary neoplasm or in bone sarcomas with extensive involvement of the underlying bone.

Studies have demonstrated no differences in survival between patients treated with wide margins who undergo amputations or limb salvage procedures. Currently, limb salvage procedures are performed for most anatomic locations. More difficult anatomic locations; include the acetabulum and distal tibia or fibula as well as the foot. In these anatomic locations, a surgeon's ability to obtain wide margins is compromised by the local anatomy and amputation may be necessary.

Ewing's sarcoma is a unique sarcoma in that there remains controversy over the role of operative resection and it's potential benefits over radiation therapy. Both appear to be able to control the disease locally and current recommendations are surgical resection for expendable bone locations and radiation therapy for non-expendable bones, in addition to multi-agent chemotherapy. Of course, the definition of an expendable bone, given current limb salvage techniques and the availability of endoprosthesis, is highly controversial.

Although wide surgical resection remains curative for most low-grade bone sarcomas, most patients with high-grade bone sarcomas have microscopic or macroscopic metastatic disease at diagnosis. The true improvements in survival seen in these patients have largely been the result of adjuvant or neoadjuvant chemotherapy.

## Chemotherapy

### Osteosarcoma

Historically, osteosarcoma was considered a chemotherapy unresponsive disease. Classic objective responses to chemotherapy are generally difficult to demonstrate, in major part due to the fact that the underlying osteoid matrix of these tumors remains intact even when there is complete cellular necrosis. This is almost always true in the primary tumor and frequently also true in metastatic tumors. The view of osteosarcoma as chemotherapy resistant changed in the early 1970's with near simultaneous but independent reports of the activity of methotrexate and doxorubicin in osteosarcoma [11, 12].

Shortly thereafter, these findings lead to the use of combination chemotherapy and chemotherapy as a post-surgical adjuvant. Today, chemotherapy is generally given preoperatively and again post-operatively. Despite the difficulty demonstrating chemotherapy response by the usual objective measures, chemotherapy results in a 50% decrease in the risk of relapse or death from osteosarcoma as compared historically to patients receiving no adjuvant chemotherapy for whom long term survival rates were < 20% [15]. This difference is even greater than that seen with adjuvant chemotherapy for breast and colon cancer, the adult malignancies most commonly treated with adjuvant chemotherapy.

*Single Agents*

Four chemotherapy drugs stand out as most active in osteosarcoma; doxorubicin, methotrexate, cisplatin, and ifosfamide.

Doxorubicin. This was first reported to be active in osteosarcoma in a phase I study by Cortes in 1972 [11]. In this initial report, 4 of 13 patients achieved a radiological complete response (CR) (1 patient) or partial response (PR) (3 patients) in pulmonary metastases with doxorubicin 17.5–35 mg/m$^2$/day x 3–4 days. Subsequently, Cortes et al. of the Acute Leukemia Group B performed a trial of doxorubicin as adjuvant chemotherapy for osteosarcoma [14]. Twenty one patients underwent amputation followed by doxorubicin, 30 mg/m$^2$/day x 3 days every 4–6 weeks starting a median of 2 wks after surgery. In their initial report, 71% of patients were disease free at 18 months compared to a historical control of 30% [15]. Longer term follow up of a cohort of 88 patients treated by the same group revealed an 18 month disease free survival (DFS) of 56% and 5 year DFS of 39%. This compared very favorably to the historical control of 20% [13].

Doxorubicin is thought to demonstrate an important dose response relationship. This has been demonstrated in vitro and can be inferred as well from clinical data [15–17]. Because anthracyclines are probably more toxic in the pediatric population, both acutely and long-term, and because doxorubicin appears to be less cardiotoxic with long infusions, most regimens incorporating doxorubicin utilize infusions of 24–96 hours. Doxorubicin remains the most commonly used drug for the treatment of osteosarcoma.

Methotrexate. This was first demonstrated to be active in the landmark paper by Jaffe in 1972 [12]. In this report, 4 of 10 patients achieved a CR (2 patients) or PR (2 patients) after receiving 50–500 mg/kg methotrexate over 6 hours every 2–3 weeks with leucovorin rescue. Subsequently Jaffe et al. at the Sidney Farber Cancer Center reported early results of a trial of adjuvant methotrexate in 20 patients with non-metastatic osteosarcoma [18] and compared their results to those of a historical control group of 98 patients at their Institution. Vincristine 2 mg/m$^2$ was given just prior to 1500–7500 mg/m$^2$ methotrexate with leucovorin. Both the incidence of metastases and the overall survival at 18 months (92%) were statistically significantly better than historical controls. Long-term follow up of this group showed a relapse rate > 50% at 5 years [19].

Methotrexate appears to be much more effective in high dose regimens than in low or moderate doses [20]. Even with the high dose regimens (> 4 g/m$^2$), a dose response curve probably exists [21] which may be at least in part dependent on achieving a high peak methotrexate level [22]. In one study, a peak level of > 700 μmol was associated with 40% complete tumor necrosis compared to 15.5% of patients who did not achieve this level (p < 0.002) [23]. Methotrexate has been commonly used in adjuvant chemotherapy programs, although its use today is sometimes reserved for post-operative therapy in non-responders to other drugs.

Cisplatin. This has demonstrated high response rates near 50% as a single agent in the treatment of osteosarcoma [24, 25]. Its efficacy was first demonstrated in eight heavily pretreated patients given 80–120 mg/m$^2$ intravenous cisplatin [24] and subsequently in 11 patients receiving 150 mg/m$^2$ intraarterial cisplatin [25]. Although the intraarterial route may lead to improved tumor necrosis and possibly fewer local recurrences, the systemic efficacy is equal with the intravenous route, and therefore intraarterial routes is less commonly used today [26]. One small randomized trial demonstrated superiority of intraarterial cisplatin over methotrexate in the treatment of primary osteosarcoma [27].

Although little other comparative data exist, cisplatin is probably at least as effective as any other drug and is utilized in almost all modern osteosarcoma protocols.

Carboplatin. Despite being less toxic than cisplatin, carboplatin is less effective in the therapy of osteosarcoma than cisplatin [28, 29].

Ifosfamide. Early studies of cyclophosphamide in the 1970's demonstrated a consistent but low response rate in osteosarcoma. Ifosfamide, however, has shown a consistently high level of activity with responses in approximately one-third of patients [30, 31]. The appropriate role of ifosfamide in the adjuvant/neoadjuvant treatment of osteosarcoma remains to be seen. At minimum, it should be used post-operatively in patients with poor response to a non-ifosfamide containing regimen and it is currently being studied as part of multi drug pre-operative regimens.

Other chemotherapy drugs. Numerous other chemotherapy drugs have been utilized in the treatment of osteosarcoma. Most commonly these have included bleomycin, cyclophosphamide, dacarbazine, actinomycin D, mitomycin C, vincristine, and etoposide. The activity of most of these drugs however is limited in osteosarcoma and they are generally not incorporated into modern chemotherapy programs.

New Drug Testing. The four most active drugs against osteosarcoma (doxorubicin, methotrexate, cisplatin and ifosfamide) are extremely toxic, and their overlapping toxicities (myelosuppression and nephrotoxicity) make combination therapy difficult. As a result of this toxicity and the failure of chemotherapy to cure about 40% of patients, the identification of new active drugs is critical. The testing of new drugs for the treatment of osteosarcoma has been somewhat problematic. It is difficult to incorporate new drugs into maximally dosed aggressive regimens which already result in a 50% reduction in the risk of death. Thus the approach has been to test new drugs in the setting of relapsed osteosarcoma. Because of the rarity of this disease, however, and because most of those patients who relapsed have been pre-treated and have chemoresistant tumors, few new drugs have been adequately tested in trials of osteosarcoma. Paclitaxel was studied in a recent trial of 15 pretreated patients. No responses were seen [32]. Further research in this area is needed.

## Adjuvant Chemotherapy

The initial reports of the activity of doxorubicin and methotrexate against metastatic and primary osteosarcoma led to numerous phase II studies of adjuvant doxorubicin and methotrexate based combinations. Long-term metastasis-free survival ranged from 40–55% [33]. Despite what appeared to be a clear improvement in outcome with chemotherapy, some researchers felt that outcome without chemotherapy was also improved. This contention served as the impetus for 3 subsequent, "definitive" randomized trials [34–37]. The convincing nature of these results has precluded the use of a no chemotherapy control arm in subsequent studies.

The first trial was completed by the Mayo Clinic and published in 1984. Researchers there had contended based on review of the outcome of sequential patients at their institution, that the natural history of the disease was changing and that outcome with surgery alone was significantly better than the previously reported 20% long term survival. The Mayo Clinic study randomized 38 of 87 eligible patients to surgery only or surgery followed by 1 year of vincristine and high dose methotrexate. Ninety-seven percent of patients underwent amputation. Neither disease free survival at 5 years (control 44%, chemo group 40%) or overall survival (control 54%, chemotherapy group 50%) were improved. Eligible non-participants (10 of 54) who did receive chemotherapy fared equally well as randomized participants [34].

The results of this "negative" study remain less than fully explained, as the two studies that followed showed significant differences. One important criticism is that the dose and dose intensity of the high dose methotrexate was low by today's standard. Salvage chemotherapy with active agents may have also contributed to survival for patients developing metastases.

The next published study was the Multi-Institutional Osteosarcoma Study. The results of this study were published with early follow-up in 1986 [35], due to major differences in outcome between the chemotherapy and control groups. Significant differences in survival have persisted over time. In this trial, 36 patients were randomized to undergo either surgery alone (amputation in 28 of 16 total) or surgery followed by BCD (bleomycin, cyclophosphamide and dactinomycin) alternating with high dose methotrexate/leucovorin and doxorubicin and cisplatin. Relapse free survival at six years (11% in control arm and 61% chemotherapy arm) and overall survival (50% control vs 71 chemotherapy arm, including all 113 patients randomized or choosing one of the two arms) were significantly in favor of chemotherapy [36]. It is notable that many patients relapsing after surgery alone were cured with subsequent pulmonary metastasectomy and adjuvant chemotherapy.

The third study, randomized 59 patients at UCLA to receive "surgery" (limb salvage in 44 of 59 patients) or surgery followed by adjuvant chemotherapy [37]. All patients received pre-operative intraarterial doxorubicin, 30 mg/m$^2$ x 3 days, followed by 5 fractions of 350 cGy to the involved bone. Patients receiving adjuvant chemotherapy received high dose methotrexate and leucovorin with vincristine followed by doxorubicin, followed by BCD, with 6 week cycles repeated 4 times. Overall survival at 2 years was 80% for the chemotherapy group and 48% for the control group (p <0.01). With the results of this study, adjuvant chemotherapy became uniformly accepted in osteosarcoma.

### Neoadjuvant Chemotherapy

Practical and theoretical rationale led to the widespread use of neoadjuvant or presurgical, chemotherapy in the 1980's. From a practical standpoint, custom prostheses often took several months to produce. Chemotherapy was instituted to fill the gap of time while awaiting surgery. This was done on sound theoretical grounds. Early treatment of micrometastases might allow for a better outcome compared with waiting an addition 2–4 months until production of the prosthesis and recovery from surgery. Neoadjuvant chemotherapy could shrink or otherwise alter the tumor rendering it more easily resectable. Finally, analysis of the resected specimen allows an individual patient "in vivo" assay of the effectiveness of preoperative chemotherapy and its potential for benefit in the post-operative setting. From an analysis of the results of many phase II trials of neoadjuvant chemotherapy, one can conclude, although never compared in a randomized fashion, that neoadjuvant chemotherapy is at least equivalent to adjuvant chemotherapy [33]. Neoadjuvant chemotherapy probably improves the likelihood of successful limb salvage. Most clear is the ability of the pathological assessment of neoadjuvant chemotherapy cell kill to predict outcome. As a result of the above rationale, most patients receive their chemotherapy prior to surgery for 2–4 months and receive further chemotherapy post-operatively.

*Standard Chemotherapy*

Because of the rarity of this curable disease, a standard regimens do not exist. Most patients are and should be treated on clinical trials at tertiary care centers where orthopedic oncologic and multidisciplinary expertise is available. These clinical trials generally take many years to complete at either single institutions or in cooperative groups. Therefore, the "best" published regimens may not be those currently being used or investigated.

Most regimens include 2 or 3 of the effective drugs (doxorubicin, cisplatin, methotrexate and ifosfamide) preoperatively. Good responders (> 90% necrosis) generally continue with the same or similar regimen unless toxicity or cumulative doses warrant a change. In many programs, "non-responders" (< 90% necrosis) change to a regimen to include the drugs which they have not yet received.

For patients without access to clinical trials, a reasonable regimen includes cisplatin, 100–120 mg/m$^2$ plus doxorubicin 60–75 mg/m$^2$ (by prolonged infusion), every 3 weeks for three preoperative cycles. Good responders can receive 3 postoperative cycles of the same preoperative chemotherapy. Ifosfamide 2,500–3000 mg/m$^2$/day x 3 can be substituted for cisplatin if neuropathy or ototoxicity prohibit further cisplatin. Poor responders can receive alternating high dose ifosfamide and high dose methotrexate, with or without further doxorubicin and cisplatin.

Several studies have attempted to define prognostic variables for outcome in osteosarcoma with the goal of minimizing treatment for patients with very good prognosis and possibly intensifying treatment in poor prognostic patients. The variable which consistently is the most predictive is the degree of necrosis obtained with preoperative chemotherapy. Patients with > 90% necrosis fare significantly better than those with < 90% necrosis. All subgroups with < 90% necrosis fare significantly worse than good responders, although some studies do show improved survival for patients with near 90% necrosis [38]. Unfortunately the degree of necrosis is partially a post-treatment variable as is positive margins, which also predicts for poor survival [41]. Pre-treatment variables which have been shown to predict for worse outcome in some studies include large tumor size [38–40], male sex [42] and various anatomic sites, particularly pelvis and axial skeleton. Age is probably not a significant prognostic factor differentiating outcome between children and young adults [38], but elderly adults generally fare poorly with osteosarcoma.

*Treatment of Metastatic Disease*

The goals of treatment of metastatic disease are divided into palliative and curative intent therapy. For those with extrathoracic metastases or poor prognosis pulmonary metastases treatment is palliative. For those patients with good prognosis pulmonary metastases, including limited number of metastases, long interval from therapy to development of metastases, and no prior chemotherapy, the goal of therapy is cure, which is achieved in approximately 20–30% of patients. For patients relapsing within a year or two of chemotherapy, therapy should be limited to pulmonary metastasectomy. For those patients who have had no chemotherapy or, controversially, those who have had a long interval since chemotherapy, therapy should consist of surgery with chemotherapy given before or after surgery.

Patients who are not candidates for curative metastasectomy should receive, if appropriate, active drugs which they have not yet received. It is important too that these patients be enrolled in clinical trials to help identify new active drugs, particularly the "new" drugs of the 1990's which have yet to be adequately tested. High dose chemotherapy for osteosarcoma has not yet met with success [44].

## Other Tumor Types

Ewing's Sarcoma: Peripheral Neuroectodermal Tumor (PNET)

Prior to the era of chemotherapy, Ewing's sarcoma/PNET was cured in only 10–20% of patients, despite radical surgical procedures. In the 1960's, Ewing's sarcoma was found to be responsive to chemotherapy. The Intergroup Ewing's Sarcoma Study I (IESS-I) (1973–1978) established that approximately 60% of patients with non-pelvic, non metastatic, primaries were curable with vincristine, dactinomycin, cyclophosphamide +/– doxorubicin [44]. The IESS-2, from 1978–1982, intensified these drugs and achieved a 68% (57% pelvic) cure rate in non-metastatic disease [45]. The third intergroup study (1988–1993) established that the addition of alternating cycles of ifosfamide and etoposide to vincristine, doxorubicin, cyclophosphamide and actinomycin increased the 3 year disease free survival, including pelvic primaries, to 68% [46]. The current study is comparing the 5 drug regimen (vincristine, doxorubicin, cyclophosphamide, alternating with ifosfamide and etoposide) in a standard or intensified fashion.

In general, local therapy (radiation, surgery, or both) is performed after 3 months of chemotherapy. Chemotherapy then continues post-local therapy. It is notable that approximately 25% of patients with metastatic disease at presentation can be cured with standard therapy [44–47]. High dose chemotherapy with stern cell support has been used in several small studies with an apparent, but not definite, improvement in survival [48, 49]. All patients with these rare tumors should be treated at institutions with a multidisciplinary sarcoma treatment team, preferably on a clinical trial.

## Chondrosarcoma and Chordoma

Chondrosarcoma and chordoma are both chemotherapy refractory malignancies. Possible exceptions include mesenchymal chondrosarcoma and dedifferentiated chondrosarcoma where occasional responses may be seen [50, 51].

## *Other Spindle Cell Tumors of Bone*

Malignant fibrous histiocytoma, fibrosarcoma and leiomyosarcoma of bone are rare spindle cell tumors which occur much less frequently than osteosarcoma. Although solid data is lacking from large trials, these are generally treated like osteosarcomas rather than their soft tissue counterparts, with outcomes equal to or slightly worse than with osteosarcoma.

## Conclusions

Chemotherapy plays an essential role in the curative therapy of osteosarcoma, reducing the relapse rate by 50% and reducing the death rate by nearly the same. Further work is needed to establish the least toxic, curative regimen for osteosarcoma and to identify new drugs for its treatment. Pulmonary metastasectomy can be curative in selected patients.

Chemotherapy plays an essential role in the curative multimodality therapy of Ewing's sarcoma/PNET. Chemotherapy has little or no role in chondrosarcoma and chordoma.

## Key Questions

Key questions regarding bone tumors include:
a) Establishment optimal drug regimen for osteosarcoma.
b) Comparison of outcomes with neoadjuvant and adjuvant regimens.
c) Definition of treatment and prognosis for non-osteosarcoma spindle cell tumors of bone.
d) Definition of new active drugs for osteosarcoma.
e) Role of chemotherapy for lung metastases.
f) Optimal local and systemic therapy for PNET/Ewing's.
g) Timing of local therapy for Ewing's/PNET.
h) Identification of effective systemic therapy of chondrosarcoma and chordoma.

## References

1. Landis SH, Murray T, Bolden S, Wingo PA (1998) Cancer Statistics. In: Murphy G (ed) CA: A Cancer Journal for Clinicians, p 10
2. Mirra JM (1989) Bone Tumors. Clinical, Radiographic, and Pathologic Correlation. Lea & Febiger, p 255
3. Weis L (1998) Common Malignant Bone Tumors. In: Simon MA, Springfield DS (eds) Surgery for Bone and Soft-Tissue Tumors. Lippincott-Raven, Philadelphia, p 265–298
4. Goorin AM, Abelson HT, Frei E (1985) Osteosarcoma: Fifteen years later. N Engl J Med 313: 1637
5. Li FP, Froumeni JF (1969) Soft-tissue sarcomas, breast cancer, and other neoplasms: a familial syndrome? Ann Intern Med 71: 747–752
6. Wold LE, McLeod RA, Sim FH, Unni KK (1990) Atlas of Orthopaedic Pathology. WB Saunders, p 87
7. Demay CT (1996) Gene Rearrangements in Ewing's Sarcoma. Canc Invest 14: 83–88
8. American Joint Committee on Cancer: Bone (1997) In: Beahrs OH, Myers MH (eds) Manual for Staging 5th ed. JB Lippincott, Philadelphia, pp 143–147
9. Mankin HJ, Mankin CJ, Simon MA (1997) The Hazards of Biopsy, Revisited. J Bone Joint Surg 78: 659
10. Enneking WF, Spanier SS, Goodman MA (1990) A system for the surgical staging of musculoskeletal sarcoma. Clin Orthop 153: 106–120
11. Cortes EP, Holland JF, Wang JJ et al (1972) Doxorubicin in disseminated Osteosarcoma. JAMA 221: 1132–1138
12. Jaffe N, Paed D (1972) Recent advances in the chemotherapy of metastatic osteogenic sarcoma. Cancer 30: 1627–1631

13. Marcove RC, Mike V, Hajek JV et al (1971) Osteogenic sarcoma in childhood. NY State J Med 71: 855–859
14. Cortes EP, Holland JF, Wang JJ et al (1974) Amputation and adriamycin in primary osteosarcoma. N Engl Med 291: 998–1000
15. Cortes EP, Holland JF, Glidewill O ( 1978) Amputation and adriamycin in primary osteosarcoma: A 5-year report. Cancer Treat Rep 62: 271–277
16. Cortes EP, Holland JF, Wang JJ et al (1975) Adriamycin (NSC-123127) in 87 patients with osteosarcoma. Cancer Chemo Rep 6: 305–313
17. Bacci G, Picci P, Ferrari et al (1993) Influence of adriamycin dose in the outcome of patients with osteosarcoma treated with multidrug neoadjuvant chemotherapy: results of two sequential studies. J Chemother 5: 237–246
18. Jaffe N, Frei F, Traggis D et al (1974) Adjuvant methotrexate and citrovorum-factor treatment of osteogenic sarcoma. N Eng J Med 291: 994–997
19. Jaffe N, Frei III E, Watts H et al (1978) High-dose methotrexate in osteogenic sarcoma: A 5-year experience. Cancer Treat Rep 62: 259–264
20. Bacci G, Picci P, Ruggieri P et al (1990) Primary chemotherapy and delayed surgery (neoadjuvant chemotherapy) for osteosarcoma of the extremities. Cancer 65: 2539–2553
21. Rosen Gy, Marcove RC, Huvos AG et al (1983) J Cancer Res Clin Oncol 106: 55–67
22. Solheim OP, Saeter G, Elomaa I et al (1992) Ann Oncol 3: S7–S11
23. Bacci G, Ferrari S, Picci P et al (1996) Methotrexate serum concentration and histologic response to multiagent primary chemotherapy for osteosarcoma of the limbs. J Chemother 8: 472–478
24. Ochs JJ, Freeman AI, Douglass HO et al (1978) cis-Dichlorodiammineplatinum (II) in advanced osteogenic sarcoma. Cancer Treat Rep 62: 239–245
25. Jaffe N, Knapp J, Chuang VP et al (1983) Osteosarcoma: Intra-arterial treatment of the primary tumor with Cis-Diammine-Dichloroplatinum II (CDP). Cancer 51: 402–407
26. Bacci G, Ruggier P, Picci P et al (1996) Intraarterial versus intravenous cisplatinum in addition to systemic and high dose adriamycin and high dose methotrexate in the neoadjuvant treatment of osteosarcoma of the extremities. Results of a randomized trial study. J Chemother 9: 70–81
27. Jaffe N, Raymond AK, Avala A et al (1989) Analysis of the efficacy of intraarterial and cisdiamminedichloroplatinum-II and high dose methotrexate with citrovorum factor rescue in the treatment of primary osteosarcoma. Regional Cancer Treatment 2: 157–163
28. Ferguson W, Harris M, Link M et al (1996) Carboplatin in the treatment of newly-diagnosed metastatic or unresectable osteosarcoma: a Pediatric Oncology Group study. Proc Am Soc Clin Oncol 15: 521
29. Bieling P, Maerker I, Beron G et al. (1992) Phase II study of carboplatin (CB) in pre-treated disseminated osteosarcoma (OS). Proc Am Soc Clin Oncol 11: 414
30. Marti C, Kroner T, Remagen W et al (1985) High-dose ifosfamide in advanced osteosarcoma. Cancer Treat Rep 69: 115–117
31. Pratt CB, Horowitz ME, Meyer WH et al (1987) Phase II trial of ifosfamide in children with malignant solid tumors. Cancer Treat Rep 71: 131–135
32. Patel SR, Papadopoulos NE, Plager C et al (1996) Phase II study of paclitaxel in patients with previously treated osteosarcoma and its variants. Cancer 78: 741–744
33. Jaffe NJ, Patel SR, Benjamin RS (1995) Chemotherapy in osteosarcoma. Basis for application and antagonism to implementation: Early controversies surrounding its implementation. Heme Onc Clin N Amer 9: 825–840
34. Edmonson JH, Green SJ, Ivins JC et al (1984) A controlled pilot study of high-dose methotrexate as postsurgical adjuvant treatment of primary osteosarcoma. J Clin Oncol 2: 152–156

35. Link MP, Goorin AM, Miser AW et al ( 1986) The effect of adjuvant chemotherapy of relapse-free survival in patients with osteosarcoma of the extremity. N Engl J Med 314: 1600–1606

36. Link MP, Goorin AM, Horowitz M et al (1991) Adjuvant chemotherapy of high-grade osteosarcoma of the extremity: Update results of the multi-institutional osteosarcoma study. Clin Ortho and Rel Res 270: 8–14

37. Eilber F, Guiliano A, Eckardt J et al (1987) Adjuvant chemotherapy for osteosarcoma: A randomized prospective trial. J Clin Oncol 5: 21–26

38. Hudson M, Jaffe MR, Jaffe N et al (1990) Pediatric osteosarcoma: Therapeutic strategies, results, und prognostic factors derived from a 10-year experience. J Clin Oncol 8: 1988–1997

39. Davis AM, Bell RS, Goodwin PJ (1994) Prognostic factors in osteosarcoma: A critical review. J Clin Oncol 12: 423–431

40. Bieling P, Rehan N, Winkler P et al (1996) Tumor size and prognosis in aggressively treated osteosarcoma. J Clin Oncol 14: 848–858

41. Ward WG, Mikaelian K, Dorey F et al (1994) Pulmonary metastases of stage IIIB extremity osteosarcoma and subsequent pulmonary metastases. J Clin Oncol 12: 1849–1858

42. Petrilli AS, Gentil FC, Epelman S et al (1991) Increased survival, limb preservation, and prognostic factors for osteosarcoma. Cancer 68: 733–737

43. Colombat P, Biron P, Coze C et al (1994) Failure of high dose alkylating agents on osteosarcoma. Solid tumors working party (letter). Bone Marrow Transplant 14: 665–666

44. Nesbit ME, Gehan EA, Burgert Jr EO et al (1990) Multimodal therapy for the management of primary, nonmetastatic Ewing's sarcoma of bone: A long-term follow-up of the first intergroup study. J Clin Oncol 9: 1664–1674

45. Burgert Jr EO, Nesbit ME, Garnsey LA et al (1990) Multimodal therapy for the management of nonpelvic localized Ewing's sarcoma of bone: Intergroup study IESS-II. J Clin Oncol 8: 1514–1524

46. Grier HE, Krailo M et al (1994) Improved outcome in non-metastatic Ewing's sarcoma (EWS) and PNET of bone with the addition of ifosfamide and etoposide to vincristine, Adriamycin, cyclophosphamide and actinomycin: a Children's Cancer Group (CCG) and Pediatric Oncology Group (POG) report. Proc Am Soc Clin Oncol 113: 421

47. Cangir A, Vietti TJ, Gehan FA (1990) Ewing's sarcoma metastatic at diagnosis. Results and comparison of two intergroup Ewing's sarcoma studies. Cancer 66: 887–893

48. Burdach S, Jürgens H, Peters C et al (1993) Myeloablative radiochemotherapy and hematopoietic stem-cell rescue in poor-prognosis Ewing's sarcoma. J Clin Oncol 11: 1482–1488

49. Ladenstein R, Hartmann O, Pinkerton CR (1993)The role of megatherapy with autologous bone marrow rescue in solid tumours of childhood. Ann Oncol 4: S45–S58

50. Huvos AG (1991) Chondrosarcoma including spindle-cell (dedifferential) and myxoid chondrosarcoma; mesenchymal chondrosarcoma. In: Huvos AG (ed) Bone Tumors, 2nd. WB Sauders. Philadelphia, PA Chap 13, p 343–381

51. Fleming GF, Heimann PS, Stephens JK et al (1993) Dedifferentiated chordoma. Response to aggressive chemotherapy in two cases. Cancer 72: 714–71

# Thyroid Malignancies

# Thyroid Malignancies

K.B. Ain

## Epidemiology, Risk Factors

Thyroid malignancies comprise a broad range of neoplasms of the thyroid gland with differing biological and clinical implications. Differentiated carcinomas of thyroid epithelial (follicular) cells are the most common; while dedifferentiated (anaplastic) tumors and medullary cancers, malignancies of the parafollicular (calcitonin-secreting) cells, are quite infrequent. In addition, *extremely rare* thyroid tumors include: angiomatoid neoplasms, mucoepidermoid carcinomas, thyroid thymomas, malignant teratomas, paragangliomas, and primary thyroid lymphomas.

### Incidence and Prevalence

There are more than 17,200 thyroid carcinomas diagnosed in the United States each year, constituting just over 1% of incident cancers [1]. This is the "tip of the iceberg" of prevalent disease, since survival for differentiated thyroid cancer is considerable over several decades. Although outdated and likely low, one may grasp the magnitude of the population prevalence by noting estimates from Connecticut in 1982 of 67.7 cases/100,000 for women and 23.7 cases/100,000 for men [2]. This *clinical disease* is dwarfed by ubiquitous *occult* papillary microcarcinomas (unifocal tumors ≤1 cm diameter) found in up to one third of all individuals at autopsy [3]. Clinical thyroid cancers are less common in children (although 1.4% of childhood cancers) with a female yearly incidence and prevalence of 0.22 cases and 3.6 cases per 100,000, respectively, and male values at 0.09 and 1.5 cases, respectively (before age 15) [4].

**Differentiated Epithelial Carcinomas.** Nearly 90% of thyroid cancers are considered differentiated neoplasms of the follicular cells responsible for iodide uptake and thyroid hormone synthesis. Just under 90% of differentiated epithelial cancers are classified as papillary and the remainder considered follicular [5], based on histologic and cytologic features. Historically, follicular variants of papillary carcinomas were often misclassified as follicular or mixed papillary/follicular cancers; however they can be clearly distinguished as papillary cancers based upon nuclear features [6]. Distinctive variants of both papillary and follicular cancers are associated with adverse clinical behaviors and outcomes (described in Pathology section, below).

**Uncommon and Rare Thyroid Cancers.** Anaplastic carcinomas are rare terminal dedifferentiations of papillary and follicular carcinomas, with an estimated annual incidence of less than 300 cases in the United States, based on its proportion of 1.6% of incident thyroid cancers [7]. With typical survival less than 3 months, the prevalence of this disease is far less than the yearly incidence. Medullary thyroid cancers constitute 5%–10% of thyroid cancers; although familial clusters are seen in 20% of the cases, due to an autosomal dominant expression of the associated oncogene mutations. Around 1%–5% of thyroid malignancies are primary thyroid lymphomas [5, 8], constituting less than 1% of all lymphomas. The remaining rare thyroid cancers, mentioned above, are unusual enough "zebras" to warrant case reports.

Race, Sex, Age Distribution, Predisposition

Differentiated thyroid cancers are typically sporadic or related to environmental exposures; however familial concentrations have been described [9, 10]. A couple of studies have associated this with Histocompatability markers HLA-B7 and DR1 [10] or HLA-DR7 [11]. Recent analyses have described three translocations involving the RET proto-oncogene on chromosome 10, RET/PTC1 [12], RET/PTC2 [13], and RET/PTC3 [14], which are associated with papillary thyroid carcinomas. Most cases do not appear to be connected to these factors.

There are different incidence rates associated with different ethnic or racial groups in similar environments. Higher rates of differentiated cancers are seen in Chinese, Hawaiian, and Filipino groups than in

Caucasians, with lower rates in African Americans and Puerto Ricans [15].

Approximately 20% of medullary carcinomas are inherited as highly penetrant autosomal dominant traits, consequent to assorted mutations of the RET proto-oncogene [16]. These include patients with the multiple endocrine neoplasia (MEN) syndromes, MEN IIa (parathyroid hyperplasia, pheochromocytomas, and medullary cancer) and MEN IIb (marfanoid habitus, gastrointestinal ganglioneuromatosis, mucosal neuromas, pheochromocytomas, and medullary cancer), or simple familial medullary carcinomas. Conditions associated with occurrence of differentiated thyroid cancers include Gardner's syndrome (familial adenomatosis polyposis) [17], Carney's complex [18], Cowden's disease [19], and Alagille syndrome [20].

Differentiated thyroid cancers predominate in women over men by at least 2.2- to 2.7-fold [1, 21]. Despite this, male sex appears to be an independent prognostic risk factor for thyroid cancer mortality [22]. Basic researchers have failed to identify biological mechanisms for these epidemiological findings. Anaplastic cancers are also more often found in women, probably reflecting the greater prevalence of progenitor differentiated thyroid cancers in the female population.

Age at time of diagnosis has continually reaffirmed itself as an independent prognostic risk factor in diverse studies of differentiated thyroid cancer. Older patients have significantly increased risks of mortality than younger adults, with the cut-off age set at age 41 years [23] to 50 years [24] in different analyses. Children manifest distinctly different tumor behavior for unknown reasons (nearly all are papillary cancers), with greater rates of local invasion, local recurrence, and distant metastases [25].

Risk Factors and Etiology

There is a definite association between exposure to external radiotherapy or substantial radioactive fallout and the development of differentiated thyroid carcinomas. Such exposure increases the incidence of thyroid nodules, as well as the risk that a nodule is malignant [26]. The estimated incidence rate of thyroid cancer is 0.5%/year in populations exposed to thyroid doses of 200–500 rads (no lower threshold defined) [27] and young children are more susceptible to this effect. This is most evident in the dramatic increase of aggressive papillary thyroid carcinomas in Belarussian children exposed to the radioactive fallout from the Chernobyl reactor explosion [28, 29]. Tumorigenic effects persist at least 40 years from exposure [30]. This remains an area of intense interest, particularly in view of recent analyses of potential American thyroid cancer cases caused by domestic nuclear fallout [31]. There is no evidence that diagnostic radiation doses (from diagnostic xrays or radioiodine thyroid scanning) or therapeutic I-131 therapy of Graves' disease can induce thyroid cancer [32].

Other environmental factors contributing to development of thyroid cancer are poorly defined and speculative. There is a geographic association of higher incidence of thyroid cancer in regions of the globe with significant volcanic activity [33]. Industrial exposures to chlorophenol and creosote [34], hexachlorobenzene [35], and dioxins [36] have been implicated. Dietary iodine supplementation reduces the proportion of follicular (and possibly anaplastic) carcinomas relative to papillary carcinomas [37]. Most thyroid carcinoma cases are not able to be associated with any known causative environmental exposure.

## Pathology and Staging

As mentioned, it is helpful to classify thyroid cancers into three broad categories based upon progenitor cell type: follicular (epithelial) thyroid cells, parafollicular (calcitonin-secreting) cells, and other cell types (e.g. endothelial, thymic, lymphoid, and solid cells). These are further divided into common histologic groups.

### Differentiated Epithelial Thyroid Cancers

Thyroid oncologic pathology, particularly in discriminating unusual cancer variants, is one of the most difficult areas in the field of surgical pathology. Even among pathologists skilled in thyroid pathology, there is poor agreement in histologic diagnoses [38]. For this reason, it is common to require additional pathology consultations to confirm the diagnostic classification.

*Papillary Carcinomas*

Around 80% of primary thyroid malignancies are papillary carcinomas, of which 75% are "usual" papillary cancers with slow growth and regional lymphatic spread, and the remainder consisting of several subtypes, some with distinct clinical behaviors [18]. Although many demonstrate a classic feature of "complex branching papillae that have a fibrovascular core" [39] and some may have gross features typical of follicular cancers, their nuclear features define them as papillary cancers [6, 40] rather than mixed papillary and follicular cancers.

Varieties of papillary carcinoma with typically good clinical outcomes encompass 90% of papillary cancers and include: usual papillary carcinoma, encapsulated papillary carcinoma, and follicular variant of papillary carcinoma (previously mistaken as follicular carcinomas). Papillary microcarcinomas (≤1.0 cm diameter and unifocal) constitute the "occult" thyroid cancer found in around one third of the entire population and have virtually no clinical significance.

Aggressive papillary cancer subtypes are noted for their invasive growth, local recurrence, distant spread, risk of eventual loss of radioiodine uptake (rendering them untreatable with I-131), and increased mortality. They include: tall cell variant (3%–12% of papillary cancers) [18, 41–43], columnar cell variant (0.2%) [44–46], diffuse sclerosing variant (2%–6%) [47–49], diffuse follicular variant (1.6%) [50], and Hürthle (oxyphilic) cell variant (2%–4%) [51, 52].

*Follicular Carcinomas*

Follicular thyroid carcinomas share identical cytologic features with benign follicular adenomas, differing only by the presence of vascular &/or tumor capsular invasion [53], suggesting that some adenomas may be carcinomas "in situ" [54, 55]. For this reason, efforts to identify adenomas in order to avoid surgical resection are misdirected. Follicular cancers can spread hematogenously to lung, bone, brain, and liver; resulting in a more aggressive clinical course and higher mortality than usual papillary carcinomas [24, 56, 57]. Two particular subtypes of follicular carcinoma, insular (previously misclassified as anaplastic) [58–61] and Hürthle (oxyphilic) cell, are felt to be clinically aggressive with poorer outcomes than typical follicular cancers.

*Anaplastic (Dedifferentiated) Carcinomas*

These are the most aggressive solid tumors of any organ and have uniformly fatal outcomes despite all therapeutic efforts. The three major histological patterns often coexist in the same tumor: spindle cell (53%), giant cell (50%), and squamoid (19%) [58, 62]. Much of the older literature is invalidated by including "small cell" anaplastic carcinoma, now correctly classified as lymphoma, as a chemotherapy-responsive subtype in clinical reviews [63]. Anaplastic carcinomas are believed to be resulting from terminal dedifferentiation of pre-existing papillary and follicular carcinomas, accounting for the presence of coexisting areas of such cancers [64, 65]. Considering the aggressive course of the anaplastic component, with mortality approaching 100% within several months, the clinical impact of differentiated components can be ignored.

*Medullary (Parafollicular) Carcinomas*

Medullary thyroid carcinomas derive from the parafollicular ("C") cells and usually secrete calcitonin and carcinoembryonic antigen (CEA). Immunohistochemistry complements and confirms a thorough pathologic analysis. Tumors are usually found in the lateral upper two-thirds of the gland in the regions of highest C-cell concentration. Sporadic tumors are usually unifocal and large at time of diagnosis in 40–60 year-old patients; whereas inherited tumors are seen in younger patients and nearly always bilateral and associated with diffuse pre-neoplastic C-cell hyperplasia [66]. Genetic testing has permitted prophylactic thyroidectomies in patients with germline RET mutations, revealing only C-cell hyperplasia or microscopic foci of medullary cancer, long before outmoded calcitonin stimulation tests become positive [67]. In addition, some medullary thyroid cancers considered sporadic by clinical assessment have been found to be index cases of familial disease, warranting genetic testing in most cases [16]. A key clinical feature is the recognition of associated inherited neoplasms and clinical features of MEN 2 syndromes. Prognosis, even in the face of widespread distant metastases, is extremely variable since some patients have been known to survive for decades with large, slow-growing tumor burdens.

## Other Uncommon Thyroid Malignancies

Thyroid lymphomas are primarily B-cell type while T-cell lymphomas are distinctly rare [68]. Over 80% show a diffuse histologic pattern with 70%–80% considered large cell lymphomas (histiocytic lymphomas). Around 5%–10% are intermediate grade (poorly differentiated), 10%–12% are low grade (small cell), and very rarely do they manifest as Hodgkin's disease [5]. Over 70% reveal characteristic lymphoepithelial lesions, indicative of mucosa-associated lymphoid tissue (MALT) malignancy. This reflects autopsy findings of concurrent tumors in the gastrointestinal tract, typical of MALT lymphomas [69].

With a little over 20 reported cases, mucoepidermoid cancers are exceedingly rare. They are believed to develop from ultimobranchial-derived solid cell nests in the thyroid [70]. Likewise, thyroid cancers with thymic differentiation are though to develop from rests of thymus cells in the thyroid gland. They have been subdivided into four categories: ectopic hamartomatous thymomas, ectopic cervical thymomas, spindle epithelial tumors with thymus-like differentiation (SETTLE), and carcinomas showing thymus-like differentiation (CASTLE) [71]. The rarity of malignant adult thyroid teratomas is exceeded only by the mortality of such tumors. On the other hand, malignant thyroid hemangioendotheliomas and angiosarcomas were frequently seen in Alpine regions prior to iodine prophylaxis [72], but are currently extremely rare in the United States. They are typically aggressive tumors and prove lethal after a few months [73].

## Staging of Papillary and Follicular Cancers

There are several tumor features with prognostic significance, based upon multivariate analyses of large, retrospective studies, without controlling for treatments administered. The prognostic effects of age at time of diagnosis and sex are discussed above. Additional prognostic criteria include histologic findings of: primary tumor size, presence of extrathyroidal invasion, and clinical evidence of local or distant metastatic disease. As in many malignancies, the larger the primary tumor, the more aggressive is the clinical course. Unifocal papillary microcarcinomas (≤1.0 cm diameter) have the least best prognostic consequences as suggested by their classification as occult tumors. These effects are not relevant to multifocal disease, with multifocality serving as an independent risk factor for development of local and distant metastases [74]. Follicular cancers do not reveal a minimum diameter associated with absence of mortality, although prognosis worsens with larger tumors [75]. Vascular invasion seems to be a negative prognostic factor [76], although this is controversial [77]. On the other hand, all studies agree that extrathyroidal invasion is a critical prognostic feature of an aggressive clinical course [78]. Likewise, distant metastases to soft tissues and bone have important negative prognostic consequences [77], while the negative effect of local metastases is quite low in papillary [18] and follicular [55] cancers.

A variety of prognostic staging systems have been developed for differentiated thyroid carcinomas. Many of them are helpful for use in epidemiological studies, statistical analyses of large patient populations, and as stratification tools for designing prospective therapeutic trials. *None of them are sufficiently predictive of outcome to permit their use for determining therapy in individual patients* [79, 80]. The most valuable staging system for thyroid cancer uses the pTNM classification system [81–83], as shown in Table 1. In addition to the common features of: size of tumor, associated regional nodes, and presence of distant metastases, this system distinguishes pathologic types between papillary or follicular cancers, medullary cancers, and anaplastic cancers. Recent pTNM modifications describing the location of local nodal metastases [84] may be of significance in surgical management [85]. Major shortcomings of

**Table 1.** Clinical staging of thyroid cancer: method of the American Joint Committee on Cancer [81] using the pTNM classification of the Union of Internationale Centre de Cancer [82] as later modified [84].

| Stage | Papillary or follicular Age <45 years | Age ≥45 years | Medullary | Anaplastic |
|---|---|---|---|---|
| I | Any T any N M0 | T1 N0 M0 | T1 N0 M0 | |
| II | Any T any N M1 | T2-3 N0 M0 | T2-4 N0 M0 | |
| III | | T4 N0 M0, or Any T N1 M0 | Any T N1 M0 | |
| IV | | T2-3 N0 M0 | Any T any N M1 | All cases |

Tumor (T): T1, intrathyroidal ≤1 cm; T2, intrathyroidal >1–4 cm; T3, intrathyroidal >4 cm; T4, extrathyroidal of any size; TX, cannot be assessed; a, solitary focus; b, multifocal; (i), grossly encapsulated; (ii), grossly nonencapsulated. Nodes (N): N0, no regional lymph node metastases; N1, regional lymph node metastasis; NX, cannot be assessed. N1 site location: N1a, ipsilateral node(s); N1a (i), ipsilateral central; N1a (ii), ipsilateral lateral; N1b, other than (may include) ipsilateral node(s); N1b (i), contralateral central (or midline)± any ipsilateral node(s); N1b (ii), contralateral lateral± any ipsilateral node(s); N1b (iii), mediastinal site. Distant metastases (M): M0, none; M1, present; MX, cannot be assessed.

this, and other, thyroid cancer staging systems are the failure to consider histologic subtypes with poorer clinical outcomes and the lack of any prospective clinical trials defining the interaction of different therapeutic protocols on patient outcome.

It is not possible to provide meaningful survival times or percentages for patients with differentiated thyroid carcinoma. There are important reasons for this. First, deaths and recurrences from differentiated thyroid cancers manifest over the course of several decades from initial disease diagnosis. For that reason, all studies with sufficient follow-up time are retrospective reviews and those prospective studies with shorter follow-up have little value. Second, patients with similar stages of disease receive widely differing treatments, invalidating evaluations of clinical outcomes in retrospective reviews. Even the most recent consensus treatment guidelines for thyroid cancer management [86] are diffuse and ambiguous, reflecting the absence of any useful standard of care. The only exception appears to be the excellent survival of unifocal, non-metastatic, papillary microcarcinomas [87], which require little more than surgical resection and thyrotropin-suppressive levothyroxine therapy.

## Initial Work-up and Follow-up Evaluations

Most thyroid carcinomas present as an asymptomatic thyroid mass, usually discovered by looking in the mirror, being noted by a family member, or on routine medical evaluation. Alternatively, the first evidence of cancer may be a palpable cervical lymph node or an incidental finding on a radiological study for some other purpose (e.g. carotid ultrasonography). Occasionally, thyroid cancer is first discovered as a distant metastasis. Immunohistochemistry of a fine needle aspirate or of surgical samples may reveal staining for thyroglobulin [88], a marker for papillary or follicular cancer. The flow chart in Figure 1 provides an overview of the evaluation and therapy of differentiated thyroid epithelial carcinomas.

Evaluation of a Thyroid Nodule and Thyroid Surgery

The most efficient evaluation of a thyroid nodule begins with a clinical history for evidence of familial thyroid cancers or therapeutic radiation

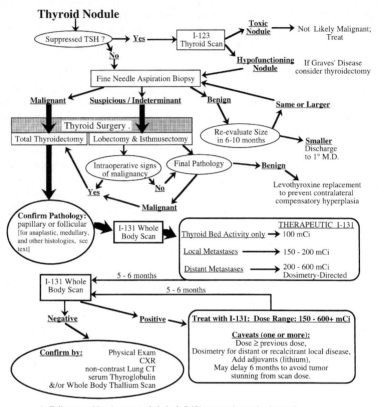

**Thyroid Nodule**

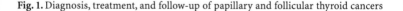

**Fig. 1.** Diagnosis, treatment, and follow-up of papillary and follicular thyroid cancers

(or nuclear fallout) exposure, as well as an evaluation for the presence of thyrotoxicosis. Thyrotoxic patients should undergo radioiodine thyroid scanning to reveal autonomously functioning ("hot") thyroid nodules, which are nearly never cancers, as well as the unusual hypofunctioning ("cold") nodule in the context of Graves' disease (which should be biopsied). *In nonthyrotoxic patients, thyroid nuclear scans should not be performed since they cannot distinguish benign from malignant nodules* [89]. Proper assessment of such a patient requires fine-needle aspiration biopsy of the nodule with cytology evaluated by a specialist. Expert cytologic interpretation of biopsy samples with sufficient follicular cells reveals nodules to be benign (which should be re-evaluated after 8 months and re-biopsied if not spontaneously smaller), malignant, or indeterminate/suspicious. There is no role for attempts at diagnostic suppression of suspicious thyroid nodules with thyroid hormone. Malignant nodules should be treated by a total thyroidectomy and suspicious nodules should be evaluated by an ipsilateral lobectomy with isthmusectomy (*never a nodulectomy or partial lobectomy*) which is always followed by a completion thyroidectomy (except for occult microcarcinomas) if cancer is confirmed by pathologists. Thyroidectomy should be accompanied by appropriate local node resection in all cases of differentiated thyroid cancers [85].

Nodule cytology demonstrating anaplastic cancer or lymphoma may be supplemented by open biopsy or, for lymphoma, repeat aspiration biopsy with B-cell immunotyping by flow cytometry. Complete surgical resection of anaplastic cancers should be attempted (if possible), but lymphomas can be treated without resection. Medullary carcinomas require the most aggressive surgical treatment and show best results following compartment-oriented microdissection of regional lymph nodes [90].

Additional Initial Evaluations

The typical thyroid nodule does not require any radiological evaluation prior to fine needle biopsy and surgical thyroidectomy, if indicated. Ultrasonography has been advocated to enhance the diagnostic yield of biopsies, however this is unnecessary in most cases. *It is critical to avoid any radiologic studies using iodinated contrast, since stable iodine will compromise any diagnostic or therapeutic use of I-131 for up to 10 months.* There are no such restrictions for anaplastic cancers, lymphomas, medullary cancers, or other non-epithelial thyroid cancers which benefit by contrast CT or MR scans for staging evaluations.

Radioiodine Whole Body Scanning for Differentiated
Papillary or Follicular Carcinomas

Differentiated thyroid carcinomas often demonstrate tissue-specific
expression of the sodium-iodide symporter [91], accounting for their
ability to concentrate iodide in response to sufficient thyrotropin (TSH)
stimulation, evoked by thyroid hormone withdrawal or administration
of recombinant human TSH (rhTSH, newly released in 1999 [92]).
Traditional preparation for I-131 whole body scans after complete surgical thyroidectomy requires administration of liothyronine (Cytomel¨, 25
µg twice daily) for 4 wks, which is discontinued for 2 wks along with
implementation of a strict low-iodine diet [93, 94]. This causes sufficient
TSH elevation (TSH <30 mU/l) to stimulate I-131 uptake in normal and
malignant residual thyroid tissue, permitting imaging with a suitable
gamma-camera and assessment of residual or metastatic disease [95].
These scans follow the thyroidectomy by 6 wks to permit therapeutic I-
131 dose planning. In addition, at 2–7 days after therapeutic I-131 administrations, a whole body scan is obtained using the therapy dose as the
scan dose; permitting a sensitive assessment for metastases and detection of possible "tumor stunning" [96] as an explanation for treatment
failure (for remedy see [97]).

After I-131 treatments, scans are typically performed (with identical
preparation regimen) every 6 months (and I-131 treatments given) until
negative for evidence of thyroidal tissue (malignant or otherwise).
Subsequent scans are performed after one year, then two years, then 3
years, and then every 3–4 years, indefinitely. Since metastases have been
noted several decades after apparent resolution of disease, patients are
considered to have a "chronic disease" requiring life-long follow-up.

Some differentiated thyroid carcinomas lose iodine uptake, particularly some of the aggressive histologic subtypes. Additional nuclear imaging techniques may aid in assessing such patients. They include use of
thallium-201 [98], technetium-99m-sestamibi [99], and positron emission tomographic imaging with fluorine-18 fluorodeoxyglucose [100].

Tumor Markers

Thyroglobulin is a large glycoprotein with unique expression by thyroid follicular cell-derived tissues. TSH stimulation of residual thyroid

cancer enhances release of thyroglobulin and suppression of TSH with levothyroxine will inhibit thyroglobulin release. After surgical thyroidectomy and radioiodine ablation of residual normal and malignant thyroid tissue, there should be no detectable thyroglobulin (i.e., the "normal" level is "zero"). In this situation, thyroglobulin serves well as a tumor marker, with a rough correlation between quantity of tumor and thyroglobulin level. One problem is the 15%–30% incidence of interfering anti-thyroglobulin autoantibodies which can invalidate the thyroglobulin assay.

Thyroglobulin may serve as a parameter for presence of persistent thyroid cancer, independent of I-131 scanning, since tumor functions of iodide uptake and thyroglobulin production are not necessarily linked. Values above an arbitrary thyroglobulin cutoff of 8 ng/ml, in hypothyroid patients demonstrating a negative I-131 whole body scan, reveal the presence of thyroid cancer which may still respond to high-dose I-131 therapy [101]. When monitoring patients of TSH-suppressive levothyroxine doses, any detectable thyroglobulin levels which are significantly above the assay background should be considered clinically significant.

Calcitonin levels, particularly when stimulated by pentagastrin &/or calcium infusion, are markers which correlate with tumor burden in most medullary carcinomas. Previous reliance upon them, for screening kindreds of inherited medullary thyroid cancer, has been superseded by genetic testing. Stimulated calcitonin is still useful as a marker for persistent or recurrent disease after attempts at curative surgical resection. In patients with metastatic disease, calcitonin levels provide rough reflections of tumor burden. CEA levels may also function as a tumor marker for this disease, although relative expression of CEA in medullary cancer is extremely variable.

## Standard Treatment Options

Due to the dramatic biological and clinical differences in tumor behavior between: papillary and follicular cancers, anaplastic cancers, medullary cancers, thyroid lymphomas, and other rare thyroid cancers, it is impossible to lump all thyroid cancers into any singular treatment protocol.

## Surgical Treatment

Thyroid surgeons practice a distinctive subspecialty, requiring exceptional skills and judgment. With the advent of radioiodine therapy of Graves' disease, thyroidectomies became sufficiently uncommon to produce case-loads inadequate to maintain surgical expertise in most general surgical practices. Complication rates from this surgery are inversely proportional to the training, skill, and case-loads of the surgeon [102]. If possible, patients should be referred to regional centers with qualified endocrine surgeons.

The minimal acceptable surgery for a malignant or suspicious thyroid nodule is a total ipsilateral lobectomy and isthmusectomy. This provides sufficient tissue for pathologic diagnosis and removes any need for ipsilateral reoperation with its concomitant increased surgical risks [103, 104]. In most cases of differentiated follicular cell tumors (except for unifocal papillary microcarcinomas) confirmation of malignancy should result in completion of the total thyroidectomy. The surgical approach to thyroid tumors, other than papillary or follicular carcinomas, is different (as mentioned previously).

## Radiotherapy

### Radioiodine (I-131; Open Source)

Post-surgical radioiodine therapy of follicular and papillary carcinomas is essential in both pediatric [105] and adult patients [56, 57, 106]. Such treatment is of no value in any other types of thyroid cancer. Therapeutic efficacy is dependent upon adequate patient preparation (as for whole body scans) and sufficient administered I-131 activity. There is no role for "outpatient doses" of <30 mCi since they are insufficient to achieve the best therapeutic endpoints [97]. I advocate fixed doses of 100–150 mCi for local disease or thyroid remnant ablation (based on the preceding whole body scan results), and maximal dosimetry-directed doses of 200–600 mCi [107] for distant disease or recalcitrant tumors (for method see [97]). Treatments are repeated when subsequent follow-up whole body scans reveal persistent or metastatic disease. An important caveat is to always augment repeat therapy doses, either by increasing the activity of the dose, or by adding adjuvant lithium carbonate [108, 109] to enhance tumor retention of radioiodine. Despite unsubstantiated claims to the contrary, there is no intrinsic limit to the cumulative administered dose of I-131, provided that treatments are given for persistent or progressive cancer and proper clinical judgment is used. Unfortunately, many nuclear medicine physicians are remarkably timid in their dosing of I-131 and few are practiced in the method of radioiodine dosimetry, to determine safe maximal treatment doses, despite the safe use of this method for over three decades. For patients with recalcitrant or distantly metastatic tumors, appropriate referral to a center with expertise in high-dose radioiodine therapy is preferable to fruitless attempts with homeopathic treatments.

Some papillary and follicular cancers tend to dedifferentiate and lose the ability to concentrate iodine. This places a particular burden upon clinicians to provide speedy and efficacious radioiodine therapy while there is still a reasonable hope of response. Since there are no effective alternative systemic chemotherapies, failure to respond to radioiodine leaves suppression of TSH by levothyroxine as the only therapeutic option.

*External Radiotherapy (Sealed Source)*

External beam radiotherapy (XRT) is rarely indicated for primary post-surgical treatment of differentiated papillary and follicular cancers. This is because such treatment is able to deliver a maximum of 60 Gy to a local site; whereas I-131 can deliver doses exceeding 300 Gy, specifically to tumor deposits anywhere in the body [110]. Some studies have suggested a beneficial therapeutic response to adjuvant XRT, given as 55 Gy to the neck region following post-surgical I-131 ablation [111]; however this approach is certainly controversial. The most reasonable indication for XRT of differentiated thyroid cancer is in patients with localized disease and demonstrated inability to concentrate iodine. Alternatively, XRT is occasionally useful for palliation of unresectable, painful bone metastases.

Anaplastic thyroid carcinoma is uniformly lethal. Aggressive XRT to the neck and superior mediastinum may be of value by improving local disease control and delaying inevitable death from distant metastatic disease [112]. Two innovations in XRT are hyperfractionation and radiosensitization (usually with low-dose doxorubicin). Both were applied to a cohort of anaplastic cancer patients by Kim and Leeper [113], with claims of enhanced local disease control and enhanced length of survival; however, the study relied upon historical controls and patients had significant local morbidity. Although additional investigators have also reported benefits of hyperfractionated radiosensitized XRT [114], others report little benefit and potentially increased risks [115].

Chemotherapy, Combined Modality Therapy

Chemotherapy is ineffective in differentiated thyroid carcinomas and should not even be considered if the tumor retains sufficient ability to concentrate radioiodine, is surgically resectable, or is amenable to XRT. Patients with dedifferentiated distantly metastatic thyroid cancer, which is progressive, are sometimes given single-agent or combination chemotherapy in lieu of effective alternative treatments. With extremely rare exception, this is of no value. The exceptional patient with a partial response may have slightly delayed mortality [116]; however, this is exceedingly unusual [117]. There are no specific agents with any increased likelihood of eliciting a tumor response.

Anaplastic thyroid carcinoma is inevitably metastatic at multiple distant sites. Most patients ultimately receive some sort of chemotherapy and only rare patients show, at most, partial responses. Although a variety of agents have been used, they have generally included doxorubicin and cisplatin, with little beneficial effect [116, 118]. Recent laboratory investigations have suggested significant antineoplastic activity of paclitaxel in multiple human anaplastic thyroid carcinoma cell lines [119]. Preliminary data from a phase II clinical trail suggest a response rate far in excess of 50% (unpublished data), making this a preferred agent for chemotherapeutic efforts. Multimodality treatments, using surgery and XRT for local disease control, and chemotherapy for distant disease, are the best available plans for treatment of a lethal neoplasm.

As in other types of thyroid malignancies, medullary carcinomas are notably unresponsive to chemotherapy. Dacarbazine (DTIC) is the most frequently reported agent, and rare patients have partial responses [120]. On the other hand, thyroid lymphomas are remarkably responsive to multimodal therapy with chemotherapy and XRT. Matsuzuka et al [8] reported an 8-year survival of 100% with one course of CHOP, followed by 40–60 Gy of local XRT, and concluding with five additional courses of CHOP chemotherapy.

## Hormone Therapy

Lifelong suppression of endogenous TSH with levothyroxine is a mainstay of the treatment of papillary and follicular thyroid carcinomas. This requires daily administration of sufficient levothyroxine to maintain low TSH levels (<0.10 mU/l) without thyrotoxic symptoms (mean dose 2.0 μg/kg per day [121]). Suppressive therapy appears to be an important modality in a number of studies [122, 123] and is well tolerated by most patients. Some patients with resting tachycardia or palpitations are aided with long-acting -adrenergic blocking agents [124] and initial concerns of accelerating osteoporosis are probably unfounded in premenopausal patients [125]. Patients with other thyroid cancers should receive sufficient daily levothyroxine to maintain TSH within the normal range, since they are not TSH-responsive. There are no known roles for any other hormonal agents in any type of thyroid cancer, except for the response of thyroid lymphomas to glucocorticoids.

## Current Key Questions

The thyroid follicular cell has the capacity to become transformed into either the least aggressive human cancer (occult papillary microcarcinoma) or the most aggressive human cancer (anaplastic carcinoma). Although much progress has been made concerning the underlying biological etiologies for such distinctions, fundamental answers await discovery. Likewise, the unique insensitivity of thyroid cancers to chemotherapy agents presents a major roadblock to devising alternative systemic therapies. In addition, thyroid autoimmunity is extraordinarily common, suggesting the potential for immunotherapeutic approaches [126]. Such questions provide important investigative opportunities for thyroid oncologists.

## References

1. Landis SH, Murray T, Bolden S, Wingo PA (1998) Cancer statistics, 1998. Ca Cancer J Clin 48 (1):6–29
2. Feldman AR, Kessler L, Myers MH, Naughton MD (1986) The prevalence of cancer: estimates based on the Connecticut tumor registry. N Engl J Med 315 (22):1394–1397

3. Harach HR, Franssila KO, Wasenius V-M (1985) Occult papillary carcinoma of the thyroid. Cancer 56 (3):531–538
4. Parkin DM, Stiller CA, Draper GJ, Bieber CA, Terracini B, Young JL (eds) (1988) International Incidence of Childhood Cancer (Vol. No. 87). International Agency f or Research on Cancer, Lyon
5. LiVolsi VA (1990) Surgical Pathology of the Thyroid. In Major Problems in Pathology, Bennington JL ed W. B. Saunders Co., Philadelphia
6. Tielens ET, Sherman SI, Hruban RH, Ladenson PW (1994) Follicular variant of papillary thyroid carcinoma. Cancer 73 (2):424–431
7. Gilliland FD, Hunt WC, Morris DM, Key CR (1997) Prognostic factors for thyroid carcinoma: a population-based study of 15,698 cases from the Surveillance, E pidemiology and End Results (SEER) Program 1973–1991. Cancer 79 (3):564–573
8. Matsuzuka F, Miyauchi A, Katayama S, Narabayashi I, Ikeda H, Kuma K, Sugawara M (1993) Clinical aspects of primary thyroid lymphoma: diagnosis and treatment based on our experience of 119 cases. Thyroid 3 (2):93–99
9. Lote K, Andersen K, Nordal E, Brennhovd IO (1980) Familial occurrence of papillary thyroid carcinoma. Cancer 46 (5):1291–1297
10. Ozaki O, Ito K, Kobayashi K, Suzuki A, Manabe Y, Hosoda Y (1988) Familial occurrence of differentiated, nonmedullary thyroid carcinoma. World J Surg 12 (4):565–571
11. Sridama V, Hara Y, Fauchet R, DeGroot LJ (1985) Association of differentiated thyroid carcinoma with HLA-DR7. Cancer 56 (5):1086–1088
12. Pierotti MA, Santoro M, Jenkins RB, Sozzi G, Bongarzone I, Grieco M, Monzini N, Miozzo M, Herrmann MA, Fusco A, Hay ID, Della Porta G, Vecchio G (1992) Characterization of an inversion on the long arm of chromosome 10 juxtaposing D10S170 and RET and creating the oncogenic sequence RET/PTC. Proc Natl Acad Sci USA 89:1616–1620
13. Sozzi G, Bongarzone I, Miozzo M, Borrello MG, Butti MG, Pilotti S, Della Porta G, Pierotti MA (1994) A t (10, 17) translocation creates the RET/PTC2 chimeric transforming sequence in papillary thyroid carcinoma. Genes Chromo Cancer 9:244–250
14. Santoro M, Dathan NA, Berlingieri MT, Bongarzone I, Paulin C, Grieco M, Pierotti MA, Vecchio G, Fusco A (1994) Molecular characterization of RET/PTC3; a novel rearranged version of the RET proto-oncogene in a human thyroid papillary carcinoma. Oncogene 9 (2):509–516
15. Spitz MR, Sider JG, Katz RL, Pollack ES, Newell GR (1988) Ethnic patterns of thyroid cancer incidence in the United States, 1973–1981. Int J Cancer 42:549–553
16. Wohllk N, Cote GJ, Evans DB, Goepfert H, Ordonez NG, Gagel RF (1996) Application of genetic screening information to the management of medullary thyroid carcinoma and multiple endocrine neoplasia type 2. Endocrinol Metab Clin N Amer 25 (1):1–25
17. Bell B, Mazzaferri EL (1993) Familial adenomatous polyposis (Gardner's syndrome) and thyroid carcinoma: a case report and review of the literature. Digest Dis Sci 38 (1):185–190
18. Ain KB (1995) Papillary thyroid carcinoma: etiology, assessment, and therapy. Endocrin Metab Clin N Amer 24 (4):711–760
19. Thyresson HN, Doyle JA (1981) Cowden's disease (multiple hamartoma syndrome). Mayo Clin Proc 56 (3):179–184
20. Kato Z, Asano J, Kato T, Yamaguchi S, Kondo N, Oril T (1994) Thyroid cancer in a case with the Alagille syndrome. Clin Genet 45:21–24
21. Correa P, Chen VW (1995) Endocrine gland cancer. Cancer 75 (1, Suppl):338–352

22. Cunningham MP, Duda RB, Recant W, Chmiel JS, sylverter J, Fremgen A (1990) Survival discriminants for differentiated thyroid cancer. Am J Surg 160:344–347
23. Carcangiu ML, Zampi G, Pupi A, Castagnoli A, Rosai J (1985) Papillary carcinoma of the thyroid: a clinicopathologic study of 241 cases treated at the University of Florence, Italy. Cancer 55 (4):805–828
24. Shah JP, Loree TR, Dharker D, Strong EW, Begg C, Vlamis V (1992) Prognostic factors in differentiated carcinoma of the thyroid gland. Am J Surg 164:658–661
25. Zimmerman D, Hay ID, Gough IR, Goellner JR, Ryan JJ, Grant CS, McConahey WM (1988) Papillary thyroid carcinoma in children and adults: long-term follow-up of 1039 patients conservatively treated at one institution during three decades. Surgery 104 (6):1157–1166
26. Schneider AB (1990) Radiation-induced thyroid tumors. Endocrinol Metab Clin N Amer 19 (3):495–508
27. DeGroot LJ (1989) Diagnostic approach and management of patients exposed to irradiation to the thyroid. J Clin Endocrinol Metab 69 (5):925–928
28. Demidchik EP, Kazakov VS, Astakhova LN, Okeanov AE, Demidchik YE (1994) Thyroid cancer in children after the Chernobyl accident: clinical and epidemiological evaluation of 251 cases in the Republic of Belarus. In: Nagataki S (ed) Nagasaki Symposium on Chernobyl: Update and Future. Elsevier, Amsterdam, pp 21–30
29. Baverstock KF (1993) Thyroid cancer in children in Belarus after Chernobyl. World Health Stat Q 46 (3):204–208
30. Schneider AB, Ron E, Lubin J, Stovall M, Gierlowski TC (1993) Dose-response relationships for radiation-induced thyroid cancer and thyroid nodules: evidence for the prolonged effects of radiation on the thyroid. J Clin Endocrinol Metab 77 (2):362–369
31. National Cancer Institute (1997). Estimated exposures and thyroid doses received by the American people from iodine-131 in fallout following Nevada atmospheric nuclear bomb tests. National Cancer Institute
32. Franceschi S, Boyle P, Maisonneuve P, La Vecchia C, Burt AD, Kerr DJ, MacFarlane GJ (1993) The epidemiology of thyroid carcinoma. Crit Rev Oncogenesis 4 (1):25–52
33. Kung T-M, Ng W-L, Gibson JB (1981) Volcanoes and carcinoma of the thyroid: a possible association. Arch Environ Health 36 (5):265–267
34. Hallquist A, Hardell L, Degerman A, Boquist L (1993) Occupational exposures and thyroid cancer: results of a case-control study. Eur J Cancer Prev 2:345–349
35. Grimalt JO, Sunyer J, Moreno V, Amaral OC, Sala M, Rosell A, Anto JM, Albaiges J (1994) Risk excess of soft-tissue sarcoma and thyroid cancer in a community exposed to airborne organochlorinated compound mixtures with a high hexachlorobenzene content. Int J Cancer 56:200–203
36. Pesatori AC, Consonni D, Tironi A, Zocchetti C, Fini A, Bertazzi PA (1993) Cancer in a young population in a dioxin-contaminated area. Int J Epidemiol 22 (6):1010–1013
37. Franceschi S, Talamini R, Fassina A, Bidoli E (1990) Diet and epithelial cancer of the thyroid gland. Tumori 76:331–338
38. Fassina AS, Montesco MC, Ninfo V, Denti P, Masarotto G (1993) Histological evaluation of thyroid carcinomas: reproducibility of the ÇWHOÈ classification. Tumori 79:314–320
39. Hedinger CE, Williams ED, Sobin LH (1988) Histological Typing of Thyroid Tumours. In Internationl Histological Classification of Tumours, no. 11; World Health Organization, Springer-Verlag, Berlin

40. Harach HR, Zusman SB (1992) Cytologic findings in the follicular variant of papillary carcinoma of the thyroid. Acta Cytol 36 (2):142–146

41. Johnson TL, Lloyd RV, Thompson NW, Beierwaltes WH, Sisson JC (1988) Prognostic implications of the tall cell variant of papillary thyroid carcinoma. Am J Surg Pathol 12 (1):22–27

42. Ostrowski ML, Merino MJ (1996) Tall cell variant of papillary thyroid carcinoma: a reassessment and immunohistochemical study with comparison to the usual type of papillary carcinoma of the thyroid. Am J Surg Path 20 (8):964–974

43. Rüter A, Nishiyama R, Lennquist S (1997) Tall-cell variant of papillary thyroid cancer: disregarded entity? World J Surg 21 (1):15–21

44. Evans HL (1986) Columnar-cell carcinoma of the thyroid: a report of two cases of an aggressive variant of thyroid carcinoma. Am J Clin Pathol 85 (1):77–80

45. Sobrinho-Sim›es M, Nesland JM, Johannessen JV (1988) Columnar-cell carcinoma. Another variant of poorly differentiated carcinoma of the thyroid. Am J Clin Pathol 89 (2):264–267

46. Wenig BM, Thompson LDR, Adair CF, Shmookler B, Heffess CS (1998) Thyroid papillary carcinoma of columnar cell type. Cancer 82 (4):740–763

47. Soares J, Limbert E, Sobrinho-Sim›es (1989) Diffuse sclerosing variant of papillary thyroid carcinoma: a clinicopathologic study of 10 cases. Path Res Pract 185:200–206

48. Carcangiu ML, Bianchi S (1989) Diffuse sclerosing variant of papillary thyroid carcinoma: clinicopathologic study of 15 cases. Am J Surg Pathol 13 (12):1041–1049

49. Rosai J (1993) Papillary Carcinoma. Monographs in Pathology 1993 (35):138–165

50. Sobrinho-Sim›es MA, Soares J, Carneiro F, Limbert E (1990) Diffuse follicular variant of papillary carcinoma of the thyroid: report of eight cases of a distinct aggressive type of thyroid tumor. Surg Pathol 3 (3):189–203

51. Herrera MF, Hay ID, Wu PS-C, Goellner JR, Ryan JJ, Ebersold JR, Bergstralh EJ, Grant CS (1992) Hürthle cell (oxyphilic) papillary thyroid carcinoma: a variant with more aggressive biologic behavior. World J Surg 16 (4):669–675

52. Sobrinho-Sim›es MA, Nesland JM, Holm R, Sambade MC, Johannessen JV (1985) Hürthle cell and mitochondrion-rich papillary carcinomas of the thyroid gland: an ultrastructural and immunocytochemical study. Ultrastruct Pathol 8:131–142

53. Franssila KO, Ackerman LV, Brown CL, Hedinger CE (1985) Session II: follicular carcinoma. Sem Diag Pathol 2 (2):101–122

54. Schürmann G, Mattfeldt T, Feichter G, Koretz K, M_ller P, Buhr H (1991) Stereology, flow cytometry, and immunohistochemistry of follicular neoplasms of the thyroid gland. Hum Pathol 22 (2):179–184

55. Grebe SKG, Hay ID (1995) Follicular thyroid cancer. Endocrinol Metab Clin N Amer 24 (4):761–801

56. Robbins J, Merino MJ, Boice Jr JD, Ron E, Ain KB, Alexander HR, Norton JA, Reynolds J (1991) Thyroid cancer: a lethal neoplasm. Ann Int Med 115 (2):133–147

57. Mazzaferri EL, Jhiang SM (1994) Long-term impact of initial surgical and medical therapy on papillary and follicular thyroid cancer. Am J Med 97:418–428

58. Rosai J, Sax_n EA, Woolner L (1985) Session III: Undifferentiated and poorly differentiated carcinoma. Sem Diag Pathol 2 (2):123–136

59. Justin EP, Seabold JE, Robinson RA, Walker WP, Gurll NJ, Hawes DR (1991) Insular carcinoma: a distinct thyroid carcinoma with associated iodine-131 localization. J Nucl Med 32 (7):1358–1363

60. Carcangiu ML, Zampi G, Rosai J (1984) Poorly differentiated ("insular") thyroid carcinoma: a reinterpretation of Langhans' "wuchernde Struma". Am J Surg Pathol 8 (9):655–668

61. Hassoun AAK, Hay ID, Goellner JR, Zimmerman D (1997) Insular thyroid carcinoma in adolescents: a potentially lethal endocrine malignancy. Cancer 79 (5): 1044–1048

62. Carcangiu ML, Steeper T, Zampi G, Rosai J (1985) Anaplastic thyroid carcinoma: A study of 70 cases. Am J Clin Pathol 83 (2):135–158

63. Nusynowitz ML (1991) Differentiating anaplastic thyroid carcinomas. J Nucl Med 32 (7):1363–1364

64. Aldinger KA, Samaan NA, Ibanez M, Hill Jr CS (1978) Anaplastic carcinoma of the thyroid: a review of 84 cases of spindle and giant cell carcinoma of the thyroid. Cancer 41 (6):2267–2275

65. Nishiyama RH, Dunn EL, Thompson NW (1972) Anaplastic spindle-cell and giant-cell tumors of the thyroid gland. Cancer 30 (1):113–127

66. Schr_der S, Holl K, Padberg BC (1992) Pathology of sporadic and hereditary medullary thyroid carcinoma. Rec Res Cancer Res 125:19–45

67. Cote GJ, Wohllk N, Evans D, Goepfert H, Gagel RF (1995) RET proto-oncogene mutations in multiple endocrine neoplasia type 2 and medullary thyroid carcinoma. Baillieres Clin Endocrinol Metab 9 (3):609–630

68. Abdul-Rahman ZH, Gogas HJ, Tooze JA, Anderson B, Mansi J, Sacks NP, Finlayson CJ (1996) T-cell lymphoma in Hashimoto's thyroiditis. Histopathol 29:455–459

69. Anscombe AM, Wright DH (1985) Primary malignant lymphoma of the thyroid – a tumour of mucosa-associated lymphoid tissue: review of seventy-six cases. Histopathol 9:81–97

70. Harach HR, Vujanic GM, Jasani B (1993) Ultimobranchial body nests in human fetal thyroid: an autopsy, histological, and immunohistochemical study in relation to solid cell nests and mucoepidermoid carcinoma of the thyroid. J Pathol 169: 465–469

71. Chan JKC, Rosai J (1991) Tumors of the neck showing thymic or related branchial pouch differentiation: a unifying concept. Hum Pathol 22 (4):349–367

72. Hedinger C (1981) Geographic pathology of thyroid diseases. Path Res Pract 171:285–292

73. Mills SE, Gaffey MJ, Watts JC, Swanson PE, Wick MR, LiVolsi VA, Nappi O, Weiss LM (1994) Angiomatoid carcinoma and 'angiosarcoma' of the thyroid gland: a spectrum of endothelial differentiation. Am J Clin Pathol 102 (3):322–330

74. Carcangiu ML, Zampi G, Rosai J (1985) Papillary thyroid carcinoma: a study of its many morphologic expressions and clinical correlates. Pathol Ann 20:1–44

75. DeGroot LJ, Kaplan EL, Shukla MS, Salti G, Straus FH (1995) Morbidity and mortality in follicular thyroid cancer. J Clin Endocrinol Metab 80 (10):2946–2953

76. Coburn MC, Wanebo HJ (1992) Prognostic factors and management considerations in patients with cervical metastases of thyroid cancer. Am J Surg 164:671–676

77. Ozaki O, Ito K, Sugino K (1993) Clinico-pathologic study of pulmonary metastasis of differentiated thyroid carcinoma: age-, sex-, and histology-matched case-control study. Int Surg 78:218–220

78. McCaffrey TV, Bergstralh EJ, Hay ID (1994) Locally invasive papillary thyroid carcinoma: 1940–1990. Head Neck 16 (2):165–172

79. Loh K-C, Greenspan FS, Gee L, Miller TR, Yeo PPB (1997) Pathological tumor-node-metastasis (pTNM) staging for papillary and follicular thyroid carcinomas: a retrospective analysis of 700 patients. J Clin Endocrinol Metab 82 (11):3553–3562

80. DeGroot LJ, Kaplan EL, Straus FH, Shukla MS (1994) Does the method of management of papillary thyroid carcinoma make a difference in outcome? World J Surg 18 (1):123–130

81. Beahrs OH, Henson DE, Hutter RVP, Kennedy BJ (eds) (1992) Manual for Staging of Cancer; American Joint Committee on Cancer (4th ed). J. B. Lippincott Co, Philadelphia

82. Hermanek P, Sobin LH (eds) (1987) TNM classification of malignant tumours (4th ed). Springer-Verlag, Berlin

83. Brierley JD, Panzarella T, Tsang RW, Gospodarowicz MK, O'Sullivan B (1997) A comparison of different staging systems predictability of patient outcome. Thyroid carcinoma as an example. Cancer 79 (12):2414–2423

84. Hermanek P, Henson DE, Hutter RVP, Sobin LH (eds) (1993) TNM supplement 1993: a commentary on uniform use; International Union Against Cancer. Springer-Verlag, Berlin

85. Scheumann GF, Gimm O, Wegener G, Hundeshagen H, Dralle H (1994) Prognostic significance and surgical management of locoregional lymph node metastases in papillary thyroid cancer. World J Surg 18 (4):559–567

86. Singer PA, Cooper DS, Daniels GH, Ladenson PW, Greenspan FS, Levy EG, Braverman LE, Clark OH, McDougall IR, Ain KB, Dorfman SG (1996) Treatment guidelines for patients with thyroid nodules and well-differentiated thyroid cancer. Arch Intern Med 156:2165–2172

87. Yamashita H, Noguchi S, Murakami N, Mochizuki Y, Nakayama I (1986) Prognosis of minute carcinoma of thyroid: follow-up study of 49 patients. Acta Pathol Jpn 36 (10):1469–1475

88. Pacini F, Fugazzola L, Lippi F, Ceccarelli C, Centoni R, Miccoli P, Elisei R, Pinchera A (1992) Detection of thyroglobulin in fine needle aspirates of nonthyroidal neck masses: a clue to the diagnosis of metastatic differentiated thyroid cancer. J Clin Endocrinol Metab 74 (6):1401–1404

89. Ashcraft MW, Van Herle AJ (1981) Management of thyroid nodules. II: Scanning techniques, thyroid suppressive therapy, and fine needle aspiration. Head Neck Surg 3:297–322

90. Dralle H, Damm I, Scheumann GF, Kotzerke J, Kupsch E, Geerlings H, Pichlmayr R (1994) Compartment-oriented microdissection of regional lymph nodes in medullary thyroid carcinoma. Surg Today 24 (2):112–121

91. Venkataraman GM, Yatin M, Ain KB (1997) Cloning of the human sodium-iodide symporter promoter and characterization in a differentiated human thyroid cell line, KAT-50. Thyroid in press

92. Meier CA, Braverman LE, Ebner SA, Veronikis I, Daniels GH, Ross DS, Deraska DJ, Davies TF, Valentine M, DeGroot LJ, Curran P, McEllin K, Reynolds J, Robbins J, Weintraub BD (1994) Diagnostic use of recombinant human thyrotropin in patients with thyroid carcinoma (phase I/II study). J Clin Endocrinol Metab 78 (1):188–196

93. Lakshmanan M, Schaffer A, Robbins J, Reynolds J, Norton J (1988) A simplified low iodine diet in I-131 scanning and therapy of thyroid cancer. Clin Nucl Med 13 (12):866–868

94. Ain KB, DeWitt PA, Gardner TG, Berryman SW (1994) Low-iodine tube-feeding diet for iodine-131 scanning and therapy. Clin Nucl Med 19 (6):504–507

95. Goldman JM, Line BR, Aamodt RL, Robbins J (1980) Influence of triiodothyronine withdrawal time on 131I uptake postthyroidectomy for thyroid cancer. J Clin Endocrinol Metab 50 (4):734–739

96. Park H-M, Perkins OW, Edmondson JW, Schnute RB, Manatunga A (1994) Influence of diagnostic radioiodines on the uptake of ablative dose of iodine-131. Thyroid 4 (1):49–54

97. Ain KB (1997) Management of thyroid cancer. In: Braverman LE (ed) Diseases of the thyroid. Humana Press, Inc., Totowa, N.J., pp 287–317

98. Hoefnagel CA, Delprat CC, Marcuse HR, de Vijlder JJM (1986) Role of thallium-201 total-body scintigraphy in follow-up of thyroid carcinoma. J Nucl Med 27 (12):1854–1857

99. Yen T-C, Lin H-D, Lee C-H, Chang SL, Yeh SH (1994) The role of technetium-99 m sestamibi whole-body scans in diagnosing metastatic Hürthle cell carcinoma of the thyroid gland after total thyroidectomy: A comparison with iodine-131 and thallium-201 whole-body scans. Eur J Nucl Med 21 (9):980–983

100. Scott GC, Meier DA, Dickinson CZ (1995) Cervical lymph node metastasis of thyroid papillary carcinoma imaged with fluorine-18-FDG, technetium-99m-pertechnetate and iodine-131-sodium iodide. J Nucl Med 36 (10):1843–1845

101. Pineda JD, Lee T, Ain KB, Reynolds JC, Robbins J (1995) Iodine-131 therapy for thyroid cancer patients with elevated thyroglobulin and negative diagnostic scan. J Clin Endocrinol Metab 80 (5):1488–1492

102. Demeure MJ, Clark OH (1990) Surgery in the treatment of thyroid cancer. Endocrinol Metab Clin N Amer 19 (3):663–683

103. Soh EY, Clark OH (1996) Surgical considerations and approach to thyroid cancer. Endocrinol Metab Clin N Amer 25 (1):115–139

104. Pasieka JL, Rotstein LE (1993) Consensus conference on well-differentiated thyroid cancer: a summary. Can J Surg 36 (4):298–301

105. Samuel AM, Sharma SM (1991) Differentiated thyroid carcinomas in children and adolescents. Cancer 67 (8):2186–2190

106. Wong JB, Kaplan MM, Meyer KB, Pauker SG (1990) Ablative radioactive iodine therapy for apparently localized thyroid carcinoma: a decision analytic perspective. Endocrinol Metab Clin N Amer 19 (3):741–760

107. Benua RS, Leeper RD (1986) A method and rationale for treating metastatic thyroid carcinoma with the largest safe dose of 131I. In: Medeiros-Neto G, Gaitan E (eds) Frontiers in Thyroidology (Vol. 2). Plenum Medical Book Co, New York, pp 1317–1321

108. Gershengorn MC, Izumi M, Robbins J (1976) Use of lithium as an adjunct to radioiodine therapy of thyroid carcinoma. J Clin Endocrinol Metab 42 (1): 105–111

109. Pons F, Carri I, Estorch M, Ginjaume M, Pons J, Milian R (1987) Lithium as an adjuvant of iodine-131 uptake when treating patients with well-differentiated thyroid carcinoma. Clin Nucl Med 25 (8):644–647

110. Maxon HR, Thomas SR, Hertzberg VS, Kereiakes JG, Chen I-W, Sperling MI, Saenger EL (1983) Relation between effective radiation dose and outcome of radioiodine therapy for thyroid cancer. New Eng J Med 309:937–941

111. Phlips P, Hanzen C, Andry G, Van Houtte P, Früuling J (1993) Postoperative irradiation for thyroid cancer. Eur J Surg Oncol 19:399–404

112. Levendag PC, De Porre PMZR, van Putten WLJ (1993) Anaplastic carcinoma of the thyroid gland treated by radiation therapy. Int J Radiation Oncology Biol Phys 26 (1):125–128

113. Kim JH, Leeper RD (1987) Treatment of locally advanced thyroid carcinoma with combination doxorubicin and radiation therapy. Cancer 60:2372–2375

114. Tennvall J, Lundell G, Hallquist A, Wahlberg P, Wallin G, Tibblin S (1994) Combined doxorubicin, hyperfractionated radiotherapy, and surgery in anaplastic thyroid carcinoma. Cancer 74 (4):1348–1354

115. Wong CS, Van Dyk J, Simpson WJ (1991) Myelopathy following hyperfractionated accelerated radiotherapy for anaplastic thyroid carcinoma. Radiother Oncol 20:3–9

116. Ahuja S, Ernst H (1987) Chemotherapy of thyroid carcinoma. J Endocrinol Invest 10:303–310

117. Droz J-P, Schlumberger M, Rougier P, Ghosn M, Gardet P, Parmentier C (1990) Chemotherapy in metastatic nonanaplastic thyroid cancer: experience at the Institut Gustave-Roussy. Tumori 76:480–483

118. Asakawa H, Kobayashi T, Komoike Y, Maruyama H, Nakano Y, Tamaki Y, Matsuzawa Y, Monden M (1997) Chemosensitivity of anaplastic thyroid carcinoma and poorly differentiated thyroid carcinoma. Anticancer Res 17:2757–2762
119. Ain KB, Tofiq S, Taylor KD (1996) Antineoplastic activity of taxol against human anaplastic thyroid carcinoma cell lines in vitro and in vivo. J Clin Endocrinol Metab 81 (10):3650–3653
120. Orlandi F, Caraci P, Berruti A, Puligheddu B, Pivano G, Dogliotti L, Angeli A (1994) Chemotherapy with dacarbazine and 5-fluorouracil in advanced medullary thyroid cancer. Ann Oncol 5 (8):763–765
121. Ain KB, Pucino F, Shiver TM, Banks SM (1993) Thyroid hormone levels affected by time of blood sampling in thyroxine-treated patients. Thyroid 3:81–85
122. Mazzaferri EL, Young RL (1981) Papillary thyroid carcinoma: a 10 year follow-up report of the impact of therapy in 576 patients. Am J Med 70 (3):511–518
123. Simpson WJ, Panzarella T, Carruthers JS, Gospodarowicz MK, Sutcliffe SB (1988) Papillary and follicular thyroid cancer: impact of treatment in 1578 patients. Int J Rad Onc Biol Phys 14 (6):1063–1075
124. Fazio S, Biondi B, Carella C, Sabatini D, Cittadini A, Panza N, Lombardi G, Saccˆ L (1995) Diastolic dysfunction in patients on thyroid-stimulating hormone suppressive therapy with levothyroxine: beneficial effect of -blockade. J Clin Endocrinol Metab 80 (7):2222–2226
125. Marcocci C, Golia F, Bruno-Bossio G, Vignali E, Pinchera A (1994) Carefully monitored levothyroxine suppressive therapy is not associated with bone loss in premenopausal women. J Clin Endocrinol Metab 78 (4):818–823
126. Baker JR, Fosso CK (1993) Immunological aspects of cancers arising from thyroid follicular cells. Endocrine Rev 14 (6):729–746

# Skin Cancers

# Cutaneous Melanoma

T.F. Gajewski

Melanoma is a cancer of the pigmented cell of the skin, the melanocyte. The incidence of cutaneous melanoma is rising steadily worldwide, and the median survival of patients with metastatic disease remains less than 1 year. Nonetheless, significant advances have been made in the past several years in the diagnosis and treatment of this disease. The use of smaller surgical margins for patients with thin primary lesions, the advent of lymph node mapping and sentinel lymph node biopsy, the possibility to detect minimal residual disease using RT-PCR, the use of adjuvant interferon-$\alpha$2b (IFN-$\alpha$2b) for resected lymph node-positive patients, and the potential efficacy of new biologic therapies in patients with metastatic disease, are all approaches currently in clinical practice that are refining the therapy for melanoma.

## Epidemiology, Risk Factors

### Incidence

Skin cancer is the most common type of cancer in the United States, accounting for approximately one-third of all new cancer cases. Cutaneous melanoma constitutes only 5%–10% of skin cancer cases, but accounts for 75% of skin cancer deaths. The incidence of cutaneous melanoma has been rapidly rising since the 1930s, the rate of increase being over 1000%. In addition, the death rate from melanoma has more than doubled, indicating that early detection does not account completely for the increase in new cases observed. It is estimated that in the year 2000 the lifetime risk of an American developing melanoma will be 1/75 (Fig. 1). The reason for this increase is not clear, but it correlates with a cultural affinity for sunbathing, the popularity of a beach lifestyle, and

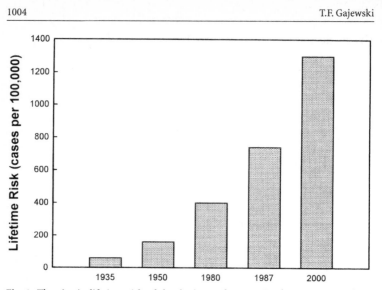

**Fig. 1.** The rise in lifetime risk of developing melanoma. By the year 2000, 1 in 75 Americans will develop melanoma at some time during their life, making it the fastest rising incidence of any cancer

the apparently eroding ozone layer, all of which increase exposure to ultraviolet light.

Race, Gender, Age Distribution

The peak incidence of melanoma is between ages 30 and 60, although there is a steady increase in incidence with increasing age. Individuals older than 15 years have a 90-fold greater risk for melanoma than do individuals younger than 15 years. Males and females can be equally affected, but the most common location of lesions differs. Melanomas most commonly occur on the back in men, but on the lower extremities in women. In addition, males are more likely to die from melanoma than are females. The risk of melanoma is 12 times greater in Caucasian than in African-American individuals, and 7 times greater than in the Hispanic population. Melanoma lesions in non-Caucasian individuals more frequently involve the nail beds, the palms and soles, or mucosal sites than they do the skin.

## Geography

In general, the incidence of melanoma in the United States increases from north to south. The highest incidence worldwide is in Queensland, Australia, where greater than 30 per 100,000 individuals have the disease. In contrast, the incidence is less than 0.8 per 100,000 in China. However, there is not a strict correlation between cumulative sun exposure and the development of melanoma. In Europe, the least number of cases is seen in central Europe, with the incidence increasing as one moves north or south.

## Risk Factors and Etiology

The risks for developing melanoma include genetic, environmental, socioeconomic, and occupational factors, as well as age and co-existing medical conditions (Table 1). Familial clusters of melanoma have been studied, and as many as 10% of melanoma patients have had a first degree relative with the disease. Mutations in the gene encoding the cyclin-dependent kinase inhibitor p16 located on chromosome 9 have been observed in several kindreds [1]. Interestingly, many patients without a documented family history of melanoma but with multiple independent primary melanoma lesions also have mutations in the p16 gene [2]. Individuals with the dysplastic nevus syndrome, who have as many as

**Table 1.** Risk factors for developing melanoma

| Risk factor | Relative risk |
| --- | --- |
| Age above 15 | 90 |
| Familial melanoma | 148 |
| Caucasian Race | 12 |
| Melanoma in first-degree relative | 8 |
| Freckling tendency | 4 |
| Red or blond hair | 2 |
| Blue eyes | 2 |
| Excessive sun exposure | 3 |
| History of blistering sunburns | 3–12 |
| Dysplastic nevi | 15 |
| History of melanoma | 9 |
| History of nonmelanomatous skin cancer | 4 |
| Congenital nevus | 21 |
| Immunosuppression | 4 |

100 pigmented cutaneous lesions, have a relative risk of greater than 100 [3]. Caucasian individuals have a 12-fold increased probability of developing melanoma, and several additional phenotypic characteristics contribute to this risk. These include fair skin, red or blond hair, blue eyes, freckling, pre-existing moles, and a tendency to sunburn.

It is generally felt that exposure to ultraviolet light plays an important causal role in the development of melanoma. It is clear that UV irradiation induces DNA damage which would increase the somatic mutation rate, and that cutaneous immunosuppression develops during UV exposure [4]. However, case-control studies of sunscreen use have not demonstrated a decreased melanoma incidence in individuals who routinely use sunscreen [5-7], and several studies of tanning salon users have failed to demonstrate an increased chance of developing a melanoma lesion [8]. This is despite the fact that non-melanomatous skin cancers are clearly affected by both of these behaviors. In addition, melanoma more commonly affects urban, white collar workers with intermittent sun exposure than blue collar employees who work outdoors. Nonetheless, a history of blistering sunburns, especially during childhood or adolescence, has been a consistently observed epidemiologic factor. It seems likely that intermittent, extreme sun exposure through sun "binging" may be more dangerous than controlled, frequent sun exposure, although a tendency toward sunburning may be only a phenotypic marker for individuals who have an associated melanoma risk. The likelihood that childhood sunburning may be a major melanoma risk factor has prompted education and primary prevention programs targeting not only adult [9] but children populations as well [6].

The presence of certain cutaneous lesions can be predictive for developing melanoma [3]. A prior history of melanoma or of non-melanomatous skin cancer, the presence of greater than 5 nevi over 5 mm in diameter, having a large congenital nevus, or having a dysplastic nevus or a changing mole, each increases the likelihood of developing melanoma.

Immunosuppression, either secondary to administration of immunosuppressive drugs or as a result of the acquired immunodeficiency syndrome, increases 4-fold the risk of developing melanoma. Inasmuch as other cancers in such patients have a viral etiology, it is conceivable that a virus may contribute to the pathogenesis of melanoma as well. However, there is no evidence to date linking a virus to this disease. The fact that immunosuppression results in increased melanoma risk has supported the notion that immune-based interventions may have utility in the treatment of this disease.

## Pathology and Staging

Macroscopic Growth Patterns

Cutaneous melanoma has generally been categorized into several growth patterns, although when depth of the lesion is controlled for, these histologic subtypes have similar prognoses [10]. The most common type is superficial spreading melanoma, accounting for 70% of cases. In this lesion, the malignant cells extend radially as they proliferate, generating an irregularly colored, slightly raised plaque with an irregular border on clinical presentation. The horizontal growth behavior often gives an opportunity for clinical detection at an earlier (thinner) stage. Superficial spreading melanoma often arises from a pre-existing nevus, and evolves over months to years.

Nodular melanoma is the next most common variety and accounts for 15% of cases. The malignant cells grow in a vertical plane, presenting as a rapidly growing nodular mass. Nodular melanomas may be ulcerated or pedunculated on presentation, and can be amelanotic. Because of the vertical growth characteristics, these lesions more often are detected at a later (deeper) stage. They usually do not arise from a pre-existing nevus, and clinically can be blue/black, gray, red, or purple, often resembling a blood blister.

Lentigo maligna melanomas account for 5% of melanoma cases and arise within lentigo maligna lesions, which are large (greater than 3 cm), flat "shoe polish" freckles occurring on sun-exposed areas of elderly individuals. These lesions are heterogeneous in shape, color, and texture, usually containing areas of regression as well as papular regions.

Acral lentiginous melanoma is the most common presentation of melanoma in non-Caucasian individuals. It characteristically occurs beneath the nail beds or on the palms or soles. These lesions account for only 8% of melanoma cases in Caucasians, but up to 60% of cases in dark-skinned patients. It usually begins as a pigmented macule that grows radially over years and then becomes raised and palpable. Subungual lesions often begin as a discoloration under the nail bed, usually involving the great toe or thumb.

Melanoma also may present within mucosal surfaces, such as the sinuses, or involving the genitals of either males or females. Such presentations are approached differently than the typical cutaneous melanoma, depending on the location, and surgical resection constitutes first line treatment. Some patients present with metastatic disease without an apparent cutaneous lesion. In these cases, the primary lesion is thought to have regressed spontaneously, perhaps via an immune-mediated mechanism. Metastatic melanoma with an unknown primary can present in virtually any organ, including the gastrointestinal tract, kidney, lung, liver, bone, brain, and subcutaneous sites. Therefore, melanoma should be considered in the differential diagnosis of any unusual metastatic carcinoma.

## Pathologic Markers

Establishing a histologic diagnosis of melanoma is usually straightforward when the primary cutaneous lesion is appropriately excised. However, immunohistochemical markers are useful when the diagnosis is unclear, such as with lesions lacking pigment or with cases that present as metastatic disease without an obvious primary lesion. The two commonly used markers are S-100 and HMB-45. S-100 is expressed by virtually all melanomas but is not specific, as it also can be present in sarcomas, nerve sheath tumors, and some carcinomas. HMB-45 is 100% specific for melanoma but is only expressed by about 80% of lesions. A metastatic carcinoma of unknown primary should be negative for cytokeratin, leukocyte common antigen, and adenocarcinoma markers such as CEA, as well as positive for S-100 and/or HMB-45, to be designated a melanoma.

The genes encoding several melanoma tumor antigens and melanocyte differentiation antigens have been cloned, which offers the possibility of performing RT-PCR to establish a melanocyte/melanoma lineage by molecular analysis. These include MAGE-1, MAGE-3, Melan-A/MART-1, gp100, and tyrosinase [11, 12]. Assessing expression of these genes is being investigated to clarify pathologic diagnosis, to detect minimal residual disease in lymph node specimens and peripheral blood, and to screen patients for participation in melanoma vaccine trials [13–15].

## Primary Lesion Thickness

The single most important prognostic indicator for early melanoma lesions is tumor thickness. Therefore, although biopsies of suspicious lesions may be incisional or excisional, they must be full-thickness. A shaving technique for tissue sampling is not used and must be avoided. The thickness of the primary lesion determines all the subsequent diagnostic and therapeutic procedures to be performed, and therefore it must be accurate and should be analyzed by a pathologist experienced in reading melanoma specimens.

The first staging system of cutaneous melanoma lesions was developed by Clark, and is based upon the extent of invasion into the architectural levels of the skin [16]. A level I lesion is confined to the epidermis (and is therefore a melanoma in situ), a level II lesion penetrates the papillary dermis, level III is up to the reticular dermis, level IV invades the reticular dermis, and level V penetrates into the subcutaneous fat. However, although depth of invasion is inversely proportional to patient survival, there are not stepwise jumps in survival rates that correlate with the dermal layer being violated. Rather, absolute depth of penetration (in millimeters) is the most accurate predictor of metastatic risk, and a microstaging system was developed by Breslow based on measured tumor thickness [17]. Both the Clark level and the absolute Breslow depth of the primary lesion should be reported by the pathologist, as a lesion with a Breslow depth of <1.0 mm has a worse prognosis if it has penetrated Clark's level IV [18].

## Staging

Although the thickness of the primary tumor carries important prognostic information, the presence of regional lymph node involvement or of distant metastases has obvious clinical significance. Thus, as with other cancer types, the AJCC has developed a four-stage TNM system for categorizing patients with melanoma. The indicated staging categorization is current as of 1998. However, there are several important prognostic factors not considered in the current classification scheme, the neglect of which has prompted a movement for updating the staging system for melanoma [19]. Thus, this information will likely evolve in the near future. Nevertheless, according to present guidelines (Table 2), stage I

**Table 2.** AJCC staging system for melanoma

| | |
|---|---|
| Primary tumor | |
| pTx | Primary tumor cannot be assessed |
| pT0 | No evidence of primary tumor |
| pTis | Melanoma in situ (Clark's level I) |
| pT1 | Tumor <0.75 mm in thickness and invading the papillary dermis (Clark's level II) |
| pT2 | Tumor more than 0.75 mm but less than 1.5 mm in thickness and/or invades to the papillary-reticular dermal interface (Clark's level III) |
| pT3 | Tumor more than 1.5 mm but less than 4 mm in depth and/or invades the reticular dermis (Clark's level IV) |
| pT3a | 1.5–3 mm thickness |
| pT3b | 3–4 mm thickness |
| pT4 | Tumor >4 mm in thickness and/or invades subcutaneous tissue (Clark's level V) and/or satellites within 2 cm of primary tumor |
| pT4a | >4 mm in thickness or Clark's level V |
| pT4b | Satellites within 2 cm |
| Regional lymph nodes | |
| Nx | Regional lymph nodes cannot be assessed |
| N0 | No regional lymph node metastasis |
| N1 | Metastasis 3 cm or less in any regional lymph nodes |
| N2 | Metastasis more than 3 cm in greatest dimension in any regional lymph node and/or in-transit metastasis |
| N2a | Metastasis more than 3 cm in any regional lymph node |
| N2b | In-transit metastasis |
| N2c | Both N2a and N2b |
| Distant metastasis | |
| Mx | Presence of distant metastasis cannot be assessed |
| M0 | No distant metastasis |
| M1 | Distant metastasis |
| M1a | Metastasis in skin, subcutaneous tissue, or lymph nodes beyond the regional lymph nodes |
| M1b | Visceral metastasis |
| Stage grouping | |
| Stage 0 | pTis N0 M0 |
| Stage Ia | pT1 N0 M0 |
| Stage Ib | pT2 N0 M0 |
| Stage IIa | pT3 N0 M0 |
| Stage IIb | pT4 N0 M0 |
| Stage IIIa | Any pT N1 M0 |
| Stage IIIb | Any pT N2 M0 |
| Stage IV | Any pT any N M1 |

patients have primary melanoma lesions less than 1.5 mm thick, while stage II patients have melanomas deeper than 1.5 mm, in each case if there has been no metastasis to lymph nodes. Stage III patients have regional lymph node involvement or local in-transit metastases, and stage IV patients have metastatic disease. The five-year survival rate is greater than 90% for patients with stage I disease, 75% for stage II, 35% for stage III, and less than 10% for stage IV.

The advent of sentinel lymph node mapping (discussed below) has allowed for the microscopic detection of minimal disease that frequently involves only the single initial lymph node draining a cutaneous lesion. Although this level of disease burden is obviously less than that of a patient with grossly palpable lymph nodes, they are both categorized as stage III. In-transit metastases are thought to arise from tumor cells trapped in draining lymphatics, and thus are categorized along with lymph node-positive patients as stage III as well. However, the treatment of in-transit metastases often poses special challenges, as lymph nodes are often easier to remove surgically despite their representing disease that is clinically more advanced.

Prognostic Factors

With respect to the primary cutaneous melanoma lesion, tumor thickness is the single most important prognostic factor, and appears to be more accurate at predicting survival and the probability of metastasis than does the Clark level [18]. Ulceration, either macroscopic or microscopic, is the next most important negative prognostic indicator [20]. In one study, patients with stage I or stage II disease without ulceration exhibited a median survival of 79% at 10 years, compared to 50% survival of patients with ulcerated lesions [21]. DNA ploidy and S-phase content also may correlate inversely with survival [22].

Although the size of the involved metastatic lymph nodes may not influence outcome, the number of involved nodes certainly does [23]. In one study, the median 3-year survival for patients with a single involved lymph node was 40%, compared to 26% survival of patients with 2–4 involved nodes and 15% survival of patients with 5 or greater involved nodes [20]. Microstaging of lymph node involvement using immunohistochemical staining and/or RT-PCR for melanoma antigen gene expression may provide for a greater accuracy in assessing node status [13, 24].

The anatomic location of metastatic deposits carries prognostic information. Patients with metastases to skin, subcutaneous regions, or non-regional lymph nodes appear to have a greater survival rate than do patients with visceral metastases. A recent report has indicated that patients with a single visceral metastasis have comparable survival to patients with soft tissue metastases, but that multiple metastases portend a worse prognosis [25]. As such, disease recurrence manifested as a single metastasis is usually treated by surgical resection [26]. In addition, normal serum levels of LDH and albumin predict a better outcome [25].

## Initial Work-up and Staging

### Patient Evaluation

The patient with melanoma often presents first to a primary care physician or dermatologist. As usual, a careful history and physical examination should be performed. Attention should be paid to the degree of sun exposure, occupation, family history of skin cancer, and possible immunosuppression, as well as the appearance of the primary lesion and other pigmented cutaneous lesions, evidence for lymphadenopathy (particularly in the likely draining lymph node basins,) and any systemic signs or symptoms that may indicate metastatic disease. A full-body skin examination should be performed, and any suspicious additional lesions also should be brought to the attention of a dermatologist. It is appropriate to recommend sun avoidance and sunscreen use to the patient and his or her family, especially children, during the initial clinic visits. A strong family history warrants referral to a cancer risk clinic.

The most critical component of staging is an optimal biopsy of the suspicious lesion. The diagnosis is established by a full-thickness biopsy, and excisional biopsy is the preferred method. Accurate determination of the Breslow thickness dictates the subsequent diagnostic and therapeutic interventions to be performed, including the recommended surgical margins for wide excision, the need for a sentinel lymph node biopsy and possible lymph node dissection, and a potential evaluation for metastatic disease. Thus, staging procedures are intimately linked to the surgical aspects of treatment, and these will be discussed together below.

### Ancillary Tests

The extent of radiologic procedures and blood tests indicated for a new patient with melanoma is perhaps controversial, but extensive imaging procedures are not cost-effective and are limited to patients with unu-sual symptoms [27]. A chest X-ray is optional, but is usually performed, for asymptomatic patients with thin melanomas less than 1 mm in depth, and a CBC and chemistries with LDH are routinely obtained. Patients with deeper lesions will be undergoing a more involved surgical proce-dure (at least a sentinel lymph node biopsy), and for those patients one routinely obtains a chest X-ray, CBC, chemistries with LDH, and PT/PTT. Body CT scanning is reserved for patients with a poor performance sta-tus, unusual symptoms, documented lymph node involvement, or deep (>4 mm) primary lesions. Brain CT scanning is reserved for patients with neurologic symptoms or with multiple documented metastases being considered for systemic therapy.

There currently are no reliable tumor markers measurable in the serum that can be used to follow the course of disease or for screening purposes. However, RT-PCR analysis for the presence of melanoma anti-gen mRNA in peripheral blood cells is being performed on an investiga-tional level, as an attempt to detect micrometastatic disease at the ear-liest possible stage. This technique is sensitive enough to pick up one tumor cell in a population of $10^6$–$10^7$ normal cells, and in some prelimi-nary studies the incidence of positive RT-PCR appears to correlate with disease stage and may predict the likelihood of relapse [14, 28, 29]. Additional investigation will be necessary to optimize and standardize this approach.

## Treatment

### Surgical Resection of the Primary Lesion

If there is no evidence of metastatic disease by history or physical exam, the course of treatment begins with analysis of the thickness of the pri-mary lesion obtained by biopsy. A wide excision is then performed in a second procedure based on the Breslow depth, but this should be coordi-nated with the sentinel lymph node biopsy or complete lymph node diss-ection if they are being performed. Thus, the re-excision is usually done by a surgical oncologist for deeper lesions. Historically, a wide excision with the most generous surgical margin possible had been carried out, but ran-domized clinical trials have allowed a safe narrowing of the required extent of this margin for lesions less than 1 mm [30–32] or 1–4 mm [33] in depth.

**Table 3.** Recommended margins for wide excision of primary melanoma lesion

| Breslow depth | Surgical margin |
|---|---|
| Melanoma in situ | 0.5 cm |
| <1 mm | 1 cm |
| 1–4 mm | 2 cm |
| >4 mm | 2–3 cm |

The current recommended surgical margins for wide excision of primary cutaneous melanoma lesions are presented in Table 3. Melanoma in situ lesions are safely excised with a margin of 0.5 cm. Lesions less than or equal to 1 mm in depth are re-excised with a surgical margin of 1 cm, and no further staging or diagnostic procedures are required, unless there is ulceration, penetration to Clark's level IV or V, or undetermined depth due to partial regression. In those instances, a sentinel lymph node biopsy is recommended at the time of wide excision. For lesions between 1 and 4 mm in depth, a sentinel lymph node biopsy is the current standard of care, along with re-excision of the primary lesion with a surgical margin of 2 cm. For lesions deeper than 4 mm, the incidence of metastasis to draining lymph nodes is approximately equal to that of distant metastases [34], so sentinel lymph node biopsy has not been routinely performed. However, recent evidence has suggested that patients with deep primary melanomas and positive lymph nodes that are treated as stage III disease may have a greater survival than those that develop distant metastases only [35]. Thus, sentinel lymph node biopsy may be appropriate for all patients with primary melanomas deeper than 1 mm, including those with lesions deeper than 4 mm. Re-excision of the primary with a margin of 2–3 cm is recommended for these patients; however, local recurrence usually is less of an issue than is metastatic disease for patients with deep primaries.

Sentinel Lymph Node Biopsy and Complete Lymph Node Dissection

Inasmuch as many patients with intermediate thickness primary melanoma lesions recur in regional lymph nodes, elective lymph node dissection of the suspected draining lymph node basin had been the standard of care for many years [36, 37]. However, this practice has become controversial [38], as several retrospective studies and 2 prospective randomized trials have failed to demonstrate a survival advantage for patients receiving lymph node dissection in addition to wide local excision [39]. In addition, lymphedema and poor wound healing are relatively common following complete lymph node dissection [40, 41], adding morbidity to the procedure. A recent study has indicated that patients who actually had microscopic lymph node involvement had a longer survival with immediate elective lymph node dissection than with delayed lymph node dissection, although overall survival for all patients studied was not significantly different whether or not lymph node dissection was performed [35]. Thus, if patients with occult stage III disease could be identified in advance, then complete lymph node dissection could be reserved for that subgroup of patients most likely to benefit. It is this rationale that underlies the principle of the sentinel lymph node biopsy.

The sentinel lymph node biopsy relies on the observation that melanoma tumor cells arising in a cutaneous site follow a stepwise progression through the particular lymph node basin draining that site, beginning with the first lymph node in the chain [42]. This first lymph node is called the sentinel node, and if the sentinel node does not contain metastatic tumor cells then the rest of that lymph node group should not be involved with disease. Only patients with a positive sentinel lymph node undergo a subsequent elective lymph node dissection. The accuracy of the sentinel node in predicting the disease status of the nodal basin has been borne out in several recent studies [42, 43].

The identification of the sentinel node has been facilitated by 3 technical advances [44]. The first is lymphoscintigraphy, which is performed by the injection of radioactive technetium sulfur colloid around the perimeter of the primary tumor site. Nuclear medicine scanning then allows for the identification of the appropriate lymph node basin to address [45, 46]. Importantly, experience with this procedure has indicated that approximately 10% of patients have drainage to unusual lymph node sites or to contralateral lymph nodes. Many patients with axial melanoma lesions have drainage to 2 or more lymph node basins, and each of these must be analyzed for possible metastases. In addition, this procedure has identified a minority of patients with lymph nodes located along the lymphatic channel en route to the lymph node basin, a location that otherwise would have been overlooked by the surgeon. The second technical procedure involves additional intraoperative lymph node mapping by injection of 1% lymphazurin blue dye around the perimeter of the primary melanoma lesion, which rapidly passes into draining lymphatics and labels the sentinel lymph node with accuracy. The third technical advance has come from the intraoperative use of a geiger counter, or gamma probe, that allows identification of the lymph node(s) containing the greatest level of radioactivity carried over from the lymphoscintigraphy procedure. A radioactivity level three times that of the background level is used to designate a sentinel node. The combination of radiolymphoscintigraphy and vital blue dye reportedly allows identification of the sentinel lymph node in 98% of cases [43]. The complications of the sentinel lymph node biopsy are few, and include tattooing of the skin and urinary excretion of blue dye. Much of the tattoo is usually removed during the wide local excision done on the primary site during the procedure. The technique is rapid, performed on an outpatient basis, and does not lead to lymphedema.

The identified sentinel node is analyzed by routine histological staining, but a greater number of sections through the node is examined. However, preliminary observations have indicated that at least 15% of patients with histologically negative sentinel nodes subsequently recur [13, 47]. More sensitive measures of potential lymph node involvement are being explored, including immunohistochemical staining for HMB-45 expression and RT-PCR analysis for the presence of melanoma antigen mRNA [13]. Interestingly, a small retrospective analysis of patients with negative sentinel lymph nodes by routine histology who subsequently recurred were found to have been PCR-positive for tyrosinase mRNA expression in those nodes [13]. Thus, the future state of the art may utilize RT-PCR as the most sensitive measure of micrometastatic disease, and studies are ongoing to determine the validity of this technique.

Patients with a positive sentinel lymph node undergo a complete lymph node dissection of the involved lymph node basin. Whether this lymphadenectomy contributes to increased survival is not yet known, but it remains the current standard of care. In addition, patients with clinically apparent stage III disease (who do not require a sentinel node biopsy) also undergo complete lymph node dissection. Documented stage III patients are then eligible for adjuvant systemic therapy.

Adjuvant Therapy for High-Risk Disease

Approximately two-thirds of patients with deep (>4 mm) primary lesions or with stage III disease recur following optimal surgical resection.

Therefore, multiple therapeutic modalities have been explored in the adjuvant setting in an attempt to decrease the likelihood of disease recurrence in these populations. Adjuvant radiation therapy to involved lymph node basins has been examined in several studies. However, melanoma cells are relatively radio-resistant, apparently secondary to very efficient mechanisms of DNA repair that might be predicted given the normal location of melanocytes in the skin conferring regular exposure to DNA-damaging agents [48]. As such, there is little evidence for an increased survival advantage conferred by adjuvant radiation therapy. One exception may be in the treatment of melanoma of the head and neck. In one study, modified neck dissection followed by large dose fractions of 24–30 Gy in 4 or 5 fractions postoperatively for patients with head and neck melanomas deeper than 1.5 mm resulted in 95% locoregional control at 2 years [49]. Thus, radiation therapy should be considered as part of a multimodality treatment plan of such patients. However, the proven efficacy of IFN-α2b in the post-surgical setting, as described below, has prompted its use in the treatment of patients with melanomas of the head and neck as well [50]. Whether radiation therapy plus IFN-α2b may be superior to either agent alone has yet to be determined.

Chemotherapeutic agents active in metastatic disease have been examined in the post-surgical adjuvant setting. However, no survival benefit has been conferred by any of these regimens. Dacarbazine, the most active single agent in metastatic disease, has shown no survival benefit using a regimen of 200 mg/m$^2$ daily for five days every 4 weeks for up to 24 cycles [51]. Combination therapy using 6 cycles of dacarbazine, vindesine, and cisplatin also conferred no prolongation in survival [52].

The only agent that has been demonstrated to benefit high-risk patients in the adjuvant setting is IFN-α2b. Kirkwood and colleagues carried out a study utilizing 4 weeks of high-dose IFN-α2b (20 MU/m2 per day intravenously for 5 days with 2 days off per week) followed by low-dose IFN-α2b (10 MU/m$^2$ subcutaneously three times per week for 48 weeks) in patients with AJCC stage IIB or IIIA melanoma [53]. Disease-free survival was increased from 26% to 37%, with overall median survival increasing from 2.8 to 3.8 years, in the treated group compared to the observation group. Toxicities were significant, and included fatigue, flu-like symptoms, myelosuppression, hepatotoxicity, and depression. With appropriate dose adjustment, 74% of patients completed the year of therapy. Quality of life assessments also support a benefit of IFN-α2b therapy [54]. Although both stage IIB and IIIA patients were included in this study, subgroup analysis failed to demonstrate benefit for the IIB patients [53]. Although only 15 stage IIB patients per group were studied, the available information does not support the routine use of adjuvant IFN-α2b in patients with deep primaries. It is conceivable that stage IIB patients with occult lymph node involvement represent a subgroup of patients that might benefit, and sentinel lymph node biopsy should be used to reveal those patients. Stage IIB patients should thus be enrolled in investigational clinical trials when possible, to establish a standard of care for this subgroup [55]. IFN-α2b is the current standard of care in the post-surgical setting for stage IIIA patients, and has been approved by the FDA for the treatment of all patient subgroups included in this study.

Melanoma immunotherapies also are being explored in the adjuvant setting. Earlier studies using post-surgical systemic administration of BCG [51, 56] or levamisole [57] failed to reveal a survival benefit. However, the technological developments in antigen-specific vaccination approaches are beginning to be examined in the clinical arena. A recent report of vaccination to induce anti-GM2 antibodies, directed against a ganglioside expressed on melanoma cells, suggested a prolongation of survival in those patients who responded immunologically to the vaccine [58]. Approaches that induce a T cell-mediated immune response also are being examined in this setting. Although still investigational, antigen-specific immunologic approaches are likely to become integrated into the post-surgical adjuvant treatment of patients with melanoma in the foreseeable future.

Treatment of Advanced Disease: Chemotherapy

It is probably fair to say that there is no standard therapy for metastatic melanoma and that patients should be encouraged to enroll in clinical trials whenever possible. This point notwithstanding, clinical responses can be achieved in some patients with chemotherapy, non-specific immunotherapy, or combination chemoimmunotherapy, and such regimens are often administered as first-line treatment.

Melanoma is only modestly sensitive to chemotherapeutic agents (Table 4). The most active single agent is dacarbazine (DTIC), giving a response rate of approximately 20% [59]. However, durable complete responses are rarely achieved (<1% of cases) using DTIC alone, and there is

**Table 4.** Single-agent chemotherapy in advanced melanoma

| Agent | n | Response rate | Reference |
|---|---|---|---|
| 2-chloroadenosine | 12 | 0% | 108 |
| Carboplatin | 27 | 11% | 109 |
| Carmustine | 20 | 20% | 110, 111 |
| Cisplatin | 36 | 19% | 112 |
| Cyclophosphamide | 13 | 8% | 113 |
| Dacarbazine | 143 | 20% | 59 |
| Docetaxel | 40 | 12% | 114 |
| Fotemustine | 153 | 24% | 115, 116 |
| Hydroxyurea | 48 | 10% | 117–119 |
| Ifosfamide | 36 | 11% | 120 |
| Lomustine | 17 | 18% | 121 |
| Mitomycin C | 15 | 0% | 122 |
| Pirarubicin | 23 | 4% | 123 |
| Piritrexim | 31 | 23% | 124 |
| Taxol | 37 | 18% | 125, 126 |
| Vinblastine | 11 | 18% | 127 |
| Vindesine | 42 | 20% | 128 |
| Zeniplatin | 21 | 9% | 129 |

no evidence that overall survival is prolonged with this treatment. Other commonly used active agents are cisplatin, the nitrosoureas, and the vinca alkaloids, all yielding response rates of approximately 15%. The taxanes have been examined and generate responses in 10%–15% of patients. Multiple additional chemotherapeutic agents have been examined in melanoma, either through patient participation in phase I studies or in dedicated phase II studies, but generally with inferior results.

Many combination chemotherapy regimens have been examined, with response rates that appear marginally superior to DTIC alone in single institution phase II studies [60–64]. Although a multitude of studies have been performed, Table 5 lists the most commonly used chemotherapy regimens. Del Prete et al. reported a regimen of BCNU, cisplatin, and DTIC (with tamoxifen) that generated a response rate of 55% among the small sample size of 20 patients treated [65]. Legha and colleagues reported a 40% overall response rate using a combination of cisplatin, vinblastine, and dacarbazine [66]. The combination of bleomycin, vincristine, lomustine, and dacarbazine was administered to a group of 91 patients, also resulting in an overall response rate of 40% [67]. Interestingly, Richards et al. treated 20 patients that had progressed following therapy with interleukin-2, using a regimen of BCNU, cisplatin,

**Table 5.** Commonly used chemotherapy regimens for metastatic melanoma

| Regimen | Dosing | Frequency |
|---|---|---|
| Dacarbazine | 250 mg/m$^2$ IV days 1–5 or 800 mg/m$^2$ IV day 1 | q 3–4 weeks |
| BCD | | q 6–8 weeks (carmustine every other cycle) |
|   Carmustine | 150 mg/m$^2$ IV day 1 | |
|   Cisplatin | 25 mg/m$^2$ IV days 1–3 | |
|   Dacarbazine | 220 mg/m$^2$ IV days 1–3 | |
| CVD | | q 3–4 weeks |
|   Cisplatin | 20 mg/m$^2$ IV days 1–5 | |
|   Vinblastine | 1.6 mg/m$^2$ IV days 1–5 | |
|   Dacarbazine | 800 mg/m$^2$ IV day 1 | |
| BOLD | | q 4–6 weeks |
|   Bleomycin | 7.5 U SC days 1 and 4 | |
|   Vincristine | 1 mg/m$^2$ IV days 1 and 5 | |
|   Lomustine | 80 mg/m$^2$ PO day 1 | |
|   Dacarbazine | 200 mg/m$^2$ IV days 1–5 | |

dacarbazine, and tamoxifen, which yielded a response rate of 55% [68]. This result suggested that chemotherapy and non-specific immunotherapy might not be cross-resistant, arguing for the combined use of these modalities.

Few randomized trials with meaningful sample sizes comparing chemotherapy regimens in advanced melanoma have been performed. A small study of less than 15 evaluable patients per group compared cisplatin/vinblastine/bleomycin to dacarbazine, demonstrating no significant difference in response rate [69]. Buzaid et al. compared cisplatin/vinblastine/dacarbazine to dacarbazine alone and observed a 24% versus 11% overall response rate, respectively [70]. In the largest reported study, Costanzi and colleagues compared bleomycin/hydroxyurea/dacarbazine plus BCG to dacarbazine plus BCG [71]. There were 256 evaluable patients in the combination group and 130 evaluable patients in the DTIC group, with overall response rates of 29% and 18%, respectively. Thus, although definitive data comparing the most commonly used chemotherapy regimens are lacking, available information suggests that combination therapy may be superior to single agent DTIC, generating overall response rates from 25%–40%. However, it is not certain that combination chemotherapy provides improved survival for treated patients.

The role of tamoxifen in the treatment of melanoma has been vigorously debated. Melanoma tumor cells appear to express estrogen receptors, and it is clear that nevi and melanoma lesions can become hyperpigmented during pregnancy. These and other observations suggested that hormonal blockade might be advantageous in the treatment of melanoma, and phase II studies incorporating tamoxifen appeared to offer more favorable response rates [72–75]. However, other less promising phase II studies have since been performed [76], and four randomized studies comparing various regimens with or without tamoxifen have been executed with only one of the four demonstrating an improved response rate in the tamoxifen-treated group [76–78]. Thus, it is likely that tamoxifen does not contribute to effective combination therapy for this disease, and its use in established combination regimens is now considered optional.

High dose chemotherapy with autologous bone marrow or stem cell support has been examined in metastatic melanoma, with higher response rates generally observed than those seen with standard doses of chemotherapy [79–81]. However, few complete responses have been seen, response duration has been short, and toxicities have been great. Thus, there is no evidence that high dose chemotherapy offers any survival advantage for patients with this disease, and this modality is generally not pursued. Allogeneic bone marrow transplantation has not been examined in melanoma, but perhaps should be considered in light of the graft-versus-tumor effect that has been observed in patients with hematologic malignancies treated by allogeneic transplantation and the responsiveness of melanoma to immune-based therapies. This avenue may be pursued in future clinical trials.

## Treatment of Advanced Disease:
## Immunotherapy and Combined Chemoimmunotherapy

Two biologic agents, interleukin-2 (IL-2) and interferon-α (IFN-α), have significant activity in melanoma, generating response rates between 15 and 20% [82, 83]. However, in contrast to the short response duration seen with chemotherapy, cytokine-based immunotherapy has resulted in durable complete responses in about 5% of patients. These observations have supported the notion that immune-based therapies, once optimized, may offer the best hope for the treatment of patients with melanoma.

IL-2 is a growth factor for T lymphocytes and natural killer cells but has no direct anti-tumor activity. The anti-tumor effect of IL-2 is thought to be mediated by amplification of immune effector cells that in turn induce tumor cell killing. IL-2 was first administered to patients by bolus intravenous (IV) infusion, but has since been given as a continuous intravenous (CIV) infusion or subcutaneously (SC), with lower toxicity. The maximally tolerated dose of bolus IV IL-2 is 720,000 U/kg every 8 h for up to 5 days, but this regimen requires intensive care unit support due to cardiovascular effects and pulmonary capillary leak. Therefore, 600,000 U/kg every 8 h is the usual bolus infusion schedule, which still requires very close observation for acute toxicity (Table 6). CIV IL-2 appears to be much better tolerated than bolus IL-2, and is generally administered as 18 MU/m$^2$ per day for 5 consecutive days. IL-2 also has been administered SC using a variety of schedules; one frequently used regimen utilizes 11 MU (straight dose) SC 4 days per week. The overall response rates with each of these regimens have ranged from 5%–25%, with a mean of 20% [84]. However, the optimal dose and schedule of IL-2 are not clear. It is conceivable that SC IL-2 may generate comparable responses with the least toxicity, but anecdotal experience

**Table 6.** Commonly used regimens of IL-2 and/or IFN-$\alpha$ in metastatic melanoma

| Regimen | Dosing | Frequency |
|---------|--------|-----------|
| Bolus IL-2 | 600,000 IU/kg q8 h by 15 min IV infusion days 1–5 for 14 total doses, 9 days rest, then repeat for 28 total doses | q 9–12 weeks |
| CIV IL-2 | 18 MU/m$^2$ per day CIV infusion for 5 days | q 4 weeks |
| SC IL-2 | 11 MU SC 4 days/week for 4 weeks | q 6 weeks |
| IFN-$\alpha$ | 9 or 10 MU SC 3–5 days/week for 4 weeks | q 6 weeks |
| IFN-$\alpha$/IL-2 | | q 4 weeks |
|   IFN-$\alpha$ | 10 MU SC qd days 1–5 | |
|   IL-2 | 18 MU/m$^2$ per day CIV infusion days 8–13, or 18 MU/m$^2$ IV over 6 h day 8, 18 MU/m$^2$ IV over 12 h day 9, 18 MU/m$^2$ IV over 24 h day 10, 4.5 MU/m$^2$ IV over 24 h days 11–13 (decrescendo schedule) | |
| IL-2/IFN-$\alpha$ | | q 3–4 weeks |
|   IL-2 | 9 MU/m$^2$ CIV infusion days 1–4 | |
|   IFN-$\alpha$ | 5 MU/m$^2$ SC days 1–5 | |
| SC IL-2/IFN-$\alpha$ | | q 6–8 weeks |
|   IL-2 | 11 MU SC days 1–4, each week x4 weeks | |
|   IFN-$\alpha$ | 9 MU SC days 1 and 4, each week x4 weeks | |

has suggested that higher doses of IL-2 may induce more durable complete responses.

IFN-α is a cytokine produced by leukocytes that has a variety of biologic effects in the setting of malignancy, including a direct anti-proliferative effect on melanoma cell lines and immunologic effects through the up-regulation of surface MHC molecule expression [85]. Two formulations are available, IFN-α2a and IFN-α2b, with no evidence to suggest that one is superior to the other. IFN-α has been administered IV, SC, and intramuscularly (IM), using a variety of doses and schedules. It appears that the minimal effective dose is 5 $MU/m^2$ 3 times per week [83]. The optimal dose and schedule for administration of IFN-α are not clear; one frequently used regimen utilizes 9–10 MU SC every Monday, Wednesday, and Friday (Table 6). Although the overall response rate using IFN-α is approximately 15%, about one-third of these are complete responses with many being durable.

Combinations of IL-2 and IFN-α have been examined, again using a variety of doses and schedules, with overall response rates in the range of 20%–40% (Table 6). The most frequently used combination regimens utilize SC IFN-α along with IL-2 delivered as a CIV infusion. The optimal regimen is not known, and it is not clear if the IFN-α should be administered before, during, or after the IL-2 to achieve maximal benefit. Interestingly, two sequential studies in Europe were performed, one which utilized IFN-α followed by CIV IL-2, and the second which used IFN-α followed by CIV IL-2 given on a decrescendo schedule. The overall response rate was 18% in the first study but 41% in the second, with the decrescendo schedule having far less toxicity [86]. Although the two regimens were not compared directly in a randomized phase III trial, the high response rate observed using the decrescendo schedule certainly warrants further investigation.

Because chemotherapy and cytokine therapy are thought to operate by distinct mechanisms, the two modalities also have been combined. Single institution phase II studies of chemoimmunotherapy have yielded the most promising results in the treatment of metastatic melanoma, routinely generating response rates from 40%–60% with approximately 10% of patients experiencing a durable complete response [63, 64, 87–89]. Thus, although still in the early stages of development, these combination regimens have provided the first evidence that overall survival of patients with metastatic melanoma can potentially be prolonged.

The most frequently employed chemoimmunotherapy regimens are depicted in Table 7. Richards et al. combined BCNU, cisplatin, DTIC, and tamoxifen with IV bolus IL-2 and SC IFN-a2a, and observed an objective response rate of 55% [90]. Legha and colleagues have added IL-2 by CIV infusion and SC IFN-α to their cisplatin/vinblastine/DTIC regimen, resulting in a 58% overall response rate including 17% complete responses [91]. A more recent study of concurrent cisplatin/vinblastine/DTIC plus IL-2 and IFN-α showed similar response rates to the sequential regimen but with less toxicity [92]. The decrescendo IL-2 schedule also is being combined with chemotherapy, with preliminary results that look quite promising [93]. Single agent cisplatin also has been combined with IL-2 and IFN-α, yielding a 54% response rate and less toxicity than that observed with the other regimens. More recently, Thompson reported on an outpatient regimen of BCNU/cisplatin/DTIC followed by SC IL-2 and

**Table 7.** Commonly used regimens of chemoimmunotherapy for metastatic melanoma

| Regimen | Dosing | Frequency |
|---|---|---|
| BCD (T)/IL-2/IFN-α | | q 6 weeks |
|   BCNU | 150 mg/m$^2$ IV day 1 | |
|   Cisplatin | 25 mg/m$^2$ IV days 1–3 and 22–24 | |
|   DTIC | 220 mg/m$^2$ IV days 1–3, 22–24 | |
|   IL-2 | 4.5 MU/m$^2$ IV q 8 h days 4–8, 17–21, 25–29, 38–42 | |
|   IFN-a | 6 MU/m$^2$ SC days 4–8, 17–21, 25–29, 38–42 | |
|   (Tamoxifen) | (20 mg po daily) | |
| | | |
| CVD/IL-2/IFN-α (concurrent) | | q 3–4 weeks |
|   Cisplatin | 20 mg/m$^2$ IV days 1–4 | |
|   Vinblastine | 1.6 mg/m$^2$ IV days 1–4 | |
|   DTIC | 800 mg/m$^2$ IV day 1 | |
|   IL-2 | 9 MU/m$^2$ per day CIV infusion days 1–4 | |
|   IFN-α | 5 MU/m$^2$ SC days 1–5 | |
| Cisplatin/IL-2/IFN-α | | q 4 weeks |
|   Cisplatin | 100 mg/m$^2$ IV day 1 | |
|   IL-2 | 18 MU/m$^2$ per day CIV infusion days 3–6, 17–21 | |
|   IFN-α | 9 MU SC days 1, 3, and 5 | |
| | | |
| Outpatient BCD/IL-2/IFN-α | | q 6–8 weeks |
|   BCNU | 150 mg/m$^2$ IV day 1 | |
|   Cisplatin | 75 mg/m$^2$ IV days 1, 22 | |
|   DTIC | 660 mg/m$^2$ IV days 1, 22 | |
|   IL-2 | 3 MU/m$^2$ SC days 3–9 and 24–30 | |
|   IFN-α | 3 MU SC day 3 and day 24, | |
| | 5 MU/m$^2$ SC days 5, 7, 9, and 26, 28, and 30 | |

IFN-α [94]. The overall response rate was 43% and the regimen was quite tolerable, with hospitalization being required for only 7% of patients to manage toxicity. The availability of a manageable outpatient chemoimmunotherapy regimen has made administration of this therapy more feasible in community oncology practices.

Although small randomized trials of single chemotherapeutic agents with and without IL-2 or IFN-α have been performed with mixed results [95, 96], there are no phase III data available that compare the commonly used combination chemotherapy regimens with or without IL-2/IFN-α. DTIC plus IFN-α does not appear to be superior to DTIC alone [97]. However, a recent phase III study in renal cell carcinoma indicated that IFN-α may act synergistically with IL-2 [98], arguing that the multiagent chemoimmunotherapy combinations may have merit. A European study of 138 patients with metastatic melanoma has compared IL-2/IFN-α with and without cisplatin, observing 35% and 18% response rates, respectively, but with no difference in overall survival. The high fraction of patients experiencing durable complete responses using the CVD/IL-2/IFN-α regimen has prompted initiation of a prospective trial to determine objectively the potential benefit of adding cytokines to chemotherapy for metastatic melanoma.

## Patient Follow-up

All patients with a documented history of melanoma should have a complete skin examination, preferably by a dermatologist, at least on an annual basis. The main purpose of this examination is to screen for the appearance of a second primary lesion. More frequent physician visits are recommended during the initial 2 years following diagnosis, either by a dermatologist or by a surgical or medical oncologist, to examine for lymphadenopathy and for evidence of recurrent metastatic disease.

For patients with treated stage I disease, clinical assessment every 6 months for the first 2 years followed by a life-long annual examination are recommended [27]. Treated stage II and stage III patients are generally examined every 3 months for the first 2 years, every 6 months through the 5 year point, then annually after that. Stage IV patients are more actively followed during the course of systemic therapy, and at least every 3 months if they achieve a complete response. In addition to the clinical assessment, a chest X-ray, complete blood count, and chemistries with LDH are usually performed every 6–12 months for patients with treated deep primary lesions and/or a documented history of lymph node involvement or distant metastases. More extensive imaging procedures are not cost-effective and are generally not performed, except for patients with a history of stage IV disease. It has been suggested that the most accurate predictor of disease relapse was patient self-assessment alone [99], indicating that even the aforementioned recommendations for follow-up may be too intensive, particularly for reliable patients having good disease insight.

## Key Questions and Investigational Approaches

The surgical treatment for thin primary melanoma lesions cures the vast majority of such patients. However, a minority of patients go on to develop recurrent disease, either in regional lymph nodes or at distant metastatic sites. The development of sensitive RT-PCR analysis provides a means by which to detect minimal residual disease, either in sentinel lymph nodes or in peripheral blood, and studies are ongoing to determine whether this sensitive molecular analysis is the best predictor of relapse.

Adjuvant administration of IFN-α2b is the first agent that improves survival in patients with resected stage III melanoma. However, the optimal dose and schedule for this treatment are not known. It is likely that the first 4 weeks of high dose therapy are important, because previous trials using lower doses of IFN-α generated a less significant survival advantage [100–102]. Whether adjuvant IFN-α2b extends the survival of patients with microscopic stage III disease as it does for patients with bulky clinically detected stage III disease is not known, and is currently being investigated in a randomized clinical trial. The role of IFN-α2b in the treatment of patients with stage IIB disease also remains an open question. In addition, the development of PEG-coupled IFN-α2b, which has a longer half-life in vivo, may allow for the more convenient administration of this drug, and most likely will be tested in prospective clinical trials.

Other agents are being explored for high-risk patients in the adjuvant setting. Clinical trials of melanoma tumor cell-based and ganglioside vaccines have been initiated in this patient population. In addition, IL-

2/chemotherapy combinations are beginning to be examined as an alternative adjuvant treatment. A six month regimen of DTIC plus SC IL-2 in high risk patients has resulted in a relapse-free survival of 65% at 2 years [103]. Thus, it is likely that adjuvant therapy for high risk melanoma will evolve over the next several years.

In metastatic melanoma, the single most important question is whether chemoimmunotherapy is superior to chemotherapy alone, and at least one major clinical trial has been initiated to address this question. If a survival advantage is indeed demonstrated, then a standard of care will have been established for the treatment of patients with stage IV disease, and the next step will be to optimize this combined modality therapy.

A large effort is being invested in the development of tumor antigen-specific immunization approaches in melanoma. The benefit that some patients experience following therapy with IL-2 alone may be due to the fact that they had already developed a weak specific T cell response that could be amplified by administration of a T cell growth factor. It is thus reasoned that the remaining patients that normally fail to respond to IL-2 might benefit from the initiation of a fresh tumor-specific CTL response, which subsequently could be expanded with IL-2 administration if necessary. Several tumor-specific antigens and melanoma/melanocyte differentiation antigens are being explored as immunogens in these studies, which are ongoing in Europe, at the NCI, at the University of Pittsburg, and at the University of Chicago, among other institutions. The most commonly used antigens are MAGE-1, MAGE-3, Melan-A/MART-1, tyrosinase, and gp100 [11, 12]. Multiple vaccination strategies are being investigated, which include peptides or proteins alone or in adjuvants, peptide-loaded antigen-presenting cells alone or in combination with cytokines, and recombinant viruses [104]. Other centers are pursuing tumor cell-based vaccination strategies. Pilot studies have already revealed major tumor responses in some patients, in many cases with very little toxicity [105–107]. It seems likely that, once optimized, active specific immunotherapy will constitute an important new approach for the treatment of established melanoma or for the prevention of disease recurrence. These modalities are reviewed in more detail in Chapter "Cancer Immunotherapy" of this volume.

# References

1. Cannon-Albright LA, Kamb A, Skolnick M (1996) A review of inherited predisposition to melanoma. Semin Oncol 23:667–672
2. Monzon J, Liu L, Brill H, Goldstein AM, Tucker MA, From L, μlaughlin J, Hogg D, Lassam NJ (1998) CDKN2 mutations in multiple primary melanomas. N Engl J Med 338:879–887
3. Seykora J, Elder D (1996) Dysplastic nevi and other risk markers for melanoma. Semin Oncol 23:682–687
4. Kripke ML, Fisher MS (1976) Immunologic parameters of ultraviolet carcinogenesis. J Natl Cancer Inst 57:211–215
5. Autier P, Dore J-F, Schifflers E, Cesarini J-P, Bollaerts A, Koelmel KF, Gefeller O, Liabeuf A, Lejeune F, Lienard D, Joarlette M, Chemaly P, Kleeberg UR (1995) Melanoma and the use of sunscreens: an EORTC case-control study in Germany, Belgium and France. Int J Cancer 61:749–755
6. Autier P, Dore J-F, Renard F, Cattaruzza MS, Gefeller O, Grivegnee A (1997) Melanoma and sunscreen use: need for studies representative of actual behaviours. Melanoma Res 7 (suppl 2):S115-S120
7. Elwood JM (1996) Melanoma and sun exposure. Semin Oncol 23:650–666
8. Swerdlow AJ, Weinstock MA (1998) Do tanning lamps cause melanoma? An epidemiologic assessment. J Am Acad Derm 38:89–98
9. Koh HK, Caruso A, Gage I, Geller AC, Prout MN, White H, O'Connor K, Balash EM, Blumental G, Rex IH, Wax FD, Rosenfeld TL, Gladstone GC, Shama SK, Koumans JA, Baler GR, Lew RA (1990) Evaluation of melanoma/skin cancer screening in Massachusetts. Cancer 65:375–379
10. Koh HK, Michalik E, Sober AJ, Lew RA, Day CL, Clark W, Mihm MC, Kopf AW, Blois MS, Fitzpatrick TB (1984) Lentigo maligna melanoma has no better prognosis than other types of melanoma. J Clin Oncol 2:994–1001
11. Boon T, Cerottini J, Van den Eynde B, Van der Bruggen P, Van Pel A (1994) Tumor antigens recognized by T lymphocytes. Ann Rev Immunol 12:337–365
12. Boon T, Gajewski TF, Coulie PG (1995) From defined human tumor antigens to effective immunization? Immunol Today 16:334–335
13. Reintgen DS, Conrad AJ (1997) Detection of occult melanoma cells in sentinel lymph nodes and blood. Semin Oncol 24 (suppl 4):S4–11-S4–15
14. Hoon DSB, Wang Y, Dale PS, Conrad AJ, Schmid P, Garrison D, Kuo C, Foshag LJ, Nizze AJ, Morton DL (1995) Detection of occult melanoma cells in blood with a multiple-marker polymerase chain reaction assay. J Clin Oncol 13:2109–2116
15. Lindauer M, Stanislawski T, Haussler A, Antunes E, Cellary A, Huber C, Theobald M (1998) The molecular basis of cancer immunotherapy by cytotoxic T lymphocytes. J Mol Med 76:32–47
16. Clark WHJ, From L, Bernardino EA, Mihm MC (1969) The histogenesis and biologic behavior of primary malignant melanomas of the skin. Cancer Res 29:705–726
17. Breslow A (1970) Thickness, cross-sectional areas and depth of invasion in the prognosis of cutaneous melanoma. Ann Surg 172:902–908
18. Morton DL, Davtyan DG, Wanek LA, Foshag LJ, Cochran AJ (1993) Multivariate analysis of the relationship between survival and the microstage of primary melanoma by Clark level and Breslow thickness. Cancer 71:3737–3743
19. Buzaid AC, Ross MI, Balch CM, Soong S, McCarthy WH, Tinoco L, Mansfield P, Lee JE, Bedikian A, Eton O, Plager C, Papadopoulos N, Legha SS, Benjamin RS (1997) Critical analysis of the current American Joint Committee on Cancer Staging system for cutaneous melanoma and promosal of a new staging system. J Clin Oncol 15:1039–1051

20. Balch CM, Soong S-J, Murad TM, Ingalls AL, Maddox WA (1981) A multifactorial analysis of melanoma. III. Prognostic factors in melanoma patients with lymph node metastases (stage II). Ann Surg 193:377–388

21. Balch CM, Wilkerson JA, Murad TM, Soong S-J, Ingalls AL, Maddox WA (1980) The prognostic significance of ulceration of cutaneous melanoma. Cancer 45:3012–3017

22. Ronan SG, Das Gupta TK (1988) Histologic prognostic indicators in cutaneous malignant melanoma. Semin Oncol 15:558–565

23. Cohen MH, Ketcham AS, Felix EL, Li S-H, Tomaszewski M-M, Costa J, Rabson AS, Simon RM, Rosenberg SA (1977) Prognostic factors in patients undergoing lymphadenectomy for malignant melanoma. Ann Surg 186:635–642

24. Wang X, Heller R, VanVoorhis N, Cruse CW, Glass F, Fenske N, Berman C, Leo-Messina J, Rappaport D, Wells K, DeConti R, Moscinski L, Stankard C, Puleo C, Reintgen D (1994) Detection of submicroscopic lymph node metastases with polymerase chain reaction in patients with malignant melanoma. Ann Surg 220:768–774

25. Eton O, Legha SS, Moon TE, Buzaid AC, Papadopoulos NE, Plager C, Burgess AM, Bedikian AY, Ring S, Dong Q, Glassman AB, Balch CM, Benjamin RS (1998) Prognostic factors for survival of patients treated systemically for disseminated melanoma. J Clin Oncol 16:1103–1111

26. Overett TK, Shiu MH (1985) Surgical treatment of distant metastatic melanoma. Indications and results. Cancer 56:1222–1230

27. Rigel DS (1997) Malignant melanoma: incidence issues and their effect on diagnosis and treatment in the 1990s. Mayo Clin Proc 72:367–371

28. Mellado B, Colomer D, Castel T, Munoz M, Carballo E, Galan M, Mascaro JM, Vives-Corrons JL, Grau JJ, Estape J (1996) Detection of circulating neoplastic cells by reverse-transcriptase polymerase chain reaction in malignant melanoma: Association with clinical stage and prognosis. J Clin Oncol 14:2091–2097

29. Curry BJ, Myers K, Hersey P (1998) Polymerase chain reaction detection of melanoma cells in the circulation: relation to clinical stage, surgical treatment, and recurrence from melanoma. J Clin Oncol 16:1760–1769

30. Veronesi U, Cascinelli N, Adamus J, Balch C, Bandiera D, Barchuk A, Bufalino R, Craig P, De Marsillac J, Durand JC, van Geel AN, Holmstrom H, Hunter JA, Jorgensen OG, Kiss B, Kroon B, Lacour J, Lejeune F, MacKie R, Mechl Z, Mitrov G, Morabito A, Nosek H, Panizzon R, Prade M, Santi P, van Slooten E, Tomin R, Trapeznikov N, Tsanov T, Urist M, Wozniak KD (1988) Thin stage I primary cutaneous malignant melanoma. Comparison of excision with margins of 1 or 3 cm. N Engl J Med 318:1159–1162

31. Kelly JW, Sagebiel RW, Calderon W, Murillo L, Dakin RL, Blois MS (1984) The frequency of local recurrence and microsatellites as a guide to reexcision margins for cutaneous malignant melanoma. Ann Surg 200:759–763

32. Veronesi U, Cascinelli N (1991) Narrow excision (1 cm margin). A safe procedure for thin cutaneous melanoma. Arch Surg 126:438–441

33. Balch CM, Urist MM, Karakousis CP, Smith TJ, Temple WJ, Drzewiecki K, Jewell WR, Bartolucci AA, Mihm MC, Barnhill R, Wanebo HJ (1993) Efficacy of 2-cm surgical margins for intermediate-thickness melanomas (1–4 mm). Ann Surg 218:262–269

34. Balch CM (1980) Surgical management of regional lymph nodes in cutaneous melanoma. J Am Acad Dermatol 3:511–524

35. Cascinelli N, Morabito A, Santinami M, MacKie RM, Belli F (1998) Immediate or delayed dissection of regional nodes in patients with melanoma of the trunk: a randomised trial. Lancet 351:793–796

36. McCarthy JG, Haagensen CD, Herter FP (1973) The role of groin dissection in the management of melanoma of the lower extremity. Ann Surg 179:156–159
37. Goldsmith HS, Shah JP, Kim D-H (1970) Prognostic significance of lymph node dissection in the treatment of malignant melanoma. Cancer 26:606–609
38. Veronesi U, Adamus J, Bandiera DC, Brennhovd IO, Caceres E, Cascinelli N, Claudio F, Ikonopisov RL, Javorski VV, Kirov S, Kulakowski A, Lacour J, Lejeune F, Mechl Z, Morabito A, Rode I, Sergeev S, van Slooten E, Szczygiel K, Trapeznikov NN, Wagner RI (1982) Delayed regional lymph node dissection in stage I melanoma of the skin of the lower extremities. Cancer 49:2420–2430
39. Veronesi U, Adamus J, Bandiera DC, Brennhovd IO, Caceres E, Cascinelli N, Claudio F, Ikonopisov RL, Javorski VV, Kirov S, Kulakowski A, Lacour J, Lejeune F, Mechl Z, Morabito A, Rode I, Sergeev S, van Slooten E, Szczygiel K, Trapeznikov NN, Wagner RI (1977) Inefficacy of immediate node dissection in stage 1 melanoma of the limbs. N Engl J Med 297:627–630
40. Urist MM, Maddox WA, Kennedy JE, Balch CM (1983) Patient risk factors and surgical morbidity after regional lymphadenectomy in 204 melanoma patients. Cancer 51:2152–2156
41. Karakousis CP, Heiser MA, Moore RH (1983) Lymphedema after groin dissection. Am J Surg 145:205–208
42. Reintgen D, Cruse CW, Wells K, Berman C, Fenske N, Glass F, Schroer K, Heller R, Ross M, Lyman G, Cox C, Rappaport D, Seigler HF, Balch C (1994) The orderly progression of melanoma nodal metastases. Ann Surg 220:759–767
43. North JH, Spellman JE (1996) Role of sentinel lymph node biopsy in the management of malignant melanoma. Oncology 10:1237–1242
44. Essner R (1997) The role of lymphoscintigraphy and sentinel lymph node mapping in assessing patient risk in melanoma. Semin Oncol 24 (suppl 4):S4–S-S4–10
45. Wanebo HJ, Harpole D, Teates CD (1985) Radionuclide lymphoscintigraphy with technecium 99 m antimony sulfide colloid to identify lymphatic drainage of cutaneous melanoma at ambiguous sites in the head and neck and trunk. Cancer 55:1403–1413
46. Albertini JJ, Cruse CW, Rappaport D, Wells K, Ross M, DeConti R, Berman CG, Jared K, Messina J, Lyman G, Glass F, Fenske N, Reintgen DS (1996) Intraoperative radiolymphoscintigraphy improves sentinel lymph node identification for patients with melanoma. Ann Surg 223:217–224
47. Wang X, Heller R, VanVoorhis N et al. (1994) Detection of submicroscopic metastases with polymerase chain reaction in patients with malignant melanoma. Ann Surg 220:768–777
48. Jenrette JM (1996) Malignant melanoma: the role of radiation therapy revisited. Semin Oncol 6:759–762
49. Ang KK, Byers RM, Peters LJ, Maor MH, Wendt CD, Morrison WH, Goepfert H (1990) Regional radiotherapy as adjuvant treatment for head and neck malignant melanoma. Arch Otolaryngol Head Neck Surg 116:169–172
50. Shaw PM, Sivanandham M, Bernik SF, Ditaranto K, Wallack MK (1997) Adjuvant immunotherapy for patients with melanoma: are patients with melanoma of the head and neck candidates for this therapy? Head and Neck 19:595–603
51. Veronesi U, Adamus J, Aubert C, Bajetta E, Beretta G, Bonadonna G, Bufalino R, Cascinelli N, Cocconi G, Durand J, De Marsillac J, Ikonopisov RL, Kiss B, Lejeune F, MacKie R, Madej G, Mulder H, Mechl Z, Milton GW, Morabito A, Peter H, Priario J, Paul E, Rumke P, Sertoli R, Tomin R (1982) A randomized trial of adjuvant chemotherapy and immunotherapy in cutaneous melanoma. N Engl J Med 307:913–916
52. Pectasides D, Alevizakos N, Bafaloukos D, Tzonou A, Asimakopoulos G, Varthalitis I, Dimitriadis M, Athanassiou A (1994) Adjuvant chemotherapy with dacarba-

zine,vindesine, and cisplatin in pathological stage II malignant melanoma. Am J Clin Oncol 17:55–59

53. Kirkwood JM, Strawderman MH, Ernstoff MS, Smith TJ, Borden EC, Blum RH (1996) Interferon alpha-2b adjuvant therapy of high-risk resected cutaneous melanoma: the Eastern Cooperative Oncology Group trial EST 1684. J Clin Oncol 14:7–17

54. Cole BF, Gelber RD, Kirkwood JM, Goldhirsch A, Barylak E, Borden E (1996) Quality-of-life-adjusted survival analysis of interferon alpha-2b adjuvant treatment of high-risk resected cutaneous melanoma: an Eastern Cooperative Oncology Group study. J Clin Oncol 14:2666–2673

55. Balch C, Buzaid AC (1996) Finally, a successful adjuvant therapy for high-risk melanoma. J Clin Oncol 14:1–3

56. Eilber FR, Morton DL, Holmes EC, Sparks FC, Ramming KP (1976) Adjuvant immunotherapy with BCG in treatment of regional-lymph-node metastases from malignant melanoma. N Engl J Med 294:237–240

57. Spitler LE (1991) A randomized trial of levamisole versus placebo as adjuvant therapy in malignant melanoma. J Clin Oncol 9:736–740

58. Livingston PO, Wong GYC, Adluri S, Tao Y, Padavan M, Parente R, Hanlon C, Calves MJ, Helling F, Ritter G, Oettgen HF, Old LJ (1994) Improved survival in stage III melanoma patients with GM2 antibodies: a randomized trial of adjuvant vaccination with GM2 ganglioside. J Clin Oncol 12:1036–1044

59. Hill GJ, Krementz ET, Hill HZ (1984) Dimethyl triazeno imidazole carboxamide and combination therapy for melanoma. Cancer 53:1299–1305

60. Icli F, Karaoguz H, Dincol D, Gunel N, Demirkazik A (1991) Treatment of metastatic malignant melanoma with 24 h continuous intravenous infusion of dacarbazine and cisplatin. J Surg Oncol 48:199–201

61. Verschraegen CF, Kleeberg UR, Mulder J, Rumke P, Truchetet F, Czarnetzki B, Rozencweig M, Thomas D, Suciu S (1988) Combination of cisplatin, vindesine, and dacarbazine in advanced malignant melanoma. Cancer 62:1061–1065

62. Lee SM, Margison GP, Woodcock AA, Thatcher N (1993) Sequential administration of varying doses of dacarbazine and fotemustine in advanced malignant melanoma. Br J Cancer 67:1356–1360

63. Kleeberg UR (1997) Wishful thinking, unicentric empiricism and the everyday world of the medical melanomologist. Melanoma Res 7 (suppl 2):S143-S149

64. Anderson CM, Buzaid AC, Legha SS (1995) Systemic treatments for advanced cutaneous melanoma. Oncology 9:1149–1158

65. Del Prete SA, Maurer LH, O'Donnell J, Forcier RJ, LeMarbre P (1984) Combination chemotherapy with cisplatin, carmustine, dacarbazine, and tamoxifen in metastatic melanoma. Cancer Treat Rep 68:1403–1405

66. Legha SS, Ring S, Papadopoulos N et al. (1989) A prospective evaluation of a triple-drug regimen containing cisplatin, vinblastine, and dacarbazine (CVD) for metastatic melanoma. Cancer 64:2024–2029

67. Seigler HF, Lucas VS, Pickett NJ, Huang AT (1980) DTIC, CCNU, bleomycin, and vincristine (BOLD) in metastatic melanoma. Cancer 46:2346–2348

68. Richards JM, Gilewski TA, Ramming K, Mitchel B, Doane LL, Vogelzang NJ (1992) Effective chemotherapy for melanoma after treatment with interleukin-2. Cancer 69:427–429

69. Luikart S, Kemealey G, Kirkwood J (1984) Randomized phase III trial of vinblastine, bleomycin, cis-dichlorodiamine-platinum versus dacarbazine in malignant melanoma. J Clin Oncol 2:164–168

70. Buzaid A, Legha S, Winn R et al. (1993) Cisplatin, vinblastine, and dacarbazine versus dacarbazine alone in metastatic melanoma: preliminary results of a phase III Cancer Community Oncology Program (CCOP) trial. Proc Am Soc Clin Oncol 12:389

71. Costanzi JJ, Al-Sarraf M, Groppe C, Bottomley R, Fabian C, Neidhart J, Dixon D (1982) Combination chemotherapy plus BCG in the treatment of disseminated malignant melanoma: A Southwest Oncology Group study. Med Ped Oncol 10:251–258

72. Creagan ET, Ingle JN, Green SJ, Ahmann DL, Jiang N-S (1980) Phase II study of tamoxifen in patients with disseminated malignant melanoma. Cancer Treat Rep 64:199–201

73. McClay EF, Mastrangelo MJ, Sprandio JD, Bellet RE, Berd D (1989) The importance of tamoxifen to a cisplatin-containing regimen in the treatment of metastatic melanoma. Cancer 63:1292–1295

74. McClay EF, Mastrangelo MJ, Bellet RE, Berd D (1987) Combination chemotherapy and hormonal therapy in the treatment of malignant melanoma. Cancer Treat Rep 71:465–469

75. Flaherty LE, Liu PY, Mitchell MS, Fletcher WS, Walker MJ, Goodwin JW, Stephens RL, Sondak VK (1996) The addition of tamoxifen to dacarbazine and cisplatin in metastatic malignant melanoma. Am J Clin Oncol 19:108–113

76. Margolin KA, Liu P-Y, Flaherty LE, Sosman JA, Walker MJ, Smith JWI, Fletcher WS, Weiss GR, Unger JM, Sondak VK (1998) Phase II study of carmustine, dacarbazine, cisplatin, and tamoxifen in advanced melanoma: a Southwest Oncology Group study. J Clin Oncol 16:664–669

77. Cocconi G, Bella M, Calabresi F, Tonato M, Canaletti R, Boni C, Buzzi F, Ceci G, Corgna E, Costa P, Lottici R, Papadia F, Sofra MC, Bacchi M (1992) Treatment of metastatic malignant melanoma with dacarbazine plus tamoxifen. N Engl J Med 327:516–523

78. Rusthoven JJ, Quirt IC, Iscoe NA, McCulloch PB, James KW, Lohmann RC, Jensen J, Burdette-Radoux S, Bodurtha AJ, Silver HKB, Verma S, Armitage GR, Zee B, Bennett K (1996) Randomized, double-blind, placebo-controlled trial comparing the response rates of carmustine, dacarbazine, and cisplatin with and without tamoxifen in patients with metastatic melanoma. J Clin Oncol 14:2083–2090

79. Steffens TA, Bajorin DF, Chapman PB, Lovett DR, Cody-Johnson BV, Templeton MA, Heelan RT, Wong GY, Portlock CS, Oettgen HF, Houghton AN (1991) A phase II trial of high-dose cisplatin and dacarbazine. Lack of efficacy of high-dose, cisplatin-based therapy for metastatic melanoma. Cancer 68:1230–1237

80. Wolff SN, Herzig RH, Fay JW, LeMaistre CF, Frei-Lahr D, Lowder J, Bolwell B, Giannone L, Herzig GP (1989) High-dose thiotepa with autologous bone marrow transplantation for metastatic malignant melanoma: Results of phase I and phase II studies of the North American Bone Marrow Transplantation Group. J Clin Oncol 7:245–249

81. Shea T, Graham M, Bernard S, Steagall A, Wiley J, Serody J, Brecher M, Bentley S, Johnston C, Vaisman A, Chaney S, Letrent S, Brouwer K (1995) A clinical and pharmacokinetic study of high-dose carboplatin, paclitaxel, granulocyte colony-stimulating factor, and peripheral blood stem cells in patients with unresectable metastatic cancer. Semin Oncol 22:80–85

82. Philip PA, Flaherty L (1997) Treatment of malignant melanoma with interleukin-2. Semin Oncol 24 (suppl 4):S4–32-S4–38

83. Legha SS (1997) The role of interferon alpha in the treatment of metastatic melanoma. Semin Oncol 24 (suppl 4):S4–24-S4–31

84. Keilholz U, Stoter G, Punt CJA, Scheibenbogen C, Lejeune F, Eggermont AMM (1997) Recombinant interleukin-2-based treatments for advanced melanoma: the experience of the European Organization for Research and Treatment of Cancer Melanoma Cooperative Group. Cancer J Sci Am 3:S22-S28

85. Wadler S (1991) The role of interferons in the treatment of solid tumors. Cancer 70:949–958

86. Keilholz U, Scheibenbogen C, Tilgen W, Bergmann L, Weidmann E, Seither E, Richter M, Brado B, Mitrou PS, Hunstein W (1993) Interferon-α and interleukin-2 in the treatment of metastatic melanoma. Comparison of two phase II trials. Cancer 72:607–614

87. Legha SS, Buzaid AC (1993) Role of recombinant interleukin-2 in combination with interferon-alpha and chemotherapy in the treatment of advanced melanoma. Semin Oncol 20:27–32

88. Pyrhonen S, Hahka-Kemppinen M, Muhonen T (1992) A promising interferon plus four-drug chemotherapy regimen for metastatic melanoma. J Clin Oncol 10:1919–1926

89. Khayat D, Borel C, Tourani JM, Benhammouda A, Antoine E, Rixe O, Vuillemin E, Bazex PA, Thill L, Franks R, Auclerc G, Soubrane C, Banzet P, Weil M (1993) Sequential chemoimmunotherapy with cisplatin, interleukin-2, and interferon alpha-2a for metastatic melanoma. J Clin Oncol 11:2173–2180

90. Richards JM, Mehta N, Ramming K, Skosey P (1992) Sequential chemoimmunotherapy in the treatment of metastatic melanoma. J Clin Oncol 10:1338–1343

91. Legha SS, Ring S, Bedikian A, Plager C, Eton O, Buzaid AC, Papadopoulos N (1996) Treatment of metastatic melanoma with combined chemotherapy containing cisplatin, vinblastine and dacarbazine (CVD) and biotherapy using interleukin-2 and interferon-α. Ann Oncol 7:827–835

92. Legha SS, Ring S, Eton O, Bedikian A, Buzaid AC, Plager C, Papadopoulos N (1998) Development of a biochemotherapy regimen with concurrent administration of cisplatin, vinblastine, dacarbazine, interferon alpha, and interleukin-2 for patients with metastatic melanoma. J Clin Oncol 16:1752–1759

93. O'Day SJ, Martin M, Boasberg P, Weisberg MC, Fawzy N, Guo M, Nguyen LT, Kristedja T, Fournier P, Nizze A, Olilia D, Essner R, Foshag L, Morton D, Hoon D, Gammon G, DeGregorio MW, Cabot M (1998) Escalating doses of tamoxifen in a phase I/II trial of concurrent biochemotherapy with decrescendo interleukin-2, and filgrastim (G-CSF) support in patients with metastatic melanoma. Proc Am Soc Clin Oncol 17:508a (Abstract)

94. Thompson JA, Gold PJ, Fefer A (1997) Outpatient chemoimmunotherapy for the treatment of metastatic melanoma. Semin Oncol 24 (suppl 4):S4–44, S4–48

95. Sparano JA, Fisher RI, Sunderland M, Margolin K, Ernest ML, Sznol M, Atkins MB, Dutcher JP, Micetich KC, Weiss GR, Doroshow JH, Aronson FR, Rubinstein LV, Mier JW (1993) Randomized phase III trial of treatment with high-dose interleukin-2 either alone or in combination with interferon alpha-2a in patients with advanced melanoma. J Clin Oncol 11:1969–1977

96. Bajetta E, Di Leo A, Zampino MG, Sertoli MR, Comella G, Barduagni M, Giannotti B, Queirolo P, Tribbia G, Bernengo MG, Menichetti ET, Palmeri S, Russo A, Cristofolini M, Erbazzi A, Fowst C, Criscuolo D, Bufalino R, Zilembo N, Cascinelli N (1994) Multicenter randomized trial of dacarbazine alone or in combination with two different doses and schedules of interferon alpha-2a in the treatment of advanced melanoma. J Clin Oncol 12:806–811

97. Falkson CI, Ibrahim J, Kirkwood JM, Coates AS, Atkins MB, Blum RH (1998) Phase III trial of dacarbazine versus dacarbazine with interferon α-2b versus dacarbazine with tamoxifen versus dacarbazine with interferon α-2b and tamoxifen in patients with metastatic malignant melanoma: an Eastern Cooperative Oncology Group study. J Clin Oncol 16:1743–1751

98. Negrier S, Escudier B, Lasset C, Douillard J-Y, Savary J, Chevreau C, Ravaud A, Mercatello A, Peny J, Mosseau M, Philip T, Tursz T (1998) Recombinant human interleukin-2, recombinant interferon alpha-2a, or both in metastatic renal-cell carcinoma. N Engl J Med 338:1272–1278

99. Shumate CR, Urist MM, Maddox WA (1995) Melanoma recurrence surveillance: Patient or physician based? Ann Surg 221:566–569
100. Cascinelli N, Bufalino R, Morabito A, MacKie R (1994) Results of adjuvant interferon study in WHO melanoma programme. Lancet 343:913–914
101. El Kassas H, Kirkwood JM (1996) Adjuvant application of interferons. Semin Oncol 23:737–743
102. Creagan ET, Dalton RJ, Ahmann DL, Jung S-H, Morton RF, Langdon RM, Kugler J, Rodrigue LJ (1995) Randomized, surgical adjuvant clinical trial of recombinant interferon alpha-2a in selected patients with malignant melanoma. J Clin Oncol 13:2776–2783
103. Miller DM, Jones D, Partin ML, Urist M, Ebbinghaus S, Mattar B, Redden D (1998) Effective interleukin-2 based adjuvant therapy for high risk malignant melanoma patients. Proc Am Soc Clin Oncol 17:507a (Abstract)
104. Gajewski TF, Fallarino F (1997) Rational development of tumour antigen-specific immunization in melanoma. Therapeutic Immunol 2:211–225
105. Mitchell MS, Harel W, Kempf RA, Hu E, Kan-Mitchell J, Boswell WD, Dean G, Stevenson L (1990) Active-specific immunotherapy for melanoma. J Clin Oncol 8:856–869
106. Marchand M, Weynants P, Rankin E, Arienti F, Belli F, Parmiani G, Cascinelli N, Bourlond A, Vanwijck R, Humblet Y, Canon J-L, Laurent C, Naeyaert J-M, Plagne R, Deraemaeker R, Knuth A, Jager E, Brasseur F, Herman J, Coulie PG, Boon T (1995) Tumor regression responses in melanoma patients treated with a peptide encoded by gene MAGE-3. Int J Cancer 63:883–885
107. Nestle FO, Alijagic S, Gilliet M, Sun Y, Grabbe S, Dummer R, Burg G, Schadendorf D (1998) Vaccination of melanoma patients with peptide- or tumor lysate-pulsed dendritic cells. Nature Med 4:328–332
108. Saven A, Kawasaki H, Carrera CJ, Waltz T, Copeland B, Zyroff J, Kosty M, Carson DA, Beutler E, Piro LD (1993) 2-chlorodeoxyadenosine dose escalation in nonhematologic malignancies. J Clin Oncol 11:671–678
109. Chang A, Hunt M, Parkinson DR, Hochster H, Smith TJ (1993) Phase II trial of carboplatin in patients with metastatic malignant melanoma. Am J Clin Oncol 16:152–155
110. Jones AL, O'Brien ME, Lorentzos A, Viner C, Hanrahan A, Moore J, Millar JL, Gore ME (1992) A randomised phase II study of carmustine alone or in combination with tumour necrosis factor in patients with advanced melanoma. Cancer Chem Pharm 30:73–76
111. Katz ME, Glick JH (1979) Nitrosoureas: a reappraisal of clinical trials. Cancer Clin Trials 2:297–316
112. Mortimer JE, Shulman S, MacDonald JS, Kopecky K, Goodman G (1990) High-dose cisplatin in disseminated melanoma: a comparison of two schedules. Cancer Chem Pharm 25:373–376
113. Gottlieb JA, Mendelson D, Serpick AA (1970) An evaluation of large intermittent intravenous doses of cyclophosphamide (NSC-26271) in the treatment of metastatic malignant melanoma. Cancer Chemother Rep 54:365–367
114. Bedikian AY, Weiss GR, Legha SS, Burris HA, Eckardt JR, Jenkins J, Eton O, Buxaid AC, Smetzer L, Von Hoff DD, Benjamin RS (1995) Phase II trial of docetaxel in patients with advanced cuteneous malignant melanoma previously untreated with chemotherapy. J Clin Oncol 13:2895–2899
115. Falkson CI, Falkson G, Falkson HC (1994) Phase II trial of fotemustine in patients with metastatic malignant melanoma. Invest New Drugs 12:251–254
116. Khayat D, Avril MF, Gerard B, Bertrand P, Bizzari JP, Cour V (1992) Fotemustine: and overview of its clinical activity in disseminated malignant melanoma. Melanoma Res 2:147–151

117. Gottlieb JA, Frei E, Luce JK (1971) Dose-schedule studies with hydroxyurea (NSC-32065) in malignant melanoma. Cancer Chemother Rep 55:277–280
118. Lerner HJ, Beckloff GL, Godwin MC (1970) Phase II study of hydroxyurea administered intermittently in malignant melanoma. Am Surgeon 36:505–508
119. Cassileth PA, Hyman GA (1967) Treatment of malignant melanoma with hydroxyurea. Cancer Res 27:1843–1845
120. Costanzi JJ, Stephens R, O'Bryan R, Franks J (1982) Ifosfamide in the management of malignant melanoma: a Southwest Oncology Group phase II study. Semin Oncol 9:93–95
121. Ahmann DL (1976) Nitrosoureas in the management of disseninated malignant melanoma. Cancer Treat Rep 60:747–751
122. Godfrey TE, Wilbur DW (1972) Clinical experience with mitomycin C in large infrequent doses. Cancer 29:1647–1652
123. Roche H, Guiochet N, Kerbrat P, Rebattu P, Fargeot P, Cattan A, Armand JP, Keiling R, Lentz MA, Van Glabeke M, Herait P, Fumoleau P (1993) Phase II trials of tetrahydropyranyl-adriamycin (Pirarubicin) on renal and colon carcinoma, melanoma, and soft tissue sarcoma. Am J Clin Oncol 16:137–139
124. Feun LG, Gonzalez R, Savaraj N, Hanlon J, Collier M, Robinson WA, Clendeninn NJ (1991) Phase II trial of piritrexim in metastatic melanoma using intermittent, low-dose administration. J Clin Oncol 9:464–467
125. Wiernik PH, Schwartz EL, Einzig A, Strauman JJ, Lipton RB, Dutcher JP (1987) Phase I trial of Taxol given as a 24-hour infusion every 21 days: Responses observed in metastatic melanoma. J Clin Oncol 5:1232–1239
126. Legha SS, Ring S, Papadopoulos N, Raber M, Benjamin RS (1990) A phase II trial of Taxol in metastatic melanoma. Cancer 65:2478–2481
127. Lokich JJ, Zipoli TE, Perri J, Bothe A (1984) Protracted vinblastine infusion. Phase I-II study in malignant melanoma and other tumors. Am J Clin Oncol 7:551–553
128. Quagliand JM, Stephens RL, Baker LH et al. (1984) Vindesine in patients with metastatic malignant melanoma: a Southwest Oncology Group study. J Clin Oncol 4:316–319
129. Olver I, Green M, Peters W, Zimet A, Toner G, Bishop J, Ketelbey W, Rastogi R, Birkhofer M (1995) A phase II trial of zeniplatin in metastatic melanoma. Am J Clin Oncol 18:56–58

# Skin Neoplasms Other than Melanoma

K. Soltani, H.D. Mandel

## Introduction

Cutaneous tumors are among the most common neoplasms found in humans. Many of these tumors are either benign or behave in a relatively nonaggressive manner. There are skin tumors, however, that if undiagnosed early in their course will invade, metastasize, and cause death.

Similar to most malignancies, cutaneous non-melanoma tumors may be classified as: (a) premalignant, (b) in-situ, and (c) malignant.

Among the premalignant lesions one may include actinic (solar) keratosis, arsenical keratosis, leukoplakia, and keratoses induced by other physical factors, such as thermal and radiation energy. The prototype of in situ lesions is Bowen's disease and its variants such as erythroplasia of Queyrat. The malignant neoplasms of skin include basal cell carcinoma (the most common tumor found in man), squamous cell carcinoma, and adnexal carcinomas (which arise from pilosebaceous units or sweat structures).

The incidence of skin tumors depends on factors such as ethnic origin, geographic location (both latitude and altitude), exposure to industrial pollutants, as well as occupational and recreational sun exposure. In cutaneous adnexal tumors the incidence increases with age, especially after the seventh decade of life. Although morphologically and histopathologically adnexal tumors resemble basal cell carcinomas, they have a more aggressive behavior and may metastasize.

In caucasians, basal cell carcinomas are by far more common than squamous cell carcinomas (4:1 ratio in U.S.). However, this ratio does not always apply to immunocompromised patients and in areas such as the ear and lower lip, where squamous cell carcinomas predominate. Similar inverse ratios may apply to patients of African and Asian origin.

In this chapter we will focus on the most common skin tumors including basal and squamous cell carcinomas, and will briefly mention features common to adnexal tumors with malignant potential.

## Premalignant Tumors of the Epidermis

Actinic Keratosis

Clinically, actinic keratoses are sharply demarcated, minimally raised plaques with variable degree of scales, on sun-exposed areas of skin such as the face, neck, bald scalp, forearms and dorsal aspects of hands. They increase in number with age and may become hypertrophic. Hypertrophic actinic keratoses are more likely to evolve into invasive tumors.

Histologically, actinic keratoses show hyperkeratosis and parakeratosis (presence of nuclear remnants in the stratum corneum), acanthosis (thickening of the epidermis), as well as loss of polarity, crowding, and nuclear atypia of the basal layer keratinocytes. Solar elastosis is noted in the dermis. Other variants of actinic keratoses include hypertrophic, lichenoid, and bowenoid types. Some lesions, especially on the hand dorsa and forearms, become inflamed with an underlying band-like inflammatory infiltrate in the dermis – the so called lichenoid actinic keratoses. The vast majority of actinic keratoses remain stable for many decades. However, some lesions, especially in immunosuppressed patients (chemotherapy, AIDS, transplantation, etc.) have a more aggressive course. For practical purposes, the age-related mild immunosuppression may be considered a promoting factor in the elderly.

The treatment of actinic keratosis may vary from periodic observation and follow-up to local destruction of individual lesions by such modalities as cryosurgery and electrosurgery. Large numbers of lesions may be treated by application of 5-fluorouracil (5-FU) 1%–5% cream BID for three to four weeks, which may cause significant temporary inflammation in the treated areas. This treatment may be modified by reducing the application to twice weekly, but prolonging the treatment course, e.g. six to eight weeks, to avoid significant inflammatory-induced discomfort. Clinically inconspicuous lesions become more visible by topical use of 5-FU, but are equally responsive to therapy. As with other multiple skin tumors, retinoids may prevent or reduce the development of actinic keratoses in susceptible individuals such as transplant recipients who are immunosuppressed [1, 2].


## Arsenical Keratosis

These keratoses are much less common, but may be encountered in people coming from areas where the sources of drinking water (usually wells) have significant levels of arsenic, or in patients with therapeutic, industrial, or incidental exposure to arsenic. They are associated with keratotic pits on the palms and soles. There is a higher incidence of other tumors, e.g. nasopharyngeal tumors, gastroesophageal carcinoma, bladder carcinoma, hepatic angiosarcoma, chronic leukemia and Bowen's disease [3–5].

Histologically, they are similar to hypertrophic actinic keratoses, except for the presence of numerous vacuolated keratinocytes.

Treatment includes application of various destructive methods such as electrosurgery, cryosurgery, laser ablation, and possibly systemic retinoids.


## Other Premalignant Keratoses

Keratoses caused by ionizing electromagnetic radiation (superficial and deep X-ray, Grenz rays, and gamma rays) occur in persons whose skins are exposed occupationally and therapeutically to these rays. Clinically and histologically they are similar to actinic keratoses. In addition, the surrounding skin shows changes of radiation dermatitis such as thinning of the skin, mottled pigmentary changes and telangiectasias. Histological preparations demonstrate evidence of radiation damage in superficial and deep dermis including degeneration of collagen, fibrosis, dilated capillaries and vascular occlusion. These keratoses should be treated as they may evolve into aggressive squamous cell carcinomas. The treatment options are similar to those for actinic keratoses.

Keratoses induced by heat energy within the infrared spectrum may occur de novo or in association with erythema ab igne, a pattern of mottled hyperpigmentation secondary to chronically applied heat energy. In patients who habitually sit in front of a fireplace, anterior aspects of lower extremities are the most commonly involved sites.

These keratoses have clinical and histological features similar to those of actinic keratoses and respond to the same treatment modalities.

## In Situ Malignancies of the Epidermis

### Bowen's Disease

These lesions are the prototype of the in situ tumors of the epidermis. Bowen's disease and its variants often affect persons over 60 years of age. Histologically some actinic keratoses which occur on sun-exposed skin have bowenoid features but behave like other actinic keratoses. True Bowen's disease, however, which is an in situ squamous cell carcinoma, has a more aggressive behavior. Although the majority remain in situ, an invasive squamous cell carcinoma will eventually develop in some of these lesions [6, 7]. Human papilloma virus may play a role in the pathogenesis of some Bowen's lesions. It remains controversial as to whether Bowen's disease is associated with a higher incidence of systemic malignancy. This association might be more germane in patients who have been exposed to arsenic.

Clinically, the characteristic lesion is a well-demarcated, hyperkeratotic, erythematous or pigmented plaque on either sun-exposed and sun-protected skin. It may involve the nail bed, or external genitalia. On mucus membranes, Bowen's disease may appear as an erythematous plaque or a white scaly patch. The lesions may clinically resemble other inflammatory and neoplastic conditions such as psoriasis, dermatitis, seborrheic keratosis, superficial basal cell carcinoma and amelanotic malignant melanoma.

Histologically, the main features are those of abnormal architecture and keratinocyte atypia throughout the epidermis including the basal layer. These abnormalities extend into the follicular infundibulum. Thus complete surgical excision of the lesion should include the underlying appendageal structures of the skin. Bowen's disease should be histologically differentiated from other intraepithelial neoplasms, such as Paget's disease of breast, extramammary Paget's disease and malignant melanoma. Erythroplasia (or erythroplakia) is a distinct variant of Bowen's disease which occurs on mucosal surfaces. When it occurring on glans penis, it is often referred to as erythroplasia of Queyrat, and is predominantly seen in uncircumcised men.

Although, when properly used, topical 5-FU, cryosurgery and radiation therapy are effective modalities, Bowen's disease is best treated by excision.

## Leukoplakia

Leukoplakia is a clinical term indicating a white patch on the oral and anal mucosae, or vulvar and cervical epithelia. HPV may be implicated in the pathogenesis of some of these lesions [6, 8, 9]. In the mouth it may be the result of heavy tobacco and alcohol use. The highest risk areas are the floor of the mouth, ventrolateral tongue, and soft palate. A 1% toluidine blue rinse or paint may help delineate the abnormal mucosa. The pathological changes in leukoplakia are benign in 80% (referred to as leukokeratosis), with 17% of specimens showing in situ carcinoma and 3% invasive squamous cell carcinoma [6, 10]. Excision is the treatment of choice for leukoplakia.

## Malignant Tumors of the Skin

### Basal Cell Carcinoma

Basal cell carcinoma (epithelioma) is the most common malignant skin tumor. In the U.S. over 400,000 cases are diagnosed each year [11, 12]. Although most patients are older than 40 years of age, basal cell carcinomas may be detected in much younger individuals. It occurs mostly on sun-exposed skin especially face and neck. Although UV radiation is the major implicating factor for basal cell carcinoma, occasional lesions appear on sun-protected areas, such as scalp and posterior to the ears [13]. Previous exposure to ionizing radiation in patients who receive radiotherapy predisposes the skin to basal cell carcinoma. Similarly, arsenic may lead to the development of superficial basal cell carcinomas [13, 14]. There is a 45% five-year cumulative rate of one or more new tumors developing in patients sho have had a basal cell carcinoma [15].

These tumors may occur as part of nevoid basal cell carcinoma syndrome, xeroderma pigmentosum, albinism and depigmented macules of vitiligo. The nevoid basal cell carcinoma syndrome (basal cell nevus syndrome) is an autosomal dominant disorder associated with multiple basal cell carcinomas starting in young adults, palmoplantar pitting, mandibular cysts, partial agenesis of the corpus callosum, bifid ribs, and hypertelorism. Other tumors, such as ovarian fibroma and medulloblastoma may also occur in these patients [13]. A mutation of the human homologue of the fruit fly patched gene has recently been found in both nevoid basal cell syndrome and sporadic basal cell carcinomas [16]. Most basal cell carcinomas are seen in light-skinned individuals. However, basal cell carcinomas can occur in darker individuals, including persons of African and Hispanic ancestry. The incidence is higher in men than women.

Typically basal cell carcinomas appear as pearly papules covered by a telangiectatic surface. Larger lesions may ulcerate and bleed. Five clinical types are known: 1) noduloulcerative; 2) pigmented; 3) morpheaform; 4) superficial; 5) basal cell carcinomas arising from underlying skin lesions such as fibroepithelioma or nevus sebaceous of Jadassohn.

Histologically, basal carcinoma lesions show basaloid collections of cells arising from the epidermis extending into the dermis with peripheral palisading. The cells have a large nucleus and scant cytoplasm. The nuclei appear uniform in size and contour. Mitotic figures are not prominent.

Treatment for basal cell carcinoma would depend on factors such as site, size and the histological features of the lesion, age, and the patient's general state of health. Fibrosing or morpheaform basal cell carcinomas often are larger than clinically appreciated and require excision, and the adequacy of surgical excision should be histologically confirmed [17, 18].

The first treatment option is either cryosurgery or curettage and electrodessication. By these methods, the recurrence rate, when properly done, is about five percent [19]. Cryosurgery employs liquid nitrogen, and thermocouples may be used to assure that the desired low temperatures are reached in the lower margins of these tumors. The disadvantage of cryosurgery and curettage is the lack of histologic sections used for determining margin control. Complete excision provides the best cure rate, with a recurrence rate of around one percent [19]. High recurrence rates, 33% or more, have been noted in incompletely excised tumors [19, 20]. Radiation therapy, either orthovoltage X-ray or electron beam, is predominantly used for tumors of the central face, including eyelids, nose, and lips [21]. Recurrence may occur even ten years or more after initial treatment [19]. Aesthetic results are excellent, especially when doses are properly fractionated [21, 22]. Radiation therapy is recommended in patients older than 60 years because of long term sequelae including atrophy, erythema, and irregularity of the skin [18]. Mohs microgaphic surgery using the fresh tissue technique is preferred for the treatment of recurrent basal cell carcinomas and for areas with a high risk of recurrence. This method provides a very high cure rate [21]. Photodynamic therapy uses a combination of a photosensitizer and long wavelength visible light and O2 to selectively destroy tumor cells. Sensitizers include porphyrin derivatives, hematoporphyrin and dihematoporphyrin ether which are injected, or 5-aminolevulinic acid which is applied topically. Superficial basal cell carcinomas have a superior cure rate than noduloulcerative lesions with this method [23, 24]. Interferon alpha-2b has been tried as a treatment option and may yield an 80% cure rate at one year following treatment [25]. Retinoids and 5-FU are mainly used for large numbers of lesions such as in patients with basal cell nevus syndrome [26–28].

## Squamous Cell carcinoma

Squamous cell carcinoma is the second most common malignant skin neoplasm, with over 100,000 new cases occurring each year in the U.S. [29, 30]. Most patients are over 40 years of age. The ratio of basal carcinoma to squamous cell carcinoma is about 4:1 [31, 32]. Predisposing factors include UV irradiation, thermal burns, ionizing radiation, exposure to hydrocarbons, arsenic ingestion, immunosuppression (organ transplantation and HIV), chronic wounds and draining sinuses, and human papilloma virus [31]. Squamous cell carcinomas are more common than basal cell carcinomas in both dark-skinned and immunosuppressed patients [29, 31].

Squamous cell carcinomas occur early in life in xeroderma pigmentosum, where the needed enzymes to repair UV-damaged DNA are deficient, oculocutaneous albinism, in which patients lack melanin pigment, and epidermodysplasia verruciformis, a rare inherited condition with high susceptibility to papilloma virus. PUVA (psoralen with ultraviolet light) therapy is an additional risk factor.

Clinically the tumor is a well-defined, flesh-colored or red, scaly, thick plaque, which may start de novo or develop on a pre-existing actinic keratosis. Lesions have a scaly surface and may be ulcerated or crusted. The most common sites are the head and neck (84%) and the sun-exposed skin of the upper extremity (13%) [33]. In tumors arising from actinic keratoses, early regional metastasis is uncommon [31]. Metastasis is more common in lesions located on the ear, scalp and extremities [33]. Squamous cell carcinomas of the lower lip, when thicker than 6 mm, have a 74% metastatic rate [31, 34]. Similarly, high rates of metastasis are noted in tumors associated with chronic inflammatory conditions such as burns and osteomyelitic sinuses [6, 35, 36]. More aggressive forms such as the spindle cell type squamous cell carcinoma may develop in transplant recipients [1, 37].

Keratoacanthoma may be considered as a special type of self-limited squamous cell carcinoma, and appears as a dome-shaped hyperkeratotic nodule with a central keratin plug on sun-exposed areas of skin in middle-aged or elderly patients, especially those with immunosuppression. It grows rapidly over 1–3 months and may subsequently undergo spontaneous regression over 6–12 months [6, 38].

Histologically squamous cell carcinomas may be characterized as well-differentiated, moderately differentiated, poorly differentiated, and the spindle cell variety. The well-differentiated type shows mature keratinocytes with individual cell keratinization and horn pearl formation. The moderately and poorly differentiated types show increasing cellular atypia and abnormal mitosis and less keratinization. Solar elastosis is often noted in the underlying dermis. The adenoid variant shows marked acantholysis of atypical keratinocytes. The Broders classification is a grading system based on the percentage of undifferentiated cells. In grade 1, more than 75%, in grade 2, more than 50%, in grade 3, more than 25%; and in grade 4, less than 25% of the keratinocytes are well-differentiated [39].

Keratoacanthomas show a horn-filled invagination of the epidermis with significantly less atypical keratinocytes. The dyskeratotic cells in these lesions have an eosinophilic, homogeneous appearance. The lesion is well-demarcated, by a collarette of the epidermis at the periphery. Immunohistochemical techniques may help the histological differential diagnosis of keratoacanthoma from squamous cell carcinoma, which is often difficult. BCL-2, a proto-oncogene that prevents apoptosis, is diminished in keratoacanthoma [40]. The P-53 proto-oncogene and the proliferating cell nuclear antigen (PCNA) are diffusely expressed in squamous cell carcinoma, while they are present only focally in keratoacanthoma [41]. Pseudocarcinomatous hyperplasia secondary to deep fungal infections or ingestion of halogenated compounds may mimic squamous cell carcinomas [31].

The treatment options for squamous cell carcinoma depend on the size, location, and depth of invasion. Small and minimally invasive lesions can be treated with superficial destructive methods. Excision is the mainstay of treatment for large and more advanced lesions, and those preceded by radiation dermatitis, scars or ulcers [31]. Margins of 1 cm or more are recommended for such excisions [33]. Mohs µgaphic surgery is recommended for recurrent tumors, as well as lesions arising in radiation sites or when the underlying bone and cartilage are invaded by the tumor [31]. Radiation may be the treatment of choice for large tumors in patients who are considered poor surgical risks. Cryosurgery may be used in selected small squamous cell carcinomas [31].

## Malignant Adnexal Tumors of Skin

These tumors derive from pilosebaceous units and eccrine sweat structures. There are dozens of entities in this category and the reader is recommended to refer to texts of dermatology and dermatopathology for their specific clinical and histopathological features [42, 43]. These tumors, however, share certain common characteristics:
– The incidence of these rare tumors sharply increases after the age of 80.
– They are difficult to diagnose clinically, and should be included in the differential diagnosis of clinically atypical skin tumors.
– The diagnosis almost always depends on the histopathological and/or immunohistochemical findings.
– Although morphologically they may resemble basal cell carcinomas, they behave aggressively like squamous cell carcinomas, and have the potential to metastasize.
– Adequate surgical excision is the treatment of choice for primary tumors. Metastatic lesions would require chemotherapy and/or radiation therapy.

## Prevention

Prevention is an essential aspect of skin cancer management. Patients who have had non-melanoma skin cancers require at least yearly follow-ups. Frequent self-examinations are helpful and should be recommended. Although often impractical, serial clinical photographs are of value in patients with multiple skin tumors. As ultraviolet plays a major role in the pathogenesis of skin keratoses and tumors, sun protection should be emphasized. A broad spectrum sunscreen (UVA/UVB) is crucial and sun protective clothing during the spring and summer months is also recommended. Patients should be reminded that skin damage occurs despite the use of sun screens and, when possible, sun exposure should be limited. Individuals with genetic syndromes such as albinism, xeroderma pigmentosum and basal cell nevus syndrome are particularly at high risk for the development of skin cancer and would have to be appropriately followed by their physician, and protected from sun light.

## References

1. Schwartz RA: The actinic keratosis: A perspective and update. Dermatol Surg 1997, 23:1009–18
2. Rook AH, Jaworsky C, Nguyen T et al.: Beneficial effect of low-dose systemic retinoid in combination with topical tretinoin for the treatment and prophylaxis of premalignant and malignant skin lesions in renal transplant recipients. Transplantation 1995, 59:714–9
3. Schwartz RA, Stoll HL: Epithelial precancerous lesions. In: Fitzpatrick TB, Eisen AZ, Wolff K et al., eds. Dermatology in General Medicine, 3rd ed. New York: μgraw-Hill; 1993. p.804–21
4. Chen C-J et al.: Arsenic and cancers. Lancet 1988; 1:414
5. Zaldivar R et al.: Arsenic dose in patients with cutaneous carcinomata and hepatic haemangio-endothelioma after environmental and occupational exposure. Arch Toxicol 1981, 47:145
6. Kirkham N: Tumors and cysts of the epidermis. In: Elder D, ed. Lever's Histopathology of the Skin. Philadelphia: Lippincott Raven; 1997. p 685–746
7. Kao GF. Editorial: Carcinoma arising in Bowen's disease. Arch Dermatol 1986; 122:1124
8. Löning T, Ikenberg H, Becker J et al.: Analysis of oral papillomas, leukoplakias, and invasive carcinomas for human papillomavirus type related DNA. J Invest Dermatol 1985, 84:417
9. Crum CP, Liskow A, Petras P et al.: Vulvar intraepithelial neoplasia: Severe atypia and carcinoma in situ. Cancer 1984, 54:1429
10. Waldron CA, Shafer WG: Leukoplakia revisited: a clinicopathologic study of 3256 leukoplakias. Cancer 1975, 36:1386
11. Hacker SM, Browder JF, Ramos-Caro FA: Basal cell carcinoma. Post Grad Med 1993, 93:101–111
12. Novick NL, Kest E, Gordon M. Advances in the biology and carcinogenesis of basal cell carcinoma. NY State J Med 1988, 88:367–70
13. Carter DM, Lin AN: Basal cell carcinoma. In: Fitzpatrick TB, Eisen AZ, Wolff K et al., eds. Dermatology in General Medicine, 3rd ed. New York: μgraw-Hill 1993. p.841–7
14. Pollack SV et al.: The biology of basal cell carcinoma: A review. J Am Acad Dermatol 1982, 7:569

15. Marghoob A, Kopf AW, Bart RS et al.: Risk of another basal cell carcinoma developing after treatment of a basal cell carcinoma. J Am Acad Dermatol 1993, 28:22–8

16. Gailani MR, Stahle-Backdahl M, Leffell DJ et al.: The role of the human homologue of Drosophila patched in sporadic basal cell carcinoma. Nat Genet 1996, 14:78–81

17. Luce EA: Oncologic considerations in nonmelanotic skin cancer. Clin Plast Surg 1995, 22:39–50

18. Stegman SJ: Basal cell carcinoma and squamous cell carcinoma: Recognition and treatment. Med Clin N Amer 1986, 70:95–107

19. Reymann F: Basal cell carcinoma of the skin recurrence rate after different types of treatment. A review. Dermatologica 1980, 161:217–26

20. Pascal R, Hobby LW, Lattes R et al.: Prognosis of "incompletely excised" versus "completely excised" basal cell carcinoma. Plastic Resconstr Surg 1968; 41:328–32

21. Leshin B, White WL: Malignant neoplasms of keratinocytes. In: Arndt KA, LeBoit PE, Robinson JK et al., eds. Cutaneous Medicine and Surgery: An Integrated Program in Dermatology. Philadelphia: W.B. Saunders; 1996. p.1379–1440

22. Mendenhal WM, Parson JT, Mendenhall NP et al.: T2-T4 carcinoma of the skin of the head and neck, treated with radical irradiation. Int J Radiation Oncol Biol Phys 1987, 13:975–81

23. Morton CA, Mackie RM: Photodynamic therapy for basal cell carcinoma: effect of tumor thickness and duration of photosensitizer application on response. Arch Dermatol 1998, 134:248–9

24. Roberts DJH, Cairnduff F: Photodynamic therapy of primary skin cancer: A review. Br J Plast Surg 1995, 48:360–70

25. Cornell RC, Greenway HT, Tucker SB et al.: Intralesional interferon therapy for basal cell carcinoma. J Am Acad Dermatol 1990, 23:694–700

26. Epstein E: Basal cell nevus syndrome. In: Arndt KA, LeBoit PE, Robinson JK et al., eds. Cutaneous Medicine and Surgery: An Integrated Program in Dermatology. Philadelphia: W.B. Saunders; 1996. p.1742–6

27. Strange PR, Lang PG: Long-term management of basal cell nevus syndrome with topical tretinoin and 5-fluorouracil. J Am Acad Dermatol 1992, 27:842–5

28. Hodak E, Ginzburg A, David M et al.: Etretinate treatment of the nevoid basal cell carcinoma syndrome. Int J Dermatol 1987, 26:606–9

29. Hacker SM, Flowers FP: Squamous cell carcinoma of the skin. Will heightened awareness of risk factors slow its increase? Post Grad Med 1993, 93:115–26

30. Johnson TM, Rowe DE, Nelson BR et al.: Squamous cell carcinoma of the skin (excluding lip and oral mucosa). J Am Acad Dematol 1992, 26:467–84

31. Schwartz RA, Stoll HL: Squamous cell carcinoma. In: Fitzpatrick TB, Eisen AZ, Wolff K et al., eds.Dermatology in General Medicine, 3rd ed. New York: μgraw-Hill; 1993. p. 821–39

32. Scotto J et al.: Incidence of nonmelanoma skin cancer in the United States. NIH Publication No. 83–2433, 1983

33. Gilliland MD, Zarem HA: Cutaneous malignancies: Basal and squamous cell carcinoma. In: Moosa AR, Schimpff, SC, Robson MC, eds. Comprehensive Textbook of Oncology (Vol 2). Baltimore: Williams and Wilkins;1991. p.1365–90

34. Frierson HF Jr, Cooper PH: Prognostic factors in squamous cell carcinoma of the lower lip. Hum Pathol 1986, 17:346

35. Sedlin ED, Fleming JL: Epidermal carcinoma arising in osteomyelitic foci. J Bone Joint Surg 1963, 45:827

36. Arons MS, Lynch JB, Lewis SR et al.: Scar tissue carcinoma: I. A clinical study with special reference to burn scar carcinoma. Ann Surg 1965, 161:170

37. Harwood CA, Proby CM, Leigh IM et al.: Aggressive spindle cell squamous cell carcinoma in renal transplant recipients. Br J Dermatol 1996, 135:(Suppl 47):23

38. Ghadially FN, Ghadially R: Keratoacanthoma. In: Fitzpatrick TB, Eisen AZ, Wolff K et al., eds. Dermatology in General Medicine, 3rd ed. New York: µgraw-Hill; 1993. p.848–72

39. Broder AC: Practical points on the microscopic grading of carcinoma. NY State J Med 1932, 32:667

40. Sleater JP, Beers BB, Stephens CA et al.: Keratoacanthoma: a deficient squamous cell carcinoma? Study of bcl-2 expression. J Cut Pathol 1994, 21:514

41. Tsuji T: Keratoacanthoma and squamous cell carcinoma: study of PCNA and Ley expression. J Cut Pathol 1997, 24:409–15

42. Soltani K, Clayman JL: Tumors of the skin appendages. In: Moosa AR, Schimpff SC, Robson MC, eds. Comprehensive Textbook of Oncology (Vol 2). Baltimore: Williams and Wilkins; 1991. p.1385–90

43. Massa MC, Medenica M: Cutaneous adnexal tumors and cysts; A review. In: Rosen PP, Fechner RE, eds. Pathology Annual. Norwalk (CT): Appleton-Century-Crofts; Part I:1985, 20:189–233; Part II:1987, 22:225–76

# AIDS-Related Malignancies

# AIDS-Related Malignancies

M. DeMario, D.N. Liebowitz

## Kaposi's Sarcoma

### Epidemiology, Risk Factors

*Incidence*

Epidemic Kaposi's sarcoma is associated with AIDS immunosuppression, and should be distinguished from the endemic (African) and classic forms of the disease. In 1985, near its peak incidence, the relative risk for KS in single young men in New York City was 1000 times that of the background population [1]. More recent epidemiologic data suggest a decline in KS incidence. The percentage of AIDS cases presenting with Kaposi's sarcoma declined from greater than 40% in 1980 to about 5% in 1994 [2]. In a cohort of 1341 HIV-positive homosexual/bisexual men in San Francisco, Lifson et al. report a decline in KS incidence from 79% in 1981 to 25% in 1989 [3].

*Race, Sex, Age Distribution, Predisposition*

The epidemiology of epidemic KS is mainly confined to a subset of the HIV-infected population, gay and bisexual men. One multi center AIDS cohort study (MACS) noted a 49% incidence of visceral or cutaneous KS in autopsies of a large cohort of homosexual men [4]. In 1990, Beral et al reported a 30% incidence of KS in homosexual/bisexual men with AIDS in metropolitan New York and Los Angeles [5]. In this population, the disease is most commonly observed between ages 25–44 years [5]. Adjusting for age and year of diagnosis, KS incidence in black male homosexuals is only half that observed in whites [2, 5]. In the U.S., the disease is uncommon among patients infected with HIV through intravenous drug usage, blood transfusion, or heterosexual contact.

## Etiology

A full discussion of KS pathogenesis is beyond the scope of this chapter, but several key etiologic factors are noted. The HIV tat gene and its Tat protein product sustain KS spindle cell growth in vitro [6]. Tumor invasiveness in response to exogenous Tat has been associated with degradation and release of radiolabeled collagen IV, a matrix metalloproteinase 2 (MMP-2) substrate [6]. The matrix metalloproteinases (MMPs) are thought to mediate the vascular invasiveness of AIDS-associated KS [7].

Kaposi sarcoma spindle cells express receptors for numerous cytokines, most notably IL-1, IL-2, IL-6, tumor necrosis factor (TNF) and platelet-derived growth factor (PDGF) [8]. Mononuclear cell-mediated cytokine secretion drives proliferation of KS spindle cells [9]. KS cells themselves secrete IL-1 and IL-6, which are paracrine growth mediators [8]. Interleukin-4 has been demonstrated to suppress KS cell growth in vitro [10].

KS spindle cells express basic fibroblast growth factor (bFGF) and vascular endothelial growth factor (VEGF) [11]. The importance of b-FGF as a mediator of KS growth is suggested by murine models, where b-FGF inhibitors block KS spindle cell formation [12]. VEGF mediates spindle cell growth through a paracrine effect [11].

The epidemiology of KS suggests its pathogenesis may be linked to a cofactor or other infectious agent. In 1994, Chang et al. noted a novel human herpesvirus, designated HHV-8, in AIDS-associated KS [13]. Though not definitively shown to induce this tumor, an etiologic role for HHV-8 is suggested by its presence in more than 85% of HIV and non-HIV associated KS [14, 15]. Seropositivity for antibodies against HHV-8 latency-associated nuclear antigen (anti-LANA) has been shown to precede the onset of KS in a longitudinal study [16]. In a cohort study, Martin et al. noted anti-LANA antibodies in 37.6% of 593 homosexual men, but in none of 195 heterosexual men, suggesting HHV-8 is transmitted through homosexual contact [17]. Longitudinally, HHV-8 seropositivity was independently associated with the development of KS in those men coinfected with HIV [17]. The mounting evidence of HHV-8 as an etiologic agent for KS has prompted novel antiviral and molecular-based therapies.

Pathology and Staging

A highly vascular tumor, KS histologically appears as bands of spindle cells, lymphatic channels, and a mononuclear cellular infiltrate. Grossly, KS lesions are present as flat violaceous or brown plaques or nodules. Lesions may arise on any cutaneous or mucosal surface. With the exception of pulmonary-based disease, biopsy of suspected lesions may be easily performed to confirm the diagnosis. Clinically, bacillary angiomatosis and extrapulmonary Pneumocystis carinii may mimic KS.

Typically multicentric at diagnosis, Kaposi's sarcoma is difficult to classify by the TNM system. In addition, the degree of immunosuppression and presence of other AIDS-associated illnesses have prognostic value and must be considered. The current AIDS clinical trial group (ACTG) staging system (Table 1), classifies patients as good risk, or poor risk: according to tumor extent (T), immune system status (I), and presence of HIV-1 associated systemic illness (S). The ability of this staging system to effectively predict disease outcome has recently been upheld in a prospective ACTG study [18].

Diagnostic Evaluation

Evaluation of a newly diagnosed KS patient should include a complete cutaneous and oral cavity examination. A baseline CD4+ count should be obtained. While typically cutaneous in its early stages, KS may occur

**Table 1.** AIDS Clinical Trials Group Kaposi's sarcoma staging classification

|  | Good risk (0) | Poor risk (1): any of the following |
|---|---|---|
| Tumor (T) | Confined to skin, lymph nodes, minimal oral disease | Tumor-associated edema or ulceration, Extensive oral-based disease |
|  |  | Gastrointestinal-based disease, KS in other nonnodal viscera |
| Immune status (I) | CD4 cells ≥200/µl | CD4 cells <200/µl |
| Systemic illness (S) | No hx opportunistic infections or thrush | hx of opportunistic infection or thrush |
|  | No B symptoms | B symptoms present |
|  | PS ≥70% (Karnofsky) | PS <70% |
|  |  | Other HIV-related disease (neuro/NHL etc.) |

at endobronchial, gastrointestinal or other visceral organ sites. Testing for fecal occult blood has been suggested as a screening test for GI involvement. Endobronchial-based disease is observed in as many as 20% of patients with KS and generally portends a median survival of less than 6 months [19]. Clinical presentations may include dyspnea, diffuse hemorrhage and hemoptosis. Radiographically, pulmonary KS may appear as coarse nodular densities, a solitary pulmonary nodule, or interstitial or alveolar infiltrates. Pleural fluid may be observed; it is typically serosanguineous, indicative of visceral pleural infiltration with KS. Hilar or mediastinal adenopathy is uncommon. CT findings typically support chest roentgenogram findings. Clinical suspicion of pulmonary KS in patients known to harbor cutaneous lesions should prompt bronchoscopy. Diagnosis by direct biopsy may be difficult for submucosal endobronchial tumor, however a presumptive diagnosis can usually be made by direct visualization of characteristic lesions [20]. Gallium and thallium imaging may be considered in patients unable to undergo bronchoscopy [21].

## Stage-Specific Standard Treatment Options

KS patients may be stratified into those with good risk or poor risk disease. Treatment for early stage/good risk disease may include local therapies, interferon, or trials of angiogenesis inhibitors or retinoids. Advanced or poor risk disease is best approached with single or multi-agent chemotherapy. Antiretroviral therapy should be implemented in either setting.

### Local Therapy

Local treatment modalities include intralesional chemotherapy, laser therapy, topical therapy, cryotherapy and radiation therapy. Vinblastine (0.2–0.5 mg/ml in 1% buffered lidocaine) may be injected intralesionally for both cutaneous and oral mucosal-based disease [22]. Response rates (CR and PR) are in excess of 70%, with an average response duration of 4–6 months. A notable side effect is injection site inflammation and pain, which is generally limited to 48 h following treatments. Liquid nitrogen cryotherapy may be used for limited localized disease, but results in permanent hypopigmentation. Topical 9-cis retinoic acid has shown disease activity and is currently under evaluation in Phase III trials.

Kaposi's sarcoma is radiosensitive, and this modality is useful for localized disease. Rapid response of tumor-related pain, lymphatic obstruction, or hemorrhage may be achieved. Very superficial skin lesions may be managed with electron beam therapy with little exposure to subdermal structures. More extensive lesions require conventional beam radiotherapy. A randomized study of 14 patients treated with a single 800 cGy fraction, 2000 cGy in 10 fractions, or 4000 cGy in 20 fractions showed significantly higher complete response rates with 4000 (83%) and 2000 (79%) cGY than with 8 cGY (50%) (p=0.04) [23]. The 40 week actuarial failure was significantly lower with 40 GY (48%) than with 20GY (62%) or 8 GY (84%). Single fraction therapy may nevertheless provide easily tolerated palliative therapy in end stage patients.

## Systemic Chemotherapy

Chemotherapeutic agents with demonstrated activity in KS include vincristine, vinblastine, doxorubicin, bleomycin, etoposide, and paclitaxel. Table 2 summarizes relevant dose, schedule, and response data for these agents.

**Table 2.** Single agent chemotherapy for AIDS-associated Kaposi's sarcoma

| Agent | Dose | Schedule | Response rate (%) | Reference |
|-------|------|----------|-------------------|-----------|
| Etoposide | 150 mg/m$^2$ | TID Q28 d | 76 | 24 |
|  | 150–400 mg | wkly (oral) | 36 | 25 |
|  | 25 mg/m$^2$ | dailyx7 Q 14 d | 14 | 26 |
| Vincristine | 2 mg | wkly x4, thenQ14d | 61 | 27 |
| Vinblastine | median 6 mg | wkly | 50 | 28 |
| Bleomycin | 5 mg | IM daily x3, Q21d | 71 | 29 |
|  | 6 mg/m$^2$ | CIx4d Q28d | 44 | 30 |
| Paclitaxel | 135 mg/m$^2$ | Q21d | 65 | 31 |
|  | 100 mg/m$^2$ | 3-h infus Q14d | 59 | 32 |
| Doxorubicin | 20 mg/m$^2$ | Q 14d | 48 | 33 |
| Liposomal daunorubicin | 50–60 mg/m$^2$ | Q14 d | 55 | 34 |
| Liposomal doxorubicin | 20 mg/m$^2$ | Q 21 d | 74 | 35 |

Single agent vincristine (2 mg) given weekly for one month, then bimonthly produced a response rate of 61%, with median duration 4 months [27]. As a single agent vinblastine has produced similar response rates and response duration [28]. The activity of paclitaxel was first reported by Saville et al in 1994, though myelosuppression necessitated dose reductions in the majority of patients on this every 3 week schedule [31, 36]. Gill et al. noted a 59% response rate with a median duration of 10.7 months using paclitaxel (100 mg/m²) on an every 2 week schedule [32].

Combination doxorubicin, bleomycin, and vincristine (ABV) is frequently utilized as a multiagent regimen for AIDS KS. Laubenstein et al. noted an 84% response rate with median duration 8 months for patients treated monthly with day 1 doxorubicin (40 mg/m2), vinblastine (6 mg/m²), and day 1 and 15 bleomycin (15 U) every 28 days [24]. An every other week, low dose ABV regimen (adriamycin 20 mg/m², bleomycin 10 mg/m², and vincristine 1.4 mg/m²) produced an 88% response rate with a lower incidence of neutropenia, nausea/emesis, peripheral neuropathy, and alopecia [33]. A similar, low-dose ABV regimen has been safely coadministered with the nucleoside analogues ddI and ddC [37].

Liposomal formulations of doxorubicin and daunorubicin might currently be regarded as front-line therapeutic agents for AIDS KS. Liposome-encapsulation confers the advantages of prolonged plasma half-life, higher intratumoral drug concentrations, and lower toxicity to cardiac and other nontumor tissues [38]. Single agent liposomal doxorubicin (20 mg/m² every 3 weeks) has produced response rates of 66%–74% in poor-risk KS [35, 39]. Major toxicities include neutropenia, stomatitis, and alopecia. Liposomal daunorubicin (DaunoXome) produced a response rate of 55% at doses of 50–60 mg/m² given every 2 weeks [34]. Neutropenia, nausea and diarrhea are common, while cardiac toxicity has not been observed at cumulative doses over 1000 mg/m² [34]. In a phase III trial, liposomal daunorubicin (40 mg/m² every 2 wks) had a response rate and response duration statistically equivalent to low-dose ABV [40].

## Biological Response Modifiers

The single agent activity of alpha-interferon has been demonstrated in multiple clinical trials [41, 42, 43]. A dose response relationship has been demonstrated; patients receiving interferon at doses of 20 million U/m² or greater are more likely to have a complete or partial response [42, 43]. The probability of response is closely correlated with CD4 count. Patients with a CD4 count under 100/mm³ respond less than 10% of the time [42]. Characteristic interferon "flu-like" symptoms such as low-grade fever, myalgias, fatigue, anorexia, and weight loss are more pronounced at higher doses. Significant tumor response is usually apparent by 4–8 weeks of therapy, although up to 6 months of therapy may be required for maximal benefit. Interferon is thus not appropriate for bulky disease which requires prompt cytoreduction. Practically, interferon may be initiated at 5 million U/day, escalating to 10–15 million U/day with tolerable side effects. Tumor relapse is typical after cessation of therapy, necessitating a prolonged therapeutic course.

## Current Key Questions

Our evolving knowledge of KS pathogenesis might allow for novel treatments in clinically advanced disease, and ultimately, prophylactic settings. Realizing that HHV-8 seropositivity portends a significant risk of the development of clinical KS, what is the role of anti-HHV-8 therapies as prophylaxis? What impact might such therapies have on clinically established disease? What is the role of angiogenesis inhibitors as therapy against established KS? As adjuvant therapy? Is there a clinical role for cytokine-based therapies?

## Current and Future Investigational Approaches

TNP-470, a fumagillin derivative with antiangiogenic properties, had an acceptable toxicity profile and 11% response rate in a phase I ACTG study [44]. Other anti-angiogenic agents under investigation include thalidomide, tecoglycan sodium, and vascular endothelial growth factor (VEGF) inhibitors. While preliminary data suggest these cytostatic agents have activity inferior to cytotoxics in gross disease, their utility for minimal residual disease has yet to be fully elucidated.

Preclinical models suggest retinoic acids may exert their antiproliferative effects on KS through an antagonism of IL-6 transcription [45]. Orally administered all-trans retinoic acid (90 mg/m²) produced a 17% response rate in KS patients [46]. Nine-cis-retinoic acid has shown promise in both topical and oral systemic formulations and is currently under investigation in the AIDS Malignancy Consortium.

The initiation of antiretroviral therapy has occasionally produced clinically significant responses in AIDS-associated KS. A reduction of inflammatory cytokines or, more directly, HIV Tat may account for these observations. Clinical trials examining antisense-Tat-based therapies are in development. Anti-HHV-8 therapies may have utility in KS prophylaxis.

Investigational, anti-cytokine-based therapies include vesnarinone, an inhibitor of IL-6 and tumor necrosis factor alpha in vitro. Interleukin-4, an antagonist to IL-6, may have clinical utility as an inhibitory cytokine. Antisense oligonucleotides to IL-6 block the autocrine effects of this cytokine and represent another therapeutic strategy [47].

## Systemic and Primary CNS Non-Hodgkin's Lymphoma

Epidemiology, Risk Factors

### Incidence

Non-Hodgkin's lymphoma, the second most common malignancy associated with AIDS immunosuppression, was formally classified as an AIDS-defining illness in 1985. In 1991, NHL was the defining illness in 3% of all newly diagnosed AIDS cases [48]. Currently, about 10% of all NHLs are AIDS-related, while the incidence of NHL in persons with AIDS is 200 times that of the general population [49, 50]. Unlike other AIDS-associated malignancies, the incidence of NHL is not strongly associated with a particular HIV risk population.

### Etiology

The pathogenesis of AIDS-associated NHL is clearly multifactorial; etiologic factors include virally mediated oncogenesis, cytokine dysregulation, oncogene activation, and loss of tumor suppressor genes. Epstein-Barr virus (EBV) infection has been noted to induce clonal B cell expansion and, ultimately, lymphomagenesis [51]. EBV is commonly present in systemic AIDS-associated NHL and essentially in all cases of AIDS-related primary CNS lymphoma (PCNSL) [52].

Cytokine dysregulation in the setting of HIV is known to promote B lymphocyte transformation. Monocyte/macrophage production of IL-6, an autocrine lymphocyte growth factor, is upregulated in the presence of HIV [53]. IL-10 promotes lymphomagenesis by inhibiting IL-2 and interferon gamma and upregulating IL-4, a cytokine stimulatory to B cell growth.

Rearrangements of *BCL6, MYC,* and mutations in P53 are frequently associated with AIDS-related NHL [54, 55, 56].

## Pathology

AIDS-associated NHLs express a B cell phenotype and are comprised of small noncleaved, large cell immunoblastic, and diffuse large cell histologies. In one large patient series, histologic frequencies were reported as immunoblastic 46%, small noncleaved cell Burkitt's or Burkitt-like 20%, and diffuse large cell 34% [57]. While formally intermediate-grade in the Working Formulation, AIDS-associated diffuse large-cell NHL clinically behaves as a high grade lesion.

## Evaluation and Staging

Histologically confirmed cases should be staged according to the Ann Arbor system (see Golomb HD chapter). A complete evaluation includes physical examination, a CBC, serum chemistries including LDH, chest, abdominal, and pelvic CT, CT or MRI of the brain, bone marrow biopsy, and lumbar puncture for CSF cytology. AIDS-associated NHL very commonly presents with extranodal sites of disease [58]. While CNS, gastrointestinal, bone marrow, and liver sites are common, disease has been reported at virtually every anatomic site. It follows that if localizing symptoms are present, studies in addition to those described above may be necessary for complete staging.

Aside from the traditional Ann Arbor staging, stratifying a patient as 'good risk' or 'poor risk' has had prognostic value. Four features have emerged as indicative of a poor prognosis: (1) a CD4 count of less than 100/µl, (2) Karnofsky performance status <70%, (3) prior AIDS-defining opportunistic infection (OI), and (4) disease involving the bone marrow.

## Stage-Specific Standard Treatment Options

### Systemic Chemotherapy

Chemotherapy trials for AIDS-related systemic NHL are summarized in Table 3. Early trials, which employed regimens similar to those used for non-HIV associated disease, were characterized by very short median survival and a high incidence of severe myelosuppression and OI [59, 60]. A modified m-BACOD regimen using 50% dose reductions of doxorubicin and cyclophosphamide was formulated in an attempt to reduce therapy-related toxicities [61]. CNS prophylaxis was employed as was zidovudine antiretroviral therapy following chemotherapy. While the median survival of all evaluable patients was only 6.5 months, patients with complete responses survived a median of 15 months. No CNS-relapses were noted in responding patients.

Sparano et al. noted an 18 month median survival in poor-risk AIDS NHL patients treated with a 96 hour continuous infusion regimen of cyclophosphamide (750 mg/m²), doxorubicin (50 mg/m²), and etoposide

**Table 3.** Clinical trials for systemic AIDS-related NHL

| Regimen | $n$ | Median CD4 | CR (%) | Median. survival (months) | Reference |
|---|---|---|---|---|---|
| m-BACOD (modified methotrexate, bleomycin, doxorubicin (50%), cytoxan (50%), vincristine, dexamethasone) | 35 | 150 | 46 | 6.5 | 61 |
| COMET-A (cytoxan, vincristine, methotrexate, etoposide, cytarabine) | 33 | 164 | 58 | 5.2 | 59 |
| LECP (CCNU, etoposide, cytoxan, procarbazine oral regimen) | 18 | 73 | 39 | 7.0 | 64 |
| ACVB and LNH84 (doxorubicin, cytoxan, vindesine, bleomycin, then MTX, leucovorin, ifosfamide, VP-16, asparaginase, ARA-C) | 141 | 227 | 63 | 9.0 | 65 |
| CHOP (cytoxan, doxorubicin, vincristine, prednisone) and GM-CSF | 24 | 230 | 67 | 9.0 | 66 |
| Infusional CDE cytoxan, doxorubicin, etoposide | 21 | 87 | 62 | 18.0 | 62 |

($240$ mg/m$^2$) (CDE) [62]. Patients with small noncleaved histology received whole brain radiotherapy and intrathecal methotrexate as CNS prophylaxis. Myelosuppression required dose reductions in 44% of the treatment cycles and OI occurred in 40% of patients. A phase II study of
infusional CDE is currently under investigation in the Eastern
Cooperative Oncology Group (ECOG).

Relapsed or primary refractory disease portends a very poor prognosis, with a less than 3 month median survival. Tirelli et al treated 19 such
patients using an every 21 day regimen of oral etoposide and prednimustine (both 80 mg/m$^2$x5d) with mitoxantrone (10 mg/m$^2$ day 1) [63].
Complete responses were noted in 26% of patients, who had a 7 month
median survival.

*Hematopoietic growth factors/Antiretrovirals/CNS Prophylaxis*

The high incidence of myelosuppression observed in AIDS NHL chemotherapeutic regimens has prompted the addition of hematopoietic
growth factors. Addition of GM-CSF to the CHOP regimen resulted in a
significantly higher mean nadir absolute neutrophil count and a shorter
duration of severe neutropenia, but not in a significant reduction of OI
[66]. A randomized trial of low dose m-BACOD versus standard m-
BACOD with GM-CSF was designed to determine the clinical advantage
of full dose chemotherapy with growth factor support [67]. Treatment
with standard dose m-BACOD/G-CSF conferred no significant response
or survival advantage over low dose m-BACOD and was associated with
a higher incidence of grade 3 hematologic toxicity.

The nucleoside analogues have been successfully integrated into AIDS
NHL cytotoxic regimens [68, 69, 70]. Didanosine reduces HIV-mediated
cytopenias and has therefore been evaluated with G-CSF in the CDE
regimen [70]. The incidence of neutropenia and RBC transfusions was
significantly reduced, however substantial corrections of CD4 or CD8
lymphopenia were not attained. The effects of coadministered chemotherapy and protease inhibitors are currently being examined in clinical
trials.

Given the high risk of CNS involvement at presentation or relapse,
prophylaxis has been suggested for AIDS NHL patients with 1) disease
involving the bone marrow or paranasal sinuses or 2) small noncleaved
histology. CNS prophylaxis may consist of either intrathecal cytarabine,

methotrexate, or a combination of intrathecal chemotherapy and brain irradiation. Intrathecal schedules commonly used are cycle 1, weeklyx4 cytarabine (50 mg), or methotrexate (12–15 mg) [61, 67]. No randomized trial has proven the benefit of prophylactic intrathecal chemotherapy, radiotherapy, or combined modality therapy. Nevertheless, failure to provide any form of CNS prophylaxis is associated with high rates of CNS relapse [71].

## Current Key Questions

Can immune restoration reverse the sequence of cytokine dysregulation that predisposes AIDS patients to NHL? Can this restoration induce clinical responses? What is the role of cytokine-directed therapies? Can cytotoxic AIDS-NHL regimens be safely and effectively administered with the protease inhibitors?

## Current and Future Investigational Approaches

Adoptive immunotherapy, the infusion of peripheral-expanded cytotoxic T lymphocytes, is currently under investigation for EBV-positive, AIDS-associated NHL. Complete clinical responses were noted in post transplant lymphoproliferative disorders (PTLD) using a similar technique [72]. Infusion of expansion autologous, EBV-specific cytotoxic T lymphocytes has shown promise for EBV-positive AIDS NHL in one small study [73]. Once feasible, large scale trials may be anticipated using this novel approach.

Cytokine-based therapies continue to be explored as an alternative to cytotoxic regimens. Administration of low-dose IL-2 reverses the TH1/TH2 cytokine imbalance seen in AIDS patients [74]. A prolonged schedule of low-dose IL-2 is currently under investigation for AIDS NHL in the AIDS Malignancy Consortium. Administration of a monoclonal antibody to IL-6 neutralized this cytokine in 9 of 11 patients with AIDS NHL and produced partial disease response in one patient [75].

Methyl-glyoxal-bisguanylhydrazine (MGBG) is a novel non-cytotoxic compound which exerts its antitumor effect at the level of polyamine synthesis. With active CNS penetration and lack of myelosuppressive effects, the agent is attractive for study in the AIDS NHL setting. MGBG produced a 23% response rate in treatment-refractory or otherwise poor prognosis AIDS NHL [76]. MGBG warrants further investigation in combined-modality regimens.

5-azacytidine represents a treatment strategy specific for EBV-positive AIDS NHL. 5-azacytidine enhances EBV lytic replication, which may subsequently render EBV-infected tumor cells susceptible to nucleoside antivirals [77]. Prolonged-infusion 5-azacytidine is currently under investigation in the AIDS Malignancy Consortium.

## Primary CNS Lymphoma

Primary CNS lymphoma (PCNSL) is observed in up to 13% of all AIDS patients during their disease course [78]. AIDS-PCNSL typically presents in the setting of profound immunosuppression; CD4 counts are frequently less than 50/μl. AIDS-related PCNSL is nearly universally associated with the Epstein-Barr virus [52]. Understanding EBV's pathogenic role in AIDS-PCNSL may have practical implications for novel treatment strategies.

The clinical presentation of PCNSL varies from subtle cognitive deficits and personality changes to focal neurologic deficits, confusion, lethargy, and seizures. Seizures and mental status changes are observed more frequently in AIDS-related than in immunocompetent PCNSL, while increased intracranial pressure is a less common finding [79]. Lesions are frequently supratentorial (75%) and within the periventricular grey matter (60%), but may be present in essentially any CNS location. AIDS-PCNSL demonstrates ring enhancement in more than 50% of cases, but up to 10% of patients may harbor disease that is not apparent with contrast-enhanced CT imaging.

CNS toxoplasmosis may appear radiographically indistinguishable from PCNSL and must be excluded from the differential diagnosis prior to initiating therapy. Following a positive CT or MRI examination, serum toxoplasmosis serologies should be obtained. AIDS PCNSL may be confirmed with CSF cytology, and lumbar puncture should be performed if not otherwise contraindicated [80]. AIDS PCNSL has been diagnosed with high sensitivity and specificity using polymerase chain reaction (PCR) to assay for the presence of EBV in CSF [81]. An empiric 2 week course of anti-toxoplasmosis therapy is generally advocated, even in the absence of elevated serum toxoplasma titers. Follow-up imaging typically demonstrates radiographic improvement with CNS toxoplasmosis; lesions which do not regress should be evaluated with stereotactic biopsy by an experienced neurosurgeon. Some investigators, recognizing the possibility for rapid clinical decompensation, recommend proceeding directly to stereotactic biopsy for CT or MRI-demonstrated lesions [82].

Whole brain radiation has been the standard therapy for AIDS-PCNSL, yet median survivals range from only 2.2–5 months with this modality [83–87]. DeAngelis et al. have noted prolonged survival in non-HIV PCNSL with a combined chemoradiotherapy regimen [88]. As such, the Eastern Cooperative Oncology Group (ECOG) has recently examined sequential CHOD (cyclophosphamide, doxorubicin, vincristine and dexamethasone) chemotherapy and whole brain radiotherapy in AIDS-PCNSL.

## Cervical Intraepithelial Neoplasia/Carcinoma

### Epidemiology, Risk Factors

#### *Incidence, Prevalence*

In January 1993 the CDC included grade II/III cervical dysplasia and invasive cervical cancer as category B and C AIDS-defining conditions, respectively. The prevalence of cervical intraepithelial neoplasia (CIN) in HIV-positive women has been estimated to be as high as 26%–50% [89–91]. In women under 50 years of age, 19% of all cervical carcinomas are currently associated with underlying HIV infection [92]. A strong association between cervical carcinoma and AIDS might be expected not solely from immunosuppression, but also from sexual practices which predispose these women to human papilloma virus (HPV). In 2 large patient series, HPV infection has been noted in 49%–58% of HIV-positive women [90, 93].

#### *Etiology*

Women recipients of solid organ transplants have a greater than 30-fold increased risk of developing cervical neoplasia [94]. HIV-induced immunosuppression would similarly be expected to increase the incidence of this disease. The association of cervical carcinoma and infection with numerous HPV subtypes is well known. Reduced immunosurveillance in the setting of HIV allows for HPV reactivation and proliferation.

## Pathology, Screening, and Staging Evaluations

Cervical cytologic atypia is observed in as many as 30%–60% of Pap smears in HIV-infected women, while frank CIN is noted in 26%–50% of such cases [89–91, 95, 96]. CIN may be staged as I – low, II – intermediate, or III – high grade. A correlation between progressive CIN and lower mean CD4:CD8 ratio has been demonstrated [89]. High grade CIN is much more frequent in HIV-positive women than in HIV-seronegative controls [92].

Studies to date suggest limitations in the ability of cytologic methods to effectively screen HIV-positive women. While Pap smears have a high positive predictive value for detecting abnormal cytology in this setting, Pap cytology correlates poorly with the severity of CIN noted at biopsy [89]. Fruchter et al. report Pap cytology failed to predict the aggressiveness of biopsied lesions in 49% of HIV-positive women in their series [97]. When cervical neoplasia was included as an AIDS-defining illness in 1993, the CDC recommended semiannual Pap smears for HIV-infected women. Given the limitations of cytology in these patients, any Pap abnormality should be followed by colposcopy and biopsy. Biannual visits should include complete examination of the vagina, vulva, and anus.

Invasive cervical carcinoma is stage II or greater twice as frequently in HIV-positive women than in seronegative patients [92]. Cervical carcinoma associated with HIV should be staged by the conventional FIGO system (see Massad cervical/vagina/vulva chapter). CT or MRI imaging, intravenous pyelogram, and chest roentgenogram should be performed to evaluate the extent of disease. In HIV-positive women, early and unusual sites of metastasis are frequently observed. It follows that additional diagnostic testing is required with suggestive physical findings or history.

## Stage-Specific Standard Treatment Options

### Surgical Treatment

Standard therapies for CIN include cryosurgery, laser ablation, loop electrosurgical excision procedure (LEEP), and cone biopsy. Unfortunately, the rate of CIN recurrence following these procedures is much higher in HIV-positive women than in those who are HIV-negative (39%–59% vs. less than 13%) [98, 99]. Rates of recurrence correlate closely with the CD4 count [98]. The time to disease recurrence is also significantly shorter in HIV-associated cases [92]. Given these dismal recurrence rates, follow-up has been advocated at 3 month intervals for Pap smear and, if indicated, colposcopy with biopsy.

Surgical therapy for invasive stage I cervical cancer may be undertaken without apparent increased morbidity in HIV-positive women [100], and should be considered as in non-HIV-associated cases.

*Radiotherapy*

Radiotherapy for stage IB-IVA carcinoma is conventionally applied with curative intent and is appropriate for similarly staged HIV-positive women. Consideration should be given to pre-existing HIV-related cytopenias, which may be compounded by radiation-induced myelosuppression.

*Chemotherapy, Combined Modality Therapy, Biological Response Modifiers*

Chemotherapeutic options for advanced (IV-B) carcinoma include cisplatin and ifosfamide, which have response rates of 21%–31% and 33%, respectively, in the non-HIV setting [101, 102]. A regimen of cisplatin, bleomycin, and vincristine has been investigated in advanced disease [103]. Chemotherapy-induced myelosuppression is more severe in this population; investigations utilizing growth factor support are warranted.

A regimen of alpha-interferon ($6 \times 10^6$ U/day x 2 months) and oral 13-cis-retinoic acid (1 mg/kg per dayx2 months) has produced a 50% response rate in non-HIV patients with locally advanced disease [104]. Interferon's immunomodulatory and antiviral properties make it appealing for investigation in advanced, HIV-associated cervical carcinoma (see below).

## Current Key Questions

What is the impact of new antiretroviral therapies on the incidence of CIN and invasive carcinoma? What is the value of 5-fluorouracil and retinoid therapies in (1) primary prevention of CIN, and (2) prophylaxis for CIN recurrence? Is a cytotoxic/interferon/antiretroviral regimen feasible for treating cervical neoplasia in HIV-positive women?

## Current and Future Investigational Approaches

The high rates of primary CIN eradication failure and recurrence observed in HIV-positive women suggest a role for adjuvant and chemoprevention studies. Two promising agents include the retinoids and 5-fluorouracil [105, 106]. The role of isotretinoin as primary therapy for AIDS-associated CIN I is under investigation. ACTG 200 is a randomized study examining the value of topical 5-FU (intravaginally Q 2 wk for 6 months) as prophylaxis following CIN II/III ablation.

For advanced cervical carcinoma, the Gynecologic Oncology Group (GOG-155) is investigating a combination regimen of isotretinoin and alpha-interferon with or without zidovudine.

## References

1. Biggar R, Horm J, Lubin J, et al (1985) Cancer trends in a population at risk of acquired immunodeficiency syndrome. J Natl Cancer Inst 74:793–797
2. Biggar R, and Rabkin C (1996) The epidemiology of AIDS-related Neoplasms. Hematol/Onc Clin N Amer 10:997–1010
3. Lifson A, Darrow W, Hessol N, et al (1990) Kaposi's sarcoma in a cohort of homosexual and bisexual men. Am J Epidemiol 131:221–213
4. Ndimbie O, Hutchins G, Variakojis D et al (1993) Skin, visceral, and skin and visceral Kaposi's sarcoma in autopsies of homosexual men in the multi center AIDS cohort center study (MACS). First Natl Conf on Hum Retroviruses 501a
5. Beral V, Peterman T, Berkelman R et al (1990) Kaposi's sarcoma among persons with AIDS: a sexually transmitted infection? Lancet 335:123–128
6. Albini A, Barillari G, Benelli R, et al (1995) Angiogenic properties of human immunodeficiency virus type 1 Tat protein. Proc Natl Acad Sci USA 92:4838–4832
7. Ensoli B, Gendelman R, Markham P, et al (1994) Synergy between basic fibroblast growth factor and HIV-1 Tat protein in induction of Kaposi's sarcoma. Nature 371:674–680
8. Miles S (1993) Kaposi's sarcoma: a cytokine responsive neoplasia? Benz C, Liu E (eds) Oncogenes and tumor suppressor genes in human malignancies. Kluwer Academic Publishers, Boston pp 129–140

9. Barillari G, Buonaguro L, Fiorelli V, et al (1992) Effects of cytokines from activated immune cells on vascular cell growth and HIV-1 gene expression: implications for AIDS-Kaposi's sarcoma pathogenesis. J Immunol 149:3727–3724

10. Gill P, Puri R (1993) Interleukin-4 receptor (IL-4R) expression on AIDS-related KS cells and inhibition of tumor cell growth and cytokine production by IL-4. Proc AACR 34:a1121

11. Masood R, Cai J, Zheng T, et al (1997) Vascular endothelial growth factor (vascular permeability factor (VEGF/VPF) is an autocrine growth factor for AIDS-KS. Proc Natl Acad Sci USA 94:979–984

12. Ensoli B, Markham P, Kao V et al (1994) Block of AIDS-Kaposi's sarcoma (KS) cell growth, angiogenesis, and lesion formation in nude mice by antisense oligonucleotide targeting basic fibroblast growth factor. J Clin Invest 94:1736–1746

13. Chang Y, Cesarman E, Pessin M, et al (1994) Identification of herpesvirus-like DNA sequences in AIDS-associated Kaposi's sarcoma. Science 266:1865–1869

14. Chang Y, Ziegler J, Wabinga H, et al (1996) Kaposi's sarcoma -associated herpesvirus and Kaposi's sarcoma in Africa. Uganda Kaposi's Sarcoma Study Group. Arch Intern Med 156:202–204

15. Gao S, Kingsley L, Li M, et al (1996) KSHV antibodies among Americans, Italians, and Ugandans with and without Kaposi's sarcoma. Nat Med 2:925–928

16. Gao S, Kingsley L, Hoover D, et al (1996) Seroconversion to antibodies against Kaposi's sarcoma-associated herpesvirus-related talent nuclear antigens before the development of Kaposi's sarcoma. N Engl J Med 335:233–241

17. Martin J, Ganem D, Osmond D, et al (1998) Sexual transmission and the natural history of human herpesvirus 8 infection. N Engl J Med 338:948–954

18. Krown S, Testa M, Huang J (1997) AIDS-related Kaposi's sarcoma: prospective validation of the AIDS Clinical Trials Group staging classification. J Clin Oncol 15:3085–3092

19. Gill P, Hamiltin A, Naidu Y (1994) Epidemic (AIDS Related) Kaposi's sarcoma: epidemiology, pathogenesis and treatment. AIDS Updates 7:1–11

20. Judson M, Sahn S (1994) Endobronchial lesions in HIV-infected individuals. Chest 105:1314–1323

21. Lee V, Fuller J, O'Brien M, et al (1991) Pulmonary Kaposi's sarcoma in patients with AIDS: Scintographic diagnosis with sequential thallium and gallium scanning. Radiology 180:409–412

22. Boudreaux A, Smith L, Cosby C, et al (1993) Intralesional vinblastine for cutaneous Kaposi's sarcoma associated with acquired immunodeficiency syndrome: A clinical trial to evaluate efficacy and discomfort associated with injection. J Am Acad Dermatol 28:61–65

23. Stelzer K, Griffin T (1993) A randomized prospective trial of radiation therapy for AIDS associated Kaposi's sarcoma. Int J Radiat Oncol Biol Phys 27:1057–1061

24. Laubenstein L, Krigel R, Odajnyk C, et al (1984) Treatment of epidemic Kaposi's sarcoma with etoposide or a combination of doxorubicin, bleomycin, and vinblastine. J Clin Oncol 2:1115–1120

25. Paredes J, Kahn J, Tong W, et al (1995) Weekly oral etoposide in patients with Kaposi's sarcoma associated with human immunodeficiency virus infection: A phase I multi center trial of the AIDS clinical trial group. J Acquir Immune Defic Syndr Hum Retrovir 9:138–144

26. Sander E, Zampese M, Prolla G, et al (1993) Phase II trial of low-dose oral etoposide in AIDS-related Kaposi's sarcoma Proc Am Soc Clin Oncol 12:19, (abstr)

27. Minzer D, Real F, Jovino L, et al (1985) Treatment of Kaposi's sarcoma and thrombocytopenia with vincristine in patients with acquired immunodeficiency syndrome. Ann Intern Med 102:200–202

28. Volberding P, Abrams D, Conant M, et al (1985) Vinblastine therapy for Kaposi's sarcoma in the acquired immunodeficiency syndrome: Ann Intern Med 103:335–338

29. Caumes E, Guermonprez G, Katlama C, et al (1992) AIDS-associated mucocutaneous Kaposi's sarcoma treated with bleomycin. AIDS 6:1483–1487

30. Lassoued K, Clauvel J, Katlama C, et al (1990) Treatment of the acquired immune deficiency syndrome-related Kaposi's sarcoma with bleomycin as a single agent. Cancer 66:1869–1872

31. Saville M, Lietzau J, Pluda J, et al (1995) Treatment of HIV-associated Kaposi's sarcoma with paclitaxel. Lancet 346:26–28

32. Gill P, Scadden D, Groopman J, et al (1997) Low dose paclitaxel (Taxol) every two weeks is highly effective in the treatment of patients with advanced AIDS-related Kaposi's sarcoma. J Acquir Immun Defic Syndr Hum Retrovirol 14: A35

33. Gill P, Rarick M, McCutchan A, et al (1991) Systemic treatment of AIDS-related Kaposi's sarcoma: results of a randomized trial. Am J Med 90:427–433

34. Gill P, Espina B, Muggia F, et al (1995) Phase I/II clinical and pharmacokinetic evaluation of liposomal daunorubicin. J Clin Oncol 13:996–1003

35. Harrison M, Tomlinson D, Stewart S, et al (1995) Liposomal-entrapped doxorubicin: an active agent in AIDS-related Kaposi's sarcoma. J Clin Oncol 13:914–920

36. Saville M, Lietzau J, Wilson W, et al (1994) A trial of paclitaxel in patients with HIV-associated Kaposi's sarcoma (KS). Proc Am Soc Clin Oncol 13:54, (abstr 20)

37. Mitsuyasu R, Gill P, Paredes J, et al (1995) Combination chemotherapy adriamycin, bleomycin, vincristine (ABV) with didanosine (ddI) or dideoxycytidine (ddC) in advanced, AIDS-related Kaposi's sarcoma (ACTG 163). Proc Am Soc Clin Oncol 14:289, (abstr)

38. Brenner D, (1993) Liposomal encapsulation: Making old and new drugs do new tricks. J Natl Cancer Inst 81:13–15

39. Thommes J, Northfelt D, Rios A, et al (1994) Open-label trial of Stealth liposomal doxorubicin in the treatment of moderate to severe AIDS-related Kaposi's sarcoma (AIDS-KS). Proc Am Soc Clin Oncol 13:55, (abstr 24)

40. Gill P, Wernz J, Scadden D, et al (1996) Randomized phase II trial of liposomal daunorubicin (DaunoXome) versus doxorubicin, bleomycin, vincristine (ABV) in AIDS-related Kaposi's sarcoma. J Clin Oncol 14:2353–2364

41. Groopman J, Gottleib M, Goodman J, et al (1984) Recombinant alpha-2 interferon therapy for Kaposi's sarcoma associated with the acquired immunodeficiency syndrome. Ann Intern Med 100:671–676

42. Real F, Oettgen H, Krown S (1986) Kaposi's sarcoma and the acquired immunodeficiency syndrome: treatment with high and low doses of leukocyte A interferon. J Clin Oncol 4:544–551

43. Volberding P, Mitsuyasu R, Golando P, et al (1987) Treatment of Kaposi's sarcoma with interferon alpha 2B (intron A). Cancer 59:620–625

44. Dezube B, von Roenn J, Holden-Wiltse J, et al (1997) Fumagillin analog (TNP-470) in the treatment of Kaposi's sarcoma: a phase I AIDS Clinical Trial Group Study. J Acquir Immun Defic Syndr Hum Retrovir 14: A35

45. Nagpai S, Cai J, Zheng T, et al (1997) Retinoid antagonism of NF-IL-6: Insight into the mechanism of anti-proliferative effects of retinoids in Kaposi's sarcoma. Molec Cell Biol 17:4159–4168

46. Gill P, Espina B, Moudgil T, et al (1995) All-trans retinoic acid for the treatment of AIDS-related Kaposi's sarcoma: results of a pilot phase II study. Leukemia 8:S26-S32

47. Miles S, Rezai A, Salazar-Gonzales J, et al (1990) AIDS-Kaposi's sarcoma derived cells produce and respond to interleukin-6. Proc Natl Acad Sci USA 87:4068–4072

48. Serriano D, Salamina G, Francesche S, et al (1992) The epidemiology of AIDS-associated non-Hodgkin's lymphoma in the World Health Organization European Region. Br J Cancer 66:912–916

49. Biggar R, and Rabkin C (1992) The epidemiology of acquired immunodeficiency syndrome-related lymphomas. Curr Opin Oncol 4:883–893

50. Biggar R, Curtis R, Cote T, et al (1994) Risk of other cancers following Kaposi's sarcoma: Relation to acquired immunodeficiency syndrome. Am J Epidemiol 139:362–368

51. Neri A, Barriga F, Knowles D, et al (1991) Epstein-Barr virus infection precedes clonal expansion in Burkitt's and AIDS-associated lymphoma. Blood 77:1092–1095

52. McMahon E, Glass J, Hayward S, et al (1991) Epstein Barr virus in AIDS-related primary central nervous system lymphoma. Lancet 338:969–973

53. Nakajima K, Martinez-Mazo O, Hirano T et al (1989) Induction of IL-6 (B cell stimulatory factor-2/IFN-beta-2) production by human immunodeficiency virus. J Immunol 142:531–536

54. Gaidano G, Lo Coco F, Ye B, et al (1994) Rearrangements of the BCL-6 gene in AIDS-associated NHL: association with diffuse large cell subtype. Blood 82:397–402

55. Subar M, Neri A, Inghirami G et al (1988) Frequent c-myc oncogene activation and infrequent presence of Epstein-barr virus genome in AIDS-associated lymphomas. Blood 72:667–671

56. Ballerini P, Gaidano G, Gong J, et al (1993) Multiple genetic lesions in AIDS-related NHL. Blood 81:166–176

57. Kaplan L, Strauss D, Testa M, et al (1995) Randomized trial of standard dose mBACOD with GM-CSF vs. Reduced dose mBACOD for systemic HIV-associated lymphoma: ACTG142. Proc Am Soc Clin Oncol 14:288

58. Gisselbrecht C, Oksenhendler E, Tirelli U, et al (1992) Non-Hodgkin's lymphoma associated with human immunodeficiency virus: treatment with the LNH 84 regimen in a selected group of patients. Leukemia 6:10S-12 S

59. Kaplan L, Abrams D, Feigel E, et al (1991) AIDS-associated NHL in San Francisco. JAMA 261:719–724

60. Dugan M, Subgar M, Odajnyk C, et al (1986) Intensive multiagent chemotherapy for AIDS-related diffuse large cell lymphoma. Blood 68:124a

61. Levine A, Werntz J, Kaplan L, et al (1991) Low-dose chemotherapy with central nervous system prophylaxis and zidovudine maintenance in AIDS-related lymphoma: a prospective multi-institutional trail. JAMA 266:84–88

62. Sparano J, Wernik P, Strack M, et al (1994) Infusional cyclophosphamide, doxorubicin, and etoposide in HIV-related non-Hodgkin's lymphoma: a follow up report of a highly active regimen. Leuk Lymphoma 14:263–271

63. Tirelli U, Errante D, Spina M, et al (1996) Second-line chemotherapy in human immunodeficiency virus-related non-Hodgkin's lymphoma. Cancer 77:2127–2131

64. Remick S, McSharry J, Wolf B, et al (1993) Novel oral combination chemotherapy in the treatment of intermediate-grade and high-grade AIDS-related Non-Hodgkin's lymphoma. J Clin Oncol 11:1691–1702

65. Gisselbrecht C, Oksenhendler E, Tirelli U, et al (1993) Human immunodeficiency virus-related lymphoma treated with intensive combination chemotherapy. Am J Med 95:188–196

66. Kaplan L, Kahn J, Crowe S, et al (1990) Clinical and virologic effects of recombinant human granulocyte-macrophage colony stimulating factor in patients receiving chemotherapy for human immunodeficiency virus-related non-Hodgkin's lymphoma: results of a randomized trial. J Clin Oncol 9:929–940

67. Kaplan L, Strauss D, Testa M, et al (1997) Low-dose compared with standard-dose m-BACOD chemotherapy for non-Hodgkin's lymphoma associated with human immunodeficiency virus infection. N Engl J Med 336:1641–1648

68. Levine A, Espina B, Tupule A, et al (1993) Low dose m-BACOD with concomitant dideoxycytidine: an effective regimen in AIDS-related lymphomas. Blood 82:387, (abstr)

69. Levine A, Tupule A, Espina B, et al (1996) Low dose methotrexate, bleomycin, doxorubicin, cyclophosphamide, vincristine, and dexamethasone with zilcitabine in patients with AIDS-related lymphoma. Cancer 78:517–526

70. Sparano J, Wiernik P, Hu X, et al (1996) Pilot trial of infusional cyclophosphamide, doxorubicin, and etoposide plus didanosine and filgastrin in patients with human immunodeficiency virus-associated non-Hodgkin's lymphoma. J Clin Oncol 14:3026–3035

71. Gill P, Levine A, Krailo M, et al (1987) AIDS-related malignant lymphoma: results of prospective treatment trials. J Clin Oncol 5:1322–1328

72. Papadopoulos E, Ladanyi M, Emanuel D, et al (1994) Infusions of donor leukocytes to treat Epstein-Barr virus-associated lymphoproliferative disorders after allogeneic bone marrow transplantation. N Engl J Med 330:1185–1191

73. Wheatley G, McKinnon K, Lilly S, et al (1997) Adoptive immunotherapy using autologous EBV specific cytotoxic T lymphocytes in an HIV infected patient with refractory Epstein Barr virus expressing B cell lymphoma. J Acq Immun Def Synd Hum Retrovir 14:A53, (abstr)

74. Khatri V, Yu F, Baiocchi R, et al (1997) Analysis of TH1/TH2 cytokine gene profile during low dose IL-2 therapy in patients with AIDS or AIDS lymphoma. J Acq Immun Def Synd Hum Retrovir 14: A41, (abstr)

75. Emilie D, Wijdenes J, Gisselbrecht C, et al (1994) Administration of an anti-interleukin-6 monoclonal antibody to patients with acquired immunodeficiency syndrome and lymphoma: effect on lymphoma and on B clinical symptoms. Blood 84:2472–2479

76. Levine A, Tulpule A, Tessman D, et al (1997) Mitoguazone therapy in patients with refractory or relapsed AIDS-related lymphoma: results from a multi center phase II trial. J Clin Oncol 15:1094–1103

77. Moore S, and Ambinder R (1997) Pharmacologic induction of Epstein-Barr virus lytic cycle: Strategies for tumor therapy. J Acq Immun Def Synd Hum Retrovir 14 (4) A41, (abstr)

78. Forsyth P, and DeAngelis L (1996) Biology and management of AIDS-associated primary CNS lymphoma. Hematol Clin N Am 10:1125–1134

79. Fine H, and Mayer R (1993) Primary central nervous system lymphoma. Ann Intern Med 119:1093–1104

80. Forsyth P, Yahalom J, and DeAngelis L (1994) Combined modality therapy in the treatment of primary central nervous system lymphoma in AIDS. Neurology 44:1473–1478

81. DeLuca A, Antinori A, Cingolani A, et al (1995) Evaluation of cerebrospinal fluid EBV-DNA and IL-10 as markers for in vivo diagnosis of primary central nervous system lymphoma. Br J Hematol 90:844–849

82. Mathews C, Barba D, and Fullerton S (1995) Early biopsy versus treatment with delayed biopsy of non-responders in suspected HIV-associated cerebral toxoplasmosis. A decision analysis. AIDS 9:1243–1250

83. Goldstein J, Dickson D, Moser F, et al (1991) Primary central nervous system lymphoma in AIDS: a clinical and pathologic study with results and treatment with radiation. Cancer 67:2756–2765

84. DeWeese T, Hazuka M, Hommell D, et al (1991) AIDS-related NHL: outcome and efficacy of radiation therapy. Int J Rad Oncol Biol Phys 20:803–808

85. Baumgartner J, Rachlin J, Beckstead J, et al (1990) Primary central nervous system lymphomas: natural history and response to radiation therapy in 55 patients with AIDS. J Neurosurg 73:206–211

86. Ling S, Roach M, Larson D, et al (1994) Radiotherapy of primary central nervous system lymphoma in patients with and without human immunodeficiency virus. Cancer 73:2570–2582

87. Formenti S, Gill P, Lean E, et al (1989) Primary central nervous system lymphoma in AIDS: results of radiation therapy. Cancer 63:1101–1107

88. DeAngelis L, Yaholom J, Thaler H, et al (1992) Combined modality therapy for primary CNS lymphoma. J Clin Oncol 10:635–643

89. Maiman M, Tarricone N, Vieira J, et al (1991) Colposcopic evaluation of human immunodeficiency virus-seropositive women. Obstet Gynecol 78:84–88

90. Feingold A, Vermund S, Burk R, et al (1990) Cervical cytology abnormalities and papilloma virus in women infected with human immunodeficiency virus. J AIDS 3:896–902

91. Schrager L, Friedland G, Maude D, et al (1990) Cervical and vaginal squamous cell abnormalities in women infected with the human immunodeficiency virus. J AIDS 2:570–575

92. Maiman M, Fruchter R, Serur E, et al (1990) Human immunodeficiency virus infection and cervical neoplasia. Gynecol Oncol 38:377–382

93. Palefsky J, Minkoff H, Kalish L, et al (1997) Cevicovaginal human papillomavirus infection in HIV-positive and high risk HIV-negative patients. J Acquir Immun Def Synd and Hum Retrovir 14: abstr S3

94. Penn I (1986) Cancers of the anogenital region in renal transplant recipients. Analysis of 65 cases. Cancer 58:611–616

95. Stratton P, Ciacco K (1994) Cervical neoplasia in the patient with HIV infection. Curr Opin Obstet Gynecol 6:86–91

96. Wright T, Ellerbrock T, Chiasson M, et al (1994) Cervical intraepithelial neoplasia in women infected with human immunodeficiency virus: Prevalence, risk factors, and validity of Papanicolaou smears. Obstet Gynecol 84:591–597

97. Fruchter R, Maiman M, Sillman F, et al (1994) Characteristics of cervical intraepithelial neoplasia in women infected with the human immunodeficiency virus. Am J Obstet Gynecol 171:531–537

98. Maiman M, Fruchter R, Serur E, et al (1993) Recurrent cervical intraepithelial neoplasia in human immunodeficiency virus-seropositive women. Obstet Gynecol 82:170–174

99. Wright T, Koulos J, Scholl F, et al (1994) Cervical intraepithelial neoplasia in women infected with the human immunodeficiency virus: Outcome after LOOP electrosurgical excision. Gynecol Oncol 55:253–258

100. DeVito J, Robinson W (1995) Gynecologic surgical outcomes among asymptomatic human immunodeficiency virus-infected women and uninfected control subjects. J La State Med Soc 147:108–112

101. Bonomi P, Blessing J, Stehman F, et al (1985) Randomized trial of three cisplatin dose schedules in squamous cell carcinoma of the cervix: A Gynecologic Oncology Group Study. J Clin Oncol 3:1079–1085

102. Coleman R, Jarper P, Gallagher C, et al (1986) A phase II study of ifosfamide in advanced and relapsed carcinoma of the uterine cervix. Cancer Chemother Pharmacol 18:280–283

103. Maiman M (1994) Cervical neoplasia in women with HIV infection. Oncology 8:82–84

104. Lippman S, Kavanagh J, Paredes-Espinoza M, et al (1992) 13-cis-retinoic acid plus interferon alpha 2a: Highly active systemic therapy for squamous cell carcinoma of the cervix. J Natl Cancer Inst 84:241–245
105. Meyskens F, Surwit E, Moon T, et al (1994) Enhancement of regression of cervical intraepithelial neoplasia II (moderate dysplasia) with topically applied all-trans-retinoic acid: A randomized trial. J Natl Cancer Inst 86:539–543
106. Sillman F, Sedis A (1987) Anogenital papillomavirus infection and neoplasia in immunodeficient women. Obstet Gynec Clin North Am 14:537–558

# Supportive Care

# Hematopoietic Growth Factors

E.M. Johnston, J. Crawford

## Introduction

Treatment related cytopenias are the most common dose limiting toxicities of chemotherapy and are often the cause of dose delay or reduction in subsequent treatment cycles. The storage compartment of the marrow contains enough maturing cells to maintain peripheral counts for approximately 8–10 days after stem cell production ceases, thus the effect of cell cycle specific chemotherapy will be notable by the tenth day after treatment, nadir counts are manifest between days 14 and 18, and recovery between days 21 and 28. If a $G^o$ active agent is used nadir and recovery counts may be delayed to 4 and 6 weeks respectively owing to the preferential effect on resting stem cells. Over recent years the hematopoietic growth factors have demonstrated the ability to lessen the severity of chemotherapy induced cytopenias and have contributed to the preservation of dose intensity in standard chemotherapy regimens. Commercially available colony stimulating factors (CSFs) include G-CSF, GM-CSF, erythropoietin and Interleukin 11. Megakaryocyte growth and development factor, thrombopoietin and a pegylated version of G-CSF are available on clinical trials. The utility of these growth factors in patients with malignancy will be reviewed in this chapter.

## Erythropoietin

Anemia is prevalent among cancer patients (>50%) and often has a multifactorial basis. Myelophthisic disease, malignancy associated hemolytic disorders, treatment related anemia, nutritional deficiencies, and anemia of chronic disease are among the common etiologies. Regardless of the cause, anemia negatively impacts quality of life resulting in fatigue,

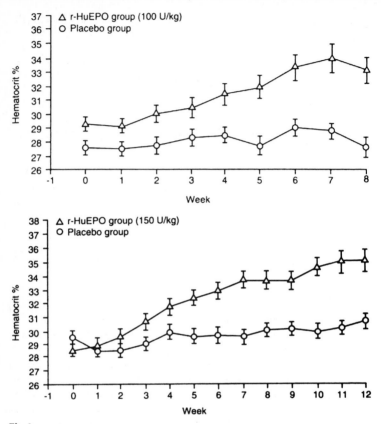

Fig. 1

dyspnea, chest pain, palpitations and diminished exercise capacity. Packed red cell transfusion has been demonstrated to improve quality of life in cancer patients with symptomatic anemia regardless of pretransfusion hemoglobin [1]. However, transfusion carries with it the risk of infectious complications, volume overload, hemolytic transfusion reactions, and perhaps, impaired immune function [2–6]. The risks and inconvenience of repeated blood product administration has prompted an interest in acceptable alternatives to red cell transfusion, most notably, therapy with recombinant human erythropoietin.

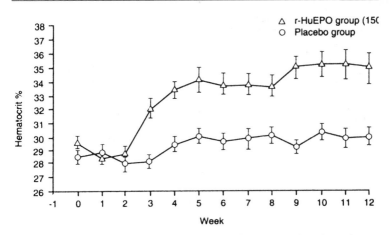

**Fig. 1.** Mean weekly hematocrit values (±SE) for patients not receiving chemotherapy (A), patients receiving non-platinum-based chemotherapy (B), and patients receiving platinum-based chemotherapy (C). Placebo and erythropoietin groups are illustrated for each stratification

Endogenous erythropoietin is produced in the peritubular interstitial cells of the kidney and in hepatocytes with "normal" serum levels displaying a wide range of variability. The viability of erythroid progenitor cells in the marrow relies on the presence of erythropoietin which is also responsible for enhancing proliferation of these progenitors in the presence of tissue hypoxia. Although erythropoietin levels are inversely related to hemoglobin levels in patients with iron deficiency anemia, this relationship is lacking in patients with anemia of chronic disease/cancer. In chronic disease Interleukin 1 and Tumor Necrosis Factor may play a role in depressing erythropoietin production and responsiveness, an effect which can be overcome by the addition of exogenous erythropoietin. Recombinant human erythropoietin became available in the 1980 s with the results of the first randomized clinical trials being published in 1992.

The utility of recombinant erythropoietin in oncology patients is best illustrated by two large randomized trials. The first trial, by Abels [7], included over 400 anemic cancer patients (hematocrit <32%) stratified by treatment with no chemotherapy, non-platinum based or platinum based chemotherapy and randomized to erythropoietin vs. placebo. Primary endpoints of the study were transfusion requirement, hemoglobin level, and quality of life. By convention, hematologic response was defined as a rise in the hematocrit by 6% or more. Hematocrit response is illustrated for each treatment group in Figure 1. After 8 weeks on study, patients not receiving chemotherapy demonstrated significantly different hematologic response rates of 32% for those on erythropoietin (100 units subcutaneously three times a week) vs. 10% in the placebo group. Those patients receiving non-platinum based regimens had erythropoietin response rates of 58% vs. 13% in placebo patients. Likewise, erythropoietin produced a response of 48% vs. 6% placebo response in the platinum treated group. Ultimately, transfusion requirements were significantly reduced in all treatment groups; this effect was seen in month 2 for the chemotherapy groups but was more gradual in the non-chemotherapy patients becoming notable in the 6 month open label follow-up portion of the trial. All quality of life parameters improved in patients demonstrating response to erythropoietin regardless of chemotherapy group. At the conclusion of the open label portion of the trial (which allowed for erythropoietin dose escalation) response rates were 40, 56 and 58% with residual transfusion requirement in 10, 13 and 12% in the no chemotherapy, non-platinum and platinum based chemotherapy arms respectively [8].

The results of the Abels trial are corroborated by Glaspy et al in an open label, non randomized, community based trial of over 2000 anemic patients with nonmyeloid malignancies who were receiving chemotherapy [9]. Patients received 150 units of erythropoietin per kilogram subcutaneously three times per week with a suggested doubling of the dose for lack of response at eight weeks. Endpoints were essentially identical to those of the Abels trial. The 2019 evaluable patients demonstrated a mean increase in hemoglobin of 1.8 g/dl with 53% of patients experiencing increases of 2 g/dl or more at the completion of the 4 month trial. Quality of life parameters improved significantly and in proportion to rise in hemoglobin in all subgroups except the group of patients with a decline in hemoglobin (Fig. 2). An initially unplanned, retrospective evaluation of tumor response revealed that improvement in quality of life was independently predicted by hemoglobin response and tumor response to chemotherapy. Finally, erythropoietin therapy resulted in a 50% reduction in the number of patients requiring transfusion as well as the number of units transfused by the second month of treatment. In both trials toxicity was minimal with less than 5% of patients discontinuing growth factor due to an adverse event.

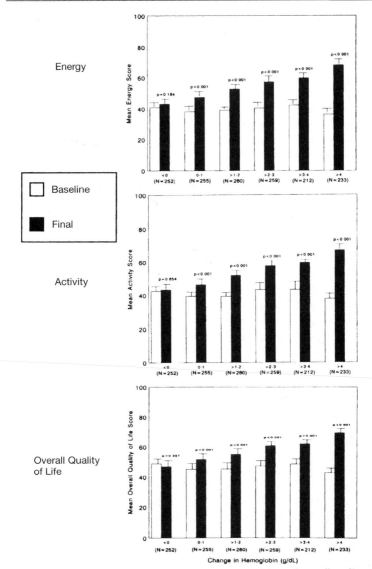

**Fig. 2.** Changes from baseline to termination in energy, activity, and overall quality of life score for subsets of patients defined by hemoglobin change from baseline to final value. Data are mean score and upper 95% confidence interval

Erythropoietin has also been evaluated in non-anemic patients initiating a course of intensive chemotherapy in an effort to primarily ameliorate the expected chemotherapy induced anemia. Patients receiving chemotherapy for small cell lung cancer [10] and patients receiving accelerated adjuvant chemotherapy for breast cancer [11] were randomized to erythropoietin vs. no growth factor during chemotherapy. In small cell lung cancer both patient groups became anemic but this was significantly delayed and less severe (fewer required transfusions) in the growth factor arm. Similarly, in the breast cancer trial 52% of patients not receiving erythropoietin developed clinically significant anemia vs. no patients in the erythropoietin arm. Likewise, preliminary studies indicate that anemia resulting from irradiation can be prevented or diminished by the initiation of erythropoietin at the outset of radiation without worsening radiation associated leukopenia and thrombocytopenia [12, 13].

Erythroid growth factors are beneficial to oncology patients demonstrating hemoglobin response to therapy with improvement in quality of life endpoints related to the hemoglobin response. Although the majority of all cancer patients are likely to respond to recombinant erythropoietin, reliable clinical predictors of response vs. non response (including pretreatment hemoglobin and erythropoietin levels, tumor type, age, gender, or disease stage) are lacking. As a rule, low pretreatment serum erythropoietin levels predict for response but a significant portion of patients with normal or elevated levels will also respond. In addition, the expected time to response and the required dose are variable among patients. Finally, the role of concurrent iron supplementation is not fully defined as several investigators have noted a "functional iron deficiency" characterized by insufficient release of stored iron in cancer patients receiving erythropoietin, a phenomenon that may be overcome by iron supplementation. A trial of erythropoietin therapy remains the only means of identifying those who will benefit from its use.

The toxicity of erythropoietin in cancer patients remains low and is generally manifest as local skin reaction or flushing. Hypertension, seizures and deep venous thrombosis have occurred on rare occasions but have typically been associated with inappropriate elevations of red cell mass. Recombinant erythropoietin is generally non-immunogenic. However, a single case has been reported in which a dialysis patient maintained on recombinant erythropoietin for anemia of end stage renal disease developed pure red cell aplasia with associated erythropoietin antibodies and no other discernible cause for the red cell aplasia. Upon withdrawal of the growth hormone the antibody titers fell over several months and hemoglobin returned to pre-erythropoietin levels [14].

The usual starting dose of erythropoietin is 150 units subcutaneously three times per week with titration to twice the starting dose for lack of response at 4–8 weeks of therapy. Based on clinical benefit seen in the surgical setting with weekly administration of 600 units/kg, trials in cancer chemotherapy patients are ongoing with weekly administration of 40,000 units with an increase to 60,000 units if no response in the first month. Most authors advocate discontinuation of the drug if there is no hemoglobin improvement after 12 weeks. Iron status should be closely monitored and many advocate a trial of iron supplementation in nonresponders regardless of iron levels before declaring erythropoietin ineffective.

## Myeloid Growth Factors

The most common dose limiting toxicity of conventional chemotherapy is neutropenia and its resultant infectious complications. The likelihood of developing fever in the setting of Grade IV neutropenia is approximately 10% per day [15] (Fig. 3). Despite intravenous antibiotics and supportive care measures mortality from neutropenic fever has been reported to be as high as 3% [16].

Efforts to mitigate the complications of neutropenia and thus preserve dose intensity have led to the development of G-CSF and GM-CSF. G-CSF is a lineage specific growth factor which stimulates proliferation and maturation of the committed myeloid progenitor pool. GM-CSF is felt to stimulate a less committed progenitor cell pool and thus results in the enhanced production of granulocytes, macrophages and eosinophils. Functionally, neutrophils produced in response to these agents have been reported to show enhanced respiratory burst, adherence, phagocytosis and bacterial killing [17].

The use of the myeloid growth factors is divided into primary prophylaxis (the preemptive initiation of growth factor prior to the occurrence of neutropenia), secondary prophylaxis (the initiation of growth factor in cycles of therapy subsequent to the occurrence of neutropenic fever or prolonged neutropenia), and therapeutic (initiation of a colony

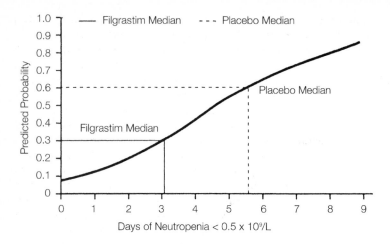

**Fig. 3.** Kaplan Meier curve representing the number of patients remaining free of fever in the setting of neutropenia during repeated cycles of cyclophosphamide, doxorubicin and etoposide. Reprinted with permission from [15]

stimulating factor in a patient with established neutropenia or neutropenic fever). Numerous randomized trials of primary prophylaxis in patients with small cell lung cancer or lymphoma have demonstrated a decrease in the duration of neutropenia (from an average of 6 days to 1 in lung cancer patients) as well as a 50% decrease in the incidence of neutropenic fever in those patients treated with G-CSF vs. placebo. Most studies also showed a decrease in the number of hospital days, antibiotic usage and confirmed infections. [18–22]. These endpoints are clearly of clinical and economic relevance and allow maintenance of planned dose and dose intensity of chemotherapy, which may also be clinically beneficial. However, the use of G-CSF specifically as a means of increasing dose intensity over that of standard regimens has not been conclusively shown to enhance overall survival and should be limited to clinical trials at present [23–24].

The primary use of G-CSF in patients receiving chemotherapy with an expected rate of neutropenia exceeding 40% in the absence of growth factor favorably impacts on clinical outcomes of neutropenia and its complications and is supported by the guidelines set forth by the American Society of Clinical Oncology (ASCO) [16]. The 40% threshold was determined by analysis of the noted randomized trials. However, cost analysis has suggested benefit for growth factors in regimens with an expected rate of hospitalization for neutropenic fever as low as 20% [25]. Special circumstances such as advanced stage of disease, comorbid illnesses, prior chemotherapy, and local organ/tissue factors may also lower the clinicians' threshold for G-CSF use.

The role of GM-CSF for primary prophylaxis in non-leukemic malignancies is less clear than that of G-CSF. GM-CSF has been evaluated in patients with small cell lung cancer, lymphoma, germ cell tumors and breast cancer. Effects of the growth factor on depth and duration neutropenia have been inconsistent among trials with beneficial effects often limited to the first cycle of therapy [26–31]. Intention to treat analysis shows improvement in hospitalization rates and antibiotic use only in those patients with HIV associated lymphoma [26]. In addition, Bunn et al noted increased rates of infection, longer hospitalizations, more toxic deaths and more severe thrombocytopenia in patients receiving concurrent chemoradiation with GM-CSF than in those not receiving growth factor, likely as a result of the combination of GM-CSF and radiation [32] post chemotherapy. A greater percentage of patients discontinued growth factor due to toxicity in the GM-CSF trials as compared to G-CSF trials although reactions were usually local and not life threatening. A possible explanation of the apparent diminished efficacy of GM-CSF compared to G-CSF is that the rates of neutropenic complications on the placebo arms in the GM-CSF trials were generally lower (four trials <10%) than in the G-CSF trials making it more difficult to detect a positive effect. Alternatively the differences seen in study results may be a result of the distinct biological effects of these two cytokines. A randomized trial comparing the two growth factors in primary prophylaxis of chemotherapy related neutropenia has not been published.

Secondary prophylaxis using granulocyte growth factors is a common clinical practice although prospective trials are limited. A single prospective trial randomized patients with lymphoma who experienced neutropenia with the first cycle of CHOP to GM-CSF versus no growth factor in the second cycle of chemotherapy. The GM-CSF patients experienced a shorter duration of neutropenia but the empiric use of antibiotics actually increased in this group apparently due to GM-CSF induced fever [33]. The data for the secondary use of G-CSF is limited to the U.S. multicenter trial of primary prophylaxis [18]. However, this trial was designed such that placebo patients experiencing febrile neutropenia during cycle 1 received open label G-CSF with subsequent cycles of therapy. With the addition of G-CSF the rate of neutropenic fever in this cohort declined from 100% in cycle 1 to 23% in cycle 2 with 50% decrease in duration of grade IV neutropenia. These data for clinical benefit, although limited, are supported by a large clinical practice experience, and the ASCO guidelines.

Prescription of growth factors for patients with established neutropenia with or without fever is more controversial. In the setting of afebrile neutropenia in cancer chemotherapy patients, G-CSF treatment compared to placebo decreased the duration of Grade IV neutropenia, but did not impact the rates of neutropenic fever (15% in both groups), hospitalization or antibiotic use [34]. The lesser impact in this setting may relate to the delay in administration compared to prophylactic strategies. At any rate, routine use of a CSF in the asymptomatic chemotherapy patient with neutropenia is not recommended.

In the case of neutropenia with fever, several trials are published in which patients with various malignancies were randomized to placebo or one of the two growth factors [35–42]. Again, the duration of neutropenia was shortened in most trials. However, the duration of hospitalization was shortened in only 2 of the 7 trials in which the use of growth factor was evaluated on an empiric basis (i.e. all patients with neutropenic fever were treated and analyzed for study endpoints regardless of their ultimate culture results) and there was no impact on duration of fever or survival. One trial analyzed only patients who ultimately developed positive cultures and did show improvement in clinical endpoints including mortality [42]. While routine use of CSFs in the treatment of febrile neutropenia is not recommended the selective use in patients at high risk for bacterial or tissue infection, or prolonged neutropenia is reasonable.

The role of CSFs in acute leukemia deserves special mention. Investigators have used two main rationales for the use of myeloid growth factors in this disease. One rationale is that growth factor delivered before and/or during chemotherapy will drive leukemic cells into the more chemosensitive S phase and may perhaps enhance remission and ultimately, overall survival rates. The second rationale is to use growth factors after chemotherapy as a means of decreasing chemotherapeutic toxicity thereby decreasing early death rates and perhaps increasing overall survival. These hypotheses have been tested in several randomized clinical trials which are somewhat difficult to interpret given variable trial design but which are summarized below. Also evaluated in these trials was a concern based on in vitro data that outcomes may be worsened by a growth factor induced stimulation of leukemia. This last concern has clearly not been borne out in clinical trials.

There are at least seven published trials of induction chemotherapy for acute myelogenous leukemia in which patients were randomized to receive growth factor before and/or during chemotherapy in an effort to enhance leukemic cytotoxicity [43–49]. There was no improvement in remission rate, overall survival or early death in any trial. The majority of these trials (5 of 7) demonstrated more rapid neutrophil recovery with growth factor but this had no impact on duration of hospitalization or infectious complications. Of concern, several investigators reported delayed platelet recovery with GM-CSF presumably due to growth factor sensitization of stem cells during chemotherapy.

CSFs have also been evaluated post chemotherapy in patients with myelogenous leukemia in an effort to reduce the infectious complications of this treatment. Six randomized trials (4 with G-CSF and 2 with GM-CSF) are published although the timing and mode of administration varies somewhat between studies as does patient population [50–55]. Consistent findings in these studies were a decrease in duration of neutropenia (decrease ranging from 2–7 days) and a lack of benefit on early death rates. One trial demonstrated enhancement of complete remission rates [52] and a second showed improvement in median survival [51] with growth factor but in both instances this effect seems to be the result of a unexpectedly poor outcome in the placebo arm. Although several investigators reported improvement in documented infection rates, days with fever and/or antibiotic use this translated into shorter hospitalization only in the Heil trial [55].

This randomized, double-blind, placebo-controlled, Phase III Trial compared G-CSF to placebo during induction and consolidation therapy in a group of 521 adult patients with De Novo acute myeloid leukemia [55]. After the first induction treatment, neutrophil recovery occurred five days earlier in the G-CSF group (p<.001) with a reduction in fever duration from 8.5 to 7 days (P=.009), parenteral antibiotic use from 18.5 to 15 days (P=.0001) and hospitalization from 25 to 20 days (P=.001). In the G-CSF group there was a decrease in the use of systemic antifungal therapy from 43% to 34% (P=.04). As in other trials, there was no negative impact of G-CSF on remission rate of survival.

The inconsistent results of growth factor support in the setting of myeloid malignancies is likely multi-factorial. Certainly the use of CSFs before or during chemotherapy for AML has not resulted in significant clinical benefit at present and should not be utilized except in the setting of a clinical trial. In the post-chemotherapy setting, the use of either G or GM-CSF appears to be safe with no negative impact on response or survival. In addition the larger trials do suggest that the reduction in neutropenia from these agents may be associated with clinically significant improvement in duration of antibiotic use, use of antifungal therapy and shortened hospitalizations, particularly in the elderly population. Based on these data, both GM-CSF and G-CSF have received FDA approval for use in this setting. To optimize clinical benefit of these agents, comparative trials would be useful as well as a study designed to evaluate the best timing for initiation of CSFs post-induction.

## Platelet Growth Factors

The widespread use of granulocyte growth factors with resulting decrease in the incidence of neutropenic complications and maintenance of dose intensity has made chemotherapy induced thrombocytopenia a common cause of chemotherapy dose reduction and/or delay. In recent years the use of platelet transfusions in oncology patients has risen considerably but this practice carries with it the risks of infection and alloimmunization as well as the costs of transfusion. Many agents (including interleukins 1, 3, 6 and 11 as well as PIXY 321, megakaryocyte growth and development factor [MGDF], and thrombopoietin) have been investigated in clinical trials in an effort to identify a growth factor capable of ameliorating chemotherapy induced thrombocytopenia in a clinically significant manner. Thus far only IL-11 is FDA approved for this indication having shown efficacy in a randomized, placebo controlled trial of secondary prophylaxis of platelet transfusion. MGDF and thrombopoietin are still early in clinical trials and may ultimately prove beneficial as well.

Interleukin 11 (IL-11) is a growth factor (discovered from a primate bone marrow stromal cell line) which results in proliferation of stem cells and megakaryocyte precursors as well as stimulation of megakaryocyte maturation. Preclinical trials demonstrated safety and efficacy in non human primates with the production of ultrastructurally normal platelets in the normal and myelosuppressed host.

Instrumental in the acquisition of FDA approval for IL-11 was a multi-institutional trial by Tepler et al in which patients with a variety of cancers, receiving a variety of chemotherapy regimens were randomized to placebo or one of two doses of IL-11 (25 or 50 µg/kg subcutaneously daily) for 14–21 days or until platelet count > 100,000/microliter [56]. Study participation required the administration of at least one platelet transfusion in the previous cycle of chemotherapy and the administration of the same chemotherapy without dose reduction after study enrollment and randomization. Prophylactic platelet transfusions were utilized for platelet count less than 20,000/microliter. The use of G-CSF was permissible (all but 3 patients received this growth factor) but GM-CSF was not due to its lack of lineage specificity. The trial included 93 patients receiving 24 different chemotherapy regimens. Intention to treat analysis and analysis of evaluable patients demonstrated that significantly fewer patients receiving the higher dose of IL-11 required platelet transfusions than those receiving placebo. However, the number of required transfusions per patient and the duration of thrombocytopenia were not statistically different among groups. There was no effect of therapy on the incidence or severity of neutropenic fever, the need for red cell transfusion, days of hospitalization, and importantly, no difference in the incidence of bleeding complications. One can conclude that in the setting of secondary prophylaxis, IL-11 reduces the likelihood of prophylactic platelet transfusion. The clinical impact, although modest, may be important in selected patients, and will be clarified in clinical practice, with FDA approval of the agent for secondary prophylaxis.

A second randomized placebo-controlled trial of IL-11 has been reported by Isaacs et al [57]. The design was similar to the above noted trial but this study was of primary prophylaxis with IL-11 in patients who received a dose intensive chemotherapy regimen for breast cancer. Prophylactic transfusions were again given for platelet counts <20,000/microliter. Patients were assessed for transfusion requirement, number of transfusions and duration of thrombocytopenia over two blinded cycles of chemotherapy with IL-11 vs. placebo. Seventy-seven patients were enrolled with 67 being assessable. Intention to treat analysis (but not analysis by treatment received) revealed that fewer patients required platelet transfusion in the IL-11 vs. placebo group during both cycles of therapy combined. There was no difference in transfusion incidence during cycle one but the difference become apparent during cycle two (Fig. 4). However, only the analysis of assessable patients revealed

**Fig. 4.** Requirement for platelet
transfusions among placebo (closed
boxes) and rhIL-11 treated patients
(open boxes) after the first and second
chemotherapy courses

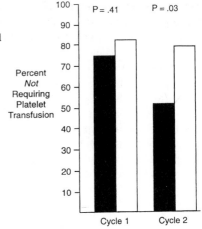

reduction in mean number of transfusions and a shorter duration of
thrombocytopenia for IL-11 treated patients. No severe adverse bleeding
events were noted. These data are difficult to interpret given differences
among the intention to treat analysis and analysis by treatment received
as well as a lack of impact on clinically relevant endpoints. IL-11 has not
been given FDA approval for primary prophylaxis of thrombocytopenia.
Toxicity of IL-11 (in both trials) was usually mild but included
edema/volume retention and atrial arrhythmias. Headache and asymptomatic conjunctival injection were also noted.

The clinical benefits of IL-11 in reduction of thrombocytopenia sets a
benchmark for testing the recombinant forms of thrombopoietin, the
primary regulator of platelet production. The search for this elusive
agent has been extensive. In 1990 a murine retrovirus was discovered
which induced a myeloproliferative disease in mice with the cloned
transforming gene termed v-mpl. A homologous gene from a human
erythroleukemia cell line, coding for a receptor called c-mpl was discovered to have characteristics shared with known cytokines and growth
factors. The ligand for this receptor was cloned and has been developed
for use in humans. This c-mpl ligand maps to chromosome 3 and in vivo
levels of the cytokine have been shown to vary inversely with platelet
count. The c-mpl ligand increases megakaryocyte number and ploidy,
increases mean platelet volume, induces maturation of the mega-

karyocyte ultrastructure and alters expression of platelet specific membrane proteins. Knockout mice for either c-mpl receptor loss or c-mpl ligand loss typically have platelet counts 15% of normal but are not lethal mutants. This suggests that this cytokine, while not essential, represents the most important regulator of platelet production. Two forms of the cytokine are available in clinical trials at the current time. Recombinant thrombopoietin (TPO) is the full length protein. Recombinant MGDF (Megakaryocyte Growth and Development Factor) represents a truncated form of the protein which is conjugated with polyethylene glycol (PEGylated) resulting in greater potency and a longer half-life than the unconjugated protein.

Mice and subhuman primates myelosuppressed by chemotherapy and radiation showed decreased mortality, decreased duration of thrombocytopenia and higher platelet nadirs when treated with thrombopoietin vs. placebo in preclinical studies. In humans, MGDF has been administered both pre and post chemotherapy in an effort to define its safety, clinical efficacy, and optimal dosing. In the prechemotherapy model, MGDF administration to patients with advanced cancers resulted in a dose dependent increase in platelet count with peak counts ranging between 51 and 584% over baseline [58]. Increases over baseline counts were notable by day 6 and peaked between days 12 and 18. Platelet appearance and aggregation were normal with normal expression of activation markers and glycoproteins [59]. One of 17 patients experienced a superficial thrombophlebitis that may or may not have been related to MGDF therapy. No other significant adverse reactions were noted although 2 patients had platelet peaks over 1000 x 10$^9$ with no clinical sequelae.

Fanucchi et al have done a randomized phase I dose escalation study of MGDF in patients with lung cancer receiving carboplatin and paclitaxel [60]. Patients receiving MGDF over a broad range of doses and duration of therapy demonstrated reduced severity and duration of platelet nadirs as compared to controls. Although the study demonstrated proof of platelet effect, there was no impact on transfusion requirement or bleeding events as the doses of chemotherapy used were not adequate to result in severe thrombocytopenia even in the placebo group. Two patients on the treatment arm developed thrombotic complications, one deep venous thrombosis with pulmonary embolus (platelet count of 243,000 per cubic millimeter) and one superficial thrombosis of the saphenous vein (platelet count of 468,000 per cubic millimeter). No other significant adverse events attributable to study drug were noted.

Basser et al also investigated the role of variable doses of MGDF after dose intensive chemotherapy with cyclophosphamide and carboplatin in patients with advanced cancers [61]. Results were similar to those of the

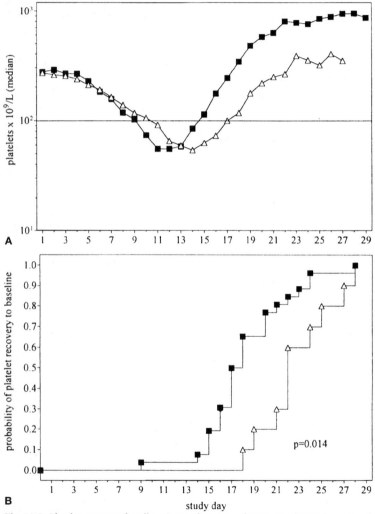

**Fig. 5A,B.** Platelet recovery for all patients administered PEG-rHuMGDF (boxes) and those given placebo (triangles) after chemotherapy

Fanucchi trial with patients receiving MGDF exceeding doses of 0.1 microgram/kg/day demonstrating earlier platelet nadirs and more rapid platelet recovery without effect on the depth of the nadir when compared to placebo patients (Fig. 5). Again there was no effect of study drug on platelet transfusion requirements, clinically significant bleeding, episodes of febrile neutropenia, or hematocrit and pertinent toxicities were limited to two episodes of thrombosis.

Clinical trials of multi-cycle, dose intensive chemotherapy supported with MGDF are ongoing. Optimal doses and dosing schedules are yet to be delineated and beneficial effects on clinically relevant endpoints are yet to be defined. Similar trials utilizing the full protein, thrombopoietin, are also ongoing with initial pre and post chemotherapy administration results very similar to those of MGDF [62].

## References

1. Gleeson C, Spencer D (1995) Blood transfusion and its benefits in palliative care. Palliative Medicine 9:307–313
2. Chung M, Steinmetz OK, Gordon PH (1993) Perioperative blood transfusion and outcome after resection for colorectal carcinoma. Br J Surg 80:427–432
3. Vamvakas E, Moore SB (1993) Perioperative blood transfusion and colorectal cancer recurrence: A qualitative statistical overview and meta-analysis. Transfusion 33:754–765
4. Vamvakas EC (1993) Perioperative blood transfusion and cancer recurrence: meta-analysis for explanation. Transfusion 35:760–768
5. Busch ORC, Hop WCJ, Hoynck van Papendrecht MAW, Marquet RL, Jeekel J (1993) Blood transfusions and prognosis in colorectal cancer. N Engl J Med 328:1372–1376
6. Houbiers JGA, Brand A, van de Watering LMG, Hermans J, Verwey PJM, Bijnen AB, Pahlplatz P, Eiftinck Schattenkerk M, Wobbes T, de Vries JE, Klementschitsch P, van de Maas AHM, van de Velde CJH (1994) Randomized controlled trial comparing transfusion of leukocyte-depleted or buffy-coat-depleted blood in surgery for colorectal cancer. Lancet 344:573–578
7. Abels RI (1992) Use of recombinant human erythropoietin in the treatment of anemia in patients who have cancer. Sem Oncol 19 (3 Suppl 8): 29–35
8. Henry DH, Abels RI (1994) Recombinant human erythropoietin in the treatment of cancer and chemotherapy-induced anemia: Results of a double-blind and open-label follow-up studies. Sem Oncol 21 (2 Suppl 3): 21–28
9. Glaspy J, Bukowski R, Steinberg D, Taylor C, Tchekmedyian S, Vadhan-Raj S (1997) Impact of therapy with Epoetin Alfa on clinical outcomes in patients with nonmyeloid malignancies during cancer chemotherapy in community oncology practice. J Clin Oncol 15:1218–1234
10. de Campos E, Radford J, Steward W, Milroy R, Dougal M, Swindell R, Testa N, Thatcher N (1995) Clinical and in vitro effects of recombinant human erythropoietin in patients receiving intensive chemotherapy for small cell lung cancer. J Clin Oncol 13:1623–1631

11. Del Mastro L, Venturini M, Lionetto R, Garrone O, Melioli G, Pasquetti W, Sertoli MR, Bertelli G, Canavese G, Costantini M, Rosso R (1997) Randomized phase III trial evaluating the role of erythropoietin in the prevention of chemotherapy-induced anemia. J Clin Oncol 15:2715–2721

12. Lavey RS, Dempsey WH (1993) Erythropoietin increases hemoglobin in cancer patients during radiation therapy. Int J Radiat Oncol Biol Phys 27:1147–1152

13. Vijayakumar S, Roach M, Wara W, Chan SK, Ewing C, Rubin S, Sutton H, Halpern H, Awan A, Houghton A, Quiet C, Weichselbaum R (1993) Effect of subcutaneous recombinant human erythropoietin in cancer patients receiving radiotherapy: preliminary results of a randomized open-labeled, phase II trial. Int J Radiat Oncol Biol Phys 26:721–729

14. Prabhakar SS, Muhlfelder T (1997) Antibodies to recombinant human erythro-poietin causing pure red cell aplasia. Clin Nephrol 47:331–335

15. Blackwell S, Crawford J (1994) Filgrastim (r-metHuG-CSF)in the chemotherapy setting. In: Morstyn G, Dexter TM (eds) Filgrastim (r-metHuG-CSF) in Clinical Practice. Marcell Dekker Inc, New York, pp 103–116

16. ASCO Ad Hoc Colony-Stimulating Factor Guidelines Expert Panel (1994) American Society of Clinical Oncology recommendations for the use of hematopoietic colony stimulating factors: evidence based, clinical practice guidelines. J Clin Oncol 12:2471–2508

17. Spiekermann K, Roesler J, Emmendoerffer A, Elsner J, Welte K (1997) Functional features of neutrophils induced by G-CSF and GM-CSF treatment: differential effects and clinical implications. Leukemia 11:466–478

18. Crawford J, Ozer H, Stoller R, Johnson D, Lyman G, Tabbara I, Kris M, Grous J, Picozzi V, Rausch G, Smith R, Gradishar W, Yahanda A, Vincent M, Stewart M, Glaspy J (1991) Reduction by granulocyte colony-stimulating factor of fever and neutropenia induced by chemotherapy in patients with small-cell lung cancer. N Engl J Med 325:164–170

19. Trillet-Lenoir V, Green J, Manegold C, Von Pawel J, Gatzemeier U, Lebeau B, Depierre A, Johnson P, Decoster G, Tomita D. (1993) Recombinant granulocyte colony stimulating factor reduces the infectious complications of cytotoxic chemotherapy. Eur J Cancer 29 A: 319–324

20. Pettengell R, Gurney H, Radford JA, Deakin DP, James R, Wilkinson PM, Kane K, Bentley J, Crowther D (1992) Granulocyte colony-stimulating factor to prevent dose-limiting neutropenia in non-Hodgkin's lymphoma: A randomized controlled trial. Blood 80:1430–1436.

21. Zizani PL, Pavone E, Storti S, Moretti L, Fattori PP, Guardigni L, Falini B, Gobbi M, Gentilini P, Lauta VM, Bendandi M, Gherlinzoni F, Magagnoli M, Venturi S, Aitini E, Tabanelli M, Leone G, Liso V, Tura S. (1997) Randomized trial with or without granulocyte colony-stimulating factor as adjunct to induction VNCOP-B treatment of elderly high grade non-Hodgkin's lymphoma. Blood 89:3974–3979

22. Gisselbrecht C, Haioun C, Lepage E, Bastion Y, Tilly H, Bosly A, Dupriez B, Marit G, Herbrecht R, Deconinck E, Marolleau JP, Yver A, Dabouz-Harrouche F, Coiffer B, Reyes F (1997) Placebo controlled phase III study of lenograstim (glycosylated recombinant human granulocyte-stimulating factor) in aggressive non-Hodgkin's lymphoma: factors influencing chemotherapy administration. Leuk Lymphoma 25:289–300

23. Negro S, Masuda N, Furuse K, Saijo N, Fukoaka M (1997) Dose-intensive chemotherapy in extensive stage small-cell lung cancer. Cancer Chemother Pharmacol 40: S70–73

24. Woll PJ, Hodgetts J, Lomax L, Bildet F, Cour-Chabernaud V, Thatcher N (1995) Can cytotoxic dose intensity be increased by using granulocyte colony-stimulating factor? A randomized controlled trial of lenograstim in small cell lung cancer. J Clin Oncol 13:652–659

25. Lyman GH, Kuderer NM, Balducci L (1996) Thresholds for the use of recombinant human colony stimulating factors (CSFs) based on revised cost estimates incorporating indirect medical, nonmedical and intangible cost considerations. Blood 88:10 Suppl 1:346a (abst)

26. Kaplan LD, Kahn JO, Crowe S, Northfelt D, Neville P, Grossberg H, Abrams DI, Tracey J, Mills J, Volberding PA (1991) Clinical and virologic effects of recombinant human granulocyte-macrophage colony-stimulating factor in patients receiving chemotherapy for human immunodeficiency virus-associated non-Hodgkin's lymphoma: results of a randomized trial. J Clin Oncol 9:929–940

27. Jones SE, Schottstaedt MW, Duncan LA, Kirby RL, Good RH, Mennel RG, George TK, Snyder DA, Watkins DL, Denham CA, Hoyes FA, Rubin AS (1996) Randomized double-blind prospective trial to evaluate the effects of sargramostim versus placebo in a moderate-dose fluorouracil, doxorubicin, and cyclophosphamide adjuvant chemotherapy program for stage II and III breast cancer. J Clin Oncol 14:2976–2983

28. Gerhartz HH, Engelhard M, Meusers P, Brittinger G, Wilmanns W, Schlimok G, Mueller P, Huhn D, Musch R, Siegert W, Gerhartz D, Hartlapp JH, Thiel E, Huber C, Peschl C, Spann W, Emmerich B, Schadek C, Westerhausen M, Pees HW, Radtke H, Engert A, Terhardt E, Schick H, Binder T, Fuchs R, Hasford J, Brandmaier R, Stern AC, Jones TC, Ehrlich HJ, Stein H, Parwaresch M, Tiemann M, Lennert K (1993) Randomized, double-blind, placebo-controlled, phase III study of recombinant human granulocyte-macrophage colony stimulating factor as adjunct to induction treatment of high-grade malignant non-Hodgkin's lymphomas. Blood 82:2329–2339

29. Hamm JT, Schiller JH, Oken MM, Gallmeier Wm, Rusthoven J, Israel RJ. (1991) Granulocyte-macrophage colony stimulating factor in small cell carcinoma of the lung: Preliminary analysis of a randomized controlled trial. Proc Am Soc Clin Oncol 255 (abst)

30. Yau JC, Neidhart JA, Triozzi P, Verma S, Nemunaitis J, Quick DP, Mayernik DG, Oette DH, Haynes FA, Holcenberg J (1996) Randomized placebo-controlled trial of granulocyte-macrophage colony-stimulating factor support for dose intensive cyclophosphamide, etoposide, and cisplatin. Am J Hematol 51:289–295

31. Bajorin DF, Nichols CR, Schmoll HJ, Kantoff PW, Bokemeyer C, Demetri GD, Einhorn LH, Bosl GJ (1995) Recombinant human granulocyte-macrophage colony-stimulating factor as an adjunct to conventional dose ifosfamide-based chemotherapy for patients with advanced or relapsed germ cell tumors: A randomized trial. J Clin Oncol 13:79–86

32. Bunn PA, Crowley J, Kelly K, Hazuka MB, Beasley K, Upchurch C, Livingston R. (1995) Chemoradiotherapy with or without granulocyte-macrophage colony-stimulating factor in the treatment of limited-stage small-cell lung cancer: a prospective phase III randomized study of the Southwest Oncology Group. J Clin Oncol 13:1632–1641

33. Kaku K, Takahashi M, Moriyama Y, Nakahata T, Masaoka T, Yoshida Y, Shibata A, Kaneko T, Miwa S (1993) Recombinant human granulocyte-macrophage colony-stimulating factor (rhGM-CSF) after chemotherapy in patients with non-Hodgkin's lymphoma; a placebo-controlled double blind phase III trial. Leuk Lymphoma 11:229–238

34. Hartmann LC, Tschetter LK, Habermann TM, Ebbert LP, Johnson PS, Malliard JA, Levitt R, Suman VJ, Witzig TE, Wieand HS, Miller LL. Moertel CG. Granulocyte colony-stimulating factor in severe chemotherapy-induced afebrile neutropenia. NEJM 336 (25): 1776–1780, 1997.

35. Maher DW, Lieschkle GJ, Green M, Bishop J, Stuart-Harris R, Wolf M, Sheridan WP, Kefford RF, Cebon J, Olver I, McKendrick J, Toner G, Bradstock K, Lieschke M, Cruickshank S, Tomita DK, Hoffman EW, Fox RM, Morstyn G (1994). Filgrastim in patients with chemotherapy-induced febrile neutropenia. Ann Intern Med 121:492–501

36. Mitchell PLR, Morland BJ, Dick G, Easlea D, Meyer LC, Stevens MCG, Pinkerton CR (1995) Clinical benefits and cost savings of interventional G-CSF therapy in patients with febrile neutropenia following chemotherapy. Blood 86 Suppl 1:500 (abst)

37. Mayadormo JI, Rivera F, Diaz-Puente MT, Lianes P, Colomer R, Lopez-Brea M, Lopez E, Paz-Ares L, Hitt R, Garcia-Ribas I, Cubedo R, Alonso S, Cortes-Funes H (1995) Improving treatment of chemotherapy-induced neutropenic fever by administration of colony stimulating factors. JNCI 87:803–808

38. Biesma B, deVries EGE, Willemse PHB, Sluiter W, Postmus PE, Limburg PC, Stern AC, Vellenga E (1990) Efficacy and tolerability of recombinant human granulocyte-macrophage colony-stimulating factor in patients with chemotherapy-related leukopenia and fever. Eur J Cancer 26:932–936

39. Anaissie EJ, Vartivarian S, Bodey GP, Legrand C, Kantarjian H, Abi-Said D, Karl C, Vadhan-Raj S (1996) Randomized comparison between antibiotics alone and antibiotics plus granulocyte-macrophage colony-stimulating factor (Eschericia coli-derived) in cancer patients with fever and neutropenia. Am J Med 100:17–23

40. Vallenga E, Uyl-de Groot CA, deWit R, Keizer HJ, Lowenberg B, ten Haaft MA, de Witte TJM, Verhagen CAH, Stoter GJ, Rutten FFH, Mulder NH, Smid WM, de Vries EGE (1996) Randomized placebo-controlled trial of granulocyte-macrophage colony-stimulating factor in patients with chemotherapy-related febrile neutropenia. J Clin Oncol 14:619–627

41. Ravaud A, Chevreau C, Bonichon F, Mihura J, Bui BN, Tabah I (1995) A phase III trial of recombinant granulocyte-macrophage colony stimulating factor (GM-CSF) as corrective treatment in patients with neutropenic fever following antineoplastic chemotherapy. Proc ASCO 14:261 (abst)

42. Aviles Agustin, Guzman R, Garcia E, Talavera A, Diaz-Maqueo JC (1996) Results of a randomized trial of granulocyte colony-stimulating factor in patients with infection and severe granulocytopenia. Anti-Cancer Drugs 7:392–397

43. Ohno R, Naoe T, Kanamaru A, Yoshida M, Hiraoka A, Kobayashi T, Ueda T, Minami S, Morishima Y, Saito Y, Furusawa S, Imai K, Takemoto Y, Miura Y, Teshima H, Hamajima N, and the Kohseisho Leukemia Study Group (1994) A double-blind controlled study of granulocyte colony-stimulating factor started two days before induction chemotherapy in refractory acute myeloid leukemia. Blood 83:2086–2092

44. Buchner T, Hiddemann W, Wormann B, Rottmann R, Zuhlsdorf M, Maschmeyer G, Ludwig W-D, Sauerland MC, Frisch J, Schultz G (1994) GM-CSF multiple course priming and long-term administration in newly diagnosed AML: hematologic and therapeutic effects. Blood 84 (Suppl 1): 96 (abst)

45. Zittoun R, Suciu S, Mandelli F, de Witte T, Thaler J, Stryckmans P, Hayat M, Peetermans M, Cadiou M, Solbu G, Petti MC, Willemze R (1996) Granulocyte-macrophage colony-stimulating factor associated with induction treatment of acute myelogenous leukemia: a randomised trial by the European Organization fro Research and Treatment of Cancer Leukemia Cooperative Group. J Clin Oncol 14:2150–2159

46. Heil G, Chadid L, Hoelzer D, Seipelt G, Mitrou P, Huber C, Kolbe K, Mertelsmann R, Lindemann A, Frisch J, Nicolay U, Gaus W, Heimpel H (1995) GM-CSF in a double-blind, randomised, placebo controlled trial in therapy of adult patients with de-novo acute myeloid leukemia. Leukemia 9:3–9

47. Lowenberg B, Suciu S, Archimbaud E, Ossenkoppele G, Verhoef GE, Vallenga E, Wijermans P, Berneman Z, Dekker AW, Stryckmans P, Schouten H, Jehn U, Muus P, Sonneveld P, Dardenne M, Zittoun R. (1997) Use of recombinant GM-CSF during and after remission induction chemotherapy in patients aged 61 years and older with acute myeloid leukemia: final report of AML-11, a phase III randomized study of the Leukemia Cooperative Group of European Organisation for the Research and Treatment of Cancer and the Dutch Belgian Hemato-Oncology Cooperative Group. Blood 90:2952–2961

48. Lowenberg B, Boogarts MA, Vallenga E, Ossenkoppele G, Dekker AW, vander Lelie J, Schouten HC, Fopp M, Gratwohl A, Fey M, Gmur J, van Putten W (1995) Various modalities of use of GM-CSF in the treatment of acute myelogenous leukemia (AML): a HOVON-SAAK randomised study (HOVON-4 A) Blood 86 (Suppl 1): 2035 (abst)

49. Witz F, Sadoun A, Perrin M-C, Berthou C, Briere J, Cahn J-Y, Lioure B, Witz B, Francois S, Desablens B, Pignon B, Le Prise P-Y, Audhuy B, Caillot D, Casassus P, Delain M, Christian B, Tellier Z, Polin V, Hurteloup P, Harousseau J-L for the Groupe Ouest Est Leucemies Aigues Myeloblastiques (1998) A placebo-controlled study of recombinant human granulocyte-macrophage colony-stimulating factor administered during and after induction treatment fro de novo acute myelogenous leukemia in elderly patients. Blood 91:2722–2730

50. Ohno R, Tomonaga M, Kobayashi T, Kanamaru A, Shirakawa S, Masaoka T, Dohy H, Niho Y, Hamajima N, Takaku F (1990) Effect of granulocyte colony-stimulating factor after intensive induction therapy in relapsed or refractory acute leukemia. N Engl J Med 323:871–877

51. Rowe JM, Anderson JW, Mazza JJ, Bennett JM, Paietta E, Hayes FA, Oette D, Cassileth PA, Stadtmauer EA, Wiernik PH (1995) A randomized placebo-controlled phase III study of granulocyte-macrophage colony-stimulating factor in adult patients (>55 to 70 years of age) with acute myelogenous leukemia: A study of the Eastern Cooperative Oncology Group (E1490). Blood 86:457–462

52. Dombert H, Chastang C, Fenaux P, Reiffers J, Bordessoule D, Bouabdallah R, Mandelli F, Ferrant A, Auzanneau G, Tilly H, Yver A, Degos L for the AML Cooperative Study Group (1995) A controlled study of recombinant human granulocyte colony-stimulating factor in elderly patients after treatment for acute myelogenous leukemia. AML Cooperative Study Group. N Engl J Med 332:1678–1683

53. Stone RM, Berg DT, George SL, Dodge RK, Paciucci PA, Schulman P, Lee EJ, Moore JO, Powell BL, Schiffer CA (1995) Granulocyte-macrophage colony-stimulating factor after initial chemotherapy for elderly patients with primary acute myelogenous leukemia. Cancer and Leukemia Group B. N Engl J Med 332:1671–1677

54. Godwin JE, Kopecky KJ, Head DR, Hynes HE, Balcerak SP, Appelbaum FR. (1994) A double-blind placebo controlled trial of G-CSF in elderly patients with previously untreated acute myeloid leukemia. A Southwest Oncology Group Study. Blood 86 (Suppl 1): 1723 (abst)

55. Heil G, Hoelzer D, Sanz MA, Lechner K, Liu Yin JA, Papa G, Noens L, Szer J, Gasner A, O'Brien C, Matchum J, Barge A for the International Acute Myeloid Leukemia Study Group (1997) A randomized, double-blind, placebo-controlled, phase III study of Filgrastim in remission induction and consolidation therapy for adults with de novo acute myeloid leukemia. Blood 90:4710–4718

56. Tepler I, Elias L, Smith JW, Hussein M, Rosen G, Chang AYC, Moore JO, Gordon MS, Kuca B, Beach KJ, Loewy JW, Garnick MB, Kaye JA (1996) A randomized placebo-controlled trial of recombinant human interleukin-11 in cancer patients with severe thrombocytopenia due to chemotherapy. Blood 87:3607–3614

57. Isaacs C, Robert NJ, Baily A, Schuster MW, Overmoyer B, Graham M, Cai B, Beach KJ, Loewy JW, Kaye JA (1997) Randomized placebo-controlled study of recombinant human interleukin-11 to prevent chemotherapy-induced thrombocytopenia in patients with breast cancer receiving dose-intensive cyclphosphamide and doxorubicin. J Clin Oncol 15:3368–3377

58. Basser RL, Rasko JEJ, Clarke K, Cebon J, Green Md<Hussein S, Alt C, Menchaca D, Tomita D, Marty J, Fox RM, Begley CG. (1996) Thrombopoietic effects of pegylated recombinant human megakaryocyte growth and development factor (PEG-rHuMGDF) in patients with advanced cancer. Lancet 348:1279–1281

59. O'Malley CJ, Rasko JEJ, Basser RL, McGrath KM, Cebon J, Grigg AP, Hopkins W, Cohen B, O'Byrne J, Green MD, Fox RM, Berndt MC, Begley CG. (1996) Administration of pegylated recombinant human megakaryocyte growth and development factor to humans stimulates the production of functional platelets that show no evidence of in vivo activation. Blood 88:3288–3298

60. Fanucchi M, Glaspy J, Crawford J, Garst J, Figlin R, Sheridan W, Menchaca D, Tomita D, Ozer H, Harker L. (1997) Effects of polyethylene glycol-conjugated recombinant human megakaryocyte growth and development factor on platelet counts after chemotherapy for lung cancer. N Engl J Med 336:404–409

61. Basser RL, Rasko JEJ, Clarke K, Cebon J, Green MD, Grigg AP, Zalcberg J, Cohen B, O'Byrne J, Menchaca DM, Fox RM, Begley CG. (1997) Randomized, blinded placebo-controlled phase I trial of pegylated recombinant human megakaryocyte growth and development factor with filgrastim after dose-intensive chemotherapy in patients with advanced cancer. Blood 89:3118–3128

62. Vadhan-Raj S, Murray LJ, Bueso-Ramos C, Patel S, Reddy SP, Hoots WK, Johnston T, Papadopolous NE, Hittelman WN, Johnston DA, Yang TA, Paton VE, Cohen RL, Hellman SD, Benjamin RS, Broxmeyer HE. (1997) Stimulation of megakaryocyte and platelet production by a single dose of recombinant human thrombopoietin in patients with cancer. Ann Int Med 126:673–681

# Pain Management

F. M. Boyle, S. A. Grossman

Pain is defined as "an unpleasant sensory and emotional experience associated with actual or potential tissue damage, or described in terms of such damage" [1]. Approximately 80% of patients with cancer will experience significant pain as a result of their disease and/or its treatment [2]. Optimal management of pain at all stages of the therapeutic pathway will reduce the suffering associated with cancer, enhancing quality of life and physiological adaptation. Techniques for assessment of pain and evaluation of its underlying cause allow a precise diagnosis in most instances, allowing treatment to be tailored to individual needs. Pharmacological and non-pharmacological techniques described in this chapter are applicable to the management of both acute and chronic pain in cancer patients.

## Barriers to cancer pain management

Despite the availability in developed countries of a plethora of pain relieving strategies, there is evidence that cancer pain is frequently undertreated [3]. The difficulties lie in part with health professionals, who may lack education about pain assessment and treatment [4]. Persisting attitudes that only patients who are terminal should receive maximal analgesia [5], or that patients are not good judges of their pain [6], inhibit provision of pain relief particularly in early stage disease or for treatment induced pain. Physicians may excessively fear opiate toxicity or iatrogenic opiate addiction [7]. These concerns are frequently shared by patients and families who may also under-report pain to avoid confirmation of disease progression. Multimodality approaches may not be readily accessible or affordable, and restrictions on opiate prescribing occur in most countries, to the detriment of cancer patients [4]. Changes to health care systems and patient and professional education will be required if this most feared of all consequences of cancer is to be controlled.

## Evaluation of patients with cancer pain

Pain is always a subjective experience [1] and although acute pain may be accompanied by signs of sympathetic overactivity (restlessness, tachycardia, tachypnea, hypertension, sweating and pallor), chronic pain is more likely to be accompanied by depression, inactivity and withdrawal [2]. An accurate assessment of severity, and nature of the pain will be required in order to establish an etiological framework and management plan, bearing in mind that many cancer patients will have more than one pain [2]. Frequent reassessment will be required to monitor the success of therapeutic endeavours, and this necessitates some measure of the patient's subjective experience.

Quantitative pain scales suitable for routine use in oncological settings include visual analogue or numerical rating scales, where pain intensity is scored between 0 and 10 (worst imaginable pain), and verbal descriptor scales (mild to excruciating) [8]. Evidence suggests poor correlation between staff and patient ratings [9], which may lead to under treatment of pain [6]. Such scales may also be used to plot relief achieved with various measures and facilitate communication within the multidisciplinary team. These scales measure only severity of pain. More complex instruments such as the McGill Pain Questionnaire [10] are useful in differentiating the various causes of pain described below but are impractical for routine use. Validated instruments exist for use in children of various ages [11] and may also be of benefit in adults experiencing communication difficulties.

A thorough history and physical examination, followed by appropriate investigations are required to tailor pain therapy to the patients needs. As this may take some time, it is important to begin treating the pain, especially if severe, in order to gain the patients confidence and cooperation. In the face of a pain emergency (pain intensity of at least 8 out of 10 sustained for more than 6 hours) [12] rapid titration of intravenous or oral short acting opiates (usually morphine) is required. In the acute setting, rapid pain relief facilitates rather than impedes assessment [13].

It is important to determine the underlying cause of the pain. A new back pain in a patient with metastatic malignancy may be due to bony involvement, retroperitoneal node enlargement, epidural metastases with nerve root or spinal cord compression, a crush fracture resulting from steroid induced osteoporosis, or a leaking aortic aneurysm. Each will be at least partially opiate responsive. Opiates might be appropriate alone in the last days of life, but definitive treatment for patients with a longer life expectancy requires an accurate diagnosis if permanent sequelae such as paraplegia are to be avoided.

Underlying causes of pain in cancer patients include:
**Direct effect of tumour**
– Acute e.g. pathological fracture,
– Chronic e.g. infiltration of bones, nerves or viscera
**Diagnostic/therapeutic procedures**
– Post mastectomy or thoracotomy pain syndromes
– Adhesive bowel obstruction
– Chemotherapy or radiation induced mucositis
– Peripheral neuropathy due to chemotherapy
– Osteoporotic crush fractures
**Cancer related physiologic or biochemical alterations**
– Muscle wasting and weakness
– Paraneoplastic neuropathy, myopathy or arthropathy
– Venous thrombosis, pulmonary emboli
– Infection
**Non-cancer disease or injury**
– Osteoarthritis
– Vascular disease

The site, temporal sequence, radiation and quality of the pain along with a detailed history of previous oncologic therapy will assist in determining the mechanism of pain (Table 1), thereby aiding selection of appropriate therapy.

Other factors to consider in a comprehensive pain assessment include:
– Potential utility of anti-neoplastic therapy (surgery, radiotherapy or chemotherapy)
– Other cancer related disorders such as infection, hypercalcaemia, bone marrow failure

**Table 1.** Mechanism of cancer pain and implications for treatment

| Type | Mechanism | Character | Example(s) | Treatment |
|------|-----------|-----------|------------|-----------|
| Nocioceptive somatic | Activation of nocioceptors in cutaneous and deep tissues | Well localised gnawing, aching, worsened by movement | Bone mets, incisional pain, pleurisy | Responds to NSAIDS, acetaminophen, opiates |
| Nociceptive Visceral | Activation of nociceptors by infiltration, compression or distension of viscera | Poorly localised, ± referred to cutaneous sites, deep, squeezing, colicky | Gut obstruction, liver distension, pancreatic cancer | Responds to NSAIDs, acetaminophen, opiates, antispasmodics, nerve blocks |
| Neuropathic peripheral | Damage to nerve or plexus by tumor or cancer therapy – may lead to irreversible changes in spinal cord and central nervous System (deafferentation) | Burning, tingling, shock like paroxysms radiates in dermatomal or plexus distribution, or glove and stocking if polyneuropathy. Associated sensory and/or motor loss | Brachial plexopathy, herpes zoster, cytotoxic neuro-pathy | Relatively opiate resistant, requires coanalgesics e.g. anticonvulsants, antidepressants, early referral for consideration of blocks/surgery before de-afferentation occurs |
| Neuropathic sympathetic | Damage to sympathetic nerves or ganglia by tumor or therapy | Burning, allodynia, hyperpathia, hyperalgesia, dysesthesia, oedema, osteoporosis | Pancoast (superior sulcus) tumor | Responds to sympathetic block |

- Other cancer related symptoms, including nausea, dyspnea, constipation, fatigue or insomnia
- Coexisting medical disorders
- Other non-cancer related pain disorders such as arthritis, and the prior pain and medication history
- History of substance abuse
- Other current medications
- Prior therapy for the cancer pain, and its effectiveness or otherwise.
- Patient and family beliefs and attitudes to pain and pain relief
- Effects of pain on functional status, including employment, activities of daily living, mood, sleep and relationships
- Social and family support, medical support and financial resources
- Psychiatric history

## Treatment of Cancer Pain

Aims

The goal of all professionals involved in care of the cancer patient should be relief from pain and other distressing symptoms at all times during the illness, not merely when prognosis is very limited. Psychological and spiritual support for patient and family will also be required to maintain quality of life and activity, independence and dignity. Multidisciplinary care will be required to achieve these aims, founded on appropriate communication between team members, and inpatient and outpatient settings.

Multimodality Therapy

Although analgesic medications are required by most patients with cancer pain, it is important to consider other options at every stage, to enhance pain control and reduce side effects.

*Modification of Disease Process*

Wherever possible, the best treatment for cancer pain is that which will target the underlying disease process. Surgery, chemotherapy and hormonal therapy should be considered.

Radiotherapy has a particular role in managing localized painful bony metastases, and short courses are appropriate in patients with a limited prognosis [14]. Widespread bony involvement from prostate or breast cancer can be effectively treated by radionuclide therapy with Strontium 89 [15]. Both of these approaches impact on bone marrow reserve. Prophylactic fixation followed by radiotherapy for lytic disease with a high fracture risk (> 50% cortical loss in a weight bearing bone) maintains mobility [14]. Bisphosphonates, including clodronate [16] and pamidronate [17, 18], control pain and reduce fracture risk in patients with lytic bony metastases, by inhibiting osteoclastic bone resorption. They control hypercalcemia, are well tolerated and do not impair bone marrow function. Cost may be an issue with all of these approaches.

Pain from intracranial tumors or from epidural spinal cord compression often responds well to steroids which reduce edema. Dosing is empirical and high doses may be used safely in patients with a limited life expectancy [19].

## Psychological approaches

Depression and anxiety are common in the cancer population as a response to the stress of illness, being identifiable in up to 50% of patients [20]. A strong correlation has been noted between psychiatric diagnoses and significant pain [21]. Treatment of emotional states improves pain control but is no substitute for other pain relieving measures, as psychiatric disturbance is usually a consequence rather than a cause of uncontrolled pain. Recent guidelines emphasise that placebos must not be used even if psychological overlay is suspected [13].

The diagnosis of depression in cancer patients rests not upon vegetative somatic symptoms, as these are common to both disorders, but rather psychological symptoms such as dysphoric mood, feelings of helplessness, loss of self esteem and thoughts of suicide [21]. Both tricyclic antidepressants and selective serotonin reuptake inhibitors are effective in cancer patients, although anorexia and nausea may be a limiting factor with the latter [21]. Anxiety is responsive to both behavioral therapies and benzodiazepines [21].

Behavioral techniques have a wider role in symptom management in cancer patients, and include relaxation, visualization and distraction. These are best taught at an early stage of the illness when concentration is good, and thereafter may be used by the patient to promote a sense of control by reducing helplessness [13, 22]. Hypnosis may be effective in suceptible individuals, and particularly in children and for control of procedure related pain. Cognitive-behavioral therapies [22] and supportive/expressive group therapies [23] may also be of value in maintaining quality of life, dealing with fears and promoting effective interaction with carers.

## Invasive techniques

Only a small proportion of cancer patients require invasive techniques for management of pain, after simpler measures have failed [24]. The support of anaesthesiologists is required and early referral to a comprehensive pain clinic should be considered for patients with severe neuropathic pain, particularly if it is associated with a long life expectancy and fails to respond rapidly to conventional therapy with opiates and adjuvants as described below [13]. Both regional analgesic techniques and neuroablative procedures are of value.

Non-neurolytic nerve blocks are performed with local anesthetic, both peripherally and centrally, for immediate suppression of nocioceptive neuronal activity and to assist in planning of definitive therapy. Temporary local anesthetic blocks may be useful in patients with limited life expectancy (< 1 month) with severe localized pain, and in providing temporary relief of herpes zoster pain.

Definitive neurolytic blocks with phenol or alcohol are of particular value in managing celiac plexus related pain in cancer of the pancreas or upper gastrointestinal tract, and have been shown to prevent deterioration in quality of life [25]. The superior hypogastric plexus may be blocked for relief of pelvic pain. Intrathecal neurolytic block for unilateral segmental pain compares favorably in efficacy with neurosurgical cordotomy, with fewer complications described [26]. Neurolytic sympathectomy arrests sympathetically mediated pain in upper or lower limbs and has largely replaced surgical techniques. Ablation of dorsal roots or trigeminal ganglia may be considered in unilateral head and neck pain. Intercostal nerve block or rhizotomy for localized chest wall pain is without disabling consequences.

The use of epidural or intraspinal opiates and local anaesthetics may be of benefit in carefully selected patients with localized pain and difficulty tolerating systemic opiates. With careful dose titration motor and sympathetic block can be minimized, but pruritis and nausea may be increased [24]. Clonidine may be of additional benefit in intractable neuropathic pain. Intraventricular opiates are of value in more diffuse pain or head and neck pain and in a recent meta-analysis had a favorable side effect profile and complication rate compared with spinal opiates [27].

## Specific Pharmacological Approaches

### The Analgesic Ladder

In 1986 the World Health Organisation released guidelines promoting the use of analgesics for cancer pain, on the premise that most cancer patients world wide would have adequate relief of pain with the optimal use of small number of relatively inexpensive drugs, given orally on a regular basis, and titrated to individual needs [28].

A recent large prospective study found this approach to be effective in 88% of patients with cancer pain [29]. Despite more than a decade of dissemination, no controlled studies have evaluated the effectiveness of the "ladder" in comparison with other approaches or previous practice [30]. The implicit assumption that most cancer pain will be diagnosed when it is mild may delay recognition of the patients who present with rapid onset of severe pain requiring immediate use of strong opiates [12].

The pharmacologic treatment of cancer pain is presented in Table 2.

## Non-opiates

Acetaminophen, aspirin and non-steroidal-anti-inflammatory agents (NSAID) can be considered in mild to moderate pain. They may be particularly useful in musculoskeletal and bone pain. Tolerance and physical dependence are not seen, but dose ceilings, gastrointestinal intolerance, antipyretic and antiplatelet effects may limit their use in cancer patients, particularly those receiving chemotherapy. These agents will frequently be continued along with opiates as they may assist in dose sparing, particularly in bone pain, pleurisy, tissue infiltration and lymphangitis (Table 3) [2, 31].

## Opiates

Opiates recommended for use in cancer pain are listed in Table 4.

**Table 2.** Pharmacologic treatment of cancer pain

| Mild Pain | Moderate pain | Severe Pain |
|---|---|---|
| Non opiates ± adjuvants | Weak opiates ± adjuvants | Strong opiates ± adjuvants |
| aspirin, NSAIDS Acetaminophen | codeine oxycodone | morphine |
| | Pain persists ----> or increases | Pain persists ----> or increases |

**Table 3.** Non-opiate analgesics for use in mild cancer pain

| Drug | Oral dose range | Side effects |
|------|-----------------|--------------|
| Acetaminophen | 1000 mg q 4–6 h | Hepatotoxicity |
| Aspirin | 650 mg q 4–6 h | Dyspepsia, bleeding, antiplatelet, allergy |
| Indomethacin | 25–50 mg q 6 h | Dyspepsia, bleeding, confusion, depression, nephrotoxicity |
| Naproxen | 250 mg q 12 h | Dyspepsia, bleeding, nephrotoxic |
| Ibuprofen | 600 mg q 6 h | Dyspepsia, bleeding, nephrotoxic |
| Piroxicam | 20–40 mg daily | Higher incidence of GIT side effects with chronic use |
| Ketorolac | 30 mg q 6 h oral or IM/SC | Dyspepsia, bleeding, nephrotoxic |

Codeine is useful in mild to moderate pain, particularly in combination with acetaminophen. Its ceiling for analgesia limits its use in severe pain. Oxycodone offers greater flexibility as it has no analgesic ceiling and has a better side effect profile. Recently developed controlled release preparations may allow greater exploitation of this agent in the future [32].

Oral morphine is the most widely used opiate for severe pain, and offers the flexibility of immediate release liquid or tablets (duration of analgesia approximately 4 hours) and sustained release preparations (12 hourly or 24 hourly dosing). Initial dose titration is usually with an immediate release formulation, given every four hours "around the clock". The same dose is given for breakthrough pain, as often as required [33]. Once a stable fourth hourly regime is established, transfer may be made to a twice daily or daily controlled release preparation of the same total dose [33, 34]. If patients experience breakthrough pain after stabilisation, a dose equivalent to one sixth of the total daily dose may be taken as immediate release morphine. Consistent return of pain within the usual dosing period signifies a need to reassess the underlying disease and usually increase the dose rather than shorten the interval. There is no ceiling dose of morphine. The use of "as required" rather than regular morphine is discouraged in patients with chronic pain as it results in avoidable pain and anxiety when analgesia fluctuates as blood levels fall, and unnecessary toxicity at peak blood levels [33].

In patients unable to take morphine orally, the bioavailability and duration of action of immediate release oral morphine by the rectal

**Table 4.** Opiates recommended for treatment of moderate to severe cancer pain (from [48])

| Drug | Route | Equi-analgesic dose[a] | Peak effect (HR) | Duration of effect (HR) | Comments |
|------|-------|------------------------|------------------|-------------------------|----------|
| Codeine | PO | 200 mg | 0.5 | 3-6 | Mild-moderate pain only |
| | IV | 130 mg | 0.5 | 3-6 | as ceiling for analgesia 240 mg/day More constipating than morphine Enzyme deficiency prevents activation to morphine |
| Oxycodone | PO (IR) | 30 mg | 0.5 | 3-6 | better tolerated than |
| | PO (SR) | 30 mg | 0.5 | 8-12 | codeine/ morphine |
| Morphine | PO (IR) | 30-60 mg | 1.5-2 | 4-6 | IR for initial titration or |
| | PO (SR) | 30-60 mg | 2-3 | 8-12 | breakthrough |
| | SC/IV | 10 mg | 0.5-1 | 3-6 | SR for stable pain Parenteral if oral route not tolerated, less constipating |
| Hydro-morphone | PO/PR | 7.5 mg | 1-2 | 3-4 | Useful at high doses as more potent |
| | SC/IV | 1.5 mg | 0.5-1 | 3-4 | Lower volume required SC |
| Fentanyl | TD | 0.1 mg (?) | 72 | 12+ | Titration of patch |
| | SC/IV | 0.1 mg | < 1 | 0.5-1 | Requires formation of SC depot over 2-3 days, other analgesia required during this time Less sedation, constipation, pruritis |
| Methadone | PO | 20 mg | ? | 4-6 | Long half life requires |
| | IV | 10 mg | 0.5-1.5 | 4-6 | slow titration Accumulation may occur |
| Levor-phanol | PO | 4 mg | 1-2 | 6-8 | Long half life requires |
| | IV | 2 mg | 1-1.5 | 6-8 | slow titration Accumulation may occur |
| Bupre-norphine | SL | 0.4 mg | 0.5-1 | 6-9 | SL in dysphagia partial agonist-may precipitate withdrawal |

[a] Approximate potency compared with 10 mg of parenteral morphine. PO, oral; SL, sublingual; PR, per rectum; SC, subcutaneous; IV, intravenous; IM, intramuscular; TD, transdermal; IR, immediate release; SR, sustained release; ?, insufficient data.

route are equivalent. Sustained release preparations are unreliable when given rectally [33]. Both morphine and the more potent opiate hydro-morphone may be given either subcutaneously (SC) or intravenously (IV), and patient controlled pumps offer greater flexibility during initial titration [35]. Conversions should be made using an opiate equivalency nomogram to guide initial dosing [36]. Continuous SC infusions or fourth hourly dosing via a "butterfly" needle are manageable in the outpatient setting with appropriate support. Hydromorphone allows the use of lower volumes which may be valuable when high doses are given SC [37]. When morphine is being delivered by SC infusion it can be useful to combine other medications in a syringe driver. Metoclopramide for nausea, haloperidol or midazolam for sedation, clonazepam as an anticonvulsant, and buscopan as an antispasmodic are compatible [38]. Subcutaneous administration of opiates may not be practical in patients with generalised oedema, local skin reactions, coagulation disorders or poor peripheral circulation [33]. The intramuscular route is not appropriate for use in chronic cancer pain due to the discomfort of injections [33].

These approaches with morphine produce effective control of chronic cancer pain in approximately 80% of patients [33]. In the remainder, other drugs or routes of administration are required because of intolerable side effects or inadequate analgesia [33]. Buprenorphine is well absorbed sublingually for patients with difficulty swallowing, but may precipitate withdrawal [13]. Rotation of opiates may be of value in some patients with intolerable side effects [39]. Transdermal fentanyl provides drug release over 72 hours. During the initial period of stabilisation oral drugs are gradually reduced, and will continue to be required for breakthrough pain. Pruritis, constipation and sedation are reportedly less problematic than with morphine [40]. Methadone may produce less central nervous system disturbance due to its lack of active metabolites. Its low cost and high potency are attractive for long term maintainance therapy. Incomplete cross tolerance occurs between opiates, requiring introduction of new agents at a lower than equianalgesic dose [39, 41].

The following opiates are not recommended for use in cancer pain [2]:
- Pentazocine and Butorphanol (mixed agonist and antagonist properties)
- Meperidine (toxic metabolite which reduces seizure threshold).
- Dextropropoxyphene (dysphoria and confusion).

Side effects of opiates should be anticipated. Initial effects of nausea and sedation usually wane, but constipation persists and an appropriate laxative regime must be instituted from the outset, including softeners, stimulant laxatives, attention to fluid intake and mobility, stimulants such as cisapride, or suppositories [37]. Pruritis may be managed by opiate rotation or antihistamines. Respiratory depression is unusual in patients with pain, unless accumulation occurs [13]. Myoclonus and seizures may occur at very high doses, requiring benzodiazepines and opiate rotation [42].

Although tolerance to opiates will gradually develop, increasing opiate requirements in patients with advanced cancer are most frequently due to progressive disease [2]. Addiction is almost unknown in this population but physical dependence occurs, requiring slow reduction in doses (50% on alternate days) if pain is relieved by another means, in order to avoid precipitating withdrawal symptoms [13].

## Adjuvant Analgesics for Neuropathic Pain

A number of non-opiate drugs are useful in the management of neuropathic pain. In general they should be introduced along with an optimal opiate schedule, because they have a slower onset of action and require careful dose titration to avoid adverse effects. In acute neuropathic pain exacerbations nerve blocks may be more appropriate [43].

The analgesic efficacy of tricyclic antidepressants (including amitryptyline, doxepin, imipramine, desipramine) is well established in prevention and treatment of post herpetic neuralgia, a common problem in immunosuppressed cancer patients. Other neuropathic syndromes, such as continuous dysesthesias resulting frorn plexopathy or drug induced neuropathy, respond more often than do lancinating or paroxysmal pains [43]. Sedation, most pronounced with amitryptyline, and mood elevation may be beneficial side effects. Anticholinergic and hypotensive effects should be considered and monitored. If unsatisfactory analgesia is obtained the drug should be withdrawn slowly to avoid withdrawal effects on sleep or mood [43].

Anticonvulsants may be of more benefit in lancinating pain, trigeminal neuralgia and post herpetic neuralgia. Carbamazepine, valproate, phenytoin and clonazepam have all been successfully used at anticonvulsant doses, with slow titration and monitoring of side effects and blood levels. Sedation and bone marrow effects may be limiting, particularly with carbamazepine. Gabapentin has been more recently used in this setting although no controlled trials have been published [43].

Topical capsaicin and local anaesthetics are of benefit in neuropathic pains with a strong peripheral input including post surgical pain syndromes. Systemic administration of mexiletene in patients with stable cardiac status can also be considered in refractory neuropathic pain. Nausea and dizziness are frequently limiting [43]. Sequential trials of all of these agents may be required in refractory pain, as failure to respond to one agent does not rule out benefit from another drug even within the same class.

## Special Populations

### The Elderly

It is recognized that the elderly experience greater drug sensitivity and side effects, due to concurrent medical problems and social difficulties. The tendency to under-report pain, and the problems of isolation and cognitive impairment contribute to poor compliance [44].

### Children

Assessment of pain in young children requires a high index of suspicion, as pain of more than a few days duration is likely to lead to passivity and withdrawal rather than complaint [11]. Procedure related pain is rated as a major concern by children with cancer, and behavioral techniques such as distraction and imagery, coupled with analgesia and sedation given by non painful routes help to overcome this source of distress [45]. Analgesic doses in children need to be adjusted for weight, but under 6 months of age initially lower doses are required [46].

### Substance abuse

Patients with a history of opiate abuse may experience rapid development of tolerance and require dose escalation to maintain therapeutic effects [13]. There may be concerns about the veracity of pain reports in this population, but the possibility of drug diversion must not be over-emphasised as this often leads to denial of adequate analgesia and a viscous cycle of mistrust. Frequent monitoring, use of long acting oral or transdermal opiates, and early consideration of non-drug, invasive or alternative pharmacological approaches will be of assistance. These patients will frequently require additional support due to other medical problems, family and employment difficulties [47].


## Conclusions

Pain is a common clinical problem in patients with cancer, which is usually underrecognised and undertreated despite the availability of adequate therapies. Attention to the etiology of pain is vital if appropriate therapy is to be selected and permanent sequalae such as paralysis from unrecognised epidural cord compression are to be avoided. Most cancer pain can be controlled by oral analgesics and adjuvants combined with simple non-drug measures. Support from a multidisciplinary pain service allows apropriate use of nerve blocks or alternative routes of drug delivery in selected patients, particularly those with severe neuropathic pain. Continual reassessment and adjustment will be required in order to tailor therapy to patients changing needs and maintain quality of life at all stages of the clinical pathway.


## References

1. Merskey H (1979) Pain terms: a list with definitions and notes on usage. Recommended by the IASP Subcommittee on Taxonomy. Pain 6: 249-252
2. Bonica JJ (1990) The management of pain, 2nd Ed. Lea and Febiger, Philadelphia
3. Cleeland CS, Gonin R et al. (1994) Pain and its treatment in outpatients with metastatic cancer. N Engl J Med 330: 592-596
4. Grossman S (1993) Undertreatment of cancer pain: barriers and remedies. Support Care Cancer 1: 74-78
5. Von Roenn JH, Cleeland CS et al. (1993) Physician attitudes and practice in cancer pain management. A survey from the Eastern Cooperative Oncology Group. Ann Intern Med 119: 121-126
6. Au E, Loprinzi CL et al. (1994) Regular use of a verbal pain scale improves the understanding of oncology inpatient pain intensity. J Clin Oncol 12: 2751-2755
7. Marks RM, Sachar EJ (1973) Undertreatment of medical inpatients with narcotic analgesics. Ann Intern Med 78: 173-181
8. Vallerand AH (1997) Measurement issues in the comprehensive assessment of cancer pain. Semin Oncol Nurs 13: 16-24
9. Grossman S, Sheidler V et al. (1991) Correlation of patient and caregiver ratings of cancer pain.. J Pain Symptom Manage: 6-53
10. Melzack R, Katz J (1992) The McGill Pain Questionnaire : appraisal and current status. In: Turk D, Melzack R (eds) The handbook of Pain Assessment. Guilford, New York, pp 152-190

11. Beyer JE, Wells N (1989) The assessment of pain in children. Pediatr Clin North Am 36: 837-854
12. Hagen NA, Elwood T et al. (1997) Cancer pain emergencies: a protocol for management. J Pain Symptom Manage 14: 45-50
13. Foley KM (1985) The treatment of cancer pain. N Engl J Med 313: 84-95
14. Mercadante S (1997) Malignant bone pain: pathophysiology and treatment. Pain 69: 1-18
15. Patel BR, Flowers WM Jr. (1997) Systemic radionuclide therapy with strontium chloride Sr 89 for painful skeletal metastases in prostate and breast cancer. South Med J 90: 506-508
16. Ernst DS, Brasher P et al. (1997) A randomized, controlled trial of intravenous clodronate in patients with metastatic bone disease and pain. J Pain Symptom Manage 13: 319-326
17. Hortobagyi GN, Theriault RL et al. (1996) Efficacy of pamidronate in reducing skeletal complications in patients with breast cancer and lytic bone metastases. N Engl J Med 335: 1785-1791
18. Berenson JR, Lichtenstein A et al. (1996) Efficacy of pamidronate in reducing skeletal events in patients with advanced multiple myeloma. N Engl J Med 334: 488-493
19. Ettinger AB, Portenoy RK (1988) The use of corticosteroids in the treatment of symptoms associated with cancer. J Pain Symptom Manage 3: 99-103
20. Derogatis L, Morrow G et al. (1983) The prevalence of psychiatric disorders among cancer patients. JAMA 249: 751-757
21. Massie MJ, Holland JC (1992) The cancer patient with pain: psychiatric complications and their management. J Pain Symptom Manage 7: 99-109
22. Loscalzo M. (1996) Psychological approaches to the management of pain in patients with advanced cancer. Hematol Oncol Clin North Am 10: 139-155
23. Spiegel D, Moore R (1997) Imagery and hypnosis in the treatment of cancer patients. Oncology Huntingt 11: 1179-1189
24. Cherny NI, Arbit E et al. (1996) Invasive techniques in the management of cancer pain. Hematol Oncol Clin North Am 10: 121-137
25. Kawamata M, Ishitani K et al. (1996) Comparison between celiac plexus block and morphine treatment on quality of life in patients with pancreatic cancer pain. Pain 64: 597-602
26. Lamacraft G, Cousins MJ (1997) Neural blockade in chronic and cancer pain. Int Anesthesiol Clin 35: 131-153
27. Ballantyne JC, Carr DB et al. (1996) Comparative efficacy of epidural, subarachnoid, and intracerebroventricular opioids in patients with pain due to cancer. Reg Anesth 21: 542-556
28. World Health Organisation (1990) Cancer Pain relief. Geneva, Switzerland. World Health Organisation, pp 804
29. Zech D, Grond S et al. (1995) Validation of World Health organisation guidelines for cancer pain relief a 10-year prospective study. Pain 63: 65-76
30. Jadad AR, Browman GP (1995) The WHO analgesic ladder for cancer pain management. Stepping up the quality of its evaluation . JAMA 274: 1870-1871
31. Mercadante S, Sapio M et al. (1997) Opioid-sparing effect of diclofenac in cancer pain. J Pain Symptom Manage 14: 15-20
32. Hagen NA, Babul N (1997) Comparative clinical efficacy and safety of a novel controlled-release oxycodone formulation and controlled-release hydromorphone in the treatment of cancer pain. Cancer 79: 1428-1437
33. Expert Working Group of the European Association for Palliative Care (1996) Morphine in cancer pain: modes of administration. BMJ 312: 823-826

34. Broomhead A, Kerr R et al. (1997) Comparison of a once-a-day sustained-release morphine formulation with standard oral morphine treatment for cancer pain. J Pain Symptom Manage 14: 63-73
35. Swanson G, Smith J et al. (1989) Patient-controlled analgesia for chronic cancer pain in the ambulatory setting: a report of 117 patients J Clin Oncol 7: 1903-1908
36. Grossman S, Sheidler V (1987) An aid to prescribing narcotics for the relief of cancer pain. World Health Forum 8: 525-529
37. Levy MH (1996) Pharmacologic treatment of cancer pain. N Engl J Med 335: 1124-1132
38. Woodruff R (1996) Cancer Pain. Adelaide: Asperula
39. de Stoutz ND, Bruera E et al. (1995) Opioid rotation for toxicity reduction in terminal cancer patients. J Pain Symptom Manage 10: 378-384
40. Payne R, Chandler S et al. (1995) Guidelines for the clinical use of transdermal fentanyl. Anticancer Drugs 6 Suppl 3: 50-53
41. Bruera E, Pereira J et al. (1996) Opioid rotation in patients with cancer pain. A retrospective comparison of dose ratios between methadone, hydromorphone, and morphine. Cancer 78: 852-857
42. Hagen N, Swanson R (1997) Strychnine-like multifocal myoclonus and seizures in extremely high-dose opioid administration: treatment strategies. J Pain Symptom Manage 14: 51-58
43. Portenoy RK (1996) Adjuvant analgesic agents. Hematol Oncol Clin North Am 10: 103-119
44. Gagliese L, Melzack R (1997) Chronic pain in elderly people. Pain 70: 3-14
45. Zeltzer LK, Jay SM et al. (1989) The management of pain associated with pediatric procedures. Pediatr Clin North Am 36: 941-964
46. McGrath PA (1996) Development of the World Health Organization Guidelines on Cancer Pain Relief and Palliative Care in Children. J Pain Symptom Manage 12: 87-92
47. Passik SD, Portenoy RK (1998) Substance abuse issues in palliative care. In: Berger A, Portenoy RK, Weissman DE (eds) Principles and Practice of Supportive Oncology. Lippincott-Raven, Philadelphia
48. Grossman SA, Gregory RE (1994) In: Kirkwood JM, Lotze MT, Yasko JM (eds) Current Cancer Therapeutics, 1st edn. Current Medicine, Philadelphia

# Chemotherapy-Induced Nausea and Vomiting

D.E. Morganstern, P.J. Hesketh

## Scope of the Problem, Risk Factors

Despite considerable progress in the management of chemotherapy associated nausea and vomiting, these symptoms remain among the most feared by patients beginning cytotoxic chemotherapy. The relative likelihood of significant emesis in a given individual is dependent upon both patient and treatment related factors. Patient factors with predictive value for decreased emesis include heavy alcohol consumption and male sex [1]. A number of other factors including younger age, [2, 3] poor performance status, [2] severe emesis during pregnancy [4], and susceptibility to motion sickness [5] have all been noted to be predictive of increased emesis with chemotherapy. Treatment related factors include the intrinsic emetogenicity of the cytotoxic agent(s), the dose and schedule, treatment setting, as well as additive effects of combinations [6].

At least three distinct syndromes of chemotherapy related nausea and vomiting are encountered in clinical practice: acute chemotherapy-induced emesis, delayed emesis, and less commonly, anticipatory emesis.

## Acute, Delayed, and Anticipatory Emesis

Acute emesis is defined as emesis occuring during the first 24 h following administration of chemotherapy. In the absence of effecive antiemetic prophylaxis, it typically begins between one and two hours after receiving chemotherapy. Acute emesis has been the most widely studied of the three emetic syndromes.

Delayed emesis, as first described by Kris et al with high dose cisplatin [7] has arbitrarily been defined as emesis occuring more than 24 h after chemotherapy. While the frequency and number of episodes of emesis may be less during this period compared with acute emesis, it remains a formidable problem occuring in 43%–89% of patients recieving cisplatin therapy [8]. The mechanisms of delayed emesis from cisplatin may differ from those underlying acute chemotherapy-induced emesis, and as such, the optimal antiemetic approaches to these two syndromes differ (see below). While most often associated with cisplatin therapy, delayed emesis may also occur with carboplatin, cyclophosphamide, and anthracyclines, but this has been studied less extensively.

Anticipatory emesis is a conditioned response in patients who have experienced severe nausea and vomiting with previous cycles of chemotherapy and is triggered by cues and cognitive activity related to subsequent chemotherapy [9].

## Mechanisms of Chemotherapy-Induced Vomiting

Although the precise mechanisms underlying chemotherapy-induced emesis remain incompletely defined, considerable progress has been made in recent years. A number of areas in the central and peripheral nervous systems and gastrointestinal tract all appear to play important roles (Fig. 1). Two critical areas in the brain stem include the emetic or "vomiting center" and the chemoreceptor trigger zone (CTZ). The vomiting center is an anatomically indistinct collection of receptor and effector nuclei located primarily in the nucleus tractus solitarius which is responsible for coordinating the efferent gastrointestinal respiratory and autonomic activity associated with nausea and vomiting [10, 11]. It serves as the final effector pathway through which a variety of afferent stimuli can initiate the emetic reflex.

One source of afferent input to the vomiting center is also located within the brainstem and is known as the chemoreceptor trigger zone (CTZ). It is located in the area postrema in the floor of the fourth ventricle, lies outside the blood-brain barrier and is accessible to emetic stimuli borne either in the blood or cerebrospinal fluid [12]. Two other important sources of afferent input to the vomiting center with chemotherapy-induced emesis include higher brain stem and cortical structures which appear to be involved in anticipatory emesis and input from the gastrointestinal tract along the vagus and splanchnic nerves [13].

The neurochemical mechanisms underlying the process of emesis have gradually been elucidated. Thirty or more neurotransmitters have

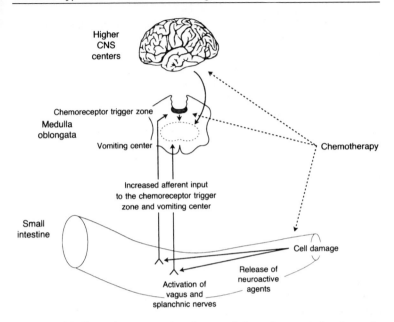

**Fig. 1.** Model illustrating proposed pathways of chemotherapy induced emesis. (Adapted from [82])

been associated with the peripheral and central nervous system sites involved in emesis caused by chemotherapy [14]. The most significant insights into the mechanisms of chemotherapy-induced emesis followed the clinical observation that very high doses of metoclopramide effectively prevented cisplatin-induced emesis. Metoclopramide at conventional doses functions as a dopamine D-2 receptor antagonist. It also is a weak antagonist of the type 3 serotonin or 5 hydroxytryptamine (5-HT3) receptor. Speculation that the antiemetic effectivenes of high-dose metoclopramide derived primarily from its ability to antagonize serotonin and not its anti dopaminergic effect led to the development of many selective 5-HT3 receptor antagonists [15]. Through pre-clinical studies with the selective 5-HT3 receptor antagonists, it is now recognized that the primary mechanism by which cisplatin and perhaps other chemotherapy agents induce emesis is through serotonin dependent mechanisms targeting the gastrointestinal tract. The current working hypothesis proposes: 1) chemotherapy induces the release of serotonin from the enterochromaffin cells in the small bowel; 2) released serotonin binds to 5-HT3 receptors on vagal and splanchnic afferent fibers within the wall of the gastrointestinal tract; 3) the stimulated vagal and splanchnic afferents project to the CTZ and emetic center resulting in activation of the emetic reflex arc; 4)5-HT3 receptor antagonists work primarily by antagonizing the latter process [16].

Clearly, mechanisms involving additional neurotransmitters such as dopamine, noradrenaline and substance P likely play a role in chemotherapy-induced emesis as evidenced by the antiemetic utility of antagonists of these substances in a number of clinical [17] and pre-clinical situations [18]. Much remains to be elucidated on the role of individual neurotransmitters and their interaction in the process of chemotherapy-induced emesis.

## Classes of Antiemetic Agents

### Phenothiazines

The antiemetic properties of phenothiazines were first discovered over thirty years ago by a group of investigators who demonstrated decreased emesis with prochlorperazine and thiopropazate compared with placebo in patients receiving fluorouracil chemotherapy [19]. These agents are believed to exert their antiemetic effect via antagonism of dopaminergic type 2 receptors $(D_2)$. Their utility is limited to chemotherapy that is mild-moderately emetogenic. At conventional doses however, phenothiazines are no better than placebo in preventing emesis induced by highly emetogenic drugs such as high-dose cisplatin [20]. Perhaps the most common and troubling side effect observed clinically is akathisia; other side effects include sedation, hypotension and acute dystonic reactions.

### Butyrophenones

These agents include haloperidol, droperidol, and domperidone. They also act as dopaminergic antagonists and hence have side effect profiles similar to the phenothiazines. Butyrophenones are only moderately effective antiemetic drugs although one study showed near equivalent efficacy to metoclopramide with high dose haloperidol in patients receiving cisplatin chemotherapy [21]. Butyrophenones may have a role as an alternative therapy in patients failing front-line antiemetic regimens.

## Substituted Benzamides

Metoclopramide is the most extensively studied agent in this class, and as noted above is both a dopaminergic antagonist and a weak 5-HT3 receptor antagonist. It has both potent antiemetic activity at higher doses (1–3 mg/kg), and potential extrapyramidal side effects. Prior to the development of the specific 5-HT3 antagonists, metoclopramide was the most important agent for control of high dose cisplatin-induced acute emesis, with a major response rate (0–2 episodes of vomiting) as a single agent of 33%–67% in patients receiving cisplatin doses >100 mg/m$^2$ [22], and approximately 60% major response rate in patients receiving a somewhat lower cisplatin dose [23].

Diphenhydramine appears to decrease the incidence of acute dystonic reactions with metoclopramide but confers no intrinsic antiemetic activity [22]. The primary role of metoclopramide at present is as an adjunctive agent for the prevention of cisplatin-induced delayed emesis [24].

## Corticosteroids

The mechanism and site of action of corticosteroids remains unclear. Dexamethasone has been studied most extensively, and as a single agent is fairly effective with both non cisplatin [25] and cisplatin [26] containing regimens. In one double blind multicenter trial comparing dexamethasone to the 5-HT$_3$ receptor antagonist ondansetron, dexamethasone was as effective as ondansetron in patients receiving anthracycline/cyclophosphamide based therapy and was actually superior in control of delayed nausea [27]. Corticosteroids, combined with the 5-HT$_3$ receptor antagonists are an integral component of current antiemetic therapy for the control of acute emesis with chemotherapy of moderate to high emetogenic potential. In addition, corticosteroids play an important role in the combination treatment of delayed emesis. Given their non overlapping toxicity, corticosteroids are ideal agents for combination with several other antiemetics.

## Benzodiazepines

Benzodiazepines are relatively weak antiemetics. Their beneficial effects may be related mostly to their anxiolytic and amnestic properties. When used with dexamethasone and metoclopramide, lorazepam can help reduce anxiety and akathisia [28] and may also be helpful in counteracting dexamethasone related insomnia.

## Cannabinoids

Cannabinoids, including the plant extract dronabinol, and semisynthetic preparations (nabilone and levonantradol) have been shown to have antiemetic activity superior to placebo and in some studies superior to prochlorperazine [29]. However dronabinol has been shown to be significantly less effective than metoclopramide in a randomized double blinded trial with highly emetogenic chemotherapy [30] The use of these drugs is limited by their side effects of vertigo, xerostomia, fatigue, disorientation, hypotension and dysphoria, particularly in older patients. As such, this class of drugs are not first line agents for any identified group of patients.

## Serotonin Receptor Antagonists

These agents, along with corticosteroids, have the highest therapeutic index among the known antiemetics, and are extremely useful with moderately high and highly emetogenic chemotherapy regimens. The most frequent side effect is mild headache in approximately 15%–20% of patients. Other potential adverse effects include constipation, especially with protracted use and transient, clinically insignificant transaminase elevations [31, 32]. Extrapyramidal effects have generally not been observed. For the four most widely approved drugs in this class (granisetron, ondansetron, dolasetron and tropisetron) comparable efficacy and safety at equivalent doses has been demonstrated in cisplatin-induced emesis [33, 34, 35] and non cisplatin chemotherapy [36]. For this reason, differences in availability and cost may be the most important factors in choosing a 5-HT$_3$ receptor antagonist. While most of these drugs were initially developed for intravenous infusion, recently available oral formulations have demonstrated equivalent efficacy to the intravenous formulations when used in appropriate doses [37, 38].

## Current Management of Chemotherapy-Induced Nausea and Vomiting

Strategies for managing chemotherapy induced emesis must take into account both patient factors as previously noted, prior history of emesis with chemotherapy, as well as the emetogenicity of the chemotherapy regimen. Moreover, etiologies other than chemotherapy should be considered in all cancer patients, given their potential reversibility or palliation (Table 1). A flowchart reflecting current principles of management is presented in Figure 2. Recommended doses of the antiemetic agents are listed in Table 2; at present there is no data to support graded dosing of individual agents according to emetogenicity. A method for predicting emetogenic risk, and strategies for the most common clinical contexts are highlighted below.

Predicting the Emetogenic Risk

The most important factor in predicting the risk of emesis is the intrinsic emetogenicity of the chemotherapy. Several efforts have been made in the past to develop schemas to define the emetogenicity of cancer

Table 1. Causes of nausea and vomiting unrelated to chemotherapy

Medication related
  Opiate analgesics
  Antibiotics
Disease related
  Central nervous system metastases
  Gastrointestinal obstruction
  Hypercalcemia
Other
  Gastritis, esophagitis, infection
  Radiation induced

**Table 2.** Recommended doses of antiemetic drugs

| Drug | Dose range | Schedule |
|------|-----------|----------|
| 5-HT$_3$ Receptor antagonists | | |
| Ondansetron IV | 8 mg or 0.15 mg/kg iv | Once, prechemotherapy |
| Ondansetron PO | Oral dose not clearly defined for acute emesis, 8 mg in delayed emesis | BID in delayed emesis, x2–3 days |
| Granisetron IV | 1 mg or 0.010 mg/kg iv | Once, prechemotherapy |
| Granisetron PO | 2 mg PO | Once, prechemotherapy |
| Dolasetron IV | 100 mg or 1.8 mg/kg iv | Once, prechemotherapy |
| Dolasetron PO | 100 mg PO | Once, prechemotherapy |
| Tropisetron IV | 5 mg IV | Once, prechemotherapy |
| Tropisetron PO | 5 mg PO | Once, prechemotherapy |
| Corticosteroids | | |
| Dexamethasone IV | 8–20 mg IV | Once, prechemotherapy |
| Dexamethasone PO | Oral doses not well studied for acute emesis. For delayed emesis 4–8 mg PO | BID starting 24 h after completion of chemo-therapy for 4 days (cispla-tin) 2 days (noncisplatin) |
| Dopaminergic antagonists | | |
| Metoclopramide IV | 2–3 mg/kg IV | Prechemotherapy and 2 h postchemotherapy |
| Metoclopramide PO | 30 mg or 0.5 mg/kg PO in delayed emesis | QID starting 24 h after Completion of chemo-therapy for 3–4 days. |
| Prochlorperazine IV | 10 mg IV | Q3–4 h PRN |
| Prochlorperazine PO | 10 mg PO | Q 3–4 h PRN |

chemotherapy [39–43]. All of the existing schema have serious limitations.

Recognizing the need for a better emetogenic classification schema, a group of clinical investigators with longstanding interest in antiemetic use recently reported a new emetogenic classification system for acute emesis [6]. It is based upon a comprehensive literature search and consensus opinion. A number of predictive factors are standardized including patient age (adults), and chemotherapy dose, rate and route of administration. Individual chemotherapy agents are divided into five emetogenic levels (Table 3). The five levels are defined by the expected frequency of emesis in the absence of effective antiemetic prophylaxis: level 1 (<10%); level 2 (10%–30%); level 3 (30%–60%); level 4 (60%–90%); level 5 (>90%).

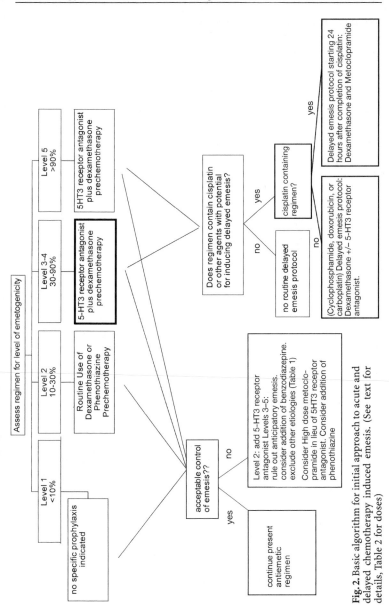

**Fig. 2.** Basic algorithm for initial approach to acute and delayed chemotherapy induced emesis. (See text for details, Table 2 for doses)

**Table 3.** Emetic potential of single chemotherapeutic agents. See Table 2 for specific dose and schedule information for antiemetics. (With permission, from [6])

| Level | Frequency of emesis (%) | Agent |
|-------|-------------------------|-------|
| 5 | >90 | Carmustine >250 mg/m$^2$<br>Cisplatin ≥50 mg/m$^2$<br>Cyclophosphamide >1500 mg/m$^2$<br>Dacarbazine<br>Mechlorethamine<br>Streptozocin |
| 4 | 60–90 | Carboplatin<br>Carmustine <250 mg/m$^2$<br>Cisplatin <50 mg/m$^2$<br>Cyclophosphamide >750 mg/m$^2$ ≤1500 mg/m$^2$<br>Cytarabine >1gm/m$^2$<br>Doxorubicin >60 mg/m$^2$<br>Methotrexate >1000 mg/m$^2$<br>Procarbazine (oral) |
| 3 | 30–60 | Cyclophosphamide ≤750 mg/m$^2$<br>Cyclophosphamide (oral)<br>Doxorubicin 20–60 mg/m$^2$<br>Epirubicin ≤90 mg/m$^2$<br>Hexamethylamine (oral)<br>Idarubicin<br>Ifosfamide<br>Methotrexate 250–1000 mg/m$^2$<br>Mitoxantrone <15 mg/m$^2$ |
| 2 | 10–30 | Docetaxel<br>Etoposide<br>5-Fluorouracil <1000 mg/m$^2$<br>Gemcitabine<br>Methotrexate >50 mg/m$^2$ <250 mg/m$^2$<br>Mitomycin<br>Paclitaxel |
| 1 | <10 | Bleomycin<br>Busulfan<br>Chlorambucil (oral)<br>2-Chlorodeoxyadenosine<br>Fludarabine<br>Hydroxyurea<br>Methotrexate ≤50 mg/m$^2$<br>L-phenylalanine mustard (oral)<br>Thioguanine (oral)<br>Vinblastine<br>Vincristine<br>Vinorelbine |

Proportion of patients who experience emesis in the absence of effective antiemetic prophylaxis

**Table 4.** Algorithm for defining the emetogenicity of combination chemotherapy (with permission, from [6])

---

1. Identify the most emetogenic agent in the combination
2. Assess the relative contribution of other agents to the emetogenicity of the combination. When considering other agents, the following rules apply:
   a) Level one agents do not contribute to the emetogenicity of a given regimen.
   b) Adding one or more level 2 agents increases the emetogenicity of the combination by 1 level greater than the most emetogenic in the combination.
   c) Adding level 3 or 4 agents increases the emetogenicity of the combination by 1 level per agent.

---

An algorithm was also proposed to define the acute emetogenicity of chemotherapy combinations (Table 4). The algorithm was partially validated by analyzing a database of patients treated with antiemetic placebos on several trials evaluating ondansetron [44–47]. In defining antiemetic treatment recommendations below, the Hesketh classification will be used to define risk categories for acute emesis.

Acute Emesis

*High Risk* (Level 5)

Highly emetogenic regimens, of which cisplatin has been most rigorously studied, impart a risk of acute emesis >90% [20, 48] in the absence of effective prophylaxis. For acute emesis, 5-HT3 receptor antagonists have shown superior efficacy to metoclopramide both as single agents [49–51] and in combination with dexamethasone [52]. Further, as the combinations of ondansetron [53–56] or granisetron [57] plus dexamethasone have consistently shown superiority to single agent therapy, *the combination of a 5-HT3 receptor antagonist and dexamethasone should be used for all patients receiving highly emetogenic chemotherapy.*

The special setting of high dose chemotherapy given as conditioning regimens for bone marrow or peripheral blood stem cell transplant appears to impart an emetic risk higher than that of conventional level 4–5 alkylator based combination regimens. In addition there are the confounding variables of multiple day regimens (see discussion below) and at times, concomitant total body irradiation. There are few randomized trials specifically studying antiemetics in the high dose setting [58–61]. However recognizing these limitations, *there is general consensus that the combination of a 5-HT3 receptor antagonist and dexamethasone is recommended for control of acute emesis in patients undergoing high dose chemotherapy.*

### Moderate to High Risk (Levels 3 and 4)

Moderate to high risk regimens are felt to cause emesis in 30%–90% of patients in the absence of effective prophylaxis. While this setting has been studied somewhat less extensively than high dose cisplatin, several contemporary studies have been completed. These randomized studies, most involving cyclophosphamide or anthracycline based chemotherapy, provide a rational basis for treatment recommendations. It is noteworthy that as single agents, 5-HT3 receptor antagonists have failed to show superiority over dexamethasone [27, 62] in patients undergoing moderately emetogenic combination chemotherapy (cyclophosphamide or anthracycline based) and may in fact be inferior with respect to control of delayed nausea and vomiting.

At least three randomized studies have looked at the combination of a 5-HT3 receptor antagonist and dexamethasone in this setting, [62–64] and the results to date are encouraging with 88%–92% of patients enjoying complete control of emesis during the first 24 h following treatment. Hence *the combination of a 5-HT3 receptor antagonist plus dexamethasone is also indicated in moderate to highly emetogic regimens.*

### Low Risk (Level 2)

This setting involves the use of single agent or combination chemotherapy regimens where the risk for acute emesis is approximately 10%–30%. Common clinical situations where this level of risk is encountered include single agent bolus 5-fluorouracil or single agent paclitaxel. Data regarding the intrinsic emetogenicity of agents in this class come solely from phase I and II studies; no formal, placebo controlled antiemetic studies have been conducted in this setting. *Given the fact that a substantial minority of patients may still develop acute emesis with level 2 regimens, routine antiemetic treatment with either dexamethasone or a dopaminergic antagonist-provided they are well tolerated-is advisable.*

*Very Low Risk* (Level 1)

No data exists on the use of antiemetics where the intrinsic risk of nausea and vomiting is less than 10%. Given the low risk coupled with the finite potential for adverse effects with any antiemetic drug, routine prophylaxis is not indicated in this setting.

Delayed Emesis

*Cisplatin*

Delayed emesis with cisplatin remains a formidable problem with on average only 50% of patients experiencing complete control regardless of the regimen used [8]. In addition to the prognostic factors noted above, the most important predictor for delayed emesis appears to be the acute antiemetic response. Prior to the development of the 5-HT3 receptor antagonists, clinical studies focussed on use of metoclopramide and/or corticosteroids for control during the delayed phase. At least two randomized placebo controlled studies demonstrate the superiority of metoclopramide and dexamethasone to single agent therapy [24] and it is apparent that the intravenous route offers no advantage over oral dosing.

Since the development of the serotonin receptor antagonists, investigators have evaluated their role in randomized studies of delayed cisplatin induced emesis.

To date, the results of these studies have been conflicting and point to a modest role for these agents in this setting. In a phase III multicenter study of patients receiving initial doses of cisplatin $\geq 100 mg/m^2$, oral ondansetron appeared only slightly more effective than placebo [65]. Further, a recent randomized comparison of dexamethasone plus ondansetron and dexamethasone plus metoclopramide during days 2–4 post platinum showed no advantage for the $5\text{-}HT_3$ receptor antagonist containing regimen [66]. *Given these findings, the combination of oral dexamethasone and metoclopramide would appear to the treatment of choice for cisplatin-induced delayed emesis, particularly when one considers the good tolerability of metoclopramide at lower doses (eg 0.5 mg/kg q6 h) and its modest cost.*

*Non-Cisplatin*

Delayed emesis can occur with carboplatin, cyclophosphamide, or anthracycline based chemotherapy, with an estimated incidence of 20%–30%. Delayed emesis following moderately emetogenic chemotherapy is an area where data from randomized studies designed specifically to address this endpoint is lacking. Only limited conclusions can be drawn from randomized studies that compare multiple day dosings of 5-HT$_3$ receptor antagonists and metoclopramide beginning on day 0 [63, 67–69], given that the different acute antiemetic regimen employed may bias the delayed results. As previously stated, the most important predictor of delayed emesis is the degree of acute antiemetic control.

The potential value of maintenance dexamethasone after standard acute treatment with granisetron/dexamethasone has been demonstrated in a randomized placebo controlled trial of patients undergoing cyclophosphamide based chemotherapy; patients randomized to receive dexamethasone on days 2–5 (4 mg po bid) had significantly better control of delayed emesis [70]. Maintenance treatment with dexamethasone may well be superior to expensive multiple day dosing of single agent 5-HT3 receptor antagonists for delayed emesis in the moderately emetogenic setting. It remains unclear whether the addition of a "maintenance" 5-HT$_3$ receptor antagonist to multiple days of dexamethasone, following standard acute treatment, is required.

Multiple Consecutive Day Regimens

When a chemotherapy regimen such as cisplatin is fractionated over multiple consecutive days, control of emesis often decreases over successive days. While the reason for this is unclear, it may be due to the compounding of acute with delayed or anticipatory emesis on subsequent days of therapy. In the moderate to high and high risk settings, repetitive daily dosing of a 5-HT$_3$ receptor antagonist with dexamethasone is indicated given the demonstrated efficacy of this combination [71–76] and its better tolerance compared to dopaminergic antagonists.

Anticipatory Emesis

Given the observation that excessive or "intolerable" post treatment vomiting is an estabished risk factor in the development of anticipatory nausea and vomiting [77], prevention of acute and delayed chemotherapy induced emesis is felt to be the most effective mode of prevention. If despite optimal management patients develop this conditioned response, non pharmacologic methods such as hypnosis and desensitization may be effective [78]. The use of benzodiazepines before and during subsequent cycles of chemotherapy may also be useful [79, 80].

## Poor Emesis Control

Chemotherapy-induced emesis will occasionally occur despite appropriate prophylaxis. Several modifications of the antiemetic regimen can be considered in these challenging and difficult cases.

Before addressing the antiemetic regimen, however, disease and medication related causes should be considered as previously outlined in Table 1. Assuming other etiologies have been excluded, the addition of a benzodiazepine such as lorazepam may prove beneficial. Other considerations include substituting high dose metoclopramide for the $5\text{-HT}_3$ receptor antagonist, or adding a dopaminergic antagonist such as prochlorperazine to the existing regimen [81].

## Conclusion and Future Directions

Marked improvements in the prevention of chemotherapy-induced emesis over the past decade can be attributed to the introduction of effective new agents, recognition of the value of combination therapy, and the application of appropriate methodologies to rigorously assess new treatment approaches. In addition, the discovery of the serotonin receptor antagonists has tremendously enhanced our understanding of the physiology underlying chemotherapy induced emesis. Presently, preclinical work implicating the role of substance P in the physiology of emesis has led to clinical trials with the tachykinin $NK_1$ receptor antagonists. Early clinical trial results point to a potentially valuable role for this new class of agents in controlling chemotherapy-induced emesis [82]. Finally, refinements made in predicting the emetogenicity of specific chemotherapy regimens, coupled with an enhanced understanding of patient factors contributing to the risk of emesis may allow for more cost effective use of current agents and more precision in the design of future antiemetic trials.

## References

1. Hesketh PJ, Plagge P, Bryson JC. (1992) Single dose ondansetron for the prevention of acute cisplatin-induced emesis: analysis of efficacy and prognostic factors. In: Bianchi L, Grelot AD, Miller GL, editors. Mechanisms and Control of Emesis. John Libby Eurotext Ltd., p. 235–236

2. Pollera CF, Giannarelli D. (1989) Prognostic factors influencing cisplatin-induced emesis. Definition and validation of a predictive logistic model. Cancer 64:1117–22

3. Pater J, Slamet L, Zee B, Osoba D, Warr D, Rusthoven J. (1994) Inconsistency of prognostic factors for post-chemotherapy nausea and vomiting. Support Care Cancer 2:161–6

4. Martin M, Diaz-Rubio E. (1990) Emesis During Past Pregnancy: a New Prognostic Factor in Chemotherapy- Induced Emesis. Ann Oncol 1:152–3 1990

5. Morrow GR. (1985) The effect of a susceptibility to motion sickness on the side effects of cancer chemotherapy. Cancer 55:2766–70

6. Hesketh PJ, Kris MG, Grunberg SM, Beck T, Hainsworth JD, Harker G et al. (1997) Proposal for classifying the acute emetogenicity of cancer chemotherapy. J Clin Oncol 15:103–9

7. Kris MG, Gralla RJ, Clark RA, Tyson LB, O'Connell JP, Wertheim MS et al. (1985) Incidence, course, and severity of delayed nausea and vomiting following the administration of high-dose cisplatin. J Clin Oncol 3:1379–84

8. Tavorath R, Hesketh PJ. (1996) Drug treatment of chemotherapy-induced delayed emesis. Drugs 52:639–48

9. Morrow GR. (1984) Clinical characteristics associated with the development of anticipatory nausea and vomiting in cancer patients undergoing chemotherapy treatment. J Clin Oncol 2:1170–6

10. Miller AD, Wilson VJ. (1983) "Vomiting Center" reanalyzed: an electrical stimulation study. Brain Research 270:154–8

11. Carpenter DO. (1990) Neural Mechanisms of Emesis. Canadian Journal of Physiol Pharmacol 68:230–6

12. Miller AD, Leslie RA. (1994) The area postrema and vomiting. Front Neuroendocrinol 15:301–20

13. Andrews PL, Rapeport WG, Sanger GJ. (1988) Neuropharmacology of emesis induced by anti-cancer therapy. Trends Pharmacol Sci 9:334–41

14. Leslie RA. (1985) Neuroactive substances in the dorsal vagal complex of the medulla oblongata: nucleus of the tractus solitarius, area postrema, and dorsal motor nucleus of the vagus. Neurochem Int 7:191–211

15. Andrews PLR, Hawthorne J. (1988) The neurophysiology of vomiting. Baillieres Clinical Gastroenterology 2:141–168

16. Andrews PLR, Davis CJ, Bingham S, Davidson HIM, Hawthorn J, Maskell L. (1990) The abdominal visceral innervation and the emetic reflex: pathways, pharmacology, and plasticity. Can J Physiol Pharmacol 68:325–45

17. Herrstedt J. (1996) New perspectives in antiemetic treatment. Support Care Cancer 4:416–9

18. Tattersall FD, Rycroft W, Hargreaves RJ, Hill RG. (1993) The tachykinin NK1 receptor antagonist CP-99,994 attenuates cisplatin induced emesis in the ferret. Eur J Pharmacol 250:R5–6

19. Moertel CG, Reitemeier RJ, Gage RP. (1963) A controlled clinical evaluation of antiemetic drugs. JAMA 186:116–8

20. Gralla RJ, Itri LM, Pisko SE, Squillante AE, Kelsen DP, Braun DW, Jr. et al. (1981) Antiemetic efficacy of high-dose metoclopramide: randomized trials with placebo and prochlorperazine in patients with chemotherapy- induced nausea and vomiting. N Engl J Med 305:905–9

21. Grunberg SM, Gala KV, Lampenfeld M, Jamin D, Johnson K, Cariffe P et al. (1984) Comparison of the antiemetic effect of high-dose intravenous metoclopramide and high-dose intravenous haloperidol in a randomized double-blind crossover study. J Clin Oncol 2:782–7

22. Kris MG, Gralla RJ, Tyson LB, Clark RA, Kelsen DP, Reilly LK et al. (1985) Improved control of cisplatin-induced emesis with high-dose metoclopramide and with combinations of metoclopramide, dexamethasone, and diphenhydramine. Results of consecutive trials in 255 patients. Cancer 55:527–34

23. Roila F, Tonato M, Basurto C, Bella M, Passalacqua R, Morsia D et al. (1987) Antiemetic activity of high doses of metoclopramide combined with methylprednisolone versus metoclopramide alone in cisplatin-treated cancer patients: a randomized double-blind trial of the Italian Oncology Group for Clinical Research. J Clin Oncol 5:141–9

24. Kris MG, Gralla RJ, Tyson LB, Clark RA, Cirrincione C, Groshen S. (1989) Controlling delayed vomiting: double-blind, randomized trial comparing placebo, dexamethasone alone, and metoclopramide plus dexamethasone in patients receiving cisplatin. J Clin Oncol 7:108–14

25. Markman M, Sheidler V, Ettinger DS, Quaskey SA, Mellits ED. (1984) Antiemetic efficacy of dexamethasone. Randomized, double-blind, crossover study with prochlorperazine in patients receiving cancer chemotherapy. N Engl J Med 311:549–52

26. Aapro MS, Plezia PM, Alberts DS, Graham V, Jones SE, Surwit EA et al. (1984) Double-blind crossover study of the antiemetic efficacy of high-dose dexamethasone versus high-dose metoclopramide. J Clin Oncol 2:466–71

27. Jones AL, Hill AS, Soukop M, Hutcheon AW, Cassidy J, Kaye SB et al. (1991) Comparison of dexamethasone and ondansetron in the prophylaxis of emesis induced by moderately emetogenic chemotherapy [see comments]. Lancet 338:483–7

28. Kris MG, Gralla RJ, Clark RA, Tyson LB, Groshen S. (1987) Antiemetic control and Prevention of Side Effects of Anti Cancer Therapy with Lorazepam or Diphehydramine when used in Combination with Metoclopramide Plus Dexamethasone. Cancer 60:2816–2822

29. Vincent BJ, McQuiston DJ, Einhorn LH, Nagy CM, Brames MJ. (1983) Review of cannabinoids and their antiemetic effectiveness. Drugs 25 Suppl 1:52–62

30. Gralla RJ, Tyson LB, Bordin LA. (1984) Antiemetic therapy: a review of recent studies and a report of a random assignment trial comparing metoclopramide with delta-9-tetrahydrocannabinol. Cancer Treatment Reports 68:163–72

31. Hesketh PJ, Murphy WK, Lester EP, Gandara DR, Khojasteh A, Tapazoglou E et al. (1989) GR 38032F (GR-C507/75) a novel compound effective in the prevention of acute cisplatin-induced emesis. J Clin Oncol 7:700–5

32. Perez EA. (1995) Review of the preclinical pharmacology and comparative efficacy of 5- hydroxytryptamine-3 receptor antagonists for chemotherapy-induced emesis. J Clin Oncol 13:1036–43

33. Hesketh P, Navari R, Grote T, Gralla R, Hainsworth J, Kris M et al. (1996) Double-blind, randomized comparison of the antiemetic efficacy of intravenous dolasetron mesylate and intravenous ondansetron in the prevention of acute cisplatin-induced emesis in patients with cancer. Dolasetron Comparative Chemotherapy-induced Emesis Prevention Group. J Clin Oncol 14:2242–9

34. Navari R, Gandara D, Hesketh P, Hall S, Mailliard J, Ritter H et al. (1995) Comparative clinical trial of granisetron and ondansetron in the prophylaxis of cisplatin-induced emesis. The Granisetron Study Group. J Clin Oncol 13:1242–8

35. Marty M, Kleisbauer JP, Fournel P, Vergnenegre A, Carles P, Loria-Kanza Y et al. (1995) Is Navoban (tropisetron) as effective as Zofran (ondansetron) in cisplatin-induced emesis? Anti-Cancer Drugs 6:15–21

36. Jantunen IT, Muhonen TT, Kataja VV, Flander MK, Teerenhovi L. (1993) 5-HT3 Receptor Antagonists in the Prophylaxis of Acute Vomiting Induced by Moderately Emetogenic Chemotherapy-A Randomized Study. European Journal of Cancer 29 A:1669–1672

37. Gralla RJ, Popovic W, Strupp J, Culleton V, Preston A, Friedman C. (1997) Can an oral antiemetic regimen be as effective as intravenous treatment against cisplatin: results of a 1054 patient randomized study of oral granisetron versus IV ondansetron (Meeting abstract). Proc Annu Meet Am Soc Clin Oncol 16:A178 1997

38. Perez EA, Hesketh P, Sandbach J, Reeves J, Chawla S, Markman M et al. (1998) Comparison of Single-Dose Oral Granisetron Versus Intravenous Ondansetron in the Prevention of Nausea and Vomiting Induced by Moderately Emetogenic Chemotherapy: A Multicenter, Double-Blind, Randomized Parallel Study. Journal of Clinical Oncology 16:754–760

39. Laszlo J. (1982) Treatment of nausea and vomiting caused by cancer chemotherapy. Cancer Treat Rev 9 Suppl B:3–9

40. Strum SB, McDermed JE, Pileggi J, Riech LP, Whitaker H. (1984) Intravenous metoclopramide: prevention of chemotherapy-induced nausea and vomiting. A preliminary evaluation. Cancer 53:1432–9

41. Craig JB, Powell BL. (1987) The management of nausea and vomiting in clinical oncology. Am J Med Sci 293:34–44

42. Lindley CM, Bernard S, Fields SM. (1989) Incidence and duration of chemotherapy-induced nausea and vomiting in the outpatient oncology population. J Clin Oncol 7:1142–9

43. Aapro M. (1993) Methodological issues in antiemetic studies. Invest New Drugs 11:243–53

44. Cubeddu LX, Hoffman IS, Fuenmayor NT, Finn AL. (1990) Antagonism of serotonin S3 receptors with ondansetron prevents nausea and emesis induced by cyclophosphamide-containing chemotherapy regimens [see comments]. J Clin Oncol 8:1721–7

45. Beck TM, Ciociola AA, Jones SE, Harvey WH, Tchekmedyian NS, Chang A et al. (1993) Efficacy of oral ondansetron in the prevention of emesis in outpatients receiving cyclophosphamide-based chemotherapy. The Ondansetron Study Group [see comments]. Ann Intern Med 118:407–13

46. Cubeddu LX, Pendergrass K, Ryan T, York M, Burton G, Meshad M et al. (1994) Efficacy of oral ondansetron, a selective antagonist of 5-HT3 receptors, in the treatment of nausea and vomiting associated with cyclophosphamide-based chemotherapies. Ondansetron Study Group [see comments]. Am J Clin Oncol 17:137–46

47. DiBenedetto J, Jr., Cubeddu LX, Ryan T, Kish JA, Sciortino D, Beall C et al. (1995) Ondansetron for nausea and vomiting associated with moderately emetogenic cancer chemotherapy. Clin Ther 17:1091–8

48. Cubeddu LX, Hoffmann IS, Fuenmayor NT, Finn AL. (1990) Efficacy of ondansetron (GR 38032F) and the role of serotonin in cisplatin-induced nausea and vomiting [see comments]. N Engl J Med 322:810–6

49. Marty M, Pouillart P, Scholl S et al. (1990) Comparison of the 5-hydroxytryptamine antagonist ondansetron (GR 38032F) with high-dose metoclopramide in the control of cisplatin-induced emesis. New England Journal of Medicine 322:816–21

50. Demulder PHM, Seynaeve C, Vermorken JB et al. (1990) Ondansetron compared with high-dose metoclopramide in prophylaxis of acute and delayed cisplatin-induced nausea and vomiting. Annals of Internal Medicine 113:834–840

51. Hainsworth J, Harvey W, Pendergrass K et al. (1991) A single-blind comparison of intravenous ondansetron, a selective serotonin antagonist, with intravenous metoclopramide in the prevention of nausea and vomiting associated with high-dose cisplatin chemotherapy. Journal of Clinical Oncology 9:721–728

52. Italian Group for Antiemetic Research. (1992) Ondansetron+dexamethasone vs metoclopramide + dexamethasone + diphenhydramine in prevention of cisplatin-induced emesis. Lancet 340:96–99

53. Hesketh PJ, Harvey WH, Harker WG et al. (1994) A randomized, double blind comparison of intravenous ondansetron alone and in combination with intravenous dexamethasone in the prevention of nausea and vomiting associated with high-dose cisplatin. Journal of Clinical Oncology 12:596–600

54. Roila F, Tonato M, Cognetti F et al. (1991) Prevention of cisplatin-induced emesis: a double-blind multicenter randomized crossover study comparing ondansetron and ondansetron plus dexamethasone. Journal of Clinical Oncology 9:675–8

55. Smith DB, Newlands ES, Rustin GJ, Begent RH, Howells N, McQuade B et al. (1991) Comparison of ondansetron and ondansetron plus dexamethasone as antiemetic prophylaxis during cisplatin-containing chemotherapy [see comments]. Lancet 338:487–90

56. Smyth JF, Coleman RE, Nicolson M, Gallmeier WM, Leonard RC, Cornbleet MA et al. (1991) Does dexamethasone enhance control of acute cisplatin induced emesis by ondansetron? BMJ 303:1423–6

57. Latreille J, Stewart D, Laberge F, Hoskins P, Rusthoven J, McMurtrie E et al. (1995) Dexamethasone improves the efficacy of granisetron in the first 24 h following high-dose cisplatin chemotherapy. Support Care Cancer 3:307–12

58. Or R, Drakos P, Nagler A, Naparstek E, Kapelushnik J, Cass Y. (1994) The anti-emetic efficacy and tolerability of tropisetron in patients conditioned with high-dose chemotherapy (with and without total body irradiation) prior to bone marrow transplantation. Support Care Cancer 2:245–8

59. Bosi A, Guidi S, Messori A, Saccardi R, Lombardini L, Vannucchi AM et al. (1993) Ondansetron versus chlorpromazine for preventing emesis in bone marrow transplant recipients: a double-blind randomized study. J Chemother 5:191–6

60. Okamoto S, Takahashi S, Tanosaki R, Sakamaki H, Onozawa Y, Oh H et al. (1996) Granisetron in the prevention of vomiting induced by conditioning for stem cell transplantation: a prospective randomized study. Bone Marrow Transplant 17:679–83

61. Gilbert CJ, Ohly KV, Rosner G, Peters WP. (1995) Randomized, double-blind comparison of a prochlorperazine-based versus a metoclopramide-based antiemetic regimen in patients undergoing autologous bone marrow transplantation. Cancer 76:2330–7

62. Italian Group for Antiemetic Research. (1995) Dexamethasone, Granisetron, or both for the prevention of nausea and vomiting during chemotherapy for cancer. New England Journal of Medicine 332:1-5

63. Soukop M, McQuade B, Hunter E, Stewart A, Kaye S, Cassidy J et al. (1992) Ondansetron compared with metoclopramide in the control of emesis and quality of life during repeated chemotherapy for breast cancer. Oncology 49:295-304

64. Carmichael J, Bessell EM, Harris AL, Hutcheon AW, Dawes PJ, Daniels S et al. (1994) Comparison of granisetron alone and granisetron plus dexamethasone in the prophylaxis of cytotoxic-induced emesis [published erratum appears in Br J Cancer 1995 May;71 (5):1123]. Br J Cancer 70:1161-4

65. Navari RM, Madajewicz S, Anderson N, Tchekmedyian NS, Whaley W, Garewal H et al. (1995) Oral ondansetron for the control of cisplatin-induced delayed emesis: a large, multicenter, double-blind, randomized comparative trial of ondansetron versus placebo [see comments]. J Clin Oncol 13:2408-16

66. Roila F, De Angelis V, Contu A, Scagliotti G, Tateo S, Massidda B et al. (1996) Ondansetron (OND) vs metoclopramide (MTC) both combined with dexamethasone (DEX) in the prevention of cisplatin (CDDP)-induced delayed emesis (Meeting abstract). Proc Annu Meet Am Soc Clin Oncol 15:A1705 1996

67. Bonneterre J, Chevallier B, Metz R, Fargeot P, Pujade-Lauraine E, Spielmann M et al. (1990) A randomized double-blind comparison of ondansetron and metoclopramide in the prophylaxis of emesis induced by cyclophosphamide, fluorouracil, and doxorubicin or epirubicin chemotherapy. J Clin Oncol 8:1063-9

68. Marschner NW, Adler M, Nagel GA, D C, Fenzl E, Upadhyaya B. (1991) Double-Blind Randomised Trial of the Antiemetic Efficacy and Safety of Ondansetron and Metoclopramide in Advanced Breast Cancer Patients Treated with Epirubicin and Cyclophosphamide. European Journal of Cancer 27:1137-1140

69. Kassa S, Kvaloy S, Dicato MA et al. (1990) A comparison of ondansetron with metoclopramide in the prophylaxis of chemotherapy-induced nausea and vomiting: a randomized double-blind study. European Journal of Cancer 26:311-4

70. Koo WH, Ang PT. (1996) Role of maintenance oral dexamethasone in prophylaxis of delayed emesis caused by moderately emetogenic chemotherapy. Ann Oncol 7:71-4

71. Hainsworth JD, Omura GA, Khojasteh A, Bryson JC, Finn AL. (1991) Ondansetron (GR 38032F): a novel antiemetic effective in patients receiving a multiple-day regimen of cisplatin chemotherapy. Am J Clin Oncol 14:336-40

72. Hainsworth JD. (1992) The use of ondansetron in patients receiving multiple-day cisplatin regimens. Semin Oncol 19:48-52

73. Nicolai N, Mangiarotti B, Salvioni R, Piva L, Faustini M, Pizzocaro G. (1993) Dexamethasone plus ondansetron versus dexamethasone plus alizapride in the prevention of emesis induced by cisplatin-containing chemotherapies for urological cancers. Eur Urol 23:450-6

74. Bremer K. (1992) A single-blind study of the efficacy and safety of intravenous granisetron compared with alizapride plus dexamethasone in the prophylaxis and control of emesis in patients receiving 5-day cytostatic therapy. The Granisetron Study Group. Eur J Cancer 28 A:1018-22

75. Rath U, Upadhyaya BK, Arechavala E, Bockmann H, Dearnaley D, Droz JP et al. (1993) Role of ondansetron plus dexamethasone in fractionated chemotherapy. Oncology 50:168-72

76. Sledge GW, Jr., Einhorn L, Nagy C, House K. (1992) Phase III double-blind comparison of intravenous ondansetron and metoclopramide as antiemetic therapy for patients receiving multiple- day cisplatin-based chemotherapy. Cancer 70:2524-8

77. Alba E, Bastus R, de Andres L, Sola C, Paredes A, Lopez Lopez JJ. (1989) Anticipatory nausea and vomiting: prevalence and predictors in chemotherapy patients. Oncology 46:26–30
78. Morrow GR, Morrell C. (1982) Behavioral treatment for the anticipatory nausea and vomiting induced by cancer chemotherapy. N Engl J Med 307:1476–80
79. Greenberg DB, Surman OS, Clarke J, Baer L. (1987) Alprazolam for phobic nausea and vomiting related to cancer chemotherapy. Cancer Treat Rep 71:549–50
80. Razavi D, Delvaux N, Farvacques C, De Brier F, Van Heer C, Kaufman L et al. (1993) Prevention of adjustment disorders and anticipatory nausea secondary to adjuvant chemotherapy: a double-blind, placebo-controlled study assessing the usefulness of alprazolam. J Clin Oncol 11:1384–90
81. Hesketh PJ, Gandara DR, Hesketh AM, Edelman M, Webber LM, McManus M et al. (1997) Improved control of high-dose-cisplatin-induced acute emesis with the addition of prochlorperazine to granisetron/dexamethasone. Cancer J Sci Am 3:180–3
82. Kris MG, Radford JE, Pizzo BA, Inabinet R, Hesketh A, Hesketh PJ (1991) Use of an NK-I receptor antagonist to prevent delayed emesis after cisplatin. J Natl Cancer Inst 89: 817–8

# Pleural Effusions

M.K. Ferguson

## Introduction

Pleural effusions, especially those that are malignant, are a common and troublesome complication of advanced malignancy. Malignant pleural effusions develop in up to 20% of patients with lung cancer prior to death and are also frequently seen in patients with advanced breast cancer. The presence of a malignant pleural effusion is usually a sign of incurability, and the therapeutic goal in such patients is palliation of symptoms from the effusion. However, some types of cancers, such as lymphomas and germ cell tumors, are potentially curable even in the presence of a malignant effusion, and the goal of therapy in these patients is therefore radically different. Benign effusions, including exudates and chylothoraces, are also diagnosed with some frequency in patients with malignancies such as lung cancer and lymphoma. As a result, appropriate assessment of the etiology of pleural effusion and the tumor type in a patient with a malignancy is important in determining optimal therapy for the effusion.

## Epidemiology

The actual number of patients with cancer who develop effusions is unknown, but it is estimated that malignant effusions develop in about 100,000 people in the United States annually, which is about 43 malignant effusions per 100,000 people [1, 2]. The chance of a cancer patient developing a malignant effusion is highest in lymphoma and leukemia (25%). The risk is also high in patients with lung cancer (10%–15%), and patients with ovarian, gastrointestinal, and breast cancers have a risk of about 3% [3]. Malignant effusions are most commonly found in patients with lung cancer and breast cancer, and an appreciable number are also due to lymphoma and leukemia (Table 1) [2, 4–10].

## Pathophysiology

Malignant pleural effusions usually arise due to factors specific to the underlying tumor but, in some patients, are the result of factors completely unrelated to the presence of the tumor (Table 2) [11]. Pleural effusions associated with malignancy can be categorized into two types [10]. Type I effusions, or true malignant effusions, are those in which the effu-

**Table 1.** The etiology of malignant pleural effusions in 2046 patients with cancer (from [2, 4–10])

| Malignancy | Incidence (%) |
|---|---|
| Lung | 35 |
| Breast | 21 |
| Lymphoma/leukemia | 12 |
| Genitourinary | 6 |
| Reproductive | 6 |
| Sarcoma/melanoma | 4 |
| Gastrointestinal | 4 |
| Other | 4 |
| Unknown | 8 |

**Table 2.** Factors associated with the development of malignant pleural effusions (from [4])

| |
|---|
| Tumor-related factors |
|   Extensive mediastinal nodal invasion |
|   Parapneumonic effusion due to an obstructing pneumonia |
|   Prior mediastinal irradiation |
|   Pericardial effusion due to malignancy or prior irradiation |
|   Malignant ascites |
|   Hypoalbuminemia |
|   Tumor- or treatment-related organ failure (heart, kidney, lungs) |
|   Pulmonary embolism |
| Factors unrelated to the tumor |
|   Parapneumonic effusion due to unrelated pneumonia |
|   Tuberculosis or fungal infection |
|   Organ failure not due to cancer or its treatment |
|   Rheumatologic or other collagen vascular disease |
|   Pulmonary embolism |

sion is the result of pleural involvement by the tumor. As a consequence, malignant cells can be recovered from the pleural fluid or by pleural biopsy. Type II effusions, or paramalignant effusions, are associated with malignancies that do not involve the pleura, and both pleural fluid cytology and pleural histology fail to yield malignant cells.

## Malignant (Type I) Effusions

In true malignant effusions a complex combination of mechanisms accounts for fluid accumulation in the pleural space. The primary mechanism relates to 1) impaired lymphatic drainage, which results from tumor involvment in the parietal pleura blocking stomata that are located between mesothelial cells; 2) enlarged mediastinal lymph nodes; and 3) malignant obstruction of the lymphatic channels that connect the stomata of the parietal pleura and the draining mediastinal lymph nodes [12, 13]. Seeding of the pleural fluid with cancer cells increases pleural fluid production due to an inflammatory response of the pleural surfaces. Involvement of the pleural surfaces by the malignant process increases capillary permeability which also releases more fluid into the pleural space. Finally, movement of fluid from the peritoneal space into the pleural space through diaphragmatic lymphatics increases total pleural space fluid. It is thought that the combination of increased pleural fluid space production and impaired lymphatic drainage are both necessary elements in the development of most malignant pleural effusions [14].

In patients with lung cancer, pulmonary arterial invasion and embolization of tumor cells to the visceral pleura accounts for most malignant pleural effusions. Tumor cells then migrate into the pleural space and seed the parietal pleura. In some patients visceral pleural invasion by a peripheral cancer may also directly seed the pleural space [1].

In patients with breast cancer the mechanisms responsible for the development of a malignant pleural effusion are direct spread of cancer through the chest wall or seeding of the pleural surface via the systemic circulation [15]. Tumors that have metastasized to the liver can enter the pleural space through the inferior vena cava, the pulmonary artery, or the right side of the heart circulation, mechanisms that help account for the presence of bilateral pleural effusions in many patients with breast cancer.

## Paramalignant (Type II) Effusions

The etiology of Type II malignant pleural effusions, which include transudates, exudates, and chylous effusions, is more multifactorial and controversial than that of true malignant effusions. Ascites, including malignant ascites, may result in excess pleural fluid without direct malignant involvement of the pleura. Malnutrition resulting in hypoalbuminemia can alter the osmotic pressure gradient across the parietal pleural surface, increasing fluid flow into the pleural space. Any tumor that causes obstruction of mediastinal lymphatics, even without direct pleural involvement by the cancer, may decrease lymphatic flow from the pleural space and lead to fluid accumulation.

Distinguishing true malignant effusions from paramalignant effusions may have important implications in the management of some malignancies, particularly lung cancers. Bronchial obstruction with associated atelectasis can produce a transudative effusion, and postobstructive pneumonia may result in an exudative effusion. Mediastinal nodal involvement can result in impaired lymphatic drainage from the pleural space causing fluid accumulation.

Chylous effusions associated with malignancy are due to obstruction of mediastinal lymphatics or, less commonly, to direct invasion of the thoracic duct by the malignant process. Nearly 80% of patients with a cancer-associated chylothorax have an underlying lymphoma, the majority of which do not have tumor cells in the pleural fluid [16, 17].

### Diagnosis

Malignant Pleural Effusions

The diagnosis of Type I, or true malignant pleural effusions, is generally straightforward. Such effusions often cause symptoms such as dyspnea, cough, and chest pain or pressure. Physical findings include dullness and egophony, and many patients also have weight loss with cachexia and other signs of advanced malignancy such as pain, clubbing, and cyanosis. A plain chest radiograph confirms the presence of fluid in the chest, and a thoracentesis is usually indicated to provide the diagnosis and to rule out other causes for pleural effusion. In a patient with a known malignancy, the fluid should be heparinized and sent for protein, lactic dehydrogenase (LDH), and cytology. Some physicians also advocate routine measurement of fluid pH and glucose levels. In the absence of a known malignancy, additional useful tests include cell count and differential, eosinophil count, and smears and culture for tuberculosis.

Malignant effusions are exudates, and thus have high LDH levels and high protein levels, both of which have good diagnostic accuracy (Table 3) [11, 18]. The finding of a transudate rules out the presence of a true malignant effusion. Cytologic findings are positive for malignancy in 80% of patients in whom the fluid pH is less than 7.30, whereas a pH >7.30 yields positive cytology in only 50% of patients. In patients with a pleural fluid glucose <60 mg/dl the cytology is positive in more than 85% of patients, whereas in those with a glucose >60 mg/dl the cytology is positive in only 50%. The presence of both a pleural fluid pH <7.30 and glucose <60 mg/dl yields positive cytology results in 90% of patients [19].

Failure to obtain positive cytologic results with thoracentesis dictates that another thoracentesis be performed. When two thoracenteses fail to achieve a diagnosis other tests may be indicated, such as blind pleural biopsy. This test usually provides little additional diagnostic yield in a patient suspected of having cancer and has been supplanted by thoracoscopy and biopsy for diagnosis and potential treatment of malignant pleural effusions. Other possible approaches include cytogenetic or flow cytometric analyses to demonstrate aneuploid populations, or, in a patient with breast cancer, hormonal analysis of the pleural fluid cellular material.

**Table 3.** Biochemical analyses in the diagnosis of malignant pleural effusion (from [11, 18])

|                          | Sensitivity (%) | Specificity (%) | Predictive value (%) Positive | Negative |
|--------------------------|-----------------|-----------------|-------------------------------|----------|
| LDH >200 U               | 70              | 100             | 100                           | 61       |
| Fluid/blood LDH >0.6     | 86              | 98              | 99                            | 77       |
| Protein >3 g             | 89              | 91              | 95                            | 79       |
| Fluid/blood protein >0.5 | 90              | 98              | 99                            | 98       |
| 1, 2 or 4 above          | 99              | 98              | 99                            | 98       |

Paramalignant Pleural Effusions

Paramalignant pleural effusions may be either transudative or exudative, as outlined in Table 3. The diagnosis of chylous effusions is made on the basis of appearance and biochemical studies. The fluid is milky white, opalescent, and odorless. It does not separate into layers when left to stand or when centrifuged. Triglyceride levels are usually >110 mg/dl, and the finding of triglyceride levels <50 mg/dl indicates that the fluid is not chylous [20]. If necessary, performing a lipoprotein analysis to demonstrate the presence of chylomicrons confirms the diagnosis.

## Treatment Options

General considerations in the management of a patient with a malignant pleural effusion include the cause of the effusion (whether malignant or paramalignant), the stage of the patient's cancer, the symptoms caused by the effusion, the performance status of the patient, and the overall treatment objectives. In malignancies such as germ cell tumors, lymphomas, and small cell lung cancers, combination chemotherapy and radiation therapy are potentially curative. In such patients, even though the presence of a malignant effusion is a sign of overall poor prognosis, an aggressive approach is appropriate. However, in most patients a malignant effusion is a sign of incurability, and treatment objectives are primarily palliative.

If the effusion is asymptomatic, specific treatment for the effusion can be deferred, and the overall therapeutic objectives can be addressed. Symptomatic effusions usually require initial therapy before the overall treatment plan can be instituted. Initial therapy may be as simple as thoracentesis, although this treatment alone is successful in managing malignant pleural effusions in only about 10% of patients, and more definitive therapy is usually necessary.

In patients with non-small cell lung cancer it is essential that the etiology of the effusion be determined in the select few individuals who might have limited-stage disease. The finding of two negative thoracenteses suggests that an effusion is paramalignant and indicates that surgical therapy may be appropriate depending on the stage of the cancer. Symptomatic malignant effusions associated with non-small cell histologies rarely respond adequately to chemotherapy or combined chemoradiotherapy alone, and usually require more specific and definitive management such as chest tube placement and sclerosis.

Patients with breast cancer and an associated malignant pleural effusion who are early in their course of therapy should undergo thoracentesis followed by systemic and/or hormonal therapy, which often prevents recurrence of the effusion [21]. Similar recommendations are appropriate for patients who suffer a relapse late after initial systemic therapy for breast cancer. In patients in whom systemic and hormonal therapy have failed and an early site of relapse is the pleural space, chest tube placement with sclerosis is generally recommended.

Patients with chylothorax due to an underlying cancer usually have lymphoma and/or extensive mediastinal nodal involvement. Systemic chemotherapy possibly combined with mediastinal irradiation is usually successful in reopening the lymphatic channels and in eliminating the chylous effusion.

## Supportive Care

In patients who have widely metastatic disease and a poor performance status, supportive measures alone are appropriate for the final weeks of life. Such supportive measures include supplemental oxygen and morphine. This recommendation is particularly appropriate for patients in a hospice setting.

## Thoracentesis

Thoracentesis alone is appropriate management for patients whose tumors are likely to respond to systemic chemotherapy, such as those with germ cell tumors, small cell lung cancer, lymphoma, and some patients with breast cancer. In addition to its diagnostic capability, thoracentesis is also appropriate as an initial step in the management of most other patients with malignant effusions to determine the symptomatic response to fluid removal and to assess whether there is any underlying component of lung entrapment. However, when used as the sole therapeutic modality for most malignant effusions, the mean time to recurrence of effusions is 4.2 days with the majority recurring in 1–3 days [5]. The concomitant risks of repeated thoracentesis, which include pneumothorax, empyema, and pleural fluid loculation, outweigh its benefits except in patients with very limited life expectancies.

Intrapleural Therapy

*Sclerotherapy*

Thoracostomy tube placement with instillation of a sclerosing agent is the standard treatment for most patients with malignant pleural effusions. Thoracostomy tube placement alone has a success rate of 11%–40% and is generally not considered effective treatment for malignant pleural effusions [22]. The addition of a sclerosing agent causes inflammation of the parietal and visceral pleural surfaces, resulting in their symphysis, elimination of the pleural space, and resolution of the effusion. Sclerosis is performed when the effusion has been completely drained and the patient's lung is completely expanded as seen on a plain chest radiograph. The actual volume of effusion that drains once these criteria are met does not appear to have an important bearing on the outcome of sclerosis, and waiting until the thoracostomy tube drainage falls below a set volume cutoff may cost additional unnecessary hospital days [23]. Routine repeated instillation of a chemical sclerosant such as tetracycline has no advantage over a single instillation in most patients [24]. Most importantly, sclerosis should not be undertaken unless complete lung expansion is achieved. Failure to achieve approximation of the visceral and parietal pleural surfaces will not permit pleural symphysis.

Tetracycline, Doxycylcline, Minocycline
The use of tetracycline for pleural sclerosis became popular in the 1970s and 1980s. When the manufacture of that drug in the United States was halted, its use was replaced by the cogeners doxycycline and minocycline. A number of nonrandomized prospective and retrospective reports have been published that demonstrate the efficacy of all of these agents to be relatively similar, with a success rate in the management of malignant pleural effusions ranging from 67% for tetracycline to 70% for doxycycline and 86% for minocycline [25–29]. Instillation through an indwelling chest tube has no apparent advantage over thoracoscopic instillation in achieving sclerosis [25]. The side effects of these agents include pain in 10%–20% and fever in 5%–15%. Repeated instillation is

necessary to achieve sclerosis more often than is required with other sclerosing agents [28]. The estimated cost of using doxycycline is in the range of $200–$400, depending on the dose used.

Talc

A common agent for sclerosis that has been in use since the 1930s is talc, which must be used in an asbestos-free form to prevent the development of mesothelioma. It can be instilled as either a powder or in the form of a slurry, the latter being a more common formulation for sclerosis through a thoracostomy tube. The efficacy of talc slurry is in excess of 90% [28, 30–32]. The side effects of this treatment include infection in 5%, fever in more than 60%, and an idiosyncratic hypoxic reaction in nearly 5% [31]. The cost of talc slurry sclerosis is substantially less than that of most other agents, averaging less than $20. Dry talc insufflation through an indwelling thoracostomy tube has similar results, although the number of patients reported is relatively small [33, 34].

Corynebacterium parvum

The use of *C. parvum* in the management of malignant pleural effusion has been popular in Europe since the 1970s. Its effect was initially attributed to its antineoplastic activity, but it appears now that its utility in the management of malignant pleural effusions is due to an inflammatory pleural reaction resulting from recruitment of neutrophils and production of an acute-phase response [35, 36]. It is effective in controlling malignant effusions in about 75% of patients, but has accompanying side effects of pain in almost 45% and fever in nearly 60% of patients [28]. Pretreatment with systemic steroids may reduce some of the side effects without preventing effective pleurodesis [37]. *C. parvum* is not available in the United States, and there is no estimated cost of therapy using it. In one randomized study comparing doxycycline to *C. parvum* the two agents were found to be equally effective in the control of malignant pleural effusion, but the side effects of *C. parvum* were substantially worse than those of doxycycline [36].

*Intrapleural Chemotherapeutic Agents*

A variety of chemotherapeutic agents have been used intrapleurally in the management of malignant pleural effusions. Although most of them act as cytoreductive agents, some also result in a chemical pleuritis and may be effective in achieving pleural sclerosis.

## Bleomycin

The most commonly used intrapleural chemotherapeutic agent is bleomycin, which appears to have both cytoreductive and chemical pleuritis effects. It is effective in controlling malignant pleural effusions in about 55% of patients [28, 38]. Its side effects include pain in almost 30%, fever in nearly 25%, and nausea in more than 10% of patients [28, 38]. One major concern with bleomycin is that it is rapidly absorbed through the pleura, possibly resulting in systemic effects and lowering the intrapleural concentration of the drug. The cost of bleomycin therapy is more than $1000. Randomized studies recently have been performed with bleomycin. Bleomycin is inferior to talc slurry (79% versus 90% success, respectively), but is more effective than tetracycline (70% versus 47% success, respectively) in the management of malignant pleural effusions [32, 39]. Bleomycin was not as effective as quinacrine in the control of malignant pleural effusions in a small randomized study [40].

## Doxorubicin, Mitoxantrone

Because of concerns over the rapid absorption of bleomycin through the pleura during intrapleural therapy, the anthracycline agents doxorubicin and mitoxantrone, which result in high intrapleural concentrations and have minimal systemic effects when administered intrapleurally, have been used in the management of pleural effusions. Their efficacy is reported to be 24%–64% [28, 41]. The side effects include pain in nearly 30%, fever in about 15%, nausea or vomiting in almost 30%, and anorexia in about 25% [28]. The cost of therapy with these agents is about $150. In randomized studies mitoxantrone was found to be similar in efficacy to bleomycin in one report and was as efficacious but had fewer side effects than quinacrine in another [41, 42].

## Other Agents

Cisplatin and cytarabine have been used in combination in the intra-pleural management of malignant pleural effusions with a success rate of about 27% but have high rates of toxicity including pain in 55%, nausea and vomiting in more than 75%, bone marrow suppression rate in excess of 50%, and renal toxicity in nearly 35% of patients [28]. The cost of therapy is estimated to be about $550. Etoposide, fluorouracil, and mito-mycin-C also have been reported to be useful in the intrapleural mana-gement of malignant pleural effusions, but the scant amount of data available precludes meaningful analysis of their efficacy [28].

## Biological Response Modifiers

### Interferon
Various preparations of interferon (interferon-$\beta$; interferon-$\alpha$-2b) have been introduced in the management of malignant pleural effusion because of their antiproliferative and immunomodulatory effects. The rate of effectiveness is about 70%, but, depending on the dosage used, side effects such as a flu-like syndrome occur in up to 70% of patients [43–45]. The estimated cost of therapy is about $200 [28].

### Other Agents
Recombinant tumor necrosis factor (TNF) and recombinant interleukin-2 (IL-2) have been used in the intrapleural management of malignant pleural effusions in phase I studies. TNF has a response rate in excess of 80%, regardless of whether the patients have had previous intrapleural therapy. Side effects include flu-like symptoms in more than 40%, fever in 35%, fatigue in nearly 25%, and chest pain or nausea/vomiting in more than 10% of patients [46]. The use of IL-2 results in control of the pleu-ral effusion in 45% of patients, the majority of the responders having pleural mesothelioma. The side effects include fluid retention in more than 35% and fever in almost 70% of patients [47].

## Radiotherapy

External beam radiotherapy has limited use in the management of mali-gnant pleural effusions. It has been shown to possibly reduce the inci-dence of ipsilateral malignant pleural effusion in patients undergoing primary treatment for breast cancer [29]. It also has utility in the mana-gement of mediastinal nodal disease that causes obstruction to lymph drainage from the chest wall and pulmonary lymphatics and in the resolution of chylothorax due to thoracic duct involvement by lym-phoma.

## Surgical Treatment

Options for surgical therapy in the management of patients with malignant pleural effusion are growing more diverse, and the boundaries between medical and surgical therapy are becoming blurred as expertise in minimally invasive surgical techniques improves. True surgical therapy for malignant effusions once consisted only of decortication or pleurectomy, options that provided excellent results at the cost of a high mortality rate. Newer thoracoscopic approaches have expanded the scope of surgical intervention, and improved perioperative management of patients with advanced cancers and symptomatic malignant pleural effusions has substantially reduced operative mortality rates in these patients.

### Thoracoscopy

Thoracoscopy is being used with increasing frequently as an adjunct to thoracostomy tube drainage and sclerosis in the management of malignant pleural effusion. The advantages include the ability to 1) lyse intrapleural adhesions; 2) thoroughly drain the pleural space; 3) optimally coat the pleural surfaces with a sclerosing agent; and 4) effectively place a pleural drain. These factors promote complete lung reexpansion and maximize the chances of successful pleurodesis. The disadvantages include the need for a general anesthetic in the hands of most physicians who perform thoracoscopy, which has associated costs and adds risk to the procedure. In retrospective reviews summarizing the treatment of nearly 600 patients in whom dry talc was insufflated at the time of thoracoscopy, the success rate of pleurodesis was greater than 85% and the operative mortality rate was less than 1% [48–51].

Two randomized trials compared the use of tetracycline or bleomycin instilled through an indwelling thoracostomy tube to talc insufflated at the time of thoracoscopy in the management of malignant pleural effusion. Talc insufflation was found to be substantially more efficacious than tetracycline instillation (more than 90% versus less than 50% success) and was also more effective than bleomycin (70% success). There was no substantial difference in the side effects experienced in the different groups of patients [52, 53]. Talc insufflation during thoracoscopy was also compared to talc slurry instillation at the bedside through a thoracostomy tube, and both had success rates in excess of 90% without important side effects [54].


## Pleurectomy

Pleurectomy is a highly successful technique for managing symptomatic malignant pleural effusions. Appropriate patient selection is very important when use of this technique is considered because of the relatively high incidence of postoperative complications and mortality. Contraindications to pleurectomy include the presence of bulky pleural disease and trapping of the lung by the neoplastic process that would prevent its complete expansion. A recent report summarizing the use of pleurectomy in 24 patients described an operative mortality rate in excess of 10%, a figure similar to those published in previous descriptions of this technique [55–57]. The success rate in these studies was in excess of 95% in survivors. Thoracoscopic techniques also have been used to perform pleurectomy with some success, although the published experience is limited [58]. The data suggest that the use of pleurectomy in the management of malignant pleural effusion should be reserved for patients whose symptoms are otherwise intractable, who have a good performance status, and whose life expectancy is likely to exceed 6 months.


## Pleuroperitoneal Shunting

The use of a shunt to move fluid in cancer patients from the pleural space to the peritoneal space was originally described in 1982 and has since found a limited place in the management of malignant pleural effusion [59]. The shunt is composed of silastic tubing forming pleural and peritoneal limbs, both of which are joined by a valved pumping chamber (Fig. 1). The limbs are inserted under local or general anesthetic into their respective body cavities, and the pumping chamber is tunnelled subcutaneously. Digital pressure applied to the pumping chamber moves fluid from the chest to the abdomen, evacuating the pleural space and reducing symptoms from the effusion.

The effectiveness of this technique in managing malignant pleural effusions is greater than 80% [49, 60, 61]. It is particularly useful in pati-

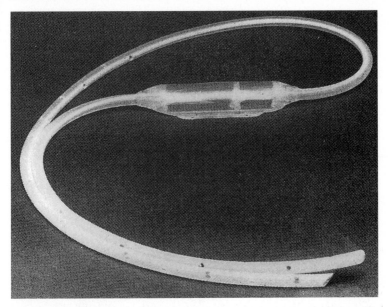

**Fig. 1.** Pleuroperitoneal shunt for management of malignant pleural effusion. The pleural and peritoneal limbs are joined by a valved pumping chamber that directs unidirectional flow from the pleural to the peritoneal space. (Reproduced from [60], with permission of Wiley-Liss, Inc., a subsidiary of John Wiley & Sons, Inc., copyright 1986, American Cancer Society)

ents who have a trapped lung due to visceral pleural fibrosis or involvement by the neoplastic process and for whom there are few other treatment options. Disadvantages include the need to place the shunt in an operating room setting, the requirement that the shunt be compressed in order to translocate fluid, and the theoretical risk of seeding the peritoneum with malignant cells. The latter occurrence is rare, considering that patients who have shunts placed have a mean survival time of less than 4 months.

*External Pleural Drainage*

The concept of pleuroperitoneal shunting of malignant pleural effusions led to the idea of shunting fluid outside of the body using a small cathe-

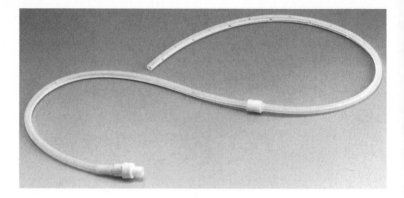

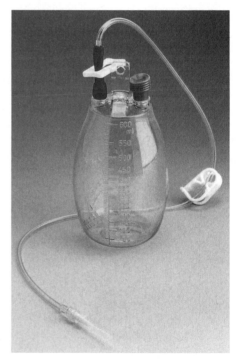

**Fig. 2a,b.** External drainage catheter (**A**) and vacuum collection system (**B**) for outpatient management of malignant pleural effusions

ter that is intermittently connected to a collection device. This permits management of the effusion at home and theoretically optimizes the patient's quality of life while minimizing the need for hospitalization. In a brief initial report this technique was utilized in 9 patients and none required additional therapy for their effusions [62]. This early success stimulated the design of a phase III trial comparing external catheter (Fig. 2) drainage to sclerosis using doxycycline instilled through a thoracostomy tube. The external catheter reduced the duration of hospitalization and provided equivalent improvement in quality of life and palliation of pleural effusion [63]. Additional clinical experience with this catheter will help define its role in the management of malignant pleural effusions.

## Current Key Questions

There are several challenges that currently confront the management of malignant pleural effusions. The optimal sclerosing agent and technique have yet to be identified. A success rate of 60%–80%, such as is reported for sclerosing agents such as doxycycline, is marginally acceptable for a condition that produces such disabling symptoms. The success rate reported for talc is substantially higher, but its administration often requires increased resource utilization and is associated with a small but important risk of respiratory distress. Traditional methods for performing pleural sclerosis usually necessitate hospital stays of 3–5 days and are accompanied by a high incidence of associated side effects. A search for new techniques that accelerate or replace the process of sclerosis is of paramount importance. Finally, the newer minimally invasive surgical techniques that potentially reduce operative morbidity need to be explored in a systematic fashion to determine whether there are relative advantages to their use.

## References

1. Lynch TJ Jr (1993) Management of malignant pleural effusions. Chest 103:385S-389 S
2. Chernow B, Sahn SA (1977) Carcinomatous involvement of the pleura: an analysis of 96 patients. Am J Med 63:695–702
3. Fenton KN, Richardson JD (1995) Diagnosis and management of malignant pleural effusions. Am J Surg 170:69–74

4. Hickman JA, Jones MC (1970) Treatment of neoplastic pleural effusions with local instillations of quinacrine (mepacrine) hydrochloride. Thorax 25:226–229

5. Anderson CB, Philpott GW, Ferguson TB (1974) The treatment of malignant pleural effusions. Cancer 33:916–922

6. Salyer WR, Eggleston JC, Erozan YS (1975) Efficacy of pleural needle biopsy and pleural fluid cytopathology in the diagnosis of malignant neoplasm involving the pleura. Chest 67:536–539

7. Storey DD, Dines DE, Coles DT (1976) Pleural effusion. A diagnostic dilemma. JAMA 236:2183–2186

8. McKenna JM, Chandrasekhar AJ, Henkin RE (1980) Diagnostic value of carcinoembryonic antigen in exudative pleural effusions. Chest 78:587–590

9. Prakash UB, Reiman HM (1985) Comparison of needle biopsy with cytologic analysis for the evaluation of pleural effusion: analysis of 414 cases. Mayo Clin Proc 60:158–164

10. Moghissi K (1990) The malignant pleural effusion: tissue diagnosis and treatment. In: Deslauriers J, Lacquet LK (eds) International Trends in General Thoracic Surgery, Volume 6, Thoracic Surgery: Surgical Management of Pleural Diseases. CV Mosby Co., St. Louis, pp 397–408

11. Ruckdeschel JC (1988) Management of malignant pleural effusion: An overview. Semin Oncol 15:24–28

12. Sahn SA (1988) State of the art. The pleura. Am Rev Respir Dis 138:184–234

13. Sahn SA (1997) Pleural diseases related to metastatic malignancies. Eur Respir J 10:1907–1913

14. Light RW, Hamm H (1997) Malignant pleural effusion: would the real cause please stand up? Eur Respir J 10:1701–1702

15. Fentiman IS (1987) Diagnosis and treatment of malignant pleural effusions. Cancer Treat Rev 14:107–118

16. Light RW (1983) Pleural diseases. Lea & Febiger, Philadelphia, p 210

17 Valentine VG, Raffin TA (1992) The management of chylothorax. Chest 102:586–591

18. Health and Public Policy Committee, American College of Physicians (1985) Diagnostic thoracentesis and pleural biopsy in pleural effusions. Ann Intern Med 103:799–802

19. Rodriguez-Panadero F, Lopez Mejias J (1989) Low glucose and pH levels in malignant pleural effusions. Am Rev Respir Dis 139:663–667

20. Staats BA, Ellefson RD, Budahn LL, Dines DE, Prakash UBS, Offord K (1980) The lipoprotein profile of chylous and nonchylous pleural effusions. Mayo Clin Proc 55:700–704

21. Perrone F, Carlomagno C, De Placido S, Lauria R, Morabito A, Bianco AR (1995) First-line systemic therapy for metastatic breast cancer and management of pleural effusion. Ann Oncol 6:1033–1043

22. Groth G, Gatzemeier U, Haussingen K, Heckmayr M, Magnussen H, Neuhauss R, Pavel JV (1991) Intrapleural palliative treatment of malignant pleural effusions with mitoxantrone versus placebo (pleural tube alone). Ann Oncol 2:213–215

23. Villanueva AG, Gray AW Jr, Shahian DM, Williamson WA, Beamis JF Jr (1994) Efficacy of short term versus long term tube thoracostomy drainage before tetracycline pleurodesis in the treatment of malignant pleural effusions. Thorax 49:23–25

24. Landvater L, Hix WR, Mills M, Siegel RS, Aaron BL (1988) Malignant pleural effusion treated by tetracycline sclerotherapy. Chest 93:1196–1197

25. Evans TRJ, Stein RC, Pepper JR, Gazet J-C, Ford HT, Coombes RC (1993) A randomised prospective trial of surgical against medical tetracycline pleurodesis in the management of malignant pleural effusions secondary to breast cancer. Eur J Cancer 29 A:316–319

26. Robinson LA, Fleming WH, Galbraith TA (1993) Intrapleural doxycycline control of malignant pleural effusions. Ann Thorac Surg 55:1115–1122
27. Heffner JE, Standerfer RJ, Torstveit J, Unruh L (1994) Clinical efficacy of doxycycline for pleurodesis. Chest 105:1743–1747
28. Walker-Renard PB, Vaughan LM, Sahn SA (1994) Chemical pleurodesis for malignant pleural effusions. Ann Intern Med 120:56–64
29. Apffelstaedt JP, Van Zyl JA, Muller AGS (1995) Breast cancer complicated by pleural effusion: Patient characteristics and results of surgical management. J Surg Oncol 58:173–175
30. Weissberg D, Ben-Zeev I (1993) Talc pleurodesis. J Thorac Cardiovasc Surg 106:689–695
31. Kennedy L, Rusch VW, Strange C, Ginsberg RJ, Sahn SA (1994) Pleurodesis using talc slurry. Chest 106:342–346
32. Zimmer PW, Hill M, Casey K, Harvey E, Low DE (1997) Prospective randomized trial of talc slurry vs bleomycin in pleurodesis for symptomatic malignant pleural effusions. Chest 112:430–434
33. Adler RH, Sayek I (1976) Treatment of malignant pleural effusion: a method using tube thoracostomy and talc. Ann Thorac Surg 22:8–15
34. Webb WR, Ozmen V, Moulder PV, Shabahang B, Breaux J (1992) Iodized talc pleurodesis for the treatment of pleural effusions. J Thorac Cardiovasc Surg 103:881–885
35. Rossi GA, Felletti R, Balbi B, Sacco O, Cosulich E, Risso A, Melioli G, Ravazzoni C (1987) Symptomatic treatment of recurrent malignant pleural effusions with intrapleurally administered Corynebacterium parvum. Clinical response is not associated with evidence of enhancement of local cellular-mediated immunity. Am Rev Respir Dis 135:885–890
36. Salomaa E-R, Pulkki K, Helenius H (1995) Pleurodesis with doxycycline or Corynebacterium parvum in malignant pleural effusion. Acta Oncol 34:117–121
37. Foresti V (1995) Intrapleural Corynebacterium parvum for recurrent malignant pleural effusions. Respiration 62:21–26
38. Patz EF Jr, McAdams HP, Goodman PC, Blackwell S, Crawford J (1996) Ambulatory sclerotherapy for malignant pleural effusions. Radiology 199:133–135
39. Ruckdeschel JC, Moores D, Lee JY, Einhorn LH, Mandelbaum I, Koeller J, Weiss GR, Losada M, Keller JH (1991) Intrapleural therapy for malignant pleural effusions. Chest 100:1528–1535
40. Koldsland S, Svennevig JL, Lehne G, Johnson E (1993) Chemical pleurodesis in malignant pleural effusions: a randomised prospective study of mepacrine versus bleomycin. Thorax 48:790–793
41. Bjermer L, Gruber A, Sue-Chu M, Sandstrom T, Eksborg S, Henriksson R (1995) Effects of intrapleural mitoxantrone and mepacrine on malignant pleural effusion-A randomised study. Eur J Cancer 31 A:2203–2208
42. Maiche AG, Virkkunen P, Kontkanen T, Moykkynen K, Porkka K (1993) Bleomycin and mitoxantrone in the treatment of malignant pleural effusions. Am J Clin Oncol 16:50–53
43. Rosso R, Rimoldi R, Salvati F, De Palma M, Cinquegrana A, Nicolo G, Ardizzoni A, Fusco U, Capaccio A, Centofanti R, et al (1988) Intrapleural natural beta interferon in the treatment of malignant pleural effusions. Oncology 45:253–256
44. Goldman CA, Skinnider LF, Maksymiuk AW (1993) Interferon instillation for malignant pleural effusions. Ann Oncol 4:141–145
45. Wilkins HE III, Connolly MM, Grays P, Marquez G, Nelson D (1997) Recombinant interferon alpha-2b in the management of malignant pleural effusions. Chest 111:1597–1599

46. Rauthe G, Sistermanns J (1997) Recombinant tumour necrosis factor in the local therapy of malignant pleural effusion. Eur J Cancer 33:226–231
47. Astoul P, Viallat J-R, Laurent JC, Brandely M, Boutin C (1993) Intrapleural recombinant IL-2 in passive immunotherapy for malignant pleural effusion. Chest 103:209–213
48. Sanchez-Armengol A, Rodriguez-Panadero F (1993) Survival and talc pleurodesis in metastatic pleural carcinoma, revisited. Chest 104:1482–1485
49. Petrou M, Kaplan D, Goldstraw P (1995) Management of recurrent malignant pleural effusions. Cancer 75:801–805
50. Viallat J-R, Rey F, Astoul P, Boutin C (1996) Thoracoscopic talc poudrage pleurodesis for malignant effusions. Chest 110:1387–1393
51. Yim APC, Chung SS, Lee TW, Lam CK, Ho JKS (1996) Thoracoscopic management of malignant pleural effusions. Chest 109:1234–1238
52. Fentiman IS, Rubens RD, Hayward JL (1986) A comparison of intracavitary talc and tetracycline for the control of pleural effusions secondary to breast cancer. Eur J Cancer Clin Oncol 22:1079–1081
53. Hartman DL, Gaither JM, Kesler KA, Mylet DM, Brown JW, Mathur PN (1993) Comparison of insufflated talc under thoracoscopic guidance with standard tetracycline and bleomycin pleurodesis for control of malignant pleural effusions. J Thorac Cardiovasc Surg 105:743–748
54. Yim APC, Chan ATC, Lee TW, Wan IYP, Ho JKS (1996) Thoracoscopic talc insufflation versus talc slurry for symptomatic malignant pleural effusion. Ann Thorac Surg 62:1655–1658
55. Fry WA, Khandekar JD (1995) Parietal pleurectomy for malignant pleural effusion. Ann Surg Oncol 2:160–164
56. Jensik R, Cagle JE Jr, Milloy F, Perlia C, Taylor S, Kofman S, Beattie EJ Jr (1963) Pleurectomy in the treatment of pleural effusion due to metastatic malignancy. J Thorac Cardiovasc Surg 46:322–330
57. Martini N, Bains MS, Beattie EJ Jr (1975) Indications for pleurectomy in malignant effusion. Cancer 35:734–738
58. Waller DA, Morritt GN, Forty J (1995) Video-assisted thoracoscopic pleurectomy in the management of malignant pleural effusion. Chest 107:1454–1456
59. Weese JL, Schouten JT (1982) Pleural peritoneal shunts for the treatment of malignant pleural effusions. Surg Gynecol Obstet 154:391–392
60. Little AG, Ferguson MK, Golomb HM, Hoffman PC, Vogelzang NJ, Skinner DB (1986) Pleuroperitoneal shunting for malignant pleural effusions. Cancer 58:2740–2743
61. Lee KA, Harvey JC, Reich H, Beattie EJ (1994) Management of malignant pleural effusions with pleuroperitoneal shunting. J Am Coll Surg 178:586–588
62. Robinson RD, Fullerton DA, Albert JD, Sorensen J, Johnston MR (1994) Use of pleural Tenckhoff catheter to palliate malignant pleural effusion. Ann Thorac Surg 57:286–288
63. Putman JB Jr, Ponn R, Olak J, Pollak J, Lee RB, Light R, Alonso A, Payne DK, Graeber G, Kovitz K, Brown B, Rodriguez M. The Pleural Catheter Study Group (1997) A phase III trial of treatment for malignant pleural effusions: Pleurx pleural catheter (PC) versus chest tube + chemical sclerosis (CT-S). Chest 112:26 S

# Miscellaneous

# Long-Term Venous Access

T. Vargish

The ability to provide long term venous access to patients afflicted with cancer has resulted in an improvement in their quality of life. The successful use of these devices is dependent on the appropriate selection of the device for each patient, technical skill in placement, and the provision of support while the patient is in the hospital and after discharge. This chapter will review all of these components and discuss the complications associated with each of these devices and their management.

## Selection

The appropriate selection of a long term venous access device is predicated upon several factors: the physical status of the patient, an accurate assessment of the patient's needs in terms of chemotherapy, nutritional support, blood product support, the frequency and quantity of blood tests for ongoing monitoring, and experience with and local availability of the different devices.

Currently there are two types of devices available for long term venous access: catheters with external access availability and implanted port systems which are surgically placed subcutaneously (Fig. 1). With each of these two types of devices, the catheter tip can be placed centrally by peripheral percutaneous access or by central venous access using the subclavian or internal jugular veins.

The peripherally introduced central catheter (PICC) for long term venous access was first described in newborn infants [1, 2]. Although the technique of using the upper extremity for right heart catheterization predates direct access to the subclavian vein through the chest wall, it is the more recent technological change in catheter composition that allowed the change in access site. The catheter is advanced through a peri-

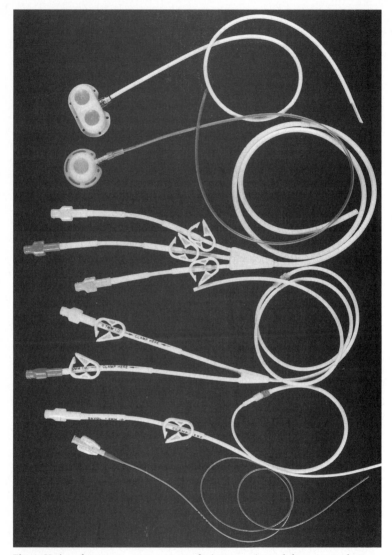

**Fig. 1.** Various long-term venous access devices are pictured from top to bottom: double lumen implantable port, single lumen implantable port, triple lumen external access catheter, double lumen external access catheter, single lumen external access catheter, and small diameter single lumen access catheter

pheral upper extremity vein into the superior vena cava. It is accessed by a hub which is fixed to the skin with sutures or tape. The indications for using the PICC (Table 1) are specifically those of short duration, low volume chemotherapy. The advantages of the PICC (Table 2) are that placement is relatively complication free, the technique can be learned quickly by a variety of health care providers, and the cost of placement is low. The disadvantages are related to the access vein size. Due to the small upper extremity access vein, the catheter must be small in diameter and multichannel devices are limited. Occlusion and phlebitis rates are higher and duration of use is lower than with centrally introduced catheter (CIC). Daily maintenance is a significant factor in the maintenance of PICC patency.

The CIC has been in use for almost 30 years. It allows direct access to the superior vena cava following needle placement in a central vein. The catheter must be directed centrally under fluoroscopic control. The cathe-

**Table 1.** Indications for device selection

| Device | Indications | Contraindications |
|---|---|---|
| PICC, PICC-implantable port | Short duration of therapy, <6 mths, Low-volume infusions Single or sequential chemotherapeutic agent planned | Multiple failed attempts at access in upper extremities Evidence of phlebitis or thrombosis in upper extremity Frequent blood testing necessary Need for multiple simultaneous infusions of blood products, TPN and chemotherapy |
| CIC implantable port | Long-term duration of therapy >6–12 mths, High-volume infusion needed Single or sequential chemotherapeutic agent planned | Chest wall or superior mediastinal tumor Radiation therapy to neck and chest Thrombosis of superior vena cava Frequent blood testing necessary Need for blood products is anticipated |
| CIC with external access | Long-term duration of therapy, >6–12 mths, High-volume infusion requirement Multiple simultaneous infusions of blood products, TPN, antibiotics, and chemotherapy High-frequency blood testing required | Chest wall or superior mediastinal tumor Radiation therapy to neck and chest Thrombosis of superior vena cava Tracheostomy |

PICC, Peripherally inserted central catheter; CIC, centrally inserted catheter.

ter is accessed through one or more hubs which are fixed to the skin of the chest wall. The indications for use of the CIC (Table 1) include the need for high volume infusions of multiple agents simultaneously and the accessibility of major veins for blood sampling. The advantages of the CIC (Table 2) are that the diameter, size and number of channels (maximum of 3) is greater, thrombosis and phlebitis rates are lower, and the duration of use is longer than with the PICC. The disadvantages of the CIC are that its placement carries a small but significant risk to the patient, the skill level required of the health care provider is much higher and the cost of placement is higher when compared with the PICC. Daily maintenance as in PICCs is a major issue and patient education concerning the management of the exit site is critical for the long term success of the catheter.

PICCs now are marketed with an associated implantable port system which can be placed subcutaneously in the upper extremity. The catheter itself must be placed in the peripheral vein as already described but the hub is attached to an access chamber which is implanted in the subcutaneous tissue of the arm. This system has many of the benefits (Table 2) associated with PICC but is currently limited to a small one channel

**Table 2.** Advantages and disadvantages of the different devices

| Device | Advantages | Disadvantages |
|---|---|---|
| PICC | Placement is relatively complication free<br>Variety of health care providers can place catheters<br>Cost of placement is low<br>Device access is easy | Longevity of catheter is limited<br>Daily maintenance is significant<br>Patient activity limited<br>Small diameter catheter limits fluid administration<br>Thrombolphlebitis rate is a concern |
| CIC-implantable port, PICC-implantable port | Patient activity is unlimited<br>Daily maintenance is minimal<br>Cosmetic appearance preferable<br>Infection rate low<br>Longevity of device better | Placement requires operation with skilled provider<br>Removal requires second procedure<br>Initial cost is high<br>For multiport system, size of device is signficant<br>Access is a concern |
| CIC with external access | Device access is easy<br>Blood sampling is facilitated<br>Large volume infusions are possible<br>Removal is easy | Placement requires operation with skilled provider<br>Initial cost is high<br>Daily maintenance is significant<br>Patient activity is somewhat limited<br>Infection rate is a concern |

PICC, Peripherally inserted central catheter; CIC, centrally inserted catheter.

device. In addition, the device must be accessed by percutaneous puncture. Complications associated with port access, usually extravasation, are magnified with the potential for significant limb injury. The cost and technical skill required for placement are increased but the patient gains the benefit of being able to bathe and participate in many activities with little or no risk of infection or catheter dislodgement.

The standard implantable port system used with CIC was first described in 1982 [3]. The indications for its use are similar to those for the CIC external access device (Table 1) and in the absence of frequent blood sampling the port system may easily substitute for the CIC with external access. The CIC implantable port system has all the advantages and disadvantages of the CIC (Table 2). Additionally, the double lumen system with a low profile access chamber is very well tolerated. In some patients, the chamber is almost undetectable and these devices can be safely left in place for many years. The disadvantages specific to implantable chambers are: they require a second procedure for removal, the access chamber must be flushed on a regular basis (usually monthly) with a dilute heparin containing solution and the process of access can induce extravasation of infusate into the access chamber pocket. As with the PICC port system, the chamber is accessed by passing a needle through the skin of the chest wall. In all of these systems, infection is always a concern, however the implantable devices seem to have a lower risk than those with external access hubs.

Patient evaluation is an additionally important component. The decision making in selecting the most appropriate device should address the following issues concerning the patient's treatment: the duration of chemotherapy; the number of intravenously administered agents and whether they will need to be given simultaneously or in close temporal proximity so as to preclude the administration of maintenance fluids and/or TPN; the need for long term TPN and/or blood and blood products during the treatment; the volume and frequency of blood testing. Some of the issues concern the patient's clinical status at the time chemotherapy is being initiated: the condition of the patient's peripheral venous system; the presence of thrombosis of central or axillary veins; the condition of the patient's chest wall and whether a tumor mass is present or whether the patient has received chest wall radiation therapy; and the presence of a tracheostomy.

From the issues just mentioned, it is evident that no two patients are alike and therefore no single device will work for everyone. In general

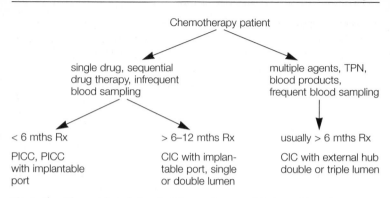

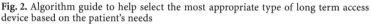

**Fig. 2.** Algorithm guide to help select the most appropriate type of long term access device based on the patient's needs

(Fig. 2), the PICC catheter or the PICC implantable chamber system are ideal for short term (less than 6 mths) single or sequential drug therapy that will not require TPN, blood product administration or frequent blood testing. As the duration of chemotherapy extends itself beyond the six month period, an access port located centrally (CIC) may be more useful allowing a longer window of use with a low infection rate. For those patients requiring long term chemotherapy, frequent blood tests, blood product administration and TPN, typical of bone marrow transplant patients, the CIC catheter with three channels is the recommended choice.

## Technique

The technique for placing either the PICC or CIC is not complicated however, appropriate training and careful supervision by experienced health care professionals are essential. The group of patients for whom these catheters are being placed can not tolerate any mistakes because of their preexistent medical problem.

The PICC can be placed under local anesthesia in a relatively clean/sterile environment. After careful skin preparation and the administration of intravenous antibiotics, a peripheral vein (basilic or cephalic) vein is accessed and the catheter with guide wire passed centrally until the catheter tip is located by measurement or fluoroscopically in the SVC just above the right atrium with the distal catheter and tip being parallel to the wall of the vessel. The catheter is then cut to length and tunneled to a new skin exit site where a hub is attached and the catheter is fixed in place. When an access chamber is used, a subcutaneous pocket is created and the catheter is tunneled to the pocket and attached to the access port. The skin is closed in routine fashion.

The CIC is placed under local anesthesia, usually with some sedation. The chest wall and neck are sterilely prepared and again intravenous antibiotics are given. The site of access is just under the clavicle at the junction of the medial and middle third. There is a nice upward curve in the clavicle at this site and one can identify the site with an index finger just below the curve. The skin and area under the clavicle are anesthetized and the zone of anesthesia is extended as far as possible towards the superior vena cava (SVC). After placing the patient in the Trendelenberg position, a finder needle is used to access the subclavian vein whereupon the Seldinger technique is used to pass a wire into the SVC. The position is confirmed with fluoroscopy. An introducer and sheath are then passed over the wire again under fluoroscopic visualization. A 5–7cm tunnel is created subcutaneously and the catheter is pulled in through the tunnel with the cuff located midway between the exit site and the point of venous access. The catheter is cut to size corresponding to the measured length to the ipsilateral end of the clavicle and the ipsilateral side of the sternum to the third intercostal space. The wire and introducer are removed and the catheter passed through the sheath into the SVC positioning the catheter tip parallel to the wall of the vessel. After confirming catheter tip position fluoroscopically and accessing all channels, the skin is closed and the catheter sutured in place.

When an access chamber is used, a pocket is created about 2 cm below and lateral to the venous access site. The access chamber is positioned and the catheter tunneled from the pocket to the venous access site. The access chamber must be secured with nonabsorbable sutures to the fascia of the chest wall (not the subcutaneous fat or breast tissue). We usually make a point of flushing all channels with a small volume of concentrated heparin at the end of the procedure. It is mandatory to confirm the position of the catheter and the absence of any surgical complication by obtaining an upright chest radiograph after the procedure.

When the neck is used for access in preference to the anterior chest wall, the procedure is preformed in similar fashion, however, the catheter is tunneled over the clavicle before being brought out through the skin. In general, we have found that this proves to be more uncomfortable for the patient when compared with the more traditional subclavicular approach although catheter function is satisfactory.

## Complications of Devices

The complications associated with any of these devices can be separated into those associated with placement and those associated with long term use. Some of the complications are device specific.

### Placement

The risks of catheter placement are most attendant with the CIC and include pneumothorax, vascular or cardiac injury, bleeding problems, and infection. All of the complications associated with placement, especially pneumothorax, seem to correlate with health care professional experience [4]. We have required our trainees to perform at least 25 of these procedures under close supervision before carrying out CIC placements independently. Nationally, the incidence of pneumothorax remains about 1%–4% [5–10]. It is almost always associated with failure to access the central vein on the first or second attempt. Documentation of the pneumothorax is usually demonstrated on an upright chest radiograph done immediately after device placement. If the pneumothorax is small and the patient is asymptomatic, we have elected to observe these patients in the hospital for several days until the pneumothorax resolves spontaneously. When the pneumothorax is large and/or the patient is symptomatic, we recommend placement of a small anterior thoracostomy tube or thoracic vent. Only rarely have we encountered situations where the patient's pneumothorax has been persistent despite tube placement. In these uncommon circumstances, it may be necessary to remove the device before the pneumothorax resolves.

Local bleeding is usually associated with platelet or clotting factor abnormalities which were present prior to the attempted placement of the device. Again this problem is a more significant one with CIC device placement. In general, I have required that the platelet count be at least 25,000/mm3 and preferably greater than 50,000/mm3 and the pro-thrombin time corrected. This can be achieved by platelet transfusion or the use of blood products just prior to and during the procedure. To avoid immediate postoperative complications, we have generally tried to keep the platelet count above 50,000/mm3 for 72 h. Usually, if this policy is followed carefully, bleeding problems are rarely an issue [11].

Injury to the vascular structures in the neck and thoracic inlet are most commonly encountered with CIC placement. This complication can be minimized by careful assessment of the blood return when accessing the vessel and by careful monitoring of the fluoroscopic image during the wire placement. Routine observation of the course of the wire should alert the observer as to whether the wire is in a venous or arterial structure. When an artery has been accessed in error, immediate removal of the finder needle and/or wire followed by 10 min of pressure over the access area is usually sufficient. When the artery has been injured by the introducer sheath and/or catheter, the catheter or sheath should be left in place and the patient should be scheduled for emergent removal of the catheter under controlled circumstances with repair of the vessel injury at the same time. Rarely, the intra pericardial superior vena cava or right atrium may be punctured, however, this is the most commonly reported health care provider (HCP) related problem recorded by the Medical Device Reporting system of the Food and Drug Administration (67% of all HCP related injuries or deaths reported) [12]. It can be avoided by careful fluoroscopic observation during the introducer placement but must be suspected whenever blood return does not occur when the introducer is removed from the sheath or the catheter is placed. In the case of hemodynamic instability, emergency pericardiocentesis must be done and a pericardial window or median sternotomy must be considered.

Occasionally, it may not be possible to access a central vein or access may be achieved but the wire may not be advanced to the appropriate location. Many of these patients have had previous CIC attempts. We try to identify these patients in advance by examining the chest wall for evidence of superficial collateral veins suggesting subclavian vein thrombosis. If this is suspected preoperatively, ultrasound evaluation of the region should be done. However, if this is discovered at the time of the CIC placement attempt, a venogram is performed on the table with the finder needle in place. Rapid disappearance of the contrast demonstrates patency, however backflow or visualization of the jugular and axillary

veins implies thrombosis more proximally and the attempted CIC placement should be abandoned on the ipsilateral side. If both sides are
obstructed, an alternative site must be selected. This will be discussed
later under special considerations.

Early thrombosis can occur with any of the catheters described in this
section. It is most commonly seen in patients with prior surgery or
radiation therapy in the region of the catheter placement or a history of
previous long term catheter placement. When placing large diameter
catheters (13.5 F or greater) we have used low dose warfarin (2.5 mg/day)
starting 36 h after the procedure. We have continued this medication
until catheter removal. For all other patients we have not routinely used
any form of anticoagulation and have infrequently had problems. In the
rare situation of extremity swelling immediately following catheter placement, we have found heparin therapy and extremity elevation helpful
in rapidly resolving the problem. In these patients, warfarin therapy is
required until device removal.

Infection is probably the most significant complication of catheter
placement and when not successfully managed early, is the most common indication for device removal. Early infections are uncommon and
imply a break in surgical technique. We use vancomycin intravenously
just prior to the placement of the catheter and do not give additional
antibiotics. Our choice is predicated on the frequency of *Staphlococcus
epidermitis* infections, however, other broad spectrum antibiotic coverage may be just as appropriate.


Late Complications

The incidence of late catheter thrombosis is reported to be as high as
50% [13–17]. Thrombolytic therapy for catheter salvage has been reported and should be considered when the need for the catheter preservation is great [18, 19]. Occasionally, we have attempted to use thrombolytic therapy to reopen an obstructed catheter but our success rate has
been disappointing. Also of concern are reports of SVC thrombosis
which can occur without symptoms [14]. For those patients who become
symptomatic and who still need the catheter, salvage should be attempted by anticoagulating the patient with heparin and then warfarin or
considering thrombolytic therapy. Catheter removal is the treatment of
choice for those patients who no longer need the catheter.

Late infections are problematic and can involve the exit site, tunnel or pocket, or the catheter tip. A compilation of the infection risk over time for long term access catheters can be seen in Table 3 [20–25]. In general, catheters which have external access sites are more prone to infections than those with implanted delivery systems. When the exit site is infected, systemic antibiotics are administered and the site monitored. Errors in management of the implanted system such as extravasation of infusate can precipitate an inflammatory reaction in the implantation pocket which can result in infection. Infections involving the tunnel or pocket usually mandate removal of the device. When a patient becomes septic and catheter sepsis is suspected, blood cultures are drawn peripherally and through the catheter. We try to manage catheter tip infections by flushing the device with the appropriate antibiotic and leaving the device catheter un-accessed for 24 h. Systemic antibiotics are routinely administered. When this fails, the device is removed. We wait for a mandatory minimum of 24 h after the patient has defervesced before placing a new long term access device.

From time to time, a device sustains a mechanical failure such as a crack or break in the device externally. When this occurs, there are kits which enable us to repair the break. Unfortunately, this is a stopgap measure and the catheter should be replaced. As long as the cause of the device failure is obstruction or mechanical failure, we have surgically isolated the catheter and passed a wire down the lumen before removing the catheter. We then proceed with placement of the introducer and sheath over the wire under fluoroscopic guidance and new catheter placement as described earlier. Antibiotics are administered during the perioperative period and we have not seen any difference in early infection rates from those catheters placed primarily with a new access attempt. Admittedly this is not done very often so experience with the technique is limited. Those devices which suffer mechanical problems in the tunnel or intravascularly must be removed.

**Table 3.** Risk of catheter infection (from [20–25]

| Device | Risk of infection/1000days |
|---|---|
| PICC[a] | 0.2 |
| CIC-implantable device | 0.4–1.2 |
| CIC external access device | 1.3–4.8 |

[a]Not usually in place for >6 months.

## Special Considerations

There are patients who require long term venous access and who have had previous long term venous devices and now present with thrombosis of the central veins in the neck and chest. These patients are a significant challenge for long term access. The two approaches we have found most useful have been by accessing the inferior vena cava through either a flank or groin approach. The flank approach is usually done under fluoroscopic guidance by our interventional radiologists. After accessing the vena cava, a wire is placed and the vein is accessed through the flank in standard percutaneous fashion using the introducer and sheath technique. The catheter tip is positioned intravascularly at the level of the diaphragm and the catheter itself tunneled around to the anterior abdomen where it is either implanted or an exit site created. The catheter is then used in routine fashion.

The groin approach involves a surgical procedure in the right or left inguinal area above the inguinal ligament. The inferior epigastric vein is identified and used to access the external iliac vein. Under fluoroscopic guidance the catheter tip is again positioned just above the diaphragm. When the inferior epigastric vein is too small, a purse string is placed in the external iliac vein and with proximal and distal control and the vein is accessed directly. We prefer to use implantable systems when in the groin however, we have also used catheters which exit the skin. Whenever possible, try to tunnel the catheter away from the incision and in the case of the implantable port system, place the access port over the iliac crest.

## Maintenance

All patients who have any of these access devices placed must participate in an intensive educational program which reviews all the necessary information about the care and maintenance of their specific access device. It is helpful to have a family member, who may be the actual caregiver, attend as well. It is beyond the scope of this chapter to address the various protocols used to dress the catheter sites and maintain patency of the various catheters. Each center should have a protocol for every device used and each patient should be familiar with his/her device's protocol. Health care providers should assure themselves that each patient is comfortable with every aspect of the management of his/her device. This is the surest way to guarantee device longevity and patient safety.

This chapter has reviewed many of the key issues surrounding long term vascular access. It is a critical component in the treatment of patients with malignancy and over time has made the quality of life for these patients much better. It is imperative that each patient be assessed carefully and that the catheters be placed by experienced individuals. Careful monitoring will turn up any complication before it becomes serious for the patient. Detailed patient education will guarantee a successful course of therapy. This portion of patient care, like other areas discussed in this book, is critical to the successful management of patients with malignant disease.

### References

1. Dolcourt J, Bose C (1982) Percutaneous insertion of silastic central venous catheters in newborn infants. Pediatrics 70:484–486
2. Loeff DS, Matlak ME, Black RE, Overall JC, Dolcourt JL, Johnson DG (1982) Insertion of a small central venous catheter in neonates and young infants. J Ped Surg 17:944–949
3. Niederhuber JE, Ensminger W, Gyves JW, Lipeman M, Doan K, Cozzi E (1982) Totally implanted venous and arterial access system to replace external catheters in cancer treatment. Surgery 92:706–712
4. Broadwater JR, Henderson MA, Bell JL, et al (1990) Outpatient percutaneous central venous access in cancer patients. Am J Surg 160:676–680
5. Mansfield PE, Hohn DC, Fornage BD, Gregurick MA, Ota DM (1994) Complications and failures of subclavian-vein catheterization. N Engl J Med 331:1735–1738
6. Morton JE, Jan-Mohamed RMI, Barker HF, Milligan DW (1991) Percutaneous insertion of subclavian Hickman catheters. Bone Marrow Transplant 7:39–41
7. Barrios CH, Zuke JE, Blaes B, Hirsch JD, Lyss AP (1992) Evaluation of an implantable venous access system in a general oncology population. Oncology 49:474–478
8. Brothers TE, Von Moll LK, Niederhuber JE, Roberts JA, Walker-Andrews S, Ensminger WD (1988) Experience with subcutaneous infusion ports in three hundred patients. Surg Gyn Obstet 166:295–301
9. Carde P, Cosset-Delaigue MF, LaPlanche A, Chareau I (1989) Classical external indwelling central venous catheter versus totally implanted venous access systems for chemotherapy administration: a randomized trial in 100 patients with solid tumors. Eur J Cancer Clin Oncol 25:939–944
10. Slater H, Goldfarb IW, Jacob HE, Hill JB, Srodes CH (1985) Experience with long-term outpatient venous access utilizing percutaneously placed silicone elastomer catheters. Cancer 56:2074–2077
11. Foster PF, Moore LR, Sankary HN, Hart ME, Ashmann MK, Williams JW (1992) Central venous catheterization in patients with coagulopathy. Arch Surg 127:273–275

12. Scott WL (1988) Complications associated with central venous catheters: a survey. Chest 94:1221–1224

13. Anderson AJ, Krasnow SH, Boyer MW, et al (1989) Thrombosis: the major Hickman catheter complication in patients with solid tumor. Chest 95:71–75

14. Horne III MK, May DJ, Alexander HR, et al (1995) Venographic surveillance of tunneled venous access devices in adult oncology patients. Ann Surg Oncol 2:174–178

15. Haire WD, Lieberman RP, Edney J, et al (1990) Hickman catheter-induced thoracic vein thrombosis: frequency and long-term sequelae in patients receiving high-dose chemotherapy and marrow transplantation. Cancer 66:900–908

16. Haire WD, Lieberman RP, Lund GB, Edney JA, Kessinger A, Armitage JO (1991) Thrombotic complications of silicone rubber catheters during autologous marrow and peripheral stem cell transplantation: prospective comparison of Hickman and Groshong catheters. Bone Marrow Transplant 7:57–59

17. Bern MM, Lokich JJ, Wallach SR, et al (1990) Very low doses of warfarin can prevent thrombosis in central venous catheters. Ann Intern Med 112:423–428

18. Gray BH, Olin JW, Graor RA, Young JR, Bartholomew JR, Ruschhaupt WF (1991) Safety and efficacy of thrombolytic therapy for superior vena cava syndrome. Chest 99:54–59

19. Seigel El, Jew AC, Delcore R, Iliopoulos JI, Thomas JH (1993) Thrombolytic therapy for catheter related thrombosis. Am J Surg 166:716–719

20. Ross MN, Haase GM, Poole MA, Burrington JD, Odom LF (1988) Comparison of totally implanted reservoirs with external catheters as venous access devices in pediatric oncology patients. Surg Gyn Obstet 167:141–144

21. Ingram, J Weitzman S, Greenberg ML, Parkin P, Filler R (1991) Complications of indwelling venous access lines in the pediatric hematology patient: A prospective comparison of external venous catheters and subcutaneous ports. Am J Pediatr Hematol Oncol 13:130–136

22. Severien C, Nelson JD (1991) Frequency of infections associated with implanted systems vs cuffed, tunneled silastic venous catheters in patients with acute leukemia. Am J Dis Child 145:1433–1438

23. Mueller BU, Skelton J, Callender DP, et al (1992) A prospective randomized trial comparing the infectious and non infectious complications of an externalized catheter versus a subcutaneously implanted device in cancer patients. J Clin Oncol 10:1943–1948

24. Pegues D, Axelrod P, McClarren C, et al (1992) Comparison of infections in Hickman and implanted port catheters in adult solid tumor patients. J Surg Oncol 49:156–162

25. Keung YK, Watkins K, Chen SC, Broshen S, Silberman H, Douer D (1994) Comparative study of infectious complications of different types of chronic central venous access devices. Cancer 73:2832–2837

# Measuring Quality of Life

M.A. List, P. Butler

## Introduction

Twenty-five years ago, when one spoke of outcomes in cancer treatment, it was assumed that the reference was to endpoints of tumor response, survival and/or disease-free survival. Over the past two decades, however, with the introduction of multi-modality treatments and the increasing number of cancer survivors, has come the growing awareness of, and concern for, the psychosocial needs of cancer patients. The loss of health and/or the consequences of treatment may result in physical or functional impairment, disruption of social and family interactions, and psychological distress, all of which affect quality of life (QOL). Accordingly, health care interventions must be judged on the basis of their effect upon quality as well as quantity of life. Extending survival does not always correlate with improvements in quality and, conversely, a treatment may not prolong life but may profoundly alter it. Understanding a patient's experience of his/her disease, its treatment and symptoms is thus critical to comprehensive cancer care and evaluation of therapeutic options.

The goal of this chapter is to discuss QOL issues in oncology and thereby to facilitate efficient and productive application of QOL measurement in both research and general clinical practice. A number of excellent historical reviews [1, 2, 3] theoretical discussions [2, 4] and papers detailing measurement development [5, 6, 7] are available. These discussions will not be repeated here; rather the chapter will highlight key concepts and then focus on when and how to utilize QOL assessment and how to interpret QOL data.

## What Is QOL?

Most people have an intuitive sense of quality of life. The subjective nature of the construct, however, has made it difficult to define, quantify and thereby study systematically. Over the past decade, investigators have arrived at the general consensus that health related QOL refers to the degree to which a disease and its treatment affect the patient's perception of his or her ability to live a satisfying life. Although environmental, economic, social and political variables also influence a person's QOL, they are not directly affected by most health care interventions and thus are excluded from the notion of health related QOL. There is also general agreement that there are two fundamental premises of health related QOL, multi-dimensionality and subjectivity. Multi-dimensionality means that QOL encompasses a broad range of domains. And, while specific definitions may vary by investigator, QOL is generally considered to include at least three and generally four dimensions: [2, 5, 8, 9, 10, 11]

- Physical/somatic (e.g., pain, nausea and fatigue);
- Functional (e.g., energy, activities of daily living);
- Social (maintenance of relationships with family and friends); and
- Psychological/emotional (e.g., mood, anxiety, depression)

Subjectivity embodies the notion that two individuals with the same disability will experience and react to their impairment differently. Individual priorities, social support and ability to adapt are only some of the factors likely to determine outcome. For example, a pianist who loses the use of a hand may suffer greater distress than a businessperson with a similar disability. Alternatively, the pianist may cope well by finding other activities, such as teaching, that give him/her pleasures while the businessperson, an avid golfer, becomes very depressed. In this way, QOL is subjective and any QOL construct must focus on the patient's perspective. These elements distinguish QOL assessment from standard toxicity ratings or global ratings of function (e.g., Karnofsky scale), both of which are made by the health care provider and summarize one area only, somatic symptoms or performance. QOL also differs from traditional outcomes such as response rates or survival in that it changes over time and the general strategy is to examine these changes over the course of disease and treatment.

## Do We Really Need To Measure It?

Studies to date support that the patient's perspective of the effects of disease and treatment is important. QOL data provide information that is more revealing than, and independent of, performance or toxicity, and patients' experience of events is at time counterintuitive. Studies have demonstrated that performance status does not generally correlate with emotional or social functioning [12–14]. Furthermore, individuals with similarly high scores on a single performance measure (e.g., Karnofsky) may be functioning very differently in other arenas such as social relationships [15]. Standard toxicity ratings also reveal nothing about a patient's experience of a particular side effect nor the degree to which it influences day to day life, issues which may, in part, affect compliance with treatment. For instance, nausea and vomiting compromises not only physical activities, but overall QOL including social, recreational and functional well-being [16, 17]. Unexpected QOL outcomes also highlight the need for inclusion of these measures. For example, a number of early studies demonstrated that, counter to investigators' expectations, aggressive therapy may be associated with better QOL than a less aggressive regimen [18–20]. In one study of women with metastatic breast cancer, the group randomized to the continuous chemotherapy arm reported better QOL than those in the intermittent chemotherapy arm [21]. These types of data underscore the importance of QOL assessment and the uniqueness of the data obtained.

## How Is Quality of Life Measured?

How then, does one go about measuring QOL? Today, it is almost universally accepted that the patient is the most appropriate source of information on his or her quality of life. By far the most common approach to obtaining this information is the use of self-assessment questionnaires. Patient-completed questionnaires can be applied in large groups of patients or busy clinical practice settings and can be given to patients directly, mailed or form the basis of a telephone or face-to-face interview.

Two basic approaches have characterized the development of QOL questionnaires: generic instruments and specific instruments. Generic instruments attempt to be inclusive and measure a very broad spectrum of QOL domains (e.g., Sickness Impact Profile, MOS-SF 36). Their advantage is that they are applicable across different diseases or conditions and thus allow for between-group comparisons. On the other hand, however, they may not provide enough data about a specific disease, condition or intervention. Specific instruments are designed to evaluate specific diseases, populations, functions or problems (e.g., cancer patients, radiation effects). They are generally more responsive to change and/or provide information on the areas of interest to clinicians. In oncology, a compromise strategy has been the development of core multi-dimensional questionnaires, appropriate for use with all cancer patients, to which disease-specific or treatment-specific modules are added. These supplemental modules include items of relevance to the disease site (e.g., breast cancer, head and neck cancer) or symptom (e.g., fatigue) of interest. For instance, while ability to swallow and be understood should be included in an instrument evaluating head and neck cancer patients, such parameters are generally irrelevant to most other cancers. The Functional Assessment of Cancer Therapy (FACT) and the European Organization for Research and Treatment of Cancer Quality of Life Questionnaire (EORTC- QLQ -C30), are two examples of this approach. The value of these measures is they provide for comparability across types of cancer as well as sensitivity to specific concerns.

At present there are a number of relatively well-developed QOL instruments appropriate for use with cancer patients. Suitable measures are those which have been rigorously constructed using input from both patients and health care workers, and demonstrated to be reliable and valid in the populations of interest. Most provide both dimension or subscale scores which describe functioning in a particular domain (e.g., social, physical) as well as a summary measure, either a single global question about overall QOL or an aggregate score, based on subscale combination.

The list of measures presented below is not exhaustive, but is illustrative of measures that generally meet these criteria. There are many review articles that describe these and other instruments in detail and discuss their development and application [7, 22, 23, 24]:

– Breast Cancer Chemotherapy Questionnaire (BCQ) [25]
– Cancer Rehabilitation Evaluation System (CARES) [26]
– European Organization for Research and Treatment of Cancer Quality of Life Questionnaire (EORTC- QLQ -C30) [27]
– Functional Assessment of Cancer Therapy (FACT) [28]
– Functional Living Index (FLIC) [29]
– McMaster University Health Index Questionnaire [30]

– Medical Outcome Study Short Form (MOS SF 36) [31]
– Multidimensional Quality of Life Scale [32]
– Nottingham Health Profile [33]
– Quality of Life Index (QL-Index) [34]
– Sickness Illness Profile [35]

The majority of these measures were developed in English. With the growing use of QOL assessment has come the increasing need for multi-lingual instruments which are acceptable and valid across cultures. Many groups have begun the process of translating and validating their instruments. At present, translations are available for a number of instruments including the CARES, EORTC-QLQ, FACT, FLIC, SF-36, SIP, McMaster Health Index and the NHP.

### For What Purpose is QOL Being Measured?

Deciding on how to measure QOL must begin with the question: for what purpose is QOL being measured and how will the results be used. There are a number of general reasons why one might collect quality of life data, the most compelling of which is as an endpoint in evaluating treatment outcomes, particularly in Phase III randomized studies. In the context of clinical trials, QOL data may also be used to describe the full range of treatment effects, to assess rehabilitation needs, and to predict future response. These uses of QOL measurement are based on groups of patients and data and are interpreted in terms of averages. Although interpretation of an individual patient's QOL scores is more difficult, QOL measures may be useful in clinical practice as a means of screening for problems or promoting patient/physician discussion.

**QOL Assessment To Describe Treatment Effects.** QOL assessment may be valuable in both randomized and non-randomized trials as a means of identifying and documenting the full range of potential treatment outcomes, including functional, physical and emotional effects. This information may be particularly valuable in the evaluation of new treatment regimens, drug combinations or schedules. The data may be used to suggest treatment modifications to minimize negative effects, to point to areas in which prophylactic interventions might be warranted or to educate and prepare patients for likely treatment outcomes.

**QOL Assessment To Identify Rehabilitation Needs.** As cancer has shifted to a more chronic disease, rehabilitation efforts have become increasingly important. Patients who have survived their cancer now must cope with the many medical, physical, and psychosocial late effects of the disease and its treatment. QOL assessment is helpful in identifying persistent late effects that may be amenable to intervention or amelioration. The same measures can then be employed to test the effectiveness of rehabilitation efforts.

**QOL as a Prognostic Variable.** Although the focus of QOL research has, to date, been on the assessment of patient outcome, there are data to suggest that pre-treatment QOL may be prognostic of survival. For example, studies in patients with advanced lung cancer [36, 37] and limited extent non-small cell lung cancer [38] have shown that baseline QOL may be a more accurate predictor of survival than performance status. This suggestion was supported in a recent study of a large, heterogeneous cancer patient population [39]. In many clinical trials, performance status rating is employed as an eligibility criterion and at times, as a stratification variable. If the above findings are confirmed in further studies, QOL ratings may become critical baseline measures to be used as a stratification variable in randomized clinical trials.

**QOL Assessment as a Screening Tool.** QOL measurement may be used for screening, that is, identification of high risk individuals for purposes of classification, determination of incidence or for subsequent study and appropriate intervention. In clinical practice, screening with multi-dimensional QOL instruments may alert health care providers to morbidities that might otherwise go undetected (e.g., unexpected physical or emotional difficulty) and thus precipitate a referral for further evaluation and/or intervention. In addition, review of a patient's responses on a QOL measure may serve as a catalyst for discussion between patient and physician about the patient's priorities and concerns.

**QOL as an Endpoint in Treatment Evaluation.** Phase III randomized trials evaluate the relative efficacy of different treatments, generally using survival advantage as the key outcome measure. Clearly, increasing survival is the primary goal of most treatment regimens. When one treatment confers a significant and substantial increase in survival it will likely be the treatment of choice regardless of morbidities or late effects. Unfortunately, however, few new treatment regimens result in such dramatic differences. More often differences in survival between treatment arms are small and other factors, including symptom alleviation, may be important in treatment selection. QOL endpoints are particularly valuable and contribute to decisions about choice of treatment when:

**Treatments Are Expected To Have Equivalent or Similar Survival Benefits but Potentially Different Effects on Physical, Emotional, Social or Other Functioning.** One illustration of this scenario is mastectomy versus lumpectomy plus radiation for appropriately selected breast cancer patients. In this example, investigators hypothesized that breast conserving surgery was better because it would confer better QOL. In fact, a decade of research has found little difference in QOL as a function of type of surgery. Rather, the factor most predictive of QOL was whether or not the woman had been offered the choice of treatment. In this instance, QOL data did not point to a specific treatment but instead to the importance of patient involvement in the decision-making process.

**Treatments Are Expected To Have Little Impact on Survival and Palliation Is the Dominant Therapeutic Consideration.** At present, there are few curative treatments for many patients with metastatic cancer and treatments are offered with the goal of palliation and/or minimal increases in survival. In these instances, QOL might be the most important and most meaningful endpoint upon which to base treatment choice. For example, Coates et al [40]. compared continuous versus intermittent chemotherapy for women with metastatic breast cancer. In contrast to their expectations that women who "got a break" from treatment would experience better QOL, the women receiving continuous chemotherapy reported better QOL. Whether these findings were related to increased response rates on the continuous therapy arm or to the sense of "continuing to do something" to combat the cancer, these QOL data were critical to selection of the preferred treatment. A recent study comparing gemcitabine to 5-FU for patients with advanced pancreatic cancer further illustrates this application of QOL data. Investigators included clinical benefit, defined as a composite measure of pain, Karnofsky performance status and weight, as a trial endpoint. While they found only a small survival advantage for gemcitabine, a greater number of gemcitabine treated patients (24% vs. 5%)

experienced a clinical benefit response. On the basis of this improvement in symptoms, gemcitabine was recently approved as a first line treatment for patients with locally advanced or metastatic pancreatic cancer [41].

**When Treatments Are Expected To Confer Different Survival Benefits but Also May Have Different Effects on QOL.** This situation may arise, for example, in trials comparing different treatment modalities or combination of modalities as exemplified in an ongoing CALGB study comparing surgery alone to neoadjuvant chemoradiotherapy followed by surgery for esophageal cancer. Investigators anticipate better survival but greater morbidity, at least short term, in the tri-modality arm. If, for example, survival differences are small, the degree to which, and for what period of time, each treatment results in declines in QOL may become an important variable in treatment selection.

**When Treatments Have Different Financial Costs as Well as Potentially Different Survival and/or Morbidities.** Treatment costs and resource allocation may play a role in selection of the preferred treatment, particularly in the current climate of health care. Rather than considering the individual's preference, however, in this context, it is society's preference that is at issue. In these cases evaluation of treatment necessitates collection of economic, QOL and survival data.

### The Logistics of QOL Assessment

Decisions about the choice of assessment instrument, the intervals and frequency of assessment, and when to start and when to stop, must be based on the purpose of the assessment. The specific research question should be formulated first, and instruments should be chosen and assessment points scheduled accordingly.

### Which Instrument?

The choice of measure depends on the QOL question being asked, the population being studied, and the group to which it is to be compared. For example, if the study goal is to document the impact of a new treatment, in order to ensure capture of unexpected outcomes, a comprehensive assessment including a broad spectrum of domains may be the approach of choice. An assessment of long-term survivors might benefit from inclusion of a generic measure that would enable comparison of the survivor cohort to population norms or individuals with other diseases. In contrast, comparisons between relatively similar treatments, as in many Phase III randomized trials, will likely require a cancer-specific and/or site-or treatment-specific instrument, selected on the basis of its inclusion of items relevant to the question being asked. Finally, at times no one instrument will contain all the information of interest and, as resources allow, a combination of two or more instruments may be necessary.

## When To Assess?

When one should measure QOL is, again, dependent upon the question of interest. All studies, however, should include a baseline (generally pretreatment) QOL assessment. The selection of additional time points must balance protocol objectives with patient, staff and analytic burdens. In addition, the risk of missing data may increase if assessments are too frequent. The timing of assessments will depend, in part, on whether it is the short-term or persistent effects of treatment that are being studied. Figure 1 presents contrived data to illustrate how study conclusions may vary as a function of when QOL is measured and for how long patients are followed.

Assume that graph lines represent two treatment arms in a randomized study, with both treatments extending over 3 months. QOL scores are presented on the Y-axis, with higher scores representing better QOL. As shown here, groups are equivalent pretreatment. As constructed, these data suggest that patients on Treatment B experience a larger decline in QOL during treatment. Were patients to be followed for 6 months post-treatment only (e.g., 9-month assessment), one would conclude that treatments result in similar QOL declines. It is not until the 24-months assessment point that differences in QOL outcome become clear, that is, confirming that Treatment B patients recover to pretreatment levels while Treatment A patients plateau below baseline.

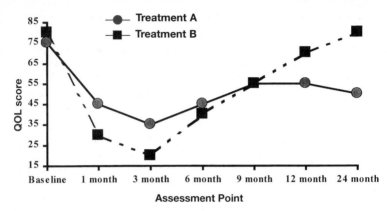

**Fig. 1.** Logistics of QOL Assessment

## Using QOL Data to Determine the Best Treatment

The discussion above provided a number of examples of how QOL data can influence choice of treatment in randomized trials. If the same treatment arm results in both increased survival and improved QOL, the choice is generally obvious. The choice is also evident if survival differences are minimal or non-existent and one treatment results in better QOL. Note that this discussion omits financial cost as a factor, but considers issues only from the patient's (versus public health) perspective. In contrast to the above examples, decisions about the "best" treatment become more complicated when a survival advantage is accompanied by significant and persistent dysfunction, (e.g., impaired speech, impotence, disfigurement) or when alternative treatments have similar survival rates but differ in their impact on certain aspects of health (e.g., surgical disfigurement versus risk of recurrence in breast cancer; likelihood of impotence versus incontinence). Do such late effects, in fact, decrease QOL; does the chance of increased survival compensate for negative sequelae; what amount of increased survival is needed to achieve a balance; what magnitude of late effects or decreased QOL are patients willing to accept? These questions can only be answered by knowing the relative value that a patient places on different outcomes or the level of importance assigned to specific impairments.

For an individual patient, these issues are addressed by providing information about the main medical and non-medical outcomes, including short and long-term QOL experiences, of alternative treatments. With information about the likelihood of different outcomes a patient can consider his or her own priorities to arrive at an informed choice. Patients may differ in the importance they attach to various outcomes and thus two patients offered the same options might choose different treatments. Decisions about which of two treatment arms should become the standard of care, however, is considerably more complicated as it involves making decisions about the best treatment for the average patient. Extensive discussion of how to formally combine quality and quantity of life to arrive at such a decision is beyond the scope of this chapter. The brief discussion below, however, will serve to illustrate the concepts involved and their application in practice.

So far this chapter has focused on QOL measures which generate health status profiles, that is, descriptions of the patient's perception of his/her life in a range of domains. These measures, however, do not provide information about the value a patient places on a given health state. Value or preference measures specifically ask patients to assign values to designated health states [42]. The underlying assumption is that for any individual the expectation of living Y years in less than full health will be equivalent to the expectation of living x years in perfect health, where $x<Y$ [43]. Values, or utilities, are generally expressed as 0–1, where 0 represents death and 1 perfect health. Thus, a health state assigned a value of 0.8 would be considered preferable to a health state assigned a value of 0.5. After a utility for a particular state has been derived, survival time can be adjusted downward to a degree proportional to the amount of disability or toxicity to arrive at Quality Adjusted Life Years (QALY's). For example, four years in a state with a utility of 0.5 would be equivalent to two years in a state with a utility of 1.0. To date, QALYs have generally been used in economic evaluations of different therapeutic options. A second approach to employing utilities to compare treatments is the calculation of Quality Adjusted Survival relative to Time without Symptoms or Toxicity (Q-TWiST). In this approach, time to survival is partitioned into QOL oriented end points, for example, time with symptoms (early and late treatment toxicities), time without symptoms, and survival time following a diagnosis of relapse. The amount of time spent in each period is then adjusted by the utility assigned to it, with time without symptoms being assigned a utility of 1.0. These concepts have

not yet been extensively used in oncology and more widespread application requires consideration of numerous methodological (e.g., whose
utilities should be used in calculating QALY's and Q-TWIST) and ethical
issues that are beyond the scope of this chapter. QALY's and Q-TWIST
are important however, in that they provide indices for combining
duration and quality of life.

## Challenges in Application and Interpretation of QOL Scores

Integration of QOL tools in clinical practice and interpretation of QOL
scores has been hampered in part by: a) the absence of a "gold standard"
against which to compare scores and b) difficulties in determining
whether a given difference, or change in QOL, is clinically meaningful.
First, each of the QOL instruments validated for use with cancer patients
has its own set of questions and scoring rules. Scores are generally not
anchored by descriptors, vary in scale across instruments and thus cannot easily be compared across measures. In response to this issue, investigators have begun to devise and test new methodologies for generating
common scores with the goal of facilitating cross study comparisons as
well as the general interpretation of QOL scores. Second, particularly
when QOL is incorporated in large clinical trials, small absolute differences in QOL outcomes may be statistically significant. But statistical
significance does not always confer clinical or subjective significance.
What magnitude of difference is, in fact, meaningful, would be noticed
by patients and thus warrants clinical attention is currently under study.
Research in the area focuses on two approaches: [44] i) a distribution-
based interpretation based on the statistical distribution of results and
ii) an anchor-based interpretation in which QOL scores are compared to
other clinical changes or results using population norms or based on a
patient or clinician global rating question. While considerably more
research is needed in this area, there are currently some preliminary guidelines available to aid in interpretation of QOL differences [45, 46, 47].

## Summary

QOL is a multidimensional, subjective construct that must be measured
over time from the patient's perspective. There is no gold standard and

instruments must be selected on the basis of the purpose of the assessment, the availability of validated measures and patient and staff burden. There are a number of well validated instruments appropriate for use with cancer patients, many of which have been validated for cross-cultural use. At present researchers in the field are focusing on the development of guidelines for determination of clinical or subjective relevance, cross-cultural validation of instruments, comparing scores across measures, integration of measures of quality and quantity, and how to manage missing data. In spite of these as yet unresolved issues, QOL data continue to provide important information that can have a substantial influence on clinical trials outcome as well as in clinical practice.

## References

1. Holland J (1991) Progress and challenges in psychosocial and behavioral research in cancer in the twentieth century. Cancer 67:767–773
2. Cella DF, Tulsky DS (1993) Quality of life in cancer: Definition, purpose and method of measurement. Cancer Invest 11:327–336
3. Kornblith AB, Holland JC (1996) Model for quality-of-life research from the Cancer and Leukemia Group B: The telephone interview, conceptual approach to measurement, and theoretical framework. JNCI Monographs 20:55–62
4. Gotay CC (1996) Trial-related quality of life: using quality-of-life assessments to distinguish among cancer therapies. JNCI Monographs 20:1–6
5. Cella D (in press) Instruments and assessments methods in psycho-oncology: quality of life. To appear in Holland JC et al (eds) Textbook of psycho-oncology. Oxford University Press, New York
6. Aaronson NK (1991) Methodologic issues in assessing the quality of life of cancer patients. Cancer 67:844–850
7. Moinpur CM, Feigl P, Metch B et al (1989) Quality of life end points in cancer clinical trials: review and recommendations. JNCI 81:475–495
8. Cella DF (1988) Quality of life during and after cancer treatment. Comprehensive Ther 14:69–75
9. Aaronson NK (1988) Quality of life:what is it? How should it be measured? Oncology 2:69–74
10. Schipper H, Levitt M (1985) Measuring quality of life: risks and benefits. Cancer Treat Rep 69:1115–1123
11. Ware JE, Kosinski MA, Bayliss MS et al (1995) Comparison of methods for scoring and statistical analysis of SF-36 health profile and summary measures: summary of results from the medical outcomes study. Med Care 33:AS264-AS279
12. Aaronson NK, Ahmedzai S, Bergman B et al (1993) The European Organization for Research and Treatment of Cancer QLQ-C30: a quality-of-life instrument for use in international trials in oncology. JNCI 85:365–376
13. Osoba D (1994) Lessons learned from measuring health-related quality of life in oncology. JCO 12:608–616
14. List MA, Mumby P, Haraf D et al (1997) Performance and quality of life outcomes in patients completing concomitant chemoradiotherapy protocols for head and neck cancer. Qual Life Res 6:274–284

15. Mackworth N (1992) Quality of life self-reports from 200 brain tumor patients: comparisons with Karnofsky performance scores. J Neurooncol 14:243–253
16. Lindley CM, Hirsch JD, O'Neill CV et al (1992) Quality of life consequences of chemotherapy-induced emesis. Qual Life Res 1:331–340
17. O'Brien BJ, Rusthoven J, Rocchi A et al (1993) Impact of chemotherapy-associated nausea and vomiting on patients' functional status and costs: survey of five Canadian centres. Can Med Assoc J 149:296–302
18. Sugarbaker PH, Barofsky I, Rosenberg SA et al (1982) Quality of life assessment of patients in extremity sarcoma trials. Surgery 91:17–23
19. Chang AE, Steinberg SM, Culnane M et al (1989) Functional and psychosocial effects of multimodality limb-sparing therapy in patients with soft tissue sarcomas. JCO 51:47–51
20. Baum M, Priestman T, West RR et al (1980) A comparison of subjective responses in a trial comparing endocrine with cytotoxic treatment in advanced carcinoma of the breast. In Mouridsen HT, Palshoff T (eds) Breast cancer. Experimental and clinical aspects. Pergammon Press, Oxford
21. Coates A, Gebski V, Bishop JF et al (1987) Improving the quality of life during chemotherapy for advanced breast cancer. N Engl J Med 317:1490–1495
22. Cella DF, Bonomi AE (1995) Measuring quality of life: 1995 update. Oncology 9 (Suppl 11):47–60
23. Kornblith AB, Holland JC (1994) Handbook of measures for psychological, social and physical function in cancer. Vol 1:quality of life. Memorial Sloan-Kettering Cancer Center, New York
24. Spilker B (ed) (1996) Quality of life and pharmacoeconomics in clinical trials (2nd ed). Lippincott-Raven, Philadelphia
25. Levine MN, Guyatt GH, Gent M et al (1988) Quality of life in stage II breast cancer: an instrument for clinical trials. JCO 6:1798
26. Schag CAC, Ganz PA, Heinrich RL (1991) Cancer Rehabilitation Evaluation System-Short Form (CARES-SF): A cancer specific rehabilitation and quality of life instrument. Cancer 68:1406–1413
27. Aaronson NK, Ahmedzai S, Bergman B et al (1993) The European Organization for Research and Treatment of Cancer QLQ-C30: A quality-of-life instrument for use in international clinical trials in oncology. JNCI 85:365–376
28. Cella DF, Tulsky DS, Gray G et al (1993) The Functional Assessment of Cancer Therapy scale: development and validation of the general measure. JCO 11:570–579
29. Schipper H, Clinch JJ, McMurray A et al (1984) Measuring the quality of life of cancer patients: the Functional Living Index-Cancer: development and validation. JCO 2:472–483
30. Chambers LW, Sackett DL, Goldsmith CH et al (1976) Development and application of an index of social function. Health Serv Res 11:430–441
31. Ware JE, Sherbourne CD (1992) The MOS 36-item short form healthy survey (SF-36) I. Conceptual framework and item selection. Med Care 30:473–483
32. Padilla GV, Mishel MH, Grant MM (1992) Uncertainty, appraisal and quality of life. Qual Life Res 1:155–165
33. Wiklund I (1990) The Nottingham Health Profile – a measure of health-related quality of life. Scan J Primary Care (Suppl 1):15–18
34. Ferrans CE, Powers MJ (1985) Quality of life index: Development and psychometric properties. Adv Nurs Sci 8:15–24
35. Bergner M, Bobbit RA, Kressel S et al (1976) The Sickness Impact Profile: Conceptual formulation and methodology for the development of a health status measure. Int J Health Services 6:393–415

36. Ganz PA, Lee JJ, Siau J (1991) Quality of life assessment. An independent prognostic variable for survival in lung cancer. Cancer 67:3131–3135
37. Ruckdeschel JC (1991) Etoposide in the management of non-small cell lung cancer. Cancer 67 (Suppl 1):250–253
38. Kaasa S, Mastekaasa A, Lund E (1989) Prognostic factors for patients with inoperable non-small cell lung cancer, limited disease. Radiother Oncol 15:235–242
39. Dancey J (1997) Quality of life scores: an independent prognostic variable in a general population of cancer patients receiving chemotherapy. Qual Life Res 6:151–158
40. Coates A, Forbes J, Simes RJ (1993) Prognostic value of performance status and quality-of-life scores during chemotherapy for advanced breast cancer. The Australian New Zealand Breast Cancer Trials Group (letter). CO 11:2050
41. Burris HA (1996) Objective outcome measures of quality of life. Oncology-Huntingt 10 (Suppl 11):131–135
42. Weeks J (1996) Taking quality of life into account in health economic analyses. JNCI Monographs 20:23–28
43. Till JE (1996) Uses (and possible abuses) of quality-of-life measures. In Spilker B (ed) Quality of life and pharmacoeconomics in clinical trials (2nd ed). Lippincott-Raven, Philadelphia
44. Lydick E, Epstein RS (1993) Interpretation of quality of life changes. Qual Life Res 2:221–226
45. Osoba D, Rodrigues G, Myles J et al (1998) Interpreting the significance of changes in health-related quality-of-life scores. JCO 16:139–144
46. Jaeschke R, Singer J, Guyatt GH (1989) Measurement of health status. Ascertaining the minimal clinically important difference. Controlled Clin Trials 10:407–415
47. Cleary PD (1996) Future directions in quality of life research. In Spilker B (ed) Quality of life and pharmacoeconomics in clinical trials (2nd ed). Lippincott-Raven, Philadelphia

# Basic Biostatistical Methods in Oncology: Principles of Clinical Research Methods

J.E. Herndon II

A scientifically logical sequence of clinical studies is conducted to investigate the value or usefulness of new oncology treatment regimens. These studies are often categorized or described in terms of their ultimate objective or purpose:

- Phase I: Initially, the toxicity profile of the new treatment regimen is examined in a phase I dose-escalation study. A reasonably safe, and not overly toxic, treatment dose is identified which will be used in later efficacy studies (e.g. phase II or III studies).
- Phase II: A small screening study or phase II study is used to identify those treatment regimens which appear promising in terms of tumor response.
- Phase III: The new treatment regimen is compared to one or more treatments in a phase III study, with the primary efficacy endpoint usually being survival or disease-free survival. One of the treatment regimens included in this comparison is typically the current standard of care.

This chapter will consider individually each of these trial types in terms of study design and basic statistical methods needed for study implementation or analysis.

## Phase I Studies

The initial decision to study a new treatment regimen and assess its clinical effectiveness is usually based upon preclinical or basic science studies which suggest that the new treatment regimen inhibits growth or recurrence of cancer tumors. These new regimens may consist of new cytotoxic drugs, new combinations of old drugs, new approaches to administering radiation treatment, or new approaches to administering radiation and chemotherapy together.

The ultimate goal of cancer treatment is to reduce the patient tumor burden or eradicate the disease from the patient. It is generally accepted that a greater biological effect (e.g. reduction of tumor burden) occurs with the administration of more intense doses of cytotoxic chemotherapy and/or radiation. Given the significant toxicities which are commonly associated with cancer treatment, the first step in examining a new regimen is to determine the maximum dose at which the regimen can be safely administered. Such is the objective of a phase I trial: To determine the maximum tolerated dose (MTD) at which a treatment regimen can be safely administered with an acceptable level of toxicity.

Phase I studies are performed by starting with a low dose at which dose-limiting toxicities (DLT) are not expected to occur. The dose for subsequent patients is increased according to prespecified dose-escalation criteria. A commonly used design involves the treatment of 3 patients at a particular dose level. If no dose-limiting toxicities are observed, the dose is escalated for the next cohort of 3 patients. If one patient is observed with DLT, then an additional 3 patients are treated at the same dose level. If no additional patients are observed to have DLT, dose escalation continues with an additional 3 patients. Otherwise dose escalation is terminated. If 2 or 3 among the initial 3 patients treated within a cohort experience DLT, then dose escalation is also terminated. It should be noted that the accrual of additional patients on a particular cohort or dose level after the initial 3 or 6 patients is not permitted until there has been adequate follow-up of these patients to determine if the dose-escalation criteria has been satisfied. For the specific phase I design described above, the maximum dose level at which 0 or 1 patient (or less than 33% of patients treated) experience dose-limiting toxicity is the maximum tolerated dose (MTD).

One of the problems associated with the commonly used phase I study design is the potential for a patient to be underdosed or severely overdose. Recently alternative designs have been proposed in an attempt to dose patients at a more optimal dose. The properties of these study designs are currently undergoing extensive examination [1, 2, 3, 4, 5].

## Phase II Designs

Objective of Phase II Design

A phase II cancer clinical trial is a small clinical study conducted to determine whether a new treatment regimen has sufficient promise in treating cancer to merit further testing in a larger group of patients. These trials, which are the first efficacy studies conducted after an MTD has been determined in phase I research, are conducted in tumor-specific patient groups, with the primary endpoint being the tumor response rate, or the percentage of patients who will have a significant reduction in the size of their cancerous tumor. These studies are typically not comparative in design. Rather, phase II studies are conducted as screening studies to determine which regimens are worthy of comparing against a standard treatment in a randomized phase III study.

Populations and Samples

The eligibility criteria of all study protocols defines the population of patients which are permitted to be accrued to the study, and describes the type of patient to which study conclusions are applicable. The study is conducted to collect data about a specific parameter or population characteristic. A sample, or small group of patients representative of the larger population, is enrolled on the protocol. Based upon this sample, a descriptive statistic describing the characteristic is calculated, and inferences or conclusions are made about the population parameter using the sample statistic.

In a phase II study, inferences about the tumor response rate among all patients with a specific tumor type are made through the use of confidence intervals and hypothesis-testing.

Estimation: Confidence Interval

A point estimate of the underlying tumor response rate is the proportion of responses observed within a sample of treated patients. A 95% confidence interval or interval estimate for the response rate, which has a 95% chance of including the true tumor reponse rate, can also be obtained.

For small sample sizes, the binomial distribution can be used to estimate a confidence interval for tumor response rate. For larger sample sizes, the 95% confidence interval can be computed as:

$$\hat{p} = 1.96\sqrt{\frac{\hat{p}\hat{q}}{n}} < p < \hat{p} + 1.96\sqrt{\frac{\hat{p}\hat{q}}{n}}$$

where p is the true response rate, $\hat{p}$ is the estimated response rate (i.e. proportion of patients responding), $\hat{q} = 1 - \hat{p}$, and n is the sample size. Consistent with intuition, the width of the confidence interval decreases with increasing sample size.

At times, the sample size for a single-stage phase II studies is chosen to insure that the width of the confidence interval is less than some maximum value L. In this case the sample size must be larger than $(1.96/L^2)$.

## Hypothesis Testing

Some phase II studies are designed with a hypothesis-testing framework in order to make a decision about the activity of the new regimen. These designs take into account decision-making errors which occur in the determination of activity or the response rate, specifically, the probability or chance of claiming activity (i.e. high tumor response rate) when the regimen is inactive and the probability of claiming inactivity (i.e. low tumor response rate) when the regimen is active. These designs assume one is interested in deciding either that the response rate p is less than some value $p_0$, selected to indicate an uninteresting response rate, or greater than some value $p_1$, chosen to indicate a response rate definitely worth further investigation. The hypothesis which is tested is:

$H_0$: $p \leq p_0$ versus $H_1$: $p \geq p_1$

where $H_0$: $p \leq p_0$ is the null hypothesis and $H_1$: $p \geq p_1$ is the alternative hypothesis.

In making a decision within this hypothesis testing framework, two types of errors can occur (see Table 1):
– A type I error occurs when the decision is made that the alternative hypothesis (i.e. treatment regimen is active) is true when in fact the null hypothesis is true (i.e. treatment regimen is not active)–someti-

**Table 1.** Truth table for hypothesis testing

| Decision based upon data | Truth | |
| | $H_0$ true | $H_1$ true |
| --- | --- | --- |
| Accept $H_0$ | Correct | Type II error |
| Reject $H_0$ and accept $H_1$ | Type I error | Correct |

mes referred to as a false positive result. The probability of a type I error occurring is designated as $\alpha$.

– A type II error occurs when the decision is made that the null hypothesis (i.e. treatment regimen is not active) is true when in fact the alternative hypothesis is true (i.e. treatment regimen is active)–sometimes referred to as a false negative result. The probability of committing a type II error is denoted as $\beta$. Power is the probability of rejecting the null hypothesis when it is false, i.e. Power=$1 - \beta$.

Typically, $\alpha$ is allowed to be 0.1, 0.05, or 0.01; and, $\beta$ is often chosen to be 0.1 or 0.2 (i.e. power is 80% or 90%). The magnitude chosen for $\alpha$ and $\beta$ is dependent upon the consequences of the error committed. For example, if the consequences of making a type II error is extremely severe, a "small" $\beta$ is preferable.

Sample size requirements are highly dependent upon the choice of $\alpha$, $\beta$, p0, p1. As demonstrated in Table 2, as $\alpha$ and $\beta$ become smaller, sample size requirements increase. Similarly, as the difference between $p_0$ and $p_1$ decreases or the average of $p_0$ and $p_1$ approaches 0.5, the sample size needs increase.

**Table 2.** Sample size requirements for various single-stage phase II studies using a hypothesis-testing framework

| $p_0$ | $p_1$ | $\alpha=0.05$ | | $\alpha=0.10$ | |
| | | $\beta=0.1$ | $\beta=0.2$ | $\beta=0.1$ | $\beta=0.2$ |
| --- | --- | --- | --- | --- | --- |
| 0.1 | 0.25 | 55 | 40 | 40 | 31 |
| 0.1 | 0.30 | 33 | 25 | 25 | 18 |
| 0.1 | 0.35 | 25 | 17 | 17 | 15 |
| 0.2 | 0.35 | 77 | 56 | 61 | 44 |
| 0.2 | 0.40 | 47 | 35 | 36 | 24 |
| 0.2 | 0.45 | 29 | 21 | 24 | 16 |
| 0.3 | 0.45 | 93 | 67 | 71 | 50 |
| 0.3 | 0.50 | 53 | 39 | 39 | 30 |
| 0.3 | 0.55 | 36 | 25 | 25 | 19 |

Often, a p-value is reported in conjunction with a hypothesis test. This p-value is the significance level at which the test statistic would have been statistically significant. Under the null hypothesis, the p-value is the probability or chance of observing study results which are more deviant from the null hypothesis than actually seen.

Multi-stage Designs

So far, only single stage studies in which no interim analysis is conducted have been described. Both ethical and practical considerations often require early termination of phase II trials if early results clearly indicate that the new regimen is not active or worthy of further investigation. Group sequential or multi-stage study designs in which interim analyses are conducted after each stage of the study are commonly utilized.

Among the many multi-stage phase II designs previously proposed, three commonly used study designs are worthy of comment here: Gehan's 2-stage design [6], and Simon's optimal and minimax designs [7]. If the target activity level is 20%, then 14 patients are accrued in the first stage of Gehan's study design. If the true response rate were 20% or less, the probability of observing no responses is less than 0.05. Therefore, if no responses are obtained among the first 14 patients, accrual is terminated and the treatment regimen is considered inactive. Otherwise, a second stage of patient accrual is needed to better estimate the response rate. The precise number of patients to be accrued during the second stage is dependent upon the width of the confidence interval desired. Gehan's design is frequently misapplied with 11 patients in the second stage-fewer patients than actually required for the desired precision for the estimate.

Simon proposes two two-stage study designs which either minimize the expected number of patients enrolled on the study or minimize the maximum number of patients required. A select few of these designs are presented in Table 3. As an example, consider the optimal two-stage study design proposed by Simon for differentiating between a tumor response rate of 10% and 30% with type I and II error rates of 0.10. Such a design is appropriate when looking at new agents for the treatment of patients with advanced non-small cell lung cancer. In that design, 12 patients are accrued to the first stage of the study. While the results of the first stage are collected and patients are evaluated for response, accrual

**Table 3.** Selected optimal phase II designs (from [7])

| | | Reject drug if response rate | | | |
|---|---|---|---|---|---|
| | | Optimal design | | Minimax design | |
| $P_0$ | $P_1$ | $\leq r_1/n_1$ | $\leq r/n$ | $\leq r_1/n_1$ | $\leq r/n$ |
| 0.10 | 0.30 | 1/12 | 5/35 | 1/16 | 4/25 |
| | | 1/10 | 5/29 | 1/15 | 5/25 |
| | | 2/18 | 6/35 | 2/22 | 6/33 |
| 0.20 | 0.40 | 3/17 | 10/37 | 3/19 | 10/36 |
| | | 3/13 | 12/43 | 4/18 | 10/33 |
| | | 4/19 | 15/54 | 5/24 | 13/45 |
| 0.30 | 0.50 | 7/22 | 17/46 | 7/28 | 15/39 |
| | | 5/15 | 18/46 | 6/19 | 16/39 |
| | | 8/24 | 24/63 | 7/24 | 21/53 |

$n_1$ is the number of patients treated during the first stage of the study; whereas, n is the total number of patients. $r_1$ is the number of responders during the first stage, and r is the total number of responders. For each value of $(P_0, P_1)$ designs are given for three sets of probability. The first, second, and third rows correspond to $(\alpha, \beta)$ of (0.10, 0.10), (0.05, 0.20), and (0.05, 0.10).

must be suspended in accordance with the specifications of the design. If at least 2 of the 12 patients respond, an additional 23 patients are accrued for a total of 35 patients. Otherwise, the new treatment regimen is rejected as being inactive after the first stage.

Multi-stage designs as described typically specify an exact number of patients at which an interim analysis is to be done. Within a multi-center setting it is very difficult to suspend patient accrual at exactly the required number of patients. The Southwest Oncology Group standardly uses a phase II study design which allows for inexact sample sizes in stage 1 and 2 [8]. The decision rules after the first and second stage are not dependent upon the number of patients accrued. Rather, after the first stage, a one-sided test of the hypothesis $H_1: p \geq p_1$ is conducted at the 0.02 level. The decision rule after both stages is based upon a one-sided test of $H_0: p \leq p_0$ at the 0.055 level.

## Randomized Phase II Trials

When there are sufficient numbers of patients available and several new treatment regimens to consider, there are advantages to a randomized phase II trial. Though randomized phase II trials are not comparative, the study design guarantees that similar types of patients have been treated with each new treatment. The choice of which treatment(s) to carry on into phase III testing will not be biased as all regimens will have been examined in an identical patient population.

## Phase III Study Designs

Objective of Phase III Study

Once the activity of a new treatment regimen has been established in a phase II study, the next logical step is to determine how it compares to the standard of care. A randomized, phase III study is conducted to compare two or more treatment groups relative to a primary endpoint such as survival or disease-free survival.

Randomization

Patients are randomized to one of the treatment arms to guarantee that treatment assignment has not been affected or influenced (i.e. biased) by a known or unknown factor. Randomization does not ensure that study patients are representative of all patients with the disease, nor does randomization guarantee that the treatment groups are equivalent clinically. Rather, randomization distributes the unknown biasing factors according to a random process which can be handled effectively in statistical analyses.

In small to moderate-sized studies major imbalances in important patient characteristics may occur by chance and complicate the study's interpretation. At times it is wise to make sure such imbalances cannot occur, by stratifying the randomization on these factors. With stratified randomization, patients are randomized separately within each strata.

Estimation of Survival Curves

Survival analysis techniques can be used to summarize most data which describe the time to a well-defined endpoint, such as time to death, time to disease recurrence, time to tissue engraftment, etc. The following methods which will be explained in terms of time to death (i.e. survival time) are applicable to all "time to event" endpoints.

For each patient treated on a clinical trial, the survival time is defined as the time from study enrollment to death. For patients remaining alive at the time of last follow-up, survival time is censored at that last follow-up. The censored observation indicates that the patient has survived the noted amount of time, and remains at risk for dying in the future.

The most common method used to estimate the survival experience of patients is the Kaplan-Meier or product limit estimate [9]. The calculations used to estimate the survival curve for the chemotherapy/radiotherapy treatment arm of CALGB 8433 [10, 11] are summarized in Table 4. (Conducted by the Cancer and Leukemia Group B, CALGB 8433 was a study of patients with stage III non-small cell lung cancer who were randomized to receive either radiation treatment alone or radiation with chemotherapy [cisplatin/vinblastine]). At time 0 or randomization, all 78 patients were at risk of dying. The first death in this treatment arm occurred at 0.197 months, with 77/78 surviving. The cumulative survival probability is 77/78=0.9872. The second death occurred at 1.869 months, with 76 of 77 patients at risk surviving. The probability of surviving 1.869 months is the product of the probability of surviving 0.97 months (0.9872) and the probability of surviving 1.869 months given that they had survived 0.97 months (76/77). Hence, the survival probability is estimated as 0.9872 x (76/77)=0.9744. The survival probability at subsequent follow-up times are computed in the same manner. The estimated survival pro-

**Table 4.** Calculation of Kaplan-Meier survival curve for the chemotherapy/radiotherapy arm of CALGB 8433

| Time (mos) | Number at risk | No. of deaths | No. of censored | Surviving fraction | | Cumulative survival |
|---|---|---|---|---|---|---|
| 0.197 | 78 | 1 | 0 | 77/78 | (77/78)= | 0.9872 |
| 1.869 | 77 | 1 | 0 | 76/77 | 0.9872x(76/77)= | 0.9744 |
| 2.721 | 76 | 1 | 0 | 75/76 | 0.9744x(75/76)= | 0.9615 |
| 3.148 | 75 | 1 | 0 | 74/75 | 0.9615x(74/75)= | 0.9487 |
| 3.869 | 74 | 1 | 0 | 73/74 | 0.9487x(73/74)= | 0.9359 |
| | | | | | | |
| 47.738 | 16 | 1 | | | | 0.2030 |
| 47.967 | 15 | 1 | 0 | 14/15 | 0.2030x(14/15)= | 0.1895 |
| 52.459 | 14 | 0 | 1 | 14/14 | | 0.1895 |
| 55.607 | 13 | 0 | 1 | 13/13 | | 0.1895 |
| 60.656 | 12 | 1 | 0 | 12/13 | 0.1895x(12/13)= | 0.1737 |
| 62.262 | 11 | 2 | 0 | 10/12 | 0.1737x(10/12)= | 0.1421 |
| 70.000 | 9 | 1 | 0 | 9/10 | 0.1421x(9/10)= | 0.1263 |

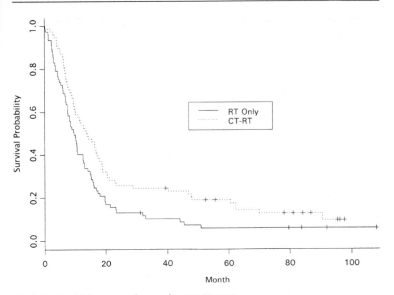

**Fig. 1.** Kaplan-Meier survival curve for CALGB 8433

babilities for both treatment arms of CALGB 8433 have been plotted in Figure 1.

Confidence intervals can be calculated for survival estimates using Greenwood' s formula [12]. The width of confidence intervals increases as survival times increase due to a decreasing number of survivors. Median survival, a statistic commonly reported with survival data, is the time point at which the survival estimate is 0.5. In other words, it is the time point at which half the patients remain alive.

Associated with a survival function is also a hazard function. The hazard, which is a function of time, is the instantaneous death rate. It may increase, decrease, remain constant, or indicate a more complicated process.

## Comparison of Survival Curves

Of primary interest in a phase III study is a comparison of the survival curve between treatment groups. A log-rank test is typically used to make this comparison [13]. The log-rank test is not a comparison of the median survival time or a comparison of the survivor fraction at a particular follow-up time. Rather, the log-rank test determines whether the treatment-specific survival curves are identical over the full-range of follow-up.

The null hypothesis is equality of treatment-specific survival distributions. The alternative hypothesis may be either a one-tailed or two-tailed alternative. If the objective of the study is to prove that the new treatment is better than the standard, a one-tailed alternative hypothesis is appropriate. However, if the study objective is to show that the two treatments are different (i.e. standard better than new, or new better than standard), then a two-tailed alternative is appropriate. The appropriateness of a one-tailed test versus a two-tailed test is controversial among statisticians.

When survival is the primary endpoint of the study, differences between treatment arms are often expressed in terms of a hazard ratio, a ratio of the hazard rate in the new arm and standard treatment arm. When the hazard ratio is 1, survival curves are identical. If the hazard rate for the new arm is greater than that with the standard arm, the hazard ratio is greater than 1 and the survival distribution within the standard arm is better than it is with the new treatment. If the underlying survival distribution in both treatment arms is exponential (i.e. has a constant hazard rate over all time), the hazard ratio is also equal to the ratio of the median survival estimates.

Sample Size Requirements

The power of statistical comparisons of survival is a function of the number of events or deaths, and not the total number of patients. Table 5 summarizes the number of deaths required to detect the noted hazard ratio with 80% power at the 0.05 level of significance (two-tailed) [14]. Please note that as the difference between treatment arms becomes small (i.e. as the hazard ratio $->1.0$), the number of events required increases dramatically.

The precise number of patients required to complete a study is dependent upon the patient accrual rate, the survival rate in each arm, accrual time, and follow-up. For example, suppose we have a 2-arm study and are interested in detecting a hazard ratio of 1.4 with 80% power at the 0.05 level of significance (two-tailed). As shown in Table 5, 278 events/deaths are needed. Let's assume further that patients will be accrued for 3 years.

**Table 5.** Number of events required to detect hazard ratio with 80% power at $p=0.05$ (two-tailed)

| Hazard ratio | Number of events |
|---|---|
| 1.1 | 3456 |
| 1.2 | 944 |
| 1.3 | 456 |
| 1.4 | 277 |
| 1.5 | 192 |
| 1.6 | 142 |
| 1.7 | 112 |
| 1.8 | 91 |
| 1.9 | 76 |
| 2.0 | 65 |
| 2.1 | 57 |
| 2.2 | 51 |
| 2.3 | 45 |
| 2.4 | 41 |
| 2.5 | 37 |

Table 6 summarizes a variety of design options which are dependent upon the survival rate in the control arm, and overall accrual rate. Several observations about Table 6 should be made: (1) If a minimal number of patients are enrolled on the study, a long follow-up period is required to observe the necessary number of events. (2) Conversely, if a large number of patients are enrolled, a minimal amount of follow-up after accrual closure is needed. (3) Patient groups with better prognosis will require larger numbers of patients as it will take longer to observe the required number of events/deaths.

Interim Monitoring

As is often the case with phase II trials, there is a need to periodically monitor the conduct and progress of phase III trials to determine whether the study can be terminated early as results clearly show a significant difference between treatment arms, or there is clearly no chance that a difference will eventually be found with additional patients and/or data.

Repeated looks at the data (or interim analyses) increase the chances that a statistically significant result will be found, and hence, increase the study's overall type I error rate. Group sequential methods, such as those

**Table 6.** Sample size requirements assuming a target hazard ratio of 1.4 and 3 years of patient accrual [assuming $\alpha=0.05$ (two-tailed) and $\beta=0.2$)]: median survival

| Control arm (years) | Accrual rate (/year) | Total no. of patients | Required follow-up (years) |
|---|---|---|---|
| 1 | 100 | 300 | 3.4 |
| 1 | 125 | 375 | 1.1 |
| 1 | 150 | 450 | 0.4 |
| 1 | 175 | 525 | 0.0 |
| 1 | 200 | 600 | 0.0 |
| 3 | 100 | 300 | 12.7 |
| 3 | 125 | 375 | 5.7 |
| 3 | 150 | 450 | 3.6 |
| 3 | 175 | 525 | 2.5 |
| 3 | 200 | 600 | 1.8 |
| 5 | 100 | 300 | 22.0 |
| 5 | 125 | 375 | 10.5 |
| 5 | 150 | 450 | 7.0 |
| 5 | 175 | 525 | 5.2 |
| 5 | 200 | 600 | 4.0 |
| 5 | 250 | 750 | 2.6 |
| 5 | 300 | 900 | 1.8 |

proposed by O'Brien and Fleming [15] and Lan and DeMets [16, 17], have been developed for conducting interim analyses while maintaining the original overall type I error rate. The O'Brien-Fleming design uses stopping boundaries that make it difficult to terminate the study early and which allows the final analysis to be conducted at nearly the conventional significance level. The sample size of a study monitored using O'Brien-Fleming stopping rules must be increased by 3%–5% to maintain the desired power [18].

Accrual to CALGB 8433 terminated early due to the discovery of significant results while the study was monitored using the Lan-DeMets analog of the O'Brien-Fleming stopping rule. Propert and Kim [18] describe the procedures which were used in monitoring CALGB 8433.

An alternative approach is to consider monitoring the study using conditional power [19, 20, 21]. Conditional power is defined as the probability of observing a statistically significant result at the end of the study given the data which has been observed to date. If the probability of eventually seeing statistical significance is small, investigators may be interested in terminating the study early.

## Other Miscellaneous Biostatistical Methods

A couple statistical methods which are commonly used in the analysis of cancer clinical trials are worth mentioning briefly: logistic regression, and Cox proportional hazards model. Both regression models are used to investigate the relationship between one or more independent variables and one dependent variable.

Logistic Regression Analysis

Logistic regression is used to examine the relationship between predictors and a binary response. The log odds of the response probability is predicted from a set of prognostic factors as:

$$\log (p/(1-p)) = \gamma_0 + \gamma_1 X_1 + \gamma_2 X_2 + \ldots$$

where p is the probability of response, $X_1, X_2, \ldots$ are the predictor variables, and $\gamma_0, \gamma_1, \gamma_2 \ldots$ are coefficients to be estimated from the data. The odds ratio estimate associated with a 1-unit change in a predictor, $X_i$, is exp $(\gamma_i)$.

Cox Proportional Hazards Model

Cox' s proportional hazards model is used to examine the joint relationship of predictors and survival. The model is defined in terms of hazard function, $\lambda$ (t):

$$\lambda(t) = \lambda_0(t) \exp (\gamma_1 X_1 + \gamma_2 X_2 + \ldots)$$

where $\lambda_0$ (t) is an arbitrary baseline hazard, $X_1, X_2, \ldots$ are the predictor variables, and $\gamma_1, \gamma_2 \ldots$ are coefficients to be estimated from the data. The risk ratio associated with a 1-unit change in a a predictor, $X_i$, is exp $(\gamma_i)$.

## Conclusion

This chapter has briefly presented some of the basic concepts and ideas associated with the design and statistical analyses of cancer clinical trials. However, the chapter has not provided the reader with the depth of understanding needed to independently design and analyze new trials. The assistance of a statistician or clinical trialist is strongly recommended.

If there is interest in gaining a greater understanding of the topics introduced in this chapter, the reader is referred to the attached reference list. These books provide more in-depth introduction to biostatistics [22–24], survival analysis [25, 26, 27], logistic regression [28, 29], clinical trials methodology [30–34], and specifically cancer clinical trial methodology [35, 36]. This list of references is not comprehensive and should be viewed as a starting point for additional reading on clinical trial design and methodology.

## References

1. Storer BE: Design and analysis of phase I clinical trials. Biometrics 1989; 45:925–937
2. O'Quigley J, Pepe M, Fisher L: Continual reassessment method: A proactical design for phase I clinical trials in cancer. Biometrics 1990; 46:33–48
3. Faries D: Practical modifications of the continual reassessment method for phase I cancer clinical trials. Journal of biopharmaceutical statistics 1994; 4:147–164
4. Korn EL, Midthune D, Chen TT, et al. A comparison of two phase I trial designs. Statistics in medicine 1994; 13:1799–1806
5. Goodman SN, Zahurak ML, Piantadosi S: Some practical improvements in the continual reassessment method for phase I studies. Statistics in medicine 1995; 14:1149–1161
6. Gehan EA. The determination of the number of patients required in a preliminary and follow-up trial of a new chemotherapeutic agent. J Chronic Dis 1961; 13:346–353
7. Simon R. Optimal two-stage designs for phase II clinical trials. Controlled clinical trials 1989; 10:1–10
8. Green S, Dahlberg S. Planned versus attained design in phase II clinical trials. Statistics in medicine 1992; 11:853–862
9. Kaplan EL, Meier P. Nonparametric estimation from incomplete observations. Journal of the American Statistical Association 1958; 53:457–481
10. Dillman RO, Seagren SL, Propert KJ, et al. A randomized trial of induction chemotherapy plus high-dose radiation versus radiation alone in stage III non-small-cell lung cancer. New England Journal of Medicine 1990; 323:940–945
11. Dillman RO, Herndon J, Seagren SL, Eaton WL, Green MR. Superiority of induction chemotherapy plus high-dose radiation therapy versus radiation therapy alone in stage III non-small cell lung cancer: long-term follow-up of CALGB 8433. Journal of the National Cancer Institute 1996; 88 (17) 1210–5
12. Greenwood M. The natural duration of cancer. Reports on public health and medical subjects 1926; 33:1–26
13. Mantel N. Evaluation of survival data and two new rank order statistics arising in its consideration. Cancer chemotherapy reports 1966; 50:163–170

14. Bernstein D, Lagakos SW. Sample size and power determination for stratified clinical trials. Journal of statistical computation and simulation 1978; 8:650–673
15. O'Brien PC, Fleming TR. A multiple testing procedure for clinical trials. Biometrics 1979; 35:549–556
16. DeMets DL, Lan, KKG. Interim analysis: the alpha spending function approach. Statistics in Medicine 1994; 1341–1352
17. Lan KK, DeMets DL. Discrete sequential boundaries for clinical trials. Biomtrika 1983; 70:659–663
18. Propert KJ, Kim K. Group sequential methods in multi-institutional cancer clinical trials: A case study. In Peace KE, editor, Biopharmaceutical sequential statistical applications. Marcel Dekker: New York, 1992
19. Lan KK, DeMets DL, Halperin M. More flexible sequential and non-sequential designs in long-term clinical trials. Commun Statist Theor Methods 1984; 13:2339–2353
20. Lan KK, Simon DL, Halperin M. Stochastically curtailed tests in long-term clinical trials. Commun. Stat.-Squential Analysis 1982; 1:207–219
21. Andersen PK. Conditional power calculations as an aid in the decision whether to continue a clinical trial. Controlled Clinical Trials 1987; 8:67–74
22. Motulsky H. Intuitive biostatistics. Oxford Press: New York, 1995
23. Matthews DE, Farewell VT. Using and understanding medical statistics. Karger: New York, 1988
24. Remington RD, Shork MA. Statistics with applications to the biological and health sciences. Englewood Cliffs, NJ: Prentice-Hall, 1985
25. Lee ET. Statistical methods for survival data analysis, 2nd ed. Belmont, CA: Wadsworth, 1996
26. Collett D. Modelling survival data in medical research. Chapman & Hall: New York, 1994
27. Marubini E, Valsecchi MG. Analysing survival data from clinical trials and observationsla studies. John Wiley: New York, 1995
28. Collett D. Modeling binary data. Chapman & Hall: New York, 1991
29. Hosmer DW, Lemeshow S. Applied logistic regression. New York: John Wiley, 1989
30. Piantadosi S. Clinical trials: a methodologic perspective. John Wiley: New York, 1997
31. Freedman LM, Furberg CD, DeMets DL. Fundamentals of clinical trials, 3rd ed. St Louis: Mosby, 1996
32. Pocock, S. Clinical trials: a practical approach, 2nd ed. New York: John Wiley, 1996
33. Meinert CL. Clinical trials: Design, conduct, and analysis. New York: Oxford University Press, 1986
34. Fleiss JL. The design and analysis of clinical experiments. New York: John Wiley, 1986
35. Leventhal BG, Wittes RE. Research methods in clinical oncology. New York: Raven Press, 1988
36. Green S, Benedetti J, Crowley J. Clinical trials in oncology. Chapman & Hall: New York, 1997

# Ethical Issues

# Ethics and the Development of New Oncologic Therapies: Informed Consent, Equipoise and the Randomized Trial

C.K. Daugherty

## Introduction

Although ethical issues are present throughout all phases of clinical research, it is randomized phase III trials which have undergone the most intense scrutiny. Indeed, it is on the randomized trial process in cancer clinical research that much of this scrutiny has centered. The overall informed consent process in phase III trials and, more specifically, how disclosure to potential subjects regarding the randomization process itself should be conducted, remain issues of controversy. In addition, a more basic and primary ethical concern is the application of the phase III trial design itself. Thus, much debate and controversy has focused on when, and if, it is ethically appropriate to perform randomized comparative trials. No ethical arguments have been made against the actual intended goals of phase III trials. Rather, it is phase III methodology, where patient-subjects are randomly assigned to receive either an investigational therapy or a standard of care, that has caused concerns for some [1–4]. Such concerns deal with a perceived dilemma for the treating physician of a specific patient, and whether the physician's therapeutic responsibilities to that individual patient overwhelm any responsibilities to clinical research and the needs to improve medical care for future patients. Some have described this as a potential conflict which arises between the physician as investigator and the physician as healer for an individual patient [5–8]. Supporters of this view have argued that the responsibilities of the physician as healer carry far greater moral weight than those of the physician as investigator, to the extent that it becomes unethical to allow a random process to be the determining factor in what therapy a patient receives. Complicating this further is the fact that in the phase III setting, the lines separating research from therapy are sometimes less clear [3, 9, 10].

The concept of informed consent, which acknowledges the rights of patients to voluntarily participate in health care, applies both to clinical practice and clinical research [11, 12]. Informed consent in clinical research is related to, but recognized as being more stringent than, informed consent outside the context of clinical trials [13]. This heightened consent standard exists for at least two reasons. First, from an ethical perspective, a patient considering clinical trial participation is always viewed as potentially vulnerable [14]. As a result of this potential vulnerability, he or she may have great difficulty in appreciating the differences between the therapeutic and research aspects of a given alternative of care or treatment. Without this distinction, patients cannot make uncoerced and autonomous health care decisions. Thus, the informed consent process, and the ethics of clinical research, require that such a clear distinction be made [9, 10]. Second, even beyond the setting of randomized trials, the physician-investigator is seen as having an intrinsic conflict of interest in their role both as a physician for an individual patient and as a scientific investigator attempting to develop improved methods of medical care and treatment in all phases of clinical research [13–15]. Within the sole context of a therapeutic relationship, the physician places his or her patient's interests above all else [16]. However, within the context of clinical research, an investigator has additional interests which may not be relative to their patients' interests [7, 15, 17–20]. From an ethical perspective, many concerns exist about the ability of clinical investigators to provide the requisite information to patients regarding participation in research as opposed, or in addition, to receiving therapy in such a way that allows patients to recognize this distinction [10, 21, 22]

In an attempt to emphasize the importance of this distinction, most ethical regulations governing clinical research have focused on the informed consent process as a means of protecting potentially vulnerable research subjects from physical and psychological harm [13, 14, 23]. These regulations have relied heavily on written informed consent documents to achieve full disclosure of the important elements of consent, including the risks of research participation, the nature of the research, and alternatives to research participation. However, from their inception to the present day, many critics have recognized the imperfect nature of the methods used to regulate the informed consent process [22, 24–28]. Empiric research on informed consent, a great proportion of which as been conducted in the cancer setting, has increasingly demonstrated that although regulations are being followed, informed consent documents have become increasingly unreadable, lengthy, and uninformative [29–31]. Indeed, they may actually be interfering with what might otherwise be an ethically appropriate informed consent process for patients, including not only those with cancer, but any patient considering therapeutic clinical trial participation.

## Informed Consent: Definition and Background

A definition of informed consent for clinical research that encompasses all relevant aspects of the process remains somewhat elusive, with varying definitions having been described [11–14]. Generally, it is viewed as a process of communication between a patient-subject and a clinician-investigator regarding an investigational or experimental treatment. Within this communication process, several elements must be disclosed. These include the disclosure of the type of research to be performed, the risks and benefits of the treatment or research, the unproven nature of the research, the alternatives other than participation in the trial, and finally, disclosure of the subject's freedom to withdraw or not to participate in the research without any detrimental effect on the patient's continued access to adequate health care. Separate from the issue of disclosure within this process, is the issue of actual understanding on the part of the patient with regard to these disclosed elements. Whether the definition of informed consent should include an actual understanding of these elements, or how much of an understanding it should include, remains a matter of controversy [11, 22, 32]. However, from an ethical standpoint it is accepted that the process of informed consent requires at least some attempt on the part of the clinician-investigator at helping a patient to understand those aspects of the consent process which have been disclosed to them, that they may truly act autonomously and voluntarily [33, 34]. Other important elements which have been described as an integral part of the informed consent process include maintaining the confidentiality of a research subject's participation and, controversially, possible disclosure of potential conflicts of interest on the part of the clinician-investigator.

Beginning in the 1960s, several events occurred which significantly changed the practice and process of informed consent in therapeutic research. One of the most important events, and clearly of greatest significance with regard to cancer and other related therapeutic research, was the publication of Henry Beecher's paper in the New England Journal of Medicine in 1966 [35]. The publication of this paper, and the subsequent discussion and debate within the medical research community and the general public [36] has arguably had more to do with the current practice of informed consent in therapeutic clinical trials than any previous event. To a great extent, Beecher's paper was a wake up call to the medical research community. As well, Beecher's cancer research examples, and the other reports described, put a great deal of the medical research process into the public limelight. The subsequent public and medical community outcry led to regulations in the late 1960s and early 1970s which resulted in greatly increased scrutiny of Government-sponsored clinical research [13, 21, 36]. Clinical researchers themselves undoubtedly became more sensitive to the issues regarding the use of patients, including those with cancer and others, as research subjects.

Other events, including the disclosure to the public regarding the United States Public Health Service Syphilis studies (otherwise known as the Tuskegee Syphilis study [37]) as well as the Thalidomide experience, and subsequent passage of the 1962 amendments to the Food, Drug, and Cosmetic Act [13] also had great impact on the regulatory requirements for informed consent in clinical research. All of these events eventually led to the creation of the National Commission for the protection of human subjects in biomedical and behavioral research. The resulting recommendations of the National Commission led to the now required and pervasive practice of formalized institutional review of clinical research protocols [14].

## Research on Consent Forms and Current Consent Practices

Soon after the implementation of modern day regulatory requirements concerning consent forms and the consent process, objective information began to become available which called into question the effectiveness of such regulations. The most comprehensive and earliest example of this was a large study of IRBs and consent forms involving 61 institutions, 2000 investigators, and more than 1000 research subjects [25]. The study included clinical research trials within, and outside of, the cancer setting. The investigators concluded that it was questionable whether subjects found consent forms useful. Moreover, these forms were found to be unreadable. Using standardized readability scales, only 7% of the consent forms were found to be readable at the periodical level, a level which has commonly been accepted as the norm by which consent forms should be measured. As well, there appeared to be no measurable impact of IRB review on the readability of consent forms or their utility.

Overall, the single largest group of consent forms reviewed by many IRBs, i.e., those used to convey information to potentially vulnerable patients making decisions about whether to become the subjects of research in clinical trials, are those employed in the cancer setting [29]. It was, in fact, cancer researchers who were some of the very first clinical investigators to make a concerted effort to conduct empiric research on the use of present day and standardized consent forms. One of the earliest of these studies was by Muss and colleagues who performed a survey of 100 breast cancer patients after they had gone through an informed consent process regarding adjuvant chemotherapy and had signed written consent documents [38]. The survey results showed that although regulatory requirements were fulfilled with regard to the use of written consent documents, these documents had little impact on patient knowledge or decision making regarding receiving adjuvant chemotherapy.

Unfortunately, based on the empiric data available, little has changed over the subsequent 2 decades since these early reports. Again, it has been in the cancer setting that much of the subsequent confirmatory empiric research on the consent process for therapeutic clinical trials has been performed. Although reviewed elsewhere [29–31], several of these studies merit highlighting and discussion. An example of one such study is that by LoVerde, where readability analyses of nearly 100 consent forms were performed by these investigators, with more than half of the consent forms pertaining to therapeutic cancer research protocols [39]. Not surprisingly, more than a full decade after the earlier reports, the authors' conclusions included the finding that consent forms were actually becoming increasingly unreadable and lengthy, with no probable impact on improving patient understanding or decision-making.

Even more recently, Grossman reported on the readability of consent forms for cancer research protocols at one institution [40]. Many of the consent forms were those used for multi-institutional and/or cooperative group trials. Only 1%–6% of the consent forms were readable at the eighth grade level, and the mean scores were measured at a level equivalent to at least two years of college education. The authors concluded that even despite the multi-level review process of consent forms by national cooperative, institutional and departmental groups, consent forms continue to be unreadable and thus potentially providing no meaningful written information to cancer patients considering research participation. A great number of other reports by investigators employing readability analyses and other empiric techniques applied to the use of cancer clinical research consent forms, have time and again supported this conclusion [41–55].

## Equipoise and the Ethics of Informed Consent in Phase III Trials

In addition to the issues related to informed consent in clinical research, much of the debate regarding ethical issues in phase III trials has centered around the issue of equipoise. As originally defined by Fried [56], equipoise is viewed as a state of genuine uncertainty on the part of a clinical investigator or treating physician regarding the comparative merits of different treatments for a specific disease process, such as cancer. Some have argued that equipoise must exist for an individual investigator or physician in regard to an individual patient, in order that he or she can ethically ask (or encourage) that patient to participate in an appropriately designed phase III trial. Others have argued that a broader definition of equipoise be accepted to justify randomized phase III trials; specifically, that clinical equipoise need not exist for an individual physician or investigator, but need only exist within a specified medical community [57, 58]. In the cancer setting, clinicians, researchers, and ethicists have debated this issue of equipoise (whether it should be applied as an individual versus a community standard), and whether randomized studies are ethical at all [3, 5, 6, 59]. The empiric research available from the cancer setting strongly suggests that the issue of equipoise remains quite unresolved for investigators, clinicians, and even patients [60–65]. The available evidence also suggests that many oncologists view the informed consent process requirements within randomized clinical trials as too cumbersome or potentially threatening to the patient and/or doctor-patient relationship to the extent that they are a significant obstacle to patient accrual to phase III trials [61, 66, 67].

Keeping this issue of equipoise in mind, and returning to the process of informed consent in phase III trials, Freedman has quite rationally argued that an individual physician or investigator is not the sole arbiter of appropriate or acceptable medical practice [57]. Rather, the medical community as a whole determines equipoise and, as long as equipoise truly exists, an individual physician can remain ethically and morally justified in consenting patients to participate in a phase III trial, even if he or she (the physician) is not in equipoise. Even more importantly, with regard to the informed consent process itself, Royal has extended this argument noting that in situations involving an autonomous patient, the decision to participate in a randomized study does not rest with the physician, but rather with the patient [68]. This is certainly the case as long as an adequate (perhaps ideal) process of informed consent can be carried out, including full disclosure of alternatives to randomized trial participation. Royal argues that what is needed for randomized trials to be justifiably conducted, beyond the presence of medical uncertainty (or equipoise) regarding particular therapies, is not physicians without preferences. Rather, it is patients who are informed of the uncertainty, i.e., the existence of perceived equipoise, and are autonomously willing to consent to randomization. Thus, within the context of phase III trials, the informed consent process becomes one of utmost importance. In the cancer setting this may be especially true because of the life-threatening nature of these diseases and the relative toxicities of potential therapies contained within the arms of many randomized trials. This importance cannot be understated.

Some efforts have been undertaken to examine different methods of obtaining consent for randomized trials and the impact of these methods on the quality of consent [69–72]. Again, much of this research has focused on phase III trials in the cancer setting. Many of these investigators have examined alternatives to the conventional methods of informed consent for phase III trials, i.e., where subjects are first consented to the trial and then randomized to either standard or experimental treatment. These alternatives to this conventional method of consent and randomization include so called preconsent randomization, where subjects are first randomized to one arm of the trial and then asked to consent to participation.

As reviewed by Altman and colleagues [72] and originally proposed by Zelen [73], these alternatives include single and double randomized consent designs. In the single randomized consent design, eligible subjects are first randomized to one of the treatment arms under study in a trial prior to consent and without their knowledge. Subjects randomized to standard treatment are simply evaluated with routine follow up and nothing is said to them about the trial or their participation, i.e., no formal consent is obtained from them. Subjects randomized to the experimental arm in such designs are consented to receive the investigational therapy. If these subjects refuse participation, they would then receive standard treatment and be followed similarly to those originally randomized to standard treatment. In the double randomized consent design, all subjects are first randomized without their knowledge then asked if they would consent to participate, receiving either the standard treatment or the experimental treatment to which they had already been randomized. Those refusing trial participation would then be offered treatment with the opposite arm to which they had been randomized, e.g., those refusing standard treatment would be treated with the experimental therapy.

Such designs were proposed in order to make the informed consent process less cumbersome and/or threatening for a participating physician-investigator. In fact, Zelen proposed such trial designs because of practical difficulties in getting physicians to participate in randomized trials, hoping to increase their willingness to participate [73]. The common theme of such designs is that patients are asked to consent to a specific treatment, rather than to participate in a randomized trial. Many statistical difficulties arise with such randomized consent designs, including an inability to blind subjects to the treatment. As well, such designs create both an underestimation and a dilution of possible differences in treatment effects, resulting in larger (and even unpredictable) accrual goals. Significant ethical issues also arise with such designs, including the fact that some subjects would be unaware that they are in a clinical trial. In addition, many subjects would likely receive biased information about the particular treatment to which they had already been prerandomized by the participating physician-investigator approaching them for inclusion in the trial.

Interestingly, even considering such criticisms, nearly a dozen cancer clinical trials have employed these consent designs [72]. Many of these trials were in the cooperative group setting, and had been initiated with conventional consent designs. They were subsequently modified to include randomized consent designs in order to improve upon slow patient accrual. Several of these trials increased their accrual rates substantially, some by a factor of 3–6 times the initial accrual rates [74–76]. Despite these improvements in accrual, these consent designs remain controversial. The ethical and statistical difficulties associated with them have prevented their implementation on a routine basis, and they have not been recommended for such use.

Gallo and colleagues formally examined the use of such trial designs and their potential impact on accrual, comparing different preconsent procedures for a hypothetical randomized trial [69]. More than 2000 subjects, who were otherwise healthy, were asked to imagine that they were ill with a life-threatening disease with some prespecified chance for 5 year survival. The subjects were first randomly assigned to three different groups with different likelihoods of five year survival, either 80%, 50%, or 20%. The groups were then randomly assigned to four different hypothetical clinical trial participation decision outcomes. Of the four consent designs, the group which was least likely to refuse clinical trial entry were those assigned to traditional one-sided informed consent, where subjects who refused trial participation would go on to receive standard treatment, with a refusal rate of 16%. Refusal to participate in the trial was highest in the group that could refuse clinical trial participation but still receive the experimental treatment, at a refusal rate of 49%. In general, the more life-threatening the disease was, the less likely subjects were to refuse clinical trial entry that allowed them to receive experimental therapy. One can then conclude that a preconsent randomization method is highly inefficient with regard to improving accrual, as subjects knowingly randomized to receive standard treatment would be likely to refuse clinical trial entry. Some of the ethical problems with randomized phase III designs and conventional consent methods described earlier are apparent in these results, as patients most likely to refuse clinical trial entry would be those that could otherwise receive experimental therapy.

Other similar research of note is that by Simes, where investigators evaluated a randomized comparison of two different consent procedures for cancer clinical trial participation [77]. They compared a consent process employing total disclosure through the use of a written consent form, i.e., the conventional process of obtaining consent in clinical trials, versus simple verbal disclosure at the discretion of a patient's individual oncologist. This latter consent process allowed oncologists to discuss with their patients the particular elements of consent according to their own (or their patients') priorities, without the use of a written consent document. The cancer patients were being asked to participate in one of several randomized clinical trials for which they were eligible. Surveys of patients were conducted at the time of subject consent to research participation, or nonconsent to participation, and then again 3–4 weeks later. The surveys were designed to measure the impact of the two different consent processes on patient understanding, patient anxiety, and the physician-patient relationship. The survey results showed that total disclosure with the use of a written consent form did lead to a better understanding on the part of the patient-subjects regarding the risks and the nature of research. In addition, there was increased anxiety on the part of the patients with regard to participating in the clinical trial. There was also less willingness on the part of patients who were randomized to the total (written) disclosure consent process to participate in a clinical trial. Interestingly, however, these differences between the 2 groups were not seen at the follow up survey 3–4 weeks later. The authors were unable to find any significant detrimental impact on the physician-patient relationship with the use of total disclosure in the consent process.

In other relevant empiric research, Fetting and colleagues have concluded that ensuring realistic patient expectations of the benefits of standard therapy is likely to be important during discussions of clinical trials [78]. Thus, any information relayed to patients in the informed consent process suggesting a preference or greater expectations of benefit for standard therapy would greatly impact on patient decisions to participate in a randomized trial.

## Conclusions

Certainly, continued study and debate regarding the complex issues surrounding the informed consent process and other related issues involved in the development of new oncologic therapies being evaluated in phase III trials is unquestionably needed. It is likely that a significant proportion of this study and debate will continue to focus on the cancer clinical research process. In considering the intense ethical issues associated with randomized phase III trials in the cancer setting, once should not be left to believe that the rate of progress in the development of new oncologic therapies should move forward more slowly or with greater caution. Indeed, society as a whole, and the cancer population at risk, would not allow a "slower pace in the conquest of disease" [34]. Rather, the rate of progress should proceed as quickly as science, technology and politics allows. However, the attention paid to the ethical difficulties and dilemmas related to therapeutic research in this setting will likely need to become even more thoughtful if the eventual conquest of cancer is to be a worthwhile and meaningful one.

## References

1. Schafer A: The ethics of the randomized clinical trial. N Engl J Med 307:719–724, 1982
2. Gifford F: The conflict between randomized clinical trials and the therapeutic obligation. J Med Philos 11:347–366, 1986
3. Kodish E, Lantos JD, Siegler M: Ethical considerations in randomized controlled clinical trials. Cancer 65 (suppl):2400–2404, 1990
4. Marquis D: Leaving therapy to chance: an impasse in the ethics of clinical trials. Hast Cen Rep 13:40–47, 1983
5. Hellman S, Hellman DS: Of mice but not men. Problems of the randomized clinical trial. N Eng J Med 324:1585–1589, 1991
6. Markman M: Ethical difficulties with randomized clinical trials involving cancer patients: Examples from the field of gynecologic oncology. J Clin Ethics 3:193–195, 1992
7. Levine RJ: Clinical trials and physicians as double agents. Yale J Biol Med 65:-74, 1992
8. Emmanual EJ, Peterson WB: Ethics of randomized clinical trials. J Clin Oncol 16:365–371
9. Freedman B, Fuks A, Weijer C: Demarcating Research in Treatment: a systematic approach for the analysis of the ethics of clinical research. Clin Res 40:655–660, 1992
10. Bok S: Shading the truth in informed consent for clinical research. J Kennedy Inst Ethics 5:1–17, 1995
11. Faden RR, Beauchamp TL, King NMP: A history and theory of informed consent. Oxford University Press; New York, 1986
12. Applebaum PS, Lindz CN, Meisel A: Informed consent: legal theory and clinical practice. Oxford University Press; New York, 1987
13. Levine RJ: Ethics and regulation of clinical research. 2nd Edition. Vurland and Schwarzenburg; Baltimore, 1986
14. National Commission for the Protection of Human Subjects of Biomedical and Behavioral Research. Belmont Report; ethical principles and guidelines for the protection of human subjects of research. Publication number (05) 78–0012. USGPO, Washington, DC, 1978
15. Pelligrino ED: Beneficence, scientific autonomy, and self-interest: Ethical dilemmas in clinical research. Cumb Q Health Ethics 1:361–369, 1992
16. Jonsen AR, Siegler M, Winslade WJ: Clinical ethics. 3rd edition, p146–149. µgraw-Hill; New York, 1992
17. Schaffner KF: Ethical problems in clinical trials. J Med Philos 11:297–315, 1986
18. Markman M: The objective clinical scientist versus the advocate: A complex ethical and political dilemma facing cancer investigators and the public. Cancer Invest 13:324–326, 1995
19. Elks ML: Conflict of interest and the physician-researcher. J Lab Clin Med 126:19–23, 1995

20. Hammerschmidt DE: When commitments and interests conflict. J Lab Clin med 126:5–6, 1995
21. Katz J: Experimentation with human beings. Russell Sage Foundation. New York, 1972
22. Annas GJ: The changing landscape of human experimentation; Nuremberg, Helsinki, and beyond. J Law-Med 2:119–140, 1992
23. The President's Commission for the Study of Ethical Problems in Medicine and Biomedical and Behavioral Research: Implementing human research regulations: The adequacy and uniformity of federal rules and their implementation. USGPO, publication number 040-000-00471-8, Washington, DC, 1983
24. Epstein LC, Lasagna L: Obtaining informed consent, form or substance. Arch Intern Med 123:682–688, 1969
25. Gray BH, Cooke RA, Tannebaum AS: Research involving human subjects. The performance of institutional review boards is assessed in this empirical study. Science 201:1094–1101, 1978
26. Hammerschmidt DE, Keanse MA: Institutional review board review lacks impact on the readability of consent forms for research. Am J Med Sci 304:341–351, 1992
27. Edgar H, Rothman DJ: The institutional review board and beyond: future challenges to the ethics of human experimentation. J Milb Q 73:489–506, 1995
28. Redshaw ME, Harris A, Baum JD: Research ethics committee audit: differences between committees. J Med Ethics 22:78–82, 1996
29. Daugherty CK, Ratain MJ, Siegler M: Ethical issues in the clinical research of cancer, in Cancer: Principles and Practice of Oncology. Devita VT Hellman S, Rosenberg SA (eds). J.P. Lippincott, Philadelphia PA. 5th ed. Pp 534–542
30. Kent G: Shared understandings for informed consent: the relevance of psychological research on the provision of information. Soc Sci Med 43:1517–1524, 1996
31. Verheggen FWSM, van Wijmen FCB: Informed consent in clinical trials. Health Policy 36:131–153, 1996
32. Katz J: Human experimentation and human rights. St. Louis Univ Law Jour 38:7–54, 1993
33. Engelhardt HT: The foundations of bioethics. 2nd edition; 330–335. Oxford University Press, New York, 1996
34. Jonas H: Philosophical reflections on experimenting with human subjects. In Paul A. Freund, ed., Experimentation with human subjects. George Brazilier; New York, 1969
35. Beecher HK: Ethics in clinical research. N Engl J Med 274:1354–1360, 1966
36. Rothman DJ: Ethics and human experimentation: Henry Beecher revisited. N Engl J Med 317:1195–1199, 1987
37. Jones JH. Bad Blood. 2nd edition. Free press; New York, 1993
38. Muss HB, White DR, Michielutte R, et al. Written informed consent in patients with breast cancer. Cancer 43:1549–1556, 1979
39. Loverde ME, Prochazka AV, Byyny RL: Research consent forms: continued unreadability and increasing length. J Gen Int Med 4:410–412, 1989
40. Grossman SA, Piantadosi S, Covahey C: Are informed consent forms that describe clinical oncology research protocols readable by most patients and their families? J Clin Oncol 12:2211–2215, 1994
41. Sutherland H: Are we getting informed consent from patients with cancer? J Royal Soc Med 83:439–443, 1990
42. Rimer B, Jones W, Keintz M, et al. Informed consent: a crucial step in cancer patient education. Health Educ Q 10:30–42, 1984
43. Aaronson N, Zittoun R: Informed consent in cancer clinical trials. In: J. Holland and R. Zittoun (eds). Psychological aspects of oncology, Springer-Verlag, 1990

44. Taub H, Baker M, Sturr H: Informed consent for research. Effects of readability, patient age, and education. J Amer Ger Soc 34:601–608, 1986
45. Morrow G, Bennet J, Carpenter P: Informed consent to treatment in clinical trials. Bio Med and Pharmacotherapy 37:10–13, 1983
46. White D, Muss H, Miechielutte R, et al. Informed consent: patient information forms in chemotherapy trials. Amer J Clin Oncol 7:183–190, 1984
47. Williams C, Zwitter M: Informed consent in European multicenter clinical trials. Are patients really informed? Euro J Cancer 7:907–910, 1994
48. Siminoff L, Fetting J, Abeloff M: Doctor-patient communication about breast cancer adjuvant therapy. J Clin Oncol 7:1192–1200, 1989
49. Penman D, Holland J, Bahna G, et al. Informed consent for investigational therapies: patients' and physicians' perceptions. J Clin Oncol 10:849–855, 1984
50. Jubelirer SJ: Level of reading difficulty in educational pamphlets and informed consent documents for cancer patients. W Virg Med J 87:554–557, 1991
51. Sutherland HJ, Lockwood GA, Tritchler BL, Sem F, Brooks L, Till JE: Communicating probabilistic information to cancer patients: is there "noise" on the line? Soc Sci Med 32:725–731, 1991
52. Lesko L, Dermatis H, Penman D, Holland J: Patients: Parents' and Oncologists' perceptions of informed consent for bone marrow transplantation. Medical and Pediatric Oncology, 17:181–187, 1989
53. Tarnowski KJ, Allen DM, Mayhall C, Kelly PA: Readability of pediatric biomedical research informed consent forms. Pediatrics 85:58–62, 1990
54. Lynoe N, Sandlund M, Dahlqvist G, et al. Informed consent: Study of quality of information given to participants in a clinical trial. Br Med J 303:610–613, 1991
55. Olver IN, Buchanan L, Ladlow C, Poulton G: The adequacy of consent forms for informing patients entering oncological clinical trials. Ann Oncol 6:867–870, 1995
56. Freid C. Medical experimentation: Personal integrity and social policy. North Holland Publishing; Amsterdam, 1974
57. Freedman B: Equipoise and the ethics of clinical research. N Engl J Med 317:141–145, 1987
58. Gifford F: Community equipoise and the ethics of randomized clinical trials. Bioethics 9:127–148, 1995
59. Freedman B: A response to a purported ethical difficulty with randomized clinical trials involving cancer patients. J Clin Ethics 3:231–234, 1992
60. Taylor KM, Margolese RG, Soskolne CL: Physicians' reasons for not entering eligible patients in a randomized clinical trial of surgery for breast cancer. N Engl J Med 310:1363–1367, 1984
61. Taylor KM, Shapiro M, Soskolne CL, et al. Physician response to informed consent regulations for randomized clinical trials. Cancer 60:1415–1422, 1987
62. Llewellyn-Thomas HK, µgreal MJ, Thiel EC: Cancer patients' decision-making and trial-entry preferences: The effects of "framing" information about short-term toxicity and long-term survival. Med Decis Mak 15:4–12, 1995
63. Silverman WA, Ultman DG: Patients' preferences and randomized trials. Lancet 347:171–174, 1996
64. Cassileth BR, Lusk ES, Hurwitz S, et al. Attitudes towards clinical trials among patients and the public. JAMA 248:968–970, 1982
65. Slevin MJ, Stubb L, Plant HJ, Wilson P, Gregory VM, Armes PJ, Downer SM: Attitudes to chemotherapy: Comparing views of patients with cancer with those of doctors, nurses, and the general public. Br Med J 300:1458–1460, 1990
66. Taylor KM, Feldstein ML, Skeel RT, Pandya KJ, Ng P, Carbone PP: Fundamental dilemmas of the randomized clinical trial process: Results of a survey of 1737 Eastern Cooperative Oncology Group investigators. J Clin Oncol 12:1796–1805, 1994

67. Lynoe N, Sandland M, Jacobson L: Cancer clinical research-some aspects on doctors' attitudes to informing participants. Acta-Oncol 35:749–754, 1996
68. Royall RM: Ignorance and altruism. J Clin Ethics 3:229–230, 1992
69. Gallo C, Perrone F, Deplando S, Giust C: Informed versus randomized consent to clinical trials. Lancet 346:1060–1064, 1995
70. Simel DL, Feussner JR: A randomized controlled trial comparing quantitative informed consent formats. J Clin Epidemiol 44:771–777, 1991
71. Baum M: New approach for recruitment into randomized controlled trials. Lancet 341:812–813, 1993
72. Altman DG, Whitehead J, Parman MK, Stenning SP, Fayers PM, Machin D: Randomized consent designs in cancer clinical trials. Eur J Cancer 31 A:1934–44, 1995
73. Zelen M: Strategy and alternate randomized designs in cancer clinical trials. Cancer Treat Rep 66:1095–1100, 1982
74. Riethmuller G, Schneider-Gadicke E, Schilmok G, et al. Randomized trial of monoclonal antibody for adjuvant therapy of resected Dukes' C colorectal carcinoma. Lancet 343:1177–1183, 1994
75. Mansour EG, Gray R, Shatila AH, et al. Efficacy of adjuvant chemotherapy of high-risk node-negative breast cancer. N Engl J Med 320:485–490, 1989
76. Fisher B, Redmond C, Poisson R, et al. Eight-year results of a randomized clinical trial comparing total mastectomy and lumpectomy with or without irradiation in the treatment of breast cancer. N Engl J Med 320:822–828, 1989
77. Simes RJ, Tattersal MHN, Coates AS, Ragahavan D, Solomon HJ, Smartt HL: Randomized comparison of procedures for obtaining informed consent in clinical trials of treatment for cancer. Br Med J 293:1065–1068, 1986
78. Fetting JH, Simonoff LA, Piantodosi S, Abeloff MD, Damron DJ, Sarsfiled AM: The effects of patients' expectations of benefit with standard breast cancer adjuvant chemotherapy on participation in a randomized clinical trial: A clinical vignette study. J Clin Oncol 8:1476–1482, 1990

# Subject Index

Printed in Italy by Legoprint S.r.l., Lavis (Trento)